# Operative Urology at the Cleveland Clinic

# Operative Urology at the Cleveland Clinic

Senior Editor

Andrew C. Novick, MD

Associate Editor

J. Stephen Jones, MD

Section Editors

Inderbir S. Gill, MD

Eric A. Klein, MD

Raymond Rackley, MD

Jonathan H. Ross, MD

*Cleveland Clinic Foundation*
*Cleveland, OH*

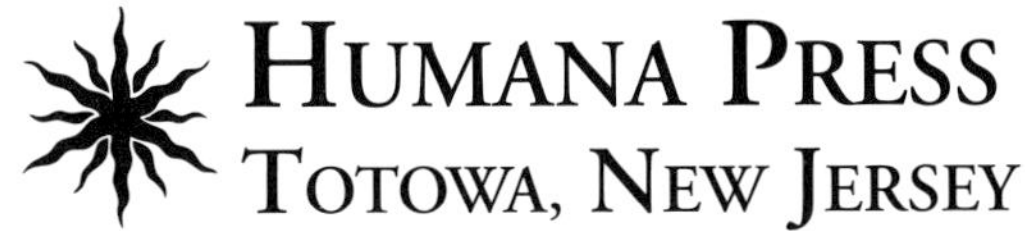
Humana Press
Totowa, New Jersey

999 Riverview Drive, Suite 208
Totowa, New Jersey 07512

**humanapress.com**

For additional copies, pricing for bulk purchases, and/or information about other Humana titles, contact Humana at the above address or at any of the following numbers: Tel.: 973-256-1699; Fax: 973-256-8341; E-mail: orders@humanapr.com; or visit our Website: www.humanapress.com



This publication is printed on acid-free paper. ∞

ANSI Z39.48-1984 (American Standards Institute) Permanence of Paper for Printed Library Materials.
Production Editor: Robin B. Weisberg
Cover Illustration: From the top down: (1) Partial nephrectomy wedge (original artwork created for the cover by the Cleveland Clinic Foundation); (2) Figure 16E, Chapter 24; (3) Open approach to bladder suspension (original artwork created for the cover by the Cleveland Clinic Foundation); (4) Figure 14, Chapter 35.
Cover design by Patricia F. Cleary



Printed in the United States of America. 10 9 8 7 6 5 4 3 2 1

eISBN 1-59745-016-2

Library of Congress Cataloging-in-Publication Data

Operative urology at the Cleveland Clinic / senior editor, Andrew C. Novick ;
associate editor, J. Stephen Jones ; section editors, Inderbir S. Gill [et al.].
p. ; cm.
Includes bibliographical references and index.
ISBN 1-58829-081-6 (alk. paper)
1. Genitourinary organs--Surgery. I. Novick, Andrew C. II. Jones,
J. Stephen, 1960- . III. Gill, Inderbir S. IV. Cleveland Clinic Foundation.
[DNLM: 1. Urologic Surgical Procedures--methods. WJ 168 O616 2006]
RD571.O6672 2006
617.4'6--dc22

2005019741

# Preface

More than 125 years have passed since the basic contributions of John Hunter, Crawford Long, and Lord Lister transformed surgery into a sound science as well as a delicate art. Several great surgeons in later decades established basic principles of management that remain valid to this day. As more knowledge was gained, surgical specialties and subspecialties evolved and grew. This has been particularly true in urology, where the surgical approach to many problems has changed significantly in recent years.

The Cleveland Clinic Glickman Urological Institute houses more than 50 full-time urological clinicians and surgeons with in-depth expertise in both general urology and every urological subspecialty area. *Operative Urology at the Cleveland Clinic* encompasses the entire field of urological surgery and is authored exclusively by our distinguished faculty. This compendium provides detailed step-by-step well-illustrated descriptions of all commonly performed inpatient and outpatient urological operations including newer approaches such as laparoscopic and minimally invasive surgery. The various chapters have been organized according to specific diseases or clinical problems. This enables the reader interested in a particular surgical problem, such as kidney cancer or bladder cancer, to find all the relevant approaches and information within a single chapter or section of the book.

This book reflects the philosophy of the Cleveland Clinic Glickman Urological Institute that urology is a broad surgical discipline that encompasses all operations that relate centrally or peripherally to the genitourinary tract and male reproductive organs. We hope that our efforts have yielded a comprehensive and practical reference source for practitioners and residents that will ultimately improve the care of patients with urological surgical problems.

A full text version of the book is available on DVD and sold separately (ISBN 1-59745-371-4).

*Andrew C. Novick,* MD
*For the editors*

# Acknowledgments

This monumental work was created through the diligence and creativity of some of the most accomplished experts in the field of urology. First and foremost are the authors whose dedication both to the science and to this book allowed us to assemble one of the most complete surgical urology atlases ever published, and certainly the largest ever published by a single institution. Second, the talented artists of the Cleveland Clinic Medical Illustrations Department have created a work of art over and above its scientific merit. More importantly, they have interpreted clinician's words and photographs into an almost life-like instrument of surgical learning. Finally, Marge O'Malley and the administrative and secretarial staff of the Glickman Urological Institute devoted endless hours to this project, allowing its smooth, timely publication.

# Contents

# Contributors


JOSEPH ABDELMALAK, MD • *Research Fellow, Section of Voiding Dysfunction and Female Urology, Glickman Urological Institute, Cleveland Clinic Foundation, Cleveland, OH*

SIDNEY C. ABREU, MD • *Section of Laparoscopic and Robotic Surgery, Glickman Urological Institute, Cleveland Clinic Foundation, Cleveland, OH*

KENNETH W. ANGERMEIER, MD • *Section of Prosthetic Surgery and Genitourethral Reconstruction, Glickman Urological Institute, Cleveland Clinic Foundation, Cleveland, OH*

JAY P. CIEZKI, MD • *Staff Physician, Department of Radiation Oncology, Cleveland Clinic Foundation, Cleveland, OH*

FIROUZ DANESHGARI, MD • *Co-Director, Center for Female Pelvic Medicine and Reconstructive Surgery, Glickman Urological Institute, Cleveland Clinic Foundation, Cleveland, OH*

GERARD A. DEOREO, JR., MD • *Glickman Urological Institute, Cleveland Clinic Foundation, Euclid, OH*

MIHIR M. DESAI, MD • *Section of Endourology and Stone Disease, Section of Laparoscopic and Robotic Surgery, Glickman Urological Institute, Cleveland Clinic Foundation, Cleveland, OH*

STUART M. FLECHNER, MD • *Director, Clinical Research, Section of Renal Transplantation, Professor of Surgery, Glickman Urological Institute, Cleveland Clinic Foundation, Cleveland, OH*

INDERBIR S. GILL, MD, MCh • *Head, Section of Laparoscopic and Robotic Surgery, Glickman Urological Institute, Cleveland Clinic Foundation, Cleveland, OH*

DAVID A. GOLDFARB, MD • *Head, Section of Renal Transplantation, Cleveland Clinic Foundation, Cleveland, OH*

HOWARD GOLDMAN, MD • *Section of Voiding Dysfunction and Female Urology, Glickman Urological Institute, Cleveland Clinic Foundation, Cleveland, OH*

J. STEPHEN JONES, MD • *Vice-Chairman, Glickman Urological Institute, Cleveland Clinic Foundation and Associate Professor of Surgery (Urology), Cleveland Clinic Lerner College of Medicine at Case Western Reserve University, Cleveland, OH*

JIHAD H. KAOUK, MD • *Section of Laparoscopic and Robotic Surgery, Glickman Urological Institute, Cleveland Clinic Foundation, Cleveland, OH*

ROBERT KAY, MD • *Chief of Staff, Cleveland Clinic Foundation, Cleveland, OH*

ERIC A. KLEIN, MD • *Head, Section of Urologic Oncology and Professor of Surgery, Glickman Urological Institute, Cleveland Clinic Foundation, Cleveland, OH*

VENKATESH KRISHNAMURTHI, MD • *Director, Kidney/Pancreas Transplantation, Section of Renal Transplantation, Glickman Urological Institute, Cleveland Clinic Foundation, Cleveland, OH*

ELROY D. KURSH, MD • *Professor of Surgery, Glickman Urological Institute, Cleveland Clinic Foundation, Cleveland, OH*

IAN C. LAVERY, MD, FACS • *Vice-Chairman, Department of Colorectal Surgery, Cleveland Clinic Foundation, Cleveland, OH*

CHARLES S. MODLIN, MD • *Co-Director, Minority Men's Health Center, Renal Transplant Surgeon, Section of Renal Transplantation, Glickman Urological Institute, Cleveland Clinic Foundation, Cleveland, OH*

ALIREZA MOINZADEH, MD • *Fellow, Section of Laparoscopic and Robotic Surgery, Glickman Urological Institute, Cleveland Clinic Foundation, Cleveland, OH*

DROGO K. MONTAGUE, MD • *Head, Section of Prosthetic Surgery and Genitourethral Reconstruction, Professor of Surgery, Glickman Urological Institute, Cleveland Clinic Foundation, Cleveland, OH*

MARK J. NOBLE, MD • *Staff Urologist, Glickman Urological Institute, Cleveland Clinic Foundation, Cleveland, OH*

ANDREW C. NOVICK, MD • *Chairman, Glickman Urological Institute, Cleveland Clinic Foundation, Associate Dean for Faculty Affairs, Professor of Surgery, Cleveland Clinic Lerner College of Medicine at Case Western Reserve University, Cleveland, OH*

RAYMOND R. RACKLEY, MD • *Co-Head, Section of Voiding Dysfunction and Female Urology, Glickman Urological Institute, Director, Urothelial Biology Laboratory, Lerner Research Institute, Cleveland Clinic Foundation, Cleveland, OH*

ANUP P. RAMANI, MD • *Fellow, Section of Laparoscopic and Robotic Surgery, Glickman Urological Institute, Cleveland Clinic Foundation, Cleveland, OH*

JONATHAN H. ROSS, MD • *Head, Section of Pediatric Urology, The Children's Hospital at the Cleveland Clinic Foundation, Cleveland, OH*

BASHIR R. SANKARI, MD, FACS • *Staff, Glickman Urological Institute, Cleveland Clinic Foundation, Charleston, WV*

MASSIMILIANO SPALIVIERO, MD • *Fellow, Section of Laparoscopic and Robotic Surgery, Glickman Urological Institute, Cleveland Clinic Foundation, Cleveland, OH*

STEVAN B. STREEM, MD • *Head, Section of Stone Disease and Endourology, Glickman Urological Institute, Cleveland Clinic Foundation, Cleveland, OH*

ANTHONY J. THOMAS, JR., MD • *Head, Section of Male Infertility, Glickman Urological Institute, Cleveland Clinic Foundation, Cleveland, OH*

OSAMU UKIMURA, MD • *Fellow, Section of Laparscopic and Robotic Surgery, Glickman Urological Institute, Cleveland Clinic Foundation, Cleveland, OH*

JAMES C. ULCHAKER, MD, FACS • *Section of Urologic Oncology/Prostate Center, Glickman Urological Institute, Cleveland Clinic Foundation, Cleveland, OH*

SANDIP P. VASAVADA, MD • *Co-Head, Section of Voiding Dysfunction and Female Urology, Glickman Urological Institute, Cleveland Clinic Foundation, Cleveland, OH*

LAWRENCE M. WYNER, MD • *Staff, Glickman Urological Institute, Cleveland Clinic Foundation, Charleston, WV*

CRAIG D. ZIPPE, MD • *Co-Director, Prostate Center, Glickman Urological Institute, Cleveland Clinic Foundation, Cleveland, OH*

# I The Kidney and Adrenal

# 1 Surgical Incisions

*J. Stephen Jones*

The purpose of any surgical incision is facilitation of the planned operation with the least possible morbidity. As most urological operations can be performed via many different approaches, the surgeon must combine understanding of all alternatives with the flexibility to choose the incision most appropriate to each clinical situation. The selection may make the difference between an easy or difficult operation, which will affect the experience of both the patient and surgeon.

## GENERAL CONSIDERATIONS

Urological organs can be approached via multiple routes. For example, the kidney can be accessed through transabdominal incisions (subcostal, midline, paramedian), flank incisions (through or between the beds of the lowest three ribs, or lumbodorsal), a combination of the two (thoracoabdominal), or laparoscopically. The surgeon should choose based on operation-specific and patient-specific factors.

Operation-specific issues depend on the surgical goals. Larger incisions, especially those that allow access to the entire coelom, give more exposure at the cost of additional morbidity and cosmetic impact. Whereas one might prioritize wide exposure and choose a thoracoabdominal incision for a large renal mass with caval involvement, an extraperitoneal flank incision gives adequate exposure with less morbidity for pyeloplasty or routine nephrectomy.

Avoidance of involving additional body cavities, particularly if infection is present, may play a role in decision making. For example, extraperitoneal flank incision for an infected renal calculus or abscess minimizes the risk of contaminating the peritoneal cavity or thorax.

Patient-specific cosmetic or anatomical considerations are often overlooked. Some patients may resist surgery if they perceive disfigurement. Other patient-specific factors to be considered include scarring or adhesions from radiation or previous surgery. Abdominal access in a patient with a stoma or neobladder may require creatively avoiding a midline incision. Artificial material (e.g., urinary prostheses, vascular grafts, or abdominal mesh) must be carefully considered prior to violating these structures.

Body habitus often influences choice of incision. The dictum, "No one is fat in the flank," results from the observation that a large pannus will fall forward when the patient is placed in the standard flank position. Therefore, nephrectomy on a morbidly obese patient can be easier to perform via a flank incision than it would be through a subcostal. Open nephroureterectomy traditionally requires both a flank and a lower abdominal incision. However, a single extended subcostal extraperitoneal flank incision may allow complete removal of the kidney, entire ureter, and bladder cuff in a thin woman with a short waist and wide pelvis. This can save time and avoid potential wound contamination during patient repositioning and draping.

Severe kyphosis or scoliosis may make surgical approaches more or less difficult. Whereas left scoliosis might make left flank incision difficult, the right side might actually be easier than usual owing to the splaying of the ribs away from the iliac crest.

Concurrent pathology may affect the decision. If a patient has gallbladder disease and a large right renal cancer, both organs may be removed through a subcostal incision. A flank incision followed by laparoscopic cholecystectomy may be chosen if the pathology is in the contralateral kidney.

Excessive incisional length increases the discomfort and cosmetic impact, whereas an undersized incision may make an otherwise easy operation a struggle. Matching the skin incision to the fascial opening assures the scar is only as long as required, but fascial closure is not compromised on either end.

Utilizing the entire incision also requires appropriate retraction. The Buchwalter retractor is useful in most flank and abdominal incisions, as it gives a fixed exposure and does not tire like a surgical assistant. Alternatively, other self-retaining retractors like the Finochietto or Balfour work well for oppositional retraction but do not offer multidirectional retraction.

From: *Operative Urology at the Cleveland Clinic*
Edited by: A. Novick et al. © Humana Press Inc., Totowa, NJ

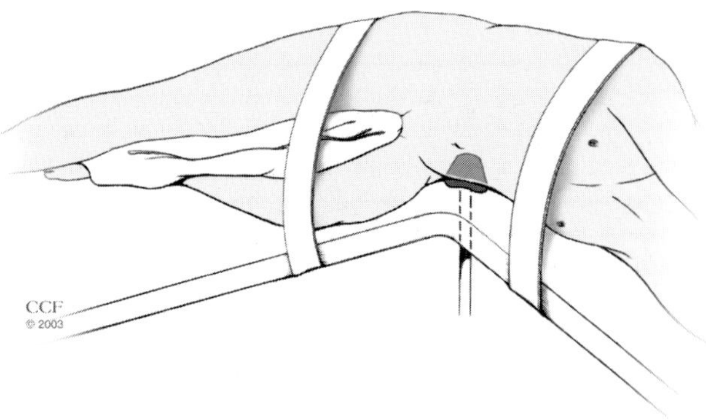


Fig. 1.1 (Front View)

## INCISIONS FOR EXPOSURE OF THE UPPER GENITOURINARY ORGANS

### Flank Approaches

A flank incision offers extraperitoneal access to the kidney and adjacent structures. However, access to the hilar structures may be limited, especially in the presence of large tumors. Experienced surgeons rarely find this limitation bothersome if exploration of other intra-abdominal structures is not required.

Nowhere is proper positioning more important than for flank incisions. This is achieved by placing the patient in the lateral decubitus position after induction of anesthesia. A towel roll or bag of intravenous fluid is placed under the axilla to protect against brachial nerve palsy. An electrically controlled surgical bed is helpful, especially during closure of the incision when a hand crank will likely hit the arm board. The dependent leg is flexed, with pillows placed between the legs to protect pressure points. The upper leg is almost straight, crossing the mid-calf of the lower leg. The lower arm is placed on an arm board. A double arm board or instrument stand may support the upper arm.

The patient's waist should be directly over the kidney rest. Extend the table at the waist only after the kidney rest is fully elevated. Correct bed extension occurs when the abdominal muscles at the waist demonstrate tension, bringing them into parallel with the floor. The ribs can be palpated and marked in all but the most obese patients.

#### ELEVENTH RIB INCISION (CLASSIC FLANK)

Although a flank incision can be made through or between the beds of the lowest three ribs, removal of the 11th rib usually offers excellent exposure and minimizes risk of entering the pleura.

The incision begins posteriorly at the angle of the rib and may extend as far as the border of the rectus abdominus. The skin and subcutaneous tissues are opened to expose the latissimus overlying the chosen rib. Transecting the overlying muscle exposes the periosteum, which can be incised along the length of the rib using the electrocautery or scalpel.

A periosteal elevator is used to remove the periosteum to the point where it wraps above and below the rib. Care must be taken caudally to stay between rib and periosteum to avoid injuring the neurovascular bundle running along the rib notch.

The opposite end of the Alexander periostial elevator is shaped to allow detachment of the intercostal fibers on the upper and lower rib margins. Because of the directional attachment of the fibers, pulling the instrument "up on the down side and down on the up side" mobilizes the rib borders.

The Doyen rib instrument slides into the plane between rib and periosteum. The instrument is then pulled in each direction along the rib to complete the rib dissection. If the instrument is placed too deeply, bleeding from the neurovascular bundle and pleural injury are likely.

A rib cutter divides the rib posteriorly. Rongeur scissors remove any bony spicules. Marrow bleeding is usually minimal.

Anteriorly the rib must be separated from the costal margin using electrocautery or heavy scissors.

Blunt dissection through the remaining fibers in the anterior rib bed exposes the retroperitoneum. Care is taken to mobilize the pleura for cephalad retraction. If

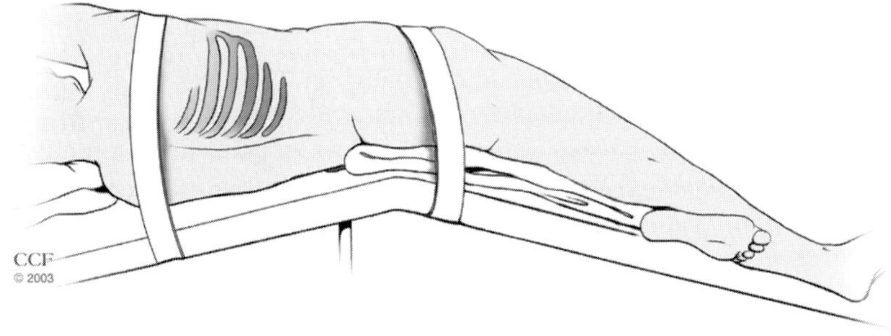


Fig. 1.2 (Back View)

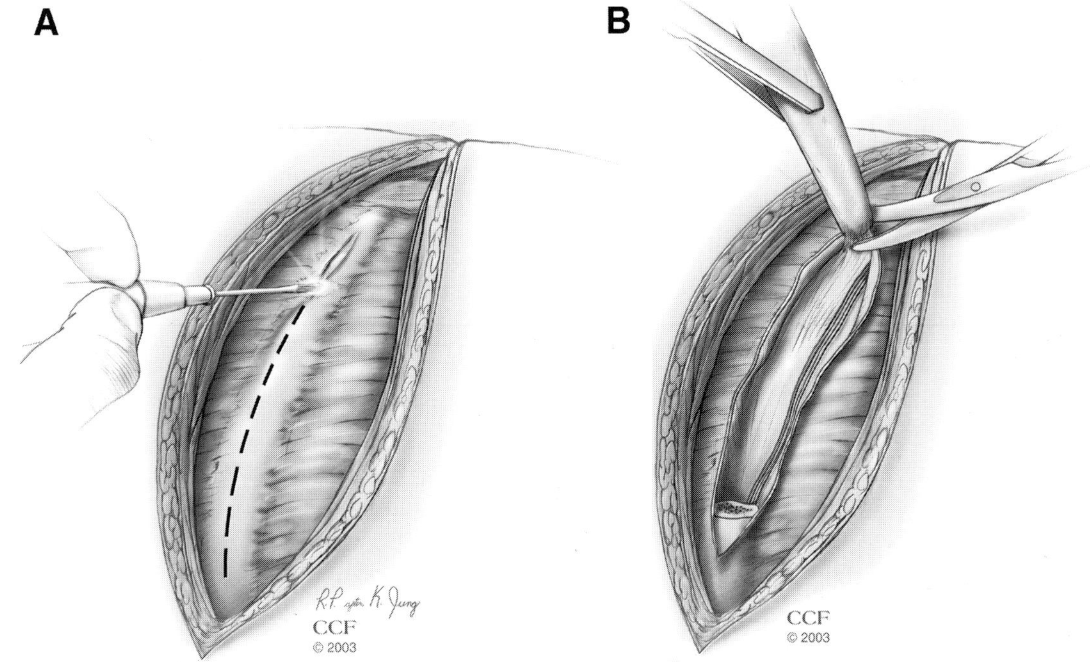


Fig. 1.3

entered, the pleura is closed at the end of the procedure after aspirating air from the thorax using a red rubber catheter.

After bluntly sweeping the peritoneum anteriorly off the abdominal wall, the muscular layers may be divided between fingers using the electrocautery.

### Subcostal Flank Incision

If there is no need for high exposure, a flank incision can be made below the 12th rib. This eliminates the risk of entering the pleural cavity, but is no less painful than a rib incision. The incision is especially useful in children.

A formal flank position is used. After marking the tips of the lower ribs with a surgical pen, it is helpful to draw the position of the 12th thoracic nerve, also known as the subcostal nerve. The incision extends from sacrospinalis muscle posteriorly to the rectus border anteriorly.

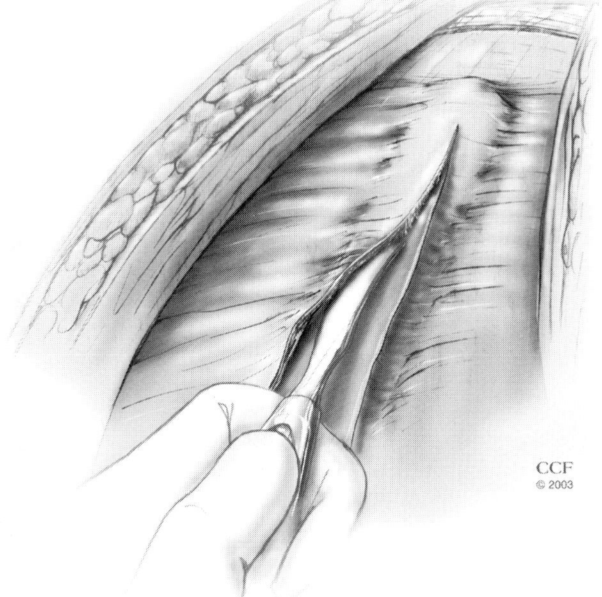


Fig. 1.4

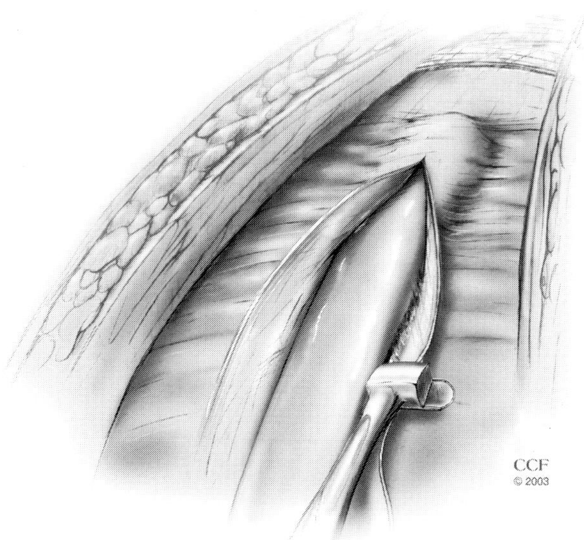


Fig. 1.5

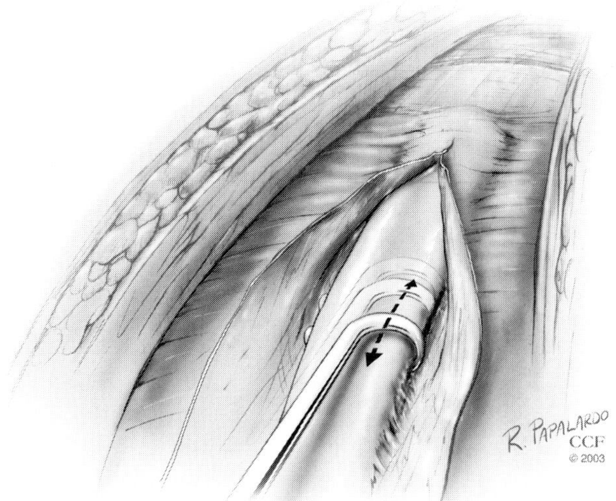


Fig. 1.6

The skin and subcutaneous tissues are opened to expose the external abdominal oblique muscle and latissimus dorsi. Care must be taken opening the internal oblique in order to avoid damaging the subcostal nerve, which lies between the internal abdominal oblique muscle and the underlying transversalis abdominus.

Careful mobilization of the subcostal nerve and vessels allows them to be retracted either cephalad or caudad. The lumbodorsal fascia (the fusion of the internal oblique and transversalis muscle sheaths posteriorly) is incised to enter the retroperitoneum. Peritoneum is then swept away from the anterior abdominal wall. The transversalis fibers are separated bluntly.

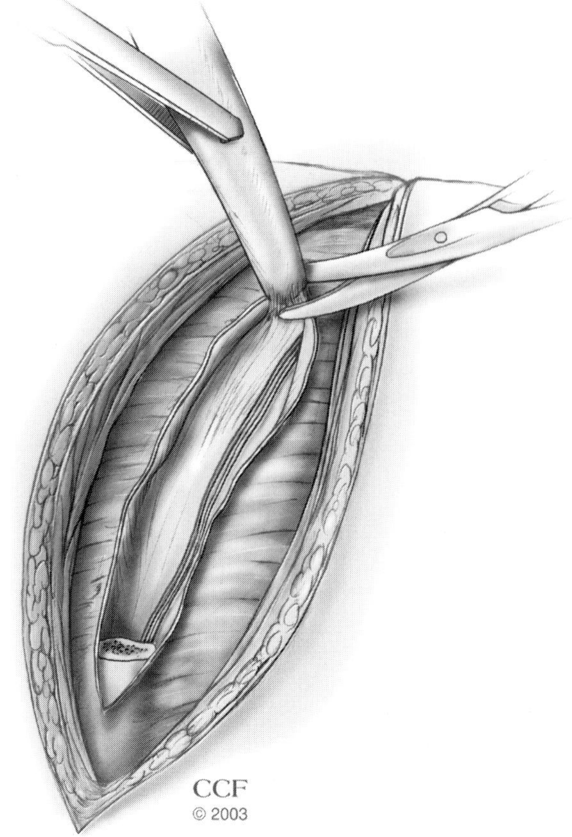


Fig. 1.8

### Dorsal Lumbotomy

This incision is used infrequently, but in properly selected thin patients it offers relatively atraumatic access to the ureteropelvic junction (UPJ). The incision is limited

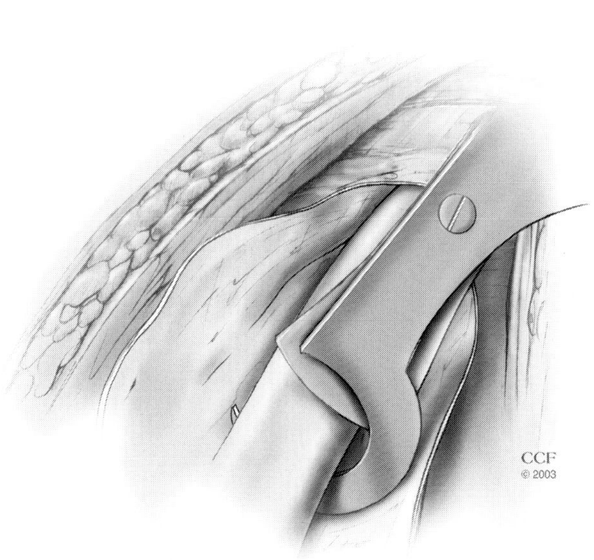


Fig. 1.7

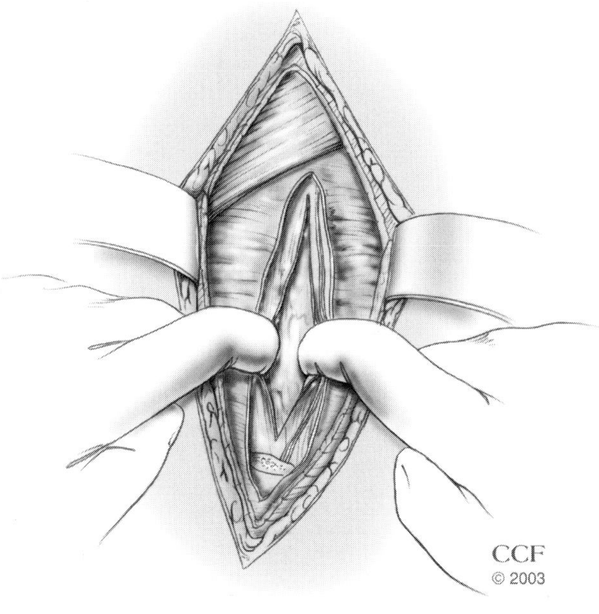


Fig. 1.9

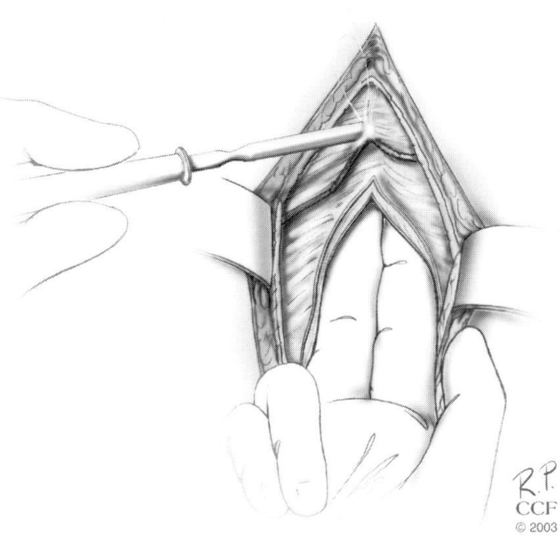

Fig. 1.10

by the 12th rib superiorly and the iliac crest inferiorly, so there is no option to extend it; therefore, it should be used only when the access needed is undoubtedly within this narrow window.

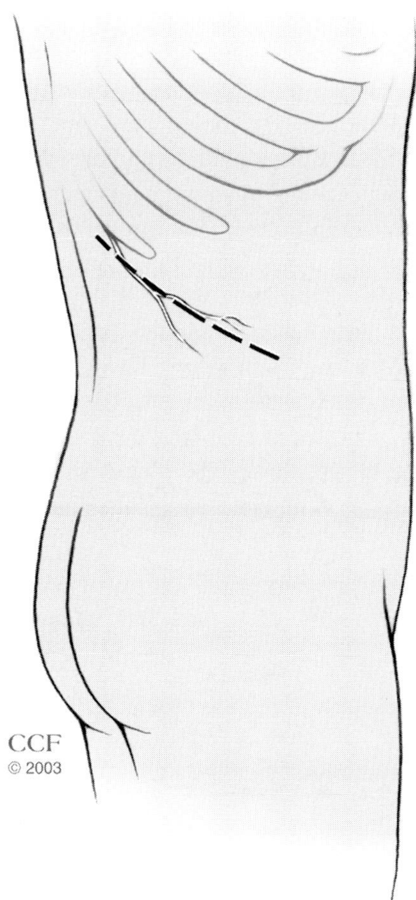

Fig. 1.11

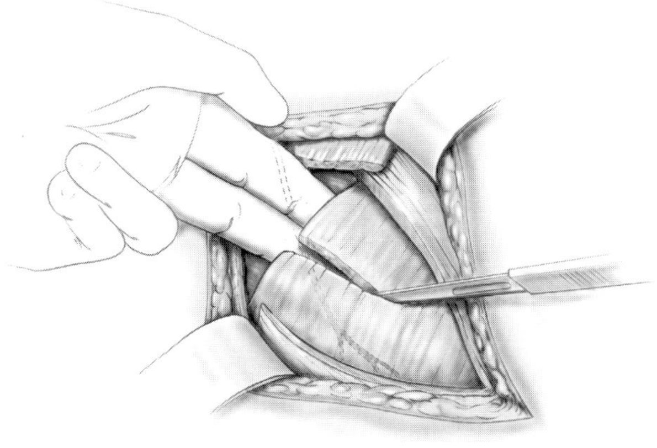

Fig. 1.12

The incision follows the lateral border of the paraspinous muscles from the 12th rib to iliac crest. Rolled sheets support the shoulders with the patient prone. A small amount of bed extension increases the distance between the bony limits.

After opening the skin and subcutaneous tissues, the lumbodorsal fascia is identified. The medial aspect is bordered by the paraspinous muscles and quadratus lumborum. The lateral aspect is bordered by the latissimus dorsi. Dividing the lumbodorsal fascia exposes Gerota's fascia. Because the space is small, the incision may be best visualized with handheld retractors. The UPJ and upper ureter are easily mobilized through a window in Gerota's fascia.

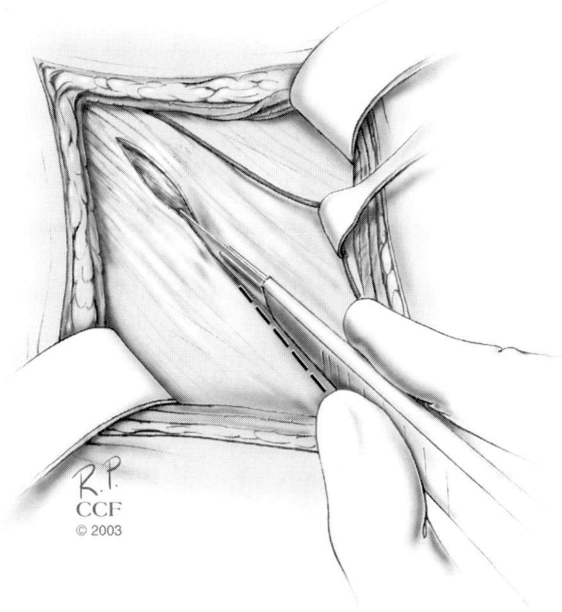

Fig. 1.13

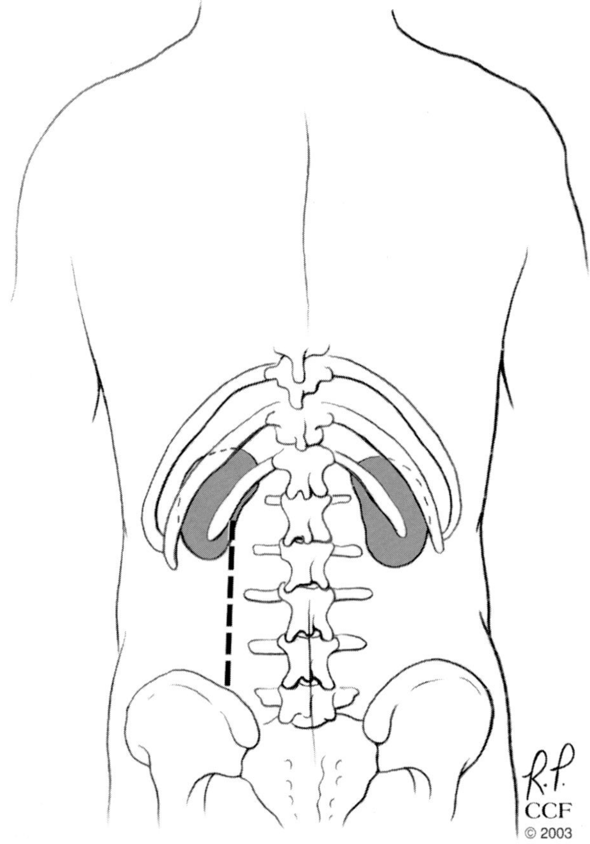


Fig. 1.14

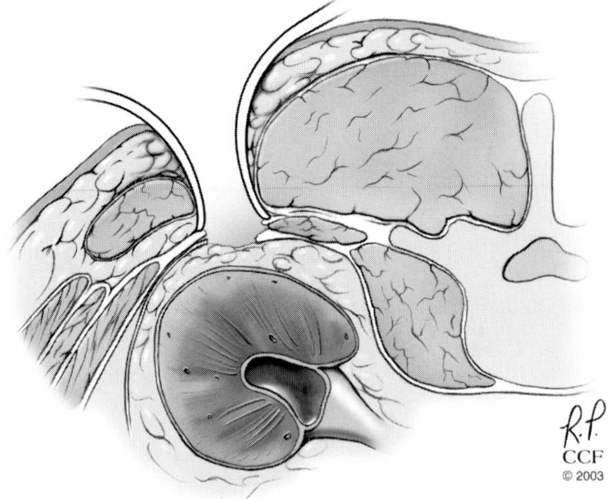


Fig. 1.15

## Anterior Approaches

Excellent exposure and ready access to the renal hilum are advantages of intra-abdominal anterior approaches. Disadvantages include the higher incidence of ileus and incisional hernia.

### Subcostal Transperitoneal Incision

The patient is placed in the supine position with the bed extended below the lumbar spine. A blanket elevating the ipsilateral shoulder enhances lateral extension. The skin is prepped all the way to the bed.

The skin incision is made two fingerbreadths below the costal margin from the anterior axillary line to slightly across the midline. The external oblique, internal oblique, and transversalis muscles are opened laterally. Their fasciae briefly join lateral to the rectus abdominus muscle. At that point, the rectus fascia splits anteriorly and posteriorly. In patients without extensive intra-abdominal scarring, an effective approach is to enter the peritoneal cavity in the midline portion of the incision under direct visualization. Properitoneal fat should be swept off the peritoneum, which is grasped with tissue forceps and held up to allow the underlying omentum and small bowel to fall away prior to cutting between the forceps (inset, Fig. 1.17).

Two fingers are placed under the abdominal wall to protect the underlying small bowel. The abdominal wall is then opened under direct vision, ligating the branches of the superior epigastric artery. The falciform ligament holds the ligamentum teres, which is the remnant of the umbilical vein. In patients with adhesion of peritoneal contents to the abdominal wall, the dissection into the abdomen should be done with a combination of blunt and sharp dissection. Lateral

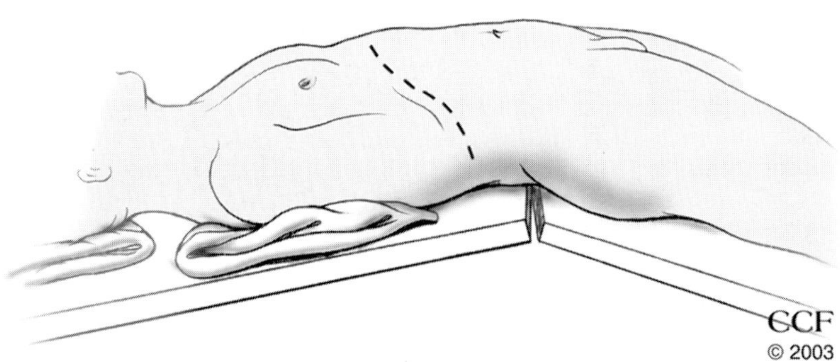


Fig. 1.16

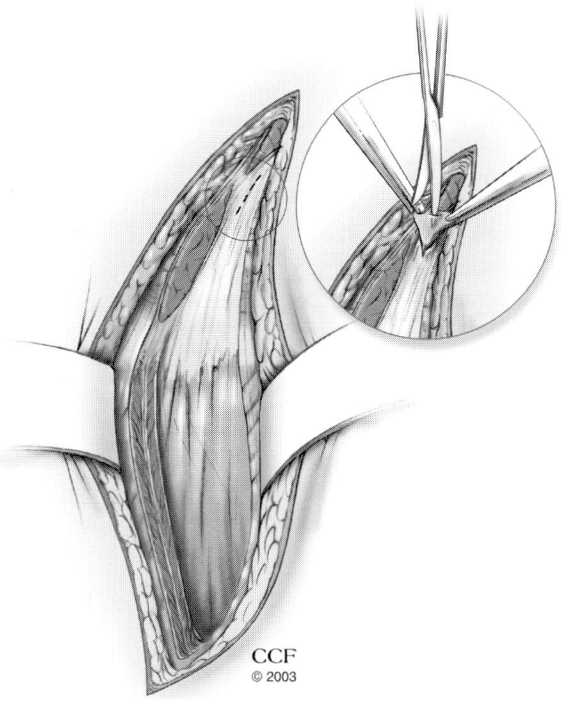


Fig. 1.17

entry sometimes avoids these adhesions. The incision ends posterolaterally near the peritoneal reflection of Toldt.

### Bilateral Subcostal Transperitoneal Incision

Excellent exposure to the upper abdominal cavity and retroperitoneum is afforded through this incision, otherwise known as a chevron or "bucket-handle" incision.

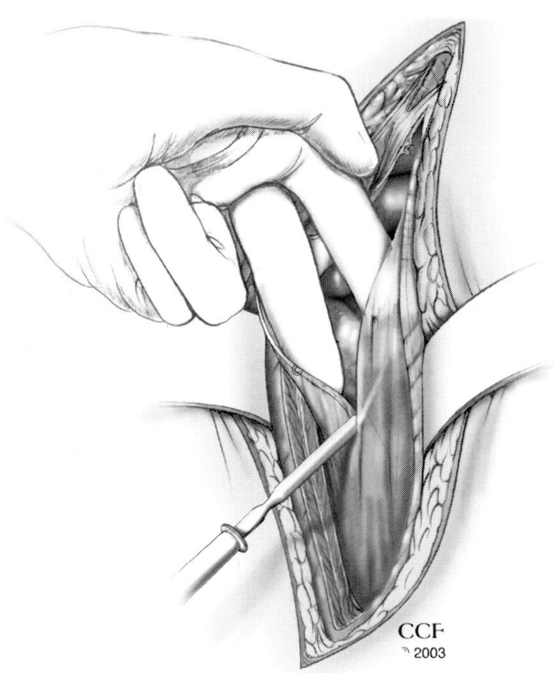


Fig. 1.18

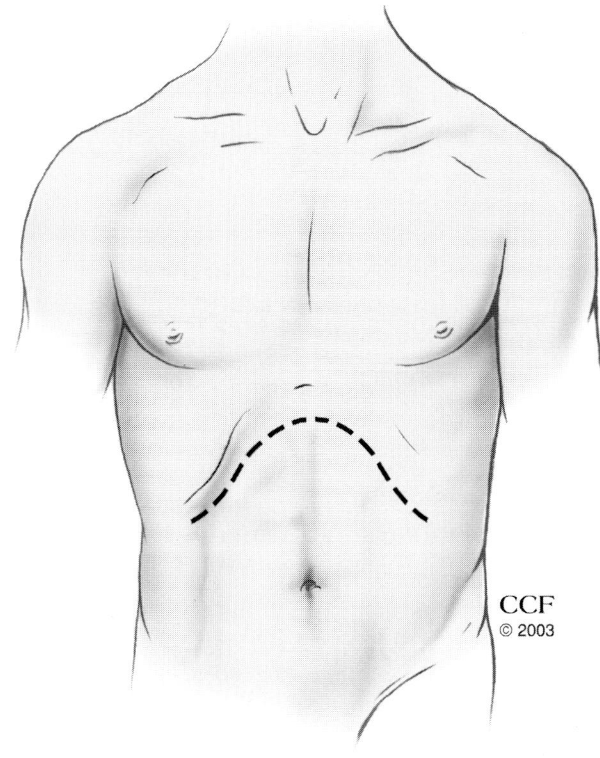


Fig. 1.19

The patient's waist is positioned over the flexion point of the surgical bed. Arms may be tucked at the patient's side, but if the dissection is planned beyond the anterior axillary line, they should be placed on arm boards. Table extension increases exposure as long as caval compression by stretching is avoided.

As with any bilateral incision, care should be taken to assure the incision is symmetrical with respect to the midline and to the costal margins. The abdomen is entered in the same manner as in the unilateral subcostal transperitoneal incision.

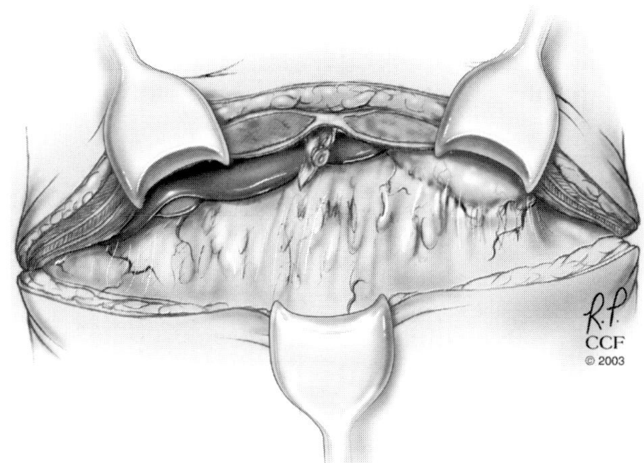


Fig. 1.20

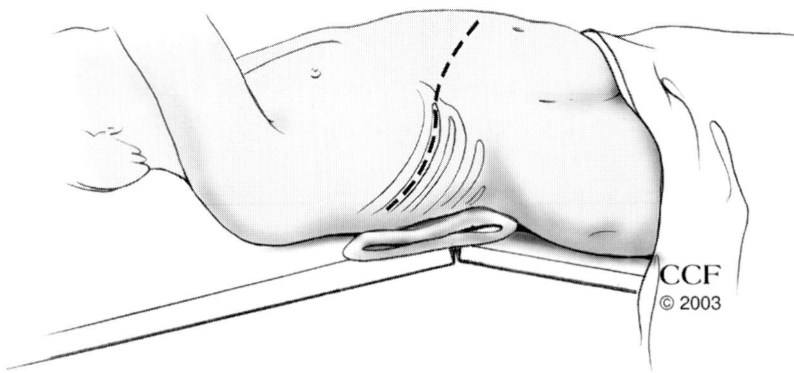


Fig. 1.21

## Thoracoabdominal Incision

Thoracoabdominal incision offers wide exposure of the upper abdomen, chest, and retroperitoneum for large renal, adrenal, or retroperitoneal tumors or when an ipsilateral lung nodule is to be removed concurrently.

With the patient in the semi-oblique position and the bed extended, an incision is made through the eighth or ninth intercostal space extending inferomedially to or across the midline. It may also be extended caudally along the midline if needed. The abdominal portion of the incision is opened first as described above if the finding of metastatic disease or tumor fixation is likely to terminate the operation.

The costal cartilage between the tips of the two ribs on either side of the incision is then divided with heavy scissors or rib cutters. Dissection is carried through the intercostal muscles along the upper border of the adjacent lower rib in order to avoid the neurovascular bundle.

The pleura is opened under direct visualization. The diaphragm is incised.

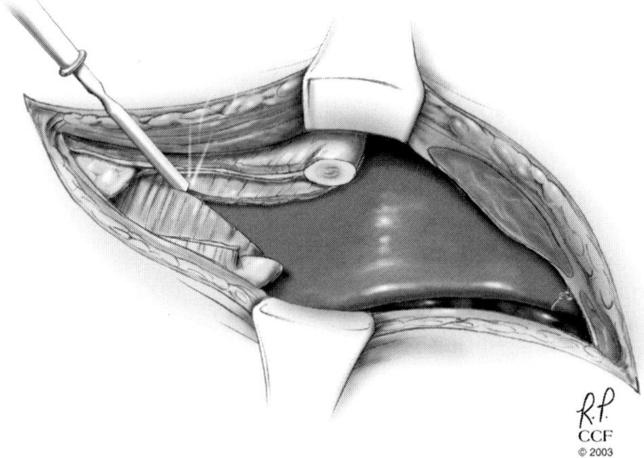


Fig. 1.23

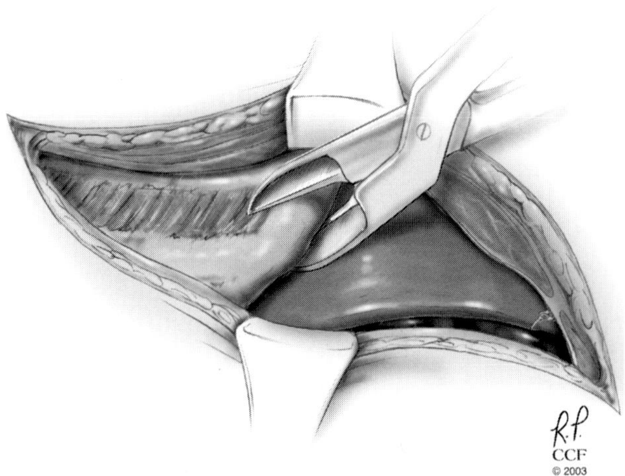


Fig. 1.22

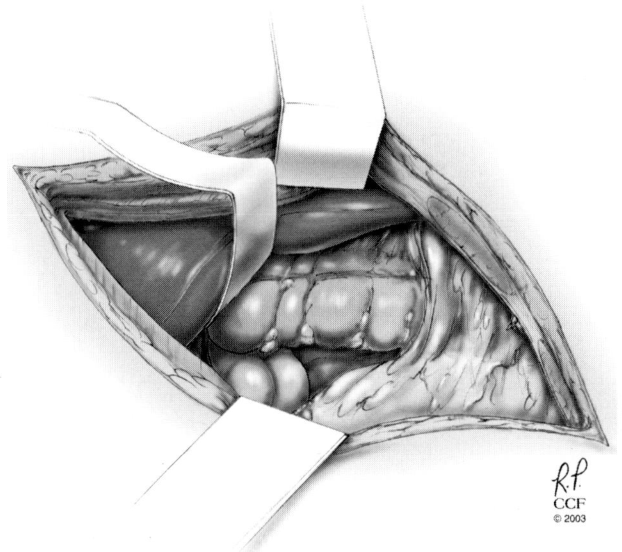


Fig. 1.24

With the diaphragm opened, the liver can be retracted into the thorax to maximize exposure of the underlying structures.

## INCISIONS FOR EXPOSURE OF UPPER AND LOWER URINARY TRACT ORGANS

### Twelfth Rib or Modified Flank Incision

A 12th rib incision carries less risk of pleural injury than entering through the bed of the 11th rib and can easily be extended inferiorly for operations involving the ureter. Although most patients will require two incisions to perform open nephroureterectomy, the procedure can be performed through a modified flank incision if extended inferiorly along the lateral border of the rectus muscle in thin patients, especially women. The time saved in repeat prep and draping is worth the effort in appropriate patients.

The positioning should be similar to an 11th rib incision, but the patient should be rotated slightly dorsad. The 12th rib is marked, and the bed developed in the same manner as the 12th rib incision. The subcostal nerve is protected as in Fig. 1.12. Below the rib bed, the incision is angled downward along the lateral border of the ipsilateral rectus muscle. If required, a "hockey stick" angulation across the recti 2 cm above the pubis can be made for better bladder exposure.

Reflecting the peritoneum medially by blunt dissection gives excellent visualization of the retroperitoneum.

### Midline Abdominal Incisions

The most versatile abdominal incision is the midline, as it can be extended in either direction if needed. This makes it the choice for diagnostic exploratory laparotomy or trauma.

Within the bony limits of the sternal xyphoid process above and pubis below, there is flexibility to use the portion needed. If the incision must extend beyond the umbilicus, we prefer to encircle it so the incision is not subject to moisture.

The midline is incised through the skin and subcutaneous tissue to expose the linea alba. This structure is identified by the decussating fibers between the bellies of the two recti abdomini. Although dissection laterally helps identify the linea alba, excessive mobilization can leave dead space that can lead to seroma or hematoma and subsequent wound infection. Understanding that there are two layers of the rectus fascia above the semilunar line (arcuate line of Douglas) is most important during wound closure.

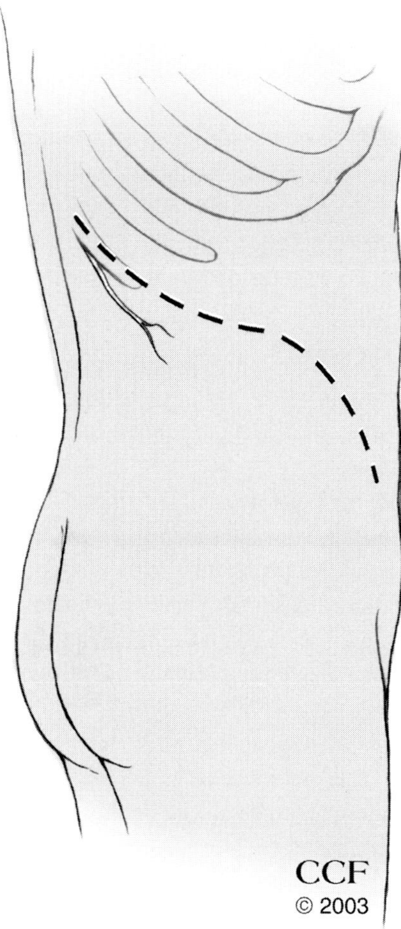


Fig. 1.25

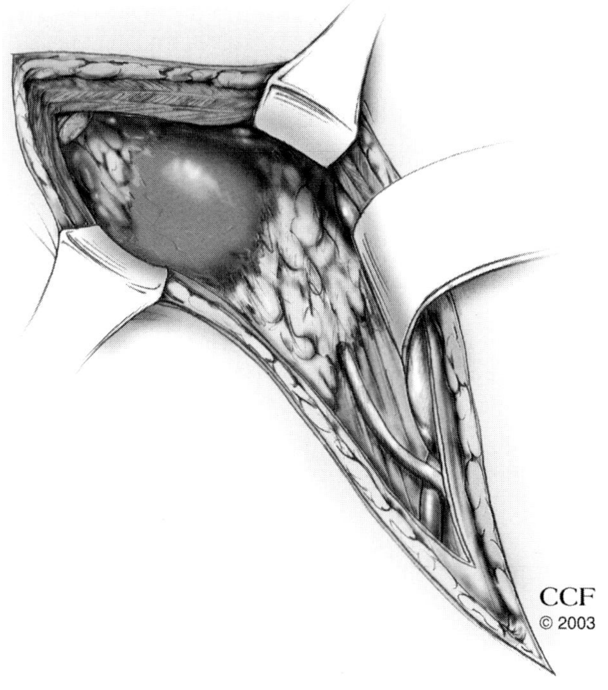


Fig. 1.26

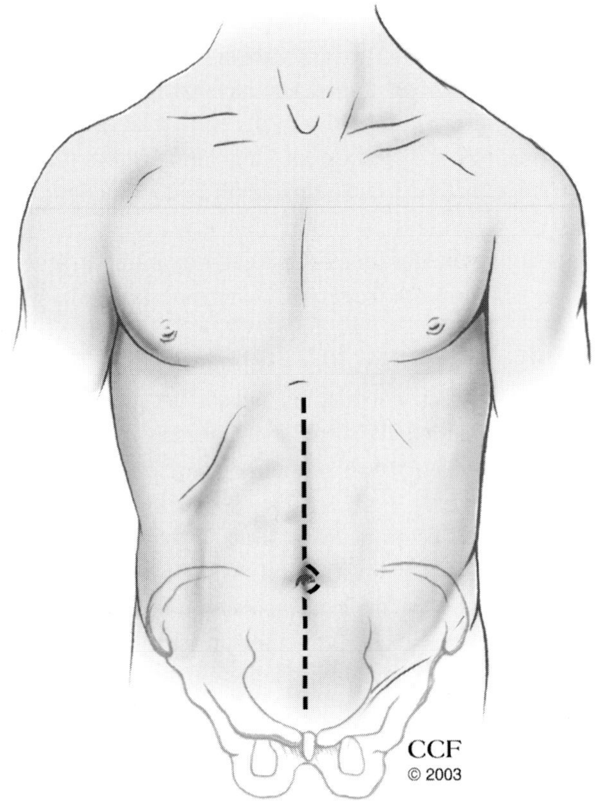


Fig. 1.27

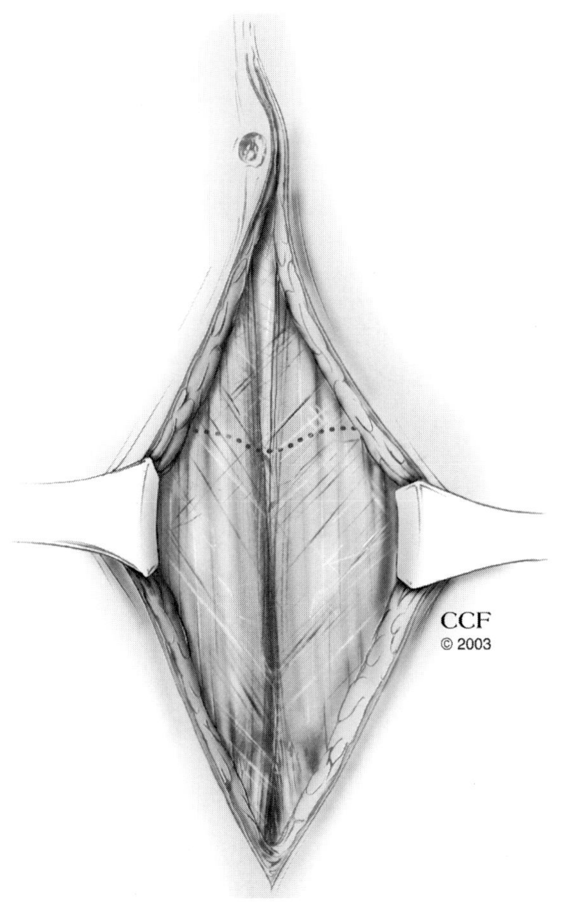


Fig. 1.28

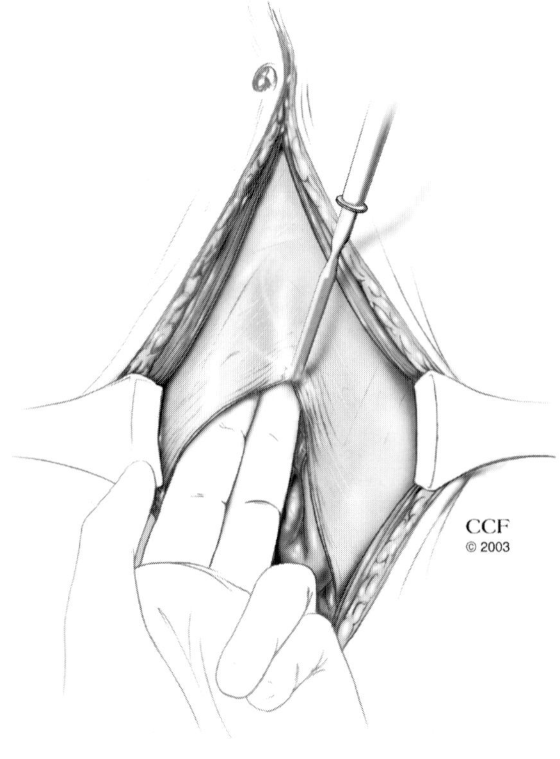


Fig. 1.29

The linea alba is wider immediately below the umbilicus than it is nearer the pubis, so it is easier to enter in this area.

Care is taken going through the linea alba, properitoneal fat, and peritoneum to prevent inadvertent injury to underlying structures if no adhesions are present. The nondominant hand can hold up the abdominal wall for protection.

## Gibson's Incision

Now used mainly for renal transplantation, the Gibson incision affords relatively atraumatic access to the iliac fossa and ureter.

In the supine position, an incision is made 2–3 cm medial to the line from the anterior superior iliac spine to the pubis. Surgeon preference will dictate whether the incision parallels that line or curves moderately. Some also prefer to make a "hockey stick" extension across the midline about 2 cm above the pubis, which gives more access to the bladder.

The external oblique aponeurosis is exposed. An incision is made along the lateral border of the rectus abdominus.

If more medial exposure is needed, the rectus may be transected across its tendinous attachment to the pubis. The inferior epigastric artery may be ligated and divided as it passes along the posterior aspect of the rectus.

The transversalis fascia is incised to expose the correct plane for blunt dissection. The peritoneum and

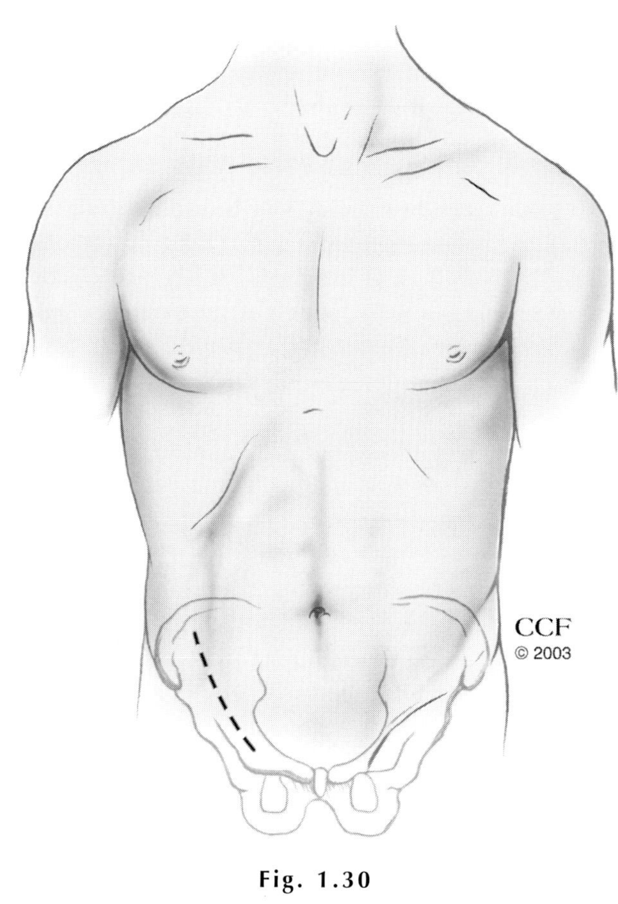


Fig. 1.30

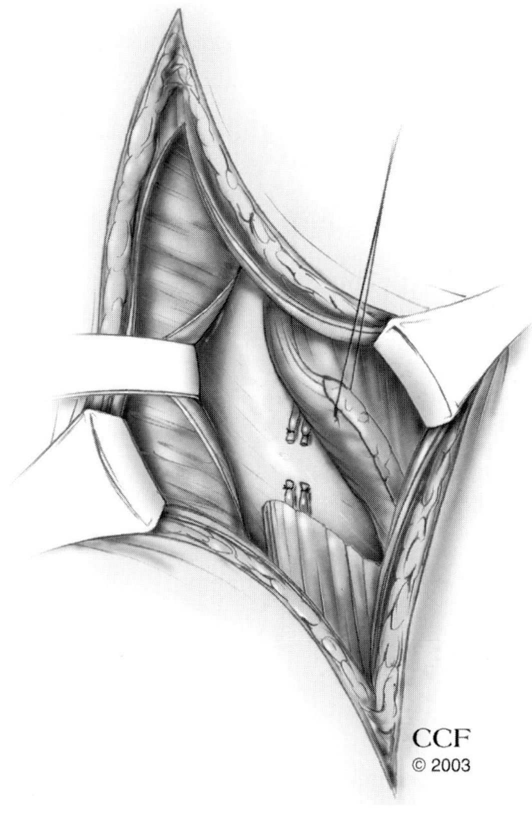


Fig. 1.32

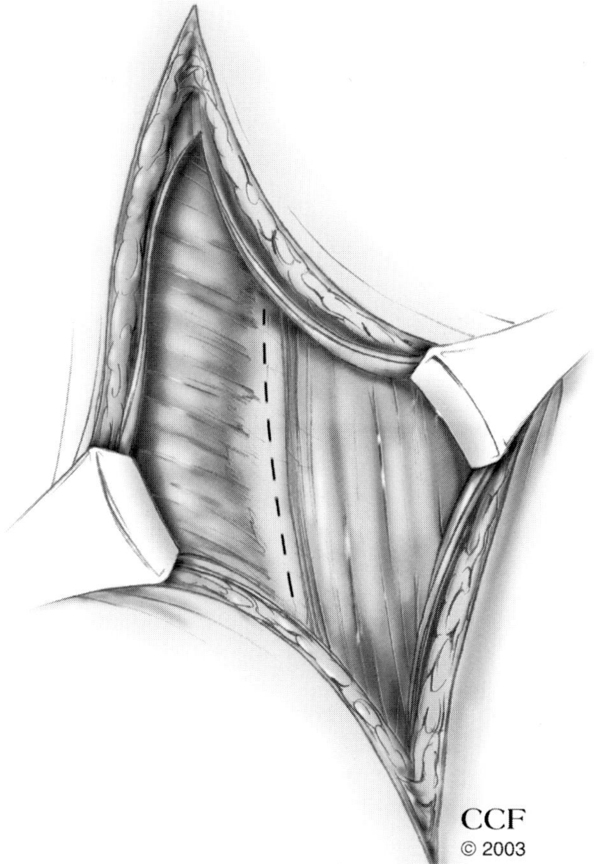


Fig. 1.31

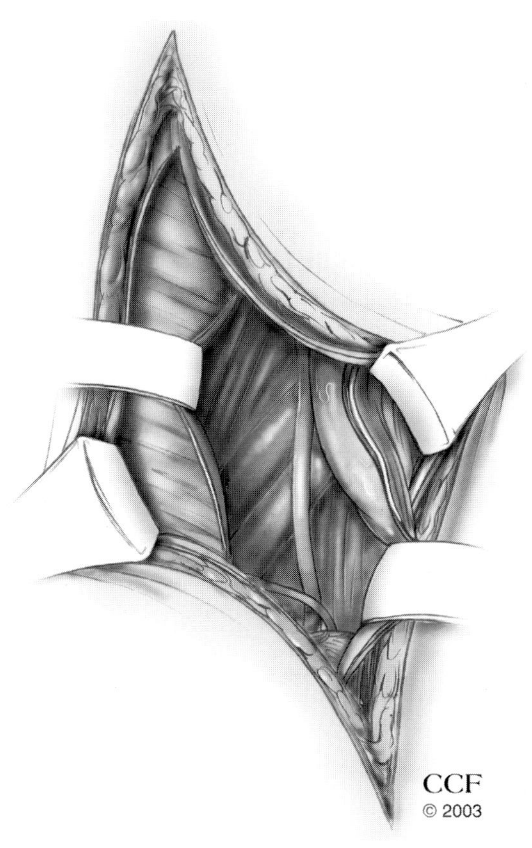


Fig. 1.33

bladder are swept medially to develop the extraperitoneal space.

## INCISIONS FOR EXPOSURE OF LOWER GENITOURINARY AND PELVIC STRUCTURES

### Infraumbilical Incision

Although it shares the same skin incision as an inferior midline incision, the infraumbilical incision is performed in a completely extraperitoneal manner.

The incision is begun below the umbilicus as in Fig. 1.27, but the peritoneum is not opened after incising the linea alba. It is easier to find the midline near the umbilicus because the linea alba is wider at this point.

Identifying the proper plane is often overlooked in developing the space of Retzius. The first plane encountered after opening the linea alba is superficial to the transversalis fascia. If this plane is developed, troublesome venous bleeding may be encountered and the inferior epigastric vessels may be injured. Opening the thin transversalis fascia allows the relatively avascular plane to be developed by sweeping two fingers along the posterior pubis. Gently pulling cephalad will expose the entire space of Retzius in two to three sweeps. Body wall retraction ventrally assists in this maneuver. This plane protects the inferior epigastric vessels, which can be retracted laterally without injury.

### Lower Abdominal Transverse Incision

Although several variations have been described, Pfannenstiel's incision is still the standard for exposure of the bladder and pelvis. The incision is strong and cosmetically acceptable. In most patients, it can be hidden below the pubic hairline. Although the skin incision is transverse, the Pfannnenstiel actually functions as a midline incision in disguise.

The patient is positioned similarly to other lower abdominal incisions unless simultaneous vaginal incision requires lithotomy. In women, it is ideal to make the incision just below or at the hairline.

The incision is carried through the skin and subcutaneous tissues to expose the rectus fascia, which has only an anterior layer at this level below the semilunar line of Douglas. Undermining the skin superiorly allows the fascia to be opened further from the pubis if needed. The fascia is incised either sharply or with the electrocautery. Ending the fascial incision at the lateral borders of the recti limits the risks of injury to the ilioinguinal nerve and contents of the inguinal canal.

Each leaf of the divided rectus fascia is grasped approx 1 cm lateral to the midline with Allis clamps and retracted

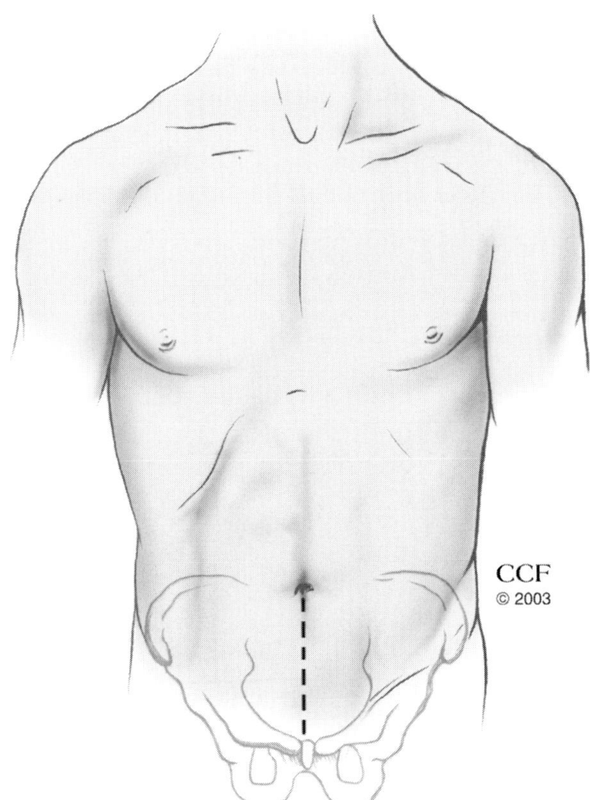


Fig. 1.34

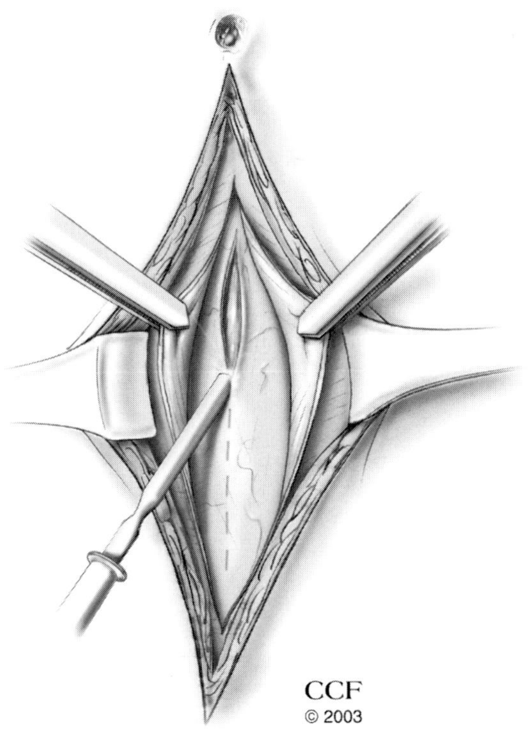


Fig. 1.35

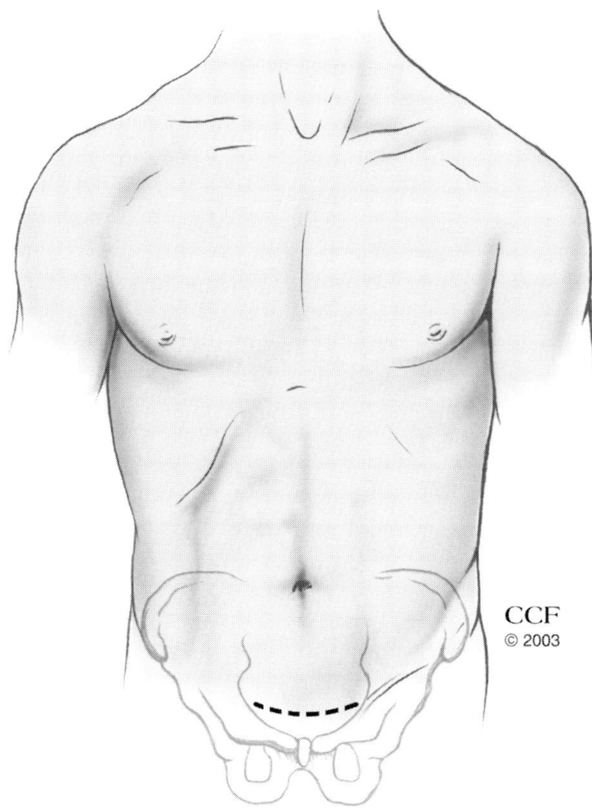


Fig. 1.36

ventrally. Countertraction is supplied by gently pushing the rectus abdominus muscle dorsally with a kuttner or sponge stick. The attaching bands can be divided under tension with the electrocautery. The limiting factor in mobilization will be the dense midline attachments. Inadequate control of penetrating vessels can lead to troublesome postoperative bleeding and possible pelvic hematoma.

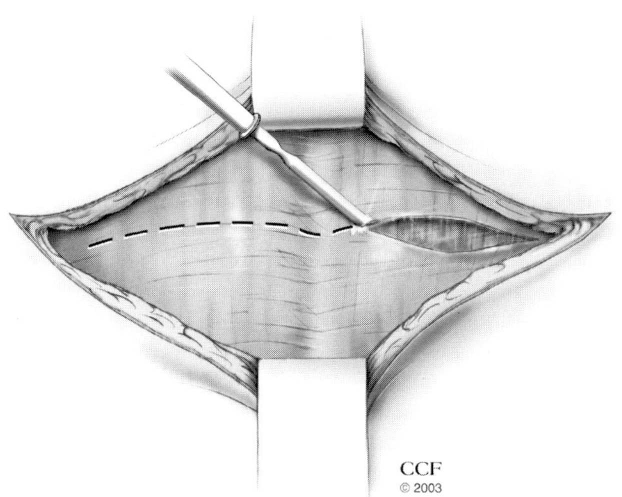


Fig. 1.37

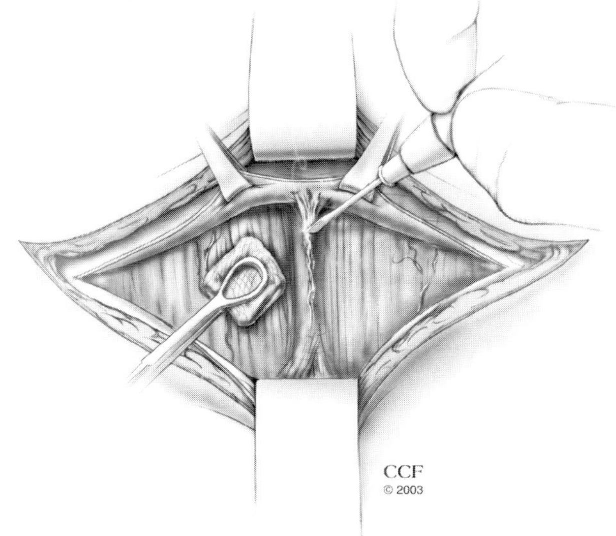


Fig. 1.38

A curved clamp bluntly separates the two recti, which are retracted laterally.

Incising the transversalis fascia, as described in Fig. 1.35, opens the proper plane of dissection. Sweeping the plane between bladder and pelvis exposes the obturator nerves and vessels.

## Inguinal Incision

Perhaps the most confusing three-dimensional anatomy urologists encounter is in the inguinal canal. The spatial relationships are best learned at the operating table.

A skin incision is created 1 or 2 cm above the inguinal ligament, identified as the line between the anterior superior iliac spine and the pubic tubercle. Making the incision

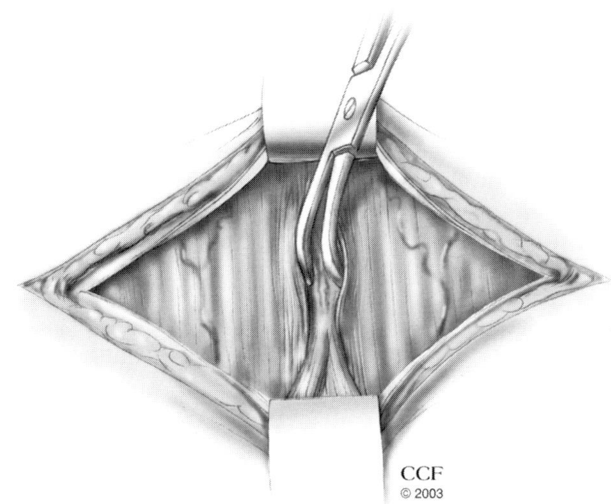


Fig. 1.39

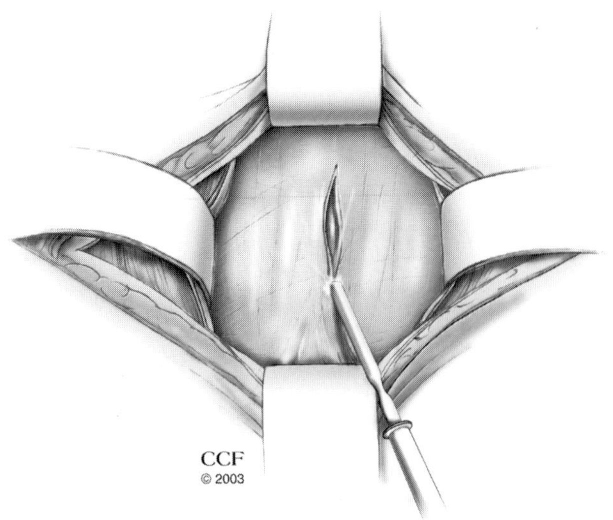


Fig. 1.40

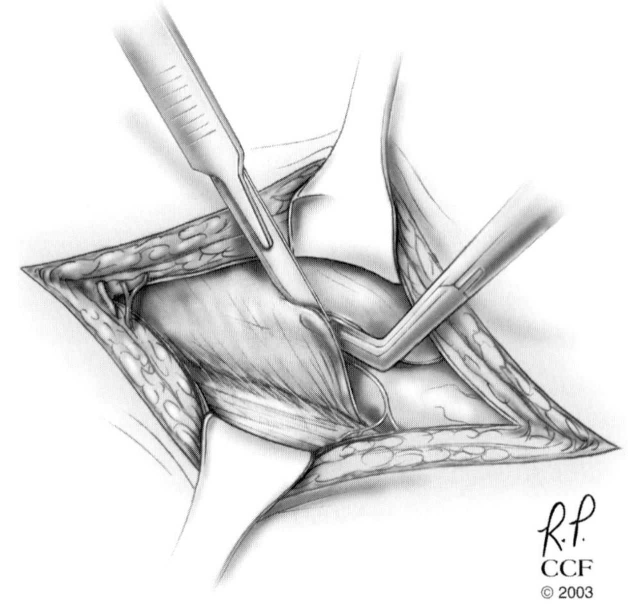


Fig. 1.42

above the inguinal (Poupart's) ligament helps avoid moisture from the groin crease.

Scarpa's (and occasionally Camper's) fascia is visualized as the dissection is carried to the external oblique aponeurosis. Care must be taken to identify and control the superficial epigastric branch of the saphenous vein. It is helpful to fully define the lower aspect of the external oblique aponeurosis, where it rolls inward to form the inguinal ligament. Just above the pubic tubercle, the aponeurosis separates around the spermatic cord to form the external inguinal ring.

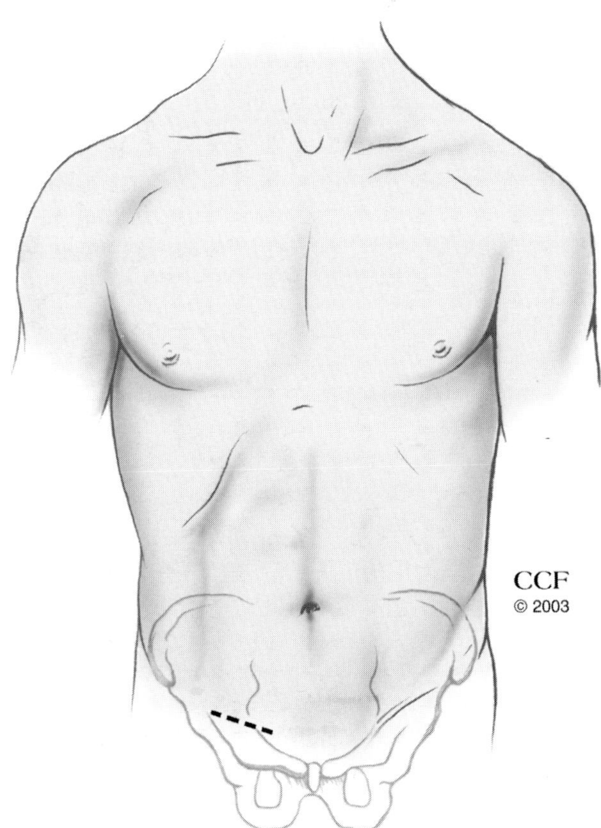


Fig. 1.41

Gentle traction on the ipsilateral testis facilitates identification of the cord. A right-angled clamp is placed through the external ring to hold the decussating fibers of the aponeurosis away from the cord. These fibers are divided sharply with a scalpel, protecting the underlying ilioinguinal nerve. Alternatively, a no. 15 scalpel blade can be used to incise the external oblique in the direction of its fibers 1.0 cm above and parallel to the inguinal ligament. Taking care to protect the underlying nerve, the spermatic cord is mobilized bluntly. The shelving edge of the inguinal ligament is identified beneath this.

# 2 Adrenal Disease

## *Open Surgery*

*Andrew C. Novick*

## SURGICAL ANATOMY

The adrenal glands are paired structures located medial to the upper poles of each kidney. The average adult adrenal weighs 3–8 g and has a characteristic shiny yellow appearance that differentiates it from the surrounding adipose tissue and pancreas. The two glands are not identical, differing with respect to size, shape, and exact location. The left adrenal is elongated and flat, whereas the right is triangular, slightly smaller, and located more superiorly than the left. The adrenals are enveloped in a compartment of Gerota's fascia and are surrounded by an adipose and connective tissue covering that forms a pseudocapsule, facilitating surgical dissection.

The arterial blood supply to the adrenal glands is multiple and variable, whereas the venous drainage is constant (Fig. 2.1). On the left side, the gland is supplied superiorly by arteries arising from the inferior phrenic artery. Along its medial aspect, branches of the middle adrenal artery originating directly from the aorta enter the gland after passing through the periaortic lymph nodes and celiac ganglia. The inferior adrenal artery arises near the origin of the left renal artery, either superiorly from the aorta or directly from the proximal left renal artery. Therefore, great care should be used when dissecting near the origin of the left renal artery to avoid transecting this branch. The venous drainage of the left adrenal gland is almost exclusively via the inferior adrenal vein, which enters the cephalic aspect of the left renal vein. This entry site occurs near the lateral margin of the aorta, which can serve as a useful landmark when dissecting the left renal vein to gain initial exposure of the adrenal vein.

As on the left side, the right adrenal gland derives its blood supply superiorly from the inferior phrenic artery. Medially, multiple middle adrenal arteries arising from the aorta course beneath the vena cava and through the pericaval lymphatics to enter the gland. The inferior adrenal artery has a relatively constant origin from the proximal portion of the right renal artery.

Some important anatomical differences pertaining to the vasculature of the right adrenal gland should be noted. First, the superior adrenal arteries on the right side lie at a higher level than on the left, even though the kidney is usually lower. This, and the presence of the overlying liver and the vena cava medially, can make the dissection of the right superior adrenal arteries more difficult than the left. Second, the drainage of the right adrenal is by a single adrenal vein, shorter and more friable than the left, entering directly into the vena cava just below the hepatic veins. This vein usually is located higher and is shorter than one might expect, and it is usually necessary to dissect surrounding tissue to gain appropriate exposure before ligating this vein.

The left adrenal gland is more elongated and situated lower on the superomedial aspect of the kidney than the right, placing it close to the renal hilum and left renal pedicle. Therefore, great care must be taken in the surgical exposure of the inferior surface of the left adrenal so as not to traumatize the left renal artery or vein. The stomach, pancreas, spleen, and splenic vessels are contiguous with the anterior surface of the left adrenal gland, while the upper pole of the kidney lies lateral and the diaphragm and pleural reflection posterosuperiorly (Fig. 2.2).

The right adrenal gland lies more cephalad than the left and is close to the liver superiorly. The kidney is lateral, the duodenum is anterior, and the diaphragmatic and pleural reflections are posterior to the gland (Fig. 2.3). Often, the medial portion of the right adrenal is retrocaval, and the adrenal vein commonly enters the posterolateral vena cava. Dense attachment of the gland to the posterior surface of the vena cava in combination with a short and friable adrenal vein makes meticulous dissection and adequate exposure a requirement to prevent troublesome hemorrhage when performing right adrenalectomy.

From: *Operative Urology at the Cleveland Clinic*
Edited by: A. Novick et al. © Humana Press Inc., Totowa, NJ

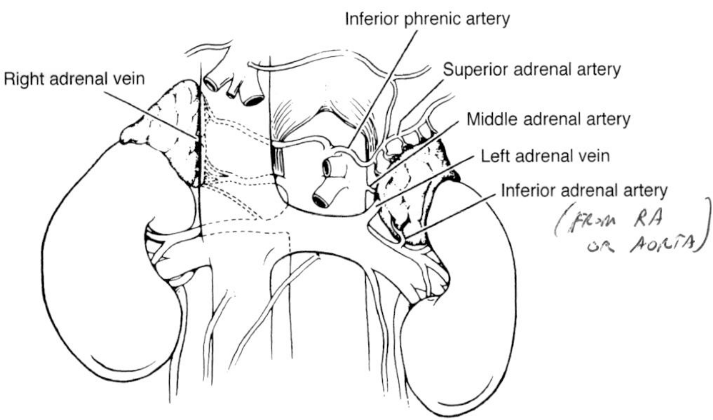


**Fig. 2.1**

Normal adrenal blood supply.

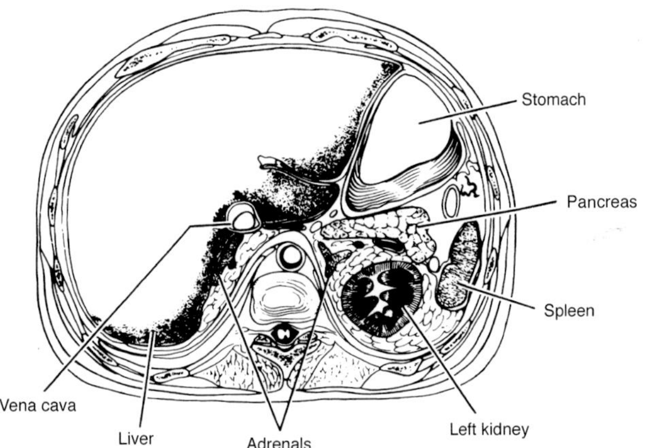


**Fig. 2.2**

Anatomical relationships of the adrenal glands, as depicted by computed tomography (CT) scan at the T1a level.

## OPERATIVE APPROACHES

There is a wide spectrum of adrenal pathology that requires surgical intervention *(1)*. One or both adrenal glands may need to be removed for either benign or malignant tumors. Adrenal hyperplasia or hormonally active adrenal tumors can be an indication for surgery.

A variety of operative approaches are available for adrenal surgery. The optimal technique must be individualized for each patient according to the adrenal pathology, the patient's body habitus and surgical history, and the familiarity of the surgeon with each operative approach *(2–4)*.

In recent years, laparoscopic adrenalectomy has become the treatment of choice for benign adrenal disorders such as (1) primary aldosteronism, (2) Cushing's disease or Cushing's syndrome caused by an adrenal adenoma *(5)*, (3) small benign pheochromocytomas, or (4) other benign lesions such as a cyst or myelolipoma *(4)*. Other indications have included small nonfunctioning adrenal masses with radiographic features suspicious for malignancy and small

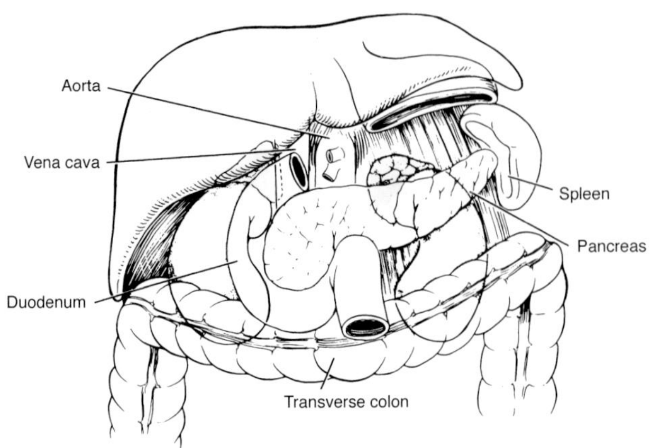


**Fig. 2.3**

Anatomical and surgical relationships of the adrenal glands viewed through an anterior abdominal approach.

solitary adrenal metastases. Open surgical adrenalectomy, the focus of this chapter, is primarily indicated in patients with large pheochromocytomas *(6)* or clinical overt adrenal cortical carcinomas *(7)*. These operations are generally performed through an anterior transabdominal approach or through a thoracoabdominal approach *(2,3)*.

### Anterior Transabdominal Approach

The anterior transabdominal approach is indicated for adrenal lesions that are either large or potentially malignant. These include suspected or proven adrenal cortical carcinomas and large adrenal pheochromocytomas. In these cases, wide exposure is necessary, which cannot be achieved to the same extent through an extraperitoneal incision. With potentially malignant adrenal masses, intra-abdominal inspection of other organs for metastatic disease is required. An anterior approach is also mandatory for adrenal malignancies that involve the inferior vena cava. The optimal anterior approach is through a bilateral subcostal or chevron incision, which provides much better exposure of the superior and lateral aspects of the adrenal gland than a midline incision. A unilateral extended subcostal incision can be used if the patient is thin and only one adrenal gland needs to be exposed. A vertical midline incision is used only if an extra-adrenal pheochromocytoma is suspected in the retroperitoneum along the great vessels or in the pelvis.

The main advantage of the transabdominal approach is that it provides excellent exposure of both adrenal glands, the vascular pedicles, the abdominal organs, and the retroperitoneum. Its principal disadvantage is that the peritoneal cavity is entered. It is not the most direct avenue to the adrenal glands, and in an obese patient exposure may be more difficult.

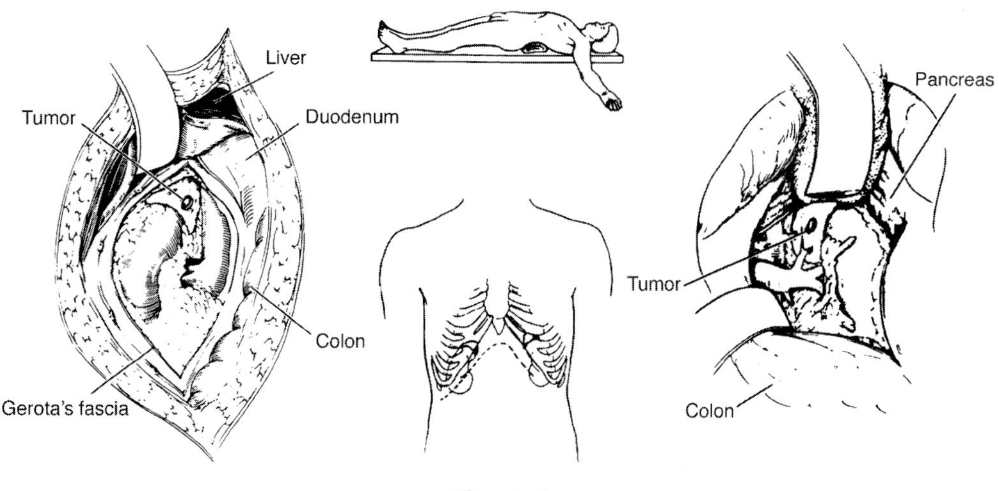


**Fig. 2.4**

Anterior transabdominal approach to the adrenal glands.

The patient is placed with a rolled sheet beneath the lumbar spine, and a unilateral extended subcostal or bilateral subcostal incision is made to enter the peritoneal cavity (Fig. 2.4). On the right side, the posterior peritoneum lateral to the ascending colon is incised, the colon and the duodenum are reflected medially, and the liver is retracted superiorly to expose the kidney and adrenal gland. The kidney is gently retracted downward to bring the anterior surface of the right adrenal gland into view. In most cases it is necessary to release the upper margin of the gland from the liver with sharp dissection to obtain complete exposure. In cases of pheochromocytoma, it is important to secure the adrenal vein as soon as possible to interrupt catecholamine release from the tumor into the systemic circulation. If the vein lies far cephalad, as it often does, division of the arterial supply medially and inferiorly may be necessary before the vein can be exposed satisfactorily and safely. Surgical exposure is facilitated by medial retraction of the inferior vena cava. In cases of suspected malignancy, it is also best to isolate the medial blood supply first and to carry out the lateral dissection later. For tumors confined to the adrenal gland, after the blood supply has been secured, the remaining lateral and inferior attachments of the gland are mobilized and divided to complete the adrenalectomy.

On the left side, the adrenal gland is exposed by incising the posterior peritoneum lateral to the descending colon and dividing the ileorenal ligament with medial retraction of the colon and superior retraction of the spleen. The left adrenal vein is identified at its entry into the left renal vein and is then ligated and divided. The inferior adrenal artery also is secured and divided at this time. The adrenal gland is mobilized posteriorly and laterally by blunt dissection. The gland is then retracted downward to expose the superior vascular attachments, which are secured and divided. The gland is then retracted laterally to expose the remaining medial arterial blood supply, which is secured and divided. Residual attachments of the gland to the upper pole of the kidney are divided into sharp dissection to complete the adrenalectomy.

In some cases an adrenal malignancy may invade the upper pole of the kidney. In this event, radical *en bloc* removal of both the kidney and adrenal gland within Gerota's fascia is the indicated procedure (Fig. 2.5). The main renal artery and vein are secured and divided in sequence, as in a radical nephrectomy; the ureter also is secured and divided. A plane is then developed posteriorly along the psoas muscle, bluntly mobilizing both the kidney and adrenal mass from behind and laterally. With downward and lateral retraction of the kidney, the medial blood supply to the tumor mass can be better identified. This exposure is facilitated by medial retraction of the vena cava. The medial adrenal arteries are secured and transected. On the right side, as the dissection proceeds upward, the adrenal vein also is identified, secured, and divided. This vein is large and friable, often lies higher than the surgeon expects, and must be carefully dissected free from surrounding structures to prevent avulsion from the vena cava. Should such an avulsion occur, the caval entry is immediately secured with Allis clamps and the defect is oversewn with a continuous 5-0 arterial suture. After the blood supply is secured, the dissection is carried upward and laterally to completely remove the tumor mass and kidney *en bloc* with Gerota's fascia. A regional lymphadenectomy is then performed from the level of the inferior mesenteric artery to the crus of the diaphragm. Splanchnic nerves and celiac ganglia may be sacrificed if adjacent nodes appear involved by neoplasm.

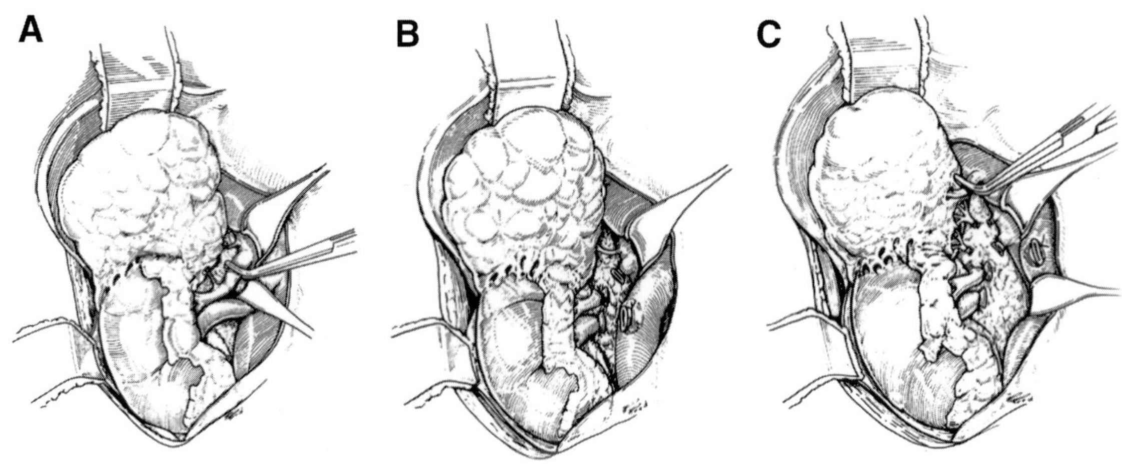


**Fig. 2.5**

Technique of radical nephroadrenalectomy on the right side.

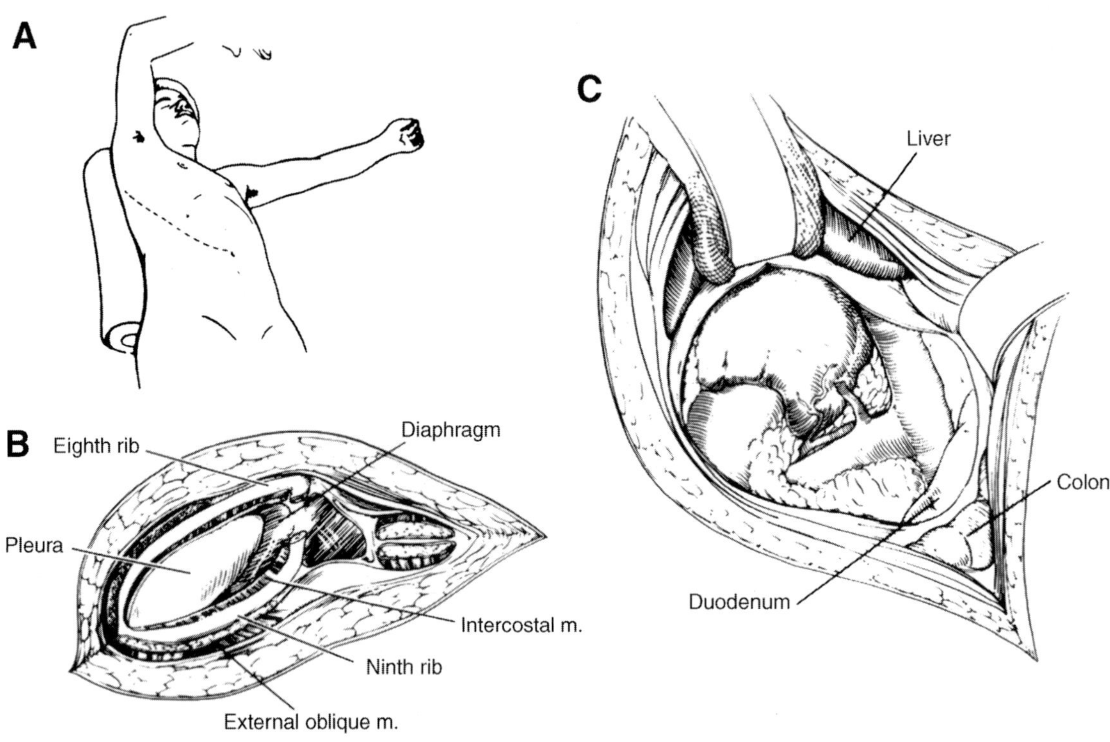


**Fig. 2.6**

Thoracoabdominal approach to the adrenal gland.

## Thoracoabdominal Approach

The thoracoabdominal approach to the adrenal gland is desirable for very large tumors that cannot be removed safely through an anterior transabdominal incision. It can be particularly advantageous for large right-sided adrenal masses, where the overlying liver and vena cava can limit exposure. There is less indication for this incision on the left side because the spleen and the pancreas usually can be elevated away from the adrenal without difficulty. The thoracoabdominal incision provides excellent exposure of the suprarenal area; however, additional operative time is required to open and close a thoracoabdominal incision. Because the thoracic cavity is entered and the diaphragm divided, potential pulmonary morbidity is greater. For these reasons, the thoracoabdominal approach is reserved for patients in whom exposure beyond that provided by an anterior subcostal incision is considered important for complete and safe tumor removal.

The patient is placed in a semi-oblique position with a rolled sheet inserted longitudinally between the flank and hemithorax (Fig. 2.6). The incision is begun in the eighth or ninth intercostal space near the angle of the rib and is carried medially across the umbilicus. The intercostal muscles are divided to reveal the pleura and diaphragm; the diaphragm is divided circumferentially. On the right side, the hepatic flexure of the colon and duodenum are reflected medially and the liver is retracted upward to expose the adrenal tumor. On the left side, the descending colon is reflected medially with superior retraction of the pancreas and spleen to expose the adrenal gland. The details of adrenalectomy or nephroadrenalectomy are the same as those described for the anterior transabdominal surgical approach.

## REFERENCES

1. Novick AC, Howards SS. The Adrenals. In Gillenwater JY, Grayhack JT, Howards SS, Mitchell ME (editors), Adult and Pediatric Urology, 4th edition, Lippincott Williams and Wilkins, Philadelphia, 2002, pp. 531–562.
2. Guz B, Straffon R, Novick AC. Operative approaches to the adrenal gland. Urol Clin N Am 16:527, 1989.
3. Novick AC. Operations upon the adrenal gland. In Novick AC, Streem SB, Pontes JE (editors), Stewart's Operative Urology, Baltimore, Williams and Wilkins, 1989, pp. 65–95.
4. Gill IS, Schweizer D, Nelson D et al. Laparoscopic vs open adrenalectomy: Cleveland Clinic experience with 210 cases. J Urol 161:21, 1999.
5. Daitch J, Goldfarb D, Novick AC. Cleveland Clinic experience with adrenal Cushing's syndrome. J Urol 158:2051, 1997.
6. Ulchaker JC, Goldfarb D, Bravo E, Novick AC. Successful outcomes in pheochromocytoma surgery in the modern era. J Urol 161:764, 1999.
7. Bodie B, Novick AC, Pontes JE. The Cleveland Clinic experience with adrenal cortical carcinoma. J Urol 141:257, 1989.

# 3 Laparoscopic Adrenalectomy

*Mihir M. Desai and Inderbir S. Gill*

## INTRODUCTION

Since the initial report by Gagner, laparoscopic adrenalectomy has rapidly emerged as the preferred approach for surgical removal of the adrenal gland. Laparoscopic adrenalectomy has been performed transperitoneally and retroperitoneally at various centers worldwide, attesting to its safety and efficacy. This chapter describes the current indications, preoperative preparation, and operative techniques of laparoscopic adrenalectomy.

## SURGICAL ANATOMY

Clear understanding of the surgical anatomy of the adrenal glands is critical to the safe performance of laparoscopic adrenalectomy. The adrenal glands are paired retroperitoneal organs, separated from the upper pole of the kidney by a fibrous layer within Gerota's fascia. Both adrenal glands are distinct in terms of anatomical position and relations, shape and size, and vascular supply.

The right adrenal gland is triangular and lies cephalad to the upper pole of the right kidney and is related to the liver superiorly, inferior vena cava (IVC) medially, duodenum and liver anteriorly, and diaphragm and pleura posteriorly. The right adrenal derives its arterial supply from the right renal artery (inferior pedicle), aorta (middle pedicle), and inferior phrenic artery (superior pedicle). The right adrenal gland is drained by a short and wide main adrenal vein that exits the superior pole of the gland and enters directly into the posterolateral aspect of the inferior vena cava.

The left adrenal gland is crescentic in shape and lies along the medial aspect of the upper pole of the left kidney, occupying a lower anatomical position in the retroperitoneum as compared to the right adrenal gland. Similar to the right side, the left adrenal gland is supplied by an upper, middle, and lower pedicle, derived from the inferior phrenic, aorta, and renal artery, respectively. The left adrenal gland, in contrast to the right side, is drained by a narrow and longer main left adrenal vein, which drains into the superior aspect of the main left renal vein. The left adrenal gland is related to the aorta medially, upper pole of the left kidney laterally, spleen superiorly, tail of pancreas anteriorly, and diaphragm and pleura posteriorly. The left adrenal gland lies at distance from the aorta, in contrast to the right adrenal gland, which is more intimately approximated to the IVC.

## INDICATIONS AND CONTRAINDICATIONS

Laparoscopic adrenalectomy is currently the standard of care for most benign hyperfunctioning adrenal tumors and the occasional localized, small adrenal cancer. Aldosteronomas are generally small and are ideally suited for laparoscopic excision. In the past, pheochromocytoma was considered a relative contraindication for laparoscopic adrenalectomy. However, worldwide data have demonstrated the efficacy of the laparoscopic approach for surgical excision of pheochromocytoma. In fact, data suggest that laparoscopic adrenalectomy may produce less intraoperative hemodynamic fluctuations as compared to the open approach. Laparoscopic adrenalectomy, unilateral and bilateral, has been successfully employed to treat Cushing's disease and syndrome. Cushingoid patients have an increased tendency to poor wound healing and increased perioperative morbidity with open adrenalectomy and may therefore benefit significantly by the laparoscopic approach. Laparoscopic adrenalectomy is also effective in excising adrenal incidentalomas that merit surgical removal. Although small, radiologically localized, noninfiltrating adrenal cancers can be excised laparoscopically, large and infiltrating cancers are best treated with open surgical wide excision.

## PREOPERATIVE EVALUATION

Apart from general preoperative laboratory testing, all patients undergoing laparoscopic adrenalectomy should undergo complete adrenal endocrinological evaluation. We prefer volume-rendered three-dimensional reconstructed computed tomography (CT) scanning for preoperative

From: *Operative Urology at the Cleveland Clinic*
Edited by: A. Novick et al. © Humana Press Inc., Totowa, NJ

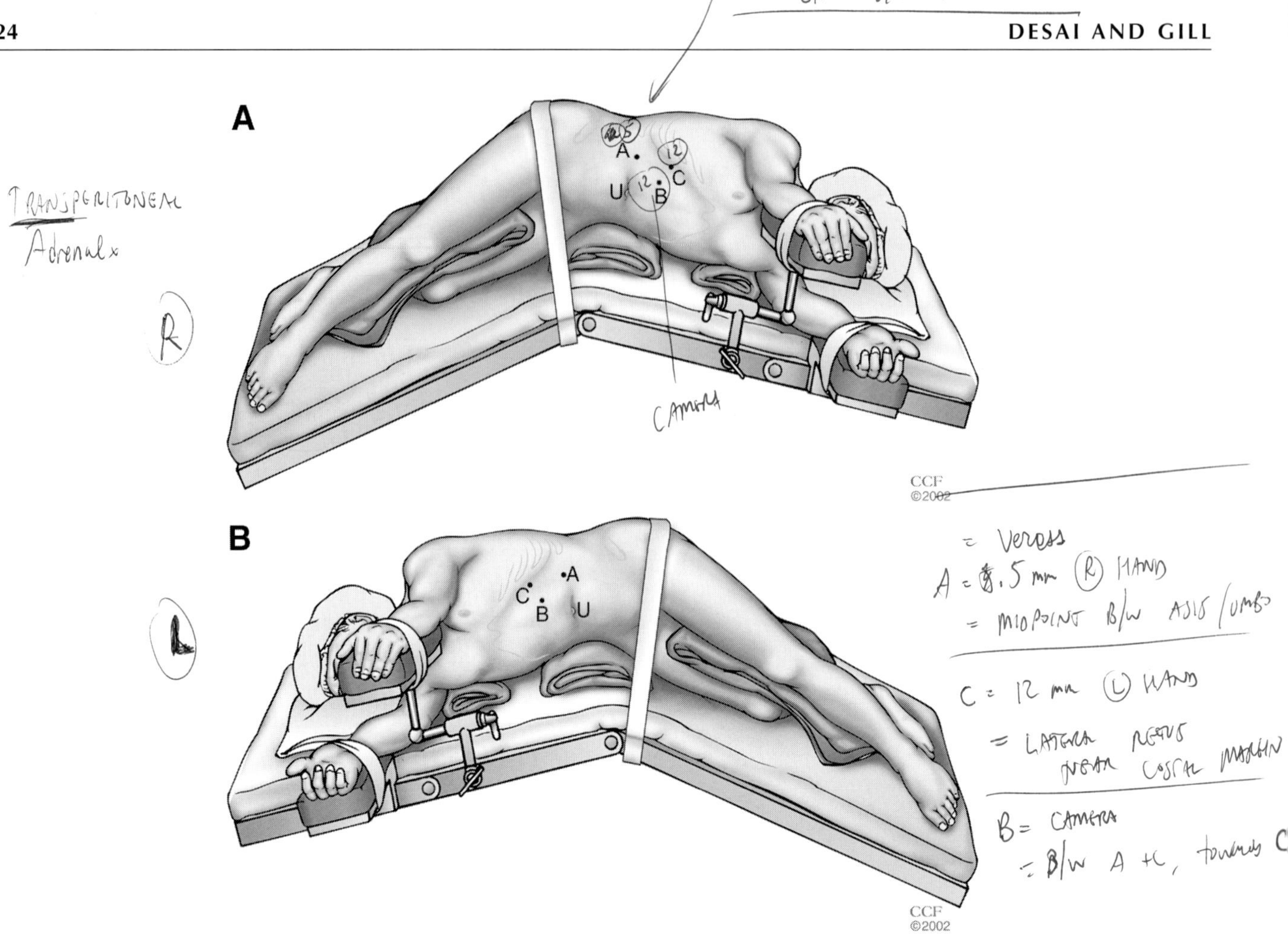


Fig. 3.1

**(A)** Patient positioning and port placement for a right transperitoneal laparoscopic adrenalectomy. **(B)** Patient position for a left-sided transperitoneal adrenalectomy is identical to that on the right side. The 5-mm port for liver retraction, however, is not required.

imaging of adrenal tumors. Thin-slice three-dimensional CT scanning provides detailed anatomical information about the adrenal tumor, vasculature, and spatial relationship of the adrenal mass to surrounding viscera and major abdominal blood vessels.

## Endocrinological Preparation

Specific preparation to correct hormonal and metabolic derangements associated with adrenal tumors is critical for a smooth operative outcome. At our institution, preoperative preparation for pheochromocytoma entails calcium channel blockers and vigorous hydration. α-Adrenergic antagonists and β-blockers are employed selectively. Patients with aldosteronoma are treated with potassium-sparing diuretics and potassium supplementation. Patients with Cushing's disease require perioperative stress steroid replacement.

## General Preparation

All patients are admitted on the morning of surgery, except patients with pheochromocytoma, who are admitted the previous day for intravenous hydration. All patients undergo a blood type and screen, but routine crossmatching is usually not carried out. Bowel preparation consists of magnesium citrate solution on the evening prior to surgery, and the patient is instructed to take only clear liquids subsequently. The patients are asked to remain nil-by-mouth from midnight preceding the day of surgery. Invasive intraoperative hemodynamic monitoring is routine for patients with pheochromocytoma and is selectively applied for patients with other adrenal tumors.

# OPERATIVE TECHNIQUE

Laparoscopic adrenalectomy can be performed transperitoneally or retroperitoneally.

## Transperitoneal Laparoscopic Adrenalectomy

### Patient Positioning (Fig. 3.1)

For transperitoneal adrenalectomy, the patient is positioned in a lateral flank position with a 45–60° tilt. The kidney rest, positioned below the iliac crest, is elevated and the table is flexed, thereby increasing the space between the

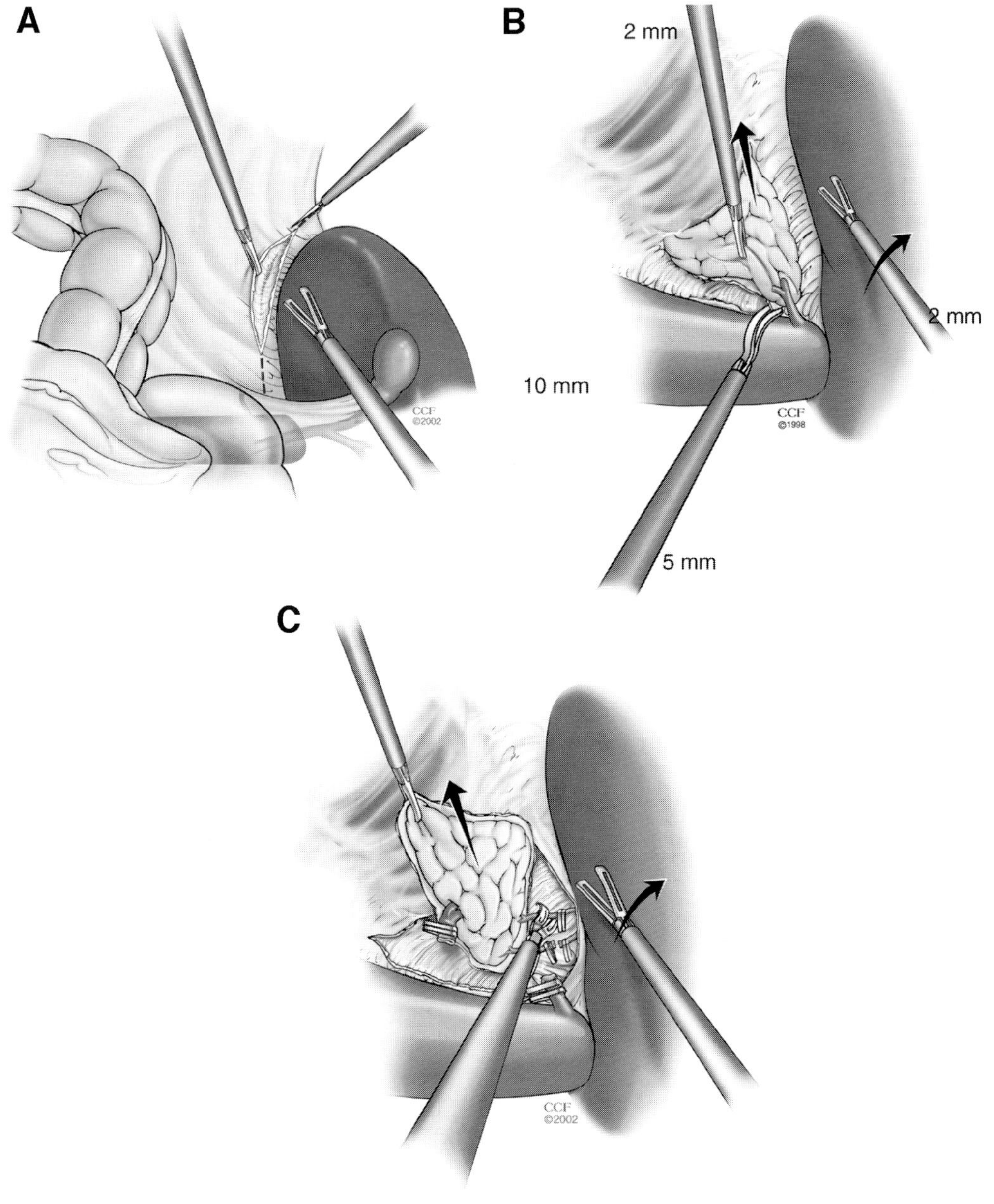


Fig. 3.2

Right transperitoneal laparoscopic adrenalectomy. **(A)** A peritoneal incision is made inferior to the liver to expose the suprarenal vena cava and main adrenal vein. **(B)** The adrenal gland is gradually dissected from the vena cava, to which it is closely approximated, to expose the main adrenal vein. **(C)** The main adrenal vein is clipped and the adrenal gland completely mobilized after dividing the superior (inferior phrenic) and inferior (renal) adrenal vascular supply.

costal margin and the iliac crest. Increased lateral flexion may be associated with an increased incidence of neuromuscular problems and also with a diminution in venous return. Unlike the retroperitoneal approach, where the flexion is critical in obtaining initial access, we currently employ a strategy of limiting the degree of lateral flexion in transperitoneal renal and adrenal surgery. The extremities are maintained in a neutral position, and all bony prominences are adequately padded using egg-crate foam and blankets. The arms are securely nestled in a double arm board, and an axillary roll is placed to prevent brachial plexus injury. Intravenous lines, arterial lines, and blood pressure cuffs are placed in the nondependent upper extremity.

## Transperitoneal Right Adrenalectomy (Fig. 3.2)

### *Step 1: Port Placement*

A right adrenalectomy is typically performed using four ports. A Verres needle placed at the midpoint of the spino-umbilical line obtains initial transperitoneal access. After creating adequate pneumoperitoneum, a 5-mm port is placed at the site of initial access. All subsequent ports are placed under laparoscopic visualization. The right-hand working port (12 mm) is placed just under the costal margin, at the lateral edge of the rectus abdominis. The primary camera port is placed between the two working ports, skewed toward the right-hand port. On the right side we routinely employ an additional 5-mm port medial and superior to the right-hand port for cephalad retraction of the liver.

#### *Step 2: Cephalad Retraction of the Liver and Exposure of the Vena Cava*

After port placement, the liver is retracted anterosuperiorly using the shaft of a 5-mm laparoscopic locking Allis clamp. The lateral parietal peritoneum is grasped by the Allis clamp, thus creating a self-retaining system to maintain constant liver retraction without the need for involving an assistant. It is critical to ensure that the shaft of the Allis clamp does not injure the liver or gallbladder. Occasionally, peritoneal bands tethering the liver may require division in order to achieve adequate upward liver retraction. Cephalad retraction of the liver provides excellent exposure to the Gerota's fascia covering the kidney and adrenal gland. A horizontal incision is made parallel and inferior to the liver dividing the inferior limb of the right coronary and triangular ligament, thereby exposing the suprarenal inferior vena cava. On the right side, significant formal mobilization of the right colon and duodenum is usually not required for obtaining adequate exposure of the adrenal gland.

#### *Step 3: Medial Dissection of the Adrenal Gland and Ligation of the Adrenal Vein*

The adrenal gland is carefully dissected away from the IVC. Small multiple aortic branches to the adrenal gland are clipped during this dissection. The dissection is carried cephalad till the main adrenal vein is seen exiting the superior pole of the adrenal gland. The adrenal vein is securely clipped and divided.

#### *Step 4: Circumferential Adrenal Mobilization*

The adrenal gland is carefully dissected from the upper pole of the right kidney by clipping the vascular supply derived from the renal artery. Subsequently, the adrenal gland is dissected from the diaphragm by clipping and dividing the vascular supply from the inferior phrenic vessels.

#### *Step 5: Specimen Entrapment and Extraction*

The completely mobilized adrenal gland is then entrapped in an impermeable 10-mm Endocatch (USSC, Norwalk, CT) bag and extracted intact. Most adrenal tumors can be extracted by minimal extension of one of the port sites.

### Transperitoneal Left Adrenalectomy (Fig. 3.3)

#### *Step 1: Port Placement*

Left transperitoneal adrenalectomy is usually performed through three ports. The port placement mirrors that used for the right side, except for the absence of the liver retraction port. An additional 2-mm port may be required for adrenal gland retraction.

#### *Step 2: Mobilization of the Colon and Spleen*

In contrast to the right side, transperitoneal left adrenalectomy requires formal mobilization of the left colon and spleen. The line of Toldt is incised and the colon retracted medially. The spleen and tail of pancreas are also mobilized cephalad and medially to expose the left adrenal gland.

#### *Step 3: Ligation of the Left Adrenal Vein*

The left main renal vein is identified. Dissecting along the superior border of the renal vein reveals the origin of the left adrenal vein. The adrenal vein is carefully dissected, clipped, and divided. This step is performed with extreme caution since an upper pole branch of the renal artery may lie immediately posterior to the main left adrenal vein.

#### *Step 4: Mobilization of the Adrenal Gland*

Once the main left adrenal vein is divided, the adrenal gland is systematically mobilized. Initially, the medial border of the adrenal gland is dissected by clipping the aortic branches. Dissection in this plane continues until the psoas muscle is identified. Subsequently, the superior aspect of the adrenal gland is mobilized by clipping the inferior phrenic vessels. Finally, the infero-lateral border of the adrenal is separated from the upper pole of the left kidney by clipping vessels that arise from the renal artery. Again, during this part of the dissection, care must be taken not to inadvertently injure an upper polar renal artery. The completely mobilized adrenal gland is entrapped in an impermeable bag and extracted intact.

## Retroperitoneal Laparoscopic Adrenalectomy

### Patient Positioning (Fig. 3.4)

Retroperitoneoscopic adrenalectomy is performed with the patient positioned in the conventional flank position. Elevation of the kidney rest and lateral flexion are important in the retroperitoneal approach during initial access. The flexion may be reversed once access has been obtained and ports adequately positioned in order to minimize neuromuscular sequelae and optimize venous return and urine output.

### Retroperitoneal Access and Port Placement

The detailed technique of obtaining retroperitoneal access has been outlined in an earlier chapter. Patient positioning and port placement are identical for right- and left-sided

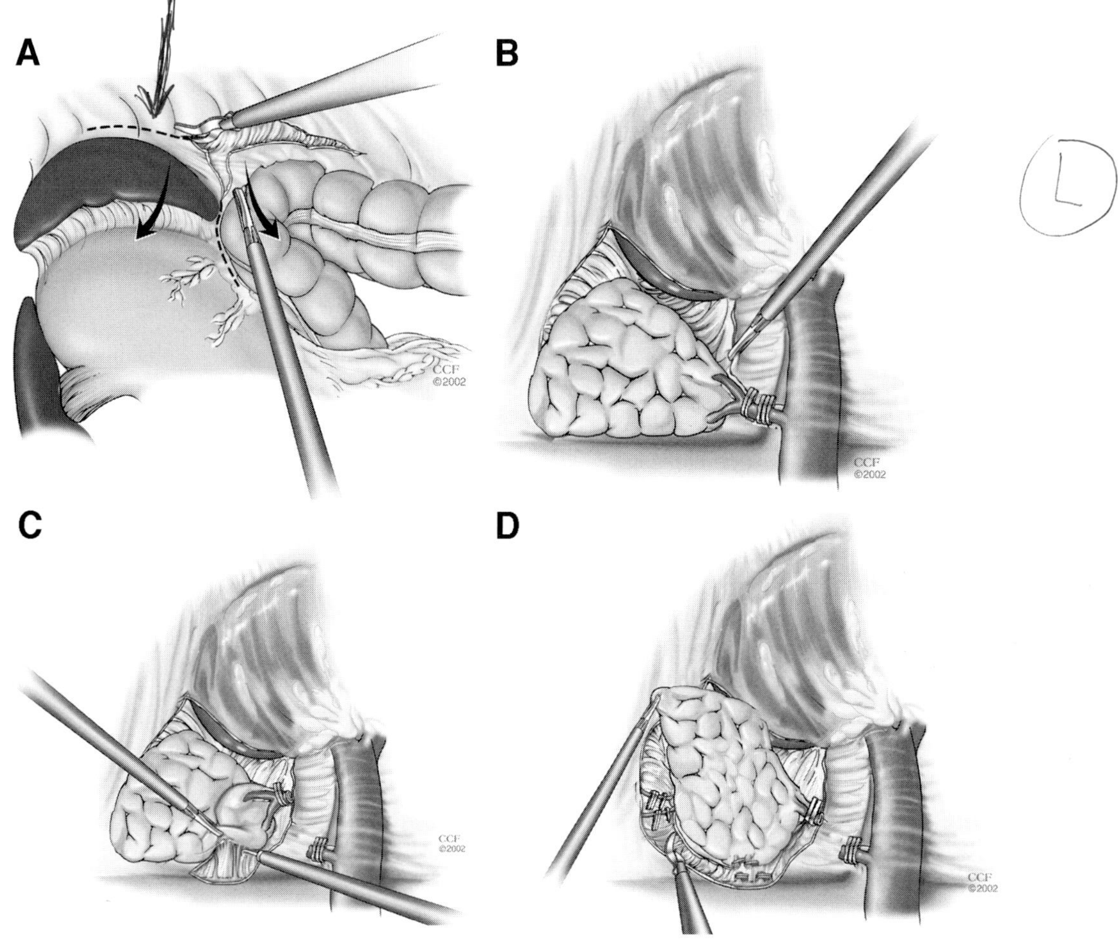


**Fig. 3.3**

Laparoscopic transperitoneal left adrenalectomy. **(A)** A T-shaped peritoneal incision is made and the left colon and spleen are mobilized. **(B)** The main adrenal vein is identified at the superior border of the main left renal vein, clipped, and divided. **(C)** The adrenal gland is dissected from the upper pole of the kidney. **(D)** The medial border of the adrenal gland is mobilized by dividing aortic branches, and the superior pole is mobilized by dividing the inferior phrenic branches, thereby completing the adrenalectomy.

*Note*: The 2-mm instruments shown in **Figs. 3.3** and **3.4** are utilized during needlescopic adrenalectomy, which is the author's preference for most transperitoneal adrenalectomies. However, 5-mm instruments may be employed in place of the 2-mm instruments for performing a transperitoneal adrenalectomy. The operative steps, as outlined above, remain the same regardless of whether or not 2-mm instruments are utilized.

retroperitoneoscopic adrenalectomy. A 1-in. incision is made below the tip of the 12th rib, and via finger dissection the retroperitoneal space is entered. An initial space is created with finger dissection in front of the psoas muscle and behind the Gerota's fascia. Further development of the retroperitoneal space is achieved by balloon inflation (PDB Balloon Dilator, Origin Medical Systems, Menlo Park, CA). Specific to retroperitoneoscopic adrenalectomy, a secondary inflation is carried out in the upper retroperitoneum by directing the shaft of the balloon dilator cephalad. An anterior port is placed approximately four finger-breadths above the anterior superior iliac spine, and a posterior port is placed in the renal angle under direct laparoscopic visualization.

## Retroperitoneal Laparoscopic Right Adrenalectomy (Fig. 3.5)

### *Step 1: Identification of Renal Artery and Suprarenal Inferior Vena Cava*

The first step in a retroperitoneoscopic right adrenalectomy is identification of the vertical sharp and bounding renal artery pulsations. Subsequently, the IVC superior to the renal artery is identified by its horizontal wavy pulsations. The adventitial tissue overlying the vena cava is carefully dissected using a monopolar J-hook. The dissection proceeds along the surface of the IVC in a cephalad direction. During this dissection, multiple small aortic branches to the adrenal gland are clipped and divided.

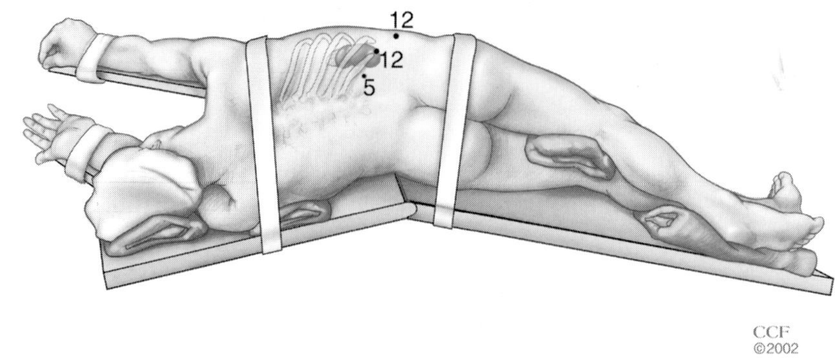


Fig. 3.4

Patient positioning and port placement for laparoscopic retroperitoneal adrenalectomy. The patient is positioned in the traditional (90°) flank position. Retroperitoneoscopic adrenalectomy is typically performed through three ports. The primary 12-mm camera port is positioned just below the tip of the 12th rib. The posterior port is placed at the renal angle, and the anterior port is placed four finger-breadths above the anterior superior iliac spine. An additional port may be required for retraction in the occasional case.

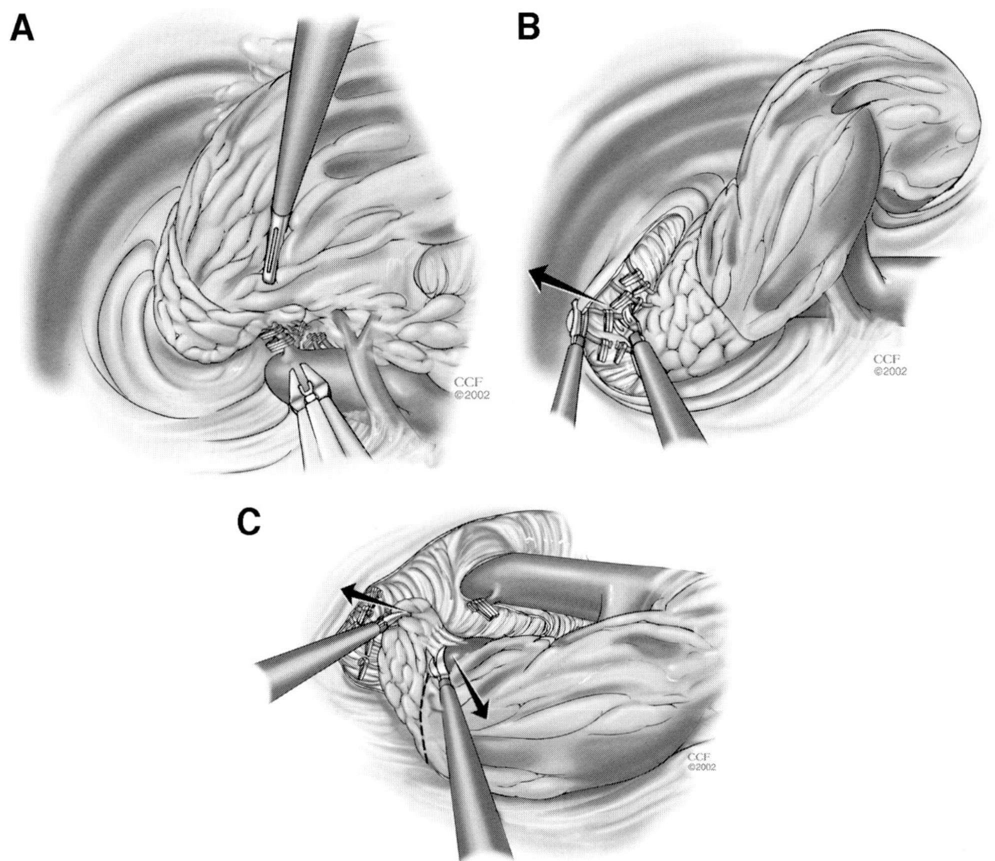


Fig. 3.5

Retroperitoneoscopic right adrenalectomy. **(A)** Identifying the suprearenal inferior vena cava. The dissection proceeds along the upper border of the vena cava, carefully dividing the aortic branches to the adrenal gland, until the main right adrenal vein is identified, clipped, and divided. **(B)** The superior attachments of the adrenal gland are divided after clipping the inferior phrenic vascular supply. **(C)** The kidney is mobilized infero-laterally, and the adrenal gland is carefully separated from the upper pole of the kidney, thereby completing the adrenalectomy.

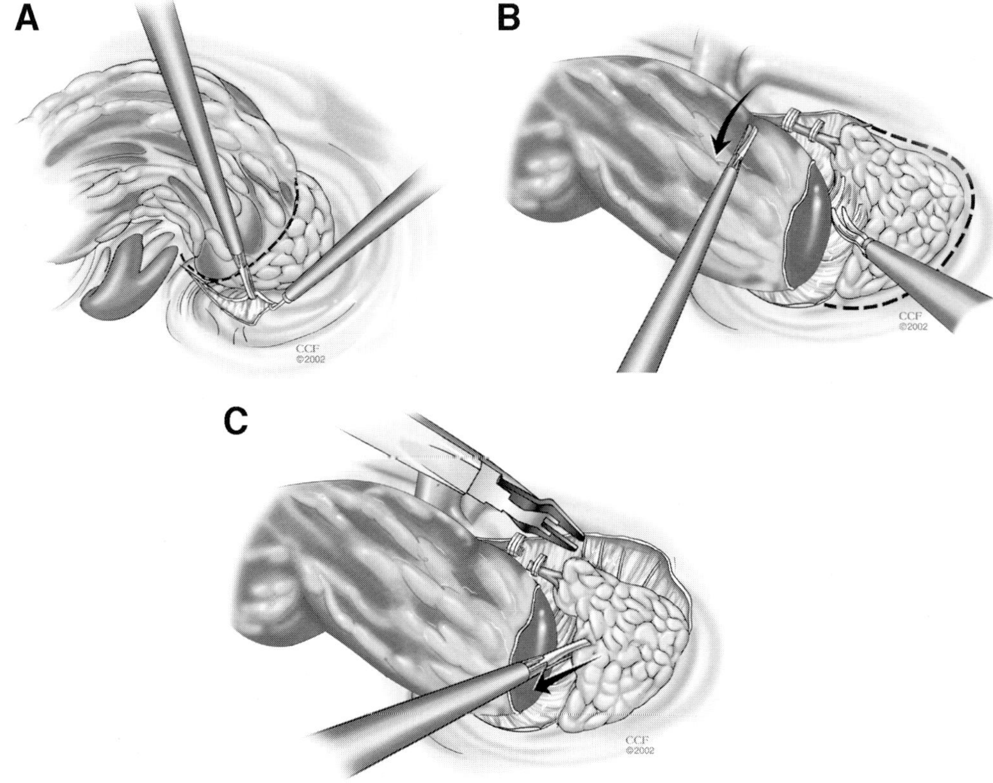


**Fig. 3.6**

Retroperitoneoscopic left adrenalectomy. **(A)** The Gerota's fascia along the upper pole is incised. **(B)** The adrenal gland is carefully mobilized from the medial border of the upper pole. **(C)** The upper pole of the kidney is mobilized laterally and inferiorly to expose the main adrenal vein. The superior attachments of the adrenal are also divided (dotted line).

### *Step 2: Control of Main Adrenal Vein*

The dissection continues until the main adrenal vein is identified as it enters the posterolateral aspect of the IVC. The main adrenal vein is clipped and divided. This step is critical because any bleeding from the IVC may be difficult to control, especially from the retroperitoneoscopic route.

### *Step 3: Adrenal Mobilization*

The superior aspect of the adrenal gland is mobilized, dissecting it away from the undersurface of the diaphragm and the liver. During the superior mobilization, the superior phrenic supply to the superior pole of the adrenal gland is clipped and divided. Subsequently, the anterior surface of the adrenal gland is mobilized from the peritoneum. Finally, the adrenal gland is carefully dissected from the upper pole of the kidney by clipping the vascular supply derived from the renal artery. During this part of the mobilization, care should be taken to avoid ligating an upper pole renal artery. The completely mobilized adrenal gland is entrapped in an impermeable bag and extracted intact.

## Retroperitoneoscopic Left Adrenalectomy (Fig. 3.6)

### *Step 1: Identification of the Left Renal Artery and Main Left Adrenal Vein*

Once retroperitoneal access is obtained and the ports placed (as described earlier), the initial step is identification of the main left renal artery. The superior aspect of the renal artery is dissected and the main left adrenal vein is identified as it courses anterior to the base of the main renal artery, clipped, and divided.

### *Step 2: Mobilization of the Medial Border of the Adrenal Gland*

After controlling the main adrenal vein, the aortic branches to the adrenal gland are clipped and divided. This mobilizes the medial border of the adrenal gland.

### *Step 3: Mobilization of the Upper Pole of the Kidney*

The left adrenal gland is located medial to the upper pole of the kidney. As such, lateral and caudal mobilization of the upper pole of the kidney is essential. After the upper pole of the kidney has been adequately mobilized, the adrenal gland is carefully dissected from the kidney surface. During this dissection extreme care is taken not to injure an upper pole renal artery. Occasionally, if the main adrenal vein is not identified at the outset (step 1), it can be identified and clipped during this part of the dissection.

### *Step 4: Mobilization of the Anterior and Superior Aspect of the Adrenal Gland*

The anterior surface of the adrenal gland can be bluntly separated from the peritoneum. A communicating vein from the inferior phrenic vein to the main adrenal vein courses along the anteromedial aspect of the adrenal gland and should be controlled. Finally, the superior pole of the adrenal gland is mobilized from the undersurface of the diaphragm, carefully ligating and dividing the superior vascular supply derived from the inferior phrenic vessels. The completely mobilized adrenal gland is entrapped and extracted intact.

## SUGGESTED READINGS

1. Bravo EL, Steward BH. The adrenal: anatomy and physiology. Urol Update Series 1:1, 1978.
2. Gill IS. The case for laparoscopic adrenalectomy. J Urol 166:429–436, 2001.
3. Gill IS, Soble JJ, Sung GT, Winfield HN, Bravo EL, Novick AC. Needlescopic adrenalectomy—the initial series: comparison with conventional laparoscopic adrenalectomy. Urology 52:180–186, 1998.
4. Sung GT, Hsu THS, Gill IS. Retroperitoneoscopic adrenalectomy: lateral approach. J Endourol 15:505–511, 2001.
5. Winfield HN, Hamilton BD, Bravo EL. Technique of laparoscopic adrenalectomy. Urol Clin North Am 24:459–65, 1997.

# 4 Renal Malignancy

## Open Surgery

*Andrew C. Novick*

## RADICAL NEPHRECTOMY

Radical nephrectomy is the treatment of choice for patients with localized renal cell carcinoma (RCC *[1]*). In many patients, a complete preliminary evaluation can be performed using noninvasive imaging modalities. Renal arteriography is no longer routinely necessary prior to performing radical nephrectomy. All patients should undergo a metastatic evaluation including a chest x-ray, abdominal computed tomography (CT) scan, and, occasionally, a bone scan; the latter is only necessary in patients with bone pain or an elevated serum alkaline phosphatase. Radical nephrectomy is occasionally done in patients with metastatic disease to palliate severe associated local symptoms, to allow entry into a biological response modifier treatment protocol, or concomitant with resection of a solitary metastatic lesion.

Involvement of the inferior vena cava (IVC) with RCC occurs in 4–10% of cases and renders the task of complete surgical excision more complicated *(2)*. Yet, operative removal offers the only hope for cure, and when there are no metastases, an aggressive approach is justified. Five-year survival rates of 40–68% have been reported after complete surgical excision *(3–6)*. The best results have been achieved when the tumor does not involve the perinephric fat and regional lymph nodes *(7)*. The cephalad extent of vena caval involvement is not prognostically important, and even with intra-atrial tumor thrombi, extended cancer-free survival is possible following surgical treatment when there is no modal or distant metastasis *(8)*. In planning the appropriate operative approach for tumor removal, it is essential for preoperative radiographic studies to define accurately the distal limits of a vena caval tumor thrombus.

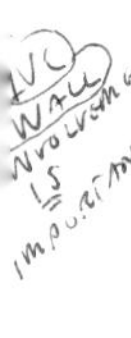

RCC involving the IVC should be suspected in patients who have lower extremity edema, a varicocele, dilated superficial abdominal veins, proteinuria, pulmonary embolism, a right atrial mass, or nonfunction of the involved kidney. Currently, magnetic resonance imaging (MRI) is the preferred diagnostic study for demonstrating both the presence and distal extent of IVC involvement *(9)*. Transesophageal echocardiography *(10)* and transabdominal color flow Doppler ultrasonography *(11)* have also proven to be useful diagnostic studies in this regard. Inferior vena cavography is reserved for patients in whom an MRI or ultrasound study is either nondiagnostic or contraindicated. Renal arteriography is particularly helpful in patients with RCC involving the IVC because distinct arterialization of a tumor thrombus is observed in 35–40% of cases. When this finding is present, preoperative embolization of the kidney often causes shrinkage of the thrombus, which facilitates its intraoperative removal. When adjunctive cardiopulmonary bypass with deep hypothermic circulatory arrest is considered, coronary angiography is also performed preoperatively *(4,12)*. If significant obstructing coronary lesions are found, these can be repaired simultaneously during cardiopulmonary bypass.

### Standard Radical Nephrectomy

Radical nephrectomy encompasses the basic principles of early ligation of the renal artery and vein, removal of the kidney outside Gerota's fascia, removal of the ipsilateral adrenal gland, and performance of a complete regional lymphadenectomy from the crus of the diaphragm to the aortic bifurcation *(1)*. Perhaps the most important aspect of radical nephrectomy is removal of the kidney outside Gerota's fascia because capsular invasion with perinephric fat involvement occurs in 25% of patients. It has recently been shown that removal of the ipsilateral adrenal gland is not routinely necessary unless the malignancy either extensively involves the kidney or is located in the upper portion of the kidney *(13)*. Although lymphadenectomy allows for more accurate pathological staging, the therapeutic value remains controversial. Nevertheless, there may be a subset of patients with micrometastatic lymph node involvement

From: *Operative Urology at the Cleveland Clinic*
Edited by: A. Novick et al. © Humana Press Inc., Totowa, NJ

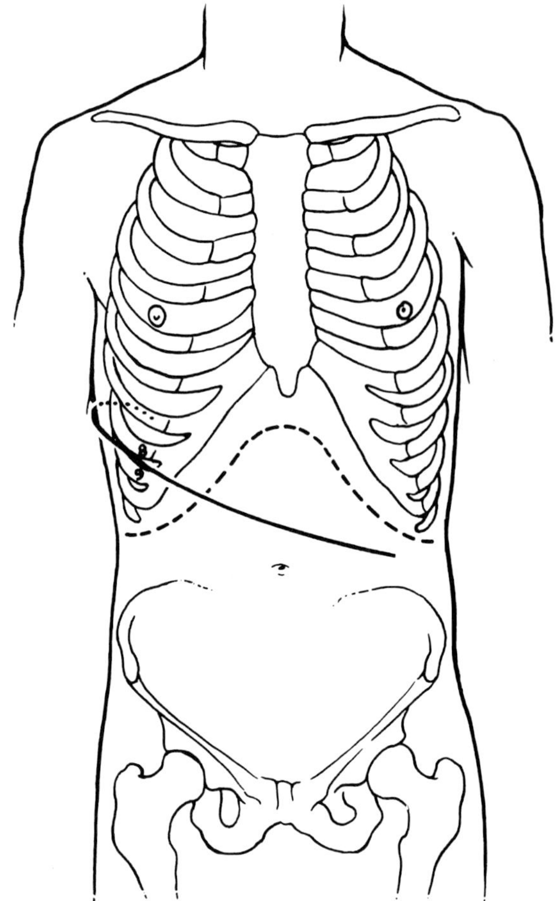

Fig. 4.1

Radical nephrectomy is performed through either a bilateral subcostal or thoracoabdominal incision.

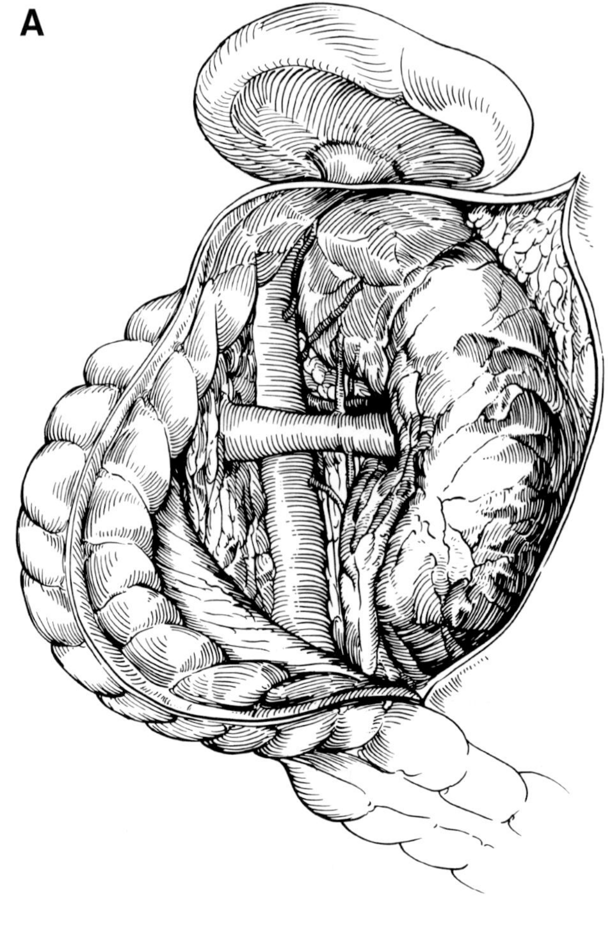


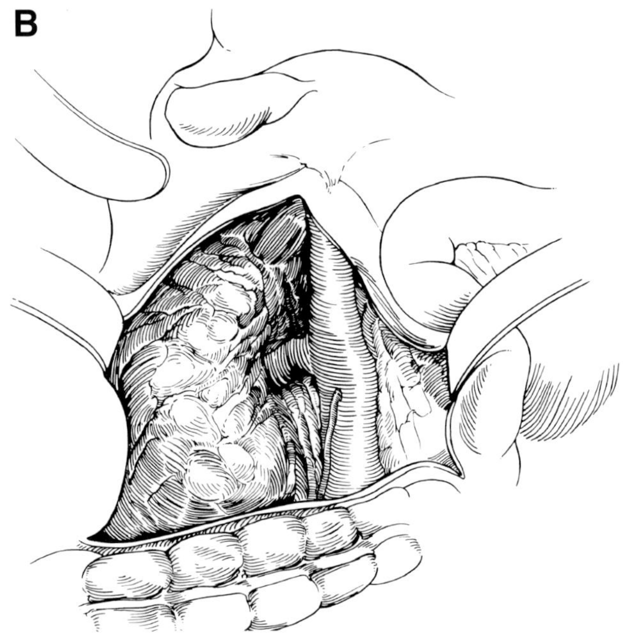


Fig. 4.2

After entering the peritoneal cavity, the colon is reflected medially to expose the left (**A**) or right (**B**) kidney and great vessels.

that can benefit from performance of a lymphadenectomy *(14)*. At the present time the need for routine performance of a complete lymphadenectomy in all cases is unresolved, and there remains a divergence of clinical practice among urologists with respect to this aspect of radical nephrectomy.

The surgical approach for radical nephrectomy is determined by the size and location of the tumor as well as the habitus of the patient. The operation is usually performed through a transperitoneal incision to allow abdominal exploration for metastatic disease and early access to the renal vessels with minimal manipulation of the tumor. The author prefers an extended subcostal or bilateral subcostal incision for most patients. A thoracoabdominal incision is used for patients with large upper pole tumors (Fig. 4.1). We occasionally employ an extraperitoneal flank incision to perform radical nephrectomy in elderly or poor-risk patients with a small tumor.

When performing radical nephrectomy through a subcostal transperitoneal incision, a thorough exploration for metastatic disease is performed after opening the abdominal cavity. On the left side, the colon is reflected medially to expose the great vessels. This is facilitated by division of the splenocolic ligaments, which also helps to avoid excessive traction and injury to the spleen. On the right side, the colon and duodenum are reflected medially to expose the vena cava and aorta (Fig. 4.2).

The operation is initiated with dissection of the renal pedicle. On the right side, the renal vein is short, and care must be taken not to injure the vena cava. The right renal artery may be mobilized either lateral to the vena cava or, with a large medial tumor, between the vena cava and the aorta (Fig. 4.3).

On the left side, the renal vein is quite long as it passes over the aorta. The vein is mobilized completely by ligating and dividing gonadal, adrenal and lumbar tributaries. The vein can then be retracted to expose the artery posteriorly which is then mobilized toward the aorta. The renal artery is ligated with 2-0 silk ligatures and divided, and the renal vein is then similarly managed (Fig. 4.4).

The kidney is then mobilized outside Gerota's fascia with blunt and sharp dissection as needed. Remaining vascular attachments are secured with nonabsorbable sutures or metal clips. The ureter is then ligated and divided to complete the removal of the kidney and adrenal gland (Fig. 4.5).

The classical description of radical nephrectomy includes the performance of a complete regional lymphadenectomy. The lymph nodes can be removed either *en bloc* with the kidney and adrenal gland or separately following the nephrectomy. The lymph node dissection is begun at the crura of the diaphragm just below the origin of the superior mesenteric artery. There is a readily definable periadventitial plane

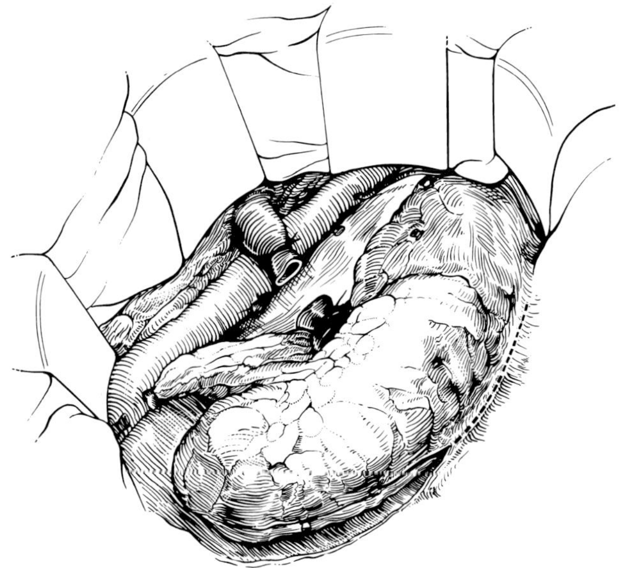

**Fig. 4.4**

After securing the pedicle and dividing the ureter, the left kidney is mobilized outside Gerota's fascia.

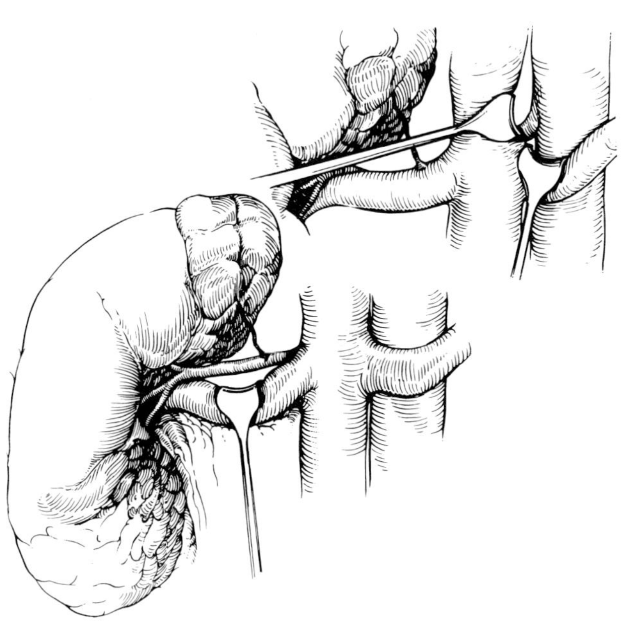

**Fig. 4.3**

The right renal artery may be mobilized either lateral to the vena cava or between the vena cava and the aorta.

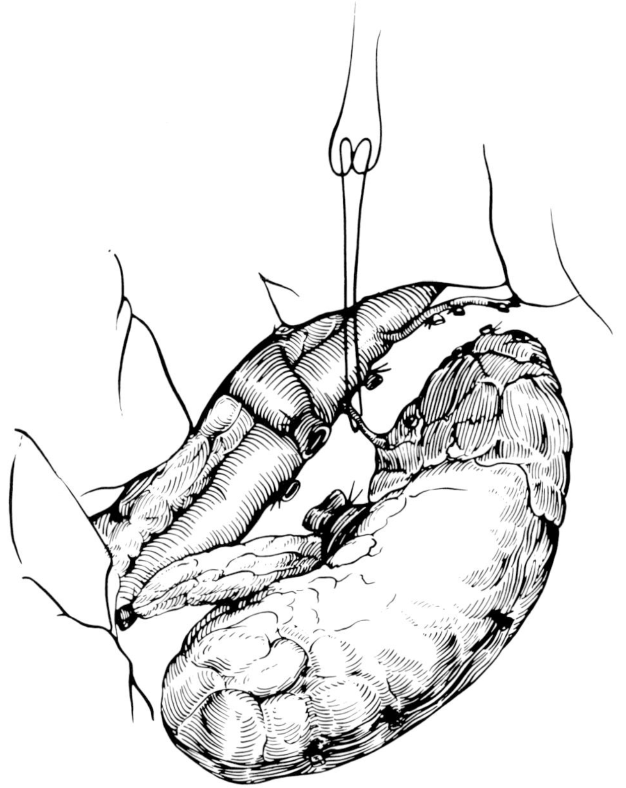

**Fig. 4.5**

Remaining medial vascular attachments are secured and divided to complete the nephrectomy.

close to the aorta that can be entered so that the dissection may be carried along the aorta and onto the origin of the major vessels to remove all of the peri-aortic lymphatic tissue. Care must be taken to avoid injury to the origins of the celiac and superior mesenteric arteries superiorly as they arise from the anterior surface of the aorta. The dissection of the peri-aortic and peri-caval lymph nodes is then carried downward *en bloc* to the origin of the inferior mesenteric artery. The sympathetic ganglia and nerves are removed together with the lymphatic tissue. The cisterna chyli is identified medial to the right crus, and entering lymphatic vessels are secured to prevent the development of chylous ascites.

A thoracoabdominal incision is preferable when performing radical nephrectomy for a large upper pole tumor. Once the liver has been retracted upward into the chest, the hepatic flexure of the colon and the duodenum are reflected medially to expose the anterior surface of the kidney and great vessels (Fig. 4.6). The renal artery is secured with 2-0 silk ligatures and divided, and the renal vein is then similarly managed (Fig. 4.7). The ureter and right gonadal vein are ligated and divided, and the kidney is mobilized outside Gerota's fascia. Downward and lateral traction of the kidney exposes the superior vascular attachments of the tumor and adrenal gland. Exposure of these vessels is also facilitated by medial retraction of the IVC (Fig. 4.8). Care is taken to preserve small hepatic venous branches entering the vena cava at the superior margin of the tumor mass. The tumor mass is then gently separated from the undersurface of the liver to complete the resection.

## Radical Nephrectomy With Infrahepatic Vena Caval Involvement

There are four levels of vena caval involvement in RCC, which are characterized according to the distal extent of the tumor thrombus (Fig. 4.9). A bilateral subcostal transperitoneal incision usually provides excellent exposure for performing radical nephrectomy and removal of a perirenal or infrahepatic IVC thrombus. For extremely large tumors involving the upper pole of the kidney, a thoracoabdominal incision may alternatively be used. After the abdomen is entered, the colon is reflected medially and a self-retaining ring retractor is inserted to maintain exposure of the retroperitoneum (Fig. 4.10A). The renal artery and the ureter are ligated and divided, and the entire kidney is mobilized outside Gerota's fascia leaving the kidney attached only by the renal vein (Fig. 4.10B,C). During the initial dissection, care is taken to avoid unnecessary manipulation of the renal vein and vena cava.

The vena cava is then completely dissected from surrounding structures above and below the renal vein, and the opposite renal vein is also mobilized. It is essential to obtain exposure and control of the supra-renal vena cava above the level of the tumor thrombus. If necessary, perforating veins to the caudate lobe of the liver are secured and divided to allow separation of the caudate lobe from the vena cava. This maneuver can allow an additional 2–3 cm length of vena cava to be exposed superiorly. The infrarenal vena cava is then occluded below the thrombus with a Satinsky venous clamp, and the opposite renal vein is gently secured with a small bulldog vascular clamp. Finally, in preparation for tumor thrombectomy, a curved Satinsky clamp is placed around the suprarenal vena cava above the level of the thrombus (Fig. 4.10D).

The anterior surface of the renal vein is then incised over the tumor thrombus and the incision is continued posteriorly with scissors, passing just beneath the thrombus (Fig. 4.10E). In most cases there is no attachment of the thrombus to the wall of the vena cava. After the renal vein has been circumscribed, gentle downward traction is exerted on the kidney to extract the tumor thrombus from the vena cava (Fig. 4.10F). After removal of the gross specimen, the suprarenal vena caval clamp may be released temporarily as the anesthetist applies positive pulmonary pressure; this

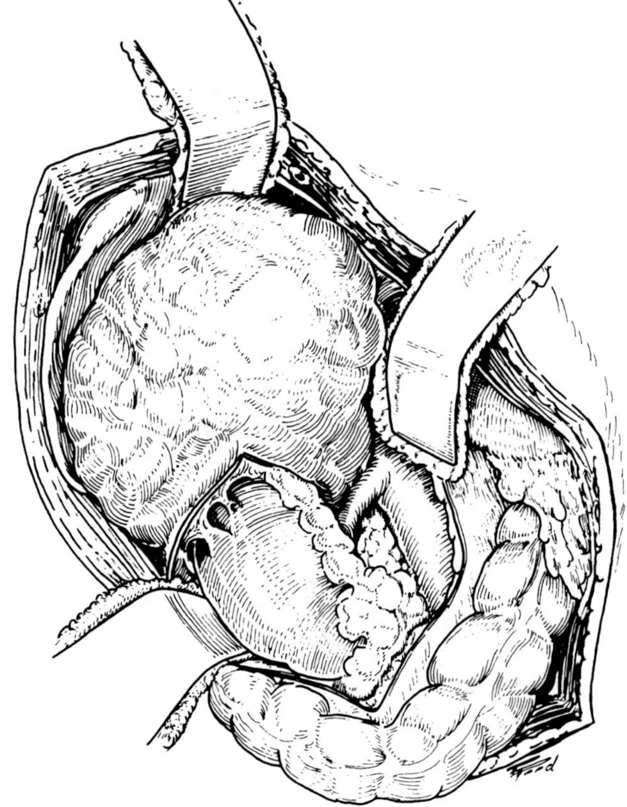

**Fig. 4.6**

Exposure of large right upper pole tumor through a thoracoabdominal incision. (The thoracoabdominal incision is depicted in Chapter 10.)

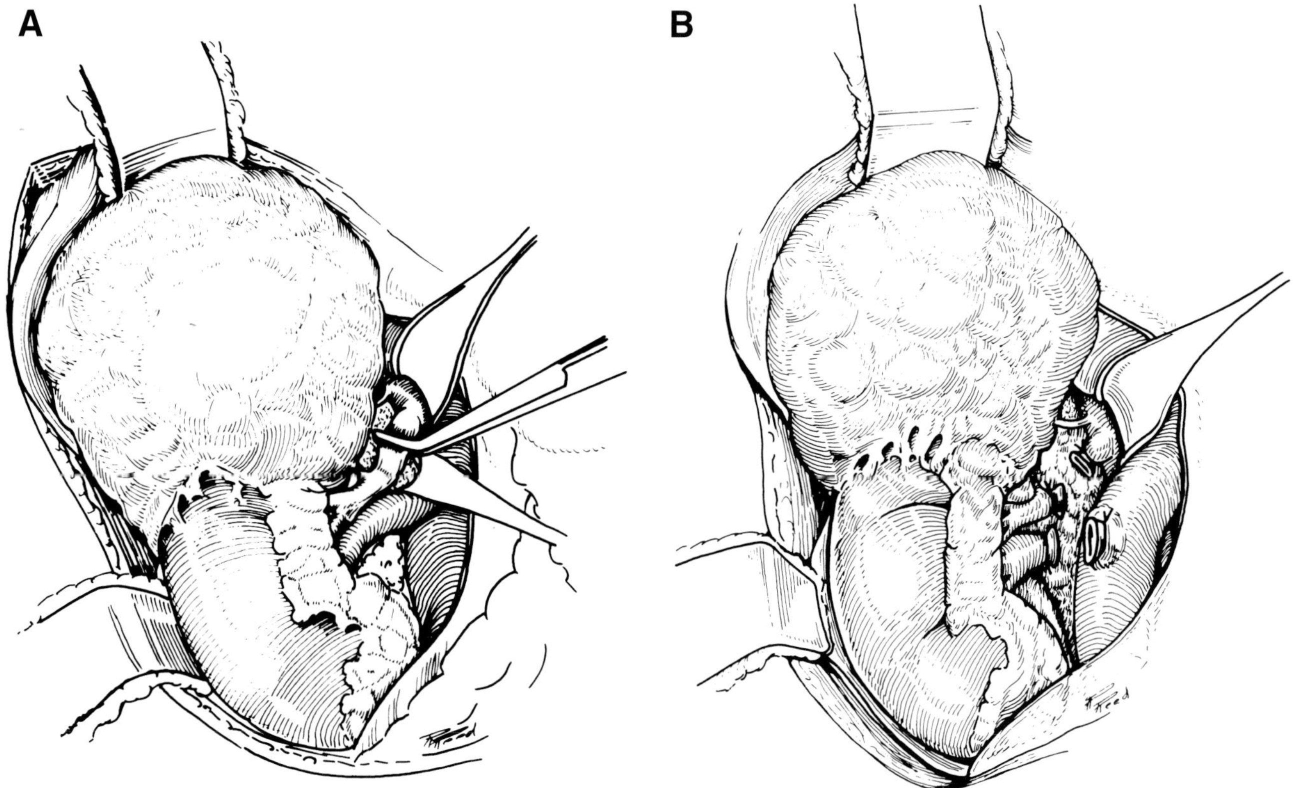


**Fig. 4.7**

The renal artery and vein are secured and divided.

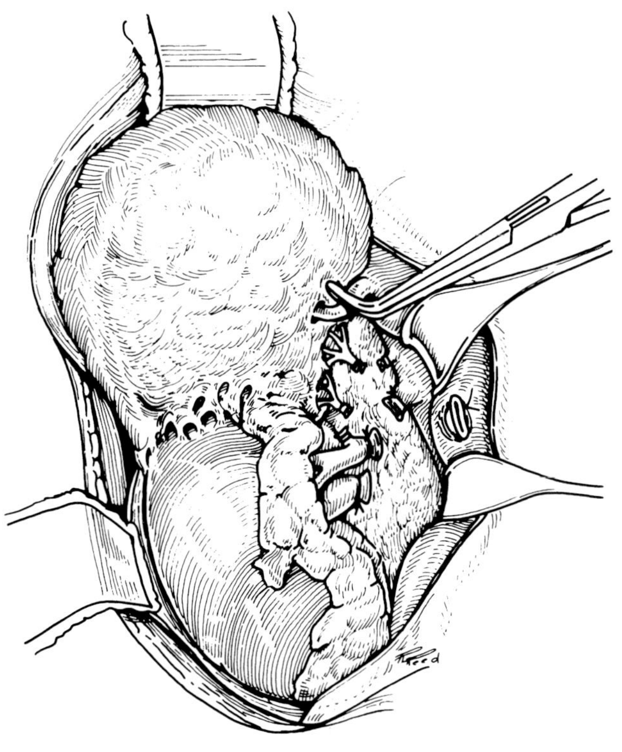

**Fig. 4.8**

The vena cava is retracted medially to expose remaining superior vascular attachments which are secured and divided.

maneuver can ensure that any small remaining fragments of thrombus are flushed free from the vena cava. When the tumor thrombectomy is completed, the cavotomy incision is repaired with a continuous 5-0 vascular suture (Fig. 4.10G).

In occasional cases, there is direct caval invasion of the tumor at the level of the entrance of the renal vein and for varying distances. This requires resection of a portion of the vena caval wall. Narrowing of the caval lumen by up to 50% will not adversely affect maintenance of caval patency. If further narrowing appears likely, caval reconstruction can be performed with a free graft of pericardium.

In some patients more extensive direct growth of tumor into the wall of the vena cava is found at surgery. The prognosis for these patients is generally poor, particularly when hepatic venous tributaries are also involved, and the decision to proceed with radical surgical excision must be carefully considered. Several important principles must be kept in mind when undertaking *en bloc* vena caval resection. Resection of the infrarenal portion of the vena cava usually can be done safely, because an extensive collateral venous supply will have developed in most cases. With right-sided kidney tumors, resection of the suprarenal vena cava is also possible provided the left renal vein is ligated distal to the gonadal and adrenal tributaries, which then provide collateral venous drainage from the left

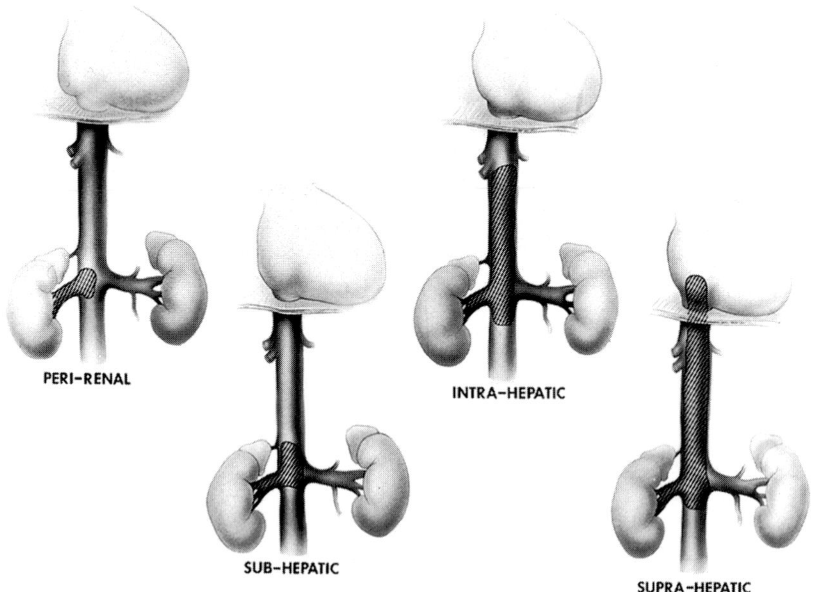


**Fig. 4.9**

Classification of inferior vena caval tumor thrombus from renal cell carcinoma, according to the distal extend of the thrombus, as perirenal, subhepatic, intrahepatic, and suprahepatic.

kidney. With left-sided kidney tumors, the suprarenal vena cava cannot be resected safely owing to the paucity of collateral venous drainage from the right kidney. In such cases, right renal venous drainage can be maintained by preserving a tumor-free strip of vena cava (Fig. 4.11), augmented, if necessary, with a pericardial patch; alternatively, the right kidney can be autotransplanted to the pelvis or an interposition graft of saphenous vein may be placed from the right renal vein to the splenic, inferior mesenteric, or portal vein.

## Radical Nephrectomy With Intrahepatic or Suprahepatic Vena Caval Involvement

In patients with RCC and an intrahepatic or suprahepatic IVC thrombus, the difficulty of surgical excision is significantly increased. In such cases, the operative technique must be modified because it is not possible to obtain subdiaphragmatic control of the vena cava above the tumor thrombus.

At the Cleveland Clinic we have preferred to employ cardiopulmonary bypass with deep hypothermic circulatory arrest for most patients with complex supradiaphragmatic tumor thrombi and for all patients with right atrial tumor thrombi. We initially reported a favorable experience with this approach in 43 patients *(4)*, and a subsequent study has shown excellent long-term cancer-free survival following its use in patients with right atrial thrombi *(8)*.

A bilateral subcostal incision is used for the abdominal portion of the operation. After confirming resectability, a median sternotomy is made. The kidney is completely mobilized outside Gerota's fascia with division of the renal artery and ureter, such that the kidney is left attached only by the renal vein. The infrarenal vena cava and contralateral renal vein are also exposed. Extensive dissection and mobilization of the suprarenal vena cava are not necessary with this approach. Adequate exposure is somewhat more difficult to achieve for a left renal tumor. Simultaneous exposure of the vena cava on the right and the tumor on the left is not readily accomplished simply by reflecting the left colon medially. We have dealt with this by transposing the mobilized left kidney anteriorly through a window in the mesentery of the left colon, while leaving the renal vein attached. This maneuver yields excellent exposure of the abdominal vena cava with the attached left renal vein and kidney. Precise retroperitoneal hemostasis is essential before proceeding with cardiopulmonary bypass owing to the risk of bleeding associated with systemic heparinization.

The heart and great vessels are now exposed through the median sternotomy. The patient is heparinized, ascending aortic and right atrial venous cannulae are placed, and cardiopulmonary bypass is initiated. When the heart fibrillates, the aorta is clamped and crystalloid cardioplegic solution is infused. Under circulatory arrest, deep hypothermia is initiated by reducing arterial inflow blood temperature as low

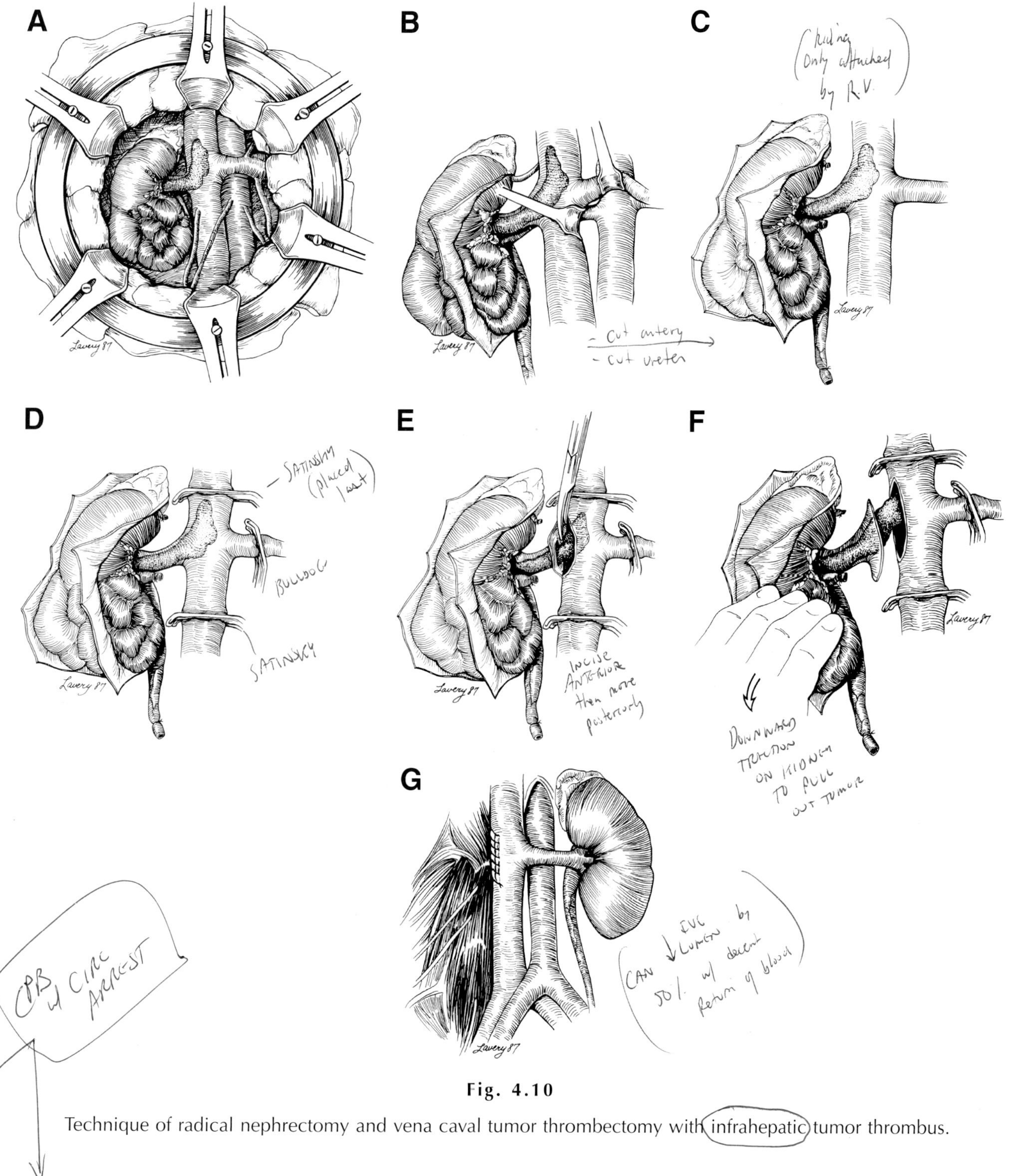


**Fig. 4.10**

Technique of radical nephrectomy and vena caval tumor thrombectomy with infrahepatic tumor thrombus.

as 10°C. The head and abdomen are packed in ice during the cooling process. After approx 30 min, a core temperature of 18–20°C is achieved. At this point flow through the perfusion machine is stopped and 95% of the blood volume is drained into the pump with no flow to any organ.

The tumor thrombus can now be removed in an essentially bloodless operative field. An incision is made in the IVC at the entrance of the involved renal vein, and the ostium is circumscribed. When the tumor extends into the right atrium, the atrium is opened at the same time (Fig. 4.12). If possible, the tumor thrombus is removed intact with the kidney. However, frequently this is not possible because of the friability of the thrombus and its adherence to the vena caval wall. In such cases, piecemeal removal

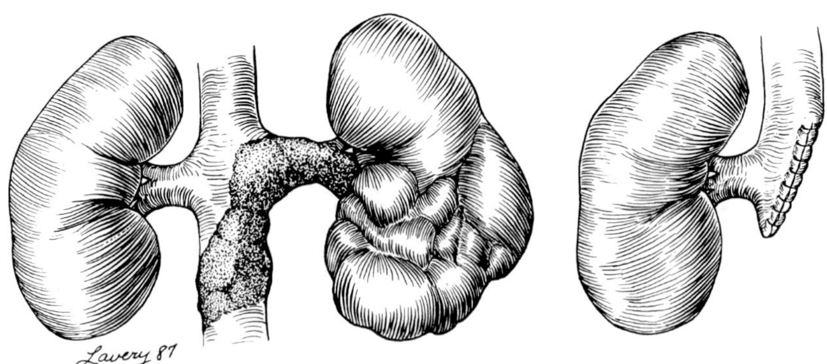


**Fig. 4.11**

With vena cava resection, right renal venous drainage can be maintained by preserving a tumor-free strip of vena cava.

of the thrombus from above and below is necessary. Under deep hypothermic circulatory arrest, the entire interior lumen of the vena cava can be directly inspected to ensure that all fragments of thrombus are completely removed. Hypothermic circulatory arrest can be safely maintained for at least 40 min without incurring a cerebral ischemic event *(15)*. In difficult cases, this interval can be extended either by maintaining "trickle" blood flow at a rate of 5–10 mL/kg/min *(16)* or by adjunctive retrograde cerebral perfusion *(17)*.

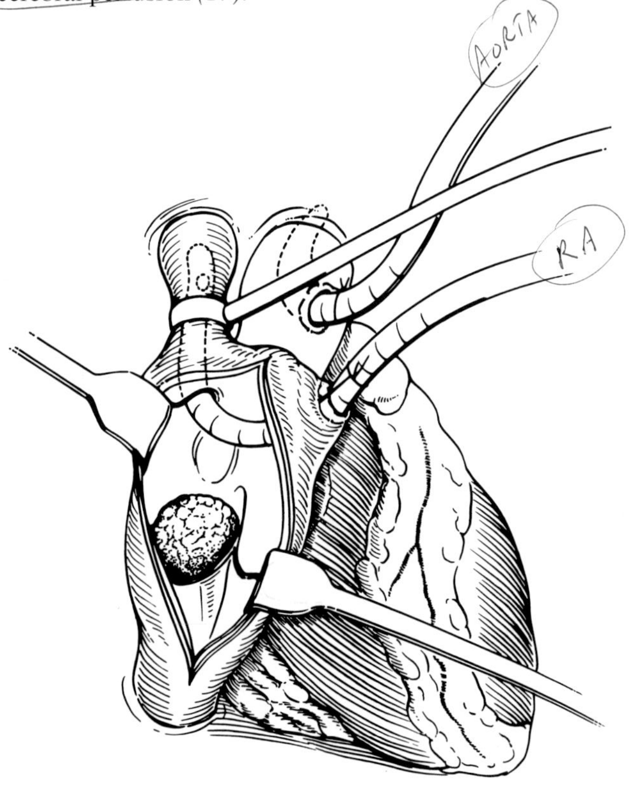

**Fig. 4.12**

Cannulas have been placed in the ascending aorta and right atrium. An atriotomy is made to expose the right atrial thrombus.

Following complete removal of all tumor thrombus, the vena cava is closed with a continuous 5-0 vascular suture and the right atrium is closed. As soon as the vena cava and right atrium have been repaired, rewarming of the patient is initiated. If coronary artery bypass grafting is necessary, this procedure is done during the rewarming period. Rewarming takes 20–45 min and is continued until a core temperature of approx 37°C is obtained. Cardiopulmonary bypass is then terminated. Decannulation takes place, and protamine sulfate is administered to reverse the effects of the heparin. Platelets, fresh-frozen plasma, desmopressin acetate, or their combination may be provided when coagulopathy is suspected. Aprotinin has also proven effective in reversing the coagulopathy associated with cardiopulmonary bypass but may induce thrombotic complications. Mediastinal chest tubes are placed but the abdomen is not routinely drained.

In patients with nonadherent supradiaphragmatic vena caval tumor thrombi that do not extend into the right atrium, veno-venous bypass in the form of a caval-atrial shunt is a useful technique *(18,19)*. In this approach the intrapericardiac vena cava, infrarenal vena cava, and opposite renal vein are temporarily occluded. Cannulas are then inserted into the right atrium and infrarenal vena cava. These cannulas are connected to a primed pump to maintain adequate flow from the vena cava to the right heart (Fig. 4.13). This avoids the obligatory hypotension associated with temporary occlusion of the intrapericardiac and infrarenal vena cava. Following the initiation of veno-venous bypass, the abdominal vena cava is opened and the thrombus is removed. If bleeding from the hepatic veins is troublesome during extraction of the thrombus, the porta hepatis may also be occluded (Pringle maneuver). After removal of the thrombus, repair of the vena cava is performed as previously described. This technique is simpler than cardiopulmonary bypass with hypothermic circulatory arrest but may entail more operative bleeding.

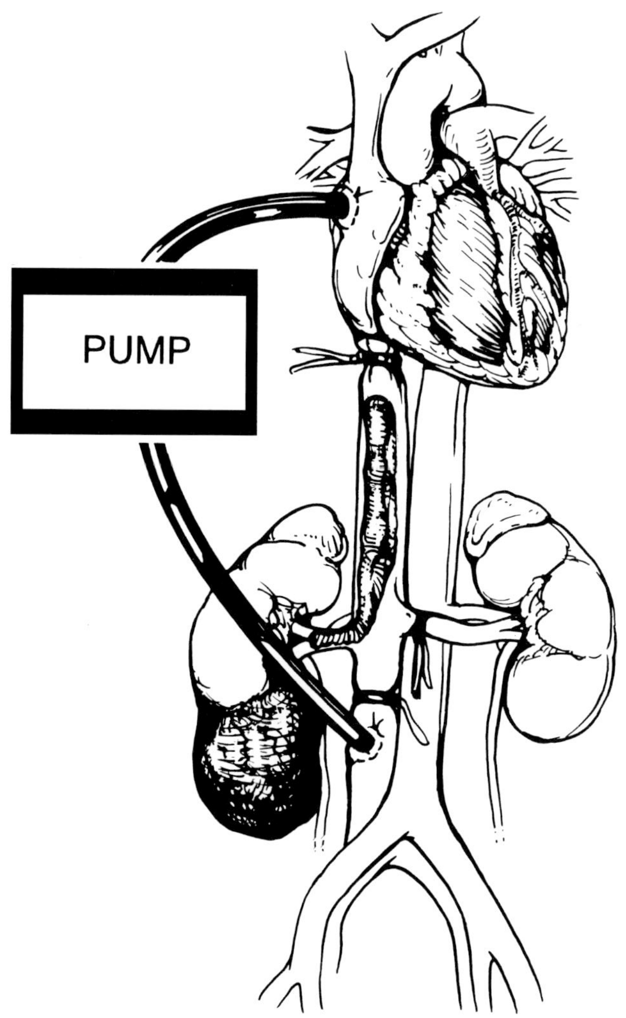


**Fig. 4.13**

Technique of veno-venous bypass for removal of supra-diaphragmatic vena caval tumor thrombus.

## RADICAL NEPHROURETERECTOMY

Radical nephroureterectomy is the standard therapy for tumors of the renal pelvis and ureter. The choice of incision depends on individual preference and the patient's habitus. The operation can be performed through two incisions: one transverse upper abdominal and one lower abdominal (Gibson) incision. Alternatively, in non-obese patients, a single midline or paramedian abdominal incision may be used.

The nephrectomy portion of this operation is similar to the one described for radical nephrectomy with the exception that the ureter is not transected. The ureter should be dissected as low as possible. The author prefers to leave the kidney and the ureter *in situ* to be removed as one anatomical piece to facilitate mapping of the specimen by the pathologist.

In many cases, removal of the distal ureter and bladder cuff can be done extravesically. The ureter is identified and

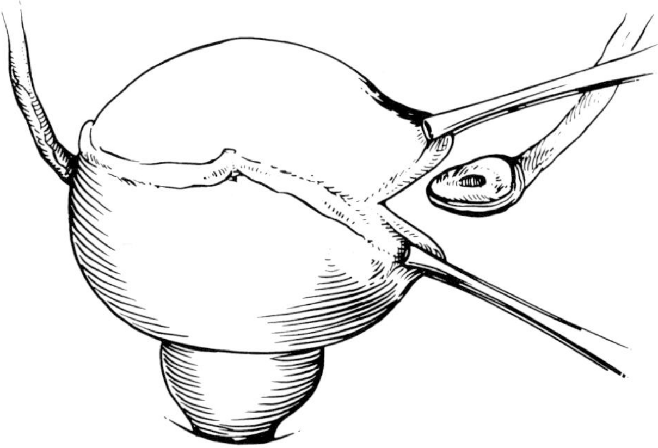

**Fig. 4.14**

Extravesical removal of the distal ureter and bladder cuff.

isolated as it crosses the common iliac artery. With blunt and sharp dissection the ureter and the periureteral tissues are freed toward the bladder. Dissection is carried out to the point of the intramural ureter. A cuff of urinary bladder is removed by applying the Ellis clamp to the bladder wall and excising a cuff around the ureter. This cuff must include the complete intramural ureter (Fig. 4.14).

If for technical reasons it is not possible to remove a cuff of bladder through an extravesical approach, an open cystostomy is performed with removal of the cuff of the bladder intravesically (Fig. 4.15). The bladder is closed using 4-0 and 3-0 polyglycolic sutures in two or three layers. The lower portion of the incision is drained using a closed drainage system. An indwelling Foley catheter is left for 7 d.

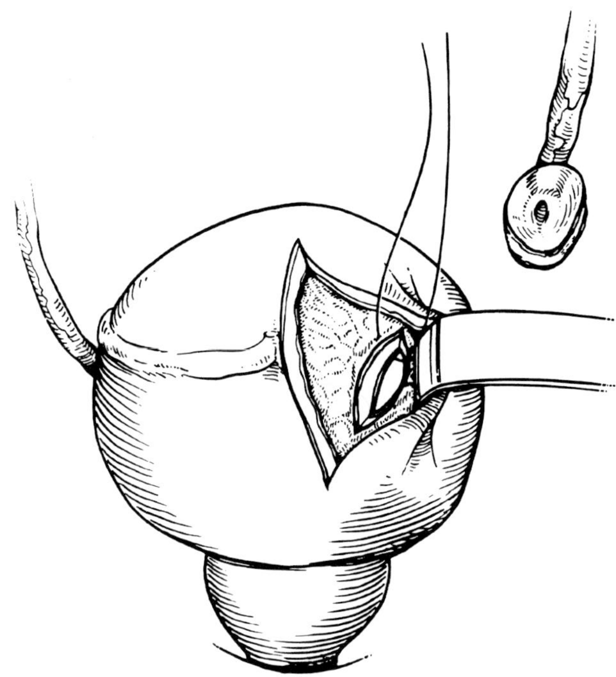

**Fig. 4.15**

Intravesical removal of the distal ureter and bladder cuff.

## PARTIAL NEPHRECTOMY

In patients with RCC, accepted indications for partial nephrectomy include situations in which radical nephrectomy would render the patient anephric with subsequent immediate need for dialysis. This encompasses patients with bilateral RCC or RCC involving a solitary functioning kidney. The latter circumstance may be present as a result of unilateral renal agenesis, prior removal of the contralateral kidney, or irreversible impairment of contralateral renal function from a benign disorder. Another indication for partial nephrectomy is represented by patients with unilateral RCC and a functioning opposite kidney, when the opposite kidney is affected by a condition that might threaten its future function, such as calculus disease, chronic pyelonephritis, renal artery stenosis, ureteral reflux, or systemic diseases such as diabetes and nephrosclerosis *(20)*.

Recent studies have clarified the role of partial nephrectomy in patients with localized unilateral RCC and a normal contralateral kidney. These data indicate that radical nephrectomy and partial nephrectomy provide equally effective curative treatment for such patients who present with a single, small (<4 cm), and clearly localized RCC *(21,22)*. The results of partial nephrectomy are less satisfactory in patients with larger (>4 cm) or multiple localized RCCs, and radical nephrectomy remains the treatment of choice in such cases when the opposite kidney is normal. The long-term renal functional advantage of partial nephrectomy with a normal opposite kidney requires further study. Partial nephrectomy is also occasionally indicated in the management of patients with renal pelvic transitional cell carcinoma of Wilms' tumor when preservation of functioning renal parenchyma is a clinically relevant consideration *(23)*.

The technical success rate with partial nephrectomy for RCC is excellent, and several large studies have reported 5-yr cancer-specific survival rates of 87–90% in such patients *(20,24,25)*. These survival rates are comparable to those obtained after radical nephrectomy, particularly for low-stage RCC. The major disadvantage of partial nephrectomy for RCC is the risk of postoperative local tumor recurrence in the operated kidney, which has been observed in 4–6% of patients *(20,24,25)*. These local recurrences are most likely a manifestation of undetected microscopic multifocal RCC in the renal remnant. The risk of local tumor recurrence after radical nephrectomy has not been studied, but it is presumably very low.

We recently reviewed the results of partial nephrectomy for treatment of localized sporadic RCC in 485 patients managed at the Cleveland Clinic before December 1996 *(26)*. A technically successful operation with the preservation of function in the treated kidney was achieved in 476 patients (98%). The overall and cancer-specific 5-yr patient survival rate in the series was 81% and 93%, respectively. Recurrent RCC developed postoperatively in 44 of 485 patients (9%). Sixteen of the patients (3.2%) developed local recurrence in the remnant kidney, whereas 28 patients (5.8%) developed metastatic disease.

More recently, we received the long-term (10-yr) results of partial nephrectomy in 107 patients with localized sporadic RCC treated before 1988 *(27)*. All patients were followed up for a minimum of 10 yr or until death. Cancer-specific survival was 88.2% at 5 yr and 73% at 10 yr. Long-term preservation of renal function was achieved in 100 patients (93%). These results attest that partial nephrectomy is an effective therapy for localized RCC that can provide both long-term tumor control and the preservation of renal function.

Evaluation of patients with RCC for partial nephrectomy should include preoperative testing to rule out locally extensive or metastatic disease. Previously, preoperative renal arteriography with or without renal venography were often necessary to delineate intrarenal vascular anatomy. Three-dimensional volume-rendered CT is a new noninvasive imaging modality that can accurately depict the renal parenchymal and vascular anatomy in a format familiar to urological surgeons *(28)*. The data integrate essential information from arteriography, venography, excretory urography, and conventional two-dimensional CT into a single imaging modality, obviating the need for more invasive vascular imaging (Fig. 4.16).

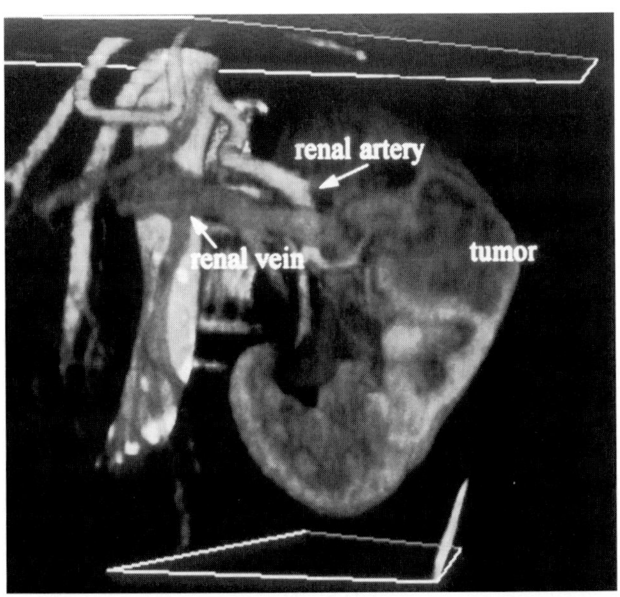


**Fig. 4.16**

Three-dimensional CT scan shows the tumor in the upper part of the left kidney with renal arterial and venous supply.

It is usually possible to perform partial nephrectomy for malignancy *in situ* by using an operative approach that optimizes exposure of the kidney and by combining meticulous surgical technique with an understanding of the renal vascular anatomy in relation to the tumor. Preoperative hydration and mannitol administration are important adjuncts to ensure optimal renal perfusion at operation. We employ an extraperitoneal flank incision through the bed of the 11th or 12th rib for almost all of these operations; we occasionally use a thoracoabdominal incision for very large tumors involving the upper portion of the kidney. These incisions allow the surgeon to operate on the mobilized kidney almost at skin level and provide excellent exposure of the peripheral renal vessels (Fig. 4.17). With an anterior subcostal transperitoneal incision, the kidney is invariably located in the depth of the wound, and the surgical exposure is simply not as good. Extracorporeal surgery is rarely necessary in these patients today.

When performing *in situ* partial nephrectomy for malignancy, the kidney is mobilized within Gerota's fascia while leaving intact the perirenal fat around the tumor. For small peripheral renal tumors, it is not necessary to control the renal artery. In most cases, however, partial nephrectomy is most effectively performed after temporary renal arterial occlusion. This measure not only limits intraoperative bleeding, but, by reducing renal tissue turgor, also improves access to intrarenal structures. When possible, it is helpful to leave the renal vein patent throughout the operation. This measure decreases intraoperative renal ischemia and, by allowing venous backbleeding, facilitates hemostasis by enabling identification of small transected renal veins. In patients with centrally located tumors, it is necessary to occlude the renal vein temporarily to minimize intraoperative bleeding from transected major venous branches.

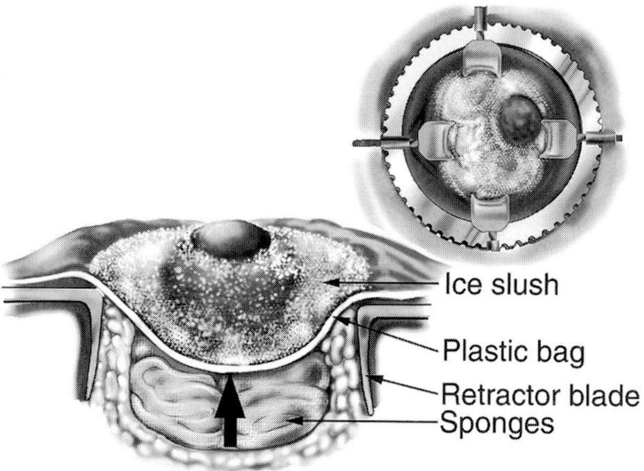


**Fig. 4.17**

Elevation of the mobilized kidney to skin level is demonstrated by placing sponges under the plastic bag containing the kidney and ice slush.

When the renal circulation is temporarily interrupted, *in situ* renal hypothermia is used to protect against postischemic renal injury. Surface cooling of the kidney with ice slush allows up to 3 h of safe ischemia without permanent renal injury. An important caveat with this method is to keep the entire kidney covered with ice slush for 10–15 min immediately after occluding the renal artery and before commencing the partial nephrectomy (Fig. 4.17). This amount of time is needed to obtain core renal cooling to a temperature (approx 20°C) that optimizes *in situ* renal preservation. During excision of the tumor, invariably large portions of the kidney are no longer covered with ice slush, and in the absence of adequate prior renal cooling, rapid rewarming and ischemic renal injury can occur. Cooling by perfusion of the kidney with a cold solution instilled via the renal artery is not recommended due to the theoretical risk of tumor dissemination. Mannitol is given intravenously 5–10 min before temporary renal arterial occlusion. Systemic or regional anticoagulation to prevent intrarenal vascular thrombosis is not necessary.

## Basic Operative Technique

A variety of surgical techniques is available for performing partial nephrectomy in patients with malignancy *(29)*. These include simple enucleation, polar segmental nephrectomy, wedge resection, and transverse resection. All of these techniques require adherence to basic principles of early vascular control, avoidance of ischemic renal damage, complete tumor excision with free margins, precise closure of the collecting system, careful hemostasis, and closure or coverage of the renal defect with adjacent fat, fascia, peritoneum, or oxycel. Whichever technique is employed, the tumor is removed with a small surrounding margin of grossly normal renal parenchyma. Intraoperative ultrasonography is helpful in achieving accurate tumor localization, particularly for intrarenal lesions that are not visible or palpable from the external surface of the kidney *(30)*.

When performing a transverse resection of the upper part of the kidney, care must be taken to avoid injury to the posterior segmental renal arterial branch, which may also occasionally supply the basilar renal segment (Fig. 4.18). Accurate preoperative vascular imaging is integral to identifying and preserving the posterior segmental artery at surgery and to thereby avoid devascularizing a major portion of the healthy remnant kidney. Midrenal resections may also be particularly complicated because the arterial supply comprises branches of anterior and posterior renal artery divisions, and the calyces often enter the same infundibula as those draining the upper and lower poles.

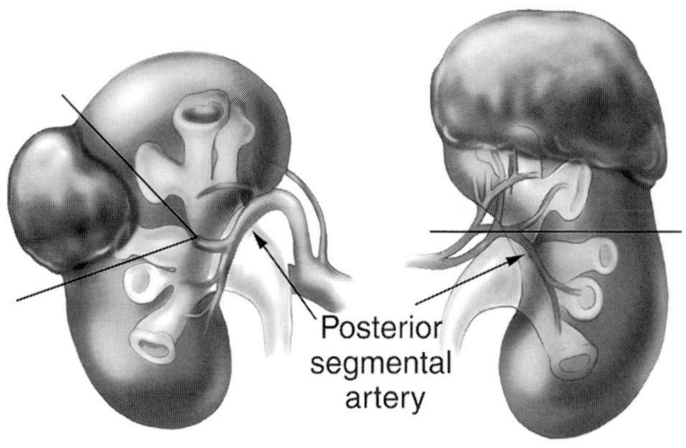


Fig. 4.18

Injury to the posterior segmental renal arterial branch must be avoided during upper or midrenal resections.

Whichever nephron-sparing technique is used, the parenchyma around the tumor is divided with a combination of sharp and blunt dissection. In many cases, the tumor extends deeply into the kidney and the collecting system is entered. Often, renal arterial and venous branches supplying the tumor can be identified as the parenchyma is being incised, and these should be directly suture-ligated at that time while they are most visible (Fig. 4.19). Similarly, in many cases, direct entry into the collecting system may be avoided by isolating and ligating major infundibula draining the tumor-bearing renal segment as the incision into the parenchyma is developed (Fig. 4.19).

After excision of the tumor, remaining transected blood vessels on the renal surface are secured with figure-of-eight 4-0 chromic sutures. Bleeding at this point is usually minimal, and the operative file can be kept satisfactorily clear by gentle suction during placement of hemostatic sutures. Residual collecting system defects are similarly closed with interrupted or continuous 4-0 chromic sutures. At this point, with the renal artery still clamped but with the renal vein open, the anesthesiologist is asked to hyperinflate the lungs and thereby raise the central and renal venous pressure. This forces blood out through residual unsecured transected veins on the renal surface and thereby facilitates their detection (Fig. 4.20). Once identified, these veins are secured with interrupted figure-of-eight 4-0 chromic sutures. The argon beam coagulator is a useful adjunct for achieving hemostasis on the transected peripheral renal surface.

In most cases, after securing the renal vasculature and collecting system, the kidney is closed on itself by approximating the transected cortical margins with simple interrupted 3-0 chromic sutures after placing a small piece of oxycel at the base of the defect. This is an important additional hemostatic measure. When this is done, the suture line must be free of tension and the blood vessels supplying the kidney must be free of significant angulation of kinking. After closure of the renal defect, the renal artery is unclamped and circulation to the kidney is restored. When the remnant kidney resides within a large retroperitoneal fossa, the kidney is fixed to the posterior musculature with interrupted 3-0 chromic sutures to prevent postoperative movement or rotation of the kidney, which may compromise the blood supply (Fig. 4.21). A retroperitoneal drain is always left in place for at least 7 d, and an intraoperative ureteral stent is placed only when major reconstruction of the intrarenal collection system has been performed.

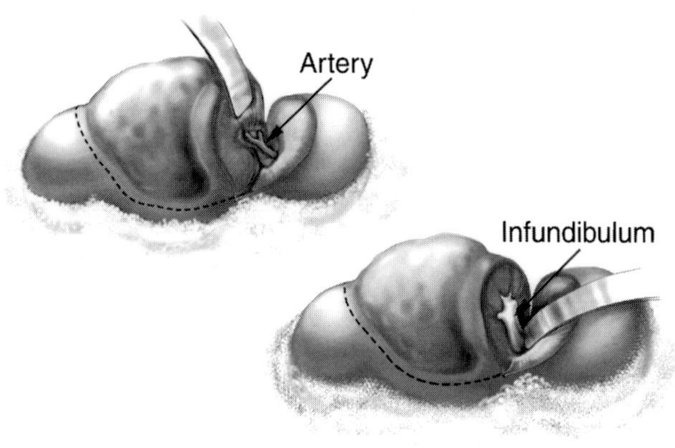


Fig. 4.19

As the parenchyma around the tumor is incised, major vessels supplying the tumor are identified and secured. Similarly, infundibula draining the tumor-bearing portion of the kidney are also identified and secured.

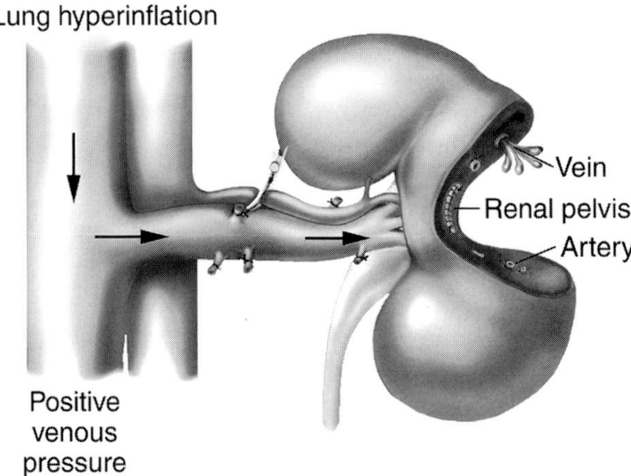


Fig. 4.20

Identification of residual unsecured transected vessels (particularly veins) on the renal surface is facilitated by increasing the renal venous pressure through hyperinflation of the lungs.

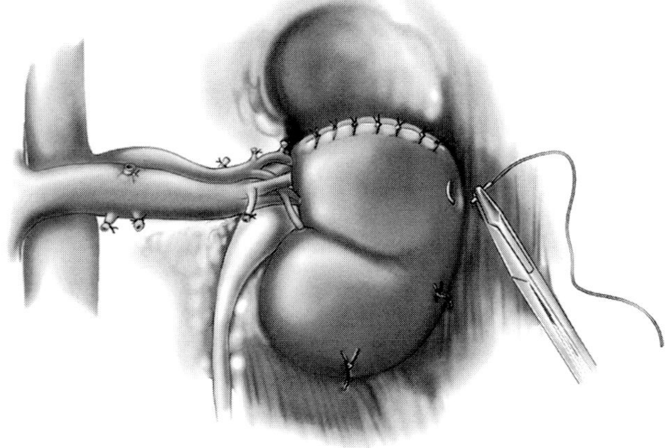


**Fig. 4.21**

Nephropexy of the remnant kidney to the retroperitoneum is achieved with several interrupted sutures.

In patients with RCC or transitional cell carcinoma, partial nephrectomy is contraindicated in the presence of lymph node metastasis because the prognosis for these patients is poor. Enlarged or suspicious-looking lymph nodes should be biopsied before initiating the renal resection. When partial nephrectomy is performed, after excision of all gross tumor, absence of malignancy in the remaining portion of the kidney should be verified intraoperatively by frozen-section examinations of biopsy specimens obtained at random from the renal margin of excision. It is usual for such biopsies to demonstrate residual tumor, but, if so, additional renal tissue must be excised.

## Segmental Polar Nephrectomy

In a patient with malignancy confined to the upper or lower pole of the kidney, partial nephrectomy can be performed by isolating and ligating the segmental apical or basilar arterial branch while allowing unrepaired perfusion to the remainder of the kidney from the main renal artery. This procedure is illustrated in Fig. 4.22 for a tumor confined to the apical vascular segment. The apical artery is dissected away from the adjacent structures, ligated, and divided. Often, a corresponding venous branch is present, which is similarly ligated and divided. An ischemic line of demarcation will then generally appear on the surface of the kidney and will outline the segment to be excised. If this area is not obvious, a few milliliters of methylene blue can be directly injected distally into the ligated apical artery to better outline the limits of the involved renal segment. An incision is then made in the renal cortex at the line of demarcation, which should be several millimeters away from the visible edge of the cancer. The parenchyma is divided by sharp and blunt dissection, and the polar segment is removed. When the collecting system and vasculature have been repaired, the edges of the kidney are reapproximated as an additional hemostatic measure using simple interrupted 3-0 chromic sutures inserted through the capsule and a small amount of parenchyma. Before these sutures are tied, perirenal fat or oxycel can be inserted into the defect for inclusion in the renal closure.

## Wedge Resection

Wedge resection is an appropriate technique for removing peripheral tumors on the surface of the kidney, particularly ones that are larger or not confined to either renal pole. Because these lesions often encompass more than one renal segment, and because this technique is generally associated with heavier bleeding, it is best to perform wedge resection with temporary renal arterial occlusion and surface hypothermia.

In performing a wedge resection, the tumor is removed with a surrounding margin of several millimeters of grossly normal renal parenchyma (Fig. 4.23). The parenchyma is divided by a combination of sharp and blunt dissection. Often, prominent intrarenal vessels are identified as the parenchyma is being incised. These may be directly

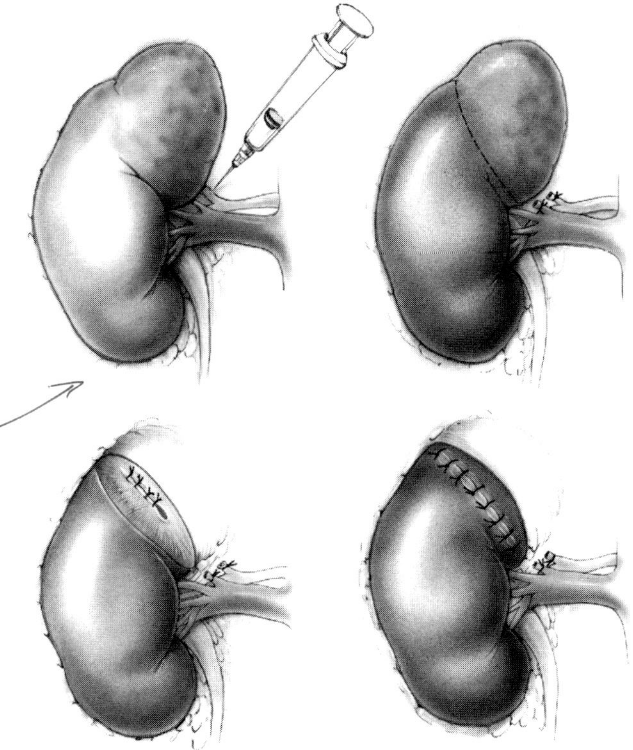

**Fig. 4.22**

Technique of segmental (apical) polar nephrectomy with preliminary ligation of apical arterial and venous branches.

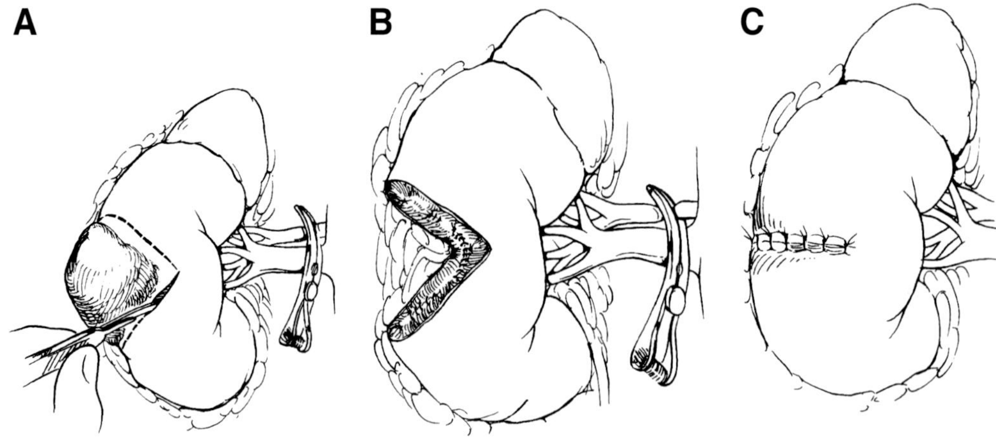


**Fig. 4.23**

Technique of wedge resection for a tumor on the lateral surface of the kidney.

suture-ligated at the time, while they are most visible. After excision of the tumor, the collecting system and vasculature are then repaired as needed. The renal defect can then be closed in one of two ways (Fig. 4.23). The kidney may be closed upon itself by approximating the transected cortical margins with simple interrupted 3-0 chromic sutures, after placing a small piece of oxycel at the base of the defect. If this is done, there must be no tension on the suture line and no significant angulation or kinking of blood vessels supplying the kidney. Alternatively, a portion of perirenal fat may simply be inserted into the base of the renal defect as a hemostatic measure and sutured to the parenchymal margins with interrupted 4-0 chromic sutures. After closure or coverage of the renal defect, the renal artery is unclamped and circulation to the kidney is restored.

## Transverse Resection

A transverse resection is done to remove large tumors that extensively involve the upper or lower portion of the kidney. This technique is performed using surface hypothermia after temporary occlusion of the renal artery. Major branches of the renal artery and vein supplying the tumor-bearing portion of the kidney are identified in the renal hilus, ligated, and divided (Fig. 4.24A). If possible, this should be done before temporarily occluding the renal artery to minimize the overall period of renal ischemia.

After occluding the renal artery, the parenchyma is divided by blunt and sharp dissection, leaving a several millimeter margin of grossly normal tissue around the tumor (Fig. 4.24B). Transected blood vessels on the renal surface are secured as previously described, and the hilus is inspected carefully for remaining unligated segmental vessels. If possible, the renal defect is sutured together with one of the techniques previously described (Fig. 4.24C). If this suture cannot be placed without tension or without distorting the renal vessels, a piece of peritoneum or perirenal fat is sutured in place to cover the defect.

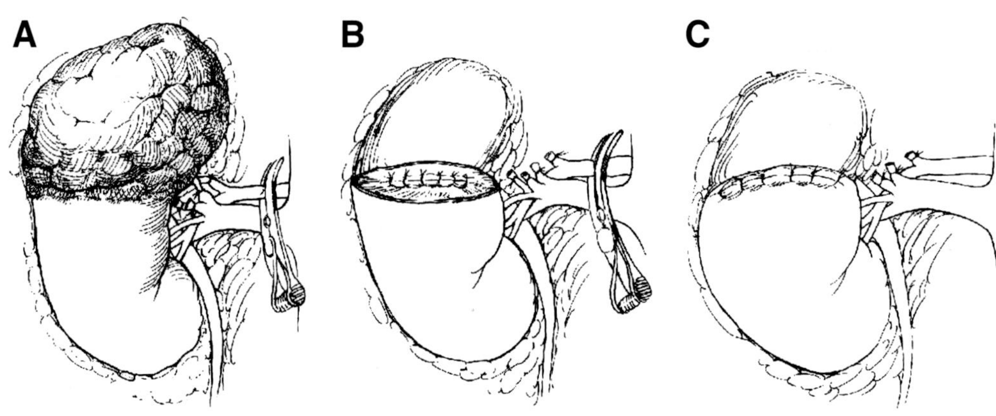


**Fig. 4.24**

Technique of transverse resection for a tumor involving the upper half of the kidney.

## Simple Enucleation

Some RCCs are surrounded by a distinct pseudocapsule of fibrous tissue. The technique of simple enucleation implies circumferential incision of the renal parenchyma around the tumors simply and rapidly at any location, often with no vascular occlusion and with maximal preservation of normal parenchyma.

Initial reports indicated satisfactory short-term clinical results after enucleation with good patient survival and low rate of local tumor recurrence *(31,32)*. However, most studies have suggested a higher risk of leaving residual malignancy in the kidney when enucleation is performed *(33,34)*. These latter reports include several carefully done histopathological studies that have demonstrated frequent microscopic tumor penetration of the pseudocapsule that surrounds the neoplasm. These data indicate that it is not always possible to be assured of complete tumor encapsulation prior to surgery. Local recurrence of tumor in the treated kidney is a grave complication of partial nephrectomy for RCC, and every attempt should be made to prevent it. Therefore, it is the author's view that a surrounding margin of normal parenchyma should be removed with the tumor whenever possible. This provides an added margin of safety against the development of local tumor recurrence and, in most cases, does not appreciably increase the technical difficulty of the operation. The technique of enucleation is currently employed only in occasional patients with von Hippel–Lindau disease and multiple low-stage encapsulated tumors involving both kidneys *(35)*.

## Partial Nephrectomy for Central Tumors

For patients with central tumors, complete delineation of the renal arterial and venous supply is mandatory for surgical planning. As stated earlier, this information can now be obtained with three-dimensional CT scanning, and invasive vascular imaging studies are no longer necessary (*28*). In patients with central tumors, nephron-sparing surgery is most effectively performed after temporary occlusion of the renal artery and vein. Renal vein occlusion is important to minimize intraoperative bleeding from transected major venous branches. The renal artery and vein are occluded separately with individual atraumatic vascular clamps.

During the preliminary dissection, the kidney is mobilized within Gerota's fascia while leaving intact the perirenal fat around the tumor. There may be relatively little perirenal fat to preserve with central tumors that extend into the renal hilus. The tumor is mobilized and isolated as much as possible by dissecting away adjacent segmental renal vessels that provide critical blood supply to the non-tumor-bearing part of the kidney that is to be preserved.

The differences between the renal arterial and venous circulations must be borne in mind and may be used to advantage in these operations. Since all segmental arteries are end-arteries with no collateral circulation, all branches supplying tumor-free parenchyma must be preserved to avoid devitalization of functioning renal tissue. However, the renal venous drainage system is different in that intrarenal venous branches intercommunicate freely between the various renal segments. Therefore, ligation of a branch of the renal vein does not result in segmental infarction of the kidney because collateral venous blood supply provides adequate drainage. This is important clinically because it enables one to obtain surgical access safely to central tumors in the renal hilus by ligating and dividing small adjacent or overlying venous branches. This allows the main renal vein to be completely mobilized and freely retracted in either direction to expose a central tumor with no vascular compromise of uninvolved parenchyma (Fig. 4.25).

At this stage, small segmental arterial branches that directly supply the tumor can also be secured and divided. If the portion of kidney or tumor supplied by a segmental artery is not readily apparent, temporary occlusion of the branch with a mini-vascular clamp can resolve this by enabling direct visualization of the ischemic supplied renal tissue. When dissecting on the posterior renal surface, particular care must be taken to avoid injury to the posterior segmental renal arterial branch, which has a variable location and may also occasionally supply the basilar renal segment; in the event of the latter, failure to identify and preserve this branch can lead to devascularization of a major portion of the healthy remnant kidney.

The object of the preliminary dissection is to isolate the tumor and secure as much of its direct blood supply as possible before clamping the main renal artery and vein, so that overall warm renal ischemia time can be minimized.

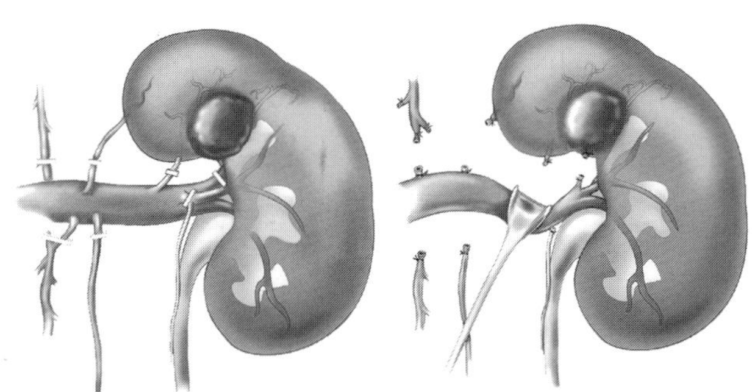

**Fig. 4.25**

Mobilization of the left renal vein to obtain better exposure of a tumor in the renal hilus by ligating and dividing small renal venous branches.

Intraoperative ultrasonography is also performed prior to temporary renal vascular occlusion for the same reason. The primary value of this adjunctive imaging modality is for localization of intrarenal tumors that are not visible or palpable from the external surface of the kidney. A recent prospective study demonstrated that intraoperative ultrasonography is of limited value for detecting occult multicentric tumors in the kidney *(30)*.

Following temporary occlusion of the renal artery and vein, the mobilized and isolated tumor is resected by incision of the attachment to the renal parenchyma. Often, small renal arterial and venous branches supplying the tumor can be identified as the parenchyma is being incised, and these should be directly suture-ligated at that time while they are most visible. Although a surrounding margin of normal parenchyma should be removed with the tumor, a wide margin of normal renal tissue is often not available for hilar tumors, which may, in part, impinge directly on the central collecting system. It is sufficient to remove these tumors with all adjacent renal sinus fat and with a 3- to 4-mm margin of surrounding normal parenchyma where this is available.

In most cases, after securing the renal vessels and collecting system, the kidney is closed on itself by approximating the transected cortical margins with interrupted sutures as an additional hemostatic measure. When this is done, the parenchymal suture line must be free of tension and the blood vessels supplying the kidney must be free of significant angulation or kinking. After closure of the renal defect, the renal artery is unclamped and circulation to the kidney is restored.

### Partial Nephrectomy for Renal Angiomyolipoma

Renal angiomyolipomas (AMLs) are benign hematomas whose course may be complicated by pain, hematuria, hemorrhage, rupture, and even death *(36)*. They may develop spontaneously or be part of the tuberous sclerosis complex, where they are often multiple and bilateral. These tumors have a propensity to grow, and treatment has been recommended for asymptomatic AMLs larger than 4 cm and symptomatic AMLs of any size *(37)*. Partial nephrectomy and selective angioembolization are two renal-preserving treatment modalities available for patients with these benign neoplasms. Currently, there are few data reporting the efficacy and ability to preserve renal function by using selective embolization, and it is therefore best suited when a distinct and accessible renal arterial branch supplies the tumor exclusively and not the adjacent normal parenchyma.

Partial nephrectomy is considered the preferred treatment in cases of bilateral tumors or tumors in a solitary kidney. Angiomyolipomas are well suited to a nephron-sparing approach for several reasons. Because these lesions are benign, the risk of residual microfocal disease is of less long-term significance. Furthermore, most AMS are exophytic and maintain a distinct pseudocapsule that is readily identified and can be dissected to a narrow base. The amount of renal parenchyma that can be spared with an open procedure is usually much greater than one would predict radiographically. There are few published studies evaluating the efficacy of partial nephrectomy for patients with AMLs. Fazeli-Matin reported the largest series of 27 patients undergoing partial nephrectomy for renal AMLs ranging in size up to 26 cm *(38)*. All kidneys maintained good function postoperatively, no patient required dialysis, and there were no recurrent AMLs or related symptoms identified at a mean follow-up time of 39 mo. When surgical treatment for renal AMLs is indicated, partial nephrectomy can be performed with a high rate of success, even in patients with larger tumors involving a solitary kidney.

## POSTOPERATIVE FOLLOW-UP AFTER RADICAL NEPHRECTOMY OR PARTIAL NEPHRECTOMY

Based on data from Levy et al. *(39)*, a stage-specific protocol for surveillance after radical nephrectomy has been proposed (Table 4.1). Following radical nephrectomy, all patients should be evaluated with a medical history, physical examination, and selected blood studies on a yearly or twice-yearly basis. Blood work should include serum calcium, liver function tests, alkaline phosphatase, blood urea nitrogen, creatinine, and electrolytes. For patients with pT1NoMo RCC, routine postoperative radiographic imaging is not necessary due to the low risk of recurrent malignancy. For patients with pT2NoMo RCC, a chest x-ray every year and an abdominal CT scan every 2 yr are recommended. Patients with pT3NoMo RCC have a higher risk of developing recurrent malignancy, particularly during the first 3 yr after radical nephrectomy, and may benefit from more frequent laboratory and radiographic follow-up including an abdominal CT scan at 1 yr, then every 2 yr thereafter.

Data from the Cleveland Clinic have shown that the need for postoperative surveillance after partial nephrectomy also varies according to the initial pathological tumor stage *(40)* (Table 4.2). All patients should be evaluated with a medical history and physical examination and selected blood studies on a yearly or twice-yearly basis. Patients who undergo partial nephrectomy for pT1NoMo RCC do not require radiographic imaging postoperatively

**Table 1**
**Postoperative Surveillance After Radical Nephrectomy for Localized RCC**

| | *Months Postop* | | | | | | | | |
|---|---|---|---|---|---|---|---|---|---|
| | *3* | *6* | *12* | *18* | *24* | *30* | *36* | *48* | *60* |
| pT1 | | | | | | | | | |
| History and exam | | | x | | x | | | x | x |
| Blood | | | x | | x | | | x | x |
| CXR | | | | | | | | | |
| Abdominal CT | | | | | | | | | |
| pT2 | | | | | | | | | |
| History and exam | | | x | | x | | x | x | x |
| Blood | | | x | | x | | x | x | x |
| CXR | | | x | | x | | x | x | x |
| Abdominal CT | | | | | x | | | x | |
| pT3 | | | | | | | | | |
| History and exam | | x | x | x | x | x | x | x | x |
| Blood | | x | x | x | x | x | x | x | x |
| CXR | | x | x | x | x | x | x | x | x |
| Abdominal CT | | | x | | | | x | | x |

CXR, chest x-ray.

**Table 2**
**Postoperative Surveillance After Partial Nephrectomy for Localized RCC**

| | *Months Postop* | | | | | | | | |
|---|---|---|---|---|---|---|---|---|---|
| | *3* | *6* | *12* | *18* | *24* | *30* | *36* | *48* | *60* |
| pT1 | | | | | | | | | |
| History and exam | | | x | | x | | | x | x |
| Blood | | | x | | x | | | x | x |
| CXR | | | | | | | | | |
| Abdominal CT | | | | | | | | | |
| pT2 | | | | | | | | | |
| History and exam | | | x | | x | | x | x | x |
| Blood | | | x | | x | | x | x | x |
| CXR | | | x | | x | | x | x | x |
| Abdominal CT | | | | | x | | | x | |
| pT3 | | | | | | | | | |
| History and exam | | x | x | x | x | x | x | x | x |
| Blood | | x | x | x | x | x | x | x | x |
| CXR | | x | x | x | x | x | x | x | x |
| Abdominal CT | | x | x | x | x | x | x | | x |

CXR, chest x-ray.

in view of the very low risk of recurrent malignancy. A yearly chest x-ray is recommended after partial nephrectomy for pT2NoMo because the lung is the most common site of postoperative metastasis. Abdominal or retroperitoneal tumor recurrence is uncommon in the latter group, particularly early after a partial nephrectomy, and these patients require only occasional follow-up abdominal CT scanning. We recommend this be done every 2 yr. Patients with pT3NoMo have a high risk of developing local tumor recurrence and metastatic disease, particularly during the first 2 yr after partial nephrectomy. They may benefit from more frequent follow-up with chest x-ray and abdominal CT scanning. Initially, we recommend that these be done every 6 mo during the first 3 yr. Thereafter, a chest x-ray is done yearly and an abdominal CT scan every 2 yr.

Postoperative bone scans, bone plain films, and head or chest CT scans are necessary only in the presence of related symptoms. The role of abdominal ultrasound in evaluating recurrent lesions of the remnant kidney is unclear. Its use may decrease the overall cost of surveillance at the risk of potentially missing other intra-abdominal recurrences. Finally, periodic blood pressure checks and urinary screening for protein are important for patients with a solitary or remnant kidney. If urinary dip reveals proteinuria, a 24-h quantitative urine protein should be obtained to screen for hyperfiltration nephropathy *(41)*.

## REFERENCES


1. Robson CJ, Churchill BM, Anderson W. The results of radical nephrectomy for renal cell carcinoma. J Urol 101:297–301, 1969.
2. Schefft P, Novick AC, Straffon RA, Stewart BH. Surgery for renal cell carcinoma extending into the vena cava. J Urol 120:28–31, 1978.
3. Libertino JA, Zinman L, Watkins E, Jr. Long-term results of resection of renal cell cancer with extension into inferior vena cava. J Urol 137:21–24, 1987.
4. Novick AC, Kaye M, Cosgrove D, et al. Experience with cardiopulmonary bypass and deep hypothermic circulatory arrest in the management of retroperitoneal tumors with large vena caval thrombi. Ann Surg 212:472–477, 1990.
5. Neves RJ and Zincke H. Surgical treatment of renal cancer with vena cava extension. Br J Urol 59:390–395, 1987.
6. Skinner DG, Pritchett TR, Lieskovsky G, Boyd SD, Stiles QR. Vena caval involvement by renal cell carcinoma: surgical resection provides meaningful long-term survival. Ann Surg 210:387–392, 1989.
7. Cherrie RJ, Goldman DG, Lindner A, deKernion JG. Prognostic implications of vena caval extension of renal cell carcinoma. J Urol 128:910–912, 1982.
8. Glazer AA and Novick AC. Long-term follow-up after surgical treatment for renal cell carcinoma extending into the right atrium. J Urol 155:448–450, 1996.
9. Goldfarb DA, Novick AC, Lorig R, et al. Magnetic resonance imaging for assessment of vena caval tumor thrombi: a comparative study with vena cavography and CT scanning. J Urol 144(5):100–104.
10. Glazer A and Novick AC. Preoperative transesophageal echocardiography for assessment of vena caval tumor thrombi: a comparative study with venocavography and magnetic resonance imaging. Urology 49:32–34, 1997.
11. McGahan JP, Blake LC, DeVere White R, Gersovich EO, Brant WE. Color flow sonographic mapping of intravascular extension of malignant renal tumors. J Ultrasound Med 12:403–409, 1993.
12. Belis JA, Pae WE, Rohner TJ, Myers JL, Thiele BL, Wickey GS, Martin DE. Cardiovascular evaluation before circulatory arrest for removal of vena cava extension of renal carcinoma. J Urol 141:1302–1307, 1989.
13. Sagalowaky AI, Kadesky KT, Ewalt DM, Kennedy TJ. Factors influencing adrenal metastasis in renal cell carcinoma. J Urol 151:1181–1184, 1994.
14. Giuliani L, Giberti C, Martorama G, Rovida S. Radical extensive surgery for renal cell carcinoma. J Urol 143:468–474, 1990.
15. Svensson L, Crawford ES, Hess K, et al. Deep hypothermia with circulatory arrest. J Thoracic Cardiovasc Surg 106(1):19–31, 1993.
16. Mault J, Ohtake S, Klingensmith M, et al. Cerebral metabolism and circulatory arrest: Effects of duration and strategies for protection. Ann Thoracic Surg 55:57–64, 1993.
17. Pagano D, Carey JA, Patel RL, et al. Retrograde cerebral perfusion: clinical experience in emergency and elective aortic operations. Ann Thorac Surg 59:393–397, 1995.
18. Burt M. Inferior vena caval involvement by renal cell carcinoma: use of venovenous bypass as adjunct during resection. Urol Clin North Am 18:437–444, 1991.
19. Foster RS, Mahomed Y, Bihrle RR, Strup S. Use of caval-atrial shunt for resection of a caval tumor thrombus in renal cell carcinoma. J Urol 140:1370, 1988.
20. Licht MR and Novick AC. Nephron-sparing surgery for renal cell carcinoma. J Urol 145:1–7, 1994.
21. Butler BP, Novick AC, Miller DP, Campbell SA, Licht MR. Management of small unilateral renal cell carcinomas: radical versus nephron-sparing surgery. Urology 45:34–41, 1995.
22. Lerner SE, Hawkins CA, Blute ML, et al. Disease outcome in patients with low-stage renal carcinoma treated with nephron-sparing or radical surgery. J Urol 155:1868–1873, 1996.

23. Ziegelbaum M, Novick AC, Streem SB, et al. Conservative surgery for transitional cell carcinoma of the renal pelvis. J Urol 138:1146–1149, 1987.
24. Morgan WR and Zincke H. Progression and survival after renal conserving surgery for renal cell carcinoma: experience in 104 patients and extended follow-up. J Urol 144:852–858, 1990.
25. Steinbach F, Stockle M, Muller SC, et al. Conservative surgery of renal tumors in 140 patients: 21 years of experience. J Urol 148:24–30, 1992.
26. Hafez KS, Fergany AF, Novick AC. Nephron-sparing surgery for localized renal cell carcinoma: Impact of tumor size on patient, survival, tumor recurrence, and TNM staging. J Urol 162:1930–1933, 1999.
27. Fergany AF, Hafez KS, Novick AC. Long-term results of nephron-sparing surgery for localized renal cell carcinoma: 10-year follow-up. J Urol 163:442–445, 2000.
28. Coll DM, Uzzo RG, Herts BR, Davros WJ, Wirth SL, Novick AC. 3-Dimensional volume rendered computerized tomography for preoperative evaluation and intraoperative treatment of patients undergoing nephron-sparing surgery. J Urol 161:1097–1102, 1999.
29. Novick AC. Anatomic approaches in nephron-sparing surgery for renal cell carcinoma. Atlas Urol Clin North Am 6:39, 1998.
30. Campbell S, Novick AC, Steinbach F, et al. Intraoperative evaluation of renal cell carcinoma: A prospective study of the role of ultrasonography and histopathological frozen sections. J Urol 155:1191–1195, 1996.
31. Graham SD Jr. and Glenn JF. Enucleation surgery for renal malignancy. J Urol 122:546–549, 1979.
32. Jaeger N, Weissbach L, Vahelensieck W. Value of enucleation of tumor in solitary kidneys. Eur Urol 11:369–373, 1985.
33. Marshall FF, Taxy JB, Fishman EK, Chang R. The feasibility of surgical enucleation for renal cell carcinoma. J Urol 135:231–234, 1986.
34. Blackley SK, Ladaga L, Woolfitt RA, Schellhammer PF. Ex situ study of the effectiveness of enucleation in patients with renal cell carcinoma. J Urol 140:6–10, 1988.
35. Spencer WF, Novick AC, Montie JE, Streem JB, Levin HS. Surgical treatment of localized renal carcinoma in von Hippel-Lindau disease. J Urol 139:507–509, 1988.
36. Steiner MS, Goldman SM, Fishman EK, et al. The natural history of renal angiomyolipoma. J Urol 150:1782–1786, 1993.
37. Oesterling JE. The management of renal angiomyolipoma. J Urol 135:1121–1124, 1986.
38. Fazeli-Matin S and Novick AC. Nephron-sparing surgery for renal angiomyolipoma. Urol 52:577–583, 1998.
39. Levy DA, Slayton JW, Swanson DA, Dinney CP. Stage specific guidelines for surveillance after radical nephrectomy for local renal cell carcinoma. J Urol 159(4):1163–1167, 1998.
40. Hafez KS, Novick AC, Campbell SC. Patterns for tumor recurrence and guidelines for follow-up after nephron-sparing surgery for sporadic renal cell carcinoma. J Urol 157:2067–2070, 1997.
41. Novick AC, Gephardt G, Guz B, Steinmuller D, Tubbs RR. Long-term follow-up after partial removal of a solitary kidney. NEJM 325(15):1058–1062, 1991.

# 5 Laparoscopic Surgery for Renal Cell Carcinoma

*Inderbir S. Gill*

## LAPARASCOPIC RADICAL NEPHRECTOMY FOR CANCER

### Introduction

Since Clayman's initial description of laparoscopic nephrectomy, this procedure has rapidly gained worldwide acceptance. At centers where such expertise is available, laparoscopic radical nephrectomy can comfortably be considered a, if not the, standard of care for the appropriate patient with an organ-confined T1 renal tumor. Either the transperitoneal or the retroperitoneal laparoscopic approach can be employed, depending on the individual patient characteristics and, particularly, the training and expertise of the laparoscopic surgeon. Contraindications for laparoscopic radical nephrectomy today include vena caval thrombus, bulky lymphadenopathy, and locally invasive tumors. Large tumor size is only a relative contraindication, dependent on the comfort level of the laparoscopic surgeon and the individual characteristics of the tumor. Although laparoscopic radical nephrectomy for pT2 tumors has been reported, the possibility of significant-sized peritumoral collateral vessels and desmoplastic reaction must be kept in mind. Contraindications include significant cardiopulmonary comorbidity, uncorrected coagulopathy, and abdominal sepsis. Significant prior surgery in the quadrant of interest and morbid obesity increase the level of technical difficulty, although we have had gratifying success in these two challenging circumstances by employing the retroperitoneal laparoscopic approach.

### Patient Preparation and Positioning

Detailed informed patient consent is obtained. Bowel preparation involves two bottles of magnesium citrate self-administered the afternoon prior to surgery. The patient reports to the hospital on the morning of the operation. Intravenous broad-spectrum antibiotics and sequential compression stockings bilaterally are routine. For the transperitoneal approach, the patient is positioned in a 60° flank position with the kidney bridge mildly elevated and the table mildly flexed. Emphasis is placed on meticulous foam padding of soft tissue and bony sites, including the head and neck, axilla, hip, knee, and ankle, along with careful ergonomically neutral positioning of the neck, arms, and legs. This is important to prevent postoperative neuromuscular strain.

### Port Placement (Fig. 5.1)

We prefer to obtain peritoneal access with the Veress needle (closed) technique. Typically, a four- to five-port approach is employed. The primary 10/12-mm trocar is inserted at the lateral border of the rectus at the level of the umbilicus. Three secondary trocars are placed: a 10/12-mm port for the laparoscope approx 2–3 finger-breadths below the costal margin at the lateral border of the rectus, a 10/12-mm port 2–3 finger-breadths lateral to the rectus muscle at the costal margin, and a 2-mm port for lateral retraction of the kidney at the anterior axillary line. For a left-sided nephrectomy, a 5-mm port is placed at the lateral border of the rectus near the costal margin. For a right-sided nephrectomy, a 5-mm port is inserted near the xiphisternum for retraction of the liver.

### Colon Mobilization

On the right side, the line of Toldt is incised to mobilize the ascending colon medially. This posterior peritoneal incision is carried transversely in a medial direction along the undersurface of the liver up to the vena cava. Blunt dissection mobilizes the ascending colon, hepatic flexure, and the duodenum medially until the anterior aspect of the inferior vena cava is clearly exposed. On the left side, more formal mobilization of the splenic flexure, spleen, and pancreas is necessary because these structures almost completely cover the anterior aspect of Gerota's fascia. As such, comparatively more mobilization of the colon is necessary on the left side compared to the right. The

From: *Operative Urology at the Cleveland Clinic*
Edited by: A. Novick et al. © Humana Press Inc., Totowa, NJ

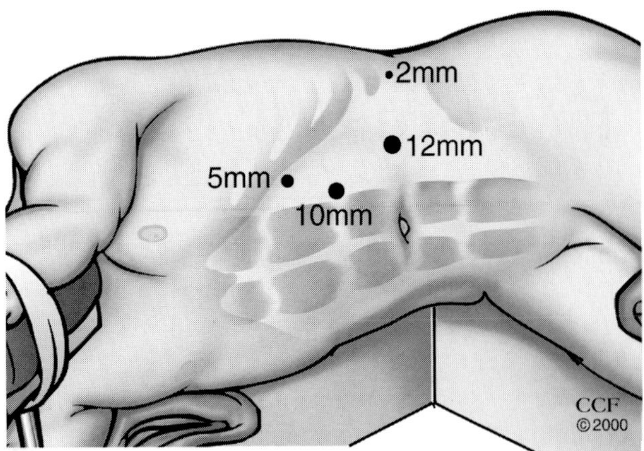


Fig. 5.1

incision along the line of Toldt is more extensive, and the splenocolic, splenorenal, and splenophrenic fascial attachments are released. The spleen is mobilized along its lateral border and is placed medially, where it typically stays by gravity alone. It is important to enter the correct avascular fascial plane between the anterior surface of Gerota's fascia and the posterior aspect of the descending mesocolon, similar to open surgery.

## Renal Hilum Control (Figs. 5.2 and 5.3)

The ureter/gonadal vein packet is identified inferior to the lower pole kidney and just lateral to the ipsilateral great vessel. Psoas muscle is identified by blunt dissection. The ureter and gonadal vein are secured and divided. Taut lateral retraction is placed on the divided ureter/gonadal vein, placing the renal hilum on stretch. Dissection along the psoas muscle and lateral border of the ipsilateral great vessel leads to the renal hilum. Antero-lateral twisting and retraction of the lower pole kidney helps to bring the posteriorly located renal artery into ready view. The renal artery is circumferentially mobilized, clipped, and divided. The renal vein is controlled with an Endo-GIA stapler (US Surgical, Norwalk, CT). A careful search must be made for any secondary renal hilar vessels, which are controlled appropriately with Weck clips.

## Concomitant Adrenalectomy

Typically, concomitant adrenalectomy is indicated if there is any alteration in size, shape, or location of the adrenal gland on preoperative computed tomography (CT) scanning. Additionally, an upper pole tumor physically abutting the adrenal gland mandates concomitant adrenalectomy. The right adrenal vein is a short, stubby vessel directly entering the infrahepatic vena cava from the supermedial aspect of the right adrenal gland. Dissection is performed along the right lateral surface of the inferior vena cava (IVC) to reach the adrenal vein, which is mobilized,

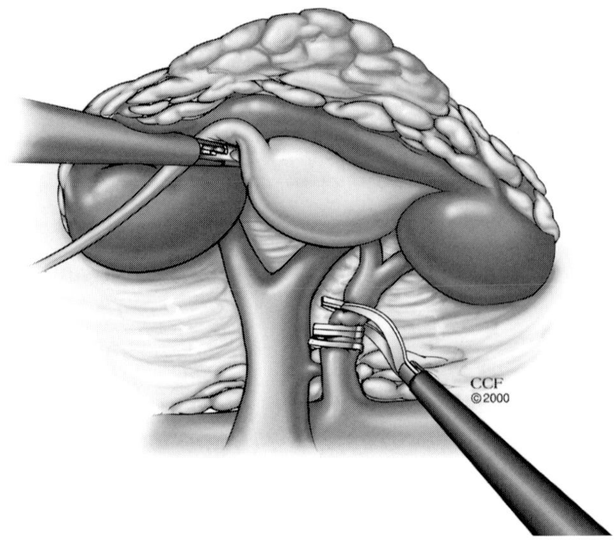


Fig. 5.2

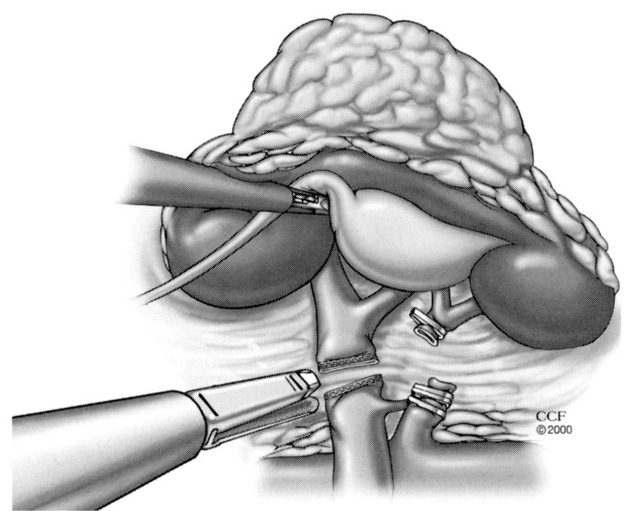


Fig. 5.3

controlled with Weck clips, and divided. On the left side, the longer, narrower main left adrenal vein arises from the inferior medial aspect of the adrenal gland and drains directly into the left renal vein. It is similarly mobilized, clipped, and divided. If concomitant adrenalectomy is indicated, the lateral surface of the ipsilateral great vessel is dissected bare, and all lymphatico-fatty tissue in this area is excised. Care must be taken to clip any suspicious lymphatic channels to avoid postoperative chylous ascites.

## Specimen Entrapment (Fig. 5.4)

We entrap the specimen in an Endo-catch bag (US Surgical, Norwalk, CT) and routinely perform intact extraction through a low Pfannenstiel's incision in the suprapubic area. For this muscle-splitting incision, the skin is incised at the level of the symphysis pubis, and the anterior rectus

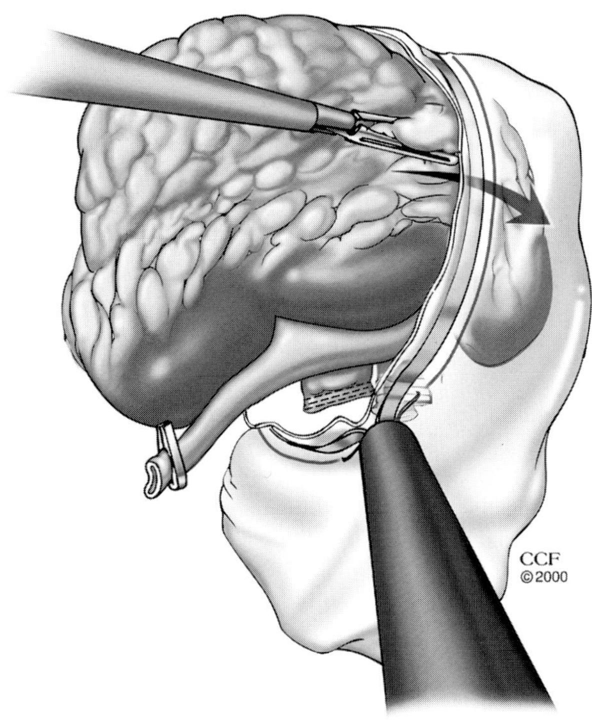


Fig. 5.4

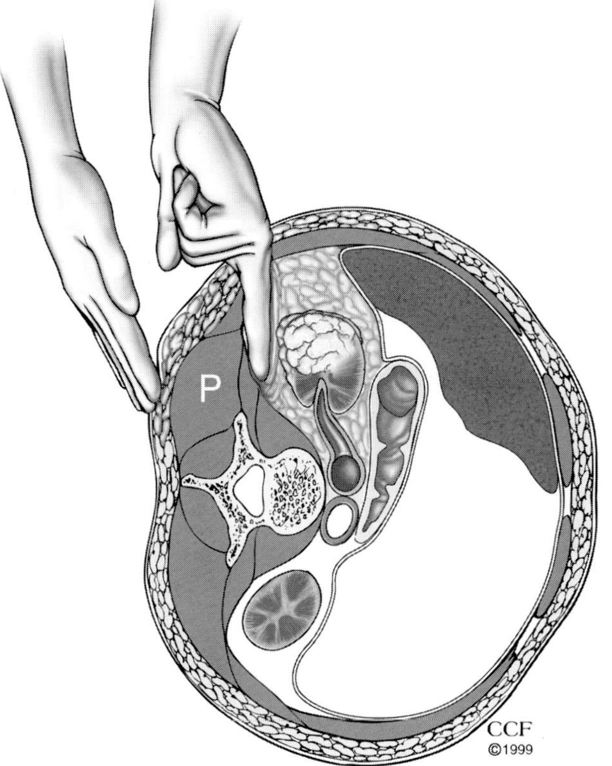


Fig. 5.5

fascia is incised obliquely somewhat higher up, thus achieving a cosmetically preferred extraction incision. The author does not perform morcellation for any cancer.

## Retroperitoneal Approach

The patient is positioned in the standard full-flank position with the kidney rest elevated and the operative table flexed. This maximizes the space between the iliac crest and the lowermost rib. However, care is taken to lower the kidney rest and straighten the operative table as soon as all laparoscopic trocars are inserted. As such, for the majority of the operation, there is virtually no flexion of the operative table.

## Retroperitoneal Access (Fig. 5.5)

The author employs the open Hasson technique. A horizontal skin incision (1.5–2 cm) is made at the tip of the 12th rib. The flank muscle fibers are separated with two S-retractors to visualize the anterior thoracolumbar fascia, which is incised to enter the retroperitoneal space with the tip of the index finger. Digital dissection is performed along the anterior surface of the psoas muscle and fascia, posterior to Gerota's fascia (to create a space for the balloon dilator).

## Balloon Dissection (Fig. 5.6)

The PDB balloon dilator (US Surgical, Norwalk, CT) is inserted into the retroperitoneum. Approximately six to eight pumps of the sphygmomanometer bulb are done to

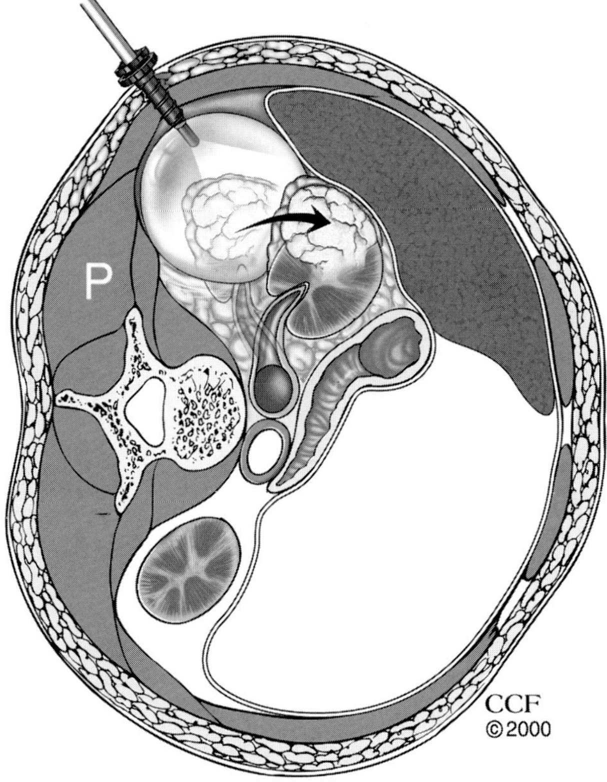


Fig. 5.6

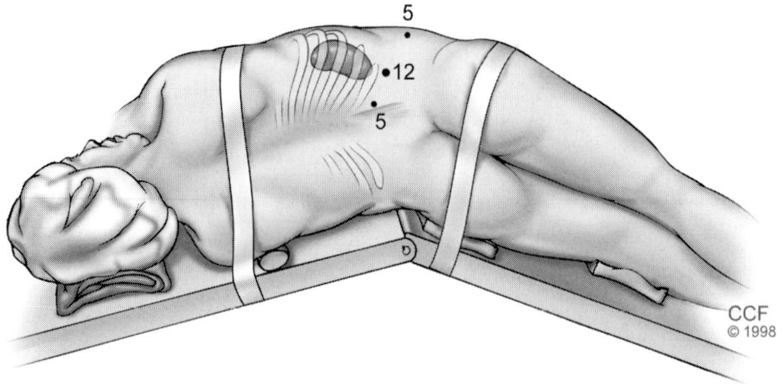


Fig. 5.7

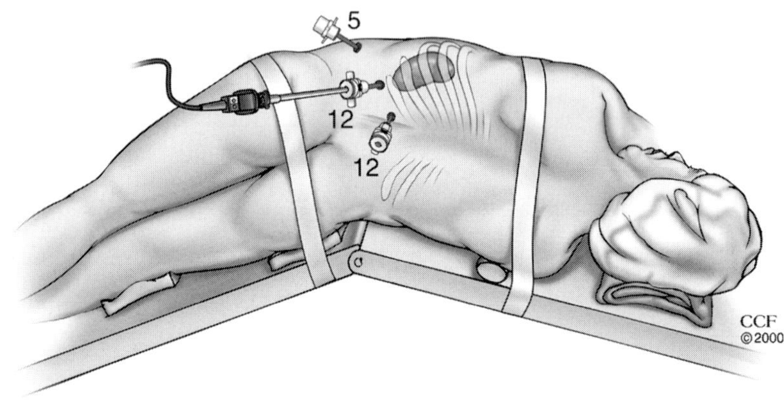


Fig. 5.8

instill approx 150 cc of air in the balloon. The shaft of the balloon dilator is now retracted outward, thereby impacting the balloon against the undersurface of the anterior abdominal wall. An additional 30 pumps of the sphygmomanometer bulb are now performed to create the retroperitoneal space. This maneuver ensures that the entire peritoneal deflection is mobilized medially, without any overhanging peritoneal shelf. In this manner, the *en bloc* kidney and surrounding Gerota's fascia are mobilized medially, thus exposing the posterior aspect of the renal hilum and the adjacent vessels to clear laparoscopic view.

## Port Placement (Figs. 5.7 and 5.8)

After removing the balloon dilator, a 10-mm blunt tip cannula (US Surgical, Norwalk, CT) is inserted as the primary port. Pneumoperitoneum (15 mm) is created and retroperitoneoscopic examination completed. An anterior port (10/12 mm) is placed 3–4 cm cephalad to the iliac crest in the anterior axillary line. A posterior port is placed at the junction of the 12th rib and the spinal muscles. Typically, we employ this standard three-port approach for all retroperitoneoscopic ablative renal and adrenal surgery. All ports are placed under clear laparoscopic visualization.

## Renal Vessel Control

Careful laparoscopic inspection reveals the pulsations of the fat-covered renal artery, which are oriented vertically and are distinct from the transversely located pulsations of the aorta (sharp pulsations) or IVC (gentle undulating pulsations). The psoas muscle must be kept horizontal at all times on the monitor and is the single most important anatomical landmark in the retroperitoneum. It is also important to maintain constant taut anterior retraction of the Gerota's fascia-covered kidney with a three-pronged retractor in the surgeon's nondominant hand inserted through the anterior port. Using the J-hook electrocautery, Gerota's fascia is incised parallel and 1–2 cm anterior to the psoas muscle directly over the renal arterial pulsations. The renal artery is circumferentially mobilized, clipped (three clips toward the aorta, two clips toward the kidney), and divided. The renal vein is usually located anteriorly and somewhat caudal to the renal artery. In a similar manner, this is circumferentially mobilized and controlled with an EndoGIA vascular stapler. Concomitant adrenalectomy is performed in a similar manner as during transperitoneal radical nephrectomy. The ureter and gonadal vein are identified as a last step, clipped, and divided.

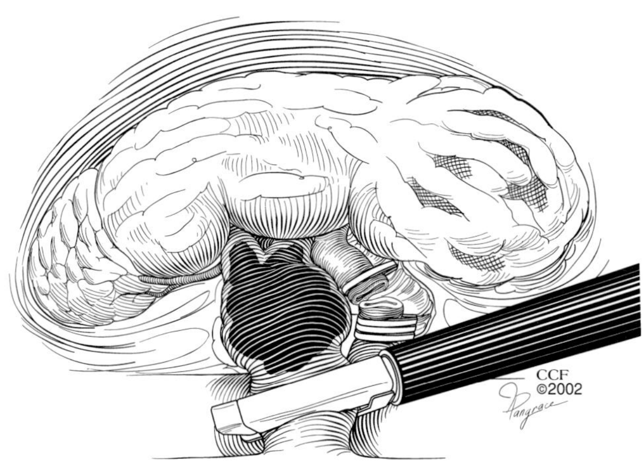


Fig. 5.9

## Renal Vein Thrombus (Fig. 5.9)

Laparoscopic radical nephrectomy for level 1 renal vein thrombus has been described. Intraoperative flexible ultrasonography is performed to specifically reveal the extent of tumor thrombus in the renal vein and make a determination as to the laparoscopic technical feasibility of complete excision and obtaining negative vascular margins. The main renal artery is secured and the renal vein completely mobilized. The proximal renal vein now typically appears flat because it is devoid of blood flow and stands clearly demarcated from the distended distal renal vein, which contains the intraluminal venous thrombus. This is typically clearly visible laparoscopically and is further confirmed by contact color Doppler ultrasonography. Using the EndoGIA stapler, the renal vein is transected proximal to the thrombus.

## Mobilization of Kidney

The inferior pole of the kidney is mobilized from the undersurface of the peritoneum. Caudal traction on the partially mobilized kidney now places the peri-renal fat around the upper renal pole on stretch. The upper pole of the kidney is mobilized from the undersurface of the adrenal gland (in adrenal-sparing nephrectomy) or from the undersurface of the diaphragm (if concomitant adrenalectomy is performed). Finally, the kidney is mobilized from the undersurface of the peritoneal envelope, completely freeing the specimen. Care is taken not to employ any electrocautery along the peritoneal surface of the kidney so as to guard against injury to intraabdominal viscerae or bowel. Remember, although out of sight, bowel loops must never be out of mind because they are separated only by the thin peritoneum, with a real potential for transmural injury.

## Specimen Extraction

The specimen is entrapped in an Endo-catch bag, as in the transperitoneal approach. Again, intact extraction is performed through a pfannensteil incision, while staying completely extraperitoneal. Typically, no drain is placed and laparoscopic exit is completed in the usual fashion.

## Postoperative Care

The patient is mobilized on the evening of surgery. Two Dulcolax suppositories are administered on the morning of postoperative day 1. In the majority of our cases, the patient is discharged on the evening of postoperative day 1, after resumption of oral fluid intake.

# LAPAROSCOPIC PARTIAL NEPHRECTOMY

In properly selected patients, open partial nephrectomy yields oncological outcomes comparable to traditional radical nephrectomy, even over the long term. There has been an increase in the detection of small (≤4 cm) incidentally diagnosed renal tumors, thus increasing the applicability of nephron-sparing techniques in contemporary patients with renal cancer. Finally, confidence and experience with reconstructive laparoscopic surgery has increased exponentially worldwide in recent years, with many complex abdominal reconstructive procedures now being addressed by minimally invasive techniques. As a result of the above three factors, significant interest has focused on laparoscopic partial nephrectomy, which has recently emerged as an attractive minimally invasive treatment alternative for select patients with a small renal mass.

Since 1999, we have performed more than 400 laparoscopic partial nephrectomies. Based on this experience, detailed herein is our technique for laparoscopic partial nephrectomy, including indications and contraindications, instrumentation, preoperative preparation, and tips and tricks. In general, the described technique is applicable to both the transperitoneal and retroperitoneal approaches. Whenever differences in technique exist, mention is made accordingly.

## Indications and Contraindications

Initially, laparoscopic partial nephrectomy (LPN) was reserved for a small, superficial, peripheral, exophytic renal mass, for which a wedge resection sufficed. With increasing experience, the indications of LPN have been carefully expanded to include more technically advanced cases: deeply infiltrating tumors requiring pelvicaliceal repair, larger tumors requiring heminephrectomy, hilar tumors, tumor in a solitary kidney, and LPN with hypothermia. LPN is an advanced minimally invasive procedure, wherein considerable laparoscopic experience and expertise are implicit. Contraindications for LPN currently include a completely intrarenal and central tumor in the midpole kidney, nephron-sparing surgery (NSS) in the presence of a renal vein thrombus, and uncorrected coagulopathy. Moderate to severe azotemia is a relative contraindication to renal hilar clamping. Finally, LPN in a morbidly obese patient increases the technical complexity and should be approached with caution.

## Instrumentation

The typical laparoscopic basic set includes, among other things, the Veress needle, blunt-tip 5-mm and 10/12-mm ports, atraumatic bowel graspers, J-hook electrocautery, disposable laparoscopic scissors, Maryland grasper, Allis clamp, disposable clip applier (10 mm, titanium) Weck hem-o-lok clips (10 mm) and applicator, right-angle clamp (10 mm), bulldog clamps, and the Carter-Thompson port-site closure device. Herein, we focus on the equipment that the author feels is particularly useful for performing LPN. The Stryker suction tip is preferred because it not only provides robust suction/irrigation, but, equally importantly, has a smooth, blunt, gently beveled tip that allows atraumatic dissection in the area of the renal hilum. The 5-mm straight Ethicon needle drivers (cat. no. E705R) are preferred because of ease of use and strong, reliable grasping. Sutured renal reconstruction is performed with a CT-1 needle 2-0 vicryl and a CTX needle 0-vicryl. The hemostatic agent Floseal (Baxter, Deerfield, IL), delivered by a reusable metal laparoscopic applicator, is used routinely. Hilar clamping is efficiently achieved with a Medtronic Satinsky vascular clamp (cat. no. CEV435-2). For retroperitoneal LPN, the working space is optimally created with the round Autosuture preperitoneal dilation balloon (OMS-PDB1000).

## Patient Preparation and Positioning

Typically, the only radiological investigation is a three-dimensional CT scan with 3-mm cuts to delineate tumor location, relation to the pelvicaliceal system, and define the renal hilar vessels as regards number, location, interrelationships, and any vascular anomaly. Anticoagulant medications (aspirin, plavix, coumadin) are discontinued at an appropriate time prior to surgery.

Preoperatively, two bottles of magnesium citrate are administered on the afternoon prior to the day of surgery. Following endotracheal general anesthesia, cystoscopy is performed to insert a 5 French open-ended ureteral catheter into the ipsilateral renal pelvis over a glidewire. The ureteral catheter, secured to the Foley catheter with silk ties, is connected to a 60-cc syringe filled with dilute indigo carmine dye (1 ampule indigo carmine in 500 cc saline) with intravenous extension tubing. The syringe and intravenous tubing are maintained sterile on the operative field for intraoperative retrograde injection. For transperitoneal LPN, the patient is placed in a 45–60° lateral position, as mentioned earlier. Retroperitonoscopic LPN is performed with the patient in the full flank position.

Selection of approach, transperitoneal vs retroperitoneal, is an important issue when performing LPN. In general, the author prefers the transperitoneal approach because it provides more working space but, even more importantly, superior suturing angles when reconstructing the partial nephrectomy defect. As such, the transperitoneal approach is employed for any anterior, anterior–lateral, or lateral tumor or a larger upper or lower pole tumor requiring polar heminephrectomy. However, for posterior tumors, the retroperitoneal approach is preferred. In deciding on the laparoscopic approach, anterior vs posterior, judgment about precise tumor location is best made on cross-sectional CT scan with 3-mm cuts. A simplistic rule of thumb in this regard is as follows: a straight line is drawn medial-to-lateral from the renal hilum to the most convex point on the lateral surface of the kidney. Any tumor located anterior to this line is approached transperitoneally, while any tumor located posterior to this line is approached retroperitoneoscopically. If the drawn line transgresses the tumor, the approach is, by default, transperitoneal.

## Intraoperative Fluid Management

Maintaining adequate intraoperative diuresis is essential. Intravenous fluid administration is tailored to the patient's baseline cardiopulmonary and renal functional status. Approximately 30–45 min before hilar clamping, we administer 12.5 g of mannitol and 10 mg of furosemide to promote diuresis. These medications are repeated just before unclamping the renal hilum, with the aim of minimizing the sequelae of renal revascularization injury, cell swelling, and free radical release and to promote diuresis.

## Port Placement (Fig. 5.10)

Pneumoperitoneum is typically obtained by the closed (Veress) needle technique. For the transperitoneal approach, the primary port (10/12 mm) is placed lateral to the rectus muscle at the level of the umbilicus. A subcostal port is placed lateral to the rectus muscle and just inferior to the costochondral margin. On the right side, this subcostal 10/12-mm port is used to facilitate passage of suture needles for the right-handed surgeon. On the left side, this subcostal port is typically a 5-mm port. A 10/12-mm port for the laparoscope is placed 3 cm inferior and medial to the subcostal port. A 5-mm port is

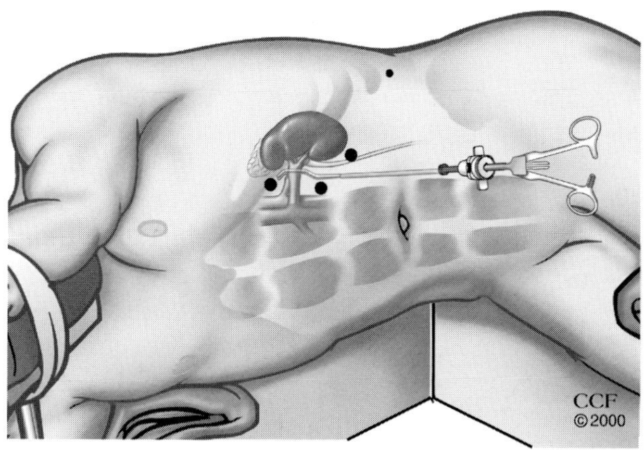


Fig. 5.10

inserted at the mid-axillary line in the vicinity of the tip of the 11th rib, and this port is employed to place lateral countertraction during renal hilar dissection and to grasp renorraphy stitches during renal parenchymal repair. Finally, a 10/12-mm port is placed in the suprapubic area lateral to the rectus muscle for insertion of the Satinsky vascular clamp.

Our standard retroperitoneal laparoscopic approach employs three ports. A 12–15 mm incision is made at the tip of the 12th rib, and entry is gained into the retroperitoneal space under direct vision. The retroperitoneal space is created as described previously with a balloon dilator, and a 10-mm blunt-tip balloon port is secured. A 10-mm port is placed anteriorly, approx 2–3 finger-widths cephalad to the anterior superior iliac spine. A posterior port (10/12 mm) is placed lateral to the erector spinae muscle along the undersurface of the 12th rib. For LPN, two additional retroperitoneal ports are employed. A 5-mm port is placed 3–4 cm superior to the anterior 10/12-mm port and is used for grasping the renorraphy sutures. Finally, a 10/12-mm port is placed in the iliac fossa just anterior to the inferior superior iliac spine and is used for inserting the laparoscopic Satinsky clamp.

## Hilar Dissection

Our essential operative strategy is as follows: renal hilar dissection first, mobilization of kidney and tumor next. On the right side, the liver is retracted anteriorly. On the left side, the spleen and pancreas are reflected medially. On either side, the ipsilateral colon is mobilized, more so on the left side than the right. The ureter and gonadal vein packet is *en bloc* dissected and lifted anteriorly off the psoas muscle. Dissection is carried towards the renal vein, which is mobilized enough to appreciate its precise location, and to visualize its anterior surface, in its entirety. We do not skeletonize the renal vein and artery individually during LPN for the following reasons: (1) it is unnecessary for achieving adequate clamping, (2) doing so may induce renal renal artery vasospasm, (3) it risks iatrogenic vascular injury, and (4) it takes approx 30 min of important operating time, which detracts from the primary mission of the procedure. Superior to the renal hilum, the adrenal gland is dissected off the medial aspect of the upper pole kidney, which is then mobilized anteriorly off the psoas muscle. Essentially, the anterior, posterior, inferior, and superior aspects of the *en bloc* renal hilum, with some hilar fat intact, are prepared. These maneuvers allow the Satinsky vascular clamp to be deployed across the *en bloc* renal hilum with safety and confidence. Care must be taken not to miss any secondary renal arteries or veins.

## Mobilization of Kidney

Gerota's fascia is entered and the kidney defatted. We prefer removing fat from most of the renal surface for the following reasons: (1) it makes the kidney more mobile, (2) it may visualize secondary satellite tumors, (3) it allows multidirectional intraoperative ultrasound viewing, and (4) it allows more versatility for tumor resection and suturing angles. However, the peri-renal overlying the tumor and its vicinity is maintained intact, thereby allowing adequate staging for potential T3a tumors and possibly serving as a handle during tumor resection.

## Intraoperative Ultrasonography

Thorough, real-time ultrasonographic examination of the tumor is performed to facilitate planning of tumor resection. The steerable, flexible, color Doppler ultrasound probe (10-mm shaft) is employed. Information is obtained regarding tumor size, invasion depth, distance of tumor from pelvicaliceal system, and identification of any large peritumoral blood vessels. Additionally, any small satellite tumors that may have been missed on preoperative CT scanning are searched for. Under real-time ultrasonographic guidance, the proposed line of tumor excision is circumferentially scored around the tumor with the tip of a monopolar J-hook electrocautery. The oncological adequacy of this scored margin is reconfirmed ultrasonographically prior to initiating tumor resection.

## Hilar Clamping (Figs. 5.11 and 5.12)

As in open surgery, a bloodless field is an essential prerequisite for a technically precise tumor excision and collecting system and parenchymal repair. This ideal surgical field is best achieved with hilar clamping. As mentioned, the author prefers to clamp the hilum *en bloc*. The Satinsky clamp must be placed on the hilum medial to the ureter and renal pelvis, thus avoiding urothelial crush injury. One

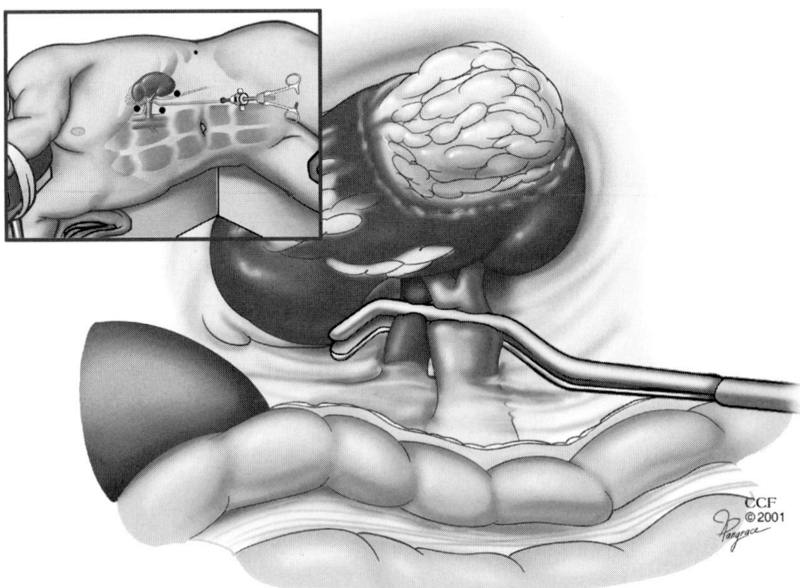


Fig. 5.11

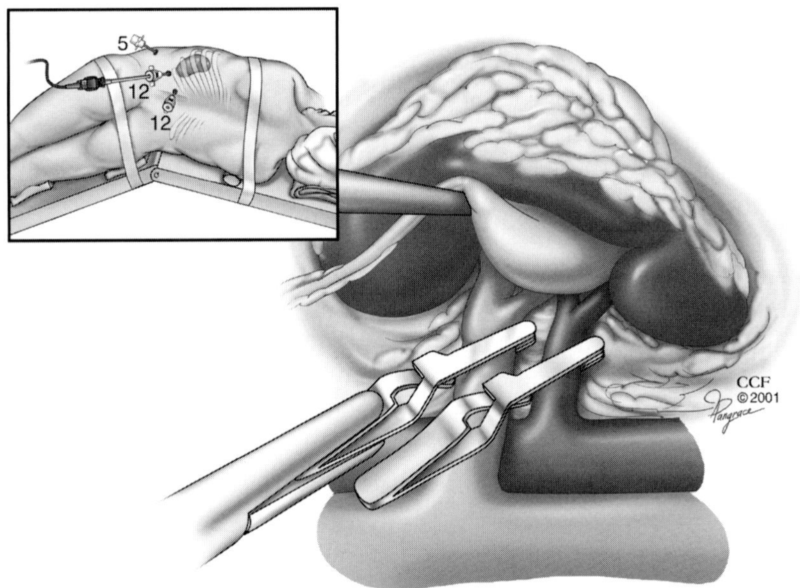


Fig. 5.12

must be certain that the entire renal hilum is enclosed within the jaws of the Satinsky. As such, the Satinsky clamp is fully opened and slowly advanced over the renal hilum in a deliberate manner, such that the jaw of the clamp facing the surgeon is anterior to the renal vein, while the posterior jaw hugs the psoas muscle. This reliably includes the renal artery and renal vein within the clamp jaws along with some hilar fat, which serves to cushion the renal vessels against clamp injury. The anesthesiologist starts a time clock to monitor the duration of warm ischemia.

In the retroperitoneal approach, the jaw of the clamp facing the surgeon lies posterior to the renal artery, while the other jaw must be anatomically anterior enough to encompass the renal vein safely. Additionally, there must be enough separation of the renal hilar structures from the peritoneum so that the clamp does not risk peritoneal entry. Alternatively, individual bulldog clamps can be placed on the renal artery and vein separately after each vascular structure has been circumferentially mobilized.

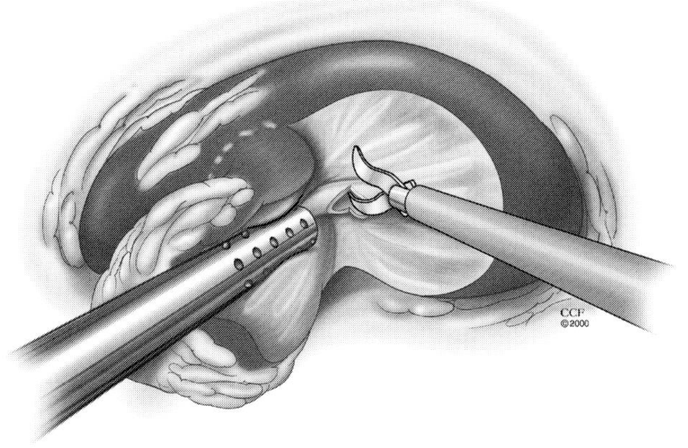


Fig. 5.13

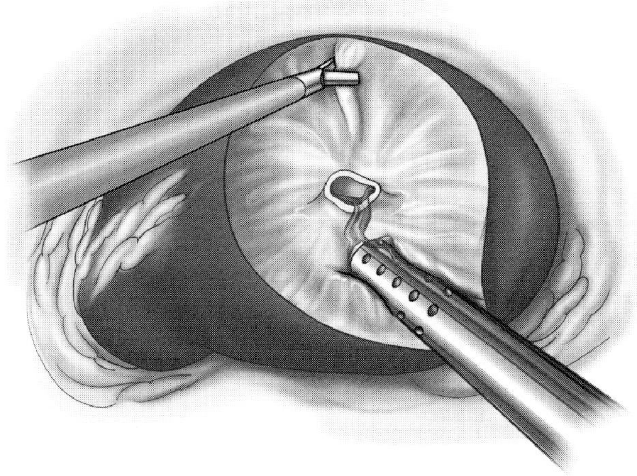

Fig. 5.14

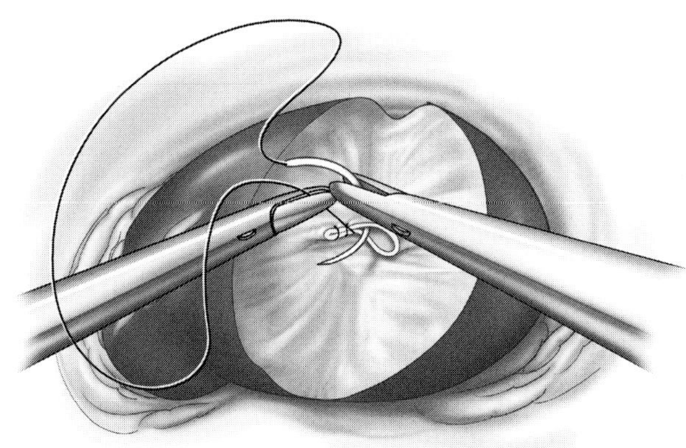

Fig. 5.15

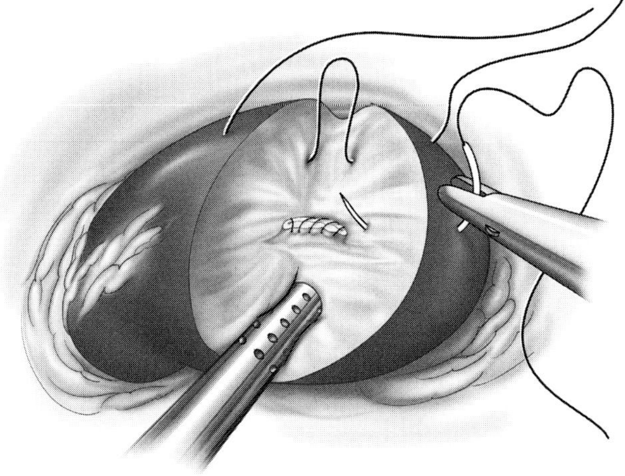

Fig. 5.16

## Tumor Resection (Fig. 5.13)

Once the hilum is clamped, tumor resection is initiated. The renal capsule is circumferentially incised with the J-hook electrocautery. Tumor resection is performed using the heavier nondisposable scissors, the jaws of which are larger than those of the disposable endoshears. Depth of tumor resection is guided by the mental map created by combining the information obtained from the preoperative CT scan, the intraoperative ultrasound examination, and laparoscopic visual cues during resection. Our aim is to obtain a margin of approx 0.5 cm around the tumor. To the uninitiated, this margin may visually appear as though an excessive amount of kidney is being excised. However, one must factor in the magnification of the laparoscope. It is most helpful for the surgeon to inspect the specimen along with the pathologist after extraction, which provides an invaluable learning experience.

## Pelvicaliceal Repair and Parenchymal Hemostasis (Figs. 5.14–5.17)

The bed of the partial nephrectomy defect is oversewn with a running 2-0 vicryl on CT-1 needle. This suturing aims to achieve two specific goals: (1) precise water-tight repair of any pelvicaliceal system entry, which is confirmed with retrograde injection of dilute indigo carmine through the ureteral catheter, and (2) oversewing of any large transected intrarenal blood vessels, the majority of which lie in the vicinity of the renal sinus. Individual suture repair with figure-of-eight stitches can be performed of any additional blood vessels, as necessary.

Parenchymal renorraphy is performed with 1-vicryl on a CTX needle. The suture is cut to port length, and a hemostatic Weck clip is preplaced 4–5 cm from the tail end of the suture to serve as a pledget. Renal parenchymal stitches are placed over a preprepared oxidized cellulose bolster (Johnson & Johnson, New Brunswick, NJ). These parenchymal stitches are placed meticulously, wherein the desired angle and depth of needle passage is preplanned to prevent multiple passages, thus minimizing possible puncture injury to the intrarenal blood vessels. This prefashioned Surgicel bolster is positioned underneath the

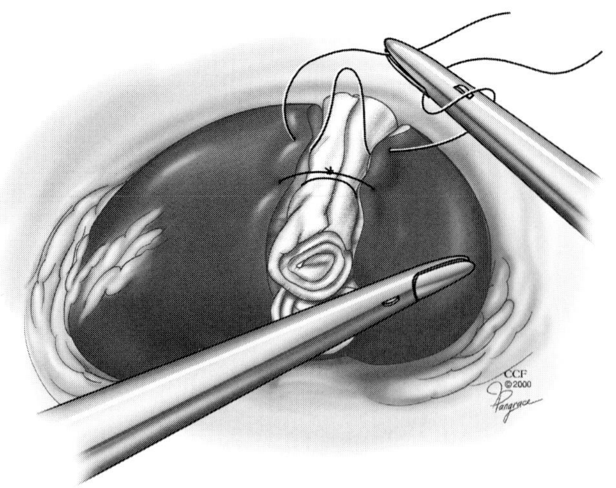


Fig. 5.17

suture loop. Using the 5-mm metal applicator, the gelatin matrix thrombin sealant Floseal (Baxter, Deerfield, IL) is layered directly onto the partial nephrectomy bed underneath the Surgicel bolster. The suture is tightened, compressing the bolster firmly onto the partial nephrectomy bed. Another Weck clip is placed on the exiting suture flush with the parenchyma, thus maintaining consistent pressure. The two suture tails are tied to one another with a surgeon's knot. With the suture cinched down, an assistant grasps the knot with the Maryland grasper to hold the suture secure at this point of maximal tension. The surgeon places two additional knots, securing the stitch. We believe that mere placement of a clip as a pledget on either end of the suture does not provide enough security of parenchymal compression, leaving the potential for bleeding from the edges of the partial nephrectomy defect. As such, tying the suture tails across the bolster over the partial nephrectomy is important to coapt the edges of the parenchymal defect. Typically, three to five parenchymal renororrhaphy sutures are required to close the entire defect.

## Hilar Unclamping

A repeat 12.5-g dose of mannitol and 10–20 mg of furosemide are administered intravenously 1–2 min before unclamping the renal hilum. The Satinsky clamp jaws are opened, but not yet removed, in order to assess the adequacy of hemostasis from the partial nephrectomy bed. Once satisfied, the clamp is slowly and carefully removed under direct vision. The entrapped specimen is extracted intact by slightly extending one of the port-site incisions. A Jackson–Pratt drain is placed during transperitoneal LPN, and a Penrose drain is placed following a retroperitoneoscopic LPN. Fascial closure of 10/12-mm port sites is achieved with the Carter–Thompson device. The partial nephrectomy bed is reinspected laparoscopically after 5–10 min of desufflation to confirm complete hemostasis.

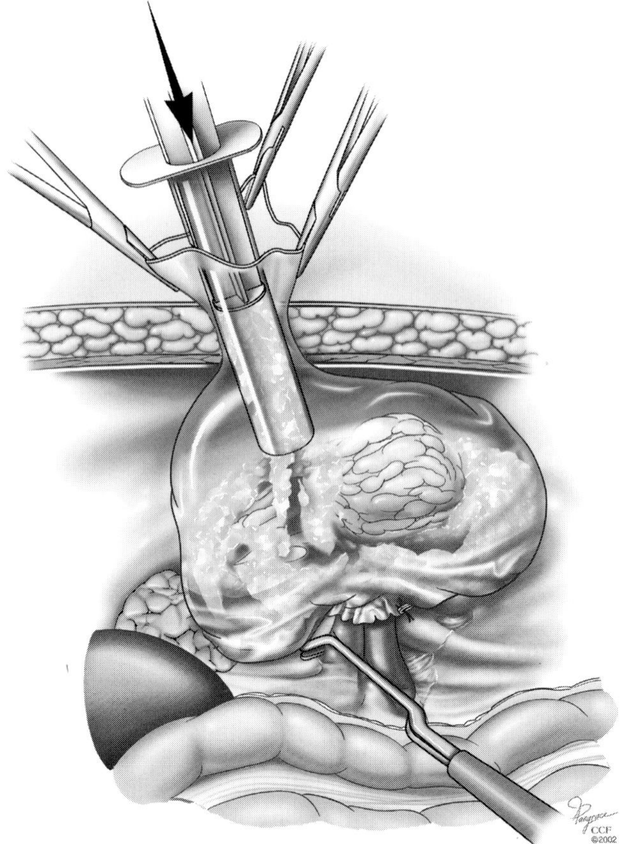


Fig. 5.18

## Renal Hypothermia (Fig. 5.18)

We recently developed the technique of laparoscopic ice-slush hypothermia during LPN. Finely crushed ice slurry is preloaded into 30-cc syringes, whose nozzle-ends have been cut off. The mobilized kidney is entrapped in an Endocatch-II bag, whose drawstring is cinched down around the intact renal hilum, thus completely entrapping the kidney. The renal hilum is clamped with a Satinsky clamp. The bottom end of the bag is retrieved outside the abdomen through the inferior para-rectal port site. The bottom end of the bag is opened, and the preloaded syringes are used to rapidly fill the intra-abdominal bag with ice slurry. Typically, 4–7 min are required to fill the bag with 600–900 cc of ice slurry, thus surrounding the entire kidney under laparoscopic visualization. After allowing 10 min for achievement of core renal cooling, the bag is incised, the ice crystals removed from the vicinity of the tumor, and partial nephrectomy completed. In 12 patients, needle thermocouples were used to document nadir renal parenchymal temperatures of 5–19°C, attesting to the efficacy of the achieved hypothermia. Recently, two additional methods of achieving renal hypothermia by either retrograde ureteric perfusion or intra-arterial profusion have been reported.

### Postoperative Care

The patient is advised strict bed rest for 24 h, followed by gradual mobilization. The ureteral and Foley catheters are removed on the morning of postoperative day 2 as the patient begins ambulation. The peri-renal drain is maintained for at least 3–5 d and removed when the drainage is less than 50 cc per day for 3 consecutive days. Following discharge from the hospital, the patient is advised restricted activity for 2 wk. Any physical activity with the potential to jar the renal remnant is inadvisable in the early postoperative period. A MAG-3 radionuclide scan is performed at 1 mo to evaluate renal function and assess pelvicaliceal system integrity. In patients with pathologically confirmed renal cancer, a follow-up CT scan and chest X-ray are obtained at 6 mo. Subsequent oncological surveillance is as per the individual pathological tumor stage.

### Complications

In our analysis of complications in the initial 200 patients undergoing LPN for renal tumor, we documented a complication rate of 33% (urological 18%, other 15%). This included hemorrhagic complications in 9.5%, urine leak in 4.5%, and open conversion in 1%, with no perioperative mortality. More recently, we have incorporated routine use of the gelatin matrix thrombin sealant Floseal during LPN. As such, in our most recent 100 patients, the rate of hemorrhagic complications has decreased to less than 3% and urine leak to less than 1.5%, mirroring current open surgical outcomes.

## LAPAROSCOPIC RENAL CRYOABLATION

### Indications

With increasing experience in laparoscopic techniques and availability of an increased number of options for NSS, our indications for renal cryoablation have become more selective. As such, at this writing, we offer renal cryoablation to only a select subgroup of patients who have a small (less than 3 cm) tumor at a nonhilar location. Such patients typically are older, may have mild to moderate baseline azotemia, and prefer NSS over watchful waiting. The patient is clearly informed about the current developmental nature of cryoablation and the consequent need for vigorous postoperative surveillance (*see* Postoperative Follow-Up).

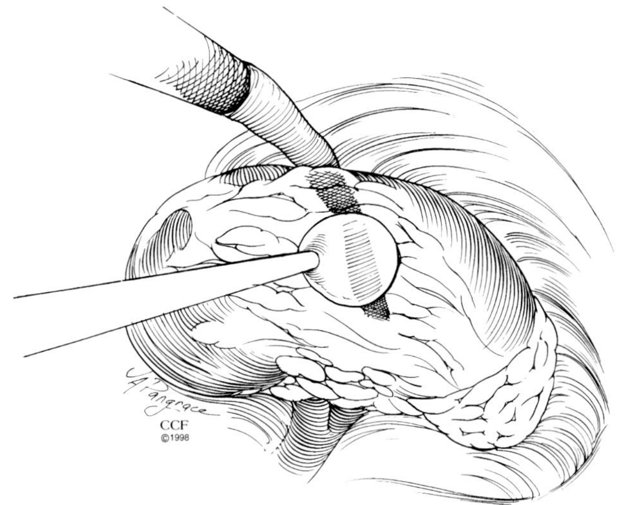


Fig. 5.19

### Patient Positioning and Port Placement

Either the transperitoneal or the retroperitoneal approach is employed depending on tumor location, considerations similar to those listed in the preceding section on laparoscopic partial nephrectomy. Port placement is also similar (port for vascular clamp is not necessary).

### Mobilization of Kidney (Fig. 5.19)

No attempt is made to dissect the renal hilar vessels. The kidney is completely mobilized within Gerota's fascia, exposing the entire renal surface, including the tumor. The peri-renal fat overlying the tumor is removed for histopathological examination. Such mobilization of the kidney has two advantages: complete ultrasound examination of entire kidney surface is feasible, and the tumor can be properly aligned for cryoprobe puncture.

### Ultrasonographic Examination

An endoscopic, steerable color Doppler ultrasound probe is inserted through an appropriate port and placed in direct contact with the kidney surface. Detailed ultrasound examination of the entire kidney is performed to evaluate the following: tumor size, margins, vascularity, distance of the deep tumor edge from the collecting system, and any satellite tumors. During real-time monitoring of the cryoablation process, the ultrasound probe is placed in contact with the kidney surface that is directly opposite to the tumor. As such, adequate renal mobilization is necessary to create space for ultrasound probe placement.

### Needle Biopsy of Tumor

A 15-gage, 15-cm Tru-Cut needle with echogenic tip (ASEP Biopsy System, Order No. 500-128, Microvasive, Boston Scientific, Watertown, MA) is employed to perform needle biopsy of the tumor prior to cryotherapy. This biopsy needle is introduced through a 2-mm port inserted specifically for this purpose. To optimize accuracy, two to three needle biopsies are taken under direct laparoscopic visualization and real-time ultrasound monitoring. The tissue is sent for permanent histopathological examination.

## Cryoprobe Puncture (Fig. 5.20)

Typically, we employ a 4.8-mm cryoprobe of an argon-gas-based system (Endocare). It is critically important to ensure that the cryoprobe enters the precise center of the tumor at right angles to the tumor surface. Also, the tip of the cyroprobe should be advanced up to, or just beyond, the inner margin of the tumor. For example, for a 2-cm tumor, the cyroprobe should be inserted approx 2.2 cm into the renal parenchyma under ultrasound and laparoscopic guidance. It is helpful to premark this length on the shaft of the cryoprobe with a marking pen. For tumors approaching 3 cm in size, one may consider using two cryoprobes instead of one.

## Cryoablation (Fig. 5.21)

A double freeze–thaw cycle is performed under real-time endoscopic ultrasound monitoring and laparoscopic visualization. A rapid initial freeze is performed (tip temperature –140°C) until the advancing hyperchoic, semilunar edge of the ice ball is noted to circumferentially extend approx 1 cm beyond the tumor margins on ultrasound. Obliteration of vascularity and blood flow within the anechoic ice ball is confirmed by color Doppler. Laparoscopic visualization confirms that the entire exophytic surface of the tumor is covered with the ice ball, including approx 1 cm of healthy margin. *Note*: It is vital that the extra-renal surface of the ice ball in its entirety is in clear laparoscopic visualization at all times. Even momentary contact of the ice ball or the active cryoprobe with the adjacent peritoneum, ureter, bowel, or other abdominal viscerae is unacceptable and likely to result in serious sequelae owing to thermal freeze injury. Upon completion of the initial freeze cycle (endpoint: ice ball completely surrounding the tumor), a passive thaw is performed. This slow complete thaw is terminated when the laparoscopically visible ice ball begins to melt. With the cryoprobe carefully maintained in position, a second rapid freeze is performed. Monitoring of the second freeze is completely by laparoscopic visualization. Ultrasonography is not helpful with the second freeze, since the ice ball created by the initial freeze renders the ablated area anechoic, and therefore ultrasonographically invisible. On completion of the second freeze, an active thaw is performed. Melting of the cryolesion releases the probe, which is removed gently without any torquing. Premature removal may create parenchymal fracture lines, which may result in hemorrhage. Upon removal of the cryoprobe, Floseal is injected into the cryopuncture site and over the entire cryoablated tumor. Hemostatic pressure is maintained with a piece of Surgicel. Argon beam coagulation is employed as necessary for hemostasis. Reinspection to confirm hemostasis is performed after 10–15 min of decreased pneumoperitoneum. Typically, no peri-renal drain is placed.

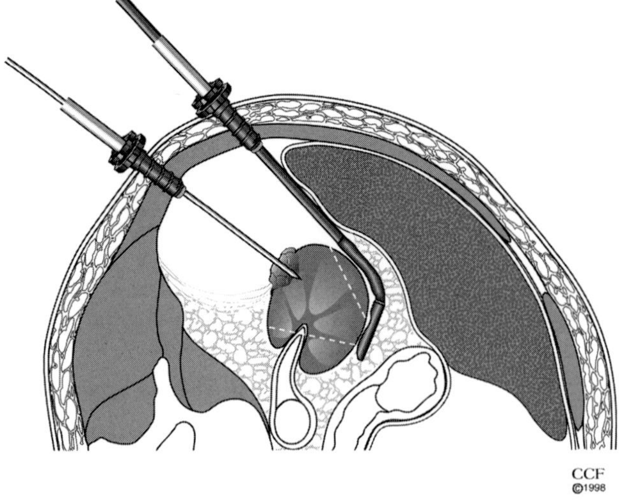


Fig. 5.20

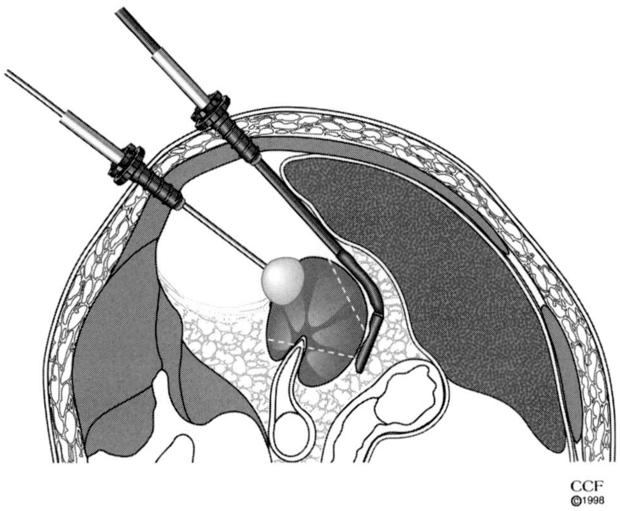


Fig. 5.21

## Postoperative Follow-Up

Given the developmental nature of cryoablation, follow-up is rigorous to ensure oncological adequacy. Our protocol comprises of biochemical, radiological, and histopathological evaluation. The aim of this follow-up is to document continuous shrinkage of the cryoablated tumor without any evidence of tumor growth, lack of shrinkage, or suspicious nodular enhancement. We obtain a magnetic resonance imaging (MRI) scan on postoperative day 1 to obtain a baseline image. Follow-up MRI scans are performed at 1, 3, and 6 mo and every 6 mo thereafter for 2 yr followed by yearly MRI scanning. Chest x-ray is performed at yearly intervals. At 6 mo postoperatively, a CT-directed percutaneous needle biopsy of the cryoablated tumor site is performed for histopathological evaluation. Complete blood count and metabolic panel, including serum creatinine, are performed.

# 6 Renal Calculus Disease

*Stevan B. Streem and J. Stephen Jones*

## INTRODUCTION

The management of urinary calculus disease has evolved dramatically. The introduction of percutaneous and ureteroscopic access to the upper tracts, along with the nearly simultaneous development of both extracorporeal and intracorporeal lithotripsy, has relegated the role of open surgery to less than 1% of patients undergoing intervention for their stone disease. This chapter reviews the indications to intervene, the basic physics of the most frequently utilized devices for both extracorporeal and intracorporeal lithotripsy, and the respective roles of extracorporeal lithotripsy, percutaneous nephrolithotomy (PCNL), ureteroscopic stone removal, and open surgery. The results and complications associated with these forms of intervention are also be reviewed.

## PATIENT EVALUATION

### Radiographic Evaluation

A thorough radiographic evaluation is an important aspect of the overall investigation of urinary stone disease. These studies are invaluable in assessing the major issues that must be addressed in order to select appropriate treatment. These issues include stone burden and location, urinary tract anatomy, and overall and ipsilateral renal function.

### Computed Tomography

Computed tomography (CT) scanning is particularly useful in identifying the etiology of otherwise radiolucent filling defects. In addition, obstruction, anatomical anomalies, and other urological problems such as a vascular insult are easily identified.

Nonenhanced spiral CT is currently the preferred diagnostic tool in the assessment of patients with acute flank pain, as it has proven more sensitive than either simple radiography or ultrasonography (US). All stones, with the exception of certain drug-related crystals, are visualized by this fast and cost-effective imaging modality.

### Plain Abdominal Radiography

More than 90% of stones within the urinary tract are radiopaque. A plain film of the abdomen (KUB) should be performed before any films that employ contrast media, because contrast may obscure the presence of calculi. Both anteroposterior (A-P) and oblique views should be included. Additionally, nephrotomograms can be employed to assist in identifying small, less radiopaque calculi within the kidneys, although nonenhanced CT is more sensitive.

### Intravenous Pyelography

An intravenous pyelogram (IVP) can be instrumental in defining the relationship of calculi to the pyelocaliceal system and ureter. Information regarding exact location of the stones and the presence of obstruction or renal or ureteral anomalies is important. Additionally, an IVP can approximate renal function in both the affected and contralateral kidney, although for more precise information on renal function, a differential renal scan should be obtained.

For patients with an apparent ureteral calculus, delayed films are obtained for as long as necessary to specifically identify their location and to prove their presence within the urinary tract. An IVP may also suggest the presence of radiolucent stones as filling defects, though such findings require further evaluation, generally with a CT scan.

### Renal Ultrasonography

US can be a screening tool for hydronephrosis or stones within the collecting system. Additional information provided include an estimate of the amount of renal parenchyma and identification of otherwise radiolucent calculi. CT scanning, however, is more sensitive.

From: *Operative Urology at the Cleveland Clinic*
Edited by: A. Novick et al. © Humana Press Inc., Totowa, NJ

## Radionuclide Evaluation

Renal radionuclide studies provide information about total and differential renal function. A differential function scan should be performed in those patients in whom an obstructing stone might have resulted in a permanent and significant reduction in renal function. Nephrectomy may be the procedure of choice for kidneys that, after relief of obstruction, contribute less than 10–15% of overall function.

# INDICATIONS FOR INTERVENTION

Although the use of newer, less invasive modalities has become standard for management of nearly all patients requiring intervention, the indications to intervene have essentially remained unchanged. These include chronic or progressive obstruction from the stone, pain, infection or hematuria associated with the stone, or active stone growth despite appropriate medical management.

# SHOCK-WAVE LITHOTRIPSY

## Historical Aspects

The first experimental lithotripters were developed in Germany during the 1970s. At that time, studies were performed, both in vitro and in vivo, examining the effects of shock waves on tissues and organs.

In 1980, Chaussy and associates successfully treated the first human patient. Since that time, thousands of scientific articles have been published detailing the use of shock-wave lithotripsy (SWL) for management of renal and ureteral calculi. Moreover, numerous second- and third-generation devices have since been introduced and are currently in use throughout the world. Ultimately, newer lithotripters may prove to both facilitate stone fragmentation and to reduce the risk of tissue injury. Even now, those goals have yet to be realized in a clinically apparent fashion.

## Lithotripsy Design

All lithotripters share four main features, including an energy source, a focusing device, a coupling medium, and a stone localization system. The original Dornier HM-3 lithotripter utilized a spark plug energy generator with an elliptical reflector for focusing the shock waves. A water bath transmitted the shock waves to the patient, while stone localization was provided by biplanar fluoroscopy. Recent modifications in some or all of these four components have resulted in the development of second- and third-generation devices.

## Shock-Wave Generation

Although all lithotripters share the four aforementioned features, the mode of shock-wave generation determines the actual physical characteristics of a particular lithotripter. The two basic types of energy sources for generating shock waves are point sources and extended sources. The electrohydraulic machines utilize point sources for energy

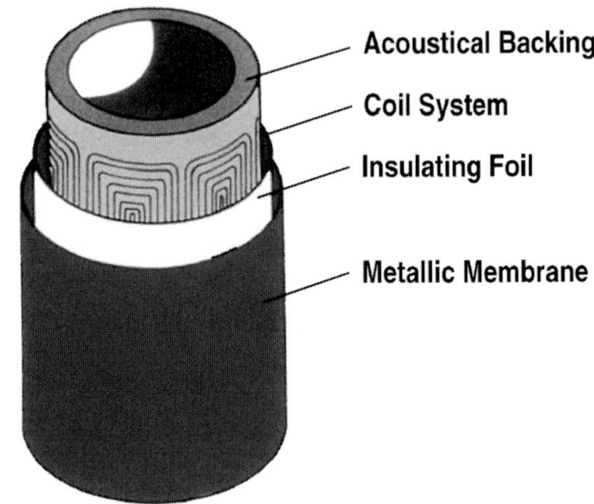


**Fig. 6.1**

In electromagnetic devices, shock waves are generated when an electrical impulse moves a thin, circular metallic membrane, which is housed within a cylindrical "shock tube."

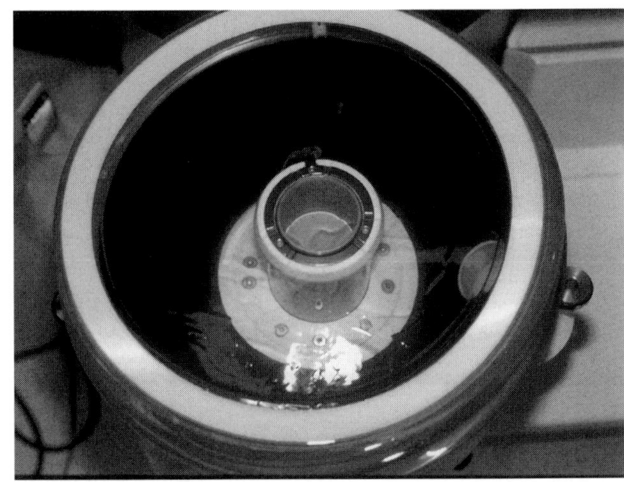

**Fig. 6.2**

The resulting shock wave, produced in the water-filled shock tube, passes through an acoustic lens and is thereby directed to the focal point, F1. The shock wave is coupled to the body surface via a water cushion.

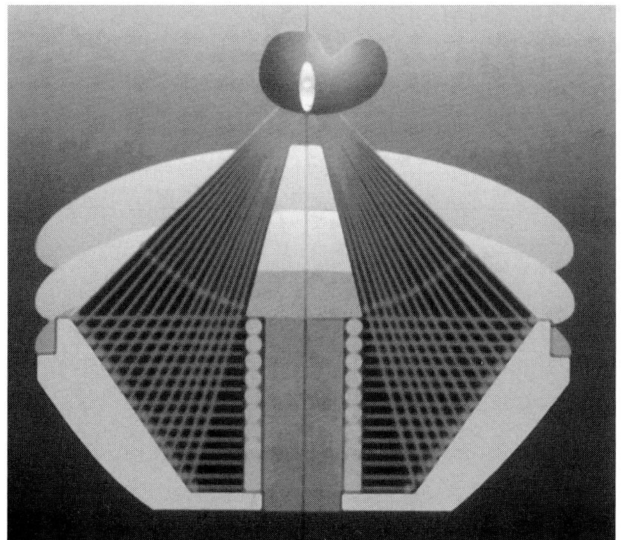

**Fig. 6.3**

Shock waves must be focused in order to concentrate their energy on a target such as a calculus. The type of shock wave generation dictates the method of focusing. For electromechanical lithotripters, the vibrating metal membranes produce an acoustical plane wave that uses an acoustic lens for focusing the shock wave at F1.

generation, whereas extended sources are incorporated in the piezoelectric and the electromagnetic devices. The latter use an electromagnetic energy source with a variable-power shock-wave generator. This allows the shock-wave energy to be tailored. The generator power can be lowered to provide significantly reduced anesthesia/analgesia requirements, or alternatively, the shock-wave intensity can be increased to allow adequate fragmentation of particularly hard or large calculi.

## SWL: Indications and Contraindications

Indications for SWL for renal calculi are the same as for any "surgical" intervention for stones. These include pain, obstruction, infection, or compromised renal function associated with obstruction. Relative contraindications to SWL include large stone size, cystine stones larger than 1 cm, active infection, proximate calcified abdominal aortic or renal artery aneurysm, distal obstruction, untreated bleeding diathesis, and pregnancy.

## Management of Large Calculi

In general, stones smaller than 1–1.5 cm do not require internal stenting. However, for some patients, such as those with solitary kidneys or otherwise compromised renal function, or for patients with a history of associated infection, internal stents are used more liberally. For stones larger than 1.5 cm, internal stenting is routinely done, with the stent placed at the time of lithotripsy.

With increasing stone volume, the efficacy of all lithotripters decreases significantly, and the stone-free rate for large calculi is less than 70%, even for patients with normal collecting system anatomy. As such, we advocate the use of PCNL as the initial form of therapy for almost any patient with a stone burden of more than 2–2.5 cm.

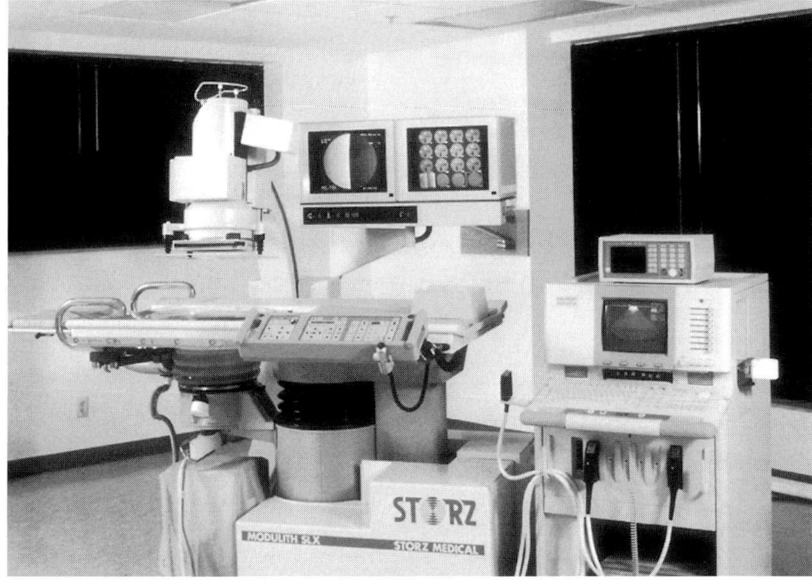


**Fig. 6.4**

Modern lithotripters alleviate the physiological, functional, and economic problems associated a large water bath. Most current models utilize a water cushion or a totally contained shock tube that allows simplified positioning and "dry" or "bathless" lithotripsy.

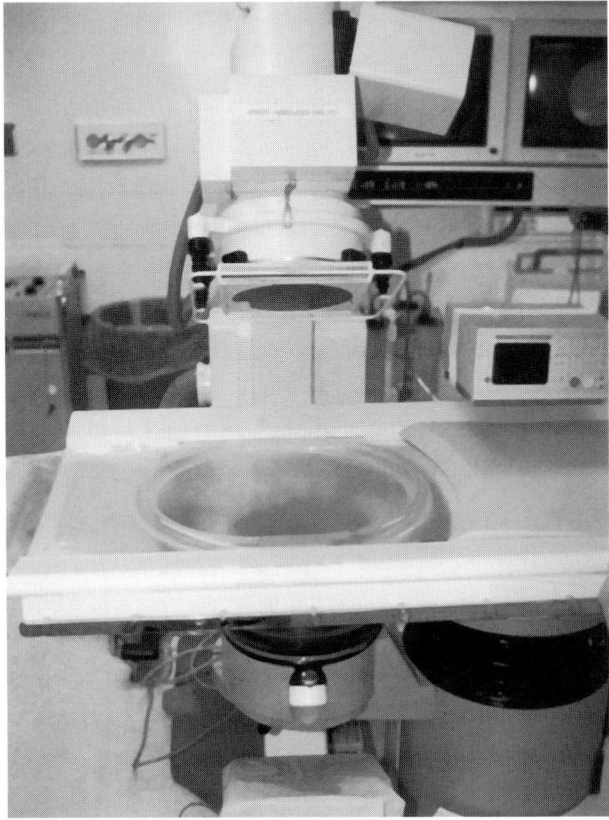

Fig. 6.5

Stone localization is accomplished with either fluoroscopy or ultrasonography. Our preference is fluoroscopy, as it is familiar to all urologists, allows the use of contrast material to delineate the anatomy of the collecting system when necessary, and is effective for ureteral stone localization, even in the absence of significant hydroureteronephrosis.

However, struvite calculi predictably tend to be "fragile," and even some larger than 2.5 cm may respond well to serial treatment with interval stenting. Our preference for serial treatments is to wait approx 4 wk between episodes.

In some situations, particularly those involving large, fully branched calculi, a combination of PCNL and SWL can be more effective than SWL alone. With this type of combination therapy, stone-free rates approaching 85–90% can be achieved, even for the most complicated calculi.

## Results

Using an "efficiency quotient," valid comparisons between different lithotripters can be made. The efficiency quotient offers a more reliable gauge for comparing the effectiveness of individual lithotripters than does a stone-free rate alone. As such, considering the need for auxiliary procedures, the efficiency quotient for the Storz SLX electromagnetic lithotripter and the Dornier MFL 5000 electrohydraulic unit has proven to be equivalent.

### Stone Location

Stone location in the collecting system is an important determinant of the outcome of SWL. Treatment of renal pelvic stones results in stone-free rates of 85–90%. In contrast, stone-free rates for patients with lower calyceal calculi may be less than 60%, compared with 75–80% for those with middle and upper calyceal stones.

Stones in calyceal diverticula are a source of treatment controversy. SWL provides improvement or resolution of symptoms in many patients, but is generally less successful in rendering such patients stone free. Published studies suggest that stones in calyceal diverticula should be managed with SWL only when specific criteria are met. These criteria include size smaller than 1 cm and a radiographically patent diverticular neck. In contrast, percutaneous management of diverticular calculi results in significantly higher stone-free rates.

### Stone Composition

As the stone composition varies, so does the efficacy of SWL. "Harder" stones such as calcium oxalate monohydrate and cystine require an increased number of shock waves at higher intensity levels to achieve adequate fragmentation. Even at these higher settings, however, results with cystine calculi have been inferior to those with calcium oxalate stones. We advocate the use of percutaneous therapy for cystine calculi larger than 1 cm.

# PERCUTANEOUS STONE EXTRACTION

## Historical Aspects

Rupel and Brown used an operatively established nephrostomy tract to extract an obstructing renal calculus

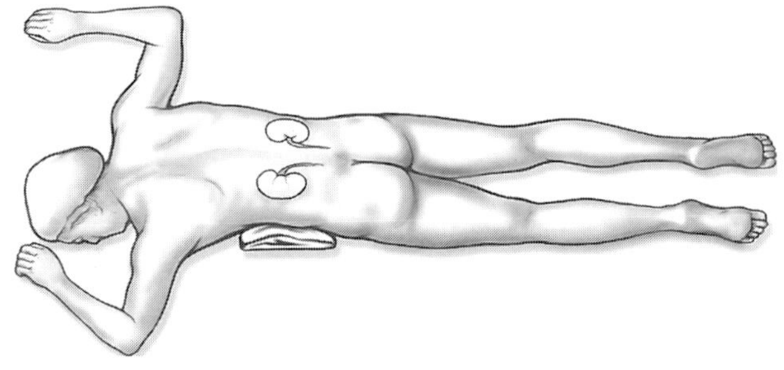

Fig. 6.6

The patient is in a prone or slightly oblique position with the ipsilateral side elevated to approx 20°. For patients with rotational anomalies such as horseshoe kidneys, the contralateral side is elevated instead to allow a more medial rotation of the otherwise anteriorly projected renal pelvis. This allows the posterior infundibula and calices to project more laterally, thus fluoroscopically simulating a more orthotopic position of the kidney.

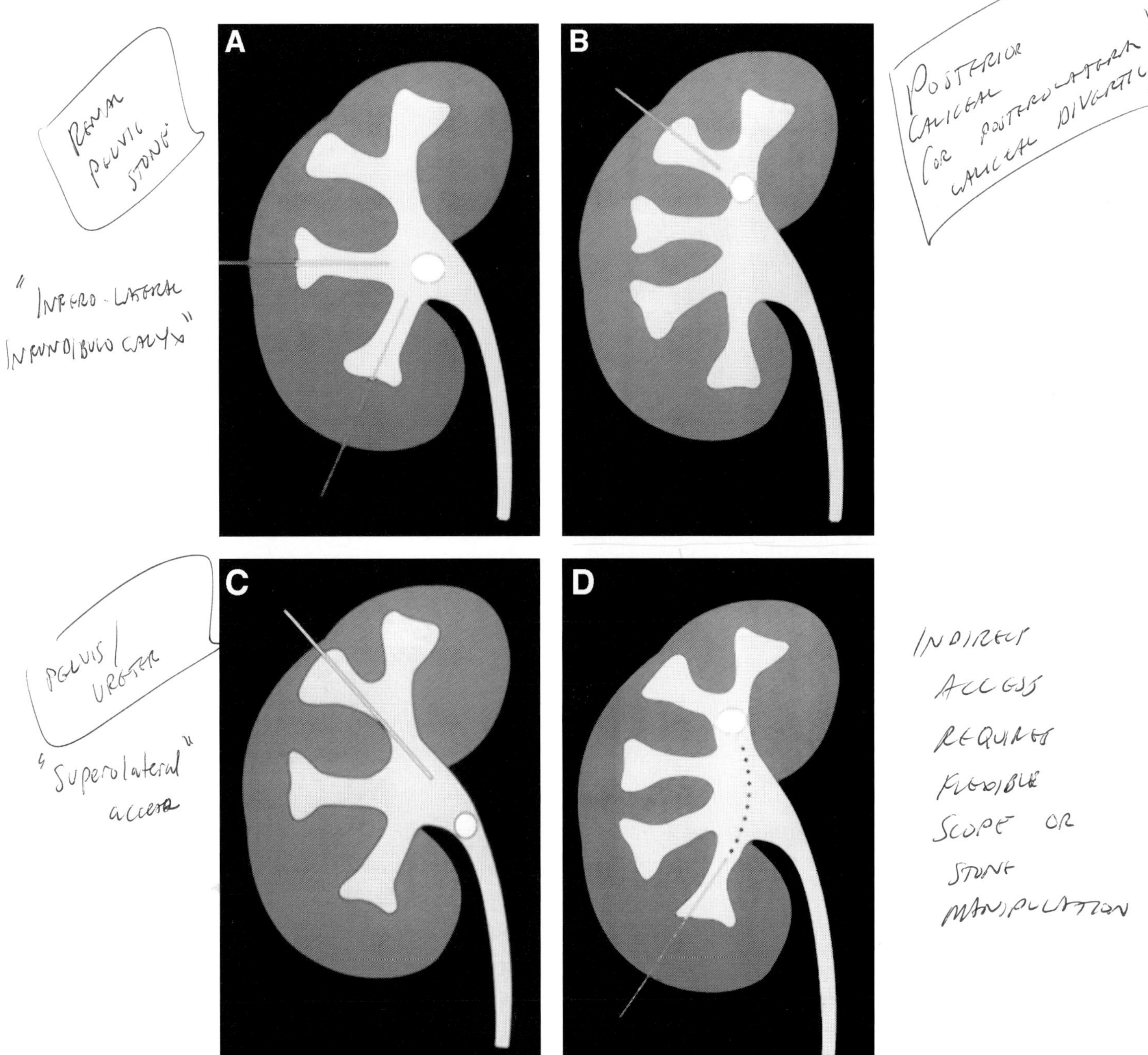


Fig. 6.7

The site of the percutaneous access is specific to the stone location. **(A)** Renal pelvic stones are generally approached via an infero-lateral infundibulocalix. **(B)** Posterior caliceal calculi, or those in posterolateral caliceal diverticula, are approached directly. Anterior caliceal calculi are never approached directly. Rather, they are visualized via access to an overlying or adjacent posterior calyx. **(C)** Stones at the ureteropelvic junction or in the proximal ureter, and some complex stones are approached with a more superolateral access. **(D)** Indirect access can be used, but then generally requires flexible instrumentation for stone manipulation and extraction.

in 1941. Fifteen years later, Goodwin reported the use of percutaneous nephrostomy drainage to provide relief of obstruction and infection. However, removal of a renal calculus via a percutaneous tract established specifically for that purpose was not performed until Fernstrom and Johansson successfully used that technique for three patients 20 yr later. Subsequently, percutaneous stone extraction gained acceptance for management of most patients with upper tract calculi in the late 1970s and early 1980s when means to fragment even large calculi were

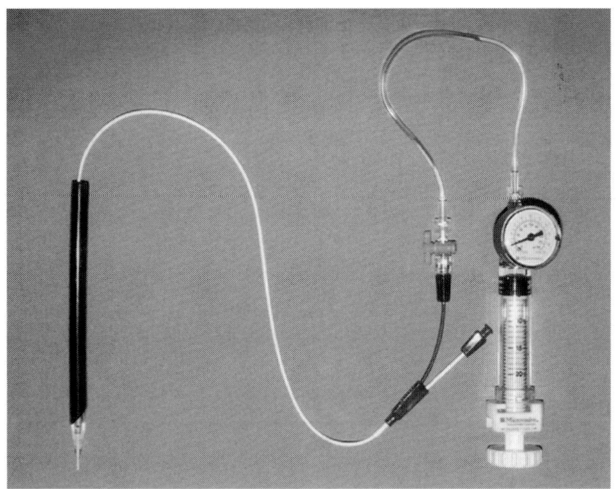

**Fig. 6.8**

A second wire is placed as a safety wire utilizing a 9 or 10 French introducer set. Over the remaining "working" wire, the tract is dilated to 30 F using a 10 F, 12-cm balloon over which is backloaded a 30 F working sheath. The working sheath is advanced over the inflated balloon using fluoroscopic guidance. At this point, a 30 F working sheath will be in place with a safety wire alongside.

introduced. During that era, any patient who would have otherwise required open stone extraction was considered a candidate for percutaneous management instead, and the indications for this procedure were essentially identical to the indications to intervene for any stone.

## Indications and Contraindications

The indications for percutaneous stone management include body habitus precluding SWL, obstruction distal to the stone, moderate to large size cystine stones, stones associated with upper tract foreign bodies, large or otherwise complex stones, and failure of or contraindication to SWL. Relative indications for percutaneous management also include the presence of an implanted cardiac defibrillator and a proximate calcified aortic or renal artery aneurysm. Currently, the only absolute contraindications to percutaneous stone extraction are an irreversible coagulopathy and, unless there are considerable extenuating circumstances, pregnancy.

## Patient Preparation

The patient is apprised of the potential risks and benefits of percutaneous lithotomy compared to applicable alternatives. In these often complex cases, these risks include the potential for secondary intervention, transfusion, infection, and, albeit very rarely, emergent open operative intervention.

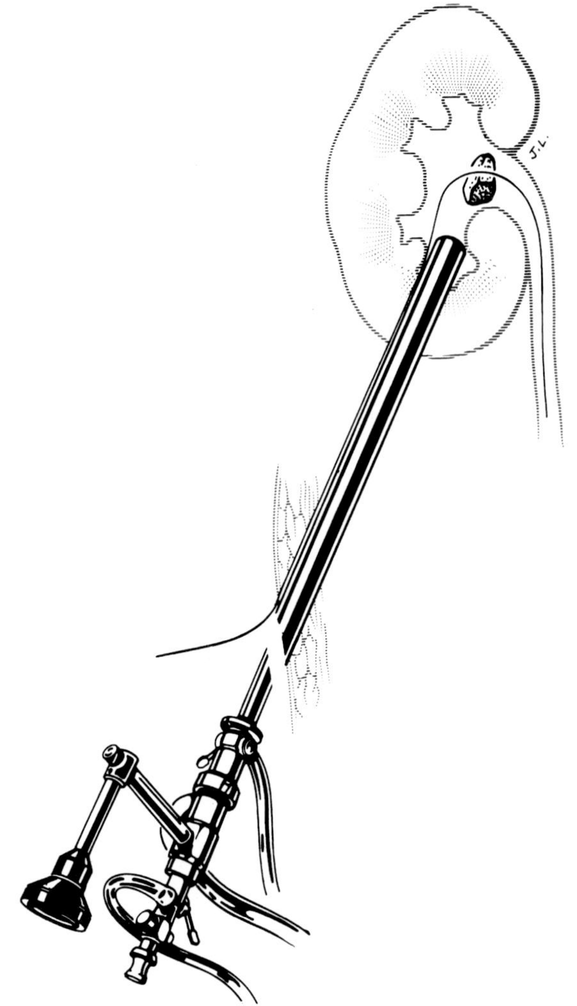

**Fig. 6.9**

In most cases percutaneous stone extraction is accomplished through direct vision using a rigid nephroscope. The nephroscope is readied by attaching the light, suction, and irrigation and is now inserted through the working sheath. Once proper positioning in the pyelocaliceal system is assured, the working wire within the sheath is removed, keeping a safety wire in place alongside the sheath. The irrigant of choice for percutaneous nephroscopy is normal saline. This prevents the possibility of hyponatremia, which might result from intravascular absorption if hyposmotic solutions are used. At the outset of nephroscopy, vision may be obscured by blood clots, which are evacuated by adjusting the irrigation and suction from the nephroscope sheath or by using suction through the ultrasound wand while ultrasonic energy is being applied to the clot.

Standard preoperative preparation includes a "type and screen," although formal cross-matching is generally not necessary. Patients with urinary tract infection are treated for approx 7–10 d with sensitively specific antibiotics on an outpatient basis, then intravenously "on call" to the

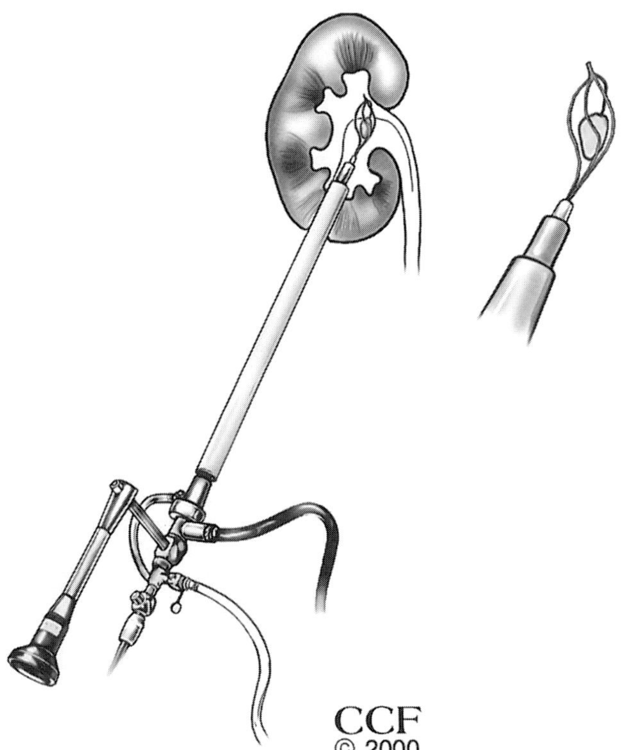


Fig. 6.10

Stones smaller than 9 or 10 mm are extracted intact through the working sheath. Such stones are simply grasped under direct vision utilizing rigid graspers passed via the working port of the nephroscope.

procedure. In the setting of sterile urine, we generally utilize a short-course antibiotic protocol consisting of a first-generation cephalosporin given just prior to percutaneous access and continued for 24 h following stone extraction.

## Technique

The procedure is always performed with the same four sequential steps that include establishing percutaneous access, dilation of the tract, stone manipulation with fragmentation and extraction, and postextraction drainage and tamponade of the tract. The specific technique is modified to the size, location, configuration, and presumed composition of the stone. At our center, percutaneous access is established the same day as the stone removal.

## Specific Indications

### Body Habitus Precluding SWL

Patients in whom body habitus precludes SWL provide some of the most challenging indications for percutaneous stone extraction. This occurs most frequently in patients with morbid obesity to the extent that the stone cannot be positioned at the focal point or within the "power path" of an extracorporeally generated shock wave. In these patients, both the percutaneous access and tract dilation are more difficult, at least in part because fluoroscopic imaging is compromised. Furthermore, once an adequate tract has been established, stone fragmentation and extraction can be severely hampered by limitations in the length of available instrumentation. However, newer "obese set" nephroscopes are now available and provide a significantly longer working instrument.

In many cases, the limitations in length of instrumentation can be overcome by allowing the tract to mature for several days following the initial dilation and placement of a large-caliber nephrostomy tube. During this time, the kidney tends to fall back posteriorly toward skin level such that access with standard nephroscopic instrumentation can be accomplished. Furthermore, a mature tract can be used to pass readily alternative instruments such as standard flexible cystoscopes that are longer than most nephroscopes.

### Cystine Stones

Although small cystine stones can at times be managed successfully with SWL, most cystinuric patients requiring intervention have larger stones at the time of presentation, and these tend to respond poorly to that modality. Fortunately, cystine stones are very amenable to most forms of intracorporeal management including ultrasonic and Holmium laser lithotripsy. At our center, percutaneous ultrasonic nephrolithotomy remains the preferred approach for the majority of cystinuric patients requiring intervention, although a ureteroscopic approach is occasionally used, even for pyelocaliceal cystine stones.

### Upper Tract Foreign Bodies

Urological practice has seen an increasingly frequent use of self-retaining stents, nephrostomy tubes, and dilating balloons, and this has led to a corresponding increase in the number of patients requiring management of "retained" upper tract foreign bodies. In some cases, these foreign bodies can be managed with retrograde endoscopy using standard ureteroscopic instrumentation. However, a ureteroscopic approach may be precluded by a prior urinary diversion, making access difficult if not impossible, or by the formation of calculi on the foreign body that are too large for ureteroscopic management. When ureteroscopic management has failed or is contraindicated, a percutaneous approach is indicated. For these patients the site of the access to the foreign body is chosen as for any stone, and this then depends on its size and location within the pyelocaliceal system. Standard nephroscopic instrumentation including forceps, graspers, or baskets may be utilized in conjunction with any form of currently available intracorporeal lithotripsy.

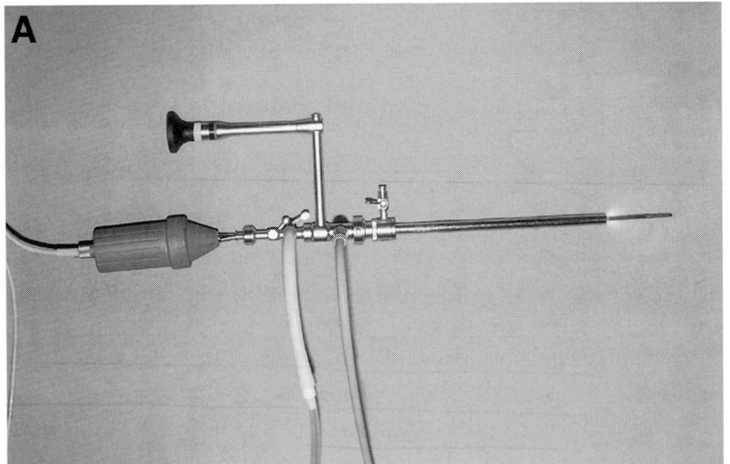


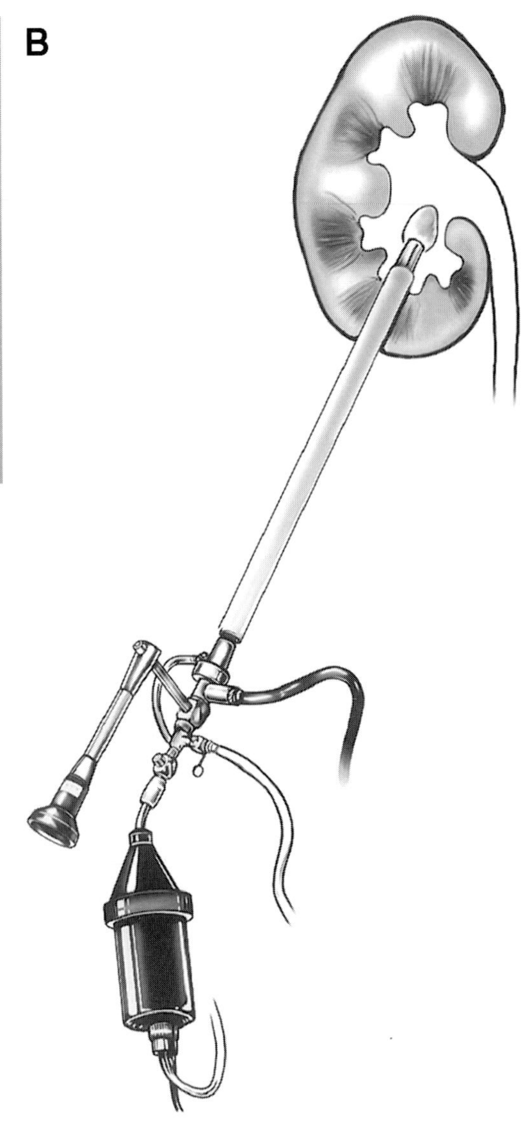


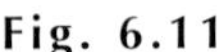
**Fig. 6.11**

Most stones managed percutaneously are too large to be extracted intact. As such, intracorporeal lithotripsy will be required, for which we generally use ultrasonic energy. The ultrasound wand (sonotrode) with its own suction attachment is introduced via the working channel of a rigid nephroscope. **(A)** Under direct vision, the tip of the sonotrode is impacted against the stone while suction is applied through the hollow sonotrode, holding the stone in place. **(B)** This allows the stone pieces to be evacuated via the sonotrode as fragmentation proceeds. Fragments that are too large to pass through the sonotrode, but now measure <9 mm, are extracted using grasping techniques via the nephroscope under direct vision, bringing the pieces out through the working sheath. The process of ultrasonic fragmentation with suctioning of fragments or forceps extraction continues until all visible stone has been removed.

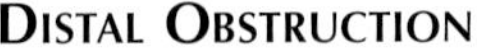
### Distal Obstruction

Successful SWL requires spontaneous passage of the resulting stone fragments. As such, obstruction distal to the targeted stone is a contraindication to SWL. For most affected patients, the distal obstruction will relate to the ureter or ureteropelvic junction (UPJ), although the same principle applies to stones in caliceal diverticula or those in calices associated with true infundibular stenosis. In these patients, percutaneous management is ideal as it provides an opportunity both to remove the stone and to provide permanent relief of the obstruction.

#### *Caliceal Diverticular Calculi*

An alternative to dilation of the diverticular neck, especially when it cannot be visualized directly nor intubated fluoroscopically, is simple fulguration. A nephrostomy tube is left in place in the diverticulum, but not across the neck. This acts to "marsupialize" the diverticulum, which does not have secretory urothelium.

#### *Infundibular Stenosis*

Stones located in calices drained by long, narrow infundibula or those in calices associated with true infundibular stenosis often require percutaneous management, and the best approach is again a direct one to the involved calyx. In contrast to management of a caliceal diverticular neck, a stenotic infundibulum should always be dilated rather than fulgurated. The infundibulum can be dilated using either sequential fascial dilators or with a balloon catheter under direct vision, fluoroscopic control, or both. Following stone extraction and dilation of the infundibulum, a large-caliber nephrostomy tube is left indwelling across the infundibulum into the renal pelvis.

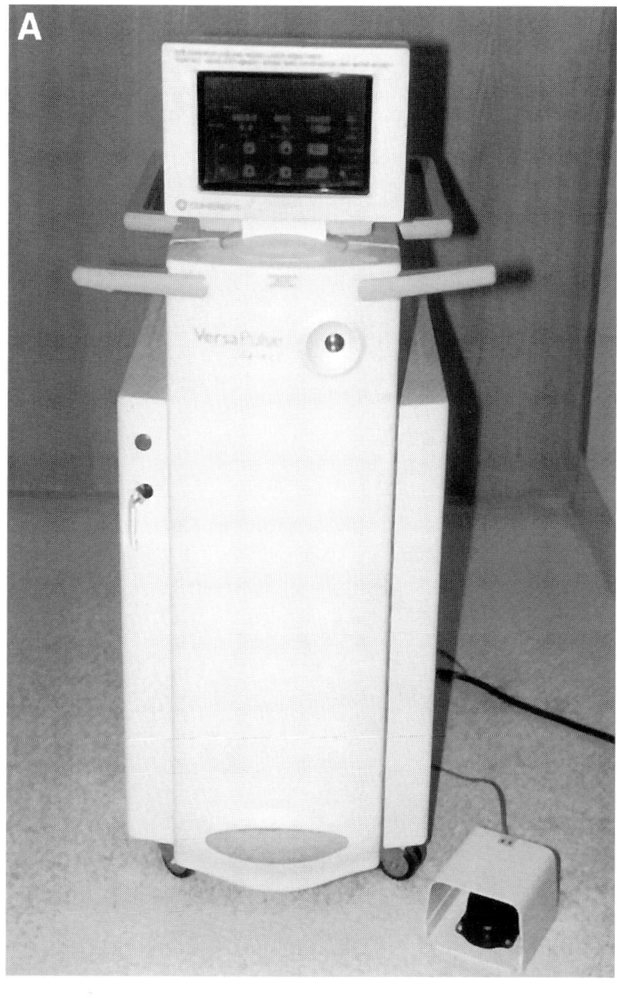


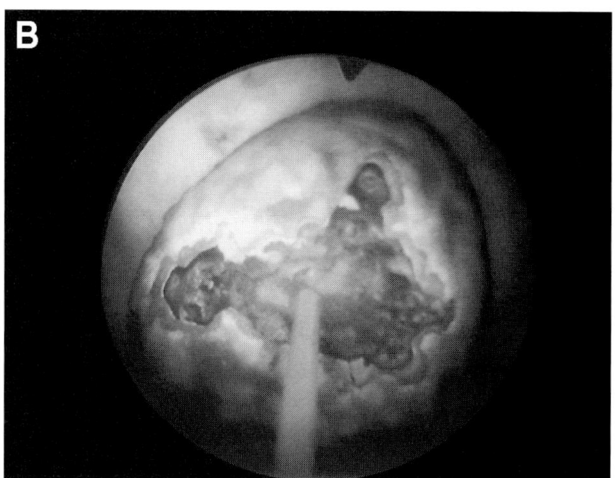


**Fig. 6.12**

Although ultrasonic lithotripsy can reliably fragment most stones, some, such as large calcium oxalate monohydrate stones, which often appear extremely dense and homogeneous on plain x-rays, and some mixed calcium oxalate/uric acid stones are physically too hard to fragment with this modality. In these cases, intracorporeal lithotripsy can be performed effectively with alternative modalities, including Holmium laser lithotripsy (shown here), electrohydraulic lithotripsy (EHL), and the Lithoclast Ultra unit that combines the power of both pneumatic and ultrasonic lithotripsy.

### *Ureteropelvic Junction Obstruction*

The association of upper tract stones with UPJ obstruction provides an ideal setting for percutaneous management as this allows simultaneous extraction of the stones and relief of obstruction. Percutaneous management of the stones is performed in a standard manner with the caveat that for this procedure percutaneous access is best accomplished via a more superolateral calyx or infundibulum that will allow direct endoscopic access to the UPJ with rigid instrumentation. However, stone extraction should precede the actual endopyelotomy incision to prevent extravasation of irrigant or stone particles during stone fragmentation and removal. At completion of the stone removal and endopyelotomy, a relatively large-caliber stent is left indwelling for approx 4 wk. Percutaneous endopyelotomy is described and illustrated in detail elsewhere in this volume.

### *Transplanted and Pelvic Kidneys*

Although small stones smaller than 1 cm may often be treated with SWL, consideration should be given to percutaneous management for even moderate-size stones in transplanted kidneys. This is because of the inherent difficulty in obtaining retrograde access in the face of potential obstruction from post-SWL fragments and the need to ensure a stone-free result in these solitary kidneys.

Management of stones in congenital pelvic kidneys poses different problems. In contrast to transplanted kidneys, congenital pelvic kidneys lie deeper within the pelvis. As such, peritoneal contents, including small and large intestines, may be interposed. In such cases, establishing percutaneous access may require laparoscopic control.

### *Large or Complex Calculi: Percutaneous Monotherapy*

Most patients with large, branched stones may be managed with a percutaneous approach alone. The best candidates are those in whom the stone burden is primarily central rather than peripheral, although multiple tracts may be required even for relatively straightforward cases.

## Postoperative Care

An estimate of the volume of irrigation and output should be kept during stone extraction. Furosemide 10–20 mg is

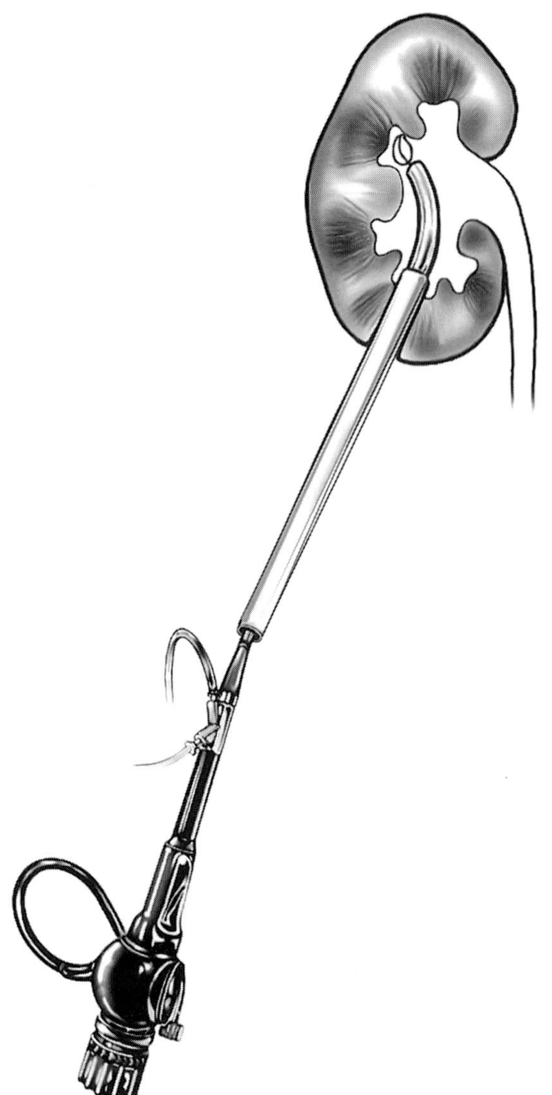

**Fig. 6.13**

For infundibular or caliceal calculi lying at acute angles to the percutaneous tract, visualization, fragmentation, and extraction often require flexible nephroscopy. Fluoroscopic guidance is important during flexible nephroscopy to assure proper orientation. When the stone is visualized, a grasping forceps, prongs, or basket can be passed through the working port of the flexible scope and the stone engaged and withdrawn. Alternatively, larger stones can be fragmented with a Holmium laser.

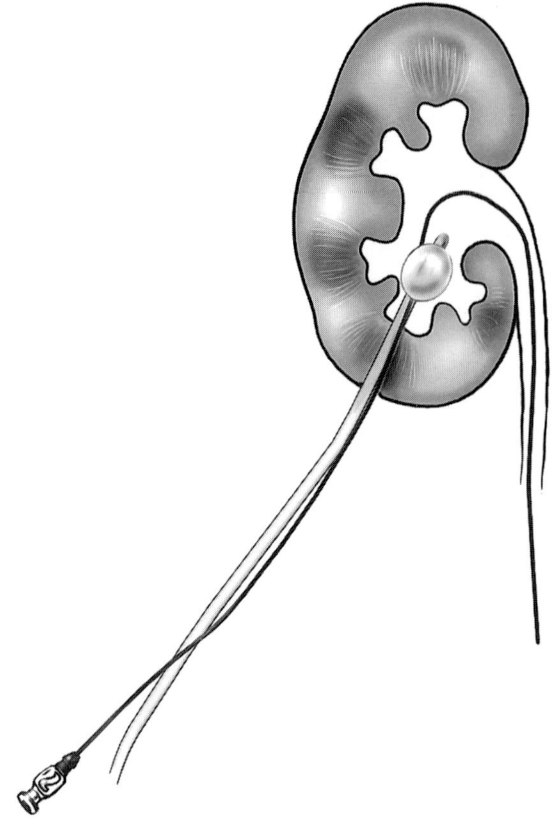

**Fig. 6.14**

When visual and x-ray control assure that all accessible stone has been extracted, nephrostomy drainage is instituted. Our preference is a 22 or 24 French nephrostomy tube passed through the working sheath and positioned fluoroscopically with its tip in the renal pelvis. The working sheath is then removed by pulling back and cutting it away from the catheter using scissors. The remaining safety wire is used to pass a pyeloureteral catheter with its distal tip in the distal one-third ureter and the proximal end coiled at skin level. The pyeloureteral catheter allows rapid access back to the pyelocaliceal system should that be required prior to elective removal of the nephrostomy tube.

given intravenously at the termination of the procedure. For the first 24 h, intravenous fluids are administered at a rate fast enough to ensure a sustained diuresis. For patients with documented infection, sensitivity-specific intravenous antibiotics are continued for at least 48–72 h while the patient is in the hospital, and then orally until the first follow-up visit. At that time, the need for chronic antibiotic prophylaxis is determined. In those patients without infection, prophylactic antibiotic coverage can be discontinued within 48 h of an uncomplicated procedure.

A nephrostogram is obtained 1 to 2 d following stone removal, although more recently, at least in uncomplicated cases, we have substituted plain radiographs for that study. Any residual fragments accessible to the percutaneous tract are managed with repeat rigid or flexible nephroscopy, often performed with light intravenous sedation. If there are no residual stones, the pyeloureteral catheter is removed and the nephrostomy tube clamped for approx 12 h. The tube is removed if there has been no flank pain, fever, or increased drainage around the tube during that time. The patient is then discharged home and allowed to return to full prehospitalization activity 10 d later.

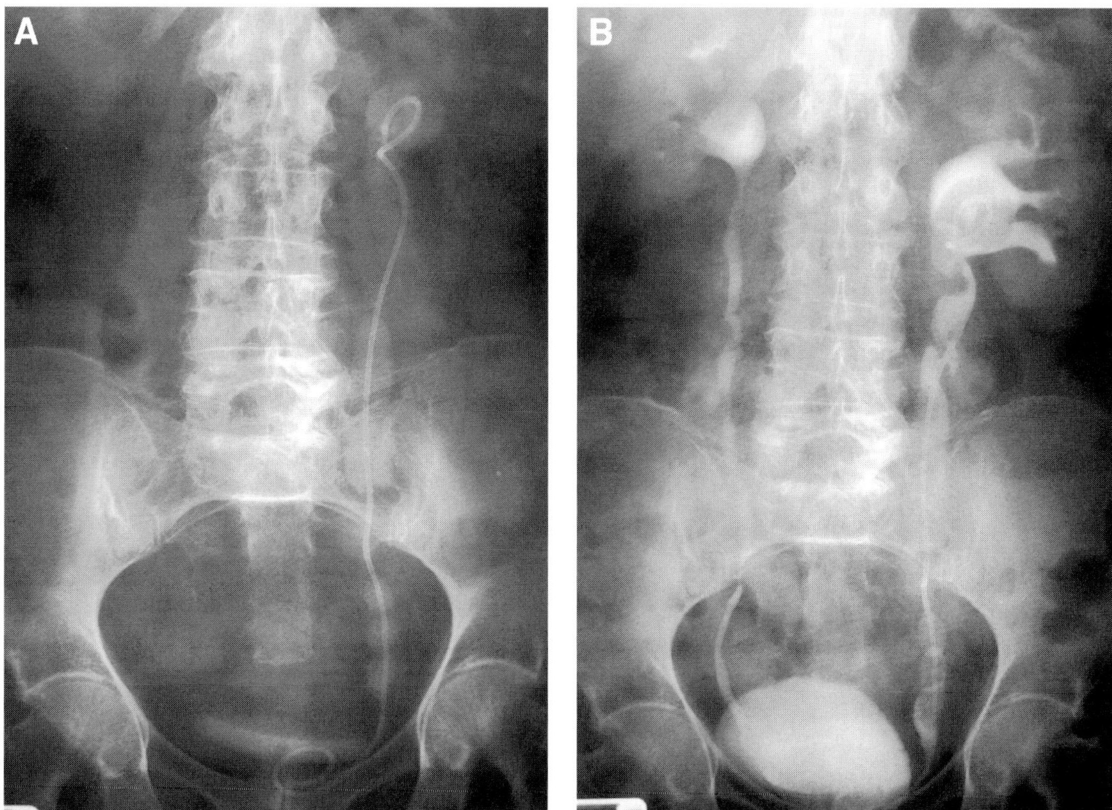


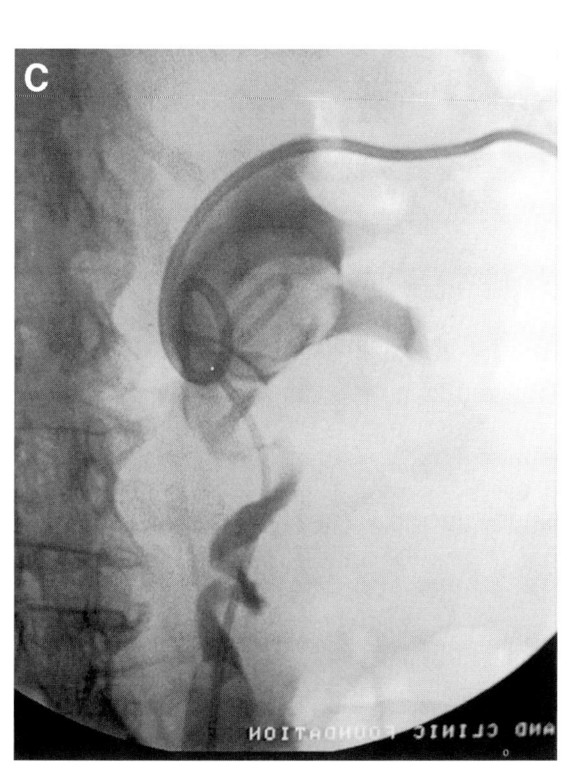


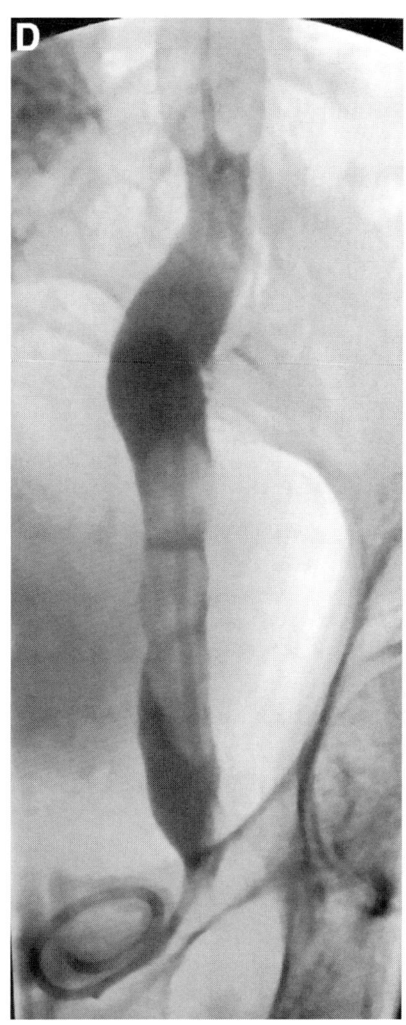


Fig. 6.15

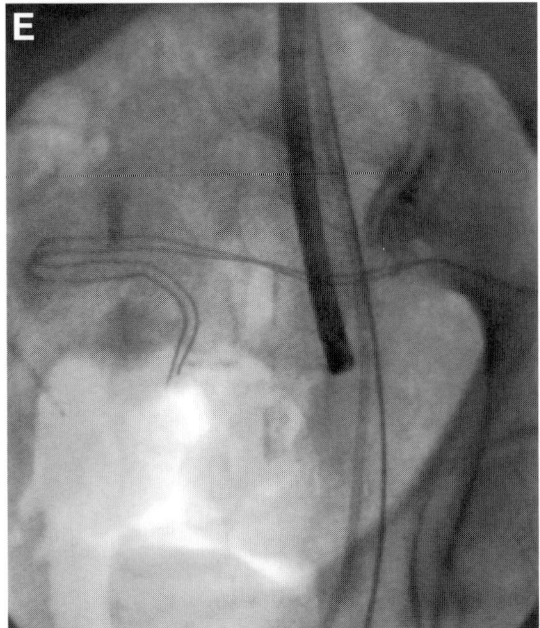


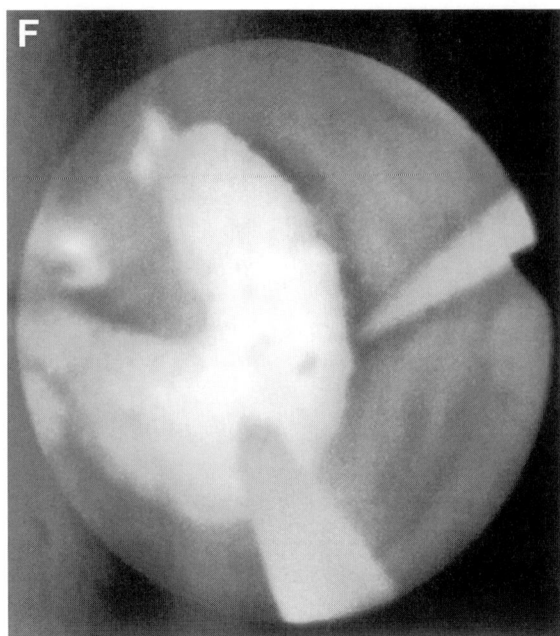


**Fig. 6.15** *(continued)*

**(A,B)** Plain film and pyelogram in a woman with a retained stent for several years. Note multiple calcifications in the renal pelvis and along the entire ureter and bladder associated with the stent. **(C)** Percutaneous access should be via a superolateral infundibulocalyx that will allow access to the pelvis as well as to the ureter in an antegrade fashion. **(D,F)** Multiple ureteral stent calcifications are managed with flexible instrumentation in an antegrade fashion all the way to the bladder. (**D**: Fluoroscopic view; **E**: antegrade passage of flexible ureteroscope; **F**: ureteroscopic view with Holmium laser fiber in place.)

If extravasation or obstruction is noted on the initial nephrostogram, the tube is left to drainage and serial studies obtained. Ureteral obstruction found at this time usually results from blood clots or edema, either of which should resolve spontaneously. Occasionally, obstruction results from small stone fragments in the ureter, which will often pass spontaneously or may be managed with antegrade or retrograde manipulation.

## Complications of Percutaneous Stone Removal

### Hemorrhage

Bleeding is one of the most significant complications. At least some bleeding is apparent in all cases and can become evident at any time during or after the procedure. Management depends on timing and severity of the bleeding. Bleeding during access or tract dilation generally responds to placement of the next size dilator that effectively tamponades the tract. Furthermore, balloon dilation, rather than sequential fascial dilation, may decrease the incidence of bleeding during this step. If significant bleeding occurs during stone manipulation, the procedure should be temporarily halted and nephrostomy drainage instituted for a couple of days.

Some bleeding through the nephrostomy tube is evident at the completion of even a relatively uncomplicated procedure. For more severe cases, successful management can often be achieved by temporarily plugging the nephrostomy tube, allowing tamponade of the collecting system. Generally, the nephrostomy tube can be safely unplugged several hours later. Bleeding that occurs during removal of the nephrostomy tube is best managed by immediate reinsertion. Delayed hemorrhage, i.e., bleeding occurring several days following removal of the nephrostomy tube, is best managed conservatively with close monitoring of vital signs, bed rest, hydration, and transfusion as necessary.

Any time that bleeding does not respond to these conservative measures, management should be renal angiography and selective arterial embolization.

### Extravasation

Some degree of extravasation occurs during all percutaneous procedure, and in a controlled setting this is generally benign and self-limiting. When significant perforation develops, it is generally at the medial pelvic wall or UPJ. This may be the result of access, tract dilation, or stone manipulation. Potential adverse effects can be minimized by maintaining a sterile urine, carefully monitoring irrigation input and output, use of a safety wire at all times, and, most importantly, use of normal saline as the irrigant of

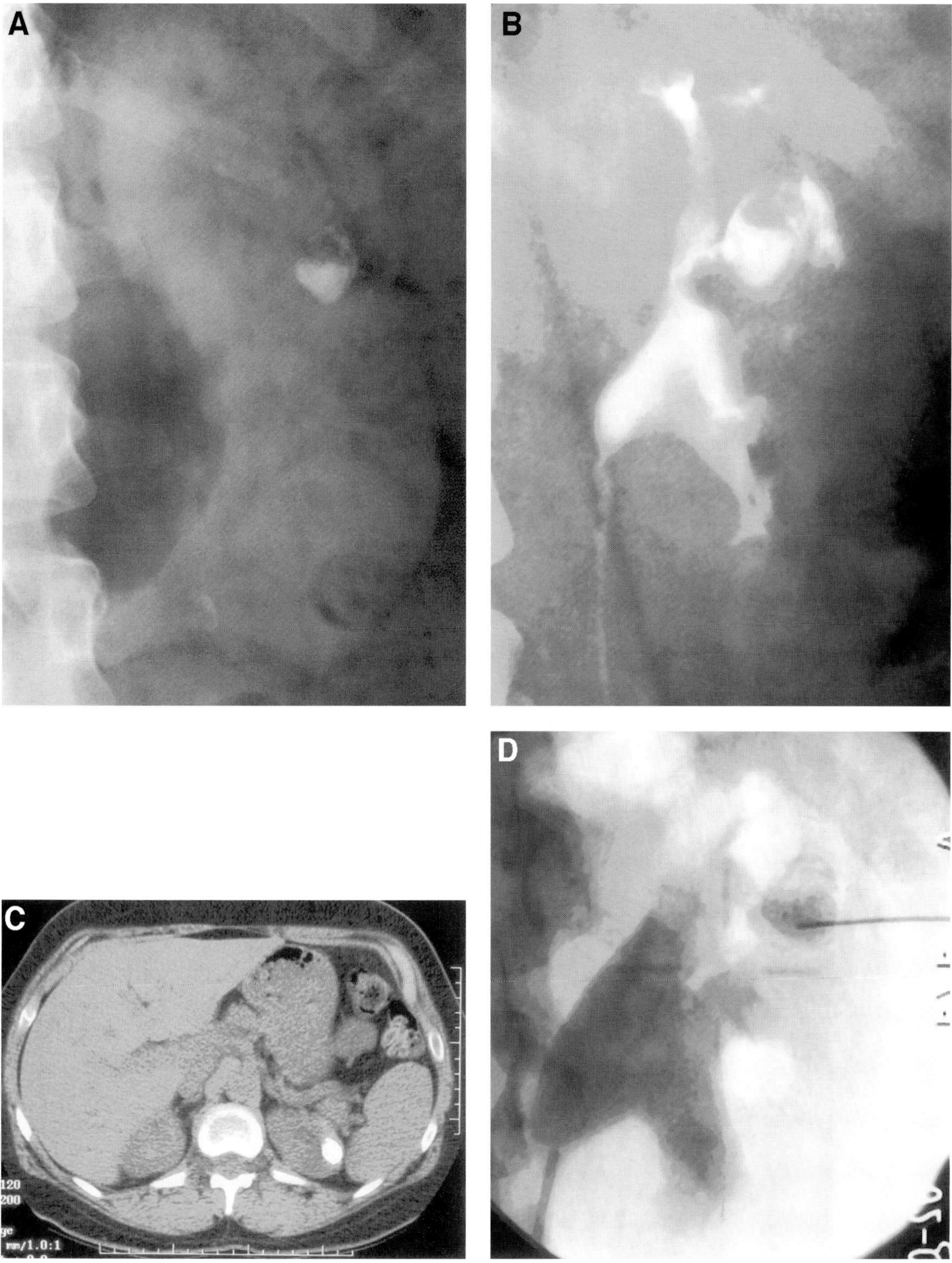


Fig. 6.16

**(A–C)** Plain film reveals calcification overlying upper lateral aspect of left kidney. Pyelogram confirms this to reside in a calyceal diverticulum. A noncontrast CT shows its posterior location, making it ideal for percutaneous access. **(D,E)** The access should involve direct puncture of the diverticulum containing the stone. Working and safety wires can either be coiled within the diverticulum or occasionally, under fluoroscopic control, passed through the diverticular neck, into the main pyelocaliceal system, and down the ureter. The tract is dilated and a working sheath placed.

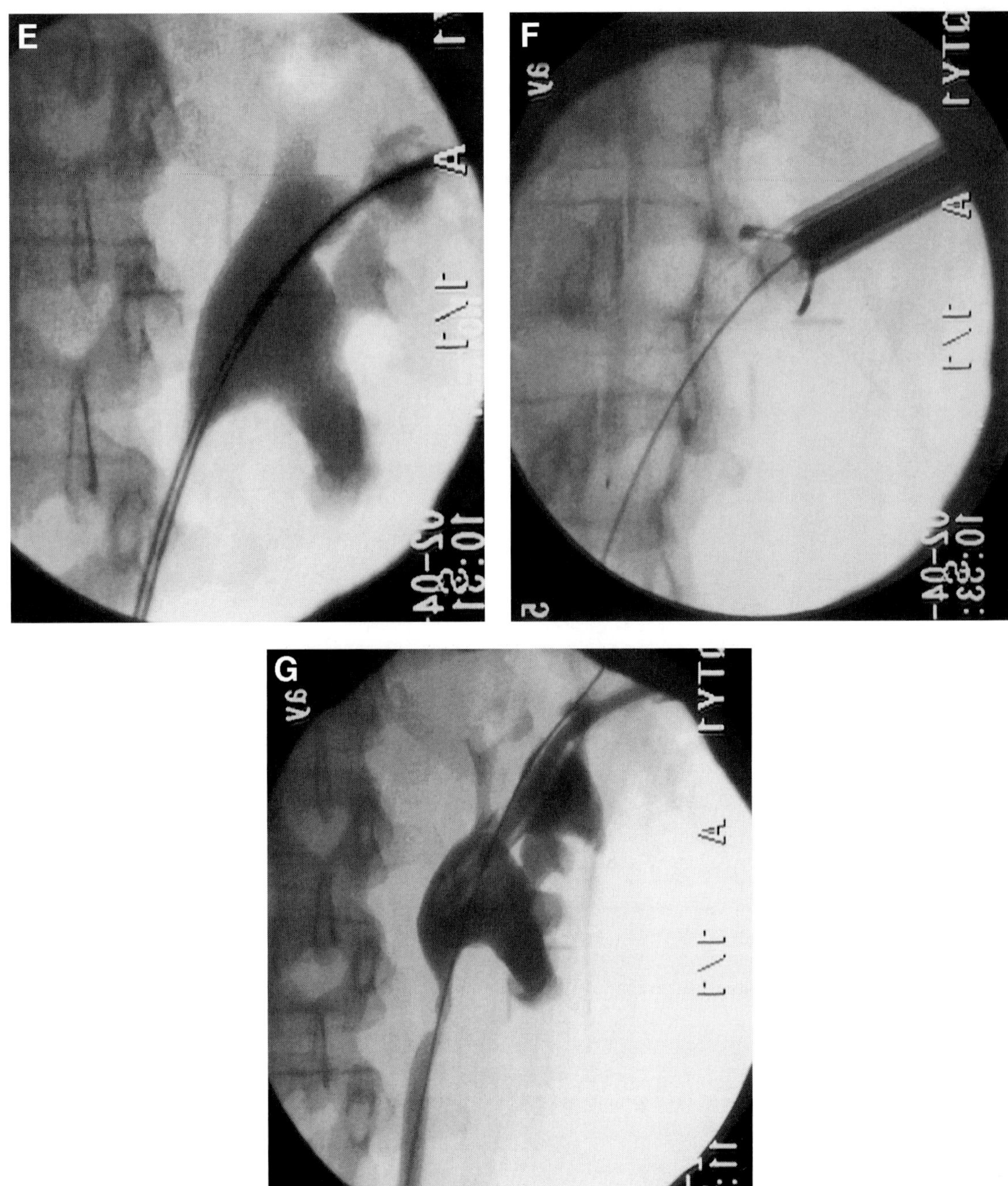

Fig. 6.16 *(continued)*

**(F)** Nephroscopic stone removal proceeds in a standard fashion, following which the diverticular neck is often better visualized. If a wire has not already been passed across the neck, it can often be done at this time and the diverticular neck subsequently dilated. **(G)** When the neck has been managed with dilation, a nephrostomy tube is left across it into the main pyelocaliceal system for several days. An adjunct to help identify the diverticular neck in these patients is cystoscopic placement of an open-end ureteral catheter up to the renal pelvis at the outset of the procedure. During nephroscopic visualization of the caliceal diverticulum, dilute methylene blue is injected in a retrograde fashion through the ureteral catheter, allowing identification of the diverticular neck.

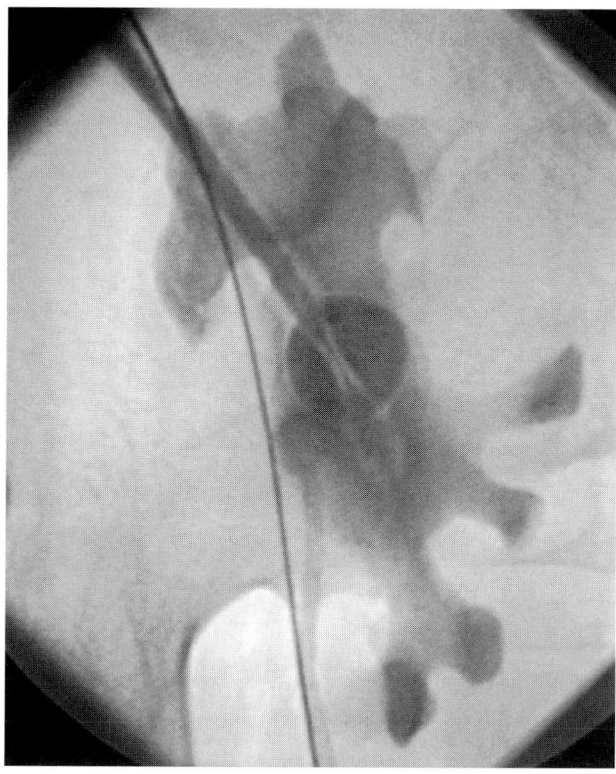

**Fig. 6.17**

Percutaneous access to transplanted kidneys is generally straightforward as the kidney lies near skin level. The only real difference from the procedure performed in native kidneys is that the patient is in a supine rather than a prone position. When renal function is adequate, access can be obtained using standard fluoroscopic imaging postintravenous injection, but initial ultrasound guidance is often preferred. Once the tract is established, the procedure proceeds as for native kidneys with standard tract dilation, stone manipulation, and nephrostomy drainage.

choice rather than distilled water. In that way the complicating effects of hyponatremia are obviated. Otherwise, large amounts of hypotonic solution may be absorbed.

All minor degrees of extravasation and even some major ones can be managed with nephrostomy drainage alone as long as the nephrostomy tube is assured to be in the collecting system, urine is egressing, and the patient is clinically stable. In such cases, especially when the injury occurs in the renal pelvis or at the UPJ, in addition to the nephrostomy tube it is preferable to have a stent across the UPJ either as a percutaneous pyeloureteral catheter or as an indwelling ureteral stent. As long as the patient is stable, serial nephrostograms can be obtained and the nephrostomy tube removed as soon as the extravasation is no longer radiographically evident and distal patency is assured. When satisfactory drainage cannot be assured, or when the patient is clinically unstable, open operative exploration and repair should be considered.

#### Extrarenal Organ Injury

Injury to a hollow or solid organ occurs in 1–5% of patients. Intraperitoneal extravasation can occur from breaching the peritoneum, and the treatment is generally conservative, although paracentesis may be required. On the right side, injury to the liver can occur, although generally this will respond to conservative measures. On the left, splenic injury can occur and initial management is again conservative, although operative exploration and repair may be required.

With the increasingly frequent use of upper pole and supracostal access, hydro-, hemo-, or pneumothorax is becoming more frequent. Management depends on the patient's clinical picture. If the patient is stable, with no ventilatory or respiratory embarrassment, observation alone may allow spontaneous resolution. Alternatively, simple aspiration on a one-time basis may be adequate, although placement of a chest tube for a few days may be required.

Duodenal or colonic injury may also occur. In some cases, even when such injury involves the colon, conservative management may be successful and consists of withdrawing the nephrostomy tube back to the colon to provide percutaneous colostomy drainage. An internal stent should also be placed into the involved collecting system to separate the colonic and urinary streams. In all cases, conservative management should also include the use of intravenous antibiotics. The patient should initially be placed NPO and this should be followed by a low-residue diet.

Another important consideration in determining whether the patient is a candidate for further conservative management vs open operative repair is whether the injury is intra- or extraperitoneal. In most cases that can be determined on the radiographic study used to initially make the diagnosis, whether it is a nephrostogram or a CT scan. Generally, extraperitoneal injuries can be managed using these nonoperative techniques. However, immediate open operative repair should be considered for injuries that are intraperitoneal.

## RENAL CALCULI: URETEROSCOPIC MANAGEMENT

Most renal calculi are currently treated with SWL. However, inadequate fragmentation or clearance of fragments may preclude successful treatment with that modality. In most cases, PCNL is then the best alternative. However, certain situations often favor ureteroscopic management, especially for a relatively small stone burden. Such factors include, but are not limited to, the coexistence of ureteral calculi, irreversible bleeding diatheses, renal anomalies, and morbid obesity.

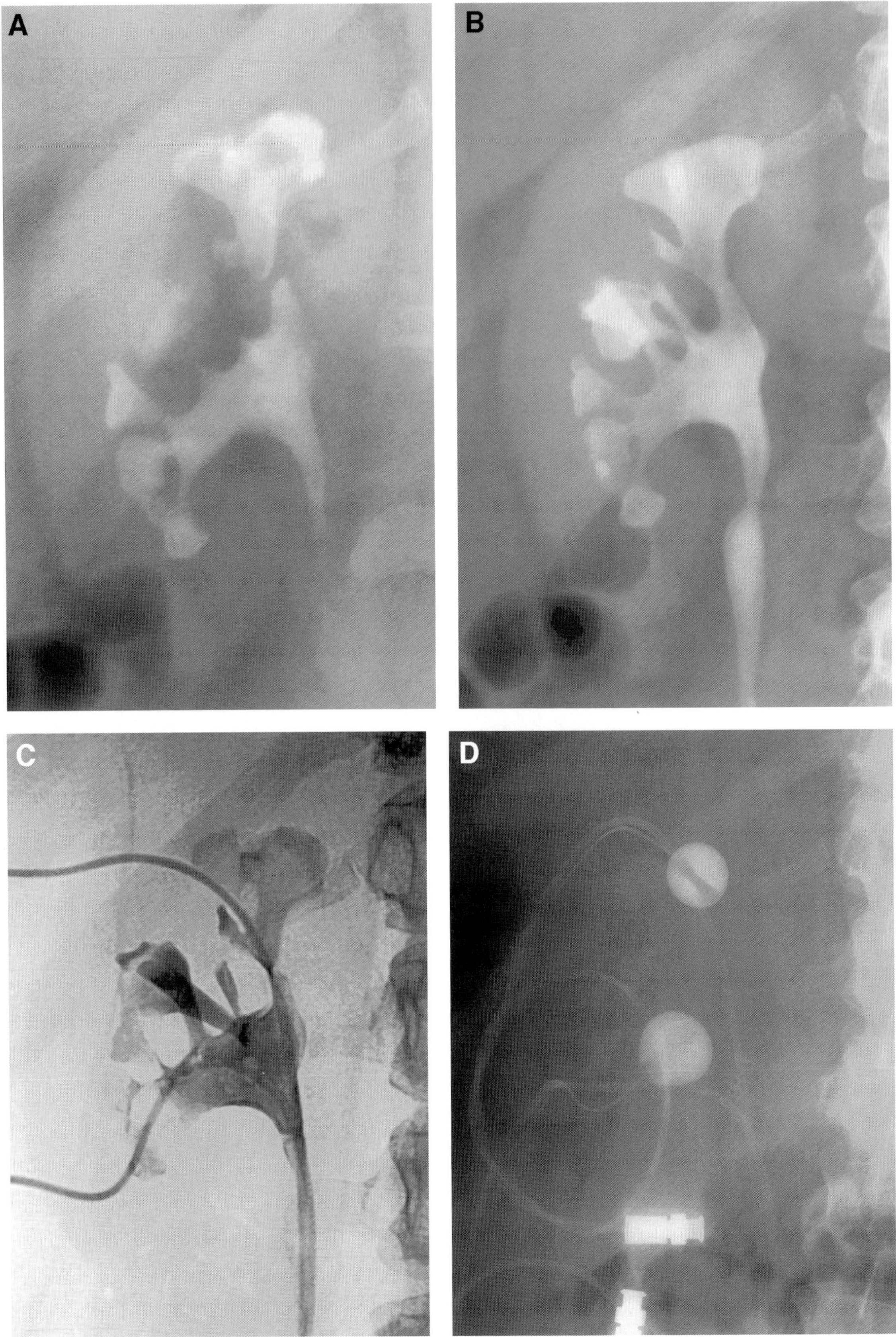


Fig. 6.18

**(A,B)** Scout film and pyelogram reveal a mature, branched calculus. **(C)** Adequate access requires two tracts for this mildly bifid system. **(D)** Post-PCNL film showing contrast in two nephrostomy tube balloons and safety wire in place.

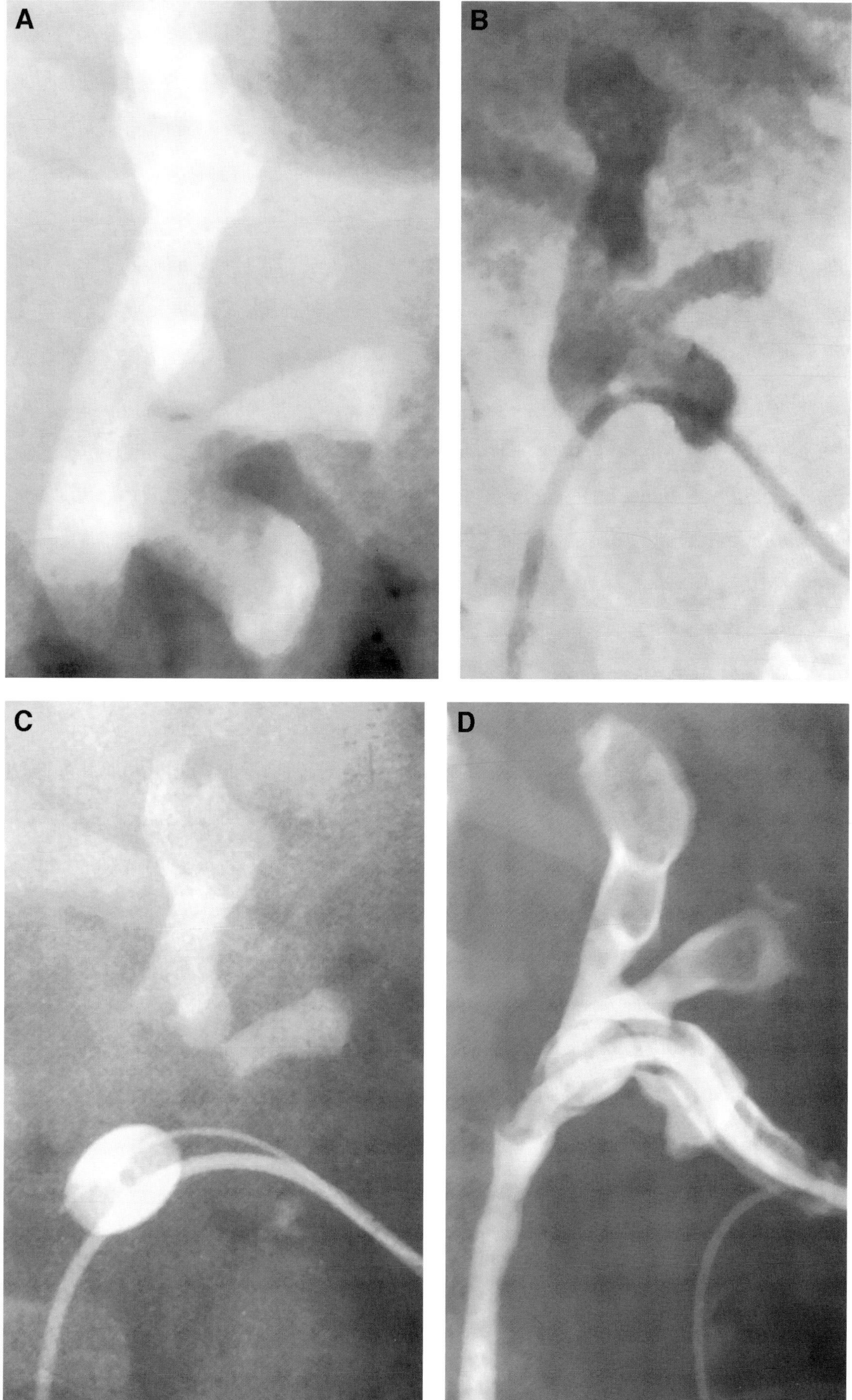


Fig. 6.19

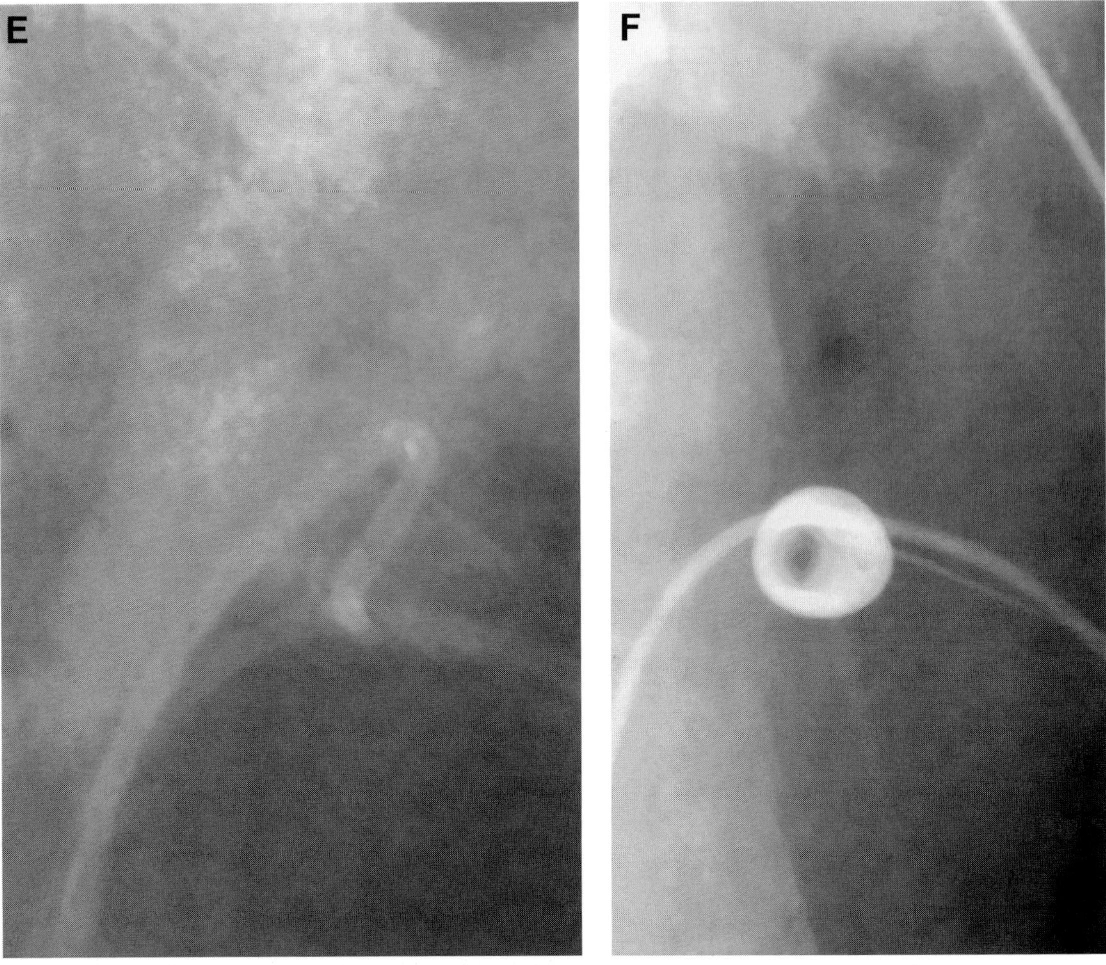


**Fig. 6.19** *(continued)*

**(A–C)** As an alternative to multiple tract percutaneous monotherapy, percutaneous management can be used for debulking prior to adjunctive SWL as part of a planned, combination sandwich approach. Percutaneous debulking reduces the stone burden for subsequent SWL. Furthermore, the placement of a large-caliber nephrostomy tube at completion of the primary percutaneous procedure allows proximal diversion with prevention of obstruction and subsequent bacteremia or sepsis from passage of post-SWL fragments. These photos demonstrate a large staghorn calculus before, during, and after debulking. **(D)** Nephrostogram shows residual calculi to be relatively inaccessible to primary percutaneous tract. SWL is then directed at the residual calculi. **(E)** Within 24–48 h of SWL, a KUB shows that the residual gravel has migrated to the pelvis, where it is now easily accessible. A secondary percutaneous procedure is done via the mature tract to hasten clearance of stone fragments and allow early nephrostomy tube removal. **(F)** Plain film confirms a stone-free result.

Another recent innovation to aid the management of renal calculi via a ureteroscopic approach is nitinol baskets and graspers. These allow nearly full deflection of the flexible ureteroscope such that even a 3 French nitinol basket or grasper can be passed through an endoscope with minimal loss of tip deflection.

A useful technique for stones that are otherwise difficult to access is utilization of a basket or grasper to reposition them. Lower pole calyceal stones can be repositioned to the renal pelvis or an upper pole calyx, allowing easier visualization and subsequent fragmentation.

A description of the techniques available for passing flexible ureteroscopes is offered elsewhere in this volume. When managing intrarenal calculi, a ureteral access sheath is preferred, as it allows repeated passage of the ureteroscope as stone fragments are broken down and removed.

## OPEN OPERATIVE INTERVENTION

### Contemporary Indications

Although the indications to intervene for stones have not changed, the indications for open operative intervention have narrowed considerably. Today these indications include an associated anatomical abnormality best managed with open operative intervention, or a failure of or contraindication to both SWL and PCNL.

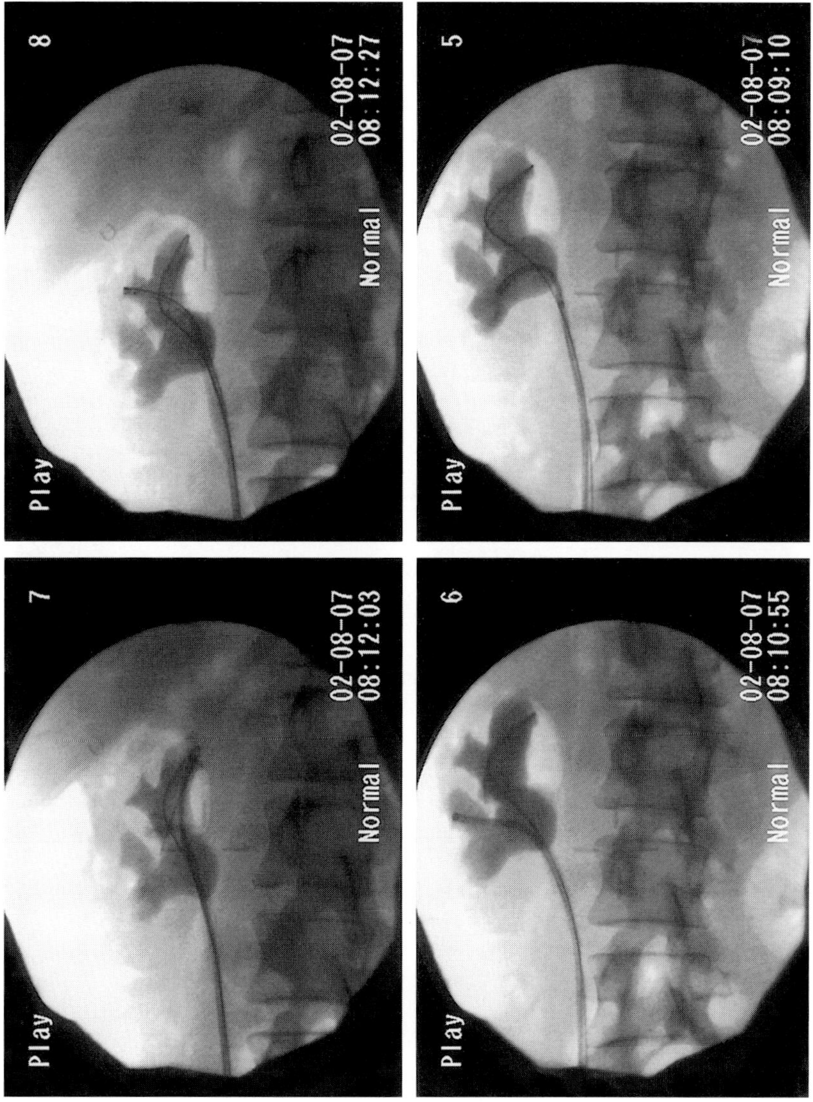


**Fig. 6.20**

Several factors now allow routine ureteroscopic management of intrarenal calculi. These include the availability of small, reliable, actively deflecting ureteroscopes that allow access to virtually any part of the pyelocalyceal system, and the Holmium laser. This efficient and relatively safe device will fragment stones of any composition. Another advantage of the Holmium laser is that the small fibers can be placed through small, flexible ureteropyeloscopes. Our preferred settings for managing intrarenal calculi with the Holmium laser are 0.6–1.0 J. In cases requiring very acute ureteroscopic deflection, small EHL probes are even more flexible and may be beneficial.

At our center, the only real contemporary indication for open operative intervention is a stone so complex that a single open operative procedure would more likely render the patient stone-free, with less risk, than would the option of a complicated, multitract percutaneous procedure with or without adjunctive SWL. As such, with very rare exception, the only open operative intervention applied to stone patients at our center is an anatrophic nephrolithotomy.

## Anatrophic Nephrolithotomy

In 1994, the American Urological Association Nephrolithiasis Clinical Guidelines Panel made recommendations regarding the management of branched, infection-related stones. In reviewing outcome probabilities for management of such stones, the panel concluded that any newly diagnosed struvite staghorn calculus was of and by itself an indication for intervention. The panel further recommended that most such stones could be

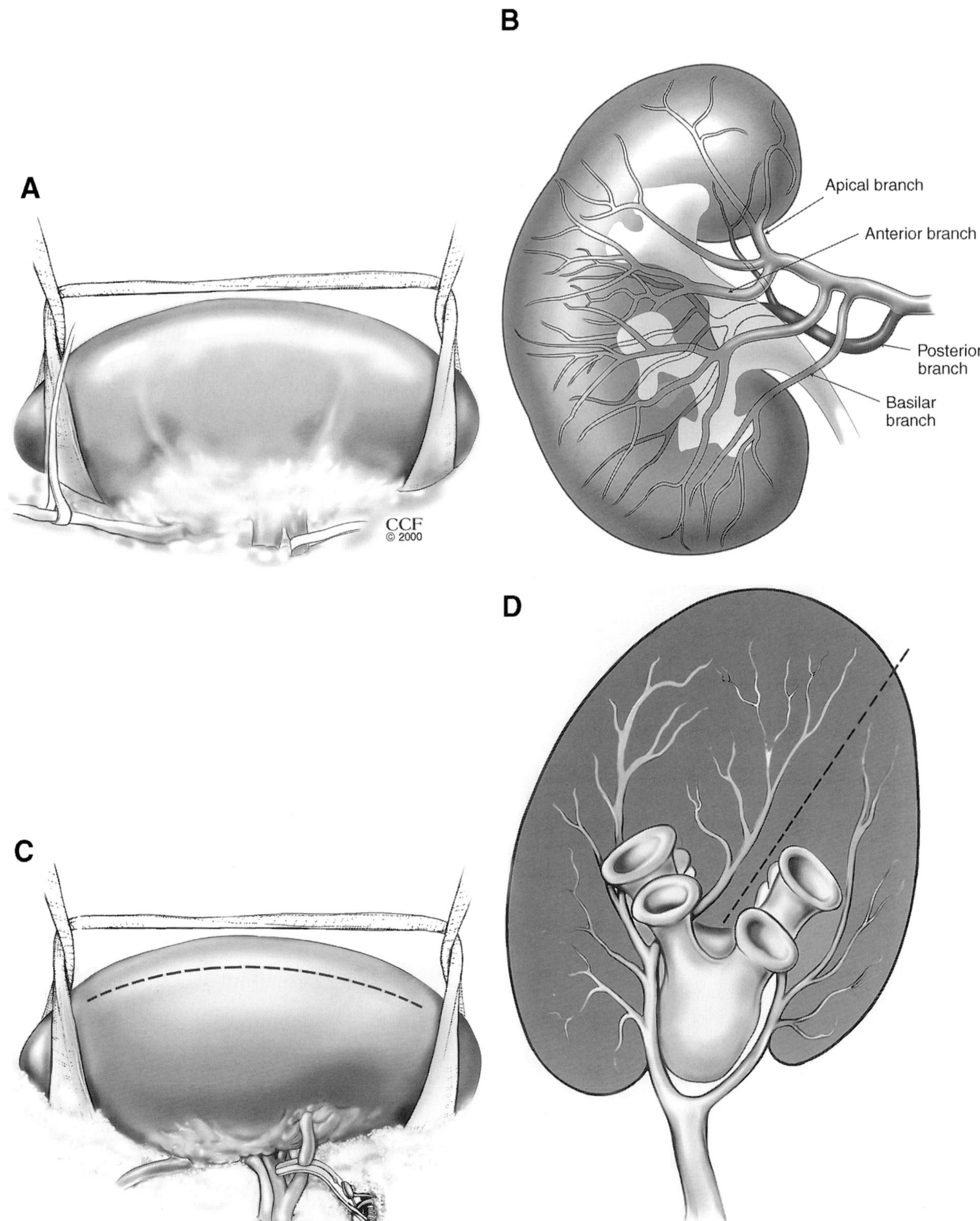


Fig. 6.21

**(A)** Our preference is a flank approach with 11th or 12th rib resection. The incision is extended medially to the lateral border of the rectus muscle. The peritoneum is reflected medially for access to the retroperitoneum. The proximal ureter is identified and surrounded with a vessel loop to prevent distal migration of stone fragments. The kidney is completely mobilized and the renal pedicle isolated. The renal artery is surrounded with a vessel loop and mannitol, 25 g, is given iv for protection during the subsequent renal ischemic episode. **(B–D)** Further dissection of the renal artery is accomplished until the anterior

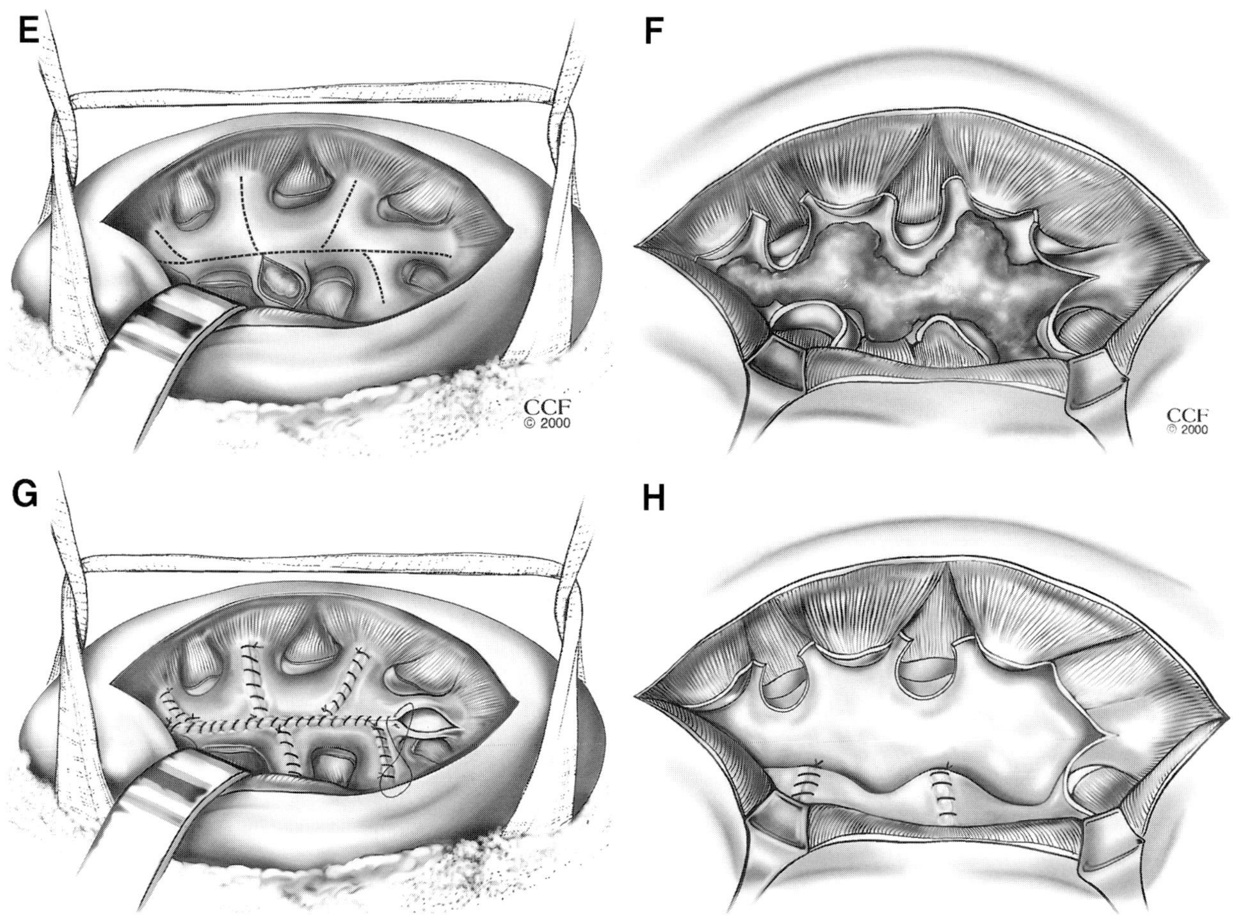


Fig. 6.21 *(continued)*

and posterior divisional branches are identified. The first major branch of the renal artery generally represents the posterior division. There is a relatively avascular plane between the junction of the blood supply to the anterior and posterior segments of the kidney. At the surface of the kidney, this generally lies on the posterior aspect approximately one third of the way from the true lateral border of the kidney to the renal hilum. This can be further delineated by temporarily placing a vascular clamp on the anterior division of the renal artery. Ten cc of methylene blue is injected iv, which results in staining of the posterior renal segment. This helps identify the appropriate line of incision and further dissection into the renal parenchyma. A bowel bag is placed beneath the kidney and wrapped around the pedicle as a reservoir for ice slush. The main renal artery is occluded with a vascular clamp. The renal vein may also be occluded to create a more blood-free surgical field. The kidney is packed with slush with a goal of obtaining a core temperature of 10°C as protection from the subsequent ischemic insult. Once the kidney has reached core temperature, the capsule is incised longitudinally between the anterior and posterior segments, with the incision extended only to the apical and basilar renal segments. The incision through parenchyma continues in a plane along the line of demarcation between the anterior and posterior arterial segments, down toward the renal pelvis. The correct plane generally runs just anterior to the posterior row of infundibula and calices. If small arterioles or venules are cut and identified during this incision or the subsequent dissection, these are ligated with fine chromic figure of eight absorbable suture. **(E)** The stone is identified by palpation in one of the involved posterior infundibula or calices, or by direct visualization. Once the initial stone-bearing infundibulocalix is open, a longitudinal infundibulotomy is performed and extended down to the renal pelvis. Every involved posterior infundibulocalix is subsequently opened longitudinally as far as necessary to extract any stone and the infundibulotomy carried down its anterior aspect toward the renal pelvis. Once the pelvic and posterior infundibulocaliceal aspects of the stone are exposed, attention is turned to the anterior and polar portions, again with sequential longitudinal infundibulotomies. These are performed on the posterior aspect of the anterior infundibula and central aspects of the polar infundibula. The infundibulotomies should begin at each infundibulopelvic junction and extend outward toward the calix as far as necessary to provide adequate exposure for stone removal. **(F)** Ultimately, the entire branched calculus is exposed and ready for removal. At times the whole stone can be delivered intact, though in practice, piecemeal extraction may be required. If infundibulocaliceal extensions of the stone are not extracted with the main portion, the involved infundibulum should be dilated or further incised out toward the calix to ensure complete visualization and stone removal.

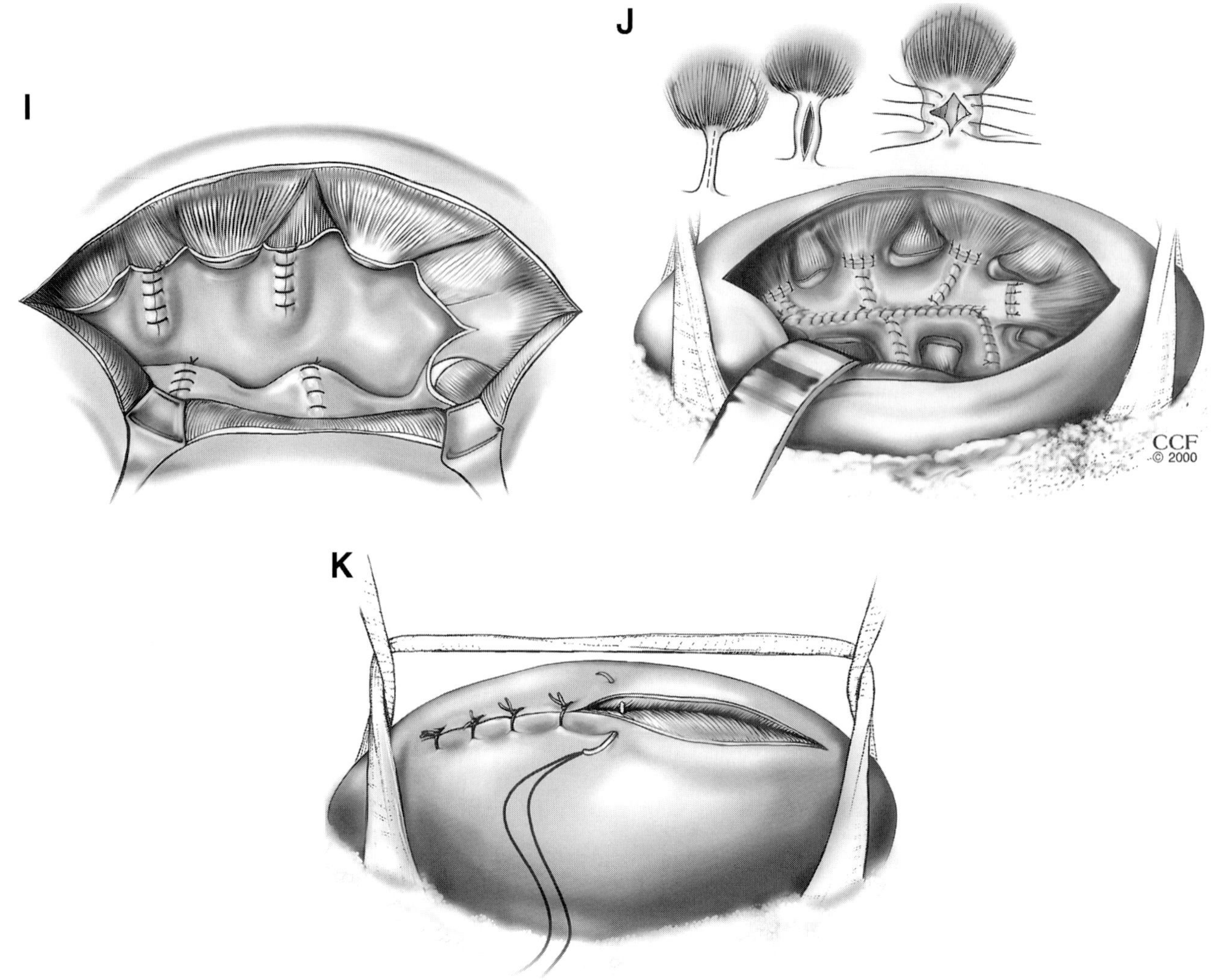


**Fig. 6.21** ***(continued)***

Once the bulk of the stone is removed, each infundibulocalix is individually explored both visually and with palpation to exclude residual fragments. Occasionally residual fragments can be palpated through thin parenchyma, but the infundibulum leading to the stone cannot be visualized. In such cases a small nephrotomy made directly over the palpable stone is acceptable. The stone is extracted, and the nephrotomy is closed with absorbable sutures. The entire collecting system should now be thoroughly lavaged with iced saline using red rubber catheters placed sequentially into each infundibulocalix. Because an optimal result requires removal of all stone fragments, there are several adjunctive maneuvers that can be performed to identify and remove any potential residual stones, including intraoperative static radiography, fluoroscopy, US, and intraoperative pyeloscopy utilizing flexible instrumentation. When all identifiable stone has been removed, a red rubber catheter is passed antegrade down the ureter and the ureter irrigated with saline. An internal stent may be placed at this time in those patients who may have residual fragments or patients with compromised renal function. Nephrostomy tubes are used even less frequently and generally only for those patients with severely compromised renal function and thinned parenchyma. **(G)** The collecting system is reconstructed using fine absorbable suture. **(H,I)** In areas of significant infundibular stenosis, infundibulorrhaphy is performed by suturing the adjacent borders of involved infundibula on their mirror image sides, thus converting two or more stenotic infundibulocaliceal systems into one larger portion of the renal pelvis. **(J)** Isolated infundibular stenosis or polar infundibular stenosis can be managed with an individual infundibulorrhaphy that involves horizontal closure of the initial vertical infundibulotomy in a Heineke–Mikulicz fashion. **(K)** The renal capsule is approximated with running or interrupted 3-0 chromic sutures incorporating only a very small bite of renal parenchyma. At this time an additional 12.5 g of mannitol is given iv and the vascular clamps are removed. Perirenal fat can be reapproximated over the nephrotomy incision, and external drainage is provided with a Penrose or closed suctioned drain placed near, but not directly on, the nephrotomy incision.

managed with PCNL or SWL, either alone or in combination. However, open operative intervention was recommended as an appropriate option in cases where the stone was so extensive that an unreasonable number of percutaneous or shock-wave procedures would be required in order to achieve a stone-free result.

## Anatrophic Nephrolithotomy: Complications

Retained calculi occur in up to 20% of patients, and when such retained stones are symptomatic or associated with infection or obstruction, further intervention is required. Almost all such retained stones can be managed with SWL or percutaneous techniques, though these procedures should be delayed at least 4–6 wk after the initial open operative intervention.

Persistent urinary drainage is uncommon and generally implies devascularization of a localized area or distal obstruction. In most cases such fistulas resolve spontaneously with conservative measures, including provision of local drainage and assurance of distal patency, at times with placement of an internal stent. A Foley catheter to minimize the likelihood of stent reflux should be considered if a stent is required.

Bleeding into the collecting system or around the kidney almost always resolves spontaneously, and conservative, supportive measures are the initial treatment. When bleeding results in the need for multiple transfusions or an unstable cardiovascular status, intervention is indicated. In most cases, the treatment of choice is selective angiographic embolization as open surgical exploration generally results in nephrectomy.

## Partial Nephrectomy

Partial nephrectomy is considered when stone disease is associated with a localized area of irrevocably poor renal function as can occur in the setting of chronic obstruction, especially with infection. In such cases removal of the diseased portion of the kidney along with the stone may be the best option, especially when localized xanthogranulomatous pyelonephritis may be present. The techniques for partial nephrectomy are addressed elsewhere in this volume.

## Nephrectomy

Nephrectomy is indicated only rarely for management of renal calculi. The specific indication is stone disease associated with a nonfunctioning or poorly functioning kidney that is irrevocably damaged and would be unlikely to support life off dialysis should it be the sole kidney. This generally implies renal function less than 10–15% of overall function, or a glomerular filtration rate of less than 15 cc/min. In these cases, salvagability of the kidney is best determined preoperatively with radiographic evaluation that includes a differential nuclear scan. We have also found CT scanning invaluable in determining the residual cortical thickness and to search for evidence of xanthogranulomatous pyelonephritis that is best managed by nephrectomy.

# SUGGESTED READINGS


1. Boyce WH, Smith MGV. Anatrophic nephrotomy and plastic calyorrhaphy. Trans Am Assoc Genitourin Surg 59:18, 1967.
2. Chaussy C, Schmiedt E, Jocham D, Brendel W, Forssmann B, Walther V. First clinical experience with extracorporeally induced destruction of kidney stones by shock waves. J Urol 127:417–420, 1982.
3. Fabrizio MD, Behari A, Bagley DH. Ureteroscopic management of intrarenal calculi. J Urol 159: 1139–1143, 1998.
4. Kessaris DN, Bellman GC, Pardalidis NP, Smith AA. Management of hemorrhage after percutaneous renal surgery. J Urol 153:604, 1995.
5. Leroy AJ, Segura JW, Williams HJ, Jr., et al. Percutaneous renal calculus removal in an extracorporeal shock wave lithotripsy practice. J Urol 138:703, 1987.
6. Meretyk S, Gofrit ON, Gafni O, et al. Complete staghorn calculi: random prospective comparison between extracorporeal shock wave lithotripsy monotherapy and combined with percutaneous nephrostolithotomy. J Urol 157:780–786, 1997.
7. Paik ML, Wainstein MA, Spirnak JP, et al. Current indications for open stone surgery in the treatment of renal and ureteral calculi. J Urol 159:374, 1998.
8. Segura JW, Preminger GM, Assimos DG, et al. Nephrolithiasis Clinical Guidelines Panel summary report on the management of staghorn calculi. The American Urological Association Nephrolithiasis Clinical Guidelines Panel. J Urol 151:1648–1651, 1994.
9. Streem SB. Contemporary clinical practice of shock wave lithotripsy. a re-evaluation of contraindication. J Urol 157:1197, 1997.
10. Streem SB, Yost A, Dolmatch B. Combination "sandwich" therapy for extensive renal calculi in 100 consecutive patients: immediate, long-term and stratified results from a 10-year experience. J Urol 158:342–345, 1997.

# 7 Renal Vascular Disease

*Andrew C. Novick*

## INTRODUCTION

Two main categories of renal artery disease, atherosclerosis and fibrous dysplasia, account for approx 80% and 20% of all such lesions, respectively. Other unusual causes of renal artery disease include an arterial aneurysm, arteriovenous fistula, neurofibromatosis, extrinsic obstruction of the renal artery, the middle aortic syndrome, and renal artery thrombosis or embolism. Intervention may be indicated in these disorders to treat associated hypertension, to preserve renal function, or to prevent rupture of an arterial aneurysm.

The role of surgical therapy in the management of these patients has changed in recent years for several reasons *(1,2)*. These include the advent of percutaneous transluminal angioplasty (PTA) and endovascular stenting as alternate effective forms of treatment for certain patients, the development of new and more effective techniques for surgical revascularization, and an enhanced appreciation of advanced atherosclerotic renal artery disease as a correctable cause of renal failure. Surgical revascularization remains the treatment of choice for patients with branch renal artery disease, with an ostial atherosclerotic lesion, with an arterial aneurysm, and in whom PTA or stenting has been unsuccessful. Surgical revascularization continues to provide excellent long-term results in properly selected patients with renal artery disease *(2,3)*.

Advances in surgical renovascular reconstruction have limited the role of total or partial nephrectomy in the management of patients with renal artery disease. These operations are occasionally indicated in patients with renal infarction, severe arteriolar nephrosclerosis, severe renal atrophy, and noncorrectable renovascular lesions. Nephrectomy may also be indicated in the elderly poor surgical risk patients with a normal contralateral kidney or after a failed revascularization procedure.

## INDICATIONS FOR TREATMENT

### Renovascular Hypertension

The coexistence of hypertension and renal artery disease does not always imply a causal relationship between the two. Renal artery disease is far more common than renovascular hypertension (RVH). Classically, RVH is a retrospective diagnosis rendered when hypertension resolves after intervention to correct a renal artery lesion. It now commonly refers to rein-mediated hypertension as a result of renal artery disease. Clinical clues to suggest RVH include age younger than 30 yr or older than 50 yr, abrupt onset and short duration of hypertension, presence of extra-renal vascular disease, end-organ damage such as left ventricular hypertrophy or high-grade hypertensive retinopathy, systolic–diastolic abdominal bruit, and deterioration of renal function in response to angiotensin-converting enzyme (ACE) inhibitors. In patients who have a moderate clinical suggestion of RVH, a number of noninvasive tests have been developed that identify patients with RVH and help to predict the outcome of interventive treatment.

For patients with RVH as a result of fibrous dysplasia, candidacy for surgical intervention is guided by the specific pathological process, as determined by angiographic findings, and its associated nature history *(4)*. Medical management of medial fibroplasia is the initial approach because loss of renal function from progressive obstruction is uncommon and intervention is reserved for those patients with difficult-to-control hypertension. Renal artery disease owing to intimal or perimedial fibroplasia is often associated with progressive obstruction, which can result in ischemic renal atrophy. Therefore, early intervention is recommended to improve blood pressure control and to preserve renal function.

The known results of PTA are important in assessing the need for surgery in patients with fibrous dysplasia.

From: *Operative Urology at the Cleveland Clinic*
Edited by: A. Novick et al. © Humana Press Inc., Totowa, NJ

Technical and clinical success rates with PTA for fibrous disease of the main renal artery are 90–95% and are no different from results obtainable with surgery *(2)*. Still, up to 30% of patients may present with branch disease or aneurysm that is not amenable to PTA. Surgery is then reserved for patients with peripheral, complex branch disease or for those who have failed PTA.

Renal artery aneurysms may require repair if they result in significant hypertension or to prevent rupture when they are larger than 2 cm and noncalcified *(5)*. This is a particular concern in women of reproductive age because of the predisposition for rupture during pregnancy.

For patients with atherosclerosis and RVH, the indications for intervention are more restrictive owing to the frequent presence of concomitant extra-renal vascular disease. More vigorous attempts at medical management for this group are warranted. Surgical revascularization is reserved for those patients whose hypertension cannot be satisfactorily controlled with medication or when renal function becomes threatened by advanced vascular disease. Whereas PTA is associated with successful blood pressure results for nonostial atherosclerosis, the long-term success rate with ostial lesions is poor owing to a higher incidence of restenosis *(2)*. The results with endovascular stenting for ostial lesions are better than those with PTA, but surgical revascularization remains the definitive long-term therapy for these patients *(3)*.

### Ischemic Nephropathy

Epidemiological studies suggest that atherosclerotic renovascular disease is common in patients with generalized atherosclerosis obliterans regardless of the presence of RVH. The development of chronic renal insufficiency from atherosclerotic renal artery disease, known as ischemic nephropathy, has become an important clinical issue that is separate and distinct from the problem of RVH. Knowledge of the natural history of atherosclerotic renal artery disease permits identification of patients at risk for ischemic nephropathy *(6)*. Those at highest risk are patients with high-grade stenosis (>75%) involving the entire renal mass (bilateral disease or disease in a solitary kidney). Intervention in these patients is for the purpose of preservation of renal function. Many of these patients are older, with diffuse extra-renal vascular disease and ostial renal artery disease. Clinical clues suggesting ischemic nephropathy include azotemia (unexplained or association with ACE inhibitor treatment), diminished renal size, and the presence of vascular disease in other sites (cerebrovascular disease, coronary artery disease, or peripheral vascular disease).

## PREOPERATIVE CONSIDERATIONS

Patients with atherosclerotic renal artery disease who are considered for surgical revascularization should undergo screening and correction of significant associated extra-renal vascular disease, such as coronary and carotid disease. With aggressive treatment of coexisting extra-renal vascular disease before surgical renal revascularization, perioperative morbidity and mortality can be minimized.

Before surgery, all patients require arteriography. For most patients we use digital subtraction angiography with iodinated contrast material because accurate anatomical information can be obtained with limited exposure to the contrast agent. In selected cases, carbon dioxide angiography can be used, which eliminates the risk for contrast-related nephrotoxicity. In addition to anteroposterior views of the renal artery and aorta, we routinely obtain a lateral aortogram to assess the celiac artery and a view of the lower thoracic aorta. These additional views are obtained in anticipation of the use of extra-anatomical bypass procedures.

All patients undergoing surgical renal revascularization are hydrated well prior to surgery. Because renovascular hypertension is associated with secondary hyperaldosteronism, potassium supplement and monitoring of serum potassium levels are needed to guard against hypokalemia. To further ensure optimal renal perfusion and an active diuresis intraoperatively, mannitol 12.5 g is given intravenously before commencing the operation; equivalent doses of mannitol are subsequently given before revascularization, immediately after revascularization, and again in the recovery room.

## AORTORENAL BYPASS

Although a variety of surgical revascularization techniques are available for treating patients with renal artery disease, aortorenal bypass with a free graft of autogenous saphenous vein or hypogastric artery remains the preferred method in patients with a nondiseased abdominal aorta *(7,8)*. Although an arterial autograft is theoretically advantageous, use of the hypogastric artery as a bypass graft is limited by its short length and frequent involvement with atherosclerosis. Therefore, autogenous saphenous vein is most often employed and excellent clinical results continue to be achieved with this type of bypass graft. This vein is extremely friable and may either rupture postoperatively or undergo severe dilatation. Currently, aortorenal bypass with a synthetic material is indicated only when an autogenous vascular graft is not

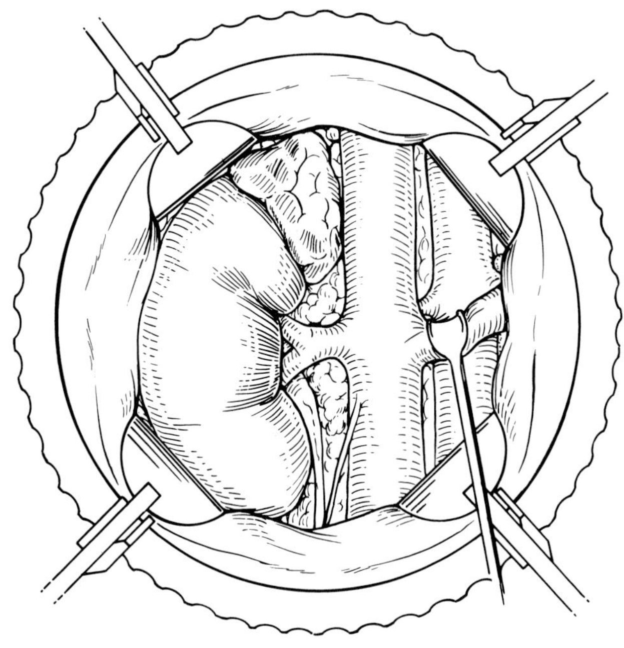

Fig. 7.1

Transperitoneal exposure of the right kidney and renal vessels for aortorenal bypass.

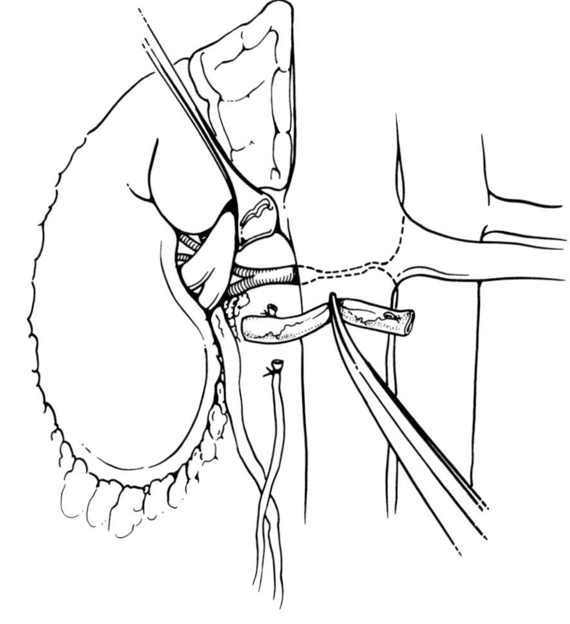

Fig. 7.2

The bypass graft is measured for alignment with the aorta and distal renal artery.

available, and polytetrafluoroethylene has become the synthetic graft of choice in such cases *(9)*.

To perform an aortorenal bypass on the right side, the kidney is exposed by reflecting the ascending colon medially and using the Kocher maneuver on the duodenum (Fig. 7.1). The liver and gallbladder are retracted upward, taking care to protect the hepatic ligament with its vessels and common bile duct. Exposure of the right renal artery, right renal vein, inferior vena cava, and the aorta is thereby obtained. The Buckwalter self-retaining ring retractor is inserted to maintain exposure. Gerota's fascia is opened laterally to expose the surface of the kidney so that its color and consistency may be observed.

The aorta is exposed from the level of the left renal vein to the inferior mesenteric artery, ligating overlying lymphatic vessels and lumbar segmental branches as necessary to gain exposure. The proximal aspect of the right renal artery is exposed by mobilizing and retracting the vena cava laterally and the left renal vein superiorly, carrying the dissection along the anterolateral aspect of the aortic wall until the renal artery origin is encountered.

The distal two-thirds of the main right renal artery is exposed by retracting the mobilized vena cava medially and the right renal vein superiorly. To accomplish this, it is often necessary to secure and divide one or more lumbar veins entering the posterior aspect of the vena cava. There are generally no significant tributaries of the right renal vein. After exposure of the right renal artery, this is then mobilized from its attached and surrounding lymphatics and nerves. Small vessels and lymphatics are secured by light electrocautery or fine suture ligatures.

The bypass graft is placed along the lateral aortic wall to determine the best position for placement of the graft (Fig. 7.2). At this point, the ring retractor blades are relaxed to allow the aorta to return to its normal position and to prevent distortion of an otherwise well-placed graft after the final retraction is released.

On the right side, it is important to bring the graft off the anterolateral aspect of the aortic wall to avoid kinking of the proximal anastomosis as the graft passes in front of the vena cava. If the aortotomy is made too far anteriorly or posteriorly, the graft may kink with subsequent development of stenosis or thrombosis. On the left side, the graft may be placed directly off the lateral aspect of the aorta.

An end-to-side anastomosis of the bypass graft to the aorta is done first to minimize the time of renal ischemia (Fig. 7.3). A DeBakey clamp is placed to occlude the aorta, taking care to avoid compression of the mesenteric and contralateral renal arteries. In most cases the lateral aortic wall is only partially occluded, thereby preserving distal aortic flow and obviating the need for systemic heparinization. In some patients (i.e., children and young females) with a small abdominal aorta, better exposure is obtained by placing the DeBakey clamp completely across the aorta; this maneuver totally interrupts aortic blood flow, and, in this event, systemic heparinization is initiated before aortic clamping.

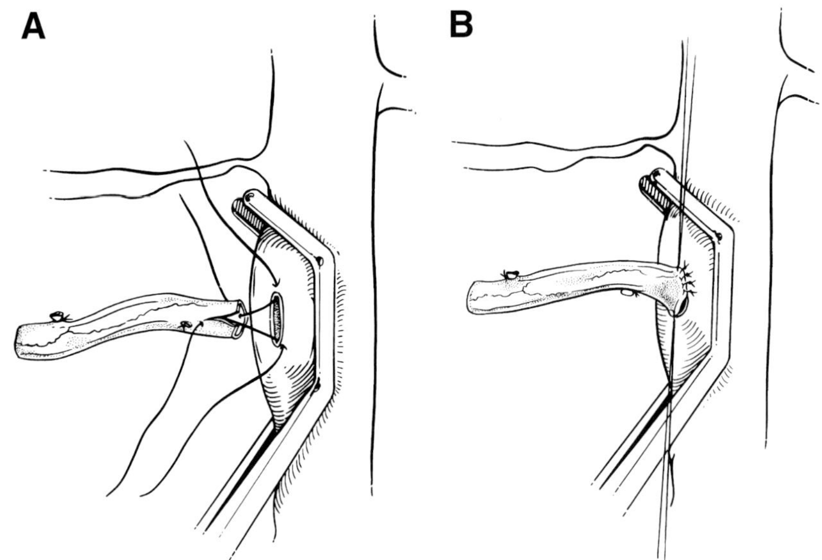


Fig. 7.3

End-to-side anastomosis of the graft to the aorta is performed.

An oval aortotomy is made on the anterolateral wall of the aorta. If significant atherosclerosis of the peri-renal aorta is present, a local endarterectomy is performed to remove atheromatous plaque from the region of the anastomosis.

The bypass graft is spatulated for a short distance, and, if length permits, the apex of the spatulation is generally placed at the caudal end of the aortotomy so that the graft can follow a gentle curve as it emerges from the aorta. If the aortotomy is located a significant distance below the distal renal artery or if the graft is short, as on the side, then the apex is reversed cephalad to avoid kinking of the aortorenal bypass graft. Two corner sutures of 6-0 silk are inserted 180° apart to begin the anastomosis.

The anastomosis is performed with interrupted 6-0 arterial sutures and the anterior wall of the anastomosis is completed first. The aorta is rotated anteriorly to expose the posterior wall of the anastomosis, which is similarly completed with interrupted 6-0 arterial sutures. The graft is occluded beyond its origin with a bulldog clamp and the aortic clamp is gently released. An arterial leakage is corrected at this time with additional sutures as needed. The bulldog clamp is intermittently released to ensure good blood flow and to flush the graft free of any athero-sclerotic fragments. The graft distal to the clamp is then irrigated with heparin solution.

The main renal artery is then mobilized in its entirety, if this has not already been done. The renal artery is ligated proximally, a bulldog clamp is placed distally, and the diseased arterial segment is excised and sent for pathological examination (Fig. 7.4). Before the distal anastomosis is performed, 10 mL of dilute heparin solution are instilled into the distal renal artery.

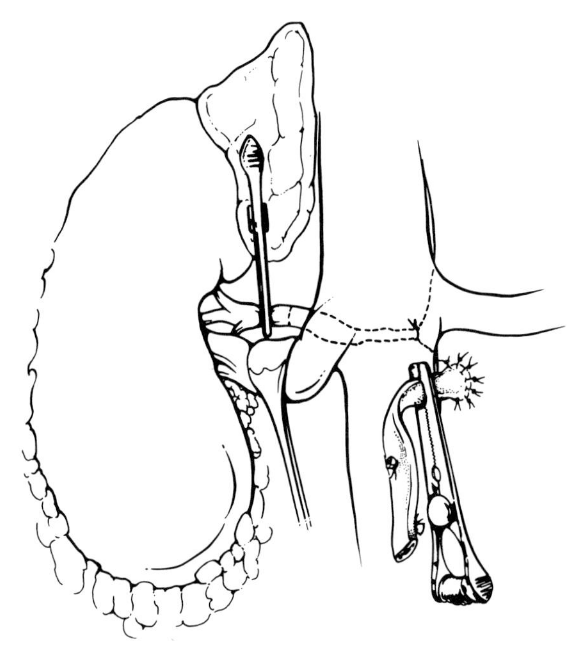

Fig. 7.4

Following completion of the proximal anastomosis, the distal renal artery is temporarily occluded prior to its division.

The bypass graft is brought anterior to the vena cava to lie in proximity to the distal renal artery. The graft is trimmed as necessary to allow a tension-free end-to-end anastomosis with no redundancy in the length of the graft. The graft and distal renal artery are spatulated to create a wider anastomosis, which minimizes the possibility for subsequent stenosis. The anastomosis is performed with 6-0 arterial sutures. Stay sutures, 180° apart, are placed in

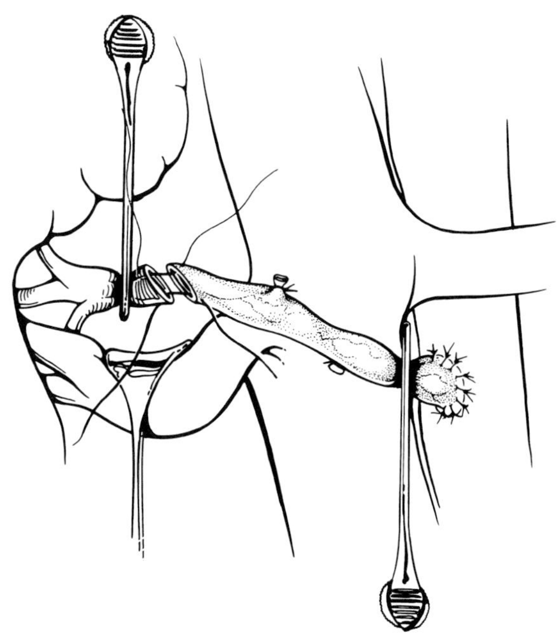

**Fig. 7.5**

Performance of end-to-end anastomosis between the graft and the distal renal artery.

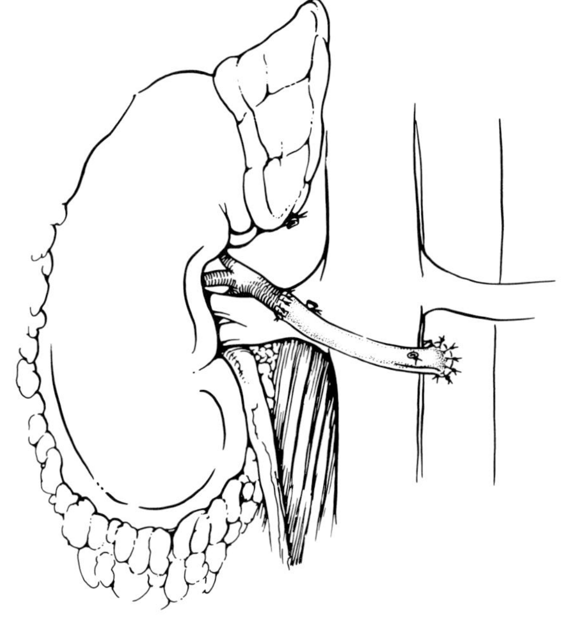

**Fig. 7.6**

Completed right aortorenal bypass operation.

the cephalic and caudal margins of the anastomosis. An end-to-end anastomosis of the graft to the renal artery is preferred over an end-to-side technique because this provides better flow rates, is easier to perform, and allows removal of the diseased renal arterial segment for pathological study. The anastomosis is performed with interrupted 6-0 arterial sutures (Fig. 7.5).

The proximal and distal bulldog clamps are released, and circulation to the kidney is restored. Adequate renal perfusion is verified by palpating the pulse in the distal renal artery and by visual inspection of the renal surface. Arterial anastomotic leakage, if present, is controlled with oxycel cotton and/or additional 6-0 interrupted arterial sutures (Fig. 7.6).

Surgical revascularization is more complicated when the disease extends into the branches of the renal artery or when vascular reconstruction is required for a kidney supplied by multiple renal arteries. When disease-free distal arterial branches occur outside the renal hilus, an aortorenal bypass operation can usually be done *in situ*. The size of the involved vessels is not a significant factor because utilizing microvascular instruments and optical magnification vessels as small as 1.5 mm in diameter can be repaired *in situ*. There are several variations of the standard aortorenal bypass technique, which may be used to repair branch renal artery disease. Because the bypass graft must be sufficiently long to reach the renal artery branches, autogenous saphenous vein is the graft of choice in these cases.

In patients with disease involving two or more renal artery branches, the author has found that aortorenal bypass with a branched saphenous vein graft offers the most useful and versatile technique for *in situ* vascular reconstruction *(10)* (Fig. 7.7). These end-to-side anastomoses are done with interrupted 7-0 arterial sutures and lead to creation of a multibranched graft that can be used to replace several diseased renal artery branches. After insertion of the proximal graft into the aorta, direct end-to-end anastomosis of

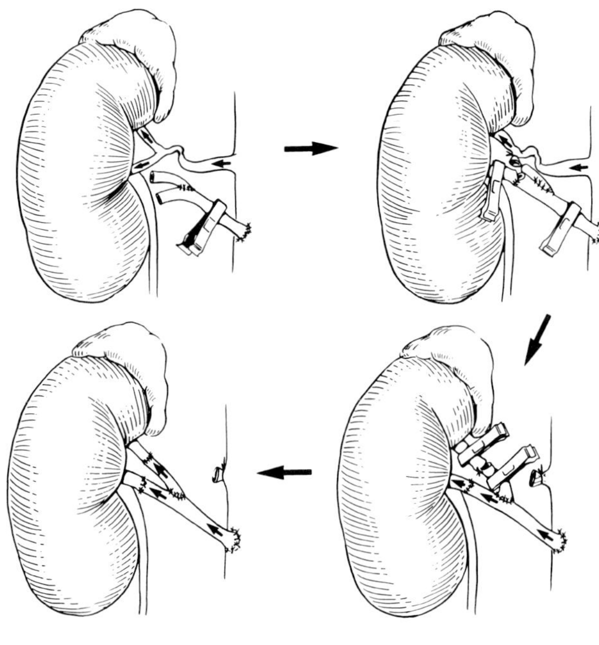

**Fig. 7.7**

Technique of aortorenal bypass with a branched graft of autogenous saphenous vein.

each graft branch to a renal artery branch is done. During performance of each individual branch anastomosis, the remainder of the kidney continues to be perfused and overall renal ischemia is thus limited to the time required for completion of a single end-to-end anastomosis (approx 15–20 min), which is an important advantage.

Renal artery aneurysms have a variable presentation, and vascular involvement may be focal or diffuse *(5,11)*. Saccular aneurysms are the most commonly encountered type of renal artery aneurysm, and these are often located at the initial bifurcation or trifurcation of the main renal artery. When the aneurysm is located outside the renal hilus, *in situ* excision may be done. If the renal artery wall at the base of the aneurysm is intact, aneurysmectomy with either primary closure or patch angioplasty with a segment of saphenous vein can be performed. If the entire circumference of the renal artery wall is diseased, then aortorenal bypass with a branched autogenous vascular graft is done as described above *(12)*.

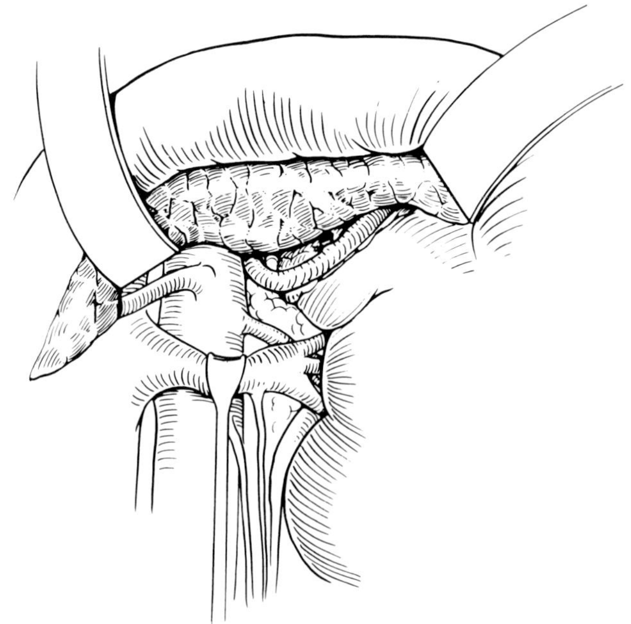

**Fig. 7.8**

The pancreas is gently retracted cephalad to expose the splenic artery. The left renal vein is retracted inferiorly to expose the left renal artery.

## ALTERNATE BYPASS TECHNIQUES

In older patients with renal artery disease, involvement of the abdominal aorta with severe atherosclerosis, aneurysmal disease, or dense fibrosis from a prior operation may render an aortorenal bypass technically difficult and potentially hazardous to perform. Simultaneous aortic replacement and renal revascularization are associated with operative mortality rates of 5–30% *(13–15)* and should be considered only in patients with a significant aortic aneurysm or symptomatic aorto-iliac occlusive disease. In the absence of a definite indication for aortic replacement, alternate bypass techniques are preferrable because they can safely and effectively restore renal arterial blood flow while avoiding the need for a more hazardous operation *(16)*. These alternate bypass operations include hepatorenal bypass, splenorenal bypass, iliorenal bypass, thoracic aortorenal bypass, and mesenterorenal bypass.

In considering patient eligibility for alternate visceral renal arterial bypass operations, the absence of occlusive disease involving the donor artery must be verified by preliminary arteriography. Candidates for hepatorenal or splenorenal bypass must be evaluated with both anteroposterior and lateral abdominal aortography to ensure that the celiac artery and its branches are unobstructed. Pelvic arteriography is a requisite study in patients considered for an iliorenal bypass. If thoracic aortorenal revascularization is contemplated, lower thoracic aortography must be obtained.

### Splenorenal Bypass

Splenorenal bypass is the preferred vascular reconstructive technique for patients with a troublesome aorta who require left renal revascularization *(17)*. Transposition of the splenic artery by retroduodenal passage for right renal revascularization has been unsatisfactory and is not recommended.

To perform splenorenal bypass, an extended left subcostal transperitoneal incision is made, and the left colon and duodenum are reflected medially. The plane between Gerota's fascia and the pancreas is developed by blunt dissection, and the pancreas and spleen are gently retracted cephalad. The left renal vein is mobilized and retracted inferiorly to expose the main left renal artery. The pancreas is gently retracted upward to permit access to the splenic vessels (Fig. 7.8). The splenic artery may be palpated posterior and superior to the splenic vein, and that portion lying closest to the distal aspect of the renal artery is chosen for mobilization. Small pancreatic arterial branches are divided and secured with fine silk sutures. The splenic artery may be quite tortuous and should be mobilized proximally as close to the celiac artery as possible, where the vessel wall is thicker and the luminal diameter larger.

After mobilization, the splenic artery is occluded proximally with a bulldog clamp, ligated distally with a 2-0 silk suture, and transected (Fig. 7.9). It is not necessary to remove the spleen, which receives adequate collateral supply from the short gastric and gastric epiploic vessels to maintain its viability. After transection, the splenic artery is often observed to be in spasm with a considerably reduced luminal size. After irrigation of the lumen

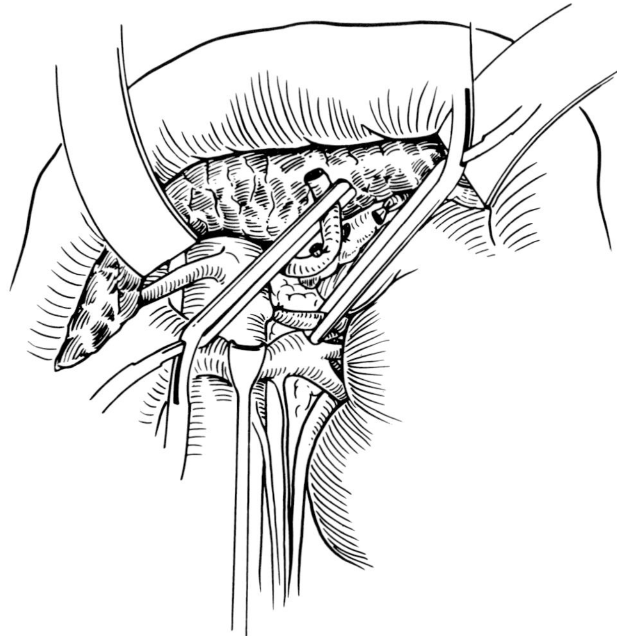

**Fig. 7.9**

The splenic artery has been transected and is temporarily occluded proximally. The left renal artery is being prepared for anastomosis to the splenic artery.

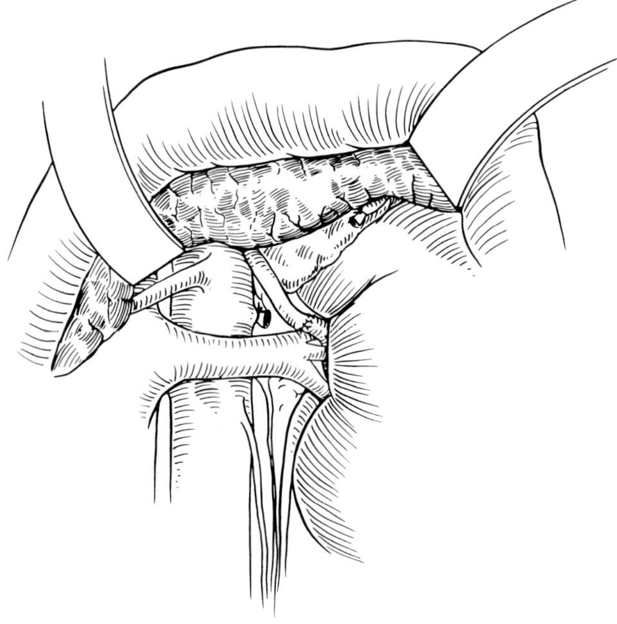

**Fig. 7.10**

Completed left splenorenal bypass operation.

with dilute heparin solution, this spasm can be relieved by gentle dilation of the splenic artery with graduated sounds. This will eliminate any disparity in the caliber of the splenic and renal arteries, and a direct end-to-end anastomosis is then performed (Fig. 7.10). The advantages of the splenorenal bypass technique are that the operation is done well away from the aorta, that only a single vascular anastomosis is necessary, and that revascularization is accomplished with an autogenous vascular graft.

## Hepatorenal Bypass

Hepatorenal bypass is the preferred vascular reconstructive technique for patients with a troublesome aorta who require right renal revascularization *(18)*. The hepatic circulation is ideally suited for a visceral right renal arterial bypass operation. The liver receives 28% of the cardiac output in resting adults and is unique in having a dual circulation from the portal vein and hepatic artery, which contribute 80 and 20% of hepatic blood flow, respectively. Hepatic oxygenation is equally derived from these two circulations. It has been well demonstrated that hepatic artery flow can be safely interrupted. When this occurs, hepatic function and morphology are maintained by increased extraction of oxygen from portal venous blood and by the rapid development of an extensive collateral arterial flow to the liver *(19)*.

The hepatic artery arises from the celiac axis and runs anterior to the portal vein and to the left of the common bile duct. The first major branch is the gastroduodenal artery, and thereafter, the hepatic artery divides into its right and left branches. In considering a hepatorenal bypass operation, one of the more clinically significant anatomical variations is origination of the right hepatic artery from the superior mesenteric artery, which occurs in about 12% of patients. The left hepatic artery arises from the gastric artery in approx 11.5% of patients.

The most common method of performing hepatorenal bypass is with an interposition saphenous vein graft anastomosed end-to-side to the common hepatic artery, just beyond the gastroduodenal origin, and then end-to-end to the right renal artery (Fig. 7.11). This technique preserves distal hepatic arterial flow and thereby reduces the risk of ischemic liver damage.

In some patients the common hepatic artery cannot be employed in this manner for hepatorenal revascularization either because it is smaller than the renal artery or because of an anatomical variation in which the right and left hepatic arterial branches have separate origins. In these situations the available major hepatic arteries are generally all of insufficient caliber to maintain adequate blood flow both to the liver and to the right kidney. It is then preferable to perform end-to-end anastomosis of either the common, right, or left hepatic arteries to the right renal artery *(20)* (Fig. 7.12). In some patients, a direct tension-free anastomosis of these vessels can be done; otherwise, an interposition saphenous vein graft is needed. Despite the resulting total or segmental hepatic dearterialization in these patients, postoperative liver

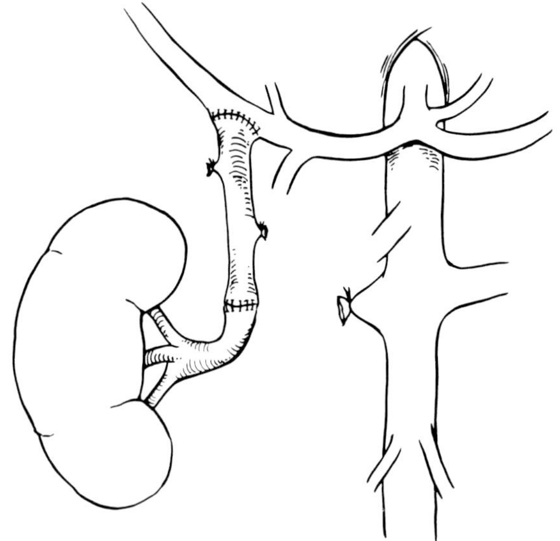

Fig. 7.11

The most common method of performing hepatorenal bypass with an interposition saphenous vein graft anastomosed end-to-side to the common hepatic artery and end-to-end to the right renal artery.

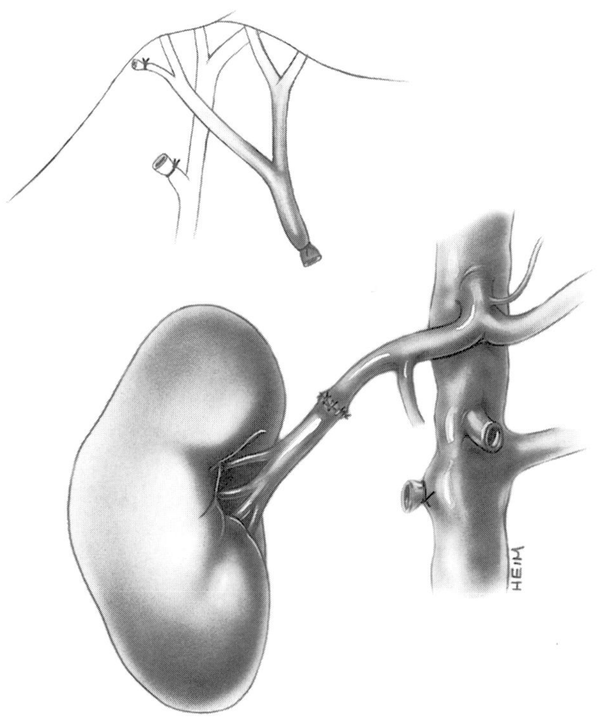

Fig. 7.12

Performance of hepatorenal bypass by direct end-to-end anastomosis of the common hepatic artery to the right renal artery.

function studies have remained normal. However, the gallbladder is more susceptible to ischemic damage in such cases and should be removed.

## Thoracic Aortorenal Bypass

Use of the thoracic aorta for renal revascularization is indicated for patients with significant abdominal aortic atherosclerosis, celiac artery stenosis, and no primary indication to replace the abdominal aorta. The subdiaphragmatic supraceliac and descending thoracic aorta are often relatively free of disease in such patients and can be used to achieve renal vascular reconstruction with an interposition saphenous vein graft *(21)*. Preoperative angiographic evaluation should include views of the supraceliac and thoracic aorta to verify their disease-free status.

For left renal revascularization, we have employed the descending thoracic aorta as a donor site because we believe that it is more readily accessible than the subdiaphragmatic supraceliac aorta (Fig. 7.13). A left thoracoabdominal incision is made below the 8th rib and extended medially across the midline. This incision provides excellent simultaneous exposure of the thoracic aorta and renal artery with no need for extensive abdominal

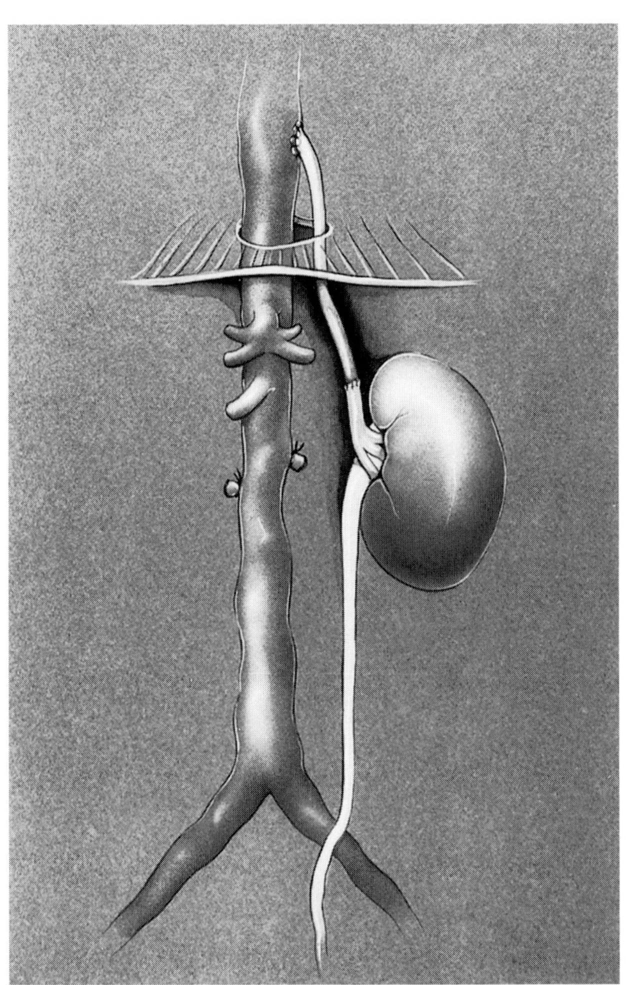

Fig. 7.13

Technique of left thoracic aortorenal revascularization.

visceral mobilization. The left colon is reflected medially to expose the kidney and renal artery. The descending thoracic aorta is exposed above the diaphragm and is partially occluded laterally with a DeBakey clamp. A small aortotomy is made, a reversed saphenous vein graft is anastomosed end-to-side to the aorta, and the aortic clamp is then removed. During performance of the proximal anastomosis, distal aortic flow is preserved and systemic heparinization is therefore not employed. A 2-cm incision is then made in the diaphragm just lateral to the aorta to enlarge the hiatus. The saphenous vein graft is passed alongside the aorta, through the diaphragmatic hiatus, posterior to the pancreas and into the left retroperitoneum. End-to-end anastomosis of the vein graft and distal left renal artery are performed to complete the operation. On the right side the subdiaphragmatic supraceliac or lower thoracic aorta are equally accessible through an anterior bilateral subcostal incision. The technique of thoracic aortorenal bypass is otherwise analogous to that described on the left side.

## Iliorenal Bypass

Iliorenal bypass is an occasionally useful technique for revascularization in patients with severe aortic atherosclerosis, provided there is satisfactory flow through the diseased aorta and absence of significant iliac disease *(22)*. The author's current approach is to consider this operation only when a splenorenal, hepatorenal, or thoracic aortorenal bypass cannot be done. This preference is based on the fact that aortic atherosclerosis may continue to progress in these patients, and, if so, this process is most likely to involve the intrarenal aorta. Such a development might then compromise flow to a revascularized kidney whose blood supply is derived exclusively from one of the iliac arteries. The suprarenal and supraceliac aorta are more often spared from progressive atherosclerosis, hence our preference for bypass procedures originating from these locations.

Iliorenal bypass is performed through a midline transperitoneal incision after harvesting a long saphenous vein graft (Fig. 7.14). The colon is reflected medially to obtain a simultaneous exposure of the ipsilateral common iliac and renal arteries. The common iliac artery is occluded proximally and distally with bulldog clamps. An oval arteriotomy is made on the anterolateral aspect of the common iliac artery. The distal clamp is temporarily released to enable 20 mL of diluted heparin solution to be instilled into the distal iliac and femoral arteries. Systemic heparinization is not routinely employed.

The proximal end of the saphenous vein graft is spatulated, and the apex of the spatulation is placed at the cephalic end of the arteriotomy. Stay sutures are placed in both cephalic and caudal margins of the anastomosis, which is then completed with interrupted 6-0 arterial sutures. A bulldog clamp is placed across the proximal portion of the vein graft, and the iliac clamps are removed, restoring circulation to the lower extremity. An end-to-end anastomosis of the saphenous vein graft to the distal disease-free renal artery is then performed with interrupted 6-0 arterial sutures. The graft is positioned to allow a tension-free distal anastomosis while avoiding angulation or kinking of the renal artery.

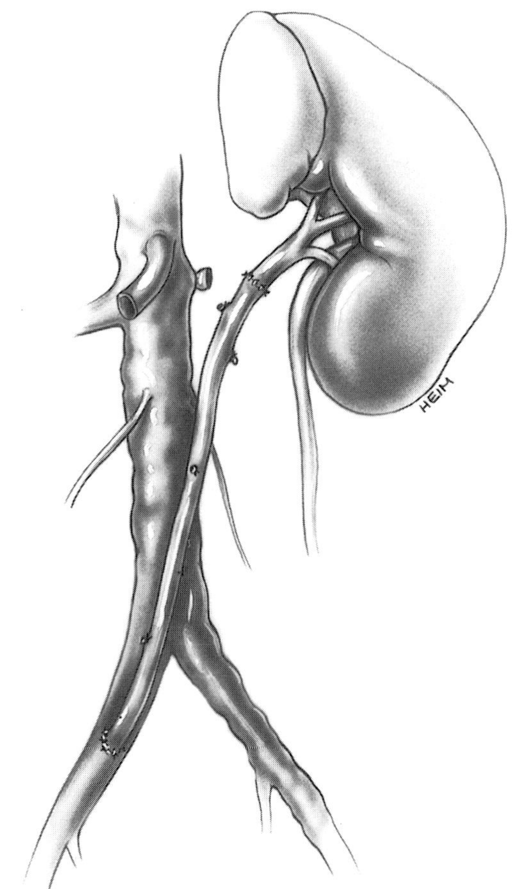

**Fig. 7.14**

Technique of iliorenal bypass with a saphenous vein graft.

## Mesenterorenal Bypass

In unusual cases, aortography reveals an enlarged superior mesenteric artery (SMA), which may then be employed for visceral arterial bypass to either kidney (Fig. 7.15). We have employed the superior mesenterorenal bypass technique in occasional patients with a troublesome aorta in whom a bypass to the kidney from the celiac or iliac arteries is not possible *(23)*. The finding of an enlarged and widely patent SMA is most often observed in patients with total occlusion of the infrarenal

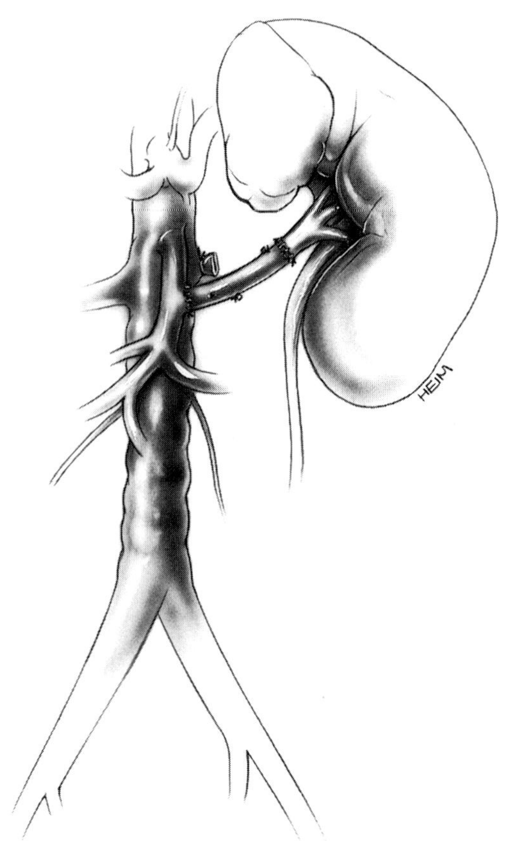


**Fig. 7.15**

Technique of superior mesenterorenal bypass to the left kidney with a saphenous vein graft.

aorta. In such cases, the SMA has a wider caliber than normal because it is supplying collateral vessels to areas ordinarily vascularized from the infrarenal aorta (i.e., the large bowel, pelvis, and lower extremities).

To perform mesenterorenal bypass, the abdomen is entered through a midline incision. During revascularization of the left kidney, the descending colon and splenic flexure are reflected medially and a plan of dissection is developed between the pancreas and first portion of jejunum cephalad, while the mesocolon is reflected medially. If necessary, additional exposure may be obtained by mobilization and evisceration of the right colon and small bowel, as is done commonly for retroperitoneal lymphadenectomy. During revascularization of the right kidney, the ascending colon and duodenum are reflected medially to gain exposure of the aorta and right renal artery. The SMA is mobilized for a distance of 2–3 cm beyond its origin, where it is most accessible and without branches. The renal artery then is exposed and isolated similarly. A reversed segment of saphenous vein is anastomosed end-to-side to the lateral aspect of the SMA with interrupted 6-0 vascular sutures. After completion of this anastomosis, which generally takes 15–20 min, blood flow through the SMA is restored immediately and the saphenous vein graft is occluded temporarily. End-to-end anastomosis of the vein graft to the renal artery then is done with interrupted 6-0 vascular sutures.

## Extracorporeal Microvascular Branch Renal Artery Reconstruction

Vascular disease involving the branches of the renal artery is most often caused by one of the fibrous dysplasias, namely, intimal, medial, or perimedial fibroplasia. Other causes of branch disease include an arterial aneurysm, arteriovenous malformation, Takayasu's arteritis, neurofibromatosis, trauma, and, rarely, atherosclerosis.

Branch renal artery lesions can often be repaired *in situ* with an aortorenal bypass when distal branches free of disease are present outside the renal hilus. Extracorporeal branch arterial repair and autotransplantation are indicated primarily when preoperative arteriography, with oblique views, demonstrates intrarenal extension of renovascular disease *(24–27)*. The advantages of employing an extracorporeal surgical approach include optimum exposure and illumination, a bloodless surgical field, greater protection of the kidney from ischemia, and more facile employment of microvascular techniques and optical magnification. Removing and flushing the kidney also causes it to contract in size, thereby enabling more peripheral dissection in the renal sinus for mobilization of distal arterial branches. Finally, the completed branch anastomosis can be tested for patency and integrity before autotransplantation.

In evaluating patients for extracorporeal revascularization and autotransplantation, preoperative renal and pelvic arteriography should be performed to define renal arterial anatomy, to ensure disease-free iliac vessels, and to assess the hypogastric artery and its branches for use as a reconstructive graft.

Extracorporeal revascularization and autotransplantation are generally performed through an anterior subcostal transperitoneal incision combined with a separate lower quadrant transverse semi-lunar incision. For non-obese patients, a single midline incision extending from the xiphoid process to the symphysis pubis may be used. Immediately after its removal, the kidney is flushed intra-arterially with 500 mL of a chilled intracellular electrolyte solution and is then submerged in a basin of ice-slush saline to maintain hypothermia (Fig. 7.16). The extracorporeal operation is completed under ice-slush surface hypothermia, and, if there has been minimal warm renal ischemia, the kidney can be safely preserved in this manner for many more hours than are needed to perform even the most complex renal

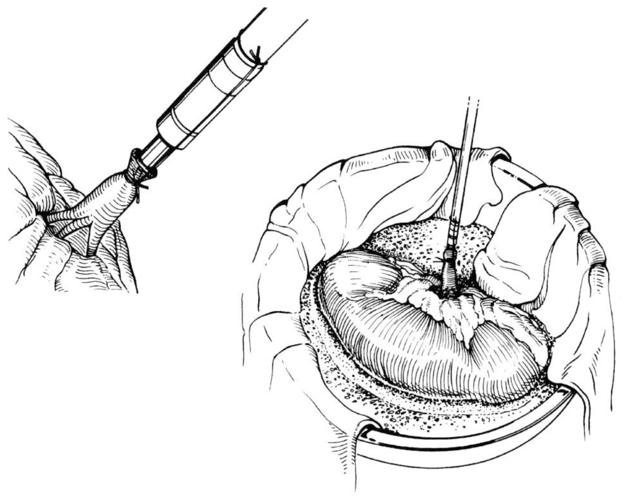

**Fig. 7.16**

The removed kidney is flushed intra-arterially with a cold electrolyte solution and is placed in a basin of ice slush to maintain hypothermia.

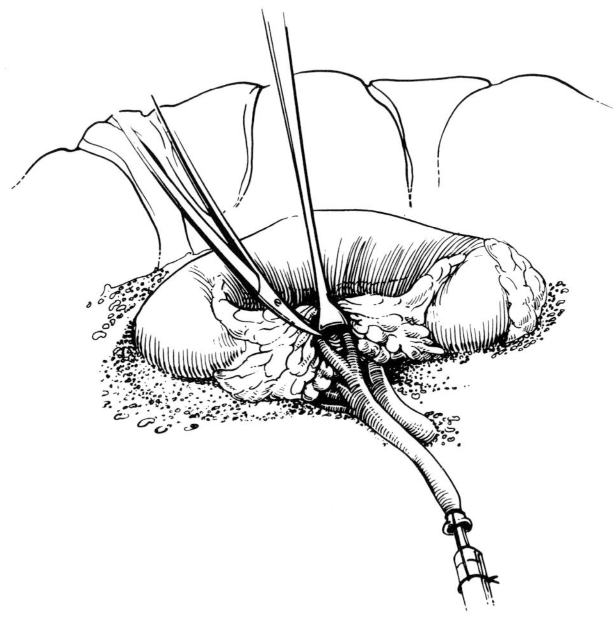

**Fig. 7.17**

Under surface hypothermia, the diseased renal artery branches are mobilized in the renal sinus.

repair. In performing extracorporeal revascularization, we have found it cumbersome to work on the abdominal wall with the ureter attached. It is preferable to divide the ureter and place the kidney on a separate workbench.

After removal and flushing of the kidney, and with maintenance of surface hypothermia, the renal artery branches are mobilized distally in the renal sinus beyond the area of vascular disease (Fig. 7.17). During this dissection, care is taken not to interfere with ureteral or renal

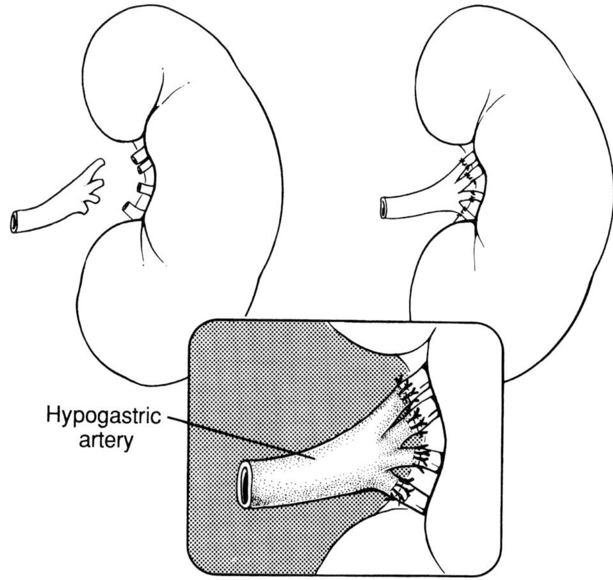


**Fig. 7.18**

Extracorporeal repair with a branched hypogastric arterial autograft.

pelvic blood supply. When the diseased renal artery branches are completely exposed, an appropriate technique for vascular reconstruction is selected.

The optimum method for extracorporeal branch renal artery repair involves the use of a branched autogenous vascular graft *(24)*. This technique permits separate end-to-end microvascular anastomosis of each graft branch to a distal renal artery branch (Fig. 7.18). A hypogastric arterial autograft is the preferred material for vascular reconstruction because this vessel may be obtained intact with several of its branches.

Occasionally the hypogastric artery is not suitable for use as a reconstructive graft because of atherosclerotic degeneration. When this occurs, a long segment of saphenous vein can be harvested and, employing sequential end-to-side microvascular anastomoses, a branched graft can be fashioned from this vessel. This branched graft is then used in a similar manner to achieve reconstruction of the diseased renal artery branches (Fig. 7.19).

Branched grafts of the hypogastric artery and saphenous vein may occasionally prove too large in caliber for anastomosis to small secondary or tertiary renal arterial branches. In these cases, the inferior epigastric artery provides an excellent alternative free graft for extracorporeal microvascular repair *(28)*. This artery measures 1.5–2.0 mm in diameter, is rarely diseased, and coapts nicely in caliber and thickness to small renal artery branches (Fig. 7.20). The inferior epigastric artery may also be employed as a branched graft, either individually or in conjunction with a segment of saphenous vein.

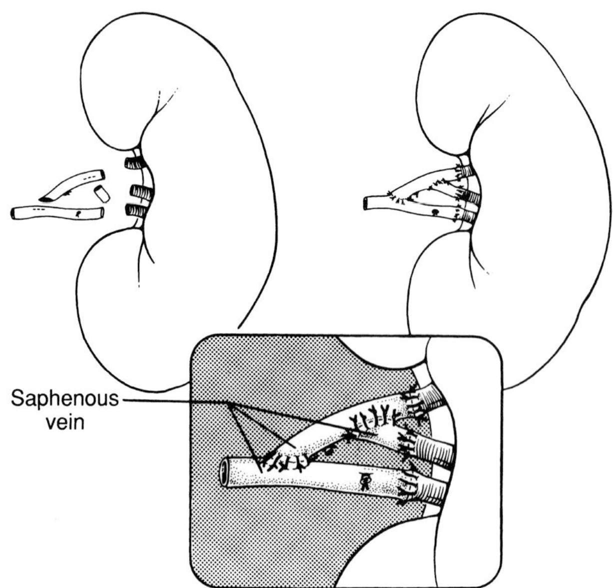


**Fig. 7.19**

Extracorporeal repair with a branched saphenous vein graft.

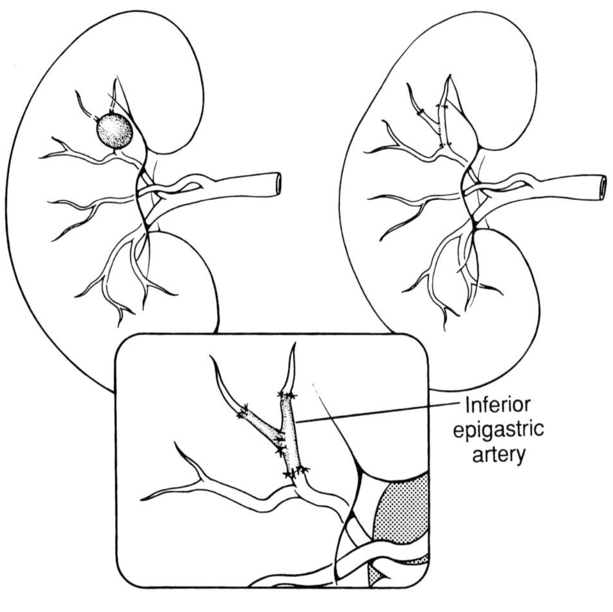


**Fig. 7.20**

Extracorporeal repair with a branched autogenous graft of the inferior epigastric artery.

Renal artery aneurysms have a variable presentation and the method of extracorporeal repair is determined by whether renovascular involvement is focal or diffuse *(25)*. If the renal artery wall at the base of an aneurysm is intact, aneurysmectomy with patch angioplasty can be performed. Aneurysms with short focal involvement of renal artery branches may also be simply resected with end-to-side branch reanastomosis or end-to-side reimplantation into an adjacent branch. In other cases, with

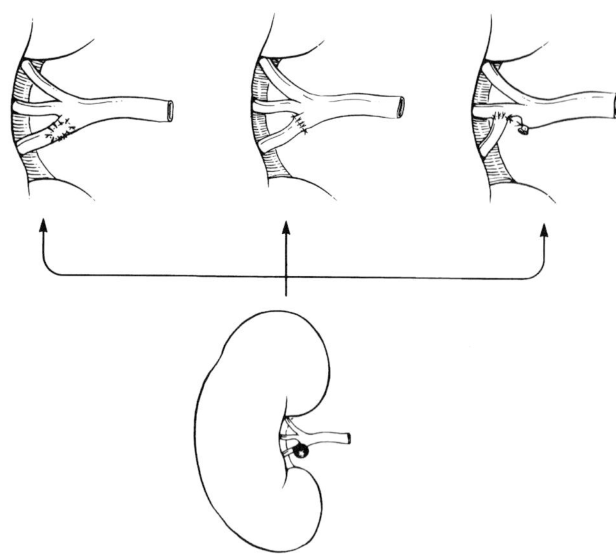

**Fig. 7.21**

Technique for renal artery aneurysmectomy with patch angioplasty (**right**), resection and reanastomosis (**middle**), or end-to-side reimplantation (**left**).

more extensive vascular disease, aneurysmectomy and revascularization with a branched autogenous graft are indicated (Fig. 7.21).

When extracorporeal revascularization has been completed, the kidney is either reflushed or placed on the hypothermic pulsatile perfusion unit to verify patency and integrity of the repaired branches. Renal autotransplantation into the iliac fossa is then performed, with anastomosis of the renal vessels to the iliac vessels and restoration of urinary continuity by ureteroneocystostomy.

## POSTOPERATIVE CARE

Patients undergoing surgical renal revascularization may experience wide fluctuations in blood pressure in the early postoperative period, with either hypotensive or hypertensive episodes, which may predispose to graft thrombosis or bleeding from vascular anastomotic sites, respectively. Therefore, these patients are placed in the intensive care unit for monitoring of the central venous pressure, urine output, pulse rate, and serum levels of hemoglobin and creatinine. During this period, the diastolic blood pressure is maintained at approx 90 mmHg to ensure satisfactory renal perfusion. If hypertensive episodes occur, they are managed with intravenous infusion of sodium nitroprusside. Within the first 24 h postoperatively, a technetium-99m renal scan is obtained to verify perfusion of the revascularized kidney. If clear evidence of perfusion is not present, then arteriography should be done immediately to examine the repaired renal artery.

If the patient's condition is stable, the nasogastric tube, central venous line, arterial line, and urethral catheter are removed 48 h postoperatively, and intensive care monitoring is discontinued. Most patients are discharged from the hospital 1 wk postoperatively. Subsequent follow-up is performed by periodic evaluation of the blood pressure, serum creatinine level, and technetium-99m renal scanning.

## REFERENCES


1. Novick AC, Ziegelbaum M, Vidt DG, et al. Trends in surgical revascularization for renal artery disease: yen year's experience. JAMA 257:498–501, 1987
2. Novick AC. Percutaneous transluminal angioplasty and surgery of the renal artery. Eur J Vasc Surg 8:1–9, 1994.
3. Steinbach F, Novick AC, Campbell S, Dykstra D. Long-term survival after surgical revascularization for atherosclerotic renal artery disease. J Urol 158:38–41, 1997.
4. Stewart BH, Dustan HP, Kiser WS, et al. Correlation of angiography and natural history in evaluation of patients with renovascular hypertension. J Urol 104:231–238, 1970.
5. Novick AC. Renal artery aneurysms and arteriovenous fistulas. In Vascular Problems in Urologic Surgery, (Novick AC, Straffon RA, eds). WB Saunders Co., Philadelphia, 1982, pp 189–204.
6. Schreiber MJ, Pohl MA, Novick AC. The natural history of atherosclerotic and fibrous renal artery disease. Urol Clin North Am 11:383–392, 1984.
7. Straffon RA, Siegel DF. Saphenous vein bypass graft in the treatment of renovascular hypertension. Urol Clin North Am 2:337–350, 1975.
8. Novick AC, Stewart BH, Straffon RA. Autogenous arterial grafts in the treatment of renal artery stenosis. J Urol 118:919–922, 1977.
9. Khauli RB, Novick AC, Coseriu GV. Renal revascularization and polytetrafluoroethylene grafts. Cleve Clin Quart 51:365–369, 1984.
10. Streem SB, Novick AC. Aotorenal bypass with a branched saphenous vein graft for in situ repair of multiple segmental renal arteries. Surg Gynecol Obstet 155:855–859, 1982.
11. Poutasse EF. Renal artery aneurysms. J Urol 113:443–449, 1976.
12. Ortenberg J, Novick AC, Straffon RA, Stewart BH. Surgical treatment of renal artery aneurysm. Br J Urol 55:341–346, 1983.
13. Tarazi RY, Hertzer NR, Beven EG, et al. Simultaneous aortic reconstruction and renal revascularization: Risk factors and late results in 89 patients. J Vasc Surg 5:707–714, 1987.
14. Shahian DM, Najafi H, Javid H, et al. Simultaneous aortic and renal artery reconstruction. Arch Surg 115:1491–1497, 1980.
15. Dean RH, Keyser JE III, DuPont WD, et al. Aortic and renal vascular disease. Ann Surg 200:336–344, 1984.
16. Fergany A, Kolettis P, Novick AC. The contemporary role of extra-anatomic surgical renal revascularization in patients with atherosclerotic renal artery disease. J Urol 153:1798–1802, 1995.
17. Khauli R, Novick AC, Ziegelbaum W. Splenorenal bypass in the treatment of renal artery stenosis: experience with 69 cases. J Vasc Surg 2:547–551, 1985.
18. Chibaro EA, Libertino JA, Novick AC. Use of hepatic circulation for renal revascularization. Ann Surg 199:406–14–17, 1984.
19. Novick AC, Palleschi J, Straffon RA, Beven E. Experimental and clinical hepatorenal bypass as a means of revascularization of the right renal artery. Surg Gynecol Obstet 148:557–561, 1979.
20. Novick AC, McElroy J. Renal revascularization by end-to-end anastomosis of the hepatic and renal arteries. J Urol 134:1089–1093, 1985.
21. Novick AC. Use of the thoracic aorta for renal arterial reconstruction. J Vasc Surg 19(4):605–609, 1994.
22. Novick AC, Banowsky LH. Iliorenal saphenous vein bypass: alternative for renal revascularization in patients with surgically difficult aorta. J Urol 122:243–245, 1979.
23. Khauli RB, Novick AC, Coseriu GV, et al. Superior mesenterorenal bypass for renal revascularization with infrarenal aortic occlusion. J Urol 133:188–190, 1985.
24. Novick AC. Management of intrarenal branch arterial lesions with extracorporeal microvascular reconstruction and autotransplantation. J Urol 162:150–154, 1981.
25. Novick AC. Extracorporeal microvascular reconstruction and autotransplantation for branch renal artery disease. In Renal Vascular Disease (Novick AC, Scoble J, Hamilton G, eds). WB Saunders Co., London, 1996. pp 497–509.
26. Dean RH, Meacham PW, Weaver FA. Ex vivo renal artery reconstructions: indications and techniques. J Vasc Surg 49:546–552, 1986.
27. Dubernard JM, Martin X, Mongin D, et al. Extracorporeal replacement of the renal artery: Techniques, indications and long-term results. J Urol 133:13–16, 1985.
28. Novick AC. Use of inferior epigastric artery for extracorporeal microvascular branch renal artery reconstruction. Surgery 89:513–517, 1981.

# 8 Surgical Technique of Cadaver Donor Nephrectomy

*Venkatesh Krishnamurthi*

## BACKGROUND

Numerous advances in surgical technique and immunosuppressive therapy have led to the current status of renal transplantation as a highly successful treatment option for patients with chronic kidney disease. Presently, more than 50,000 patients await kidney transplantation, and, despite considerable efforts to meet the increasing demand, the number of suitable cadaveric kidneys remains stable (approx 18,200 cadaveric kidney transplants in 2002). This ever-increasing disparity requires the urological surgeon to have a thorough understanding of the principles of kidney procurement for transplantation. On a broad level, the goals of cadaver donor nephrectomy are identification of suitable cadaveric kidney donors and technical performance of the operation such that the excellent organ function is achieved.

The vast majority of cadaveric donors satisfy criteria for brain death. Recent improvements in outcomes with transplantation of kidneys from donors suffering cardiac death (non-heart-beating donors) have slightly increased the pool of potential kidney donors by adding donors who may not meet strict brain death criteria. In general, cadaveric kidney donors range between the ages of 12 mo and 75 yr. The history is reviewed, and chronic conditions that affect renal function, such as hypertension or diabetes, are noted. Additionally, the hospital course both prior to and after declaration of brain death should also be reviewed. Changes in hemodynamic parameters, such as prolonged periods of hypotension, may result in acute tubular necrosis and delayed graft function posttransplantation. Furthermore vasopressor use, particularly at high doses, may result in renal vasoconstriction and add to graft dysfunction. Normal renal function is verified by clinical assessment of the urine output during the period of hospitalization and laboratory analysis of blood urea nitrogen, serum creatinine, and urinalysis.

## SURGICAL TECHNIQUE

Cadaver donor nephrectomy is most often performed in conjunction with procurement of other solid organs for transplantation. Frequently, this includes procurement of heart and lungs as well as liver and pancreas. Operative techniques of liver and pancreas procurement are not discussed in this chapter; but knowledge of the operative principles of liver and pancreas procurement are useful to the kidney procurement surgeon. The principles of abdominal organ procurement are the same regardless of the organs removed. These include wide exposure, cannulation for *in situ* perfusion, isolation of organs to be removed in continuity with their central vascular structures, and orderly removal of the organs under cold perfusion. In the setting of a combined thoracic and multiple abdominal organ donor, the initial dissection is performed by the thoracic and liver-procurement teams. After cross-clamping and perfusion, the organs are removed in the following order: heart, lungs, liver, pancreas, and kidneys. This chapter focuses on the operative technique of kidney procurement in kidney-only cadaveric organ donors.

### Exposure and Initial Dissection

Following hemodynamic stabilization, the organ donor is brought to the operating room and placed in the supine position. A small rolled towel may be placed between the shoulder blades, and the neck can then be hyperextended to facilitate median sternotomy. A long midline incision from the suprasternal notch to the symphysis pubis is utilized to obtain exposure (*see* Chapter 1). A median sternotomy is not absolutely necessary in kidney-only procurement procedures, but the improved exposure afforded by this maneuver enables easier control of proximal aorta and allows for venous outflow in the chest. The sternum is retracted with a sternal retractor, and the abdomen is widely retracted with a large Balfour retractor

From: *Operative Urology at the Cleveland Clinic*
Edited by: A. Novick et al. © Humana Press Inc., Totowa, NJ

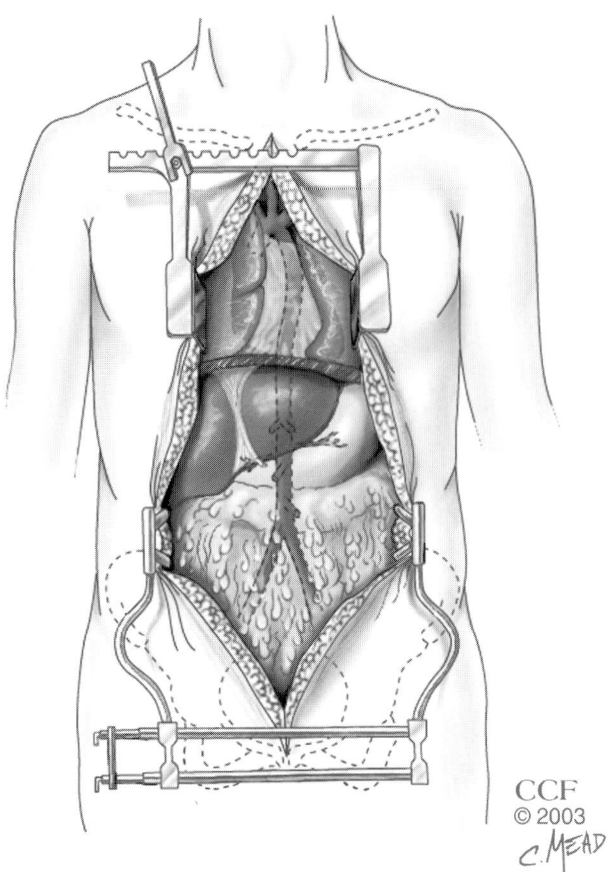


**Fig. 8.1**

Exposure for cadaver organ procurement.

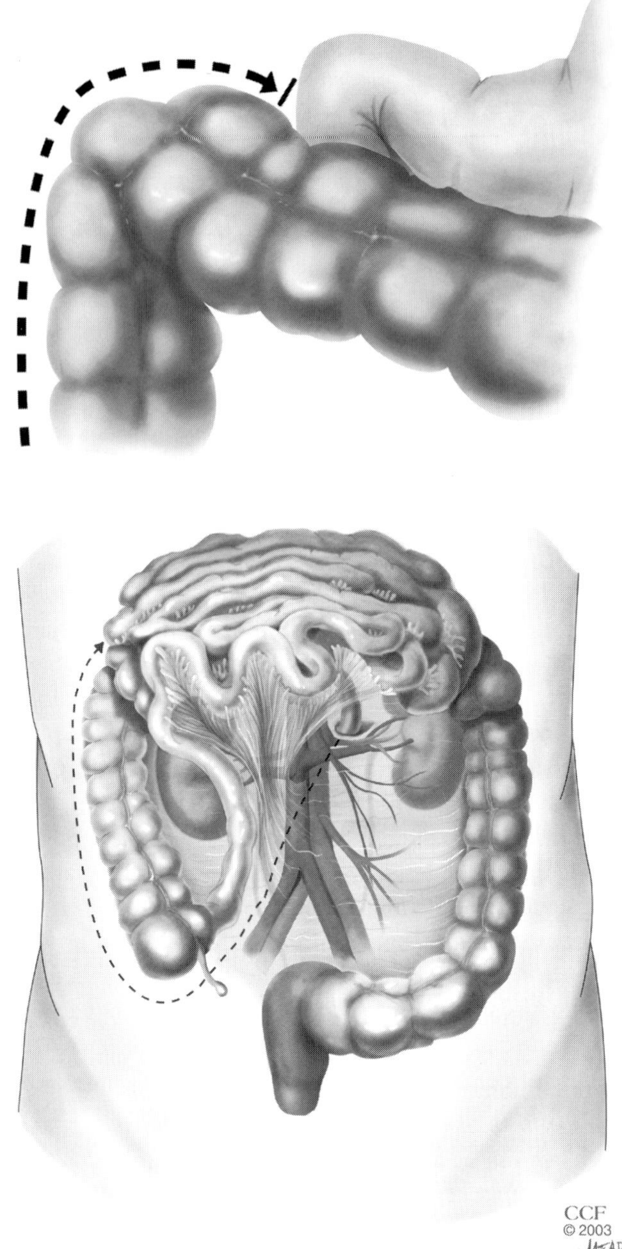


**Fig. 8.2**

Incision along peritoneal reflection for complete mobilization of small bowel and right colon.

(Fig. 8.1). Assurance of complete neuromuscular blockade is essential to maximizing exposure.

The initial steps in the abdominal dissection of all cadaveric organ donors should be directed toward exposure of the retroperitoneal structures and isolation of the distal aorta for cannulation. Performance of this step early in the operation allows for immediate cannulation should the donor become unstable. The retroperitoneum is exposed by incising the posterior peritoneum beginning near the root of the small bowel mesentery and continuing around the hepatic flexure *(1)* (Fig. 8.2). Division of the inferior mesenteric vein (IMV) allows for improved exposure of the left renal vein. The viscera are then generously retracted superiorly, and the impulse of the superior mesenteric artery (SMA) should be palpable directly superior to the left renal vein. The abundant neural and lymphatic tissue around this vessel should be divided, and the SMA should be carefully encircled at this location. It is imperative to maintain the dissection on the SMA adventitia, as attempts to encircle this vessel from the incorrect dissection plane are fraught with difficulty and may result in significant bleeding. Additionally, the SMA should be isolated near its origin from the aorta, as aberrant hepatic arterial branches may hamper dissection beyond the first 1–2 cm. Although not absolutely necessary, isolation of the SMA aids in identification of aberrant hepatic arteries when the liver and pancreas are being procured and, more importantly, for the purpose of kidney-only procurement, enables the surgeon to maximize kidney perfusion (through occlusion of the SMA).

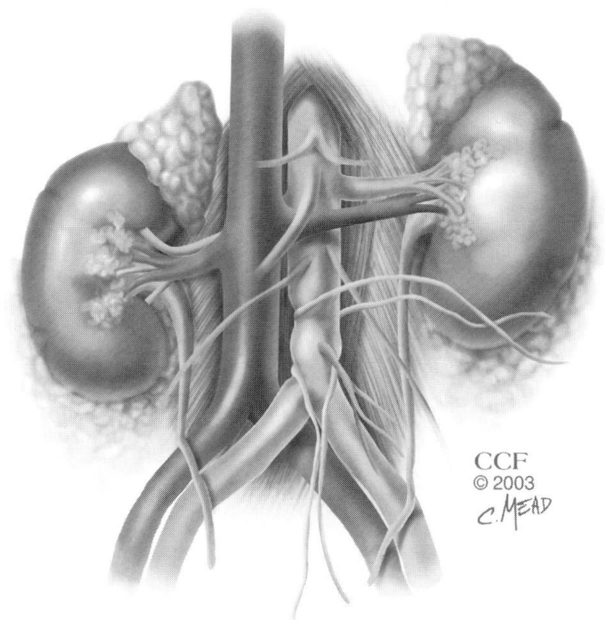


**Fig. 8.3**

Isolation of distal aorta for cannulation.

## Isolation of the Distal Aorta

The distal aorta from the inferior mesenteric artery (IMA) to the aortic bifurcation is now isolated. The aorta should be encircled with an umbilical tape at its bifurcation, and a second umbilical tape should be passed around the aorta at the level of the IMA or, if this vessel is not visible, 3–4 cm proximal to the bifurcation (Fig. 8.3). The IMA can be divided after ensuring that it is not an aberrant, low-lying renal artery. Posterior lumbar arteries along the distal aorta can be visualized by gently pulling up on the aorta with the umbilical tapes. These vessels cause troublesome bleeding during cannulation and thus should be clipped or tied. The great vessels and retroperitoneal contents on the right have already been exposed from the initial dissection, and by incising along the lateral peritoneal reflection and mobilizing the left colon medially, the left kidney is also exposed. This ensures that both kidneys will be in direct contact with iced slush. At this point no further dissection is performed on the kidneys until after cross-clamp and perfusion.

## Isolation of the Proximal Aorta

The next step involves isolation of the supraceliac aorta. Control of this segment of the aorta is most often obtained in the abdomen but supradiaphragmatic control can be obtained in certain situations. Isolation of the supraceliac aortic is begun by first mobilizing the left lateral segment of the liver. The left lateral segment is carefully retracted caudally, and the left triangular ligament is divided with the electrocautery. This dissection is continued medially, making sure not to injure the inferior phrenic vein or left hepatic vein. The left lateral segment can now be retracted towards the patient's right, and the gastrohepatic omentum (lesser omentum) is incised from the lesser curvature of the stomach to the diaphragm. The diaphragmatic crura should now be visible. The aortic impulse should palpable beneath the crural fibers and immediately to the right of the esophagus. The crural fibers are divided in a cephalad direction, which avoids potential injury to the origin of the celiac axis (Fig. 8.4). After division of the diaphragmatic crural fibers, the aortic adventitia is visualized. The anterior and lateral surfaces of the aorta are isolated. Circumferential control of the aorta can be obtained (Fig. 8.5) but is not always necessary. If circumferential aortic dissection is performed, care must be taken to avoid injury to the posterior aspect of the aorta or spinal arteries.

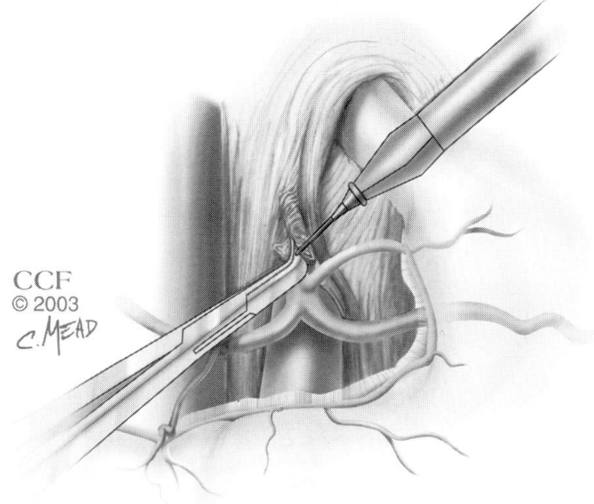


**Fig. 8.4**

Exposure of the supraceliac aorta.

Alternatively, the aortic can be controlled in a supradiaphragmatic location even in the setting of lung procurement. Collaboration with the thoracic team is essential to control the distal thoracic aorta. When the lungs are not being procured, the supradiaphragmatic aorta can be isolated by retracting the left lung and palpating the aorta at the level of the diaphragm.

## Cross-Clamping and *In Situ* Perfusion

The anesthesiologist and other organ-procurement teams are now notified that cross-clamping can proceed. Mannitol (25 g) and heparin (250–300 U/kg) are administered intravenously. A distal aorta is then exposed, and the umbilical tape along the distal aspect is secured. An aortic cannula is placed on the field and connected via tubing to

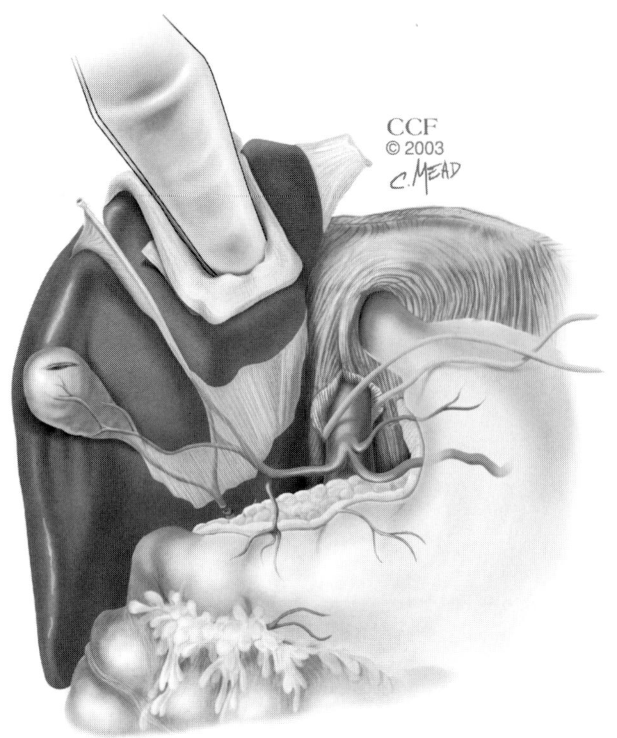


**Fig. 8.5**

Isolation of the supraceliac aorta for cross-clamping.

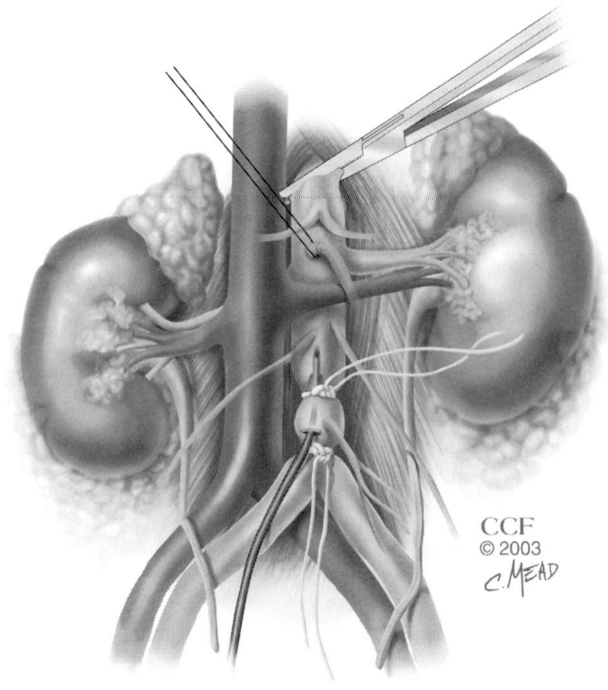


**Fig. 8.6**

Cannulation of the distal aorta.

cold preservation solution. The cannulation line should be flushed to remove any retained air. The distal aorta is controlled with the thumb and the forefinger of the nondominant hand. The anterior wall of the aorta is generously incised, and the cannula is placed within the aorta and secured by tying the proximal umbilical tape (Fig. 8.6). The cannula must be passed far enough to be secured at its flange, but passage too far proximally may prevent perfusion of lower pole renal arterial branches. Additionally, cannulation of an atherosclerotic aorta must be done with great care, as aggressive cannulation can cause an intimal dissection and thrombosis of donor organs.

When all procurement teams are ready, cross-clamping can proceed in the following manner: the umbilical tape around the SMA is now secured (for kidney-only procurement), exsanguination is achieved by the dividing vena cava at its junction with the right atrium, the supraceliac aorta is clamped, and, simultaneously, cold preservation solution is infused. Surface hypothermia is then achieved by liberally placing iced slush solution around both kidneys.

As mentioned previously, occlusion of the SMA, though not essential, improves perfusion to the kidneys. Consideration can also be given to occluding hepatic and pancreatic inflow, which can be a considerable source of perfusate loss. Placement of a large clamp across the porta hepatis (Pringle maneuver) can occlude both the common hepatic artery and the gastroduodenal artery.

Venting venous blood in the chest is preferable since this prevents warm blood from coming in contact with the kidneys. Occasionally, in the setting of heart or lung procurement, venting in the chest may not be possible. Venous blood can be vented in the abdomen by dividing the inferior vena cava (IVC) at its bifurcation. Another technique that allows for more controlled abdominal venting and avoids warm blood from coming in contact with the kidneys is cannulation of the IVC with a urinary catheter drainage bag (Dover® 4-L urinary drainage bag, Sherwood Medical, St. Louis, MO). Two umbilical tapes are passed around the IVC near its bifurcation. Proximate to the time of cross-clamping, the IVC is cannulated by securing the umbilical tape at the bifurcation, creating a small vena cavotomy through which the drainage bag tubing is passed, and then securing the more superior umbilical tape around the IVC and tubing. In this technique, which is performed identical to cannulation of the IMV, venous back bleeding is controlled during insertion of the tubing by gently pulling up on the distal (more superior) umbilical tape. Additionally, a large clamp must be placed across the tubing in order to prevent exsanguination following insertion of the drainage bag tubing. This clamp is simply removed when exsanguination is desired (immediately prior to cross-clamping the aorta). Approximately 2–4 L of preservation solution are perfused through the

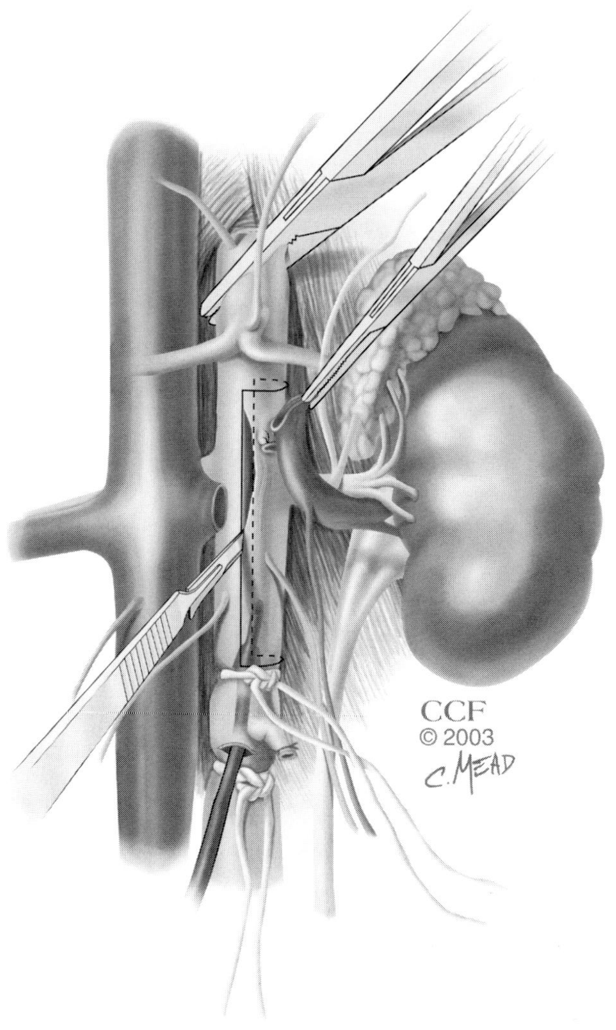


**Fig. 8.7**

*In situ* separation of right and left kidneys. The left renal vein is divided at its entrance to the IVC after which the anterior aspect of the aorta is incised.

aortic cannula. The venous efflux is evaluated, and when it is clear or slightly blood tinged, perfusion is adequate.

## Removal of Donor Kidneys

The donor nephrectomy is commenced by first isolating the distal ureters. The ureters are identified deep in the pelvis and divided. Abundant periureteral tissue should be included in the dissection of the ureters. Both ureters are freed to the level of the kidneys. The kidneys can be procured separately or in an *en bloc* manner. We favor separation of the kidneys *in situ* as optimal spatial orientation is maintained as well as easier handling of the specimen. With *in situ* splitting, the left renal vein is divided at its entrance to the vena cava (Fig. 8.7). The anterior surface of aorta is visualized by dividing the overlying lymphatic tissue and is incised immediately along its anterior aspect.

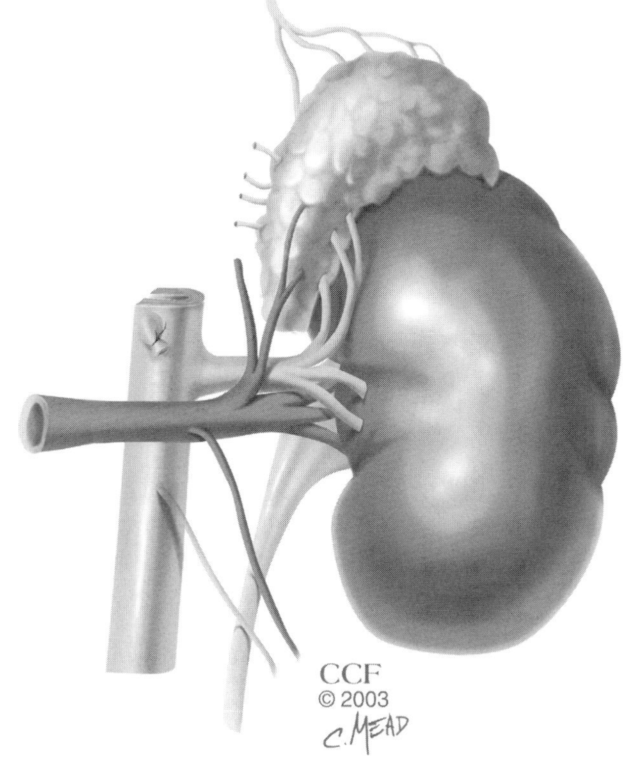


**Fig. 8.8**

Left kidney following separation.

It is essential to maintain the orientation on the anterior aspect of the aorta so as to avoid injury to the renal arteries. The posterior aspect of the aorta is similarly divided. The paired lumbar arteries can serve as a useful landmark when dividing the posterior aorta. The left kidney is then fully mobilized outside of Gerota's fascia along its posterior and superior attachments. The attachments superior to the left adrenal gland are divided so that most or all of the left adrenal gland is included with the left kidney. A large fenestration is made in the mesentery of the left colon, and the kidney is passed medially. Finally, the attachments posterior to the aorta (left half) are divided, and the kidney is removed and placed in iced slush solution (Fig. 8.8). The right kidney is similarly removed. After dividing the distal ureter, the posterior and superior attachments are freed. The kidney is then retracted laterally and upward, and attachments along the hilum are freed by sharply dividing the tissue along the posterior aspect of the right half of the aorta and the spine. The entire length of the vena cava (from bifurcation to suprarenal segment) should be preserved with the right kidney (Fig. 8.9).

*En bloc* removal of the kidneys is an equally acceptable technique and should be the preferred technique for pediatric cadaveric organ donors (<7 yr). In the *en bloc* technique both ureters are divided deep in the pelvis. The

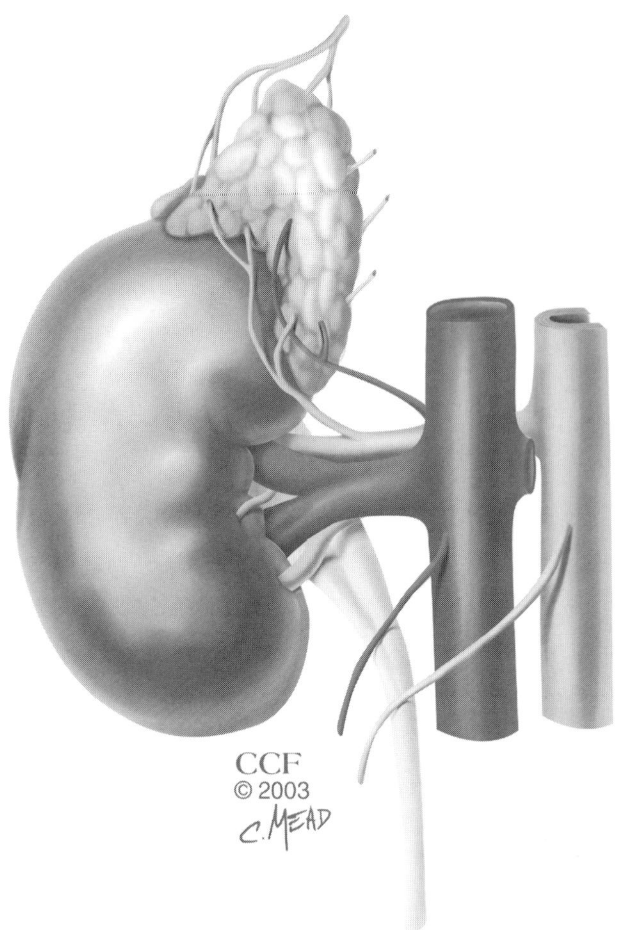


**Fig. 8.9**

Right kidney following separation. An intact IVC is included with the right kidney.

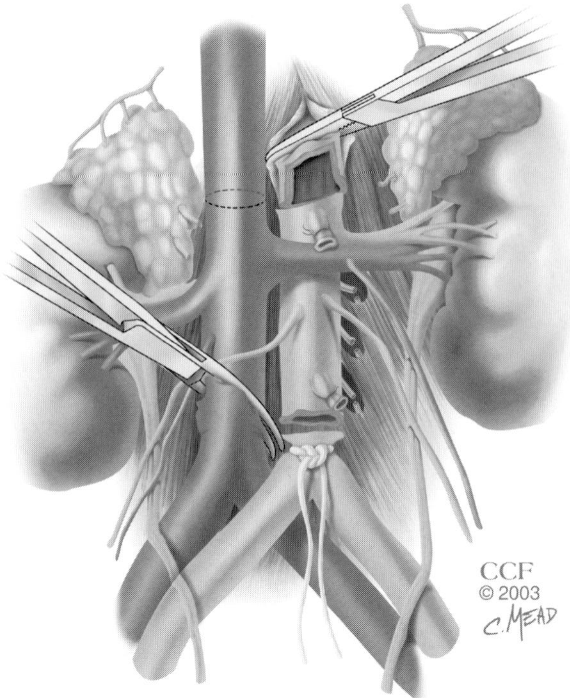


**Fig. 8.10**

Division of great vessels for *en bloc* retrieval of kidneys.

posterior and lateral attachments to the kidney are sharply divided. The attachments superior to each adrenal gland and upper pole kidney are similarly divided. A window is made in the left colon mesentery, through which the left kidney and ureter are passed medially. The proximal aorta and suprarenal vena cava are divided as are the distal aorta and vena cava (Fig. 8.10). The great vessels are freed off the spine by sharply dividing all the posterior attachments. It is important to adequately retract the great vessels as well as to frequently verify the location of the ureters and renal vessels during the *en bloc* removal. After removing both kidneys *en bloc*, they are immediately placed in an iced slush solution. The left renal vein is divided at its origin along the IVC. The posterior wall of the aorta is then divided longitudinally between the lumbar arteries (Fig. 8.11). The aorta is inspected to verify the position and number of the renal arteries. The anterior aspect of the aorta is then divided. Pediatric (<7 yr) donor kidneys should be maintained *en bloc*, as this may be the preferred method of transplantation.

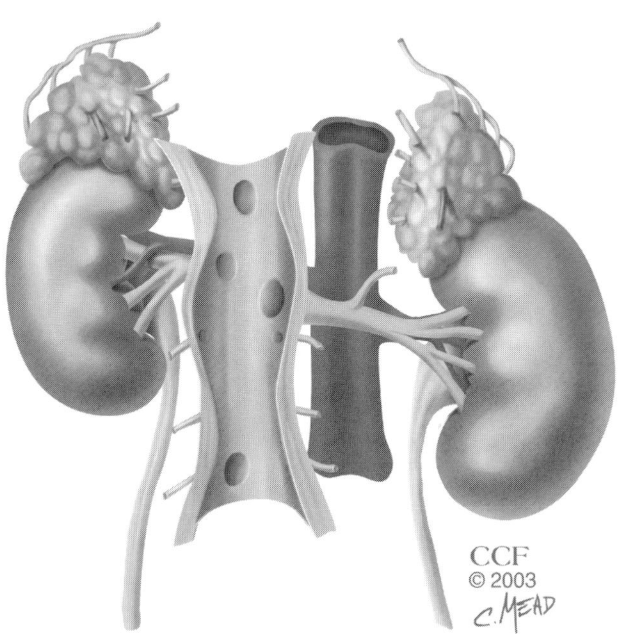


**Fig. 8.11**

Appearance of *en bloc* cadaveric kidney specimen following division of posterior aorta.

The kidneys are then individually inspected for the presence of tumors, cysts, or other abnormalities. The perinephric fat is gently removed. The number, length, and size of the vessels are verified prior to packaging. Each kidney is then placed in two sterile isolation bags and then packaged in a sterile plastic labeled container. It is helpful to remove as much air as possible from the isolation bags, as this will improve cooling.

The spleen and 10 to 15 lymph nodes are removed for histocompatibility testing. Numerous mesenteric lymph nodes can be harvested, and, if inadequate, additional lymph nodes can be found in the pelvis or mediastinum.

## RENAL PRESERVATION

Successful allograft function after transplantation is highly dependent on minimizing ischemic damage. In comparison to the other solid organs procured for transplantation, the kidneys are relatively tolerant to periods of warm and cold ischemia. Ischemic injury to numerous cellular systems begins to occur immediately after cross-clamping. Hypothermia markedly decreases the cellular metabolic demands and thus ameliorates the degree of ischemic damage. Hypothermia-induced cell swelling is a significant source of injury during preservation. For this reason, most organ preservation solutions are formulated to minimize organ damage during ischemia/reperfusion injury from oxygen-free radicals, prevent cell swelling at cold temperatures, and prevent cell membrane destruction. The addition of impermeants such as hydroxyethyl starch, lactobionate, raffinose, and gluconate helps to prevent hypothermia-induced cell swelling.

A number of other factors have also been found to be important in cell damage during preservation. Numerous cellular functions require energy in the form of adenosine triphosphate (ATP). Loss of energy-generating capabilities owing to mitochondrial injury or loss of precursors from cell membrane damage can lead to irreversible cell injury. This concept forms the basis for the addition of ATP precursors such as adenine, adenosine, and ribose to organ-preservation solution. Oxygen-free radical formation after reperfusion also plays an important role in cellular injury during preservation. The addition of free-radical scavengers such as allopurinol and mannitol may be helpful in reducing free-radical formation and oxidative damage.

Currently, the two methods of renal preservation for transplantation include cold storage or continuous machine (pulsatile) perfusion. The majority of transplant centers utilize cold storage due to its relative ease, but experience a higher rate of delayed graft function (DGF) than with pulsatile perfusion. Recent evidence suggests that early DGF significantly influences long-term graft survival. Additionally, with the increasing reliance on expanded criteria donors, pulsatile perfusion may be beneficial in assessing organ quality as well as preserving organ function. Renal hemodynamic perimeters such as perfusate flow and arterial pressure can be continuously assessed, and, from these, renal vascular resistance can be calculated.

## SUMMARY

Renal transplantation is a highly successful therapeutic option for patients with end-stage renal disease. The current level of success has been the result of improvements in surgical technique, immunosuppression, organ preservation, and patient management. The number of patients needing transplantation continues to outgrow the supply of donor organs. The techniques described in this chapter highlight the surgical aspects of organ procurement and preservation. Although these techniques have led to improvement in transplantation, their application is inherently linked to the generous gift of organ donation.

## REFERENCES

1. Cattell RB, Braasch JW. A technique for the exposure of the third and fourth portions of the duodenum. Surg Gynecol Obstet 111:379–380, 1960.

# 9 Open Donor Nephrectomy

*David A. Goldfarb*

The role of open donor nephrectomy has been diminished in the past 10 yr owing to the development of laparoscopic donor nephrectomy. Nonetheless, open donor nephrectomy remains the gold standard to which any new procurement technique must be compared. Open donor nephrectomy does not contend with the issues of pneumoperitoneum-induced renal dysfunction, warm ischemia, or shortened renal vessels (particularly right-sided procurements), compared with laparoscopic donor nephrectomy.

Although most donors will be candidates for laparoscopic donor nephrectomy, there are selected circumstances in which open donor nephrectomy is preferable. These include cases where there has been extensive prior intraperitoneal surgery and left donor nephrectomy is planned. Other circumstances include a very short right renal vein (<1.5 cm) identified by computed tomography (CT) angiography. This issue remains the surgical judgment of the entire transplant team. Even with the retroperitoneal approach to right laparoscopic donor nephrectomy, the right renal vein is transected at the level of the inferior vena cava ( IVC), without the cuff of IVC that is traditionally obtained in an open donor nephrectomy. Finally, any circumstance determined by the transplant team that would not confidently lead to a successful transplantation outcome with laparoscopic procurement should be done by the open technique. This may include situations where there are aberrant anatomical considerations in the recipient.

The development of laparoscopic donor nephrectomy has lead to improvements in the open technique. Incisions are now smaller, and resection of a rib is not mandatory. With appropriate management of patient expectation and perioperative care, the hospital convalescence may be reduced to 3 d, making the technique competitive in this regard with minimally invasive techniques.

## PREOPERATIVE EVALUATION

Preoperative evaluation ensures absence of renal disease or conditions that may affect future renal function. Glomerular filtration rate must exceed 80 mL/min, and there should be no proteinuria (<150 mg/L). Anatomical evaluation is performed using a CT angiography technique. This is an integrated exam combining features of arteriography, venography, and parenchymal assessment in one single examination. Post-CT intravenous pyelogram is used to demonstrate the collecting system. Catheter arteriography is selectively used to evaluate cases with multiple vessels to determine the territory of distribution of respective vessels. Patients are operated as a same-day surgery.

The night before surgery, patients are encouraged to take fluids liberally but are given a magnesium citrate bowel prep. On arrival to the preoperative suite, donors are administered 1 L of intravenous normal saline before anesthetic induction. At the time of renal hilar manipulation, 25 g of mannitol are given intravenously for renal protection. Following procurement, kidneys are flushed with a Euro-Collins solution and cooled in an ice bath.

## OPERATIVE PROCEDURE: RIGHT SIDE

After anesthetic induction and foley placement, the patient is placed in the classic flank position for right donor nephrectomy. The down side is supported by the kidney rest of the table, then the table is flexed and placed in slight Trendelenburg position until the flank is parallel to the floor. A roll is placed in the downside axilla to prevent brachial plexus injury. Legs are appropriately padded. A Turner–Warwick approach may be used, taking the incision between the 11th and 12th rib (*see* Chapter 1). Total incision length should be no more than 15–18 cm. The retroperitoneum is entered and the diaphragm and pleura are dissected free from under the lateral aspect of the 11th rib. The 12th rib is dissected close to its articulation with the spine so it acts like a hinged retractor for the remainder of the operation.

The retroperitoneum is then developed using blunt and sharp dissection. The ureter is identified with surrounding fibroareolar tissue (which contains its blood supply) down to the level of the ipsilateral iliac vessels. The ureter is not divided until later in the case, after confirming that the recipient is imminently transplantable.

From: *Operative Urology at the Cleveland Clinic*
Edited by: A. Novick et al. © Humana Press Inc., Totowa, NJ

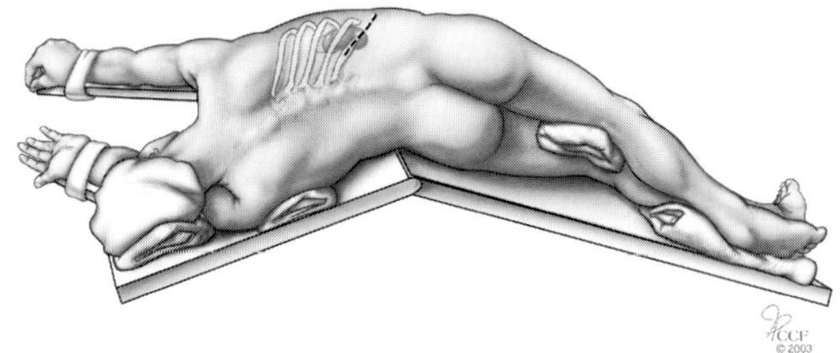


Fig. 9.1

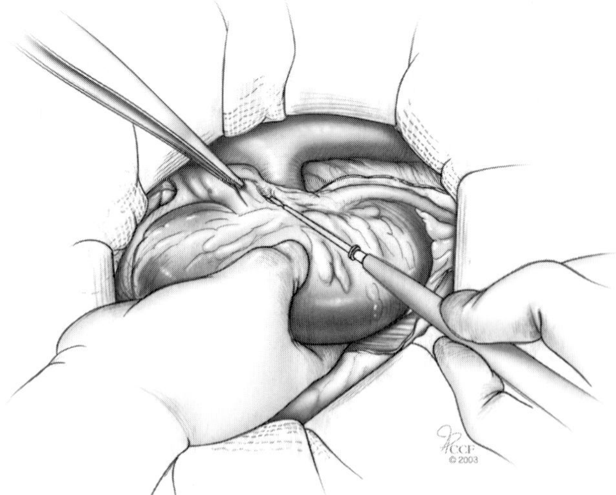


Fig. 9.4

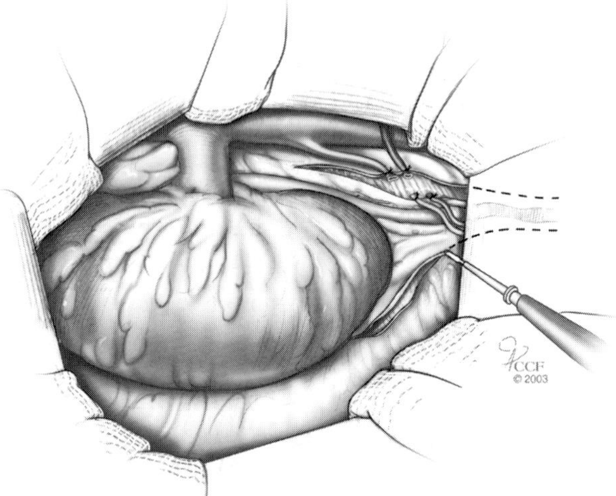


Fig. 9.2

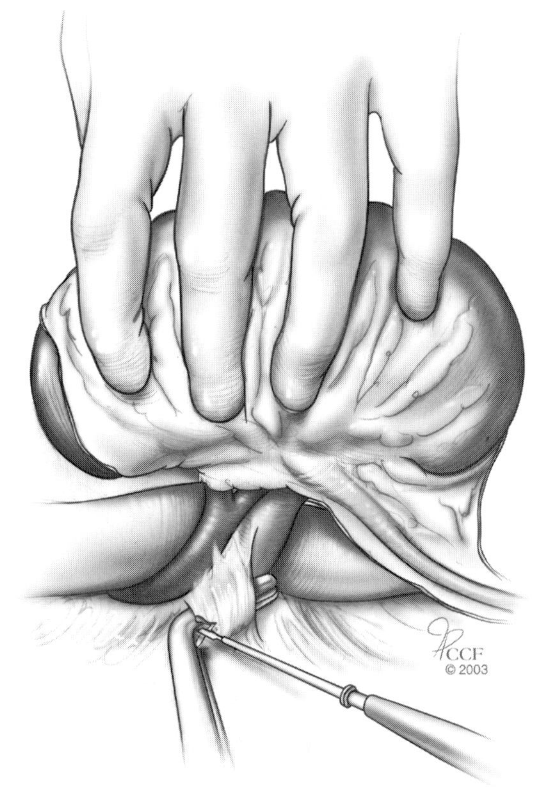


Fig. 9.5

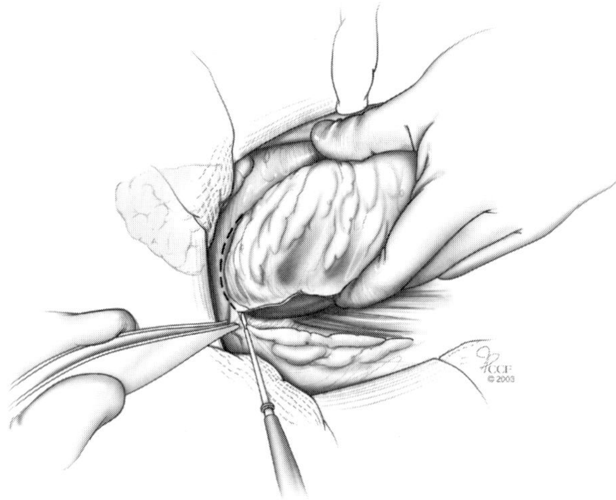


Fig. 9.3

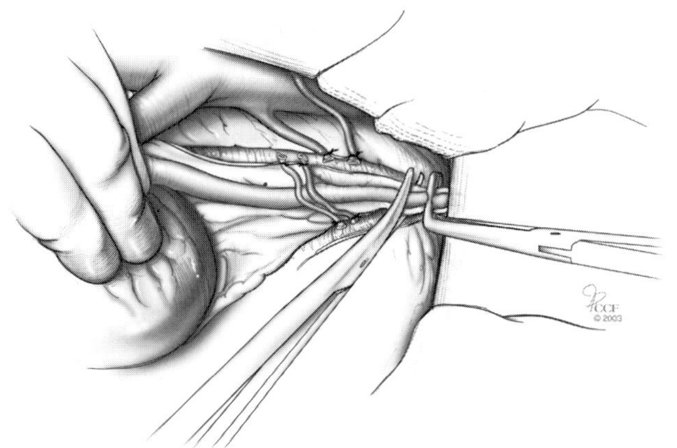


Fig. 9.6

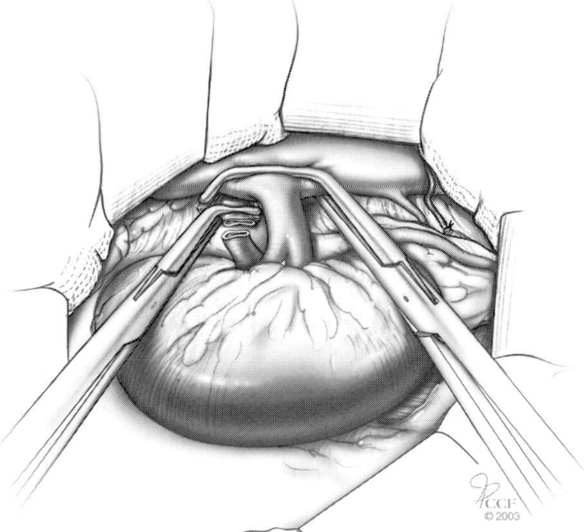


Fig. 9.7

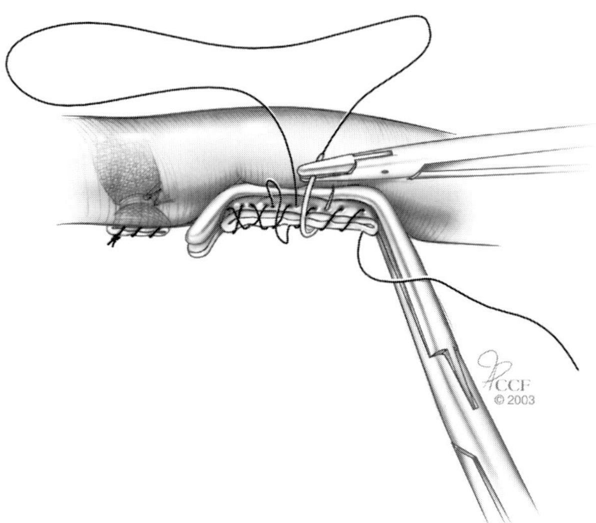


Fig. 9.8

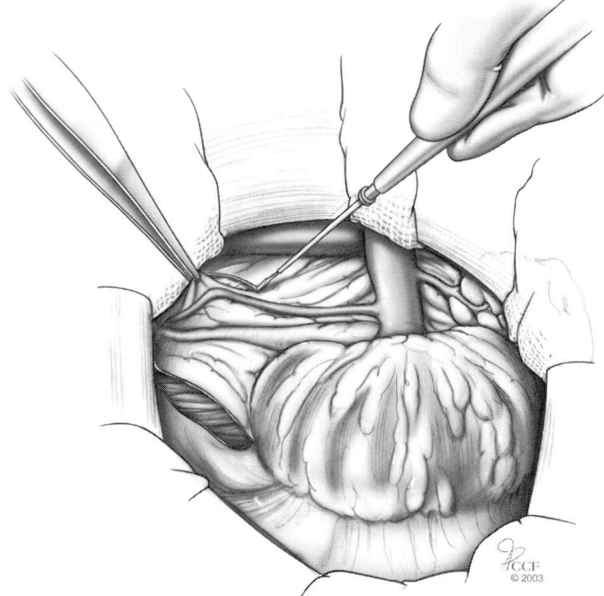


Fig. 9.9

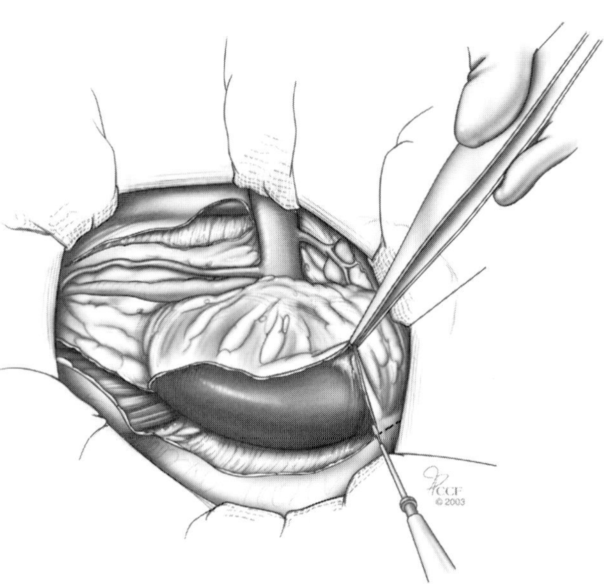


Fig. 9.10

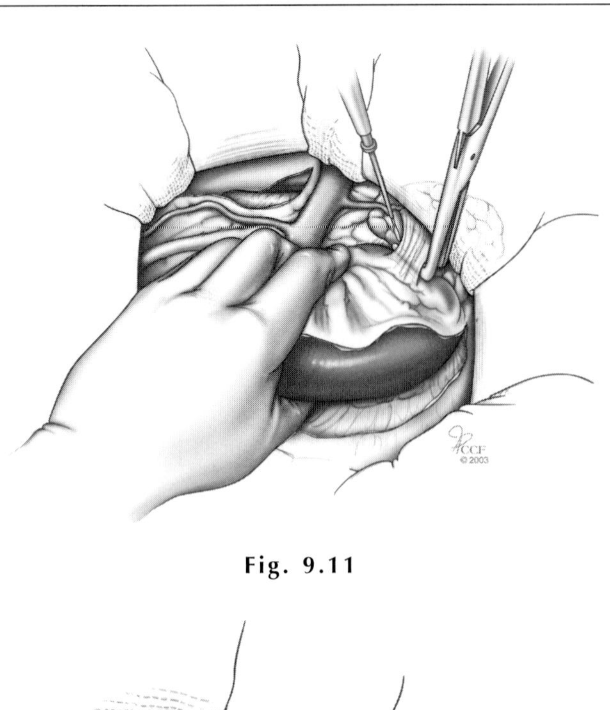


Fig. 9.11

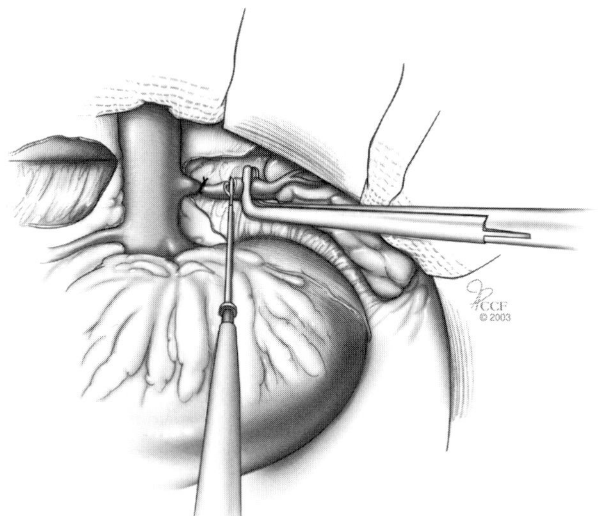


Fig. 9.12

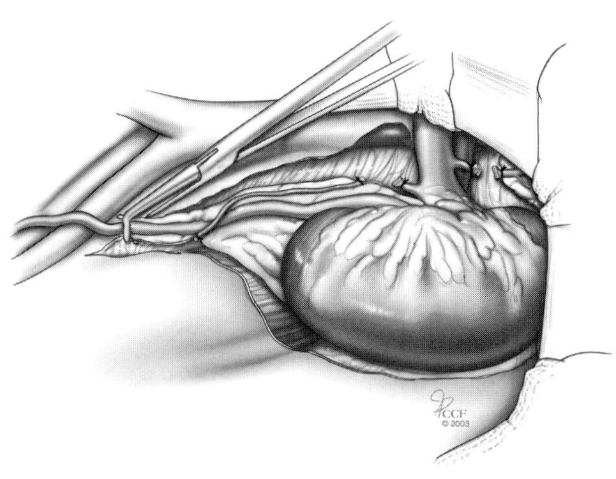


Fig. 9.13

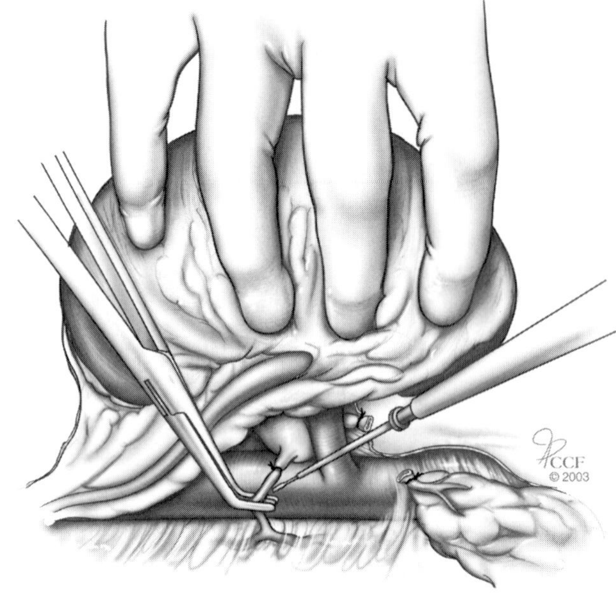


Fig. 9.14

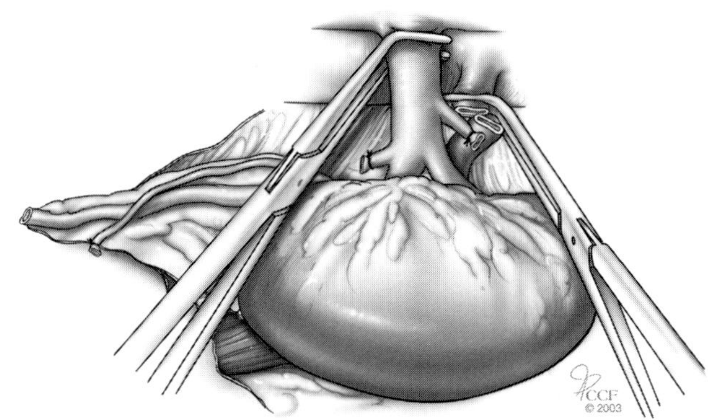


Fig. 9.15

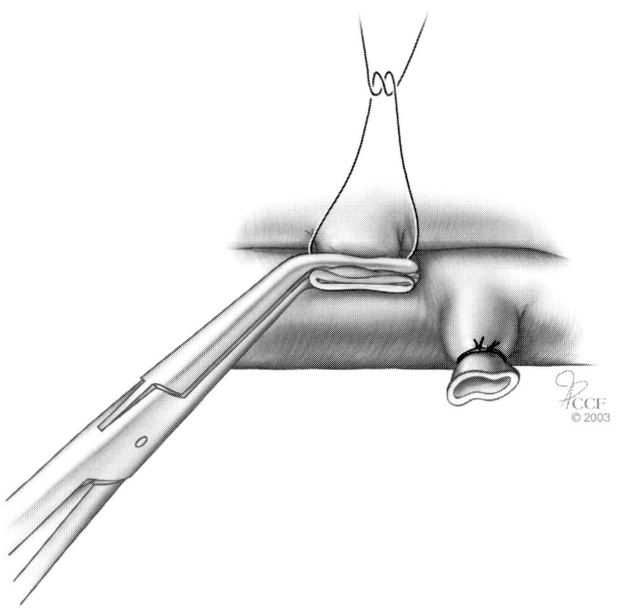


Fig. 9.16

Gerota's fascia is entered, and the kidney is mobilized. The adrenal is spared. Hilar dissection of the renal vein is then carried out. The renal artery is typically in a retro-caval position, and additional length may be achieved by dissected lateral and behind the vena cava. After confirmation with the recipient room that the recipient has favorable vasculature and is medically stable, the ureter can be divided. As much length as possible should be preserved. Also, the peri-ureteral tissues surrounding the ureter should be preserved as they contain ureteral blood supply. The triangle of tissue bordered laterally by the lower pole of the kidney, medially by the IVC and superiorly by the renal hilum represents the territory of the ureteral vasculature.

The remaining retroperitoneal attachments of the kidney are divided with electrocautery so that the kidney remains attached only by the artery and vein. The right renal artery is controlled with a right-angle clamp. The right renal vein encompassing a portion of adjacent IVC is then secured. Using a scissor, the vein is divided including a cuff of the IVC with the donor kidney. This represents an advantage to the open technique over laparoscopy.

The renal artery is doubly ligated with 0 silk ligatures. The renal vein is oversewn with a continuous 4-0 polypropylene suture. Closure of the flank incision (not shown) is in multiple layers using polydioxanone suture. Skin is approximated with clips.

## OPERATIVE PROCEDURE: LEFT SIDE

The incision for the left side is similar to the right. The retroperitoneum is developed. The ureter is identified and traced into the pelvis. The gonadal vein is identified as a landmark, and all tissue between the gonadal vein and the ureter is preserved. A tissue plane is developed between the aorta and gonadal vein, and the peritoneum is swept medially off Gerota's fascia. The gonadal vein can be ligated in the pelvis and then be used a tracer to dissect superiorly until the renal vein is visualized.

A retrorenal and lateral dissection is then carried out. Gerota's fascia may be entered to facilitate this maneuver. At the upper pole, the kidney is separated from the spleen and the adrenal gland carefully. The renal artery is then mobilized by identifying the adrenal vein, then ligating and dividing it between 4-0 silk ties.

The remainder of the renal venous dissection is completed and the gonadal vein is ligated flush near the renal vein. Then, after confirmation that there are no problems with the recipient operation, the ureter may be ligated and divided in the pelvis as far down as is comfortable. Usually this will permit ureteral length to be between 12 and 15 cm. Peri-ureteral blood supply is preserved as with the right side. Using the gonadal vein as the medial border of the dissection will ensure this.

Any lumbar veins are ligated and divided using clips or permanent suture. The renal artery is clamped as close to the aorta as feasible, ensuring adequate space for two 0-silk ties. The renal vein can be clamped over the medial aspect of the aorta to ensure a good length of vein. The artery and vein are then divided. The renal artery is doubly ligated with 0-silk ligature. The vein can be tied with 0-silk ligatures or oversewn if it is too wide. The wound is irrigated and then closed in a manner similar to the right side.

## POSTOPERATIVE CARE

Postoperative care includes early ambulation. Clear liquids can be introduced in most patients on the first postoperative day. Satisfactory intake by 3–4 d is normal. Most patients can be discharged by day 4, and some highly motivated patients by day 3. Laboratory studies to assess renal function and blood counts are monitored in the hospital, then at return office visit in 4–6 wk.

## SUGGESTED READINGS


1. El Fettouh HA, Herts BR, Nimeh T, et al. Prospective comparison of 3-dimensional volume rendered computerized tomography and conventional renal arteriography for surgical planning in patients undergoing laparoscopic donor nephrectomy. J Urol 170:57.
2. Goldfarb DA, Matin SF, Braun WE, et al. Renal outcome 25 years after donor nephrectomy. J Urol 166: 2043–2047, 2001.
3. Matas AJ, Bartlett ST, Leichtman AB, Delmonico FL. Morbidity and mortality after living kidney donation, 1999-2001: survey of United States transplant centers. Am J Transplant 3:830–834, 2003.
4. Serrano DP, Flechner SM, Modlin CS, Streem SB, Goldfarb DA, Novick AC. The use of kidneys from living donors with renal vascular disease: expanding the donor pool. J Urol 157:1587–1591, 1997.
5. Streem SB, Novick AC, Hodge E, Duriak K, Nally J. Preoperative hospitalization to hydrate living kidney donors can be omitted without sacrificing graft function. J Urol 150:1779–1781, 1993.
6. Streem SB, Novick AC, Steinmuller DR, Graneto Flank donor nephrectomy efficacy in the donor and recipient. J Urol 141:1099–1101, 1989.
7. Turner Warwick RT. The supracostal approach to the renal area. Br J Urol 37:671–672, 1965.

# 10 Living Laparoscopic Donor Nephrectomy

*Alireza Moinzadeh and Inderbir S. Gill*

## INTRODUCTION

Given the nearly 60,000 patients waiting for renal transplantation, living donor nephrectomy has become a significant source of kidney donation supplementing the shortage of available cadaveric kidneys in the United States. The first laparoscopic living donor nephrectomy (LLDN) was performed by Ratner 10 yr ago with the aim of reducing the morbidity associated with the open procedure. Since that time, more than 200 institutions worldwide have gained expertise in performing LLDN. In 2004, it was estimated that more than 10,000 kidneys had been retrieved with laparoscopic assistance.

## PATIENT SELECTION AND PREPARATION

Typically, a living donor is either an immediate blood-related family member or a spouse of the recipient who has end-stage renal failure. Recently, altruistic third-party donation has gained considerable attention. All candidates are screened preoperatively for any transmissible diseases, infection, or malignancy. Basic blood group compatibility and cross-match lymphocytic testing is performed. A thin slice (3-mm) computed tomography (CT) scan optimally assesses vascular anatomy and the integrity of both kidneys. Three-dimensional (3D) volume rendering provides details of vascular anatomy commensurate with conventional angiography. We perform an angiogram only if the 3D CT scan demonstrates vascular anomaly or multiplicity. The left kidney is preferred given its longer vein. However, in cases of complex multiple vasculature of the left kidney, the right kidney is retrieved. Similar to open surgery, the dictum of leaving the best kidney with the donor is strictly adhered to during laparoscopic donor nephrectomy.

Patients are presented a detailed discussion about the procedure, including major risks and the potential for open conversion. All patients undergo gentle bowel preparation with clear liquid diet the day prior to surgery and two bottles of magnesium citrate.

## OPERATIVE TECHNIQUE

### Transperitoneal Left Donor Nephrectomy

Although multiple techniques have been described, including hand assistance, we prefer the standard transperitoneal approach for the left kidney and the retroperitoneal approach for the right kidney. Although the right renal vein is shorter than the left, in our experience both afford adequate renal vein length for transplant anastomosis.

The patient is positioned and secured to the table using adhesive tape in a modified 45–60° lateral position (Fig. 10.1). We do not raise the kidney bar. The proposed Pfannenstiel site two finger-breadths cephalad to the pubic bone is marked. Veress pneumoperitonal access is obtained at the midway point between the anterior superior iliac spine and the umbilicus. The Veress site serves as the insertion site for the primary port. Additional ports are placed under direct vision using a 30° lens, as illustrated. During the procedure, the patient is kept well hydrated. To counteract effects of pneumoperitoneum-induced oliguria, the patient is well hydrated and mannitol/Lasix is administered.

The descending colon is reflected medially along the white line of Toldt using cold endoshears in the right hand and a small bowel atraumatic grasper in the left hand. The avascular plane between Gerota's fascia and the large bowel is developed.

The ureter and gonadal vessel are retracted anteriorly and laterally off the psoas muscle. The gonadal vein is dissected to its insertion point into the renal vein. The cephalad and inferior edges of the renal vein are dissected with J-hook electrocautery. The gonadal vein is ligated with hemolock clips and divided. A long stump of the gonadal vein attached to the renal vein facilitates its anterior retraction allowing safe dissection of the more posteriorly located lumbar vessels. Lumbar veins are dissected and

From: *Operative Urology at the Cleveland Clinic*
Edited by: A. Novick et al. © Humana Press Inc., Totowa, NJ

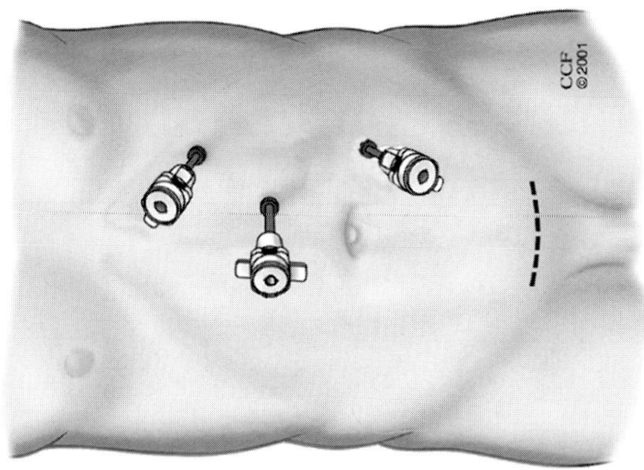


Fig. 10.1

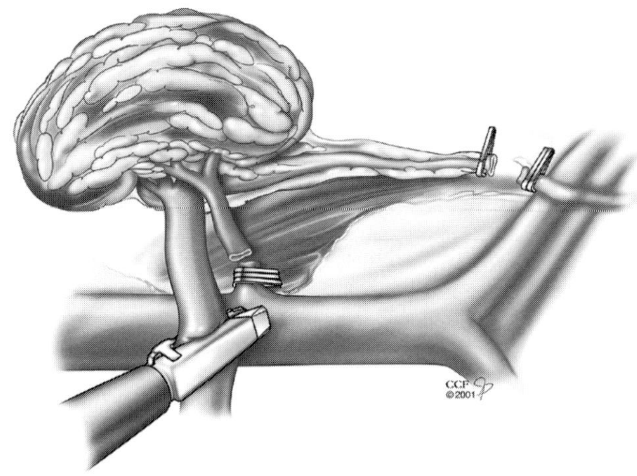


Fig. 10.2

divided with clips. Only the most proximal 2 cm of the renal artery near the aorta is dissected so as to minimize unnecessary manipulation of the renal artery, which may lead to vasospasm. Diluted papaverine is administered locally over the artery to prevent vasospasm.

The adrenal vein is identified and transected between hemlock clips at its insertion point onto the renal vein. Care must be taken not to incorporate adrenal tissue into the hemolock clip to minimize troublesome adrenal gland bleeding. Gerota's fascia is entered superiorly and the upper pole parenchyma is exposed. The attachments of the adrenal gland are dissected off the medial aspect of the upper pole kidney, taking care not to injure any arterial branches. The adrenal gland is thus preserved.

The ureter and gonadal vein are divided distally near the common iliac vessels. The proximal cut end of the ureter is not clipped to allow documentation of intraoperative urine production. The kidney is completely mobilized laterally. The previously marked modified Pfannenstiel incision site is developed in a muscle-splitting fashion down to the peritoneum. A 12-mm dilating trocar is placed in the midline of the Pfannenstiel incision for future application of the Endo-GIA vascular stapler.

Additional Lasix and mannitol are administered 5 min prior to clamping of the hilar vessels (Fig. 10.2). An assistant provides lateral traction on the kidney using a small bowel atraumatic grasper. The renal artery is ligated with two hemolock clips proximally close to the aorta and divided. The distal side of the renal artery is not clipped. The renal vein is divided with the Endo-GIA vascular stapler at an area anterior to the aorta, medial to the adrenal vein stump. The vascular stapler is fired carefully along the vein, being aware of the potential risk of inadvertent superior mesenteric artery injury. Any remaining attachment of the renal vein not divided by the Endo-GIA stapler is ligated with hemolock clips and divided.

The kidney is rapidly retrieved with the surgeon's right hand through the previously created muscle-splitting Pfannenstiel incision and transferred for bench preparation. The extraction incision is closed with a running 0-Vycril suture. After approx 5 min without pneumoperitoneum, laparoscopic inspection is performed to ensure hemostasis. Laparoscopic exit is completed.

## Retroperitoneal Right Donor Nephrectomy

Although transperitoneal laparoscopic dissection of the right kidney and renal vein length preservation using a Satinsky clamp has been described, our preference has been to perform the right donor nephrectomy by the retroperitoneal laparoscopic approach given safety concerns with the former approach. Advantages with the retroperitoneal access include early dissection of the renal vasculature as well as a more flush placement of the Endo-GIA vascular stapler alongside the inferior vena cava (IVC).

The patient is positioned in full flank 90° position (Fig 10.3). The table is flexed, but the kidney bar is not raised. All pressure points are carefully padded, and the patient is secured to the operating table.

A 1.5-cm skin incision is made at the tip of the 12th rib (Figs. 10.4 and 10.5). The lumbodorsal fascia is incised with electrocautery, and the surgeon's index finger is inserted posterior to the kidney to develop a small working space. A retroperitoneal balloon dissector is placed in the retroperitoneum posterior to the kidney and inflated to 800 cc. A blunt-tip 10-mm balloon port is placed to prevent leakage of pneumoperitoneum. A 12-mm port is placed under direct laparoscopic visualization three fingerbreadths cephalad to the anterior superior iliac spine. A 5-mm port is placed lateral to the paraspinal muscle at the junction of the 12th rib.

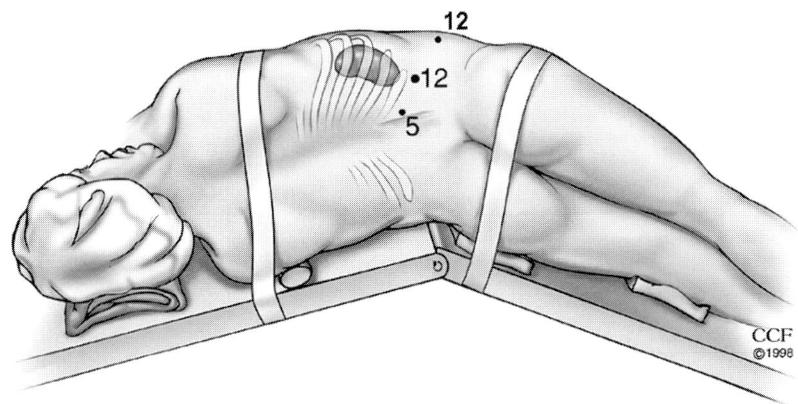


Fig. 10.3

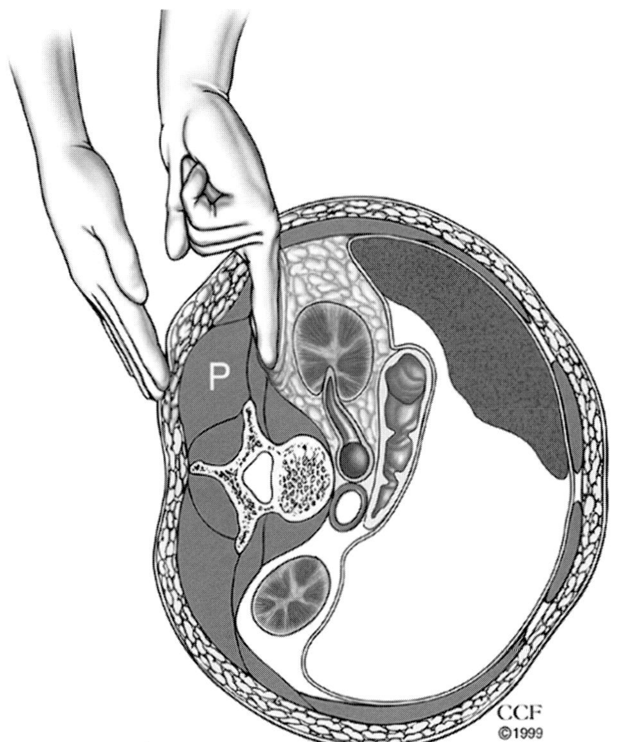


Fig. 10.4

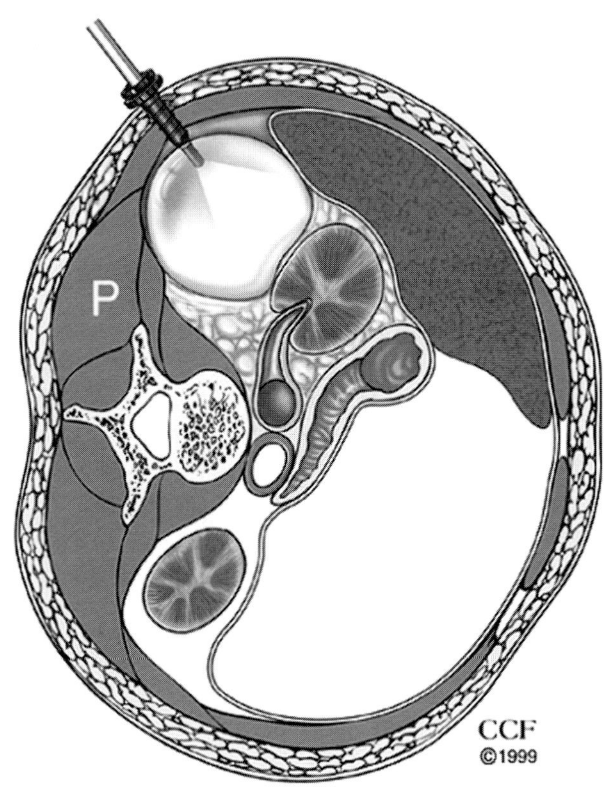


Fig. 10.5

The psoas muscle in the horizontal position serves as a key landmark during retroperitoneal surgery. Additionally, venous pulsations of the IVC may be appreciated. Minimal blunt dissection typically reveals the location of the ureter and gonadal vein caudally. Using a small bowel retractor in the left hand, the kidney is retracted anteriorly off the psoas muscle. The renal hilum is dissected with J-hook electrocautery. It is critical to dissect the junction of the renal vein and IVC to ensure that the cava has not been inadvertently lifted, leading to dangerous retro-caval dissection.

Once the hilar vessels are adequately dissected, attention is turned to the adrenal gland, which is dissected off the upper pole kidney within Gerota's fascia, allowing its preservation. During lower pole dissection, the vascular supply between the lower pole kidney and ureter is maintained intact. The ureter and surrounding fat are dissected to prevent devascularization.

A modified lateral Pfannenstiel incision is made as described previously without entry into the peritoneum (Fig. 10.6). At the time of kidney retrieval, the peritoneum is swept medially by the surgeon's hand allowing access to the retroperitoneum. Avoiding this dissection early in the case prevents loss of $CO_2$.

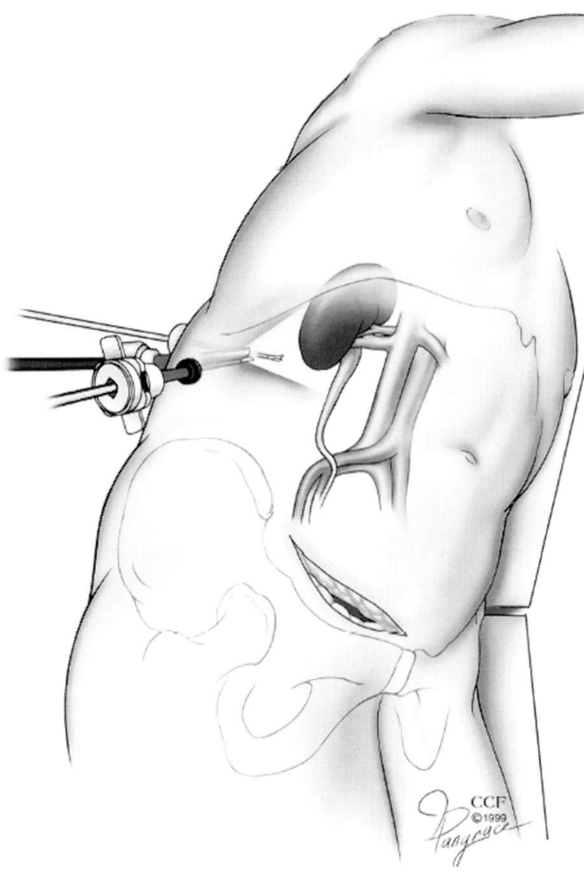

Fig. 10.6

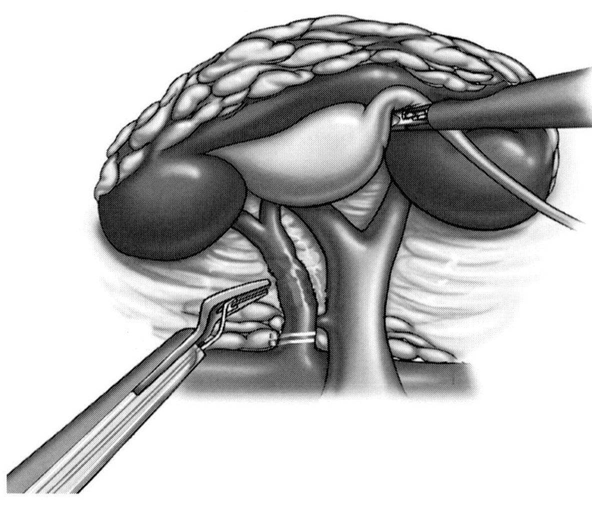

Fig. 10.7

The kidney is once again placed on anterior traction (Fig. 10.7). The renal artery is ligated proximally with hemolock clips and cut with cold endoshears. A vascular Endo-GIA stapler is placed through the right working port and fired flush with the IVC. The kidney is removed from the previously created Pfannenstiel incision and transferred for bench preparation. The extraction incision is closed with a running 0-Vycril suture. After 5 min without pneumoperitoneum, laparoscopy is performed again to ensure hemostasis. The ports are removed under direct vision. Ports measuring greater than 10 mm are closed with 0-Vycril suture.

## SUGGESTED READINGS


1. Brown SL, Biehl TR, Rawlins MC, Hefty TR. Laparoscopic live donor nephrectomy: a comparison with the conventional open approach. J Urol 165:766, 2001.
2. Cecka JM. The OPTN/UNOS Renal Transplant Registry 2003. Clin Transpl 1–12, 2003.
3. El Fettouh HA, Herts BR, Nimeh T. Prospective comparison of 3-dimensional volume rendered computerized tomography and conventional renal arteriography for surgical planning in patients undergoing laparoscopic donor nephrectomy. J Urol 170:57, 2003.
4. Giessing M. Laparoscopic living-donor nephrectomy. Nephrol Dial Transplant 19 Suppl 4:iv36, 2004.
5. Gill IS, Uzzo RG, Hobart MG, Streem SB, Goldfarb DA, Noble MJ. Laparoscopic retroperitoneal live donor right nephrectomy for purposes of allotransplantation and autotransplantation. J Urol 164:1500, 2000.
6. Handschin AE, Weber M, Demartines N, Clavien PA. Laparoscopic donor nephrectomy. Br J Surg 90:1323, 2003.
7. Ratner LE, Ciseck LJ, Moore RG, Cigarroa FG, Kaufman HS, Kavoussi LR. Laparoscopic live donor nephrectomy. Transplantation 60:1047, 1995.
8. Tooher RL, Rao MM, Scott DF, et al. A systematic review of laparoscopic live-donor nephrectomy. Transplantation 78:404, 2004.
9. Turk IA, Giessing M, Deger S. Laparoscopic live donor right nephrectomy: a new technique with preservation of vascular length. Transplant Proc 35:838, 2003.

# 11 Renal Transplantation

*David A. Goldfarb, Stuart M. Flechner, and Charles S. Modlin*

Renal transplantation has become the preferred method for renal replacement for appropriate candidates with end-stage renal disease (ESRD). It is associated with an improved quality of life and patient survival when compared with similar patients with ESRD but on dialysis. There have been improvements in patient care and immunosupression that have led to excellent outcomes. One-year graft survival for live-donor kidney recipients is 90–95%, and for deceased donor recipients is 85–90%. Overall, 1-yr patient survival is 95%.

## DONOR POOL ISSUES

With the changing demographics of US society, the number of eligible patients for renal transplantation will continue to rise. Presently, there are more than 60,000 patients awaiting renal transplantation in the United States. In 2003, approx 15,000 patients were transplanted. This disparity is a central dilemma in transplantation.

A new trend that is emerging is the significant growth in utilization of the live donor as a source for kidneys. In 2001, the number of living donors exceeded that of cadaver donors according the United Network for Organ Sharing (UNOS) for the first time.

There has been significant growth in living unrelated donation (kidneys from spouses, friends, and anonymous altruistic donors). This increase in living donation has been spurred on by several factors, first of which is the development of laparoscopic live donor nephrectomy. This new method of renal procurement is associated with less pain and a swifter recovery of the donor. This has resulted in removing some of the disincentives to donation. Many programs, including the Cleveland Clinic, have noted significant increases in rates of donation since adopting this technique. Second, long-term follow-up of renal donors (up to 20–30 yr) suggests that the procedure is safe without long-term consequences to renal function or blood pressure. Third, the renal failure community and nephrologists understand the benefits of transplantation and are more proactive in pursuing it as an option for renal replacement.

For the immediate future, increasing the number of live donors is one method of addressing the central dilemma of transplantation. Another strategy to deal with the shortage of organs is to use organs previously considered unusable for transplantation. These have come to be known as extended donor criteria kidneys and include kidneys at the extremes of age limits (<5 or >60 yr) or with concomitant diseases such as hypertension or diabetes mellitus. These are some of the solutions that our group has actively utilized.

Many older deceased donors (>65 yr) have kidneys with diminished functional nephron mass owing to senescence, hypertension, and arteriolar nephrosclerosis. These older or ischemically damaged kidneys often do not function well, which puts a further strain on donor organ supply. Each year, 5–10% of the deceased donor kidneys recovered are discarded because of concerns related to insufficient nephron mass and expectations of a poor outcome. The more common reasons are age over 65, history (generally 5 yr or less) of hypertension, history of diabetes, or severe ischemia in the donor during brain death and organ recovery. This is usually manifest as very low donor urine output, a serum creatinine over 2 mg/dL (a calculated creatinine clearance <80 cc/min), or documented glomerulosclerosis over 20% on a biopsy of the donor renal cortex. One approach to salvage some of these ischemically damaged kidneys has been to transplant both kidneys from one donor into one recipient. Two or dual kidney transplantation can provide a sufficient nephron mass to one recipient, when the expectation is that a single renal unit will not be adequate. In general, transplant centers in an organ-sharing region must first decline the use of such kidneys as single units. Our approach has been to verify the viability of such compromised kidneys using pulsatile perfusion preservation,

From: *Operative Urology at the Cleveland Clinic*
Edited by: A. Novick et al. © Humana Press Inc., Totowa, NJ

which measures the flow through these hypothermically preserved kidneys and the relative resistance required to maintain perfusion.

Kidneys from young deceased donors have been utilized successfully when transplanted into adult recipients. Experiencc has demonstrated that kidneys procured from children are not suitable for transplantation into children due to prohibitive rates of vascular complications. Kidneys from donors over the age of 2 yr may be used individually in adult recipients. The same surgical techniques used to implant adult cadaver kidneys are utilized, with the exception that an aortic Carrel patch is mandatory as well as a cuff of donor vena cava. Additional considerations taken into account when utilizing a pediatric kidney in an adult recipient are the recipient-to-donor weight relationship, the level of sensitization of the recipient, the number of prior transplants, and the anatomy of the recipient. There is concern that a very small kidney placed into a very large recipient (donor to recipient size mismatch) might provide poor results owing to hyperfiltration of the pediatric kidney. Patients highly sensitized are at greater risk for rejection and may not be the most suited to receive a small pediatric kidney, which has a diminished functional reserve. In considering utilization of kidneys from pediatric deceased donors under the age of 2 yr, experience has shown improved results using the *en bloc* technique of transplanting both donor kidneys as one unit into a single adult recipient.

## PREOPERATIVE CONSIDERATIONS

Recipients are prone to delayed wound healing and infection as a consequence of the immunosupression required to facilitate transplantation. This mandates attention to surgical detail and strict adherence to basic operative principles of asepsis and hemostasis. Anticipating surgical complications, preventing their occurrence, and prompt treatment are critical to good outcomes with this operation.

In primary transplantation, the allograft is usually transplanted into one of the iliac fossae. The right iliac fossa offers the advantage of a more horizontal course of the external iliac vein, rendering it more accessible for the venous anastamosis. For this reason it is usually preferable when available. Nonetheless, each case needs to be considered on its merits, taking into account the anticipated recipient anatomy and the anatomy of the donor organ, particularly the anteroposterior relationships of the artery, vein, and collecting system. Keep in mind that the collecting system will be the most anterior structure when a donor right kidney is placed on the left and a left donor kidney is placed on the right. This will keep the ureter off the iliac vessels, rendering it more accessible. For diabetic patients receiving a live donor kidney who are candidates for a pancreas transplant after kidney, implantation should be on the left side. This facilitates subsequent placement of the pancreas using the right common iliac artery for inflow without obligating the kidney to ischemia from vessel control. The surgical priniciple that should guide position of the kidney is a smooth geometric fit when the kidney is placed in its final resting position. This requires three-dimensional visual anticipation. The vascular and ureteral anastamoses should be on a smooth line without undue tension or kinking.

In patients with a prior failed graft, the second iliac fossa is always used. A third transplant is typically placed with the vein anastamosed to the lower vena cava and the artery to the lower aorta or common iliac artery on the right via either an intra- or extraperitoneal incision.

As part of the pretransplant evaluation process, there should be an assessment of the arterial and venous inflow by history and physical examination. Magnetic resonance angiography (for patients not yet on dialysis) or computed tomography (CT) arteriography should be carried out in patients suspected of having iliac or aortic vascular disease that would threaten the technical success of transplantation. For patients with a history of deep vein thrombosis, duplex ultrasound evaluation to determine the presence of residual iliac clot would be indicated. In the rare circumstance of the totally occluded inferior vena cava (IVC)–iliac system, consideration should be given to a portal venous anastamosis, similar to pancreas transplantation. Patients should have a bladder with an adequate capacity, acceptable compliance, and an intact continence mechanism prior to transplantation. Appropriate bladder rehabilitation or reconstruction may be neccesary and should be performed well in advance of a transplant.

## OPERATIVE PROCEDURE

At the time of anesthesia, a 20 French foley catheter is placed in the bladder. A urine sample is sent for culture or a bladder wash in the case of an anuric patient. The bladder is then filled by gravity with 100–200 cc of a 1% neomycin solution, then the catheter is clamped. The operative site and one groin is shaved and prepped with an iodine solution for 10 min. One groin is always isolated should there be need for a saphenous vein conduit.

Once the operation is completed, the wound is closed with full-thickness no. 1 polydioxanone suture. Recently

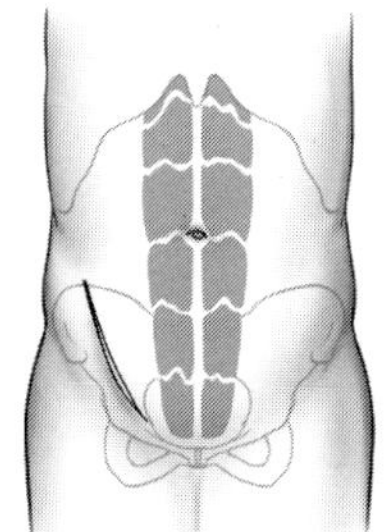

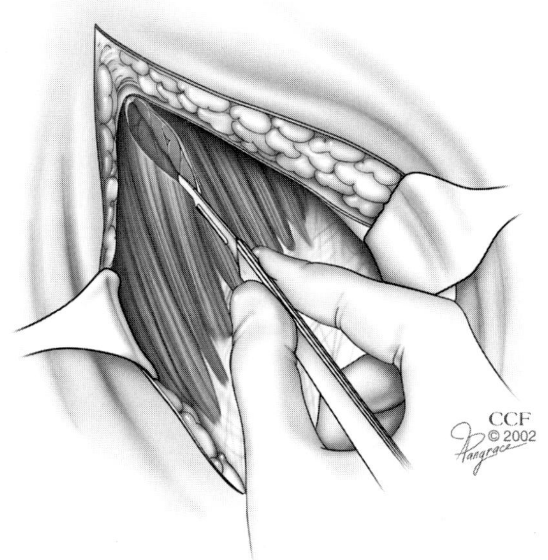


**Fig. 11.1**

A lower-quadrant Gibson incision is made extending from the midline to above the anterior–superior iliac spine. Extreme care should be taken to assure hemostasis throughout the entire operation using electrocautery, ligatures, or clips as needed. The external oblique, internal oblique, and transversus abdominus muscles are divided along the line of the incision.

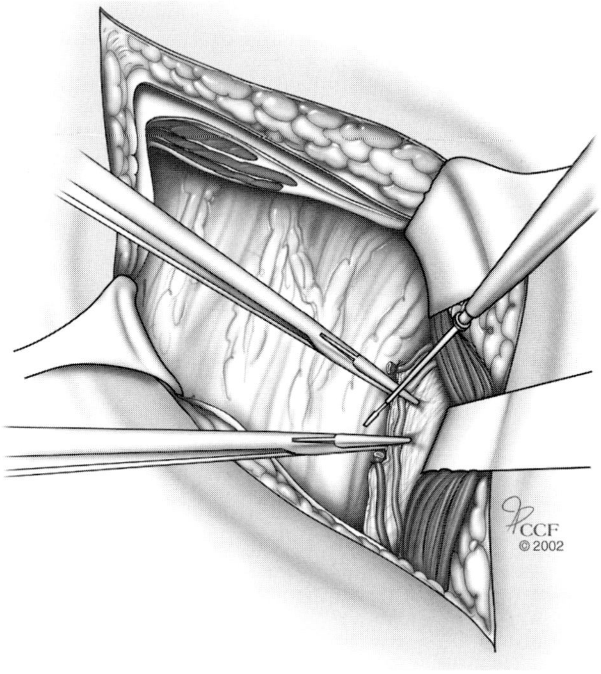


**Fig. 11.2**

The retroperitoneum is developed by rolling the peritoneum off the abdominal wall with blunt dissection. The inferior epigastric vessels are identified at the lower end of the operative field, then individually ligated and divided between 2-0 silk ties. Occasionally the epigastric artery may be preserved as an inflow source for a lower pole renal artery. In women, the round ligament of the uterus should be identified, then divided. In men, the spermatic cord should be mobilized medially and preserved.

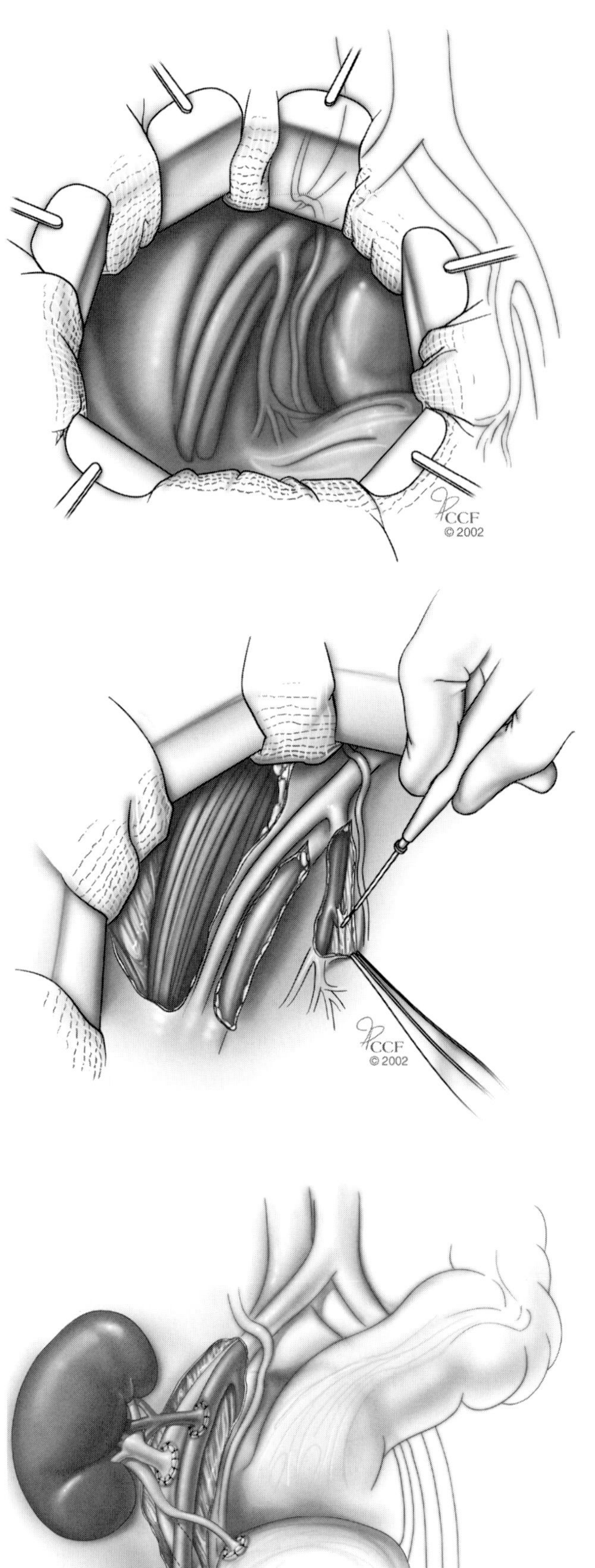


**Fig. 11.3**

Once the peritoneum is mobilized off the iliac vessels, a self-retaining retractor is used to maintain the exposure. Care should be taken to avoid compression of the ilio-psoas musculature, which contains the femoral nerve trunk. This avoids a postoperative neuropathy. Careful attention to appropriate padding laterally will prevent injury to the lateral femoral cutaneous nerves. The distal common iliac artery should be at the cephalad end of the field. The external iliac artery and vein should be visualized to the inguinal ligament caudally in the field. The lateral edge of the bladder should be seen at the medial aspect of the wound.

**Fig. 11.4**

The lympho-areolar tissues investing the iliac vessels need to be dissected. Careful control of these tissues with electrocautery needs to be obtained. Visible lymphatic trunks should be ligated and divided between 4-0 silk ligatures. These maneuvers are performed to prevent lymphocele formation. The minimal amount of arterial and venous length to facilitate vascular anastamosis should be mobilized. In most instances this will include the external iliac artery and vein, but the distal common iliac artery is often the site for proximal control and may require mobilization. In cases where the hypogastric artery will be used, a full dissection of the external iliac artery may not be necessary.

**Fig. 11.5**

Extensive mobilization and lateral transposition of the external iliac vein is a useful adjunctive maneuver when the donor kidneys vessels are shorter. This permits the surgeon to bring the recipient vessels to the donor kidney without undo tension, thus facilitating the venous anastamosis. This is particularly useful for laparoscopically procured kidneys.

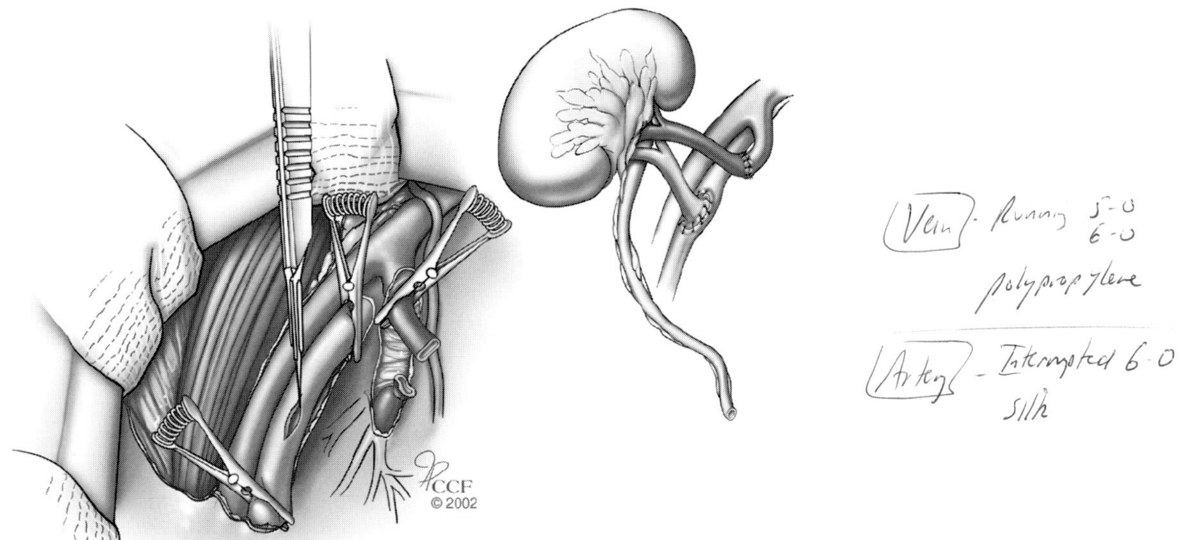


Fig. 11.6

The donor kidney is prepared on the backtable where the artery and vein are mobilized. The vasculature should be tested for its competence with injection of heparinized saline. Any leaks should be repaired with 6-0 or 7-0 suture (polypropylene or silk). The external iliac vein is controlled proximally and distally with bulldogs or a Satinsky clamp and an appropriate-sized venotomy is created with a no. 11 blade. This may be modified using a Pott's scissor. A running 5-0 or 6-0 polypropylene suture is used for the venous anastamosis. The proximal hypogastric artery is controlled with a bulldog clamp and spatulated to accept the donor artery. The arterial anastamosis for the end-to-end technique is performed using 6-0 silk interrupted sutures. The final geometry of the anastamosis should be anticipated so that when the kidney is placed into the iliac fossa there is a favorable course of the artery without kinking or twisting.

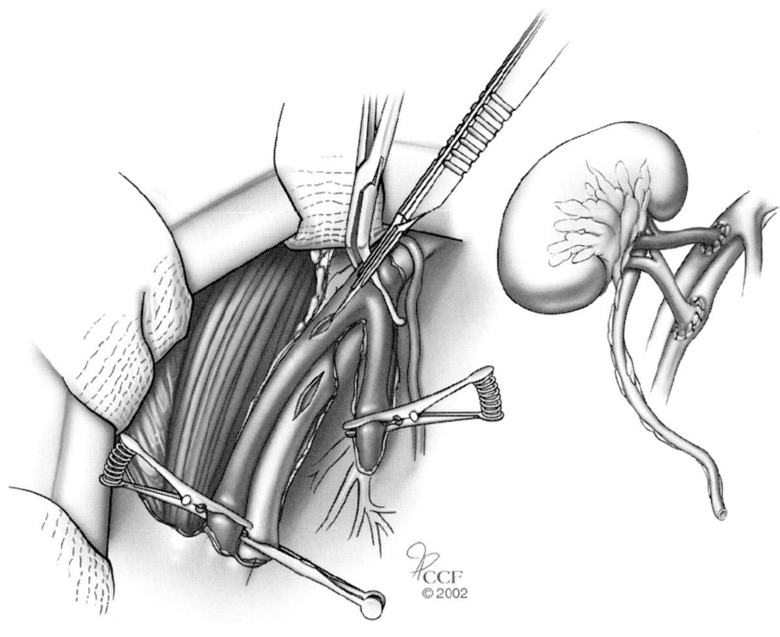


Fig. 11.7

For an end-to-side anastamosis, proximal and distal control of the external iliac artery are obtained. Sometimes this may involve clamping of the distal common iliac artery. If this is the case, as illustrated, the hypogastric artery should also be controlled to prevent backbleeding into the anastamosis. The arteriotomy is then created with a no. 11 blade and extended with a Pott's scissor to an appropriate size. The artery is usually placed slightly more cephalad on the artery compared to the vein so both sides of the artery can be anastamosed under direct vision without the vein blocking access to the medial wall. This also permits a better direct line for the artery and helps to avoid kinking.

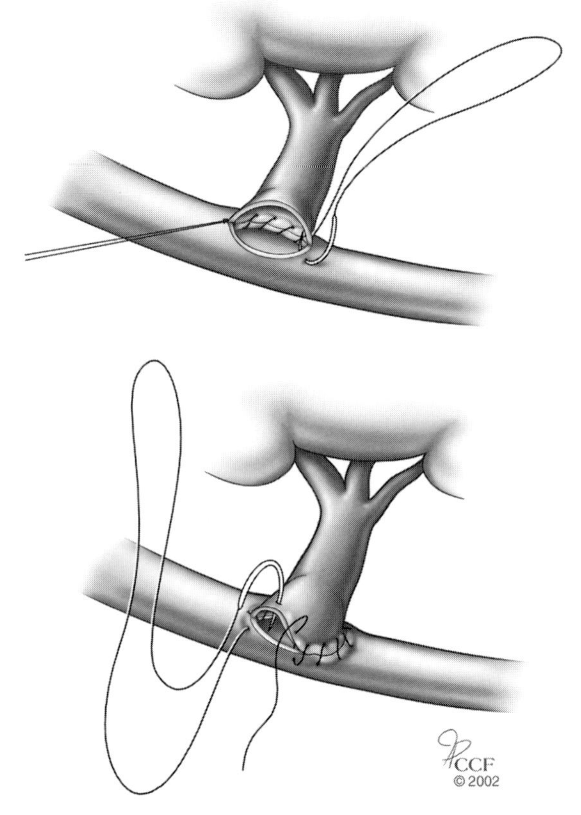


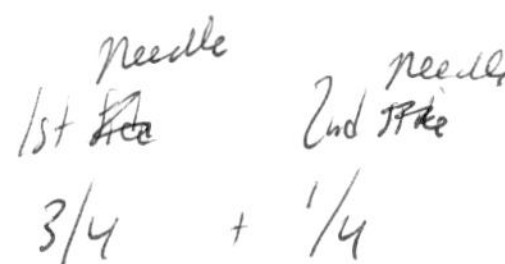

**Fig. 11.8**

The arterial end-to-side anastamosis is constructed with a double-ended 6-0 polypropylene suture on a BV or C1 needle. One continuous suture is used. The lateral wall is approximated first, then half of the medial wall. The last quarter of the suture line is then completed with the other needle. The anastamosis is then secured. The venous and arterial suture lines are tested after controlling the vessels to the kidney with bulldog clamps. Any major leaks are addressed before revascularization of the kidney.

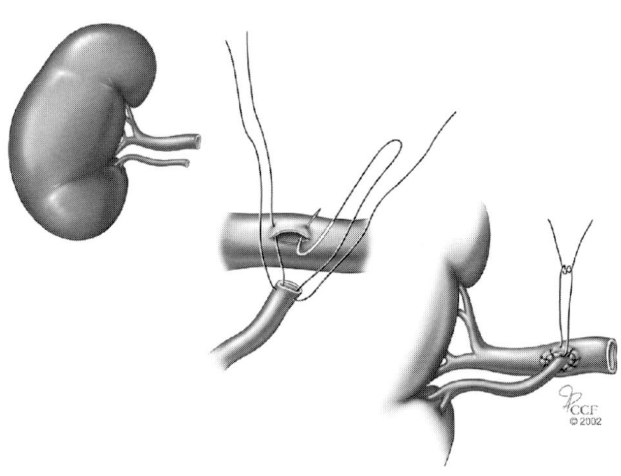


**Fig. 11.9**

When two arteries are encountered in a live donor kidney, there are several options for implantation. Widely separated arteries of disparate size may be individually anstamosed to the external iliac artery. This may slightly prolong the anastamosis time for the kidney. Another option is backtable implantation of the smaller artery into the dominant artery (end-to-side) using optical loupe magnification and 6-0 or 7-0 suture. A single anastamosis of the dominant artery into either the external iliac or hypogastric artery can then be performed.

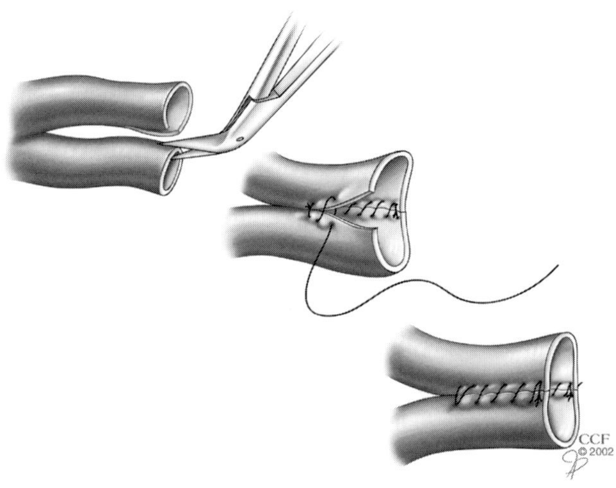


**Fig. 11.10**

If the two arteries are equal in size, as illustrated, a conjoined anastamosis may be performed. This facilitates a single anastamosis of wider caliber to the recipient external iliac artery, minimizing revascularization time. This reconstruction is also performed with loupe magnification using 6-0 or 7-0 suture.

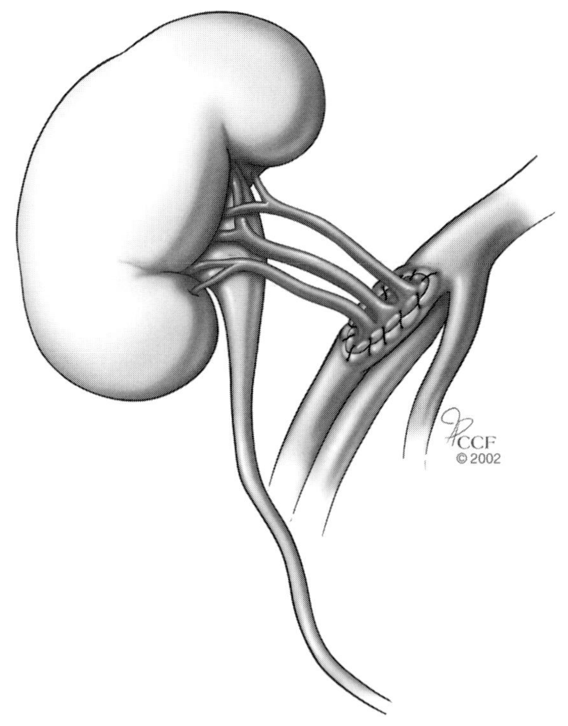

Fig. 11.11

In cadaveric kidneys with multiple arteries, a Carrel patch may be used. All arteries can be preserved on a shared cuff of donor aortic tissue. This may be anastamosed directly to the external or common iliac artery using continuous 6-0 polypropylene suture.

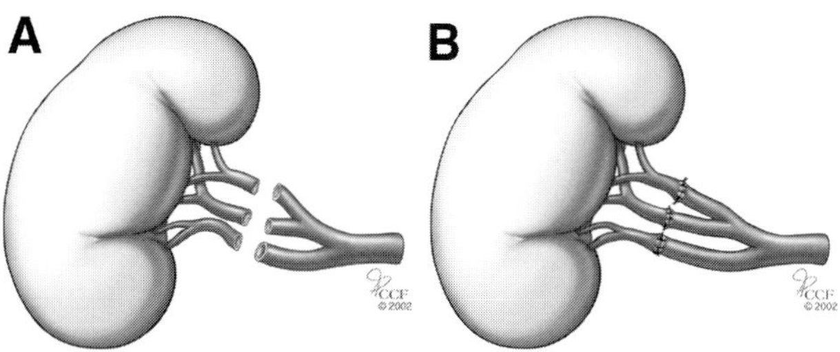


Fig. 11.12

For the unique circumstance where there are three vessels and no aortic patch as encountered in a live donor operation, utilizing a branched hypogastric artery autograft as a conduit is useful. This mandates that the recipient hypogastric artery is available, free from atherosclerosis, and branches appropriately. The major reconstruction can be performed on the backtable using optical magnification with the kidney in an iced slush basin. End-to-end anstamoses of distal branches can be performed using 7-0 suture. A single anastamosis of the conduit to either the hypogastric or external iliac artery may then be performed. The time-consuming reconstruction is performed with the kidney cooled, thus minimizing the total revascularization time.

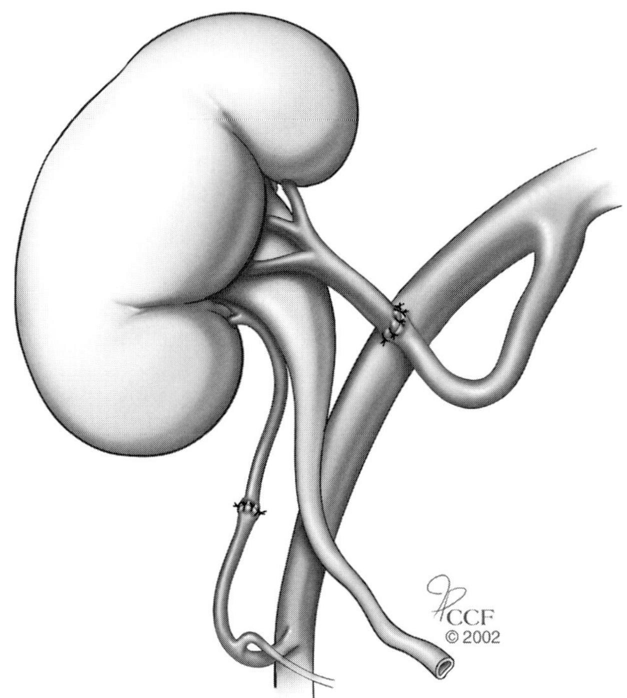

Fig. 11.13

For widely separated arteries when there is a diminuitive lower pole artery, another option is to take advantage of the epigastric artery. In live donor operations this should be planned and a longer length of the epigastric artery preserved as the incision is opened. The dominant upper pole artery can be anastamosed end-to-end as shown or end-to-side to the external iliac artery. The upper pole artery and renal vein can be unclamped and the majority of the kidney's circulation restored. A fine bulldog clamp should be placed on the lower pole artery and the epigastric artery contolled as well. The vessels are then spatulated and the anstamosis is performed using interrupted 6-0 or 7-0 suture. The lower pole circulation is then restored. This can avoid placing a small-caliber anastamosis to the external iliac artery, which can be awkward to perform.

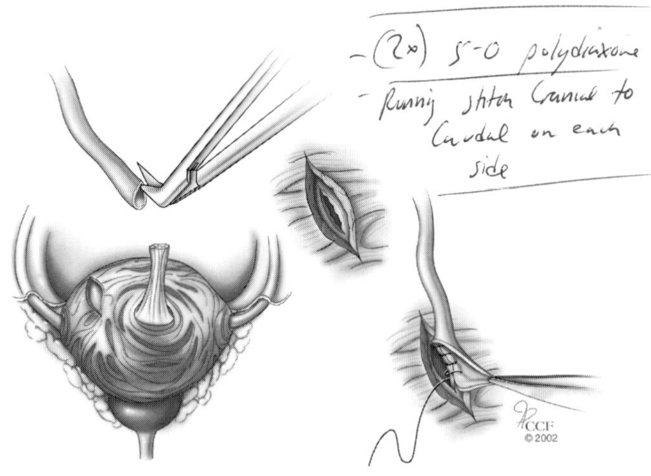


**Fig. 11.14**

The preferred ureteral reimplantation is an extravesical, Lich–Gregoire technique. First the ureter is cut to appropriate length and spatulated while ensuring adequate preservation of periureteral tissue that contains the ureteral blood supply. The lateral aspect of the bladder is mobilized and a site for the anastamosis identified. Using sharp dissection, the detrusor muscle is incised and mucosal bubble is mobilized. At the caudal end of the bubble the bladder mucosa is incised. Two 5-0 polydioxanone sutures are used to anchor the ureter (full thickness) to the bladder mucosa only. The anastamosis is then constructed with a running stitch starting from cranial to caudal on each side. At the discretion of the surgeon a double-J stent may be placed. Our group uses such a stent in the majority of cases as the evidence suggests it reduced ureteral complications.

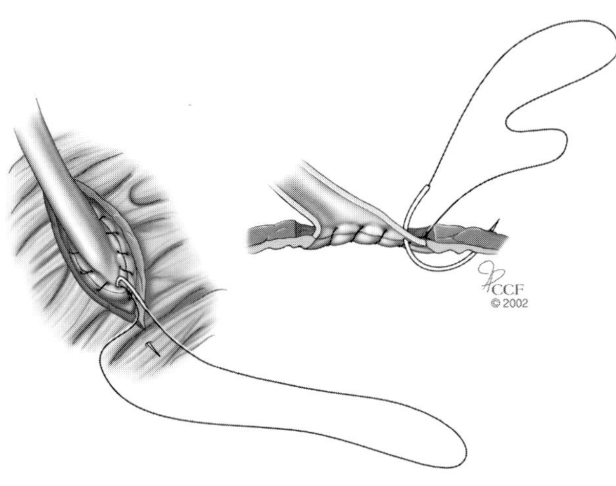


**Fig. 11.15**

After the last ureter-to-bladder mucosal stitch is placed, an advancement stitch may be used to pull the apex of the anastamosis well into to the detrusor tunnel. This can be performed using the anastamotic suture.

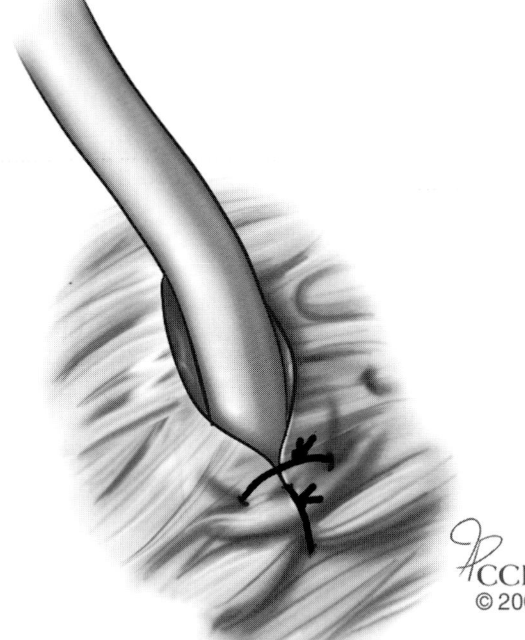


**Fig. 11.16**

The detrusor tunnel is closed with an absorbable suture (3-0 or 4-0 polyglactin).

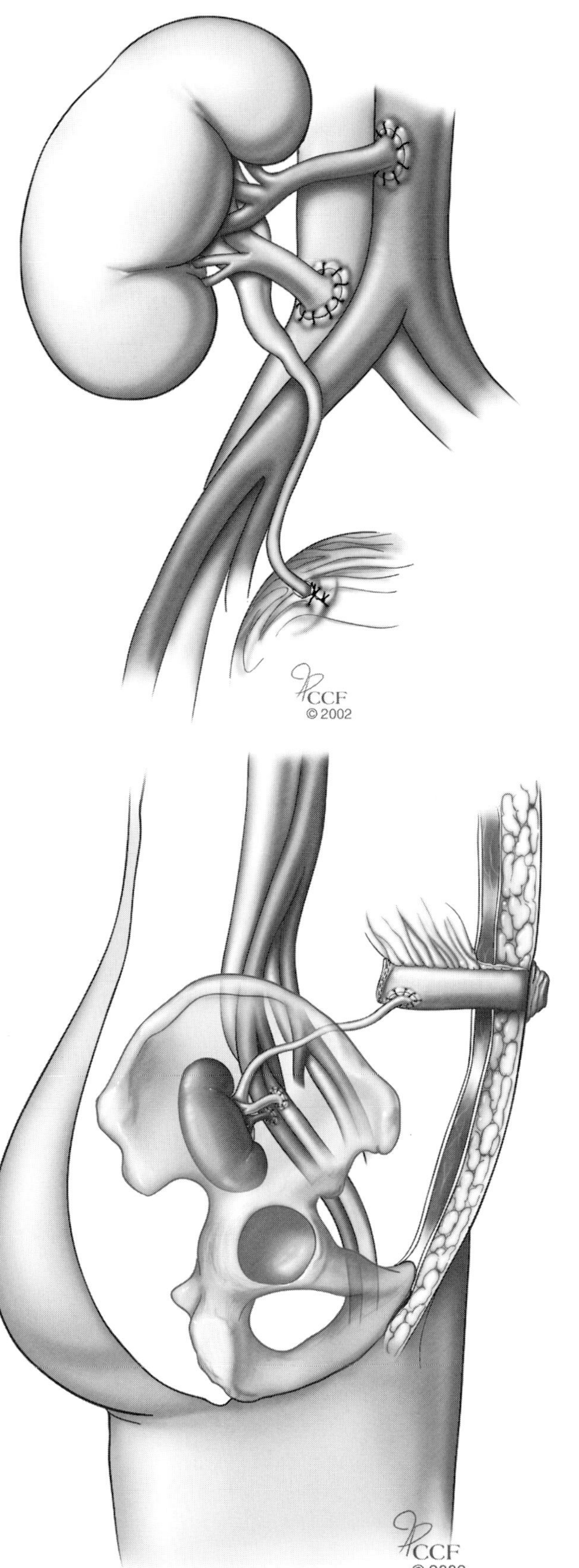


**Fig. 11.17**

In small children the vascular anastamoses are in the lower aorta or proximal common iliac for the artery and into the lower inferior vena cava for the vein. This is owing to the small-caliber vessels encountered in children. Very small children (<15 kg) may be approached using a midline transperitoneal incision. Most others will be fine with a conventional retroperitoneal approach.

**Fig. 11.18**

Kidney transplants may be placed into an ileal conduit. For these cases the kidney should be deliberately placed upside-down to direct the ureter to the ileal conduit.

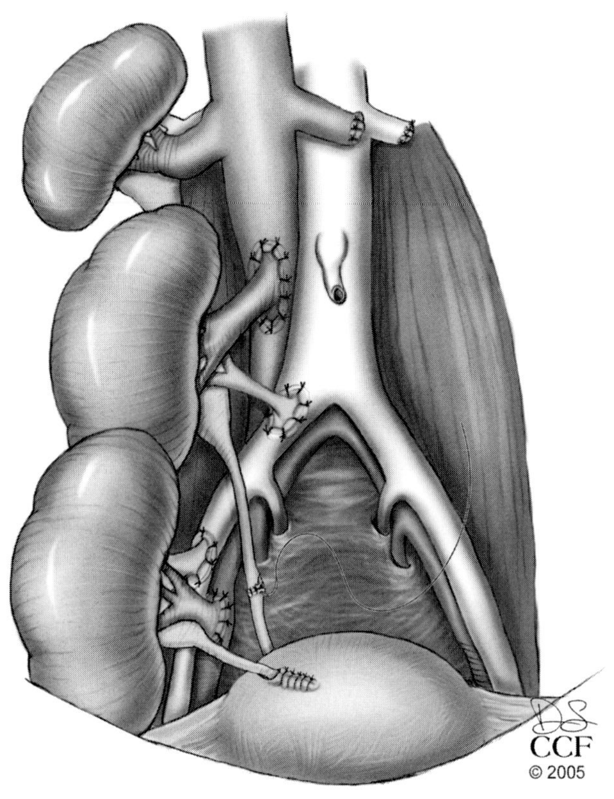


**Fig. 11.19**

Ipsilateral dual transplantation is performed through an extended Gibson incision and placed extraperitoneal. The upper renal unit is the right kidney, which is revascularized with the right renal vein end-to-side to the vena cava and the renal artery end-to-side to the common iliac artery. If available, a patch of donor aorta is useful to maximize arterial length and to facilitate anastomosis to the common iliac artery. On occasion, the right renal artery may be short and will fit best without tension when anastomosed to the lower aorta. The lower renal unit is the left kidney, which can be placed in the more typical fashion in the iliac fossa. The renal artery can be anastomosed end-to-side to the external iliac artery or rarely end-to-end to the internal iliac artery. The renal vein is anastomosed end-to-side to the external iliac vein.

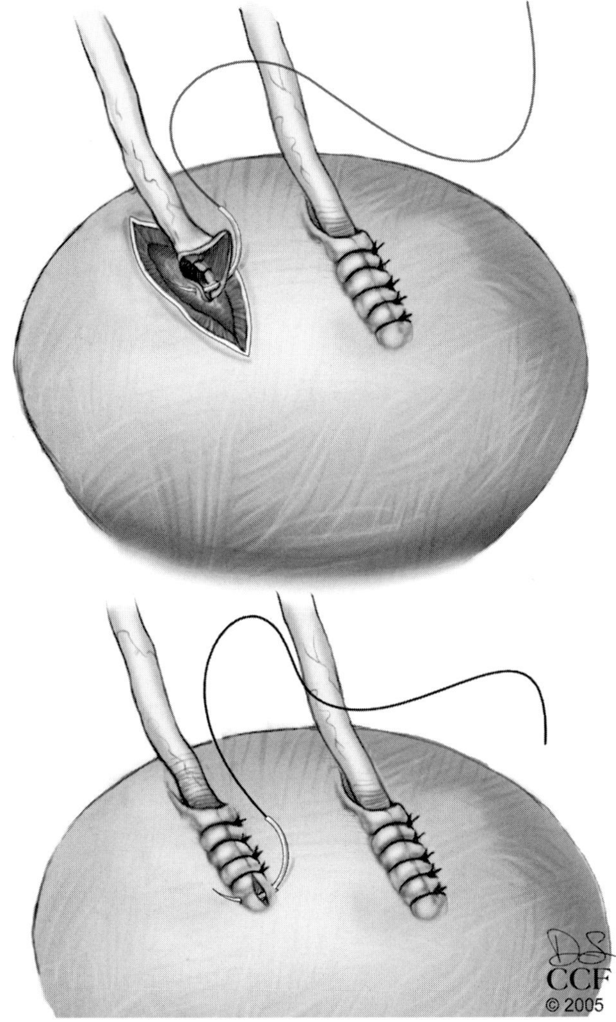


**Fig. 11.20**

Each of the two transplant ureters can be reimplanted into the bladder separately. An extravesical uretero-neocystostomy is preferred. Each ureter will have its own tunnel and is protected with an internal double-J silicone ureteral stent. It is useful to prepare each detrusor tunnel on the bladder surface before the mucosa is opened and the bladder is decompressed.

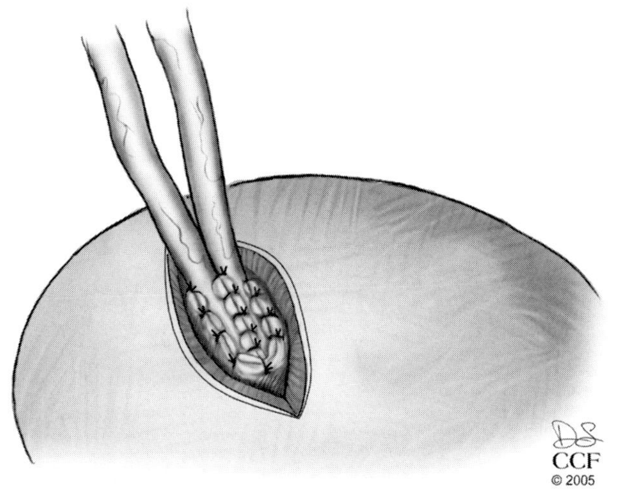


**Fig. 11.21**

If the ipsilateral approach is used, the ureters can be conjoined into one so that a single reimplantation into the bladder can be accomplished. Each ureter is incised for about 1–1.5 cm on its avascular side. The two ureters are then joined at their apex with 5-0 polyglycolic acid suture and the medial walls are run to their tip. The single ureteral ostia can then be anastomosed to the bladder mucosa in a Lich–Gregoire extravesicle uretero-neocystostomy. The ureteral anastomoses are protected with an internal double-J silicone ureteral stent placed up each ureter to the respective kidney.

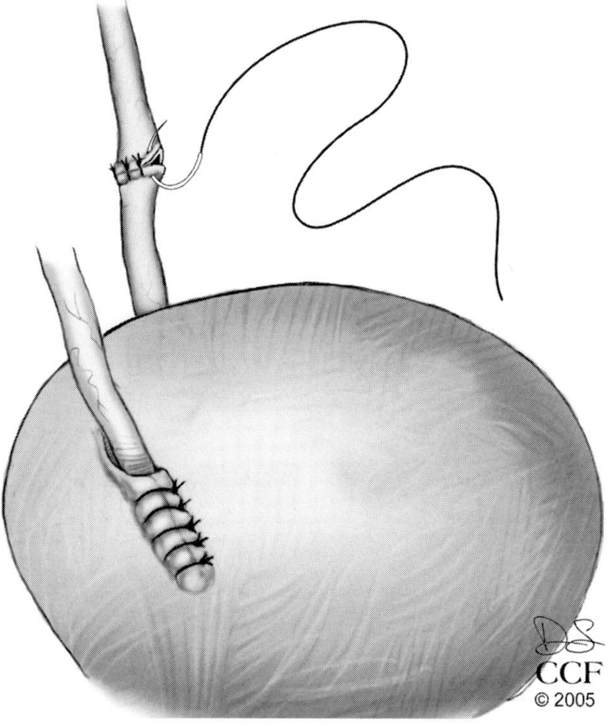


**Fig. 11.22**

An alternative for urinary tract reconstruction in the ipsilateral approach is to join the upper kidney ureter end-to-end to the native kidney ureter and then place the lower kidney ureter separately to the bladder. During ipsilateral placement the native ureter can usually be identified in the operative field. However, identification can be facilitated by the cystoscopic placement of an open-ended ureteral catheter. This catheter is also helpful in placing an antegrade guidewire to help in passage of a subsequent internal double-J ureteral stent to protect the anastomosis. The uretero-ureterostomy is completed with either running 5-0 polydioxanone or polyglycolic acid sutures. Ligation of the upper end of the native ureter does not usually cause morbidity, especially when native pretransplant urine output is negligible. If native urine output is large (liters a day), subsequent hydronephrosis could develop, necessitating native nephrectomy. However, this has not been observed in any of the dual kidney transplants that we have performed.

we have started to place a retroperitoneal closed suction drain in the deep surgical field in an effort to reduce the incidence of lymphocele formation. In selected patients with a body mass index (BMI) greater than 30, consideration is also given to placement of a subcutaneous drain to prevent seroma formation. Skin is approximated with clips that are usually kept in place for 2–3 wk. Wounds are covered until the clips are removed. Drains are removed at the discretion of the surgeon, usually when there is less than 50 cc of daily output. The ureteral stents are removed between 4 and 12 wk using flexible cystoscopy and local anesthesia.

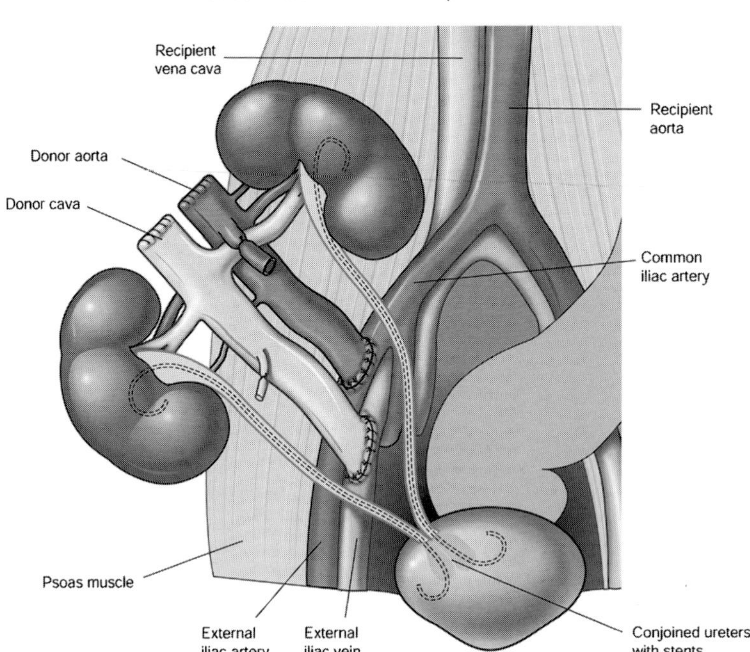


**Fig. 11.23**

For pediatric *en bloc* transplantation, backtable preparation proceeds under magnification. Lumbar veins on the undersurface of the donor vena cava are carefully identified and ligated. Care must be taken to note the location of the donor renal veins and the proximity of the renal veins and renal arteries to the cephalad portions of the donor cava and aorta. A factor determining the transplantability of pediatric *en bloc* kidneys is whether the procuring surgeon, when transecting the cephalad cava and aorta, compromised the donor renal artery or vein. If either renal artery or vein is lacerated, it usually is prudent to discard the kidneys, for attempted repair of a lacerated renal artery or vein usually results in an immediate or early postoperative vascular thrombosis of the allograft. There must be sufficient excess of cephalad donor vena cava and aorta remaining to allow closure, which is performed using a running nonabsorbable suture (6-0 or 7-0 polypropylene). Testing using a heparinized saline flush should be performed to exclude vascular leaks. For implantation, the donor vena cava is anastamosed end-to-side to the external iliac vein and the donor aorta end-to-side to the external or internal iliac artery using 6-0 or 7-0 polypropylene suture. The options for ureteral reimplantation are similar to those described previously for dual adult transplantation. Our preference is to separately anastamose the ureters so that a complication in one kidney does not affect the outcome of its mate.

## SUGGESTED READINGS

1. Alfrey EJ, Boissy AR, Lerner SM. Dual kidney transplants: long-term results. Transplantation 75:1232–1236, 2003.
2. Cecka JM. The OPTN/UNOS Renal Transplant Registry 2003. Clin Transplant 1–12, 2003.
3. Goldfarb DA, Matin SF, Braun WE, et al. Renal outcome 25 years after donor nephrectomy. J Urol 166:2043–2047, 2001.
4. Hobart MG, Modlin CS, Kapoor A, et al. Transplantation of pediatric *en bloc* cadaver kidneys into adult recipients. Transplantation 66:1689–1694, 1998.
5. Lin CH, Steinberg AP, Ramani AP, et al. Laparoscopic live donor nephrectomy in the presence of circumaortic or retroaortic left renal vein. J Urol 171:44–46, 2004.
6. Modin CS, Goldfarb DA, Novick AC. The use of expanded criteria cadaver and live donor kidneys for transplantation. Urol Clin North Am 28:687–707, 2001.
7. Modin C, Novick AC, Goormastic M, Hodge E, Mastrioanni B, Myles J. Long-term results with single pediatric donor kidney transplants in adult recipients. J Urol 890–895, 1996.
8. Ng CS, Abreu SC, Abou El-Fettouh HI, et al. Right retroperitoneal versus left transperitoneal laparoscopic live donor nephrectomy. Urology 63:857–861, 2004.
9. Patel P, Krishnamurthi V. Successful use of the inferior mesenteric vein for renal transplantation. Am J Transplant 3:1040–1042, 2003.
10. Schweitzer EJ, Wilson J, Jacobs S, et al. Increased rates of donation with laparoscopic donor nephrectomy. Ann Surg 232:392–400, 2000.
11. Serrano DP, Flechner SM, Modin CS, Wyner LM, Novick AC. Transplantation into the long-term defunctionalized bladder. J Urol 156:885–888, 1996.

# 12 Renal Trauma

*J. Stephen Jones*

Although most renal trauma can be observed nonoperatively, penetrating renal injuries and severe blunt injuries still may require surgical exploration.

## DIAGNOSIS

Renal injury may be suspected by hematuria, but the degree of hematuria correlates poorly with the degree of renal injury and should not determine clinical decision making *(1)*. Most patients with abdominal injury will be assessed with spiral computed tomography (CT) in the emergency department. The CT gives a good idea of the degree and location of renal injury, as well as information regarding nonurological injuries. The contrasted study confirms a normal contralateral kidney in case nephrectomy is a consideration.

Renal injuries are categorized according to severity as follows:

1. Contusion or subcapsular hematoma only
2. Nonexpanding peri-renal hematoma or cortical laceration less than 1 cm deep, without urinary extravasation
3. Laceration greater than 1 cm without urinary extravasation
4. Laceration into the collecting system or a segmental renal artery or vein injury with contained hemorrhage
5. Shattered kidney or avulsion of the renal pedicle

## OPERATIVE INDICATIONS

The primary indication for renal exploration after blunt trauma is uncontrollable bleeding. Otherwise, most blunt injuries may be observed even if urinary extravasation is identified. Penetrating injuries are more likely to cause significant vascular or collecting system injuries and may be associated with injury to nonurological organs. Therefore, most penetrating injuries should be explored, especially if laparotomy is required for associated injuries.

## OPERATIVE APPROACH

Because renal trauma will likely be associated with other intra-abdominal injuries, exploration through a midline incision is preferred (*see* Chapter 1). An immediate assessment is made of life-threatening bleeding, which is controlled with direct pressure or packed to stabilize the critically ill patient. Particular attention should be made to assessing and controlling hemorrhage from the liver, spleen, and major retroperitoneal vessels prior to exposing the kidney. If the patient is stabilized with these maneuvers, consideration should be made to leaving the perinephric space undisturbed. The kidney is explored if the hematoma is expanding or pulsatile, or if there is suspicion of penetrating renal injury.

The transverse colon and small bowel are retracted cephalad and to the right to expose the root of the mesentery (Fig. 12.1). Vascular control prior to exploring the kidney has been shown to minimize the likelihood that nephrectomy will be required for uncontrollable bleeding *(2)*. An incision is made in the retroperitoneum over the aorta from the level of the inferior mesenteric artery to the ligament of Treitz (dotted line). If retroperitoneal hemorrhage obscures the aorta, incision is made medial to the inferior mesenteric vein, which is readily identifiable in the mesentery.

The renal artery to the kidney of interest may be controlled as it exits the aorta (inset). The left renal vein coursing anterior to the aorta is the landmark. Sweeping the duodenum off the vena cava facilitates identification of the right renal artery. The artery and vein on the side of interest are isolated with vessel loops but not clamped unless bleeding is uncontrollable.

The colon is then reflected medially by incising the line of Toldt (Fig. 12.2). Rapid blunt dissection exposes the kidney and surrounding hematoma. If brisk bleeding ensues, the previously isolated vessels may be clamped or secured with Rummel tourniquets.

## POLAR INJURIES

Polar injuries may be managed by partial nephrectomy (Fig. 12.3). Care is taken to remove devascularized

From: *Operative Urology at the Cleveland Clinic*
Edited by: A. Novick et al. © Humana Press Inc., Totowa, NJ

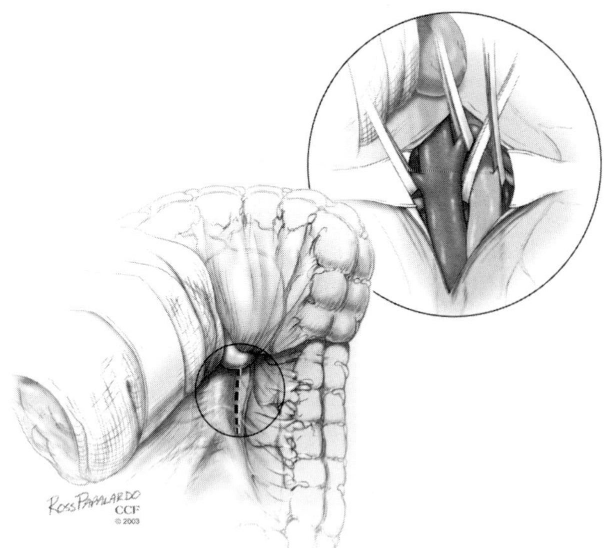


Fig. 12.1

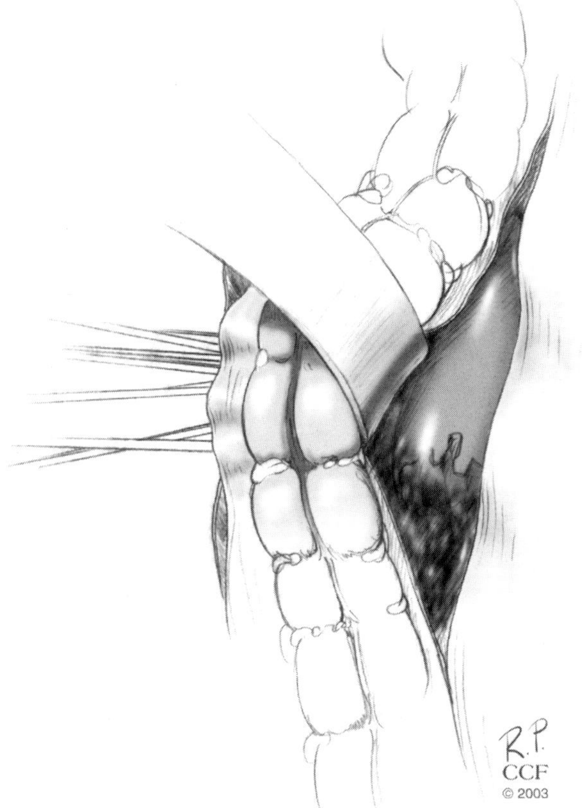


Fig. 12.2

segments in order to avoid late complications, such as urinary leakage.

The collecting system is oversewn with absorbable sutures to form a watertight closure (Fig 12.4). Significant vessels are suture ligated.

The parenchyma is closed over a pedicle of omentum or biocompatible hemostatic sponge (Fig. 12.5).

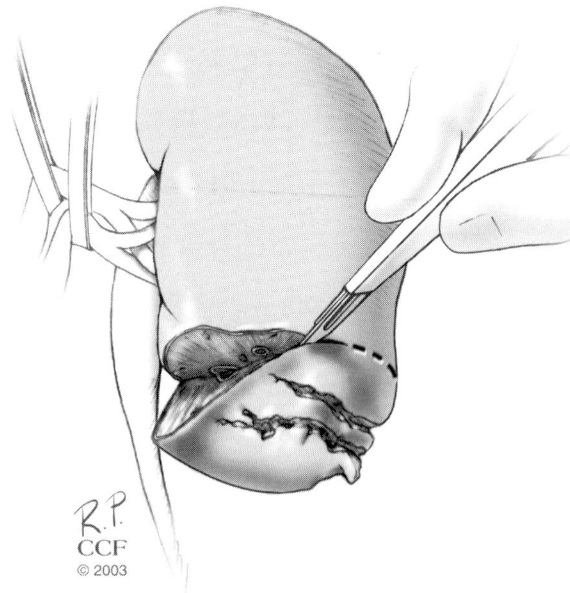


Fig. 12.3

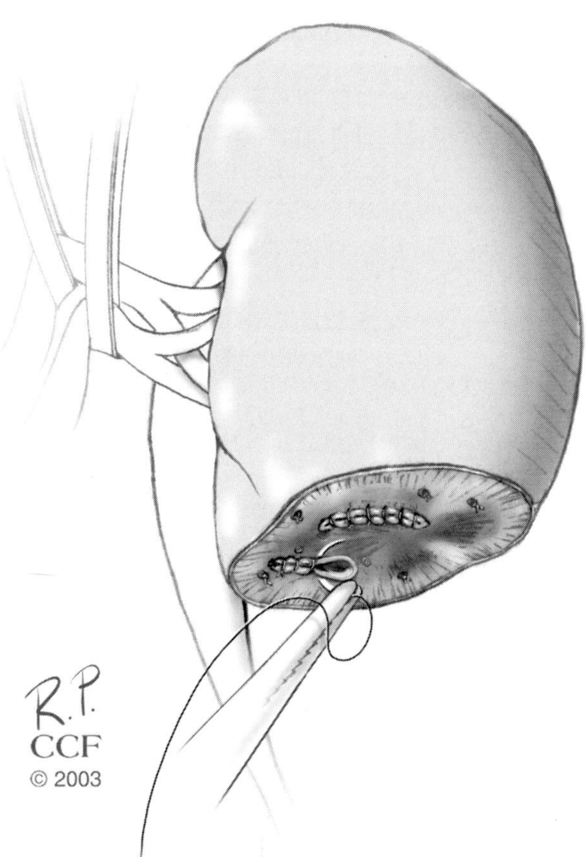


Fig. 12.4

## MID-RENAL INJURIES

Mid-renal injuries require renorrhaphy to reapproximate viable renal tissue if the kidney is explored (Fig. 12.6). All damaged tissue should be removed. A high-velocity penetrating injury (i.e., rifle bullet) causes tissue damage

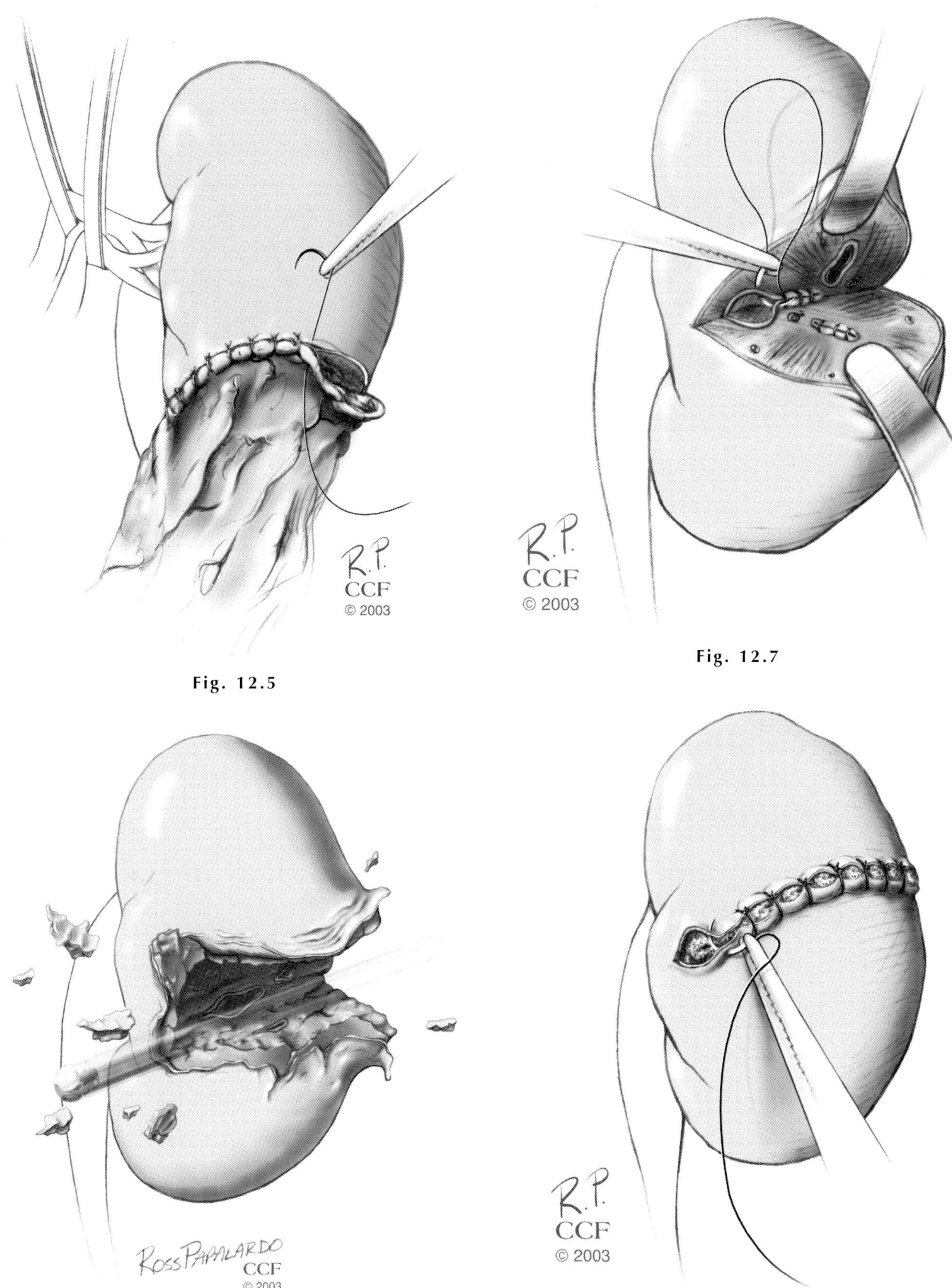


Fig. 12.5

Fig. 12.6

Fig. 12.7

Fig. 12.8

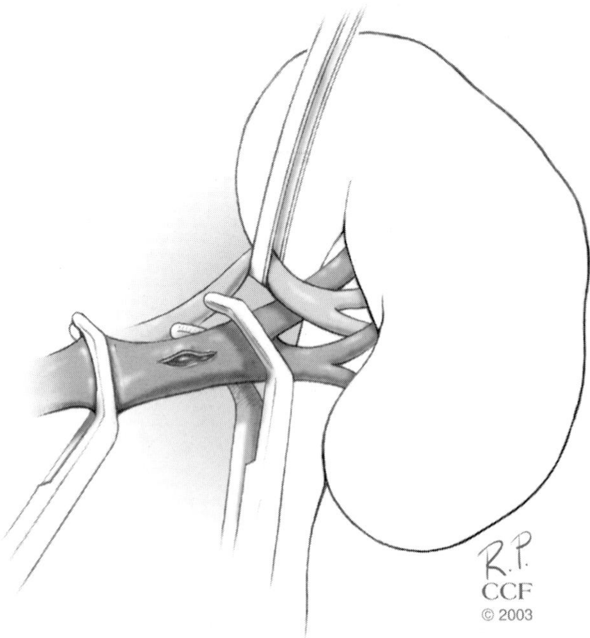


Fig. 12.9

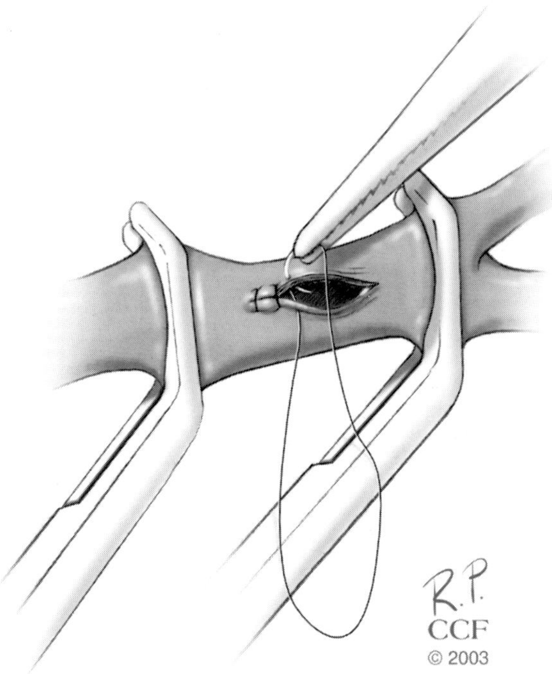


Fig. 12.10

beyond that visible, so a wider debridement should be considered.

Reconstruction following debridement involves closing the collecting system and suturing any large vessels (Fig. 12.7).

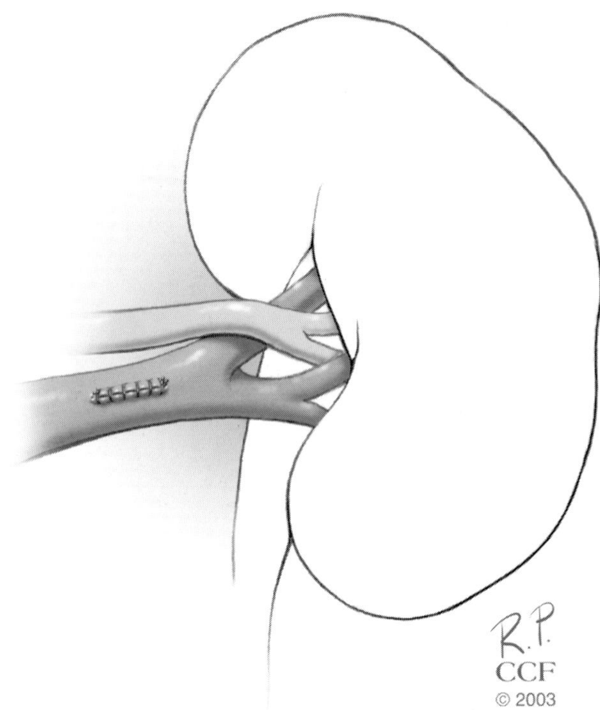


Fig. 12.11

Renorrhaphy is completed by reapproximating the renal capsule. An assistant holding the two sides in opposition while tying the interrupted absorbable sutures helps avoid suture pull-through (Fig. 12.8).

## RENAL HILUM INJURIES

Most major vascular injuries will result in ipsilateral renal loss. Nephrectomy is only required if complications occur. Partial injuries to the vein or artery may cause incomplete occlusion. If identified and isolated early, repair may be feasible (Fig. 12.9).

Polypropylene sutures are placed to make a watertight closure (Fig. 12.10).

Care must be taken to not compromise luminal diameter (Fig. 12.11).

## REFERENCES

1. Guerriero WG, Carlton CE Jr, Scorr R, Jr, et al. Renal pedicle injuries. J Trauma 11:53–62, 1971.
2. Brandes SB, McAninch JW. Reconstructive surgery for trauma of the upper urinary tract. Urol Clin North Am 26(1):3–199, 1999.

# II THE RETROPERITONUM

# 13 Nerve-Sparing Retroperitoneal Lymphadenectomy

*Eric A. Klein*

Nerve-sparing retroperitoneal lymphadenectomy (RPLND) was first described by Donohue et al. *(1)* and Jewett et al. *(2)*, representing the culmination of efforts to reduce the morbidity of extended and modified dissections in patients with testis cancer. Specifically, nerve-sparing RPLND preserves ejaculatory function in virtually 100% of patients with low-stage disease and in selected patients with more advanced stages or after chemotherapy. This technique has thus become the procedure of choice for patients in whom surgical therapy of the retroperitoneum is indicated. Appropriate candidates for nerve-sparing RPLND include (1) patients with clinical stage I disease undergoing RPLND for complete surgical staging; (2) patients with low-volume stage II disease (normal tumor markers and low-volume retroperitoneal lymphadenopathy) for both therapeutic and prognostic purposes; and (3) selected patients undergoing postchemotherapy RPLND to determine the presence of residual disease and eliminate teratoma.

Templates for performing RPLND have evolved over the past 30 yr (Fig. 13.1), reflecting improved understanding of the sequencing of chemotherapy and surgery, use of tumor markers, computed tomography (CT) and positron emission tomography (PET) scans for staging, and detailed mapping studies. The main rationale for development of the modified templates was to preserve ejaculation by avoiding disruption of the hypogastric plexus and its branches coursing over the aortic bifurcation. Although this goal is achieved in the majority of patients using modified templates, it leaves those with occult metastases on the contralateral side (about 2% for left-sided primary tumors and 10% for right-sided primary tumors) with unresected disease and at risk for both retroperitoneal and systemic recurrences. Although modified left- and right-sided templates reflecting historical practice are illustrated here, because prospective identification and preservation of the sympathetic nerves can be achieved using any template, *the current standard approach is a full bilateral nerve-sparing dissection in all patients regardless of stage.* This approach preserves ejaculation in virtually 100% of patients with low-stage disease, minimizes the risk of retroperitoneal relapse, and maximizes the chance for cure.

## RELEVANT ANATOMY

Successful performance of nerve-sparing RPLND requires a thorough understanding of the anatomy of the sympathetic chains, their branches, and their relationship to the major structures of the retroperitoneum. The key element in the surgical approach is the prospective identification of postganglionic sympathetic nerves, which arise from the lumbar sympathetic chains and form an anastomosing network (the hypogastric plexus) anterior to the abdominal aorta and surrounding the origin of the inferior mesenteric artery. Fibers from the hypogastric plexus then travel anteriorly along the aorta, across the aortic bifurcation, and descend into the pelvis to innervate the bladder neck and enter the seminal vesicles, vas deferens, prostate, and external urinary sphincter in order to subserve ejaculatory function (Fig. 13.2). The sympathetic chains run parallel to the great vessels of the abdomen on either side of the spinal column (Fig. 13.3). On the left side, the sympathetic chain is lateral and posterior to the lateral border of the aorta (Fig. 13.3A,B,D). The postganglionic fibers, which join the hypogastric plexus, leave the sympathetic chain at an oblique angle and traverse the fibrofatty and lymphatic tissue posterolateral to the aorta. Typically there are three or four postganglionic sympathetic trunks arising from ganglia L1, L2, L3, and L4. Frequently, the trunks arising from L2 and L3 ganglia fuse before reaching the anterior aorta, and other variations in anatomical configuration are common.

On the right side, the sympathetic chain lies directly posterior to the inferior vena cava (IVC; Fig. 13.3A,C). The postganglionic fibers that emerge from ganglia at L1–4

From: *Operative Urology at the Cleveland Clinic*
Edited by: A. Novick et al. © Humana Press Inc., Totowa, NJ

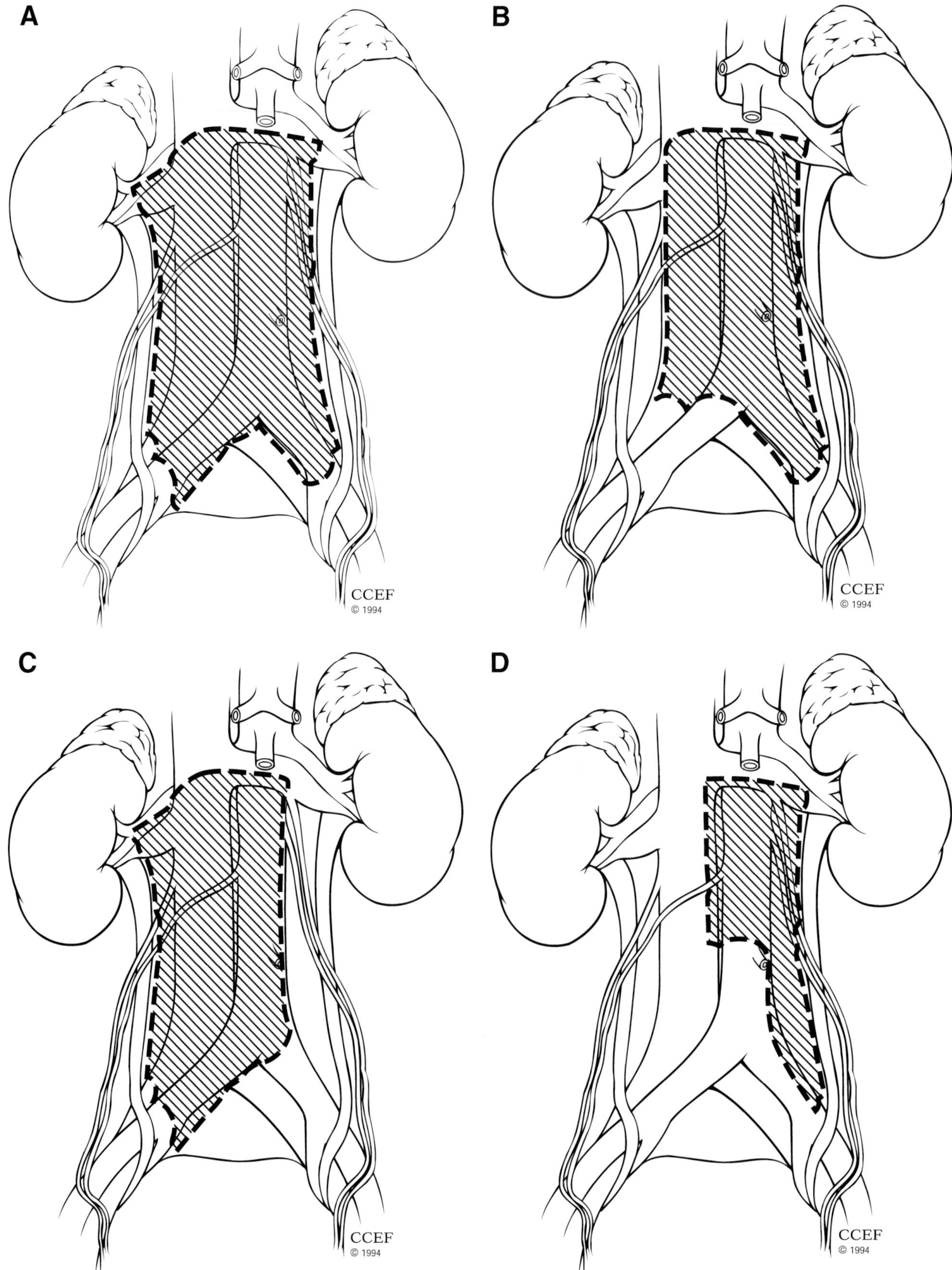


Fig. 13.1

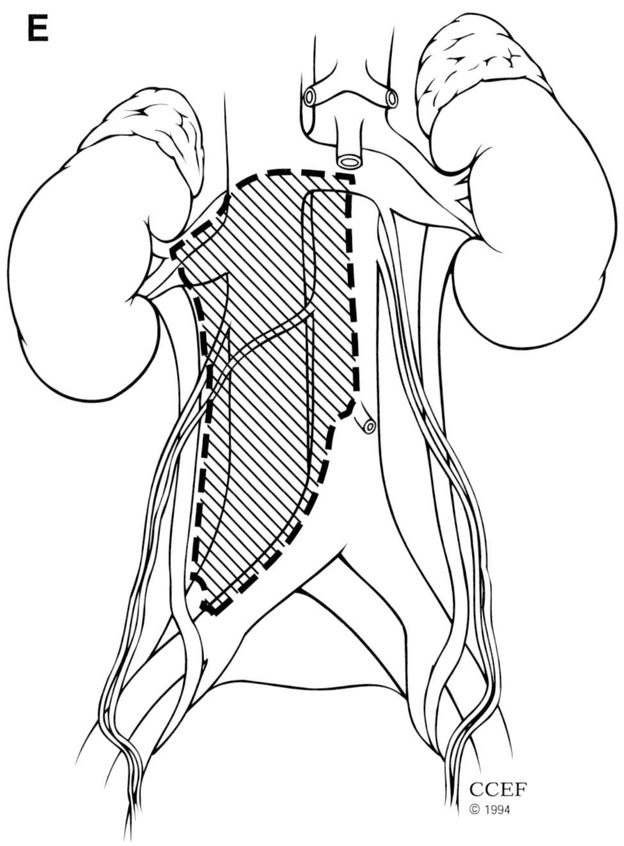


Fig. 13.1 *(Continued)*

Evolution of limits of dissection for RPLND: **(A)** Full bilateral dissection; **(B,C)**, modified right and left dissections as described by Whitmore; **(D,E)**, further evolution of modified right- and left-sided dissections. [*Because prospective identification and preservation of the sympathetic nerves can be achieved using any template, the current standard approach is a full bilateral nerve-sparing dissection in all patients regardless of stage.* (From ref. *3*.)]

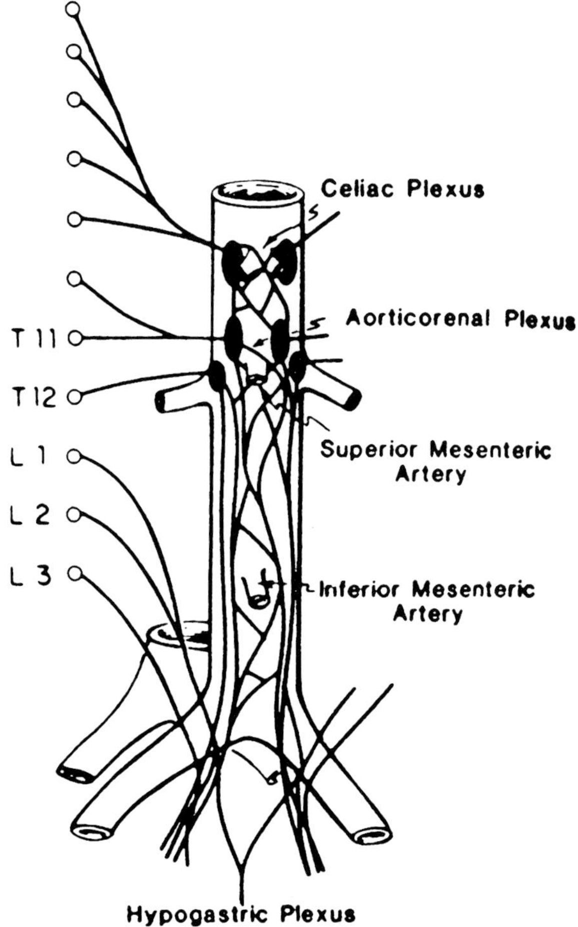


Fig. 13.2

Origin of the hypogastric plexus from the lumbar sympathetic nerves. Fibers from L1 to L4 form this plexus over the aortic bifurcation and innervate the pelvic viscera, subserving seminal emission and ejaculation. (From ref. *3*.)

course initially posterior to the vena cava and emerge from its medial edge in the interaortocaval region. Here they take an oblique and anterior course through fibrofatty and lymphatic tissue to reach the anterior aorta. Accordingly, a clean dissection along the anteromedial aspect of the IVC will not damage these fibers. However, a similar dissection along the medial border of the aorta will result in their disruption. The number of branches on the right is similar to those observed on the left. The sympathetic fibers from both sides form an anastomosing plexus on the anterior surface of the aorta, which extends from the level of the renal vessels to the aortic bifurcation and surrounds the origin of the inferior mesenteric artery (Figs. 2 and 3).

## SURGICAL TECHNIQUE

A midline transabdominal incision and a self-retaining retractor is used (*see* Chapter 1). A Foley catheter is used to drain the bladder and a nasogastric tube to decompress the stomach. For low-stage disease, the bowels are retracted within the abdomen to avoid the venous and lymphatic congestion resulting from placing them in a bag on the patient's chest; this helps minimize postoperative ileus and usually does not compromise exposure for low-stage disease. For higher stage tumors complete mobilization of the right colon and small bowel and placing them on the patient's chest may be needed for adequate exposure. When this maneuver is performed, Kocherization of the duodenum and full release of the inferior border of the pancreas is necessary to avoid traction injuries. Compression of the superior mesenteric artery by a retractor blade should be avoided.

The limits of dissection for a modified left-sided procedure include the renal hilum superiorly, the left ureter laterally, the medial border of the IVC from the level of the

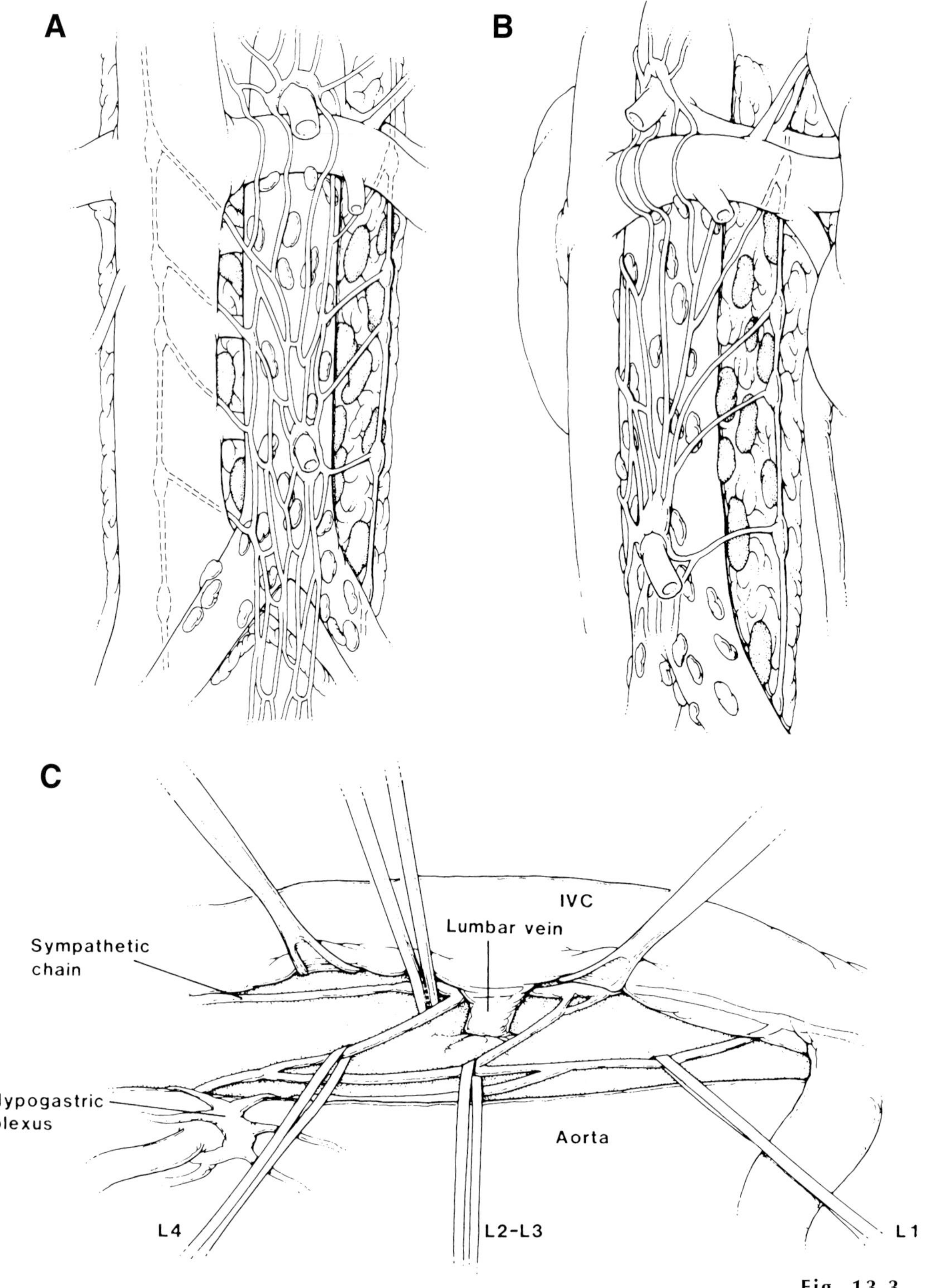


D
Hypogastric plexus
Aorta
Fused L2-L3
L1
Sympathetic chain

**Fig. 13.3**

Relationships of the sympathetic chains and nerves to the great vessels and lymphatic tissue: **(A)** anterior view; **(B)** lateral view. The left sympathetic chain runs lateral to the aorta, while the right sympathetic chain lies posterior to the inferior vena cava. **(C)** Detailed anatomy of the interaortocaval region showing branches of the right sympathetic chain in relationship to the great vessels. **(D)** Detailed anatomy of the left sympathetic chain and branches to the hypogastric plexus. (From ref. *3*.)

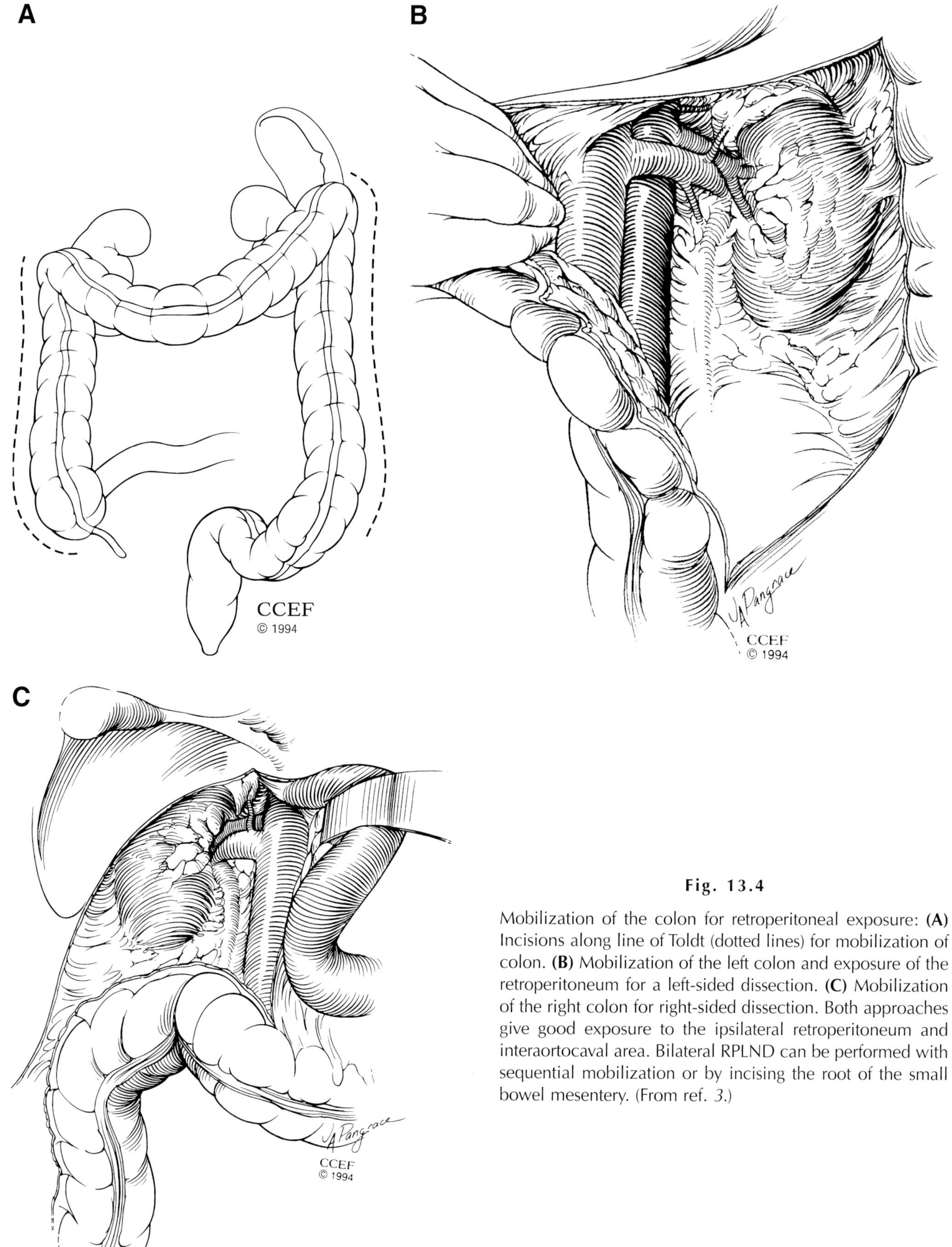


**Fig. 13.4**

Mobilization of the colon for retroperitoneal exposure: **(A)** Incisions along line of Toldt (dotted lines) for mobilization of colon. **(B)** Mobilization of the left colon and exposure of the retroperitoneum for a left-sided dissection. **(C)** Mobilization of the right colon for right-sided dissection. Both approaches give good exposure to the ipsilateral retroperitoneum and interaortocaval area. Bilateral RPLND can be performed with sequential mobilization or by incising the root of the small bowel mesentery. (From ref. *3*.)

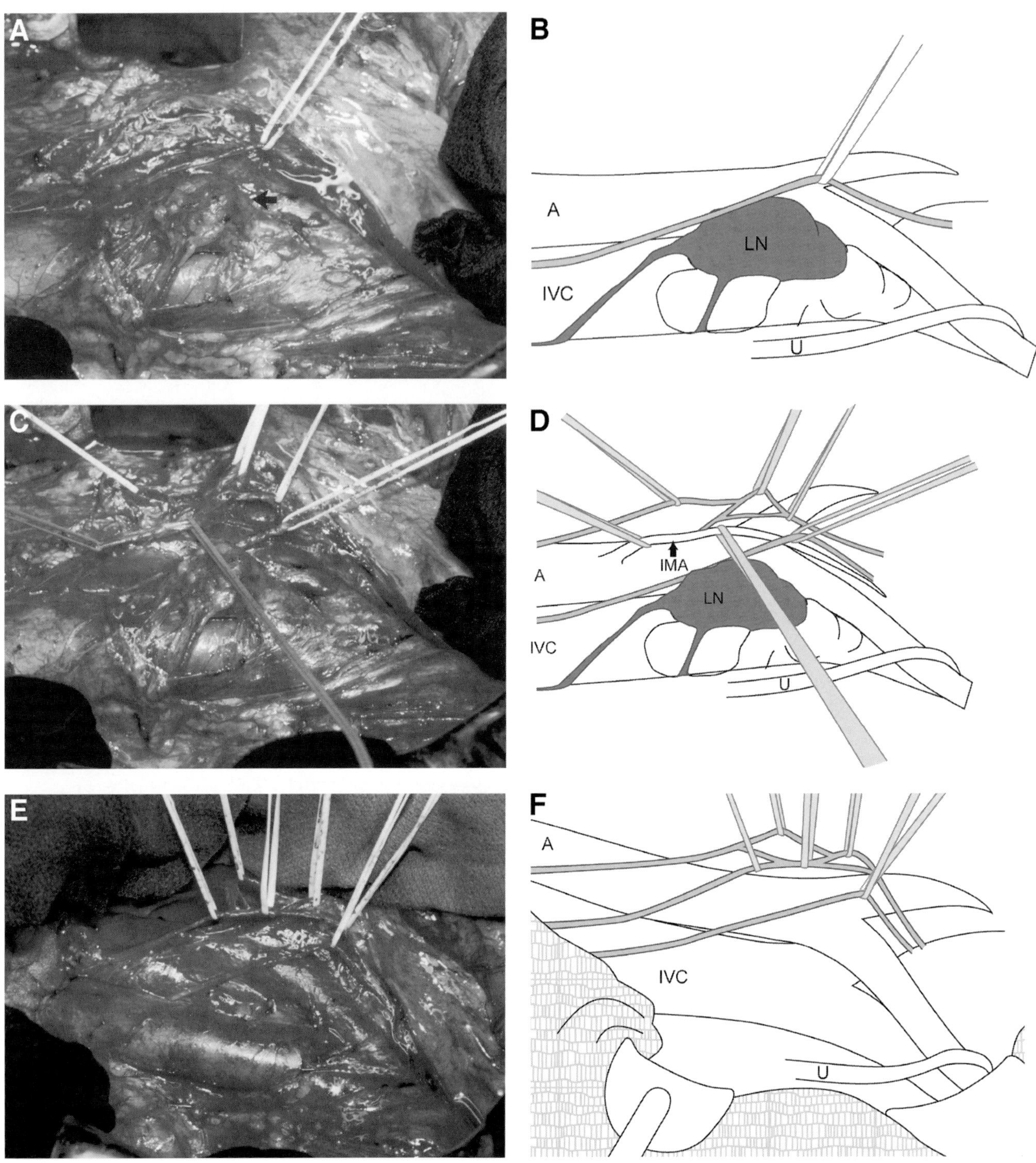


Fig. 13.5

Right-sided nerve-sparing RPLND. The patient's head is to the left. **(A)** Preliminary exposure of the retroperitoneum reveals a solitary 2-cm precaval node (arrow). A branch (probably L2) of the right sympathetic chain has been identified and encircled with a vessel loop. **(B)** Schematic diagram of the operative field shown in (A). The L2 branch of the right sympathetic trunk is shaded in gray and encircled with a vessel loop. LN, tumor-bearing lymph node; A, aorta; IVC, inferior vena cava; U, ureter. **(C)** Continued prospective identification and dissection of lumbar branches from the right sympathetic chain and hypogastric plexus. **(D)** Schematic diagram corresponding to (C). Branches off the right sympathetic chain are shaded and retracted with vessel loops. LN, tumor-bearing lymph node; A, aorta; IVC, inferior vena cava; U, ureter; IMA, inferior mesenteric artery. **(E)** Completed dissection with skeletonization of the IVC and anteromedial aorta. All lymphatic tissue in this region has been removed. Preserved nerves from the right sympathetic chain and hypogastric plexus are demonstrated. **(F)** Schematic diagram corresponding to (E). Branches off the right sympathetic chain are shaded and retracted with vessel loops. (From ref. *3*.)

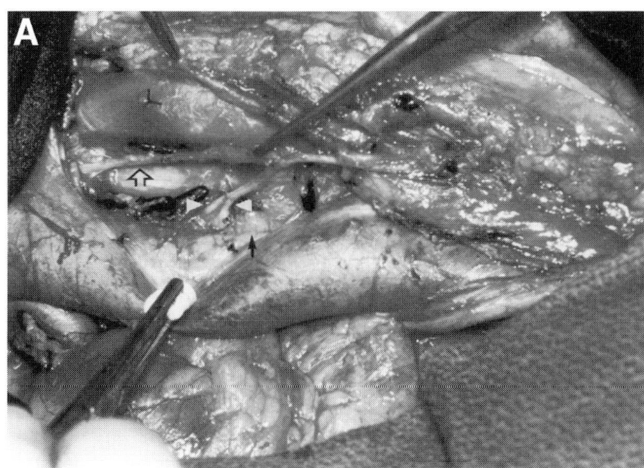


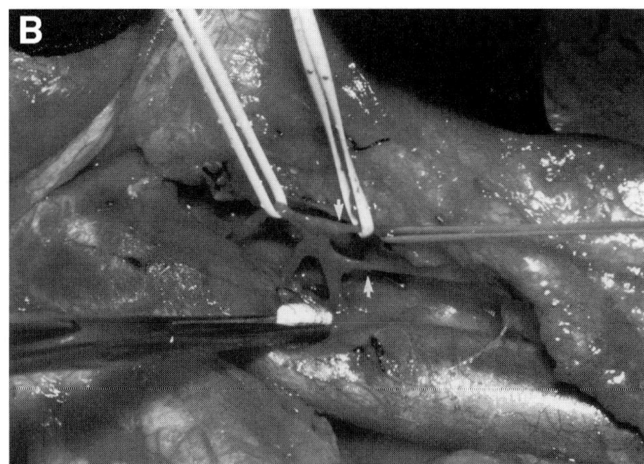


**Fig. 13.6**

Variations in the origin and configuration of lumbar sympathetic nerves: **(A)** Detail of the interaortocaval region during a right-sided nerve-sparing RPLND. The patient's head is to the left. The inferior vena cava (IVC) is retracted anteriorly to expose the right sympathetic chain (black arrow). The lower nerve trunk arises from two branches (white arrows) of the L2 ganglion and fuses with the nerve from L1 (open arrow) prior to joining the hypogastric plexus. **(B)** The branches of the right sympathetic trunk in another patient demonstrating confluence of the L1, L2, and L3 nerves just beyond the right sympathetic chain in the interaortocaval region. Two branches (arrows) travel to the hypogastric plexus. (From ref. *3*.)

renal hilum to the inferior mesenteric artery, and the lateral border of the lower aorta and common iliac artery to the level of its bifurcation, thus encompassing the left para-aortic and interaortocaval regions (Fig. 13.1E). Exposure of the retroperitoneum for a left-sided procedure is accomplished by mobilizing the left colon by incising the line of Toldt laterally and by developing the plane between the colonic mesentery and anterior surface of Gerota's fascia, as is performed for transabdominal left radical nephrectomy (Fig. 13.4A,B). The ureter is reflected laterally and defines the lateral margin of resection. The left sympathetic chain running parallel to and adjacent to the spinal column should then be identified. Individual postganglionic fibers are identified at their emergence from the sympathetic chain or as they course over the surface of the aorta and are encircled with vessel loops (Fig. 13.5). Each fiber is then dissected sharply from the surrounding tissue, proceeding from the level of the sympathetic chain to the anterior aorta. Optical loupes are helpful in identifying the nerves. Once the fibers are identified, they are lifted away from the lymphatic tissue remaining on the anterolateral surface of the aorta, which is subsequently dissected in traditional fashion to the level of the aortic adventitia (Fig. 13.5). Lumbar arteries and veins are divided as necessary. The dissection is carried cephalad, and the lymphatic tissue is removed. The gonadal vein is identified and its origin from the left renal vein divided and removed as a separate specimen.

Attention is then turned to the interaortocaval area. In this region the postganglionic sympathetic fibers are identified as they emerge from the undersurface of the medial edge of the IVC. They are dissected free from the surrounding fibrofatty and lymphatic tissue and elevated with vessel loops. The tissue in the interaortocaval area is then removed to the level of the anterior spinous ligament. Finally, the residual spermatic cord is dissected and removed.

For a right-sided modified nerve-sparing RPLND, the right colon is mobilized and retracted medially (Fig. 13.4A,C). The limits for the right-sided dissection include the renal hilum superiorly, the right ureter laterally, the lateral border of the aorta between the level of the renal hilum and the inferior mesenteric artery, and the lateral border of the common iliac artery to the level of its bifurcation (Fig. 13.1D). Because the right-sided postganglionic sympathetic nerves course underneath the vena cava (Figs. 13.2 and 13.6), it is safe to begin this dissection along the anterior or medial border of the IVC without damaging the sympathetic nerves. This is usually performed first laterally to the vena cava and the specimen removed. The interaortocaval area is then dissected following identification of the sympathetic nerve fibers emerging from the inferomedial border of the IVC (Figs. 13.5 and 13.6).

For bilateral dissections appropriate exposure is obtained by either sequential mobilization of the right and left colon or by the more traditional technique of mobilization of the small bowel mesentery with division of the inferior mesenteric vein. In either case, a similar technique of nerve identification and preservation as described for unilateral techniques is used.

Successful nerve sparing is more difficult in postchemotherapy patients because of nerve entrapment and fibrosis

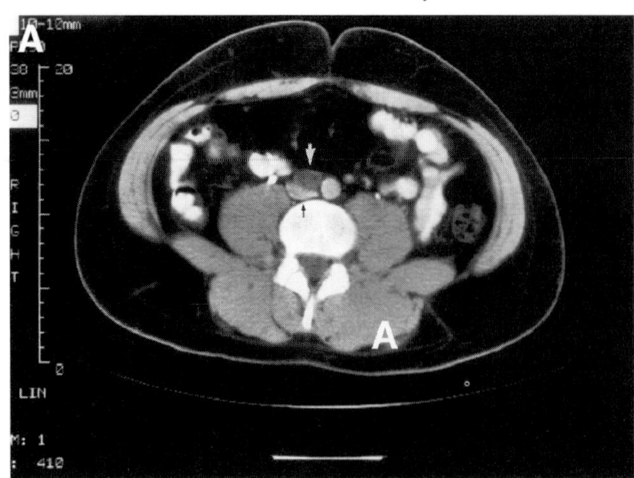

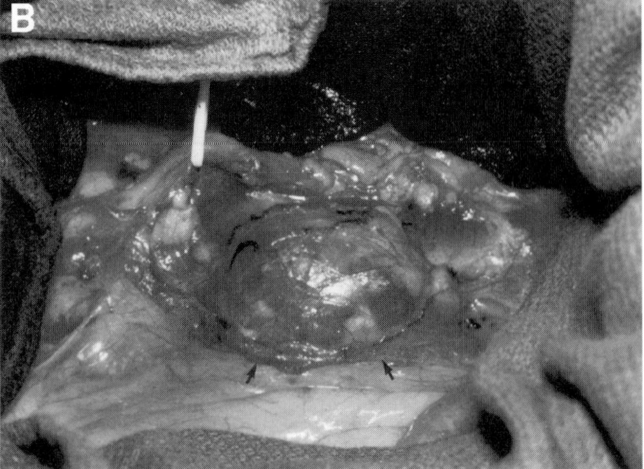

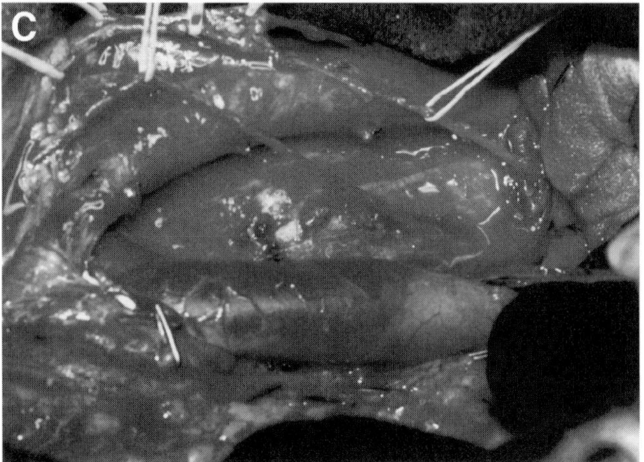

Fig. 13.7

**(A)** Computed tomography scan demonstrating a 4-cm cystic lymph node (white arrow) anterior to the inferior vena cava (IVC) (black arrow). **(B)** Intraoperative appearance of the enlarged node (arrows). A vessel loop encircles the inferior mesenteric artery. **(C)** Appearance after nerve-sparing RPLND. Node was not adherent and was easily removed from surrounding tissue. Pathology revealed mature teratoma. (From ref. *3*.)

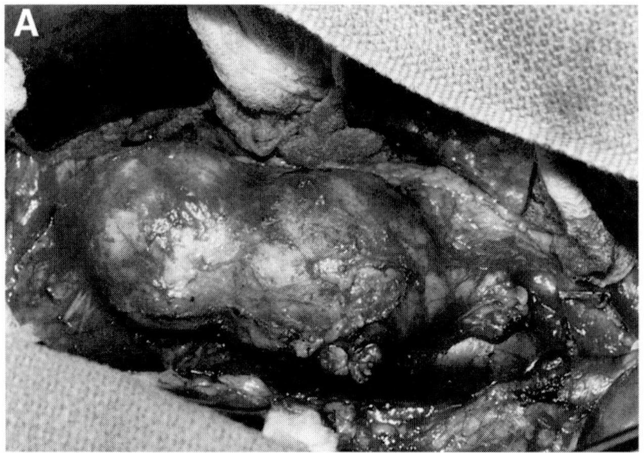

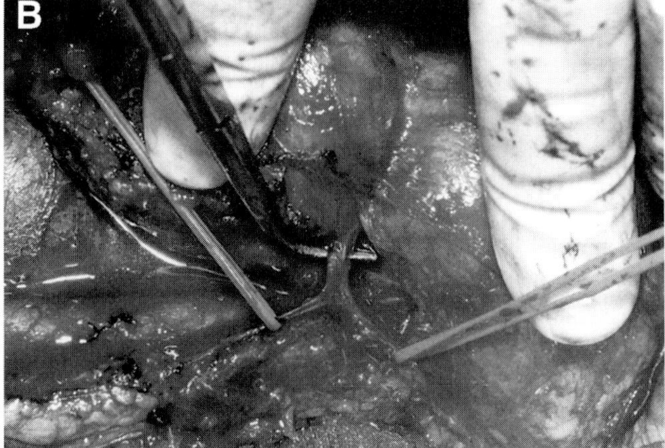

Fig. 13.8

**(A)** Midline postchemotherapy residual mass in a patient who presented with a stage III tumor. **(B)** A Lumbar sympathetic nerve (anterior to clamp) is attached to the tumor mass. The mass was adherent to most of the hypogastric plexus, and all but one nerve was sacrificed to ensure complete tumor excision. (From ref. *3*.)

between the tumor mass and great vessel adventitia. However, in patients with limited residual retroperitoneal disease, selective or unilateral nerve sparing may be attempted successfully (Figs. 13.7 and 13.8), although the reported rates of postoperative antegrade ejaculation are lower than for primary RPLND. In cases of doubt about resectability, complete excision of the tumor *always* takes precedence over nerve preservation.

Following the dissection the bowel is returned to proper position and the abdomen and is closed in a single layer using a running polyglycolic acid suture.

## POSTOPERATIVE MANAGEMENT

Patients are ambulated on the first postoperative day. In patients previously untreated with chemotherapy, the nasogastric tube is removed in the recovery room; in postchemotherapy patients it is left overnight. The Foley catheter is removed when patients are fully ambulatory. Oral intake typically begins at 48 h. The average length of stay is 5 d.

## REFERENCES

1. Donohue JP, Foster RS, Rowland RG, et al. Nerve-sparing retroperitoneal lymphadenectomy with preservation of ejaculation. J Urol 144:287, 1990.
2. Jewett MA, Kong YS, Goldberg SD, et al. Retroperitoneal lymphadenectomy for testis tumor with nerve sparing for ejaculation. J Urol 139:1220, 1987.
3. Klein EA. Nerve-sparing retroperitoneal lymphadenectomy. Atlas Urol Clin North Am 3:63–79, 1995.

# 14 Ureterolysis

*Lawrence M. Wyner*

## INTRODUCTION

Surgery for retroperitoneal fibrosis (RPF) involving the ureters may be performed for a variety of disease processes. Typically, the patient is a middle-aged or older person with idiopathic involvement of the entire retroperitoneum. Many of these patients have had prolonged exposure to analgesic medication, especially of the ergot class, which has been associated with this condition *(1)*. Symptoms of RPF may include nonspecific flank or back pain, fever, and malaise. Although severe cases manifest on intravenous pyelography with hydronephrosis and medial deviation of the ureters, in its early stages the disease process may be detected only on computed tomography or magnetic resonance imaging, with the discovery of a retroperitoneal mass. Easy ureteral catheterization is pathognomonic of RPF; thus, these patients usually have had stents placed prior to operative intervention. Although a short course of steroids may be beneficial in those with less advanced disease who may be poor surgical candidates *(2)*, most patients will come to operation for definitive diagnosis and treatment. Some of these patients ultimately will be found to have secondary RPF owing to a malignant condition, usually lymphoma. Other nonmalignant etiologies for RPF include prior abdominal irradiation, ovarian pathology, inflammatory bowel disease, and abdominal aortic aneurysm. Obviously, treatment of the underlying cause is paramount in secondary RPF.

## PREOPERATIVE PREPARATION

A full bowel prep is given. The pathology department is alerted that frozen section biopsy will be needed. Although significant blood loss is unlikely, the patient should be typed and crossed. Broad-spectrum intravenous antibiotics are given.

## OPERATIVE PROCEDURE

The patient should have had ureteral stents placed preoperatively, and if not, they should be inserted prior to making the incision. This step is crucial because the ureters are easy to catheterize in this disease process and may be difficult to dissect intraoperatively. After the induction of general or epidural anesthesia, a Foley catheter is inserted and the patient is placed in the supine position. Sequential compression device stockings are placed on both legs to prophylax for deep vein thrombosis (DVT). A nasogastric tube is placed, and a midline incision is made from the xiphoid to the symphysis pubis. The peritoneum is entered and the right colon mobilized (Fig. 14.1). The Buckwalter self-retaining retractor is placed over padded blades.

A retroperitoneal mass, if present, is usually palpable and must be biopsied to rule out a malignant process (if this is found, the patient is closed and treated for the malignancy). Assuming that the biopsy is negative for tumor, which is usually the case, the posterior peritoneum is incised from the renal hilum to the common iliac artery (Fig. 14.2). The ureter is identified as far inferiorly as possible, below the level of involvement by the disease process, since it will be difficult to identify through the thick fibrotic tissue. A plane usually can be found between the ureter and the surrounding dense inflammation and is best developed bluntly by inserting a right-angled Monaghan hemostat and gently spreading the tissue, using the cautery to cut through the fibrotic tissue overlying the ureter (Fig. 14.3). The ureter is traced as far proximally as necessary to free it from the enveloping disease process. It is unwise to manipulate uninvolved ureteral segments unnecessarily, as the ureteral blood supply may be compromised with this maneuver. Small ureteral perforations are of little consequence if stents or ureteral catheters have been placed preoperatively and may be closed with 4-0 or 5-0 chromic sutures. Once the entire involved ureter has been freed, an identical procedure is performed on the left side. The retractor blades are repositioned, and the left colon is mobilized. After both ureters have been completely freed, they must be isolated from the retroperitoneum. This is most easily accomplished by transposing them anterior to the posterior (parietal) peritoneum and sewing the cut edges of peritoneum together with interrupted 4-0 chromic suture

From: *Operative Urology at the Cleveland Clinic*
Edited by: A. Novick et al. © Humana Press Inc., Totowa, NJ

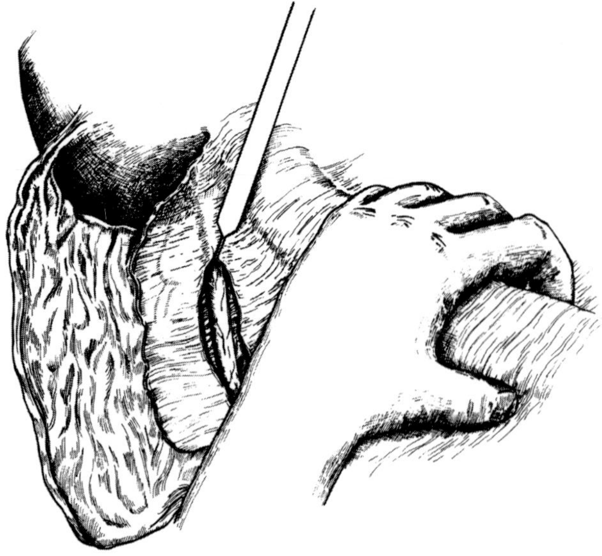

Fig. 14.1

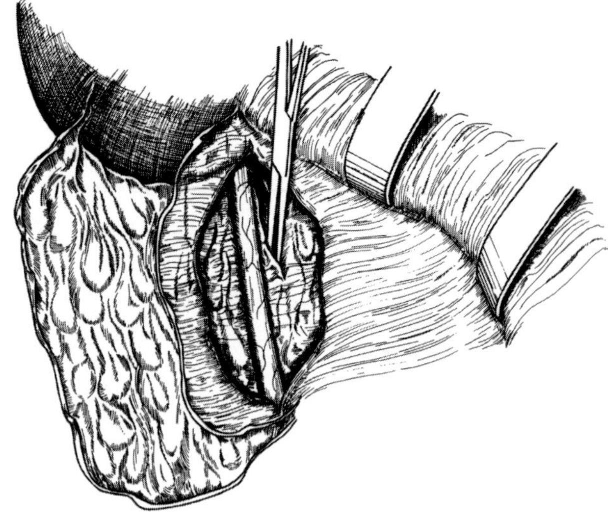

Fig. 14.3

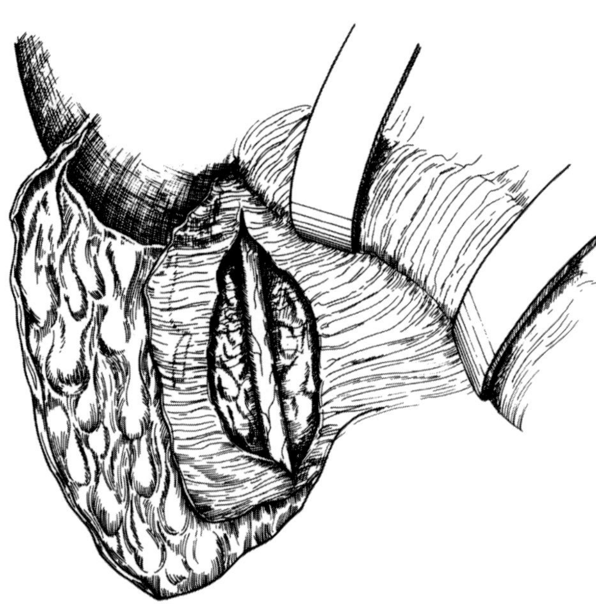

Fig. 14.2

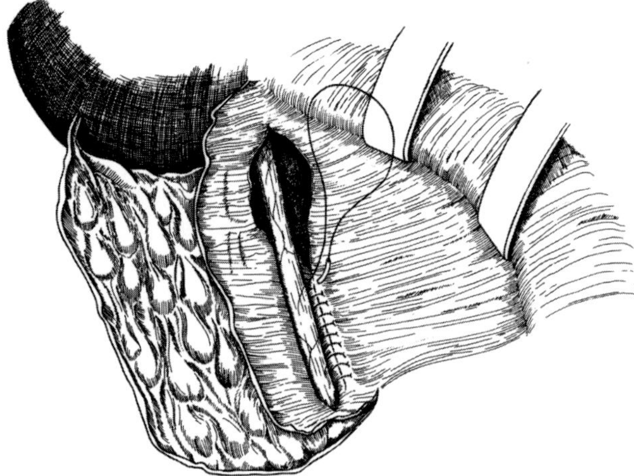

Fig. 14.4

(Fig. 14.4). Although omental wrapping is controversial *(3)*, we recommend that the ureters be surrounded with omentum to promote revascularization of the denuded ureter. This is accomplished by dividing the omentum in the midline. The short gastrics may be divided to lengthen the omentum if necessary, based on pedicles supplied by the right and left gastroepiploic arteries (Fig. 14.5). The omental tissue is then sewn to the posterior peritoneum with interrupted 4-0 chromic sutures (Fig. 14.6). The small bowel is "run" to confirm proper orientation, and a one-layer fascial closure is performed with heavy absorbable suture. No drains are placed. The skin is closed with staples.

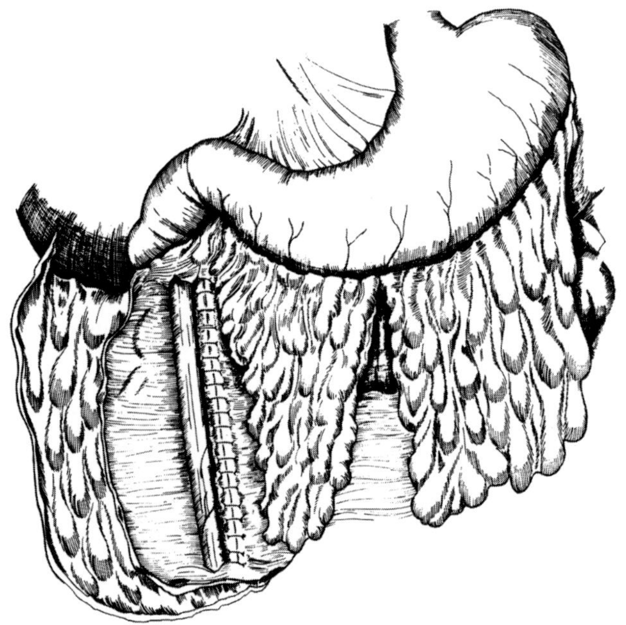

Fig. 14.5

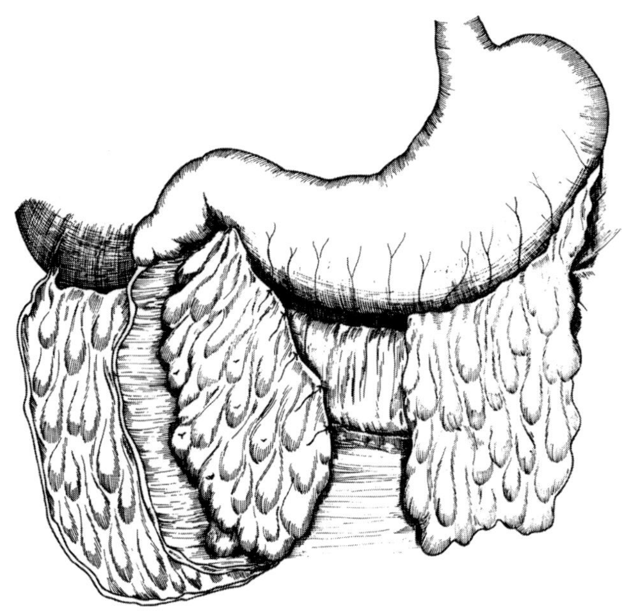

Fig. 14.6

## POSTOPERATIVE CARE

DVT prophylaxis is maintained postoperatively with daily subcutaneous low-molecular-weight heparin injections, usually after 24 h have elapsed, in order to assure hemostasis. The use of intravenous metoclopramide hastens the return of normal bowel function, along with early ambulation, and the nasogastric tube is removed after the patient's first bowel movement. The Foley catheter is taken out prior to discharge from the hospital and the patient is maintained on a prophylactic dose of antibiotics for urinary tract infection until the ureteral stents are removed 6 wk postoperatively.

## LONG-TERM FOLLOW-UP

Patients who have undergone ureterolysis should be followed with periodic renal ultrasound and serum creatinine determinations. Recurrent involvement of the ureters is rare, but strictures have been reported *(4)*, possibly as a result of localized ischemia as a result of extensive dissection. Many of these cases may be amenable to minimally invasive therapies such as ureteral dilation, repeat stenting, or laparoscopy *(3,5,6)*.

## REFERENCES

1. Koep L, Zuidema GD. The clinical significance of retroperitoneal fibrosis. Surgery 81:250, 1977.
2. Oschsner MG, Brannan W, Pond HS, Goodlet JS Jr. Medical therapy in idiopathic retroperitoneal fibrosis. J Urol 114:700–704, 1975.
3. Elashry OM, Nakada SY, Wolf JS Jr, Figenshau RS, McDougall EM, Clayman RV. Ureterolysis for extrinsic ureteral obstruction: a comparison of laparoscopic and open surgical techniques. J Urol 156:1403–1410, 1996.
4. Carini M, Selli C, Rizzo M, Durval A, Costantini A. Surgical treatment of retroperitoneal fibrosis with omentoplasty. Surgery 91:137–141, 1982.
5. Downey DB, O'Connell D, Smith J, Donohoe J. Percutaneous balloon dilatation of a mild-ureteric obstruction caused by retroperitoneal fibrosis. Br J Urol 60:84–85, 1987.
6. Ward AS, Karanjia ND, Russell AJ. Ureteral obstruction following aortobifemoral bypass: management by endoscopic balloon dilation. J Urol 147:120–122, 1992.

# 15 Pancreas Transplantation

*Venkatesh Krishnamurthi*

## BACKGROUND

Pancreas transplantation is currently the only treatment for type 1 diabetes mellitus that consistently establishes an insulin-independent euglycemic state with complete normalization of glycosylated hemoglobin levels. Since its early stages more than three decades ago, this procedure has undergone considerable evolution and expansion. According to data from the International Pancreas Transplant Registry (IPTR), more than 1000 pancreas transplants have been performed yearly at US centers since 1994. Throughout this period, graft and patient survival rates at 3 yr remain above 70 and 90%, respectively *(1)*. Along with advances in cadaveric donor management, organ preservation, and immunosuppressive medications, refinements in transplantation technique have been instrumental in driving pancreas transplantation to its current level of success.

## OPERATIVE PROCEDURE

The surgical techniques of whole-organ pancreas transplantation can be broadly classified according to the type of exocrine drainage performed. Bladder drainage (BD) remains the most common method of duct management. With improvements in immunosuppression and a reduction in the frequency of surgical complications, combined with the unique metabolic and urological complications posed by BD, increasing numbers of transplant programs are adopting enteric drainage (ED) as a primary method of duct management.

The surgical techniques described in this chapter relate to the procedures performed in the pancreas allograft recipient. Procurement of the pancreas from a cadaveric organ donor will not be discussed in this chapter but must be thoroughly understood, as proper procurement is essential to successful transplantation.

### Bench Reconstruction

Of all solid organ transplants, the pancreas allograft generally requires the greatest amount of back-table reconstruction. Some variability exists in terms of the required steps during bench preparation, depending on the manner in which the organ was procured. In the majority of instances, the pancreas, spleen, duodenum, and proximal jejunum are procured *en bloc* (Fig. 15.1). The superior mesenteric artery (SMA; transected at its origin or immediately distal to an aberrant right hepatic artery) and the splenic artery (transected immediately distal to its origin on the celiac axis) comprise the arterial inflow. The portal vein, which when shared with the liver team is divided at the level of the left gastric or coronary vein, provides the venous outflow.

Preparation of the pancreas allograft is begun by sharply excising all of the loose retroperitoneal tissue along the body and tail of the gland (Fig. 15.2). The need to maintain the dissection close to the pancreas cannot be overemphasized, as excess fatty tissue will serve as a nidus for infection. A splenectomy is then performed, making sure to secure the major splenic vessels and other small perforating vessels (Fig. 15.3). We prefer to secure these vessels with silk ties, but nonabsorbable synthetic suture (Ethibond, Ethicon™) serves equally well.

Attention is then directed toward preparation of the duodenal segment. The third and fourth portions of the duodenum and proximal jejunum are mobilized by dividing the small feeding vessels from the root of the mesentery. These vessels should not be tied directly on the mesenteric root or pancreatic head as this may impinge upon the inferior pancreaticoduodenal artery, thereby compromising the blood supply to the head of the pancreas. The duodenum is mobilized to a point approx 2 cm distal to the ampulla of Vater and then transected with a gastrointestinal stapling instrument (TLC55 or TLC75, Ethicon Endo-Surgery, Inc., Ethicon). The precise location of the ampulla can be verified by passage of a small probe via the common bile duct; but in most cases transection of the duodenum 2 cm distal to the point at which the duodenum starts to separate from the pancreatic head is satisfactory (Fig. 15.4). The proximal duodenum is also

From: *Operative Urology at the Cleveland Clinic*
Edited by: A. Novick et al. © Humana Press Inc., Totowa, NJ

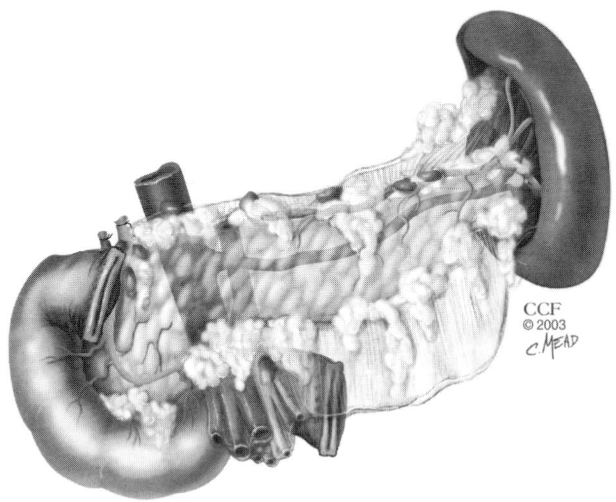


**Fig. 15.1**

Appearance of composite pancreaticoduodenosplenic specimen following procurement.

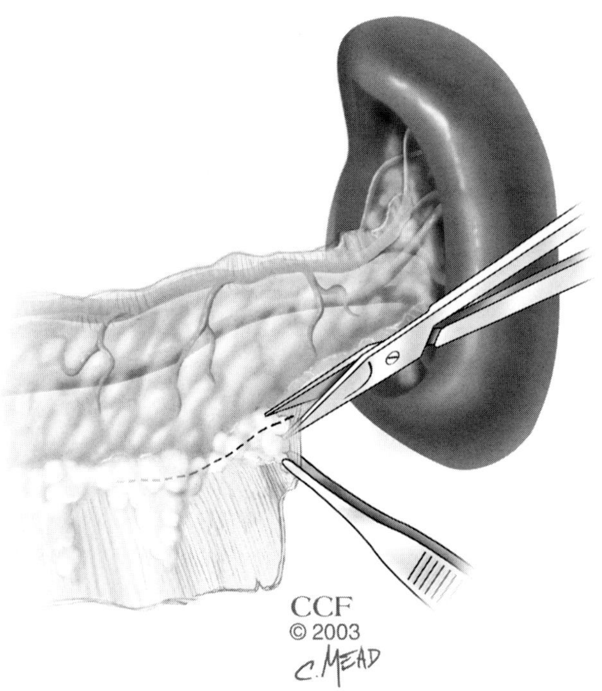


**Fig. 15.2**

Removal of excess retroperitoneal tissue from pancreatic parenchyma.

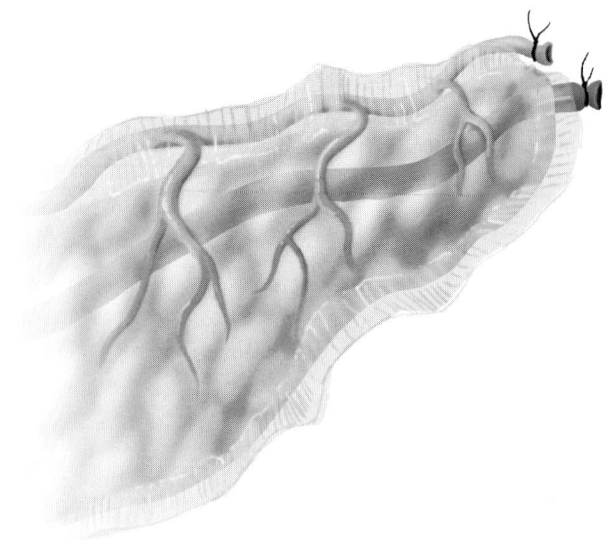

**Fig. 15.3**

Appearance of pancreatic tail following splenectomy.

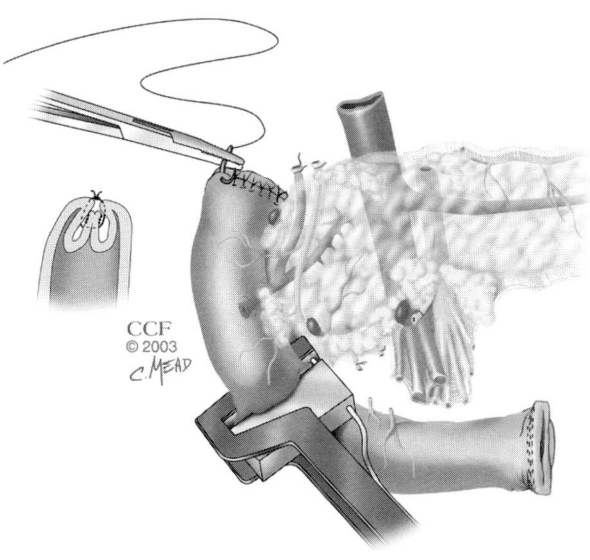


**Fig. 15.4**

Preparation of the duodenal segment.

divided (with a linear stapling instrument) immediately distal to the pylorus. The excess retroperitoneal tissue is then excised from the duodenal serosa, and the proximal and distal staple lines are inverted by placing a row of 3-0 silk interrupted seromuscular sutures (Lembert).

The mesenteric root is then controlled by securing the SMA and superior mesenteric vein (SMV) approx 1–2 cm beyond the pancreatic parenchyma. The mesenteric root can be stapled with a linear stapling instrument (TL60, Ethicon Endo-Surgery, Inc., Ethicon) (Fig. 15.5) and the staple line should be reinforced with a continuous suture. We prefer to place a 4-0 polypropylene suture in both directions immediately under the staple line (Fig. 15.6). Alternatively, if a vascular stapling instrument is used to control the root of the mesentery, a reinforcing suture is generally not necessary.

The allograft vasculature is now prepared. The donor portal vein should be fully mobilized to the confluence of the splenic and superior mesenteric branches. This often

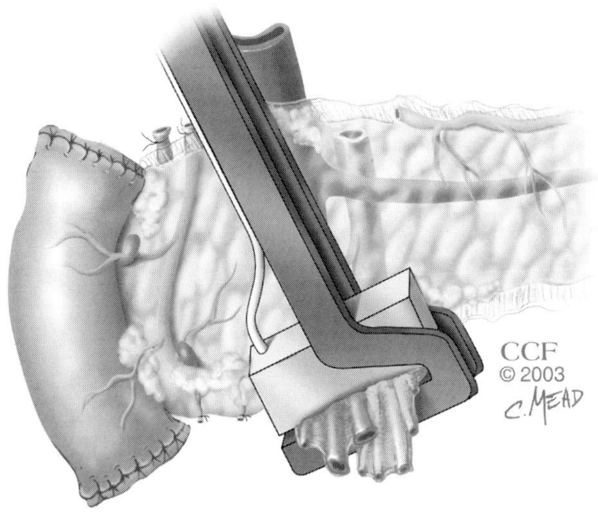


**Fig. 15.5**

Control of mesenteric vessels with stapling instrument.

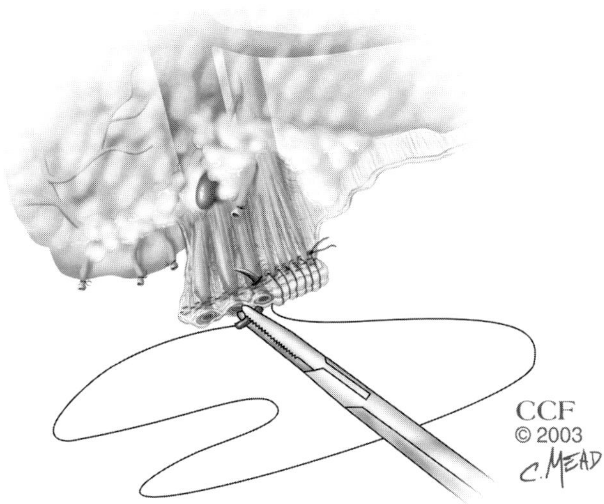


**Fig. 15.6**

Reinforcement of staple line on mesenteric vessels.

involves division of several pancreaticoduodenal branches. Venous extension grafts should generally be avoided due to the increased incidence of venous thrombosis *(2,3)*.

The neural and lymphatic tissue surrounding the proximal SMA is then sharply excised. The origin of the splenic artery is similarly mobilized (Fig. 15.7). Excessive dissection around the origin of the vessels is not necessary and should be avoided as only a very short segment of these vessels is required for arterial reconstruction. In the majority of cases, a donor Y-graft, or iliac artery bifurcation graft, is used to join the superior mesenteric and splenic arteries on the pancreas (Fig. 15.8). Most often, the hypogastric artery is similar in size to the splenic artery and is thus anastomosed in an end-to-end fashion with 7-0 polypropylene suture. The external iliac artery can then be anastomosed end-to-end to the SMA using 6-0 polypropylene suture (Fig. 15.9). The hypogastric and external iliac limbs on the Y-graft should be kept as short as possible to avoid any kinking following implantation of the allograft. In the setting of significant atherosclerosis involving the donor iliac arteries, alternate reconstruction may be considered. Other options are direct end-to-side anastomosis between the splenic artery and SMA, anastomosis between these vessels with an interposition graft, and use of the donor brachiocephalic arterial graft *(2,4,5)*. Arterial reconstruction with the donor Y-graft should be the preferred technique in whole-organ pancreas transplantation, as all other arterial reconstructive techniques are associated with an increased incidence of thrombosis *(2)* (Fig. 15.10).

## Pancreatic Allograft Implantation

Pancreas transplantation can be performed through either a lower quadrant extraperitoneal incision (identical to an incision used for renal transplantatation) or a midline intraperitoneal approach. With a retroperitoneal approach, it is recommended that the peritoneum be opened to facilitate absorption of peripancreatic secretions. In general, a midline intraperitoneal incision is preferred, as this approach allows for maximum flexibility and for the performance of concomitant procedures such as simultaneous kidney transplantation, peritoneal dialysis catheter removal, nephrectomy, and appendectomy. Additionally, the risk of wound infection appears to be lower through a single incision *(6,7)*. Following routine exposure of the abdomen, the lymphatics overlying the iliac artery and vein are divided. The right iliac artery and vein are preferred sites of implantation, as there is more favorable anatomy in the right iliac venous system.

## Venous Reconstruction

Pancreas transplantation can be performed using either of two techniques of venous reconstruction. Systemic venous (SV) drainage, the most commonly utilized technique, is an established surgical technique that is associated with excellent long-term results *(8,9)*. Portal venous (PV) drainage, a more physiological method that eliminates hyperinsulinemia, is gaining interest among pancreas transplant centers and has been shown to result in excellent graft survival rates with a reduced number of surgical complications *(10–13)*.

The technique of SV drainage involves anastomosis of the donor portal vein to the recipient iliac (common or external) vein or vena cava. The recipient common and external iliac veins should be fully mobilized by dividing all internal iliac and lumbar branches, effectively placing

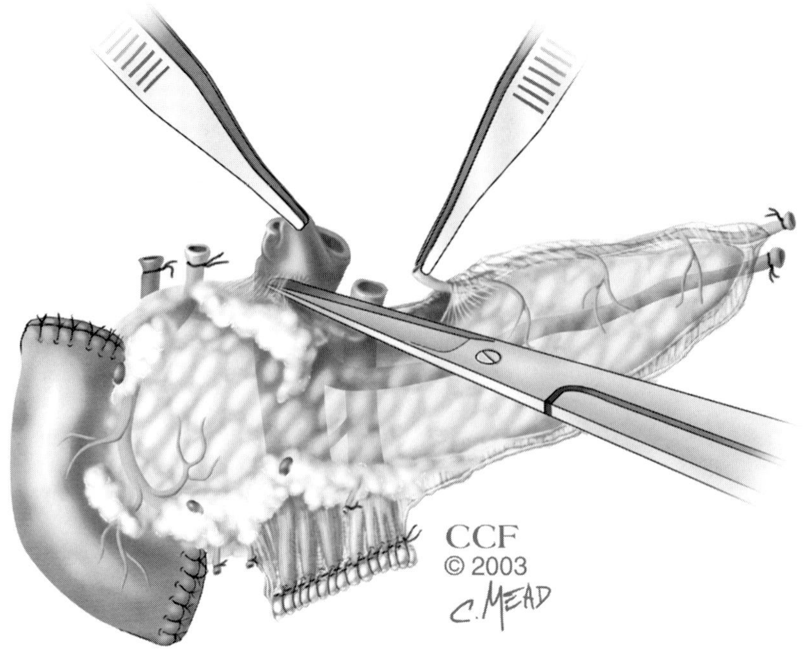


**Fig. 15.7**

Mobilization of portal vein, SMA, and splenic arteries for vascular reconstruction.

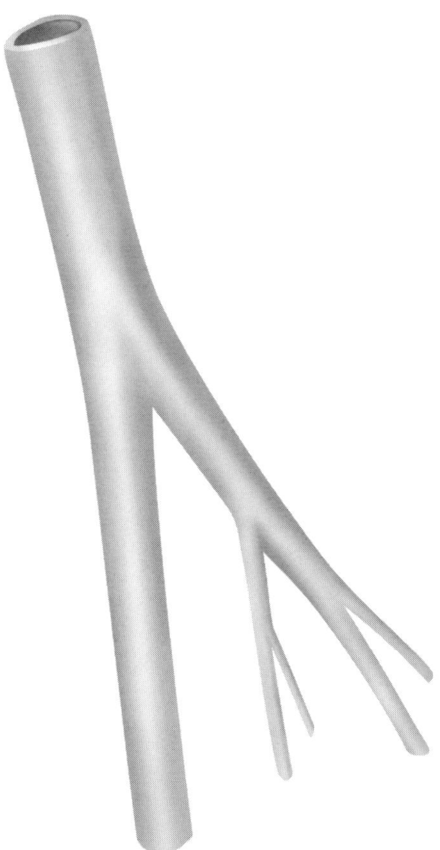

**Fig. 15.8**

Donor iliac bifurcation graft or Y-graft.

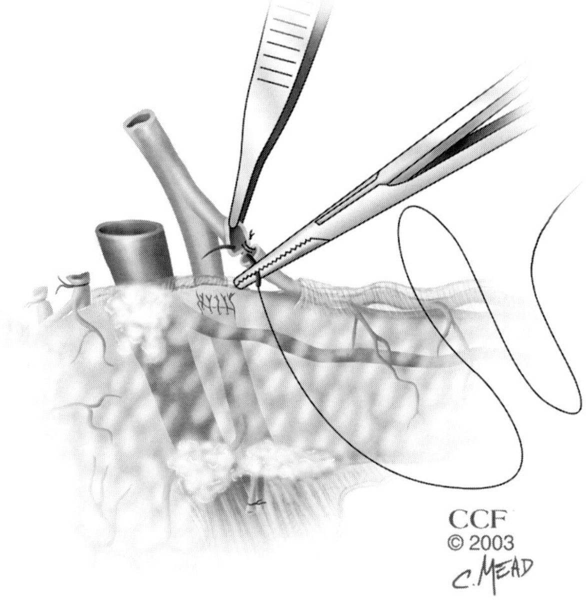


**Fig. 15.9**

Use of the Y-graft to reconstruct pancreas allograft arterial supply.

this vein anterolateral to the iliac artery on the right side and medial to the external iliac artery when performed on the left side. This maneuver decreases tension on the venous anastomosis, allows it to be performed under improved exposure, and reduces the risk of venous thrombosis

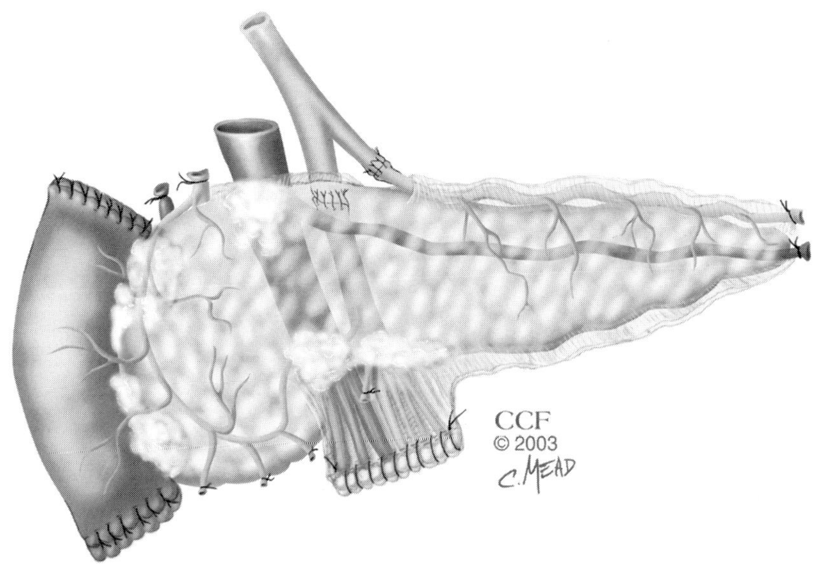


**Fig. 15.10**

Pancreas allograft following completion of back-table preparation.

*(2,3,14)*. In cases of SV drainage, we perform an end-to-side anastomosis directly between the portal vein and the iliac vein using fine (6-0) polypropylene suture.

PV drainage remains our preferred technique of venous drainage. In this technique, the transverse colon is reflected cephalad, exposing the small bowel mesentery. In many instances, the SMV or large-caliber tributary may be immediately visualized. When this is not the case, the peritoneum in the root of the mesentery is incised, the mesenteric lymphatics are divided between ligatures, and the SMV is exposed. A sufficient length (3–4 cm) of the SMV is then mobilized. Circumferential mobilization of the SMV is generally not necessary, as enough vein can be controlled with a tangentially occluding clamp. In preuremic recipients, we administer intravenous heparin (50 U/kg) prior to clamping the vein. An end-to-side anastomosis between the portal vein and the SMV is then performed using 7-0 polypropylene suture. Once the venous anastomosis is complete, we occlude the donor portal vein with a bulldog clamp and restore the venous drainage of the bowel. At this point a tunnel is made in the small bowel mesentery adjacent to the venous anastomosis and through which the arterial graft is passed to the retroperitoneum.

## Arterial Reconstruction

In selected cases, particularly when the liver is not procured, a common patch of aorta containing both the celiac and superior mesenteric orifices may be available, obviating the need for arterial reconstruction when performing a systemically drained pancreas transplant. With PV drainage however, the arterial graft must be sufficiently long to traverse the mesenteric tunnel, a feature not possible with a common aortic patch.

Arterial revascularization of the pancreas allograft is preferentially performed to the right common iliac or external iliac artery. With SV drainage, use of the right iliac vessels is technically easier because of the more superficial course of the external iliac vein and its relative ease of mobilization as compared to the left iliac vein. As indicated previously, when portal venous drainage is used, it is important to have a long Y-graft in order to comfortably reach the site of arterial anastomosis. When dictated by patient anatomy, we frequently place any excess distal external iliac artery onto the proximal common iliac artery as an extension graft during the back-table preparation of the allograft. In cases of PV drainage, the right common iliac artery is also preferred owing to its relative proximity to the mesenteric tunnel. When this vessel is not available as an inflow source, the left common iliac artery or infrarenal aorta are acceptable alternatives, which are easily reached with a long Y-graft.

## Duct Management

As indicated previously, BD remains the most common method of managing the exocrine secretions among pancreas transplant centers worldwide. When performing BD, the donor duodenum should be kept to the minimum possible length, as this avoids metabolic complications stemming from fluid and bicarbonate loss. The pancreas is oriented with the head positioned caudally, and the vascular anastomoses are completed. The bladder is mobilized by dividing the lateral attachments. A location on the dome of the bladder that provides for a tension-free anastomosis is selected. The duodenum is opened along its antimesenteric border, and the duodenocystostomy is performed with a two-layer "hand-sewn" approach or with a stapling instrument *(15)*. The hand-sewn technique is similar to a standard entero-enterostomy. The mucosal layer is performed with a running absorbable suture and the seromuscular layer with interrupted silk sutures. With both the hand-sewn and stapled techniques, it is imperative not to use permanent sutures or staples along an anastamosis that may be in contact with urine, as this will undoubtedly lead to stone formation.

As a result of improvements in immunosuppression and antimicrobial prophylaxis, enteric drainage is increasingly being utilized as a method of managing the exocrine secretions. As has been shown in recent reports comparing ED and BD, ED is associated with a significant reduction in urological and metabolic complications with no increase in septic complications *(13,16)*. For simultaneous pancreas–kidney cases, ED is now the technique of choice. For solitary transplants, BD allows monitoring of urinary amylase.

In contrast to BD, with ED the length of the donor duodenum is not as critical, as pancreatic secretions are reabsorbed in the distal bowel segment. When performing ED, reconstructive options include direct side-to-side anastomosis to the recipient small bowel or anastomosis to a diverting Roux-en-Y limb. The anastomosis to the Roux limb may be performed in either a side-to-side or an end-to-end fashion. Additionally, any enteric anastomosis can be performed by a "hand-sewn" or stapled technique. Although a diverting Roux limb has the theoretical advantage of isolating anastomotic complications from the remainder of the bowel, previous experience suggests that major complications related to the enteric anastomosis are uncommon and that creation of a Roux loop may be unnecessary *(16)*.

## SUMMARY

Since its inception more than 30 yr ago, vascularized pancreas transplantation has undergone considerable progress. Given the unique complications associated with transplantation of this organ, modifications in surgical technique have been necessary to improve outcomes. As a result of these surgical advances as well as improvements in organ preservation and immunosuppression, contemporary graft survival rates approach 90% at 1 yr. Despite this level of success, the technique of pancreas transplantation remains controversial. Future efforts to reduce morbidity and minimize immunosuppression will enable pancreas transplantation to remain an important therapeutic option for selected patients with type 1 diabetes mellitus.

## REFERENCES

1. Gruessner AC, Sutherland DE. Analysis of United States (US) and non-US pancreas transplants as reported to the International Pancreas Transplant Registry (IPTR) and to the United Network for Organ Sharing (UNOS). Clinical Transplantation 53–73, 1998.
2. Troppmann C, Gruessner AC, Benedetti E, et al. Vascular graft thrombosis after pancreatic transplantation: univariate and multivariate operative and nonoperative risk factor analysis. J Am Coll Surg 182: 285–316, 1996.
3. Sollinger HW. Pancreatic transplantation and vascular graft thrombosis. J Am Coll Surg 182:362–363, 1996.
4. Mizrahi S, Boudreaux JP, Hayes DH, Hussey JL. Modified vascular reconstruction for pancreaticoduodenal allograft. Surg Gynecol Obstet 177:89–90, 1993.
5. Ciancio G, Olson L, Burke GW. The use of the brachiocephalic trunk for arterial reconstruction of the whole pancreas allograft for transplantation. J Am Coll Surg181:79–80, 1995.
6. Douzdjian V, Gugliuzza KK. Wound complications after simultaneous pancreas-kidney transplants: midline versus transverse incision. Transplant Proc 27:3130–3132, 1995.
7. Schweitzer EJ, Bartlett ST. Wound complications after pancreatic transplantation through a kidney transplant incision. Transplant Proc 26:461, 1994.
8. Di Carlo V, Castoldi R, Cristallo M, et al. Techniques of pancreas transplantation through the world: an IPITA Center survey. Transplant Proc 30:231–241, 1998.
9. Sollinger HW, Odorico JS, Knechtle SJ, D'Alessandro AM, Kalayoglu M, Pirsch JD. Experience with 500 simultaneous pancreas-kidney transplants. Ann Surg 228:284–296, 1998.
10. Gaber AO, Shokouh-Amiri H, Hathaway DK, et al. Results of pancreas transplantation with portal venous and enteric drainage. Ann Surg 221(6): 613–624, 1995.
11. Gaber AO, Shokouh-Amiri H, Hathaway DK, et al. Pancreas transplantation with portal venous and enteric drainage eliminates hyperinsulinemia and reduces postoperative complications. Transplant Proc 25:1176–1178, 1993.
12. Bartlett ST, Kuo PC, Johnson LB, Lim JW, Schweitzer EJ. Pancreas transplantation at the

University of Maryland. Clin Transplant 271–280, 1996.

13. Stratta RJ, Gaber AO, Shokouh-Amiri MH, et al. A prospective comparison of systemic-bladder versus portal-enteric drainage in vascularized pancreas transplantation. Surgery 127:217–226, 2000.
14. Gill IS, Sindhi R, Jerius JT, Sudan D, Stratta RJ. Bench reconstruction of pancreas for transplantation: experience with 192 cases. Clin Transplant 11: 104–109, 1997.
15. Pescovitz MD, Dunn DL, Sutherland DE. Use of the circular stapler in construction of the duodenoneocystostomy for drainage into the bladder in transplants involving the whole pancreas. Surg Gynecol Obstet; 169:169–171, 1989.
16. Kuo PC, Johnson LB, Schweitzer EJ, Bartlett ST. Simultaneous pancreas/kidney transplantation—a comparison of enteric and bladder drainage of exocrine pancreatic secretions. Transplantation 63:238–243, 1997.

# 16 Ureteropelvic Junction Obstruction

*Stevan B. Streem and Jonathan H. Ross*

## INTRODUCTION

The diagnosis of ureteropelvic junction obstruction (UPJO) implies functionally significant impairment of urinary transport from the renal pelvis to the ureter. Although most cases are probably congenital in origin, the problem may not become clinically apparent until much later in life. This chapter is limited to a discussion of the treatment of congenital UPJO, although at times these techniques may be applied appropriately to the management of some related acquired conditions.

## PATIENT PRESENTATION AND DIAGNOSTIC STUDIES

UPJO, although generally the result of a congenital problem, can present at any time from prenatally to geriatrically. In older children or adults, intermittent abdominal or flank pain, at times associated with nausea or vomiting, is a frequent presenting symptom. Hematuria, either spontaneous or associated with otherwise relatively minor trauma, may also be an initial symptom. Laboratory findings of microhematuria, pyuria, or frank urinary tract infection might also bring an otherwise asymptomatic patient to the attention of a urologist. Rarely, hypertension may be a presenting finding.

Radiographic studies are performed with a goal of determining both the anatomical site and functional significance of an apparent obstruction. Excretory urography remains a cornerstone of radiographic diagnosis. Classically, findings on the affected side include delay in function associated with a dilated pyelocalyceal system. If the ureter is visualized, it should be of normal caliber. In some patients symptoms may be intermittent and intravenous pyelography between painful episodes may be normal. In such cases the study should be repeated during an acute episode when the patient is symptomatic. Alternatively, provocative testing with a diuretic urogram may allow accurate diagnosis. The patient should be well hydrated and the study then performed by injecting furosemide, 0.3–0.5 mg/kg intravenously at the time of intravenous urography.

Ultrasonography can be a valuable initial diagnostic study under any circumstances in which overall renal function is inadequate to perform intravenous urography. It may also be performed in any patient in whom an initial intravenous urogram reveals nonvisualization of the affected collecting system in order to differentiate ureteral obstruction from other causes of nonvisualization. Currently, however, computed tomography (CT) scanning is being performed in most patients in place of ultrasonography and in fact, a CT scan is now the first imaging technique generally obtained for any patient presenting with acute flank pain. Both ultrasonography and CT scanning also have a role in differentiating acquired causes of obstruction such as radiolucent calculi or urothelial tumors.

A nuclear scan will also be of value in differentiating dilated, unobstructed systems from those with functional obstruction by combining the renogram with injection of furosemide, 0.5 mg/kg, to obtain a diuretic renogram. This study will also allow quantification of the degree of obstruction.

The diagnosis of UPJO can generally be made with a high degree of certainty based on the clinical presentation and the results of any one or more of the relatively noninvasive studies just discussed here. However, retrograde pyelography retains an important role for confirmation of the diagnosis and for demonstration of the exact site and nature of obstruction prior to repair. In most cases this study is performed at the time of the planned operative intervention in order to avoid the risk of introducing infection in the face of obstruction. However, retrograde pyelography is indicated emergently whenever the UPJO requires acute decompression such as in the setting of infection or compromised renal function.

Percutaneous nephrostomy drainage is an excellent alternative to retrograde stenting for select patients requiring emergent decompression. It allows decompression of

From: *Operative Urology at the Cleveland Clinic*
Edited by: A. Novick et al. © Humana Press Inc., Totowa, NJ

the system in cases of associated infection or compromised renal function and allows assessment of recoverability of renal function following decompression. Percutaneous nephrostomy also allows the performance of antegrade studies that will help define the nature and exact anatomical site of obstruction. Finally, where there remains some doubt as to the clinical significance of a dilated collecting system, placement of percutaneous nephrostomy allows access for Whitaker pressure perfusion studies.

## INDICATIONS AND OPTIONS FOR INTERVENTION

Indications for intervention include symptoms associated with the obstruction, impairment of overall renal function or progressive impairment of ipsilateral function, development of stones or infection, or rarely, causal hypertension. When intervention is indicated, the procedure of choice had generally been open operative repair of the UPJ, i.e., a pyeloplasty. However, less-invasive endourological and laparoscopic approaches have gained a proven role, often as an initial procedure of choice, and long-term results are now available. Although success rates with most of these alternative techniques have not proven comparable to standard open pyeloplasty, the results may be significantly improved with careful patient selection. Currently, the indications for open vs endourological or laparoscopic management of UPJO are still evolving, and it is appropriate to discuss the risks and benefits of all applicable options. As such, each patient should be advised individually based on all the anatomical and functional information available preoperatively. In this setting, most patients will opt for a minimally invasive approach, even with the understanding that secondary intervention may be required. However, for secondary UPJO, it is our preference to recommend an open or laparoscopic approach to any patient who has failed primary endourological management and an endourological approach to those who have failed open or laparoscopic repair.

## ENDOUROLOGICAL MANAGEMENT

Open operative intervention for UPJO provides a widely patent, dependently positioned, well-funneled UPJ. Although the procedure has stood the test of time and offers a success rate exceeding 95%, several less-invasive alternatives to standard operative reconstruction are now available. The advantages of all these newer approaches include a significantly reduced length of hospital stay and postoperative recovery. However, for many of these procedures, the success rate does not approach that of standard open pyeloplasty. Furthermore, although open operative intervention can be applied to almost any anatomical variation of UPJO, consideration of any of the less-invasive alternatives must take into consideration individual anatomy. Factors to consider include, but are not limited to, the degree of hydronephrosis overall and ipsilateral renal function and, in some cases, the presence of crossing vessels or concomitant calculi.

Although various nuances in the technique of endopyelotomy have been described, the basic concept is constant and involves a full-thickness incision through the obstructing proximal ureter from the ureteral lumen out to the peripelvic and periureteral fat. The approach to the UPJ can be either a retrograde via the ureter or antegrade using percutaneous techniques. The incision is stented and left to heal based on the original work of Davis in 1943, who used an intubated ureterotomy in the course of an open operative procedure for UPJO. The retrograde techniques for endopyelotomy used today include a hot-wire cutting balloon, which incises the UPJ under fluoroscopic control, and a ureteroscopic approach in which the UPJ is incised using direct visual control. At our center the retrograde approach used for endopyelotomy utilizes direct ureteroscopic visual control and a Holmium laser for the endopyelotomy incision.

## URETEROSCOPIC ENDOPYELOTOMY

The main advantage of a ureteroscopic approach, compared to a fluoroscopically guided hot-wire balloon incision, is that it allows direct visualization of the UPJ and assurance of a properly sited, full-thickness endopyelotomy incision. If any major vessels are encountered, these are generally easily visualized and avoided during the procedure. Another advantage of the ureteroscopic approach is a decrease in cost compared to the use of the cautery wire balloon, assuming ureteroscopic equipment and electro-incison capability or a Holmium laser is already available.

### Indications and Contraindications

The indications for a ureteroscopic endopyelotomy include functionally significant obstruction, as defined earlier. Contraindications include relatively long areas of obstruction and the presence of upper tract stones that are best managed simultaneously with alternative approaches, described later in this chapter.

### Technique

In general, the instrument that allows the easiest retrograde access to the UPJ, as well as providing an adequate working channel, is a semi-rigid ureteroscope. In women the UPJ can often be reached with a short 6.9 French semi-rigid ureteroscope, although a standard length instrument may be required. In men a long semi-rigid ureteroscope may occassionally allow adequate access, although flexible instrumentation should be available.

General anesthesia is used in order to minimize patient movement during ureteroscopy and respiratory excursion during the incision of the UPJ. At the outset of the procedure a retrograde pyelogram is performed under fluoroscopic control. This aids in identifying the location of the ureteral insertion into the renal pelvis and the length of the obstructing segment of ureter. A hydrophilic guide wire is passed cystoscopically under fluoroscopic control and coiled in the pyelocaliceal system. The cystoscope is then withdrawn and exchanged for the semirigid ureteroscope.

When flexible ureteroscopy is used, a 10 French dual lumen catheter is passed over the initial hydrophilic guidewire. This catheter dilates the distal ureter and allows fluoroscopic passage of a second working wire, over which the flexible ureteroscope is passed. Alternatively, a second wire can be used to pass a ureteral working sheath. Once the flexible ureteroscope is passed to the UPJ, a 200-μm Holmium fiber is placed through the working channel and the UPJ incised in the appropriate location, as suggested by the radiographic studies.

Once the ureteroscope has been removed, a 10/7 French endopyelotomy stent is advanced over the remaining wire using fluoroscopic guidance. The stent and wire are then back-loaded into the cystoscope for final passage through the intramural ureter and the stent advanced until the widest portion bridges the UPJ fluoroscopically. A Foley catheter is left indwelling overnight to obviate the risk of reflux and extravasation at the site of the endopyelotomy incision. The endopyelotomy stent is subsequently removed with an office cystoscopic procedure after 4 wk and an intravenous pyelogram obtained 4–6 wk following stent removal. Clinical and radiographic follow-up is then continued at 6- to 12-mo intervals for approx 3 yr.

### Results

Several longer-term studies of the results of ureteroscopic endopyelotomy have been reported. Results have been at least comparable to those utilizing any other endopyelotomy approach, and these generally range from 70 to 85%.

### Complications

Complications of any ureteroscopic approach have diminished in frequency and severity with the refinement of ureteroscopic instrumentation over the past decade. Ureteral strictures are no longer a part of ureteroscopic management, and in contemporary series neither angiographic embolization nor nephrectomy has been experienced. Most complications are minor and relate to stent migration.

## PERCUTANEOUS ENDOPYELOTOMY

### Indications and Contraindications

As reviewed earlier, the indications to intervene for any patient with UPJO include the presence of symptoms, progressive or overall impairment of renal function, development of upper tract stones or infection, or, rarely, causal hypertension. With several alternative minimally invasive options available, a percutaneous approach is generally the most appropriate one for those patients with concomitant pyelocaliceal stones, which can then be managed simultaneously.

Contraindications to a percutaneous endopyelotomy are similar to the contraindications to any endourological approach and include a long segment (>2 cm) of obstruction, active infection, or untreated coagulopathy. Although the impact of crossing vessels is controversial, in our opinion the presence of such vessels is not by itself a contraindication to an endopyelotomy. However, significant entanglement of the UPJ by crossing vessels can occasionally be identified and, when present, will generally render any endourological approach unsuccessful. When such entanglement is suggested by intravenous or retrograde pyelography, it can be reliably proven using three-dimensional helical CT.

### Patient Preparation

Patients undergoing a percutaneous endopyelotomy should be subjected to preoperative evaluation and preparation as if they were undergoing open operative intervention. Any urinary infection should be treated, and sterile urine assured at the time of definitive intervention. If upper tract infection cannot be cleared because of obstruction, temporization should be accomplished using internal stenting or percutaneous nephrostomy drainage alone. The patient should be counseled as to the risks and benefits of the procedure including the fact that the success rate of any endourological approach, including percutaneous endopyelotomy, will be less than that of standard open operative intervention. Patients should also be apprised of the fact that bleeding requiring transfusion is a small, albeit real, risk of the procedure, and as such we obtain a "type and screen" as part of our protocol for this procedure.

### Technique

In the original descriptions of the technique both from the Institute of Urology in London (Ramsay et al., 1984) and from Long Island Jewish Hospital in New York (Badlani et al., 1986), the endopyelotomy was performed using a cold knife technique under direct vision. With one, or preferably two, wires in place across the UPJ, an endopyelotome knife is utilized. This hook-shaped cold knife is used to completely incise the UPJ in a full-thickness manner, from the ureteral lumen out to periureteral and peripelvic fat. The incision is extended for several millimeters into the normal ureter. Although some authors suggest that the incision should always be made laterally, in fact, the ureter may be inserting into the renal pelvis on the anterior or posterior wall. In such cases, the incision should instead "marsupialize" the proximal ureter into the renal pelvis so that an anterior or posterior incision may be required. When any endopyelotomy incision is made under direct vision, crossing vessels can be directly visualized and avoided.

Once the incision is complete, stenting is accomplished. A 14/7 French endopyelotomy stent may be utilized, and this is passed in an antegrade fashion with the larger diameter end of the stent positioned across the UPJ. In some cases, especially when the patient has not been prestented, passage

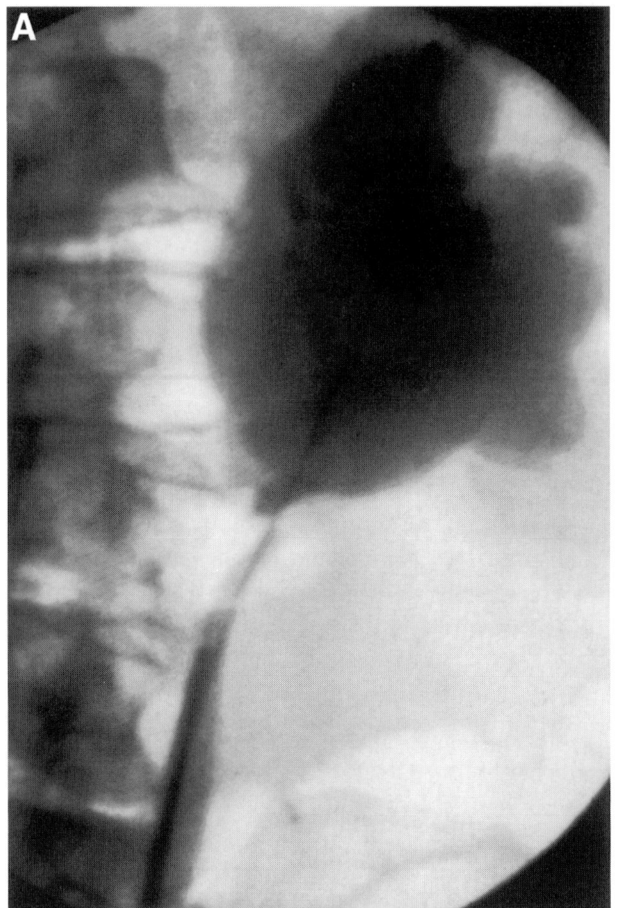


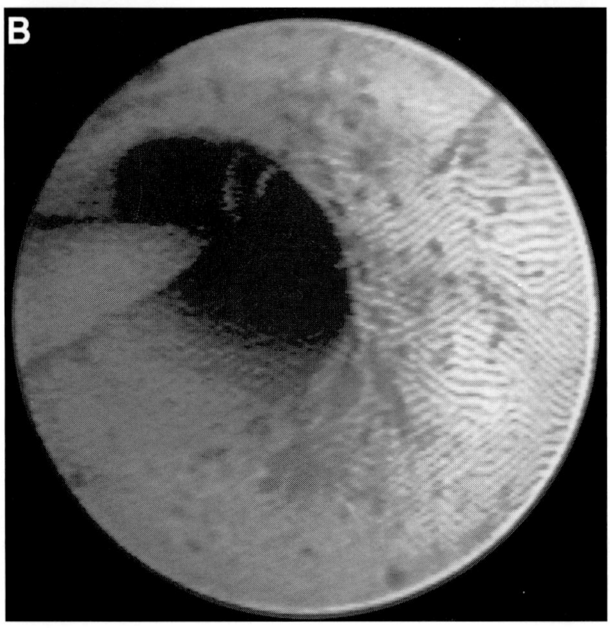


**Fig. 16.1**

Using fluoroscopic **(A)** and direct visual **(B)** control, the ureteroscope is passed alongside the guidewire to the level of the ureteropelvic junction. If the distal ureter is too narrow to allow easy passage of the ureteroscope, the intramural ureter can be dilated using a 5-mm balloon or 9 or 10 French dual lumen "introducing" catheter. If the ureter is still too narrow at any point to easily accommodate the ureteroscope, then an internal stent is placed and the procedure postponed for 5–10 d to allow "passive" ureteral dilation.

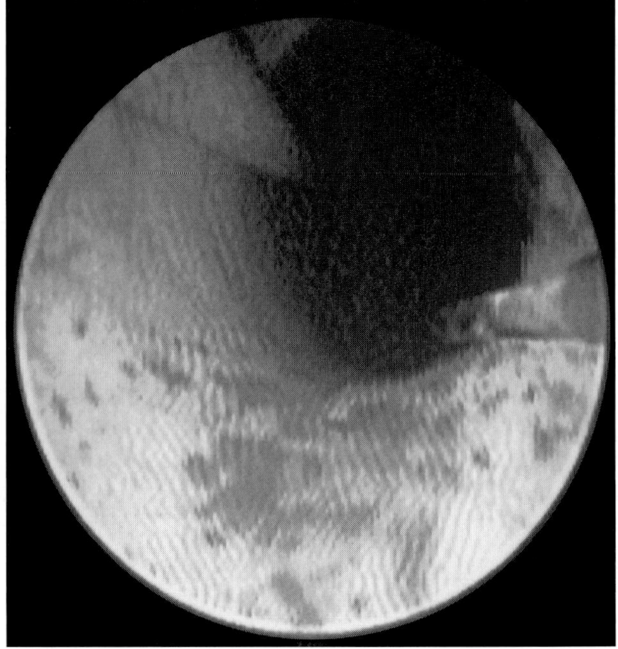

**Fig. 16.2**

When using a semi-rigid ureteroscope, once the ureteropelvic junction (UPJ) is reached, a 365-µ Holmium laser fiber is inserted through the working channel and the ureteroscope is positioned at the proximal extent of the UPJ, or preferably in the renal pelvis itself. At a setting of 1.0 J and a frequency of 10 Hz, incision of the UPJ begins, usually in a posterolateral direction, while the ureteroscope is withdrawn back down from the pelvis, across the UPJ.

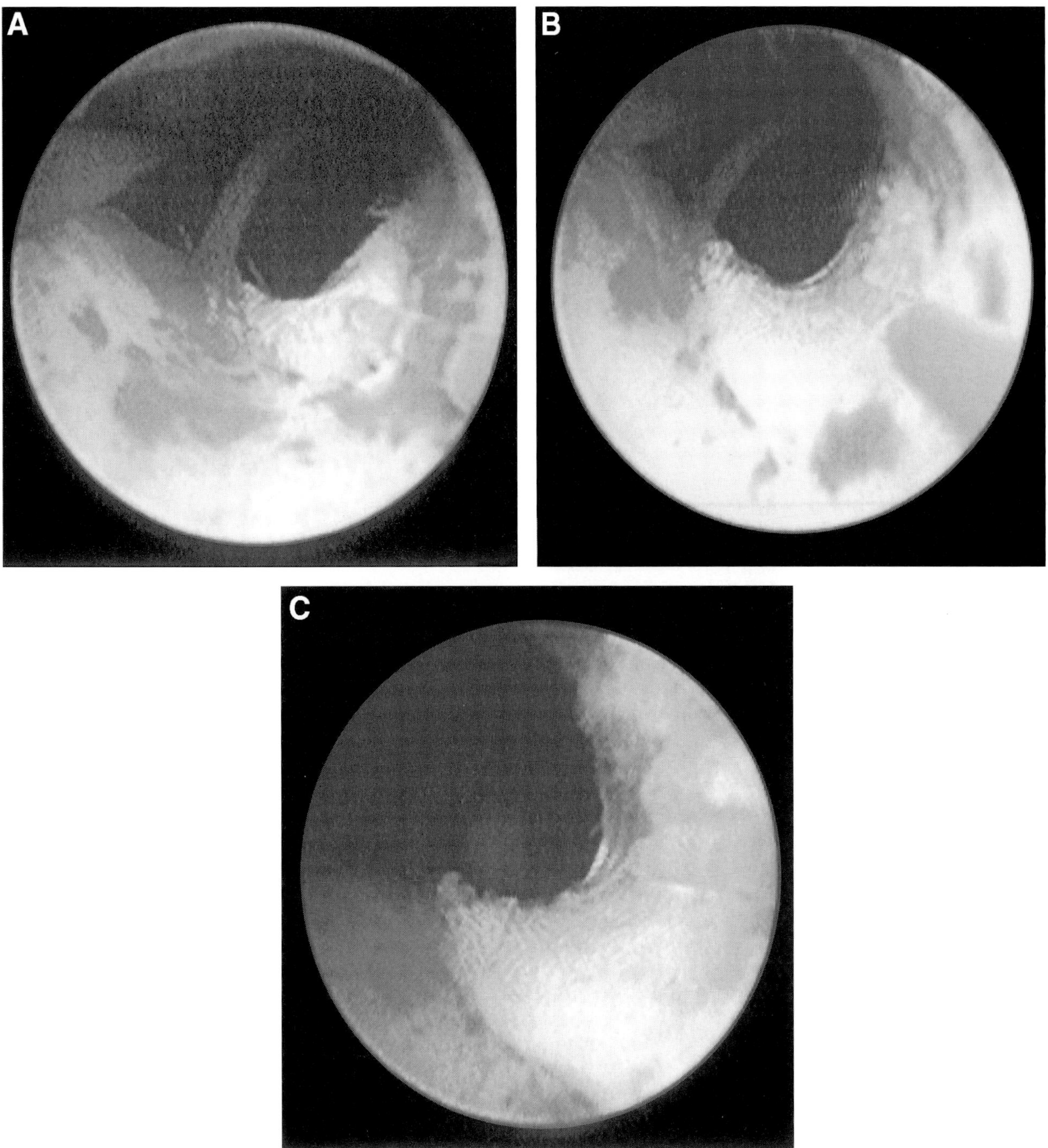


**Fig. 16.3**

This procedure is repeated and the incision gradually deepened to extend into the peripelvic and periureteral retroperitoneal space. Because this is done gradually and under direct vision, any crossing vessels, and potential significant bleeding, are avoided, though in fact, such vessels are seen only rarely at the posterolateral position. Defocusing the Holmium laser can treat small bleeding points that are visualized ureteroscopically.

of this large caliber stent may be difficult. In those instances, a 10/7 French endopyelotomy stent or even a standard 8 French internal stent may be utilized without compromising the ultimate outcome. Once proper positioning of the stent is determined fluoroscopically, any remaining safety wires are withdrawn. Our preference is to leave a nephrostomy tube indwelling for 24–48 h, after which time it is removed, with or without a brief trial of clamping.

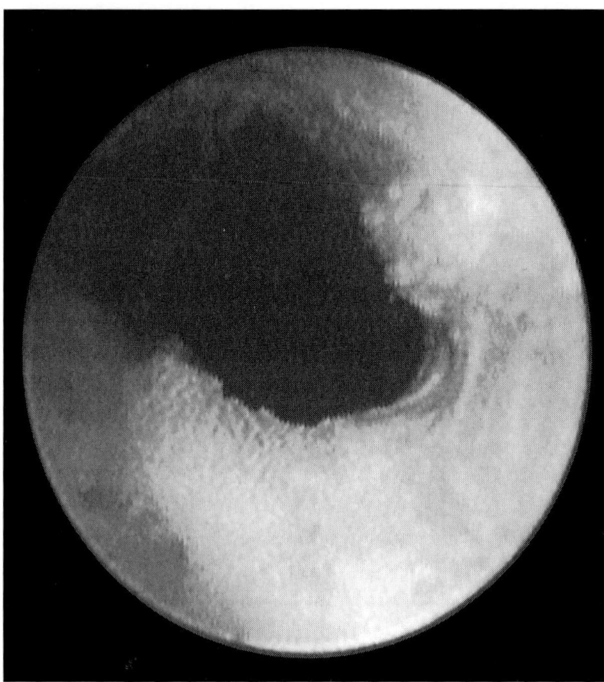

**Fig. 16.4**

The incision is carried caudally into normal ureteral tissue, until the ureteropelvic junction is widely patent. Injection of contrast through the ureteroscope can demonstrate extravasation and confirm an adequate depth of incision, although this is generally not necessary because the entire procedure has been performed under direct vision. The ureteroscope is then withdrawn from the ureter while the safety wire is left in place in the renal pelvis for subsequent passage of a stent.

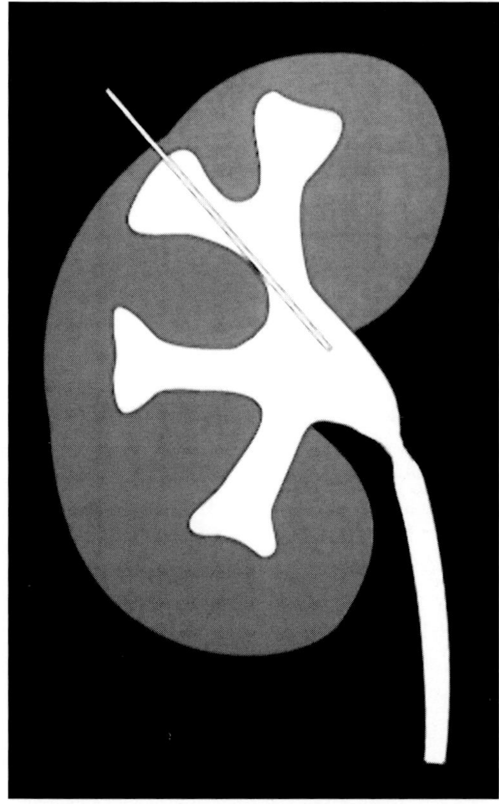

**Fig. 16.5**

With the patient in the prone position, the site for percutaneous access is chosen to allow easy access to the ureteropelvic junction utilizing rigid instrumentation. Generally, a mid-posterior or superolateral calyx is chosen. As soon as access is obtained with one wire, an introducing catheter is utilized to pass a second wire as a "safety wire" so that a working and a safety wire are both now in place. At this point, percutaneous access is complete, the tract is dilated, and the endopyelotomy is begun.

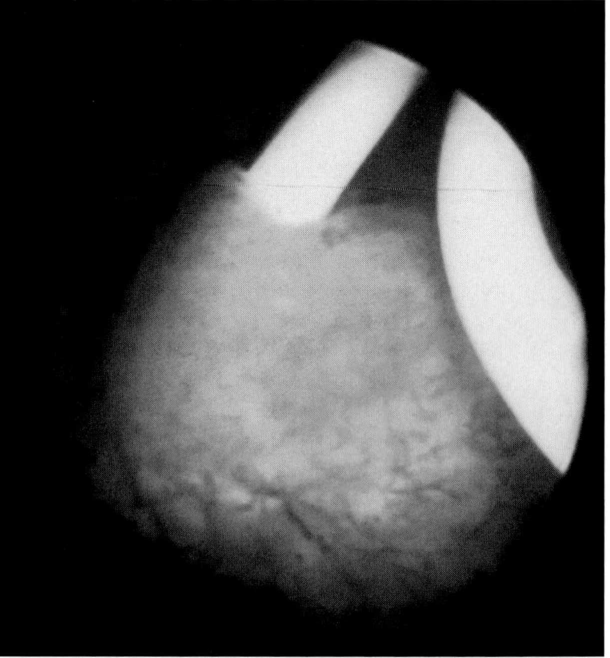

**Fig. 16.6**

For several years we have used our own modification of percutaneous endopyelotomy that is a "stent first/hot knife" technique. Again, percutaneous access is established. A wire traverses the ureteropelvic junction and passes antegrade across the ureterovesical junction into the bladder. We have found it advantageous at this point to pass a stent prior to performing the actual endopyelotomy incision. The purpose of this is twofold. First, having the stent in place at the outset of the procedure obviates concern about avulsing the ureteropelvic junction (UPJ) during placement of a stent after the UPJ has already been incised. Second, we have found that placement of the stent prior to the incision serves to better define the UPJ itself, thus allowing a more precise incision. The UPJ and proximal ureter can then often be seen to bulge into the renal pelvis, such that the subsequent endopyelotomy is equivalent to a ureteral meatotomy at the ureterovesical junction.

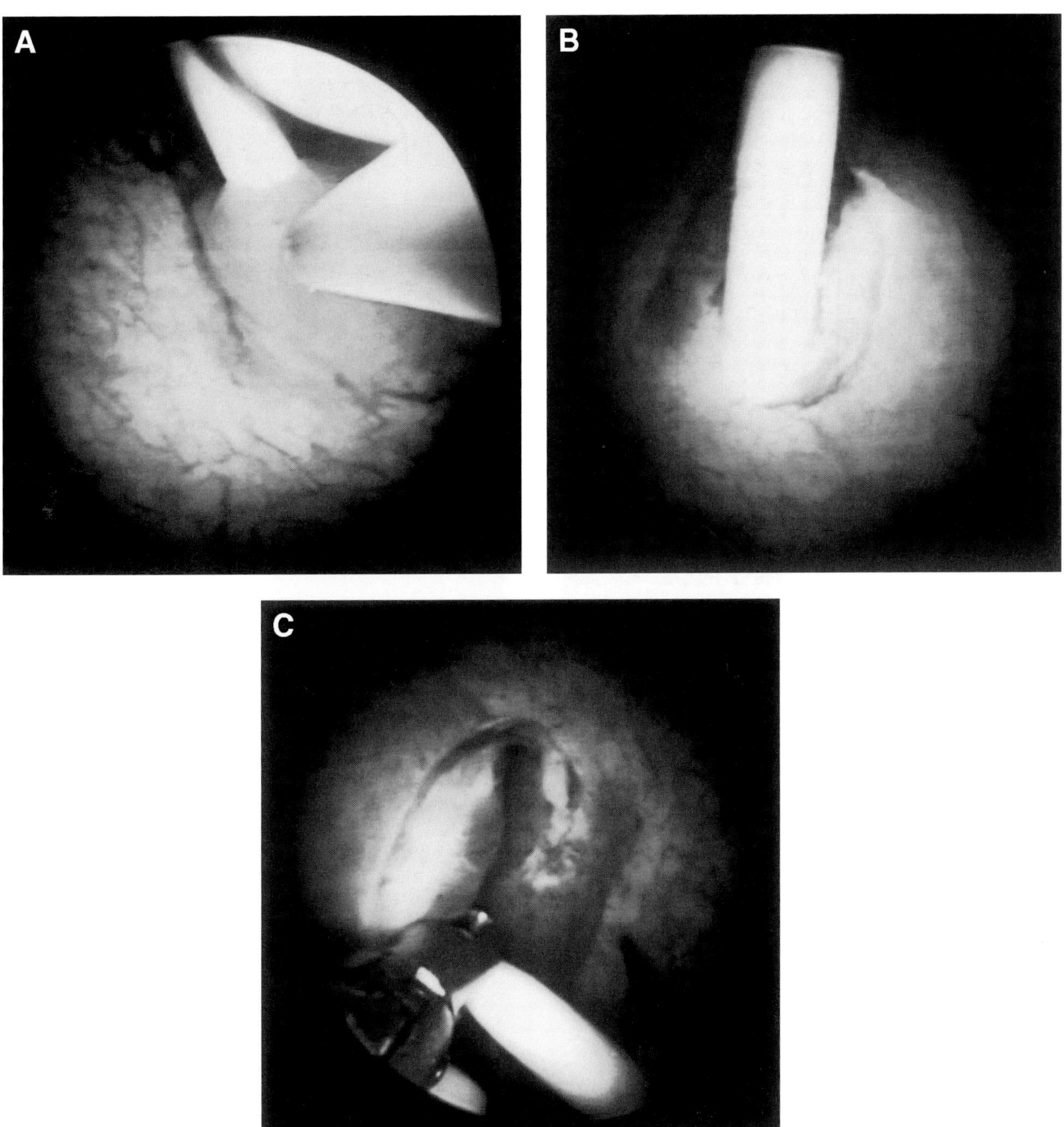


Fig. 16.7

With the stent in place, an acorn tip Bugbee electrode is used with a pure cutting current to marsupialize the proximal ureter into the renal pelvis. In the setting of a high insertion, the incision can often be extended all the way to the dependent portion of the renal pelvis. The incision also bridges the gap between the lateral wall of the ureter and the medial wall of the pelvis, across the periureteral and peripelvic fat. When using an electrode for the incision, the stent itself will insulate the remainder of the ureter from thermal injury. However, care must be taken to ensure that the safety wire used is insulated. Otherwise, this can act to transmit the current if touched by an active electrode. Once the incision is complete, the stent is already in place and the procedure is essentially done. Nephrostomy tube drainage is instituted for 24–48 h.

## Percutaneous Endopyelotomy and Rotational Anomalies

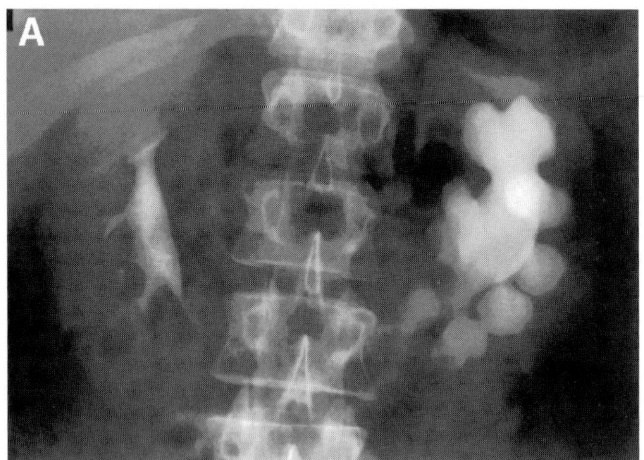


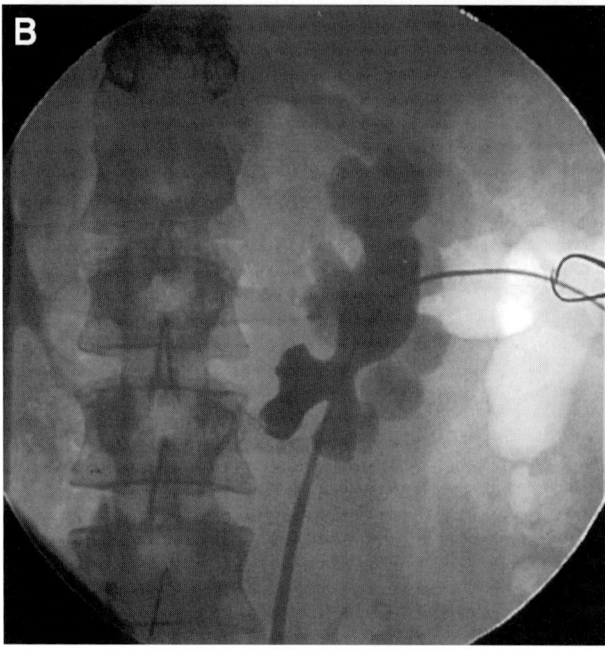


**Fig. 16.8**

Ureteropelvic junction obstruction associated with rotational anomalies such as horseshoe kidney provides an ideal setting for percutaneous management. Access is again accomplished via a superolateral infundibulocalyx. However, the calyceal system will be projected lower and more medially than that in a normally rotated kidney.

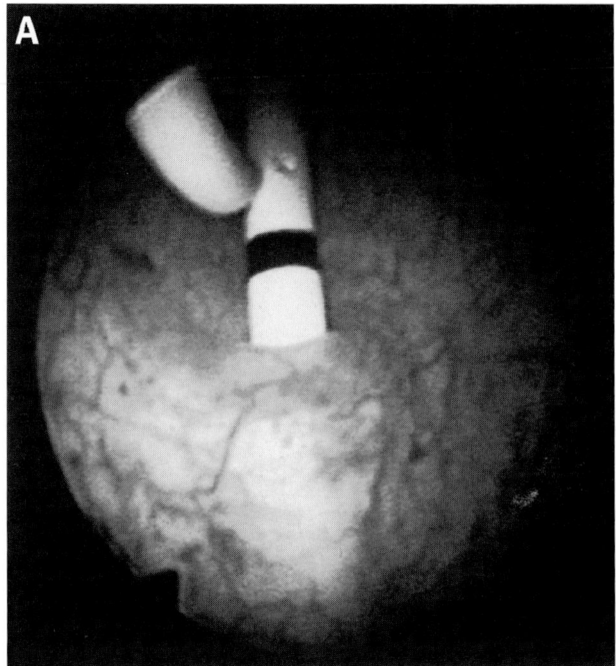


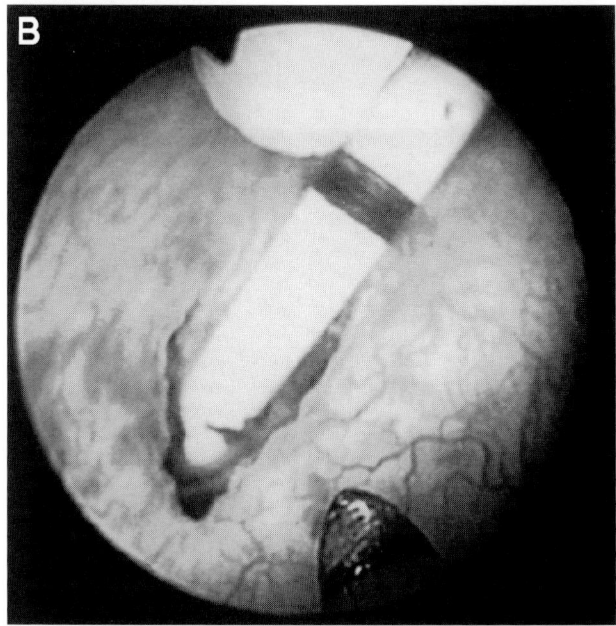


**Fig. 16.9**

During nephroscopy, the ureteropelvic junction will project almost directly anterior, and a "high insertion" will most assuredly be present. This is well suited to the "stent first/hot knife" technique.

## Simultaneous Percutaneous Nephrolithotomy/Endopyelotomy

Percutaneous management is ideal when the UPJO is associated with upper tract stone disease, as the stones can be managed concomitantly. In such cases, percutaneous access is again established with a wire across the UPJ. The stone should be removed prior to the endopyelotomy so that stone fragments do not migrate into the peripyeloureteral tissue, as can happen if the endopyelotomy is performed first. Otherwise, localized obstruction may result from fibrosis or granuloma formation.

## Postoperative Care

Avoidance of strenuous activity for 8–10 d following the procedure is recommended. The optimal time for postendopyelotomy stenting has yet to be determined, although 4 wk seems adequate. Although the need for prophylactic antibiotics is unproven while the stent is indwelling, our practice is to utilize a daily suppressive dose. Once the stent is removed, the patient is seen back after 1 mo for clinical follow-up and radiographic evaluation. This generally includes an intravenous pyelogram with or without a diuretic renogram. If the patient remains asymptomatic and the degree of calicectasis is diminished from preoperative studies, or the half-time of a diuretic renogram is in a nonobstructed range, reevaluation is performed at 6 mo and then 6- to 12-mo intervals for at least 2 yr.

## Results

The immediate and long-term results of percutaneous endopyelotomy are now well established. Clearly, percutaneous endopyelotomy compares favorably to open operative pyeloplasty in terms of postoperative pain, length of hospital stay, and return to prehospitalization activities. However, although these outcomes are important, the goal of any intervention for UPJO should be relief of obstruction as determined by relief of symptoms and stabilization, if not improvement, in ipsilateral renal function. Currently, success rates approximating 85% are being reported at experienced centers, with little difference in outcome noted in those patients undergoing the procedure for primary versus secondary UPJO.

When percutaneous endopyelotomy does fail, several options exist, including a retrograde endopyelotomy, repeat percutaneous endopyelotomy, or laparoscopic or open operative intervention. Although a repeat endopyelotomy may be offered, clearly the results in this setting will be compromised compared to a primary procedure. As such, open operative or laparoscopic intervention is generally offered to any patient who has failed an endourological approach. In this setting, the results of standard intervention will not be compromised and should exceed 95%.

## Complications

The complications associated with percutaneous endopyelotomy are analogous to those associated with percutaneous nephrolithotomy, and hemorrhage is a risk of any percutaneous procedure including endopyelotomy. However, because in patients with UPJO the renal parenchyma is generally thinner than that associated with a normal kidney, and because the collecting system is dilated, this risk seems to be less than in the general population of stone patients undergoing percutaneous manipulation. Treatment of hemorrhage in this setting should be conservative to start, and this includes bed rest, hydration, and transfusion as necessary. The nephrostomy tube should not be irrigated acutely. Rather, it is preferable to allow the pyelocaliceal system to tamponade the bleeding. When continued bleeding does not respond to these conservative measures, the next step is selective angiographic embolization. This will be almost uniformly successful and obviates the need for any open operative exploration, which may lead to nephrectomy.

Infection is a risk of any urinary tract manipulation, including percutaneous endopyelotomy, and all attempts should be made to sterilize the urinary tract prior to the procedure. Although the role of prophylactic antibiotics in the setting of sterile urine is unproven, our preference is to utilize a second-generation cephalosporin "on call" to the procedure and for two doses subsequent to it. Consideration can also be given to the use of oral prophylactic antibiotics while the endopyelotomy stent is indwelling for the month following the procedure, especially in women who are more prone to bacteruria.

Persistent obstruction is unusual in the early postoperative period because of the internal stent. Occasionally, however, the stent can be obstructed from blood clots, and continued nephrostomy drainage for a few extra days almost always allows the spontaneous lysis of any clots. In rare instances when stent obstruction persists, the stent can be changed over a wire in an antegrade or retrograde fashion, taking care not to lose access across the UPJ.

# OPEN PYELOPLASTY

## Indications

Many factors impact on the ultimate choice of approach. These factors include, but are not limited to, the presence of crossing vessels, the degree of hydronephrosis and renal pelvic size, level of ipsilateral and overall renal function, and the presence of rotational anomalies or concomitant stones. With increasing frequency, another factor impacting on this decision is a history of prior attempts at intervention and the nature of that intervention. At this time it is our practice to recommend an open operative approach to patients in whom the obstruction is associated with an especially long segment of proximal ureteral involvement and to any patient failing one or more previous attempts at any less-invasive management. It is also offered as the intervention of choice for patients in whom the most important consideration is a successful outcome without the potential need for subsequent procedures.

## Operative Approach

Adequate access to the UPJ can be achieved using a variety of incisions. An anterior extraperitoneal approach is favored by some as it allows *in situ* repair with minimal mobilization of the renal pelvis and proximal ureter. This approach may be especially valuable in patients with bilateral disease, as access is allowed to either side. This approach may also be preferred in the setting of a previous flank incision. Alternatively, a posterior lumbotomy also allows *in situ* repair with minimal mobilization of surrounding tissue and direct exposure to the UPJ. However, this approach is best utilized for relatively thin patients in whom there has been no previous ipsilateral surgery. Although a posterior lumbotomy is often embraced by pediatric urologists, it is in fact rarely used for adults, at least in the United States. At our center the approach utilized for the vast majority of patients undergoing open pyeloplasty is an extraperitoneal flank approach. Although a subcostal incision may be utilized, for adults we generally prefer an incision through the bed of the 12th rib. This is then carried anteriorly off the tip to avoid inadvertent injury to the subcostal nerve. This approach is advantageous in that it is familiar to all urologists and provides excellent exposure to the UPJ without regard to body habitus.

When a UPJO is associated with other congenital anomalies such as those of incomplete rotation or ascendance, alternative incisions are employed to allow access to a renal pelvis that is expected to be more anterior and caudal. In such cases, a more anterior, but still extraperitoneal, approach is generally preferred.

## Preoperative and Intraoperative Drainage

Preoperative drainage is required only in specific circumstances, and only rarely. Specific indications for a drainage procedure prior to open pyeloplasty include the presence of infection associated with obstruction or azotemia resulting from the obstruction such as in the setting of a solitary functioning kidney or bilateral obstruction. In such cases preoperative drainage generally allows resolution of azotemia or infection, the result being more predictable healing and less risk of complications. Preoperative drainage may also be valuable in a patient presenting with severe and unrelenting pain. For any of these indications, preoperative drainage can be achieved either by passage of an internal stent in a retrograde fashion or placement of a percutaneous nephrostomy tube.

The need for intraoperative placement of stents or nephrostomy tubes is somewhat controversial. However, in older children and adults, it is our preference to routinely place a soft, self-retaining internal stent at the time of open pyeloplasty and remove it 4 wk postoperatively. In our experience the routine use of such stents placed intraoperatively is especially advantageous in the early postoperative period. Placement of such stents decreases the amount of urinary extravasation and drainage and thereby decreases the risk of secondary fibrosis. The diminished urinary drainage during this time also allows earlier removal of any external drains and earlier hospital discharge. An internal stent may also help prevent kinking of the ureter, which could subsequently lead to secondary obstruction.

When performing an open pyeloplasty in older children and adults, the use of nephrostomy drainage is limited. Nephrostomy drainage is best reserved for especially complicated procedures such as those for secondary or even tertiary repairs. However, if a percutaneous nephrostomy tube had been placed preoperatively, at times it is left indwelling intraoperatively to allow for early proximal diversion and to provide access for postoperative radiographic studies.

Although the use of internal stents and nephrostomy drainage is always individualized, provision of external drainage from the line of repair is obligatory. This prevents urinoma formation and the potential for suture line disruption with subsequent sepsis or scarring. Such external drainage is easily accomplished with a Penrose or closed suction drain placed near, but not on, the suture line and brought out extraperitoneally through a separate stab incision.

## Historical Notes

The modem approach to dismembered pyeloplasty originated 50 yr ago. In 1949, Nesbit modified Kuster's dismembered repair by utilizing an elliptical anastomosis. This decreased the likelihood of stricture formation at the site of the repair. At about the same time, Anderson and Hynes, two English surgeons, described their modification that involved anastomosis of a spatulated ureter to a projection of the lower aspect of the renal pelvis after excision of a redundant portion of the pelvis. Thus, they performed a dismembered reduction pyeloplasty.

## General Principles

At open pyeloplasty, the application of several basic principles should ensure a successful repair. The anastomosis should be widely patent and performed in a watertight fashion without tension. Ultimately, reconstruction of the UPJ should result in a dependent, funneled-shaped transition between the renal pelvis and ureter.

## Dismembered Pyeloplasty

At our institution, the only open pyeloplasty performed is a dismembered pyeloplasty with or without renal pelvic reduction and with or without transposition of vessels. This technique is universally applicable to essentially all patients with primary UPJO. Specifically, it is appropriate for a high or dependent insertion of the ureter on the renal pelvis. Dismembered pyeloplasty also allows renal pelvic reduction in the setting of an exceptionally large, redundant renal pelvis, or straightening of a lengthy or tortuous proximal ureter. In cases in which the UPJO is associated with accessory or aberrant lower pole vessels, transposition, whether anteriorly or posteriorly, is accomplished in a straightforward fashion. Finally, a dismembered pyeloplasty, in contrast to all flap techniques, is the only approach that allows complete excision of an anatomically or functionally abnormal UPJ.

Dismembered pyeloplasty may not be applicable to patients in whom the UPJO is associated with a small intrarenal pelvis or in cases of secondary repair where the UPJ itself is not accessible as a result of intense peripelvic fibrosis. However, repair in such instances often cannot adequately be performed with any type of pyeloplasty. Rather, reconstruction in such settings is generally accomplished with a ureterocalycostomy.

### Technique

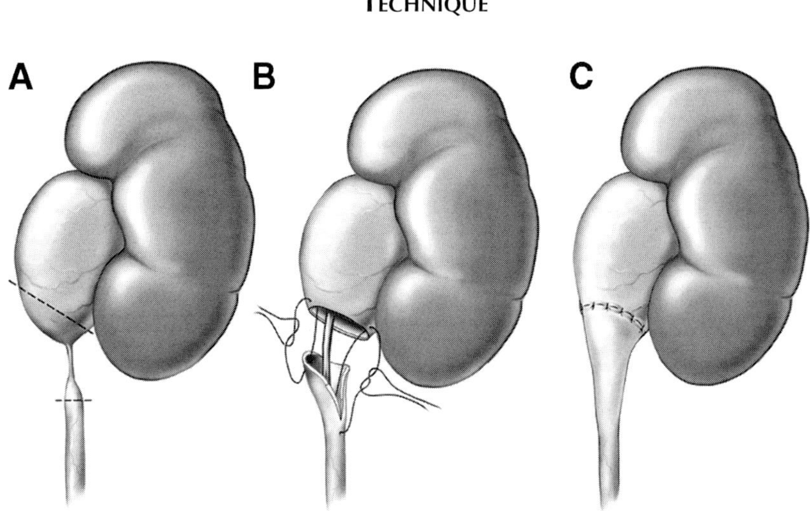


**Fig.16.10**

Exposure to the ureteropelvic junction (UPJ) is attained initially by identifying the proximal ureter in the retroperitoneum. The ureter is dissected cephalad toward the renal pelvis, preserving a large amount of periureteral tissue to ensure adequate ureteral blood supply. Once the UPJ is identified, the renal pelvis is dissected free of surrounding peripelvic tissue. **(A)** The ureteropelvic junction itself is now excised. **(B)** The lateral aspect of the proximal ureter is then marked with a fine suture placed below the level of obstruction. This marking suture will help maintain proper orientation during the subsequent repair, thus preventing torquing of the ureter. In a similar fashion, the lateral and medial aspects of the most dependent portion of the renal pelvis are delineated with marking traction sutures. The proximal portion of the ureter is then spatulated on its lateral aspect, toward the marking suture. Spatulation allows a wide, elliptical anastomosis. The apex of the spatulated, lateral aspect of the ureter is then brought to the most dependent, lateral border of the pyelotomy incision in the renal pelvis. The medial aspect of the ureter is brought to the more superior, medial aspect of the pyelotomy incision on the renal pelvis. Our preference is to place a 6 French internal stent at this time. **(C)** Completion of the anastomosis is then performed using absorbable, fine interrupted sutures placed full thickness through the renal pelvic and ureteral walls, in a watertight fashion. This interrupted technique, in contrast to a running suture, is less ischemic and avoids the potential for a "purse-string" effect, which could result in narrowing at the anastomosis.

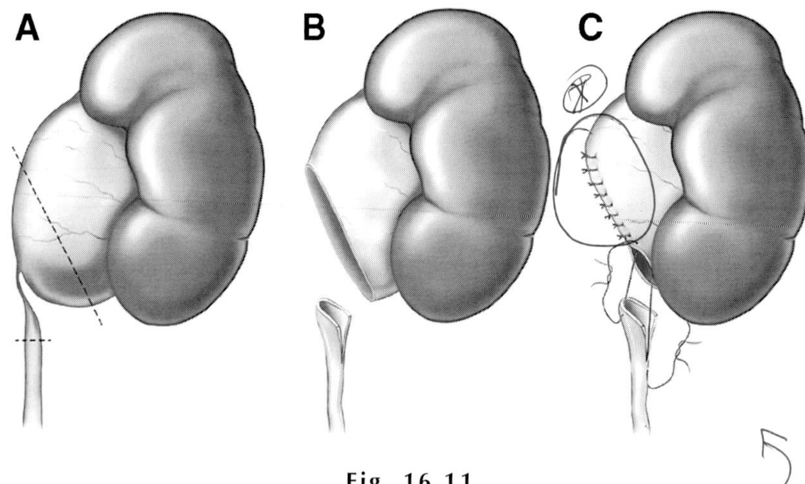


**Fig. 16.11**

In the setting of an exceptionally large or redundant renal pelvis, a renal pelvic reduction is performed as part of the dismembered repair. **(A)** Excising the redundant, medial aspect allows reduction of the renal pelvis, leaving the lateral and most caudal aspects of the renal pelvis intact. **(B)** This assures that the anastomosis can still be performed without tension, as the apex of the spatulated proximal ureter is brought to the dependent aspect of the pyelotomy incision. **(C)** The cephalad aspect of the pyelotomy is closed with running absorbable suture down to the level where the anastomosis is performed. Sutures are placed from the apex of the spatulated ureter to the dependent aspect of the pelvis, and from the highest, medial aspect of the proximal ureter to the most superior portion of the remaining open part of the pyelotomy. The anastomosis is completed with interrupted, fine absorbable suture as for a standard dismembered pyeloplasty.

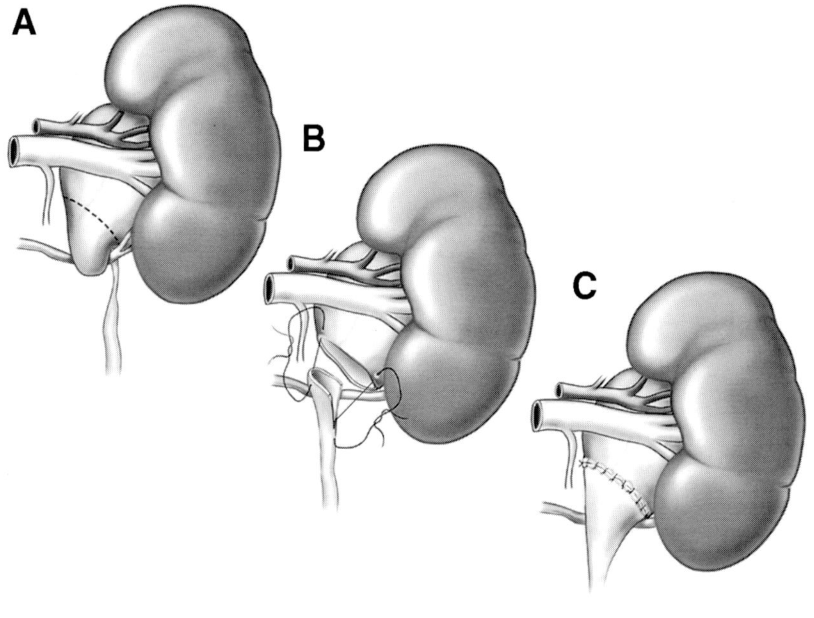

**Fig. 16.12**

Aberrant or accessory lower pole vessels are found in close association with the ureteropelvic junction (UPJ) in 30–50% of patients, although a pathophysiological relationship may not always be clear. In such cases, especially where there is significant entanglement of the UPJ with those vessels, a dismembered pyeloplasty can be combined with appropriate transposition of the UPJ in relation to the vessels. **(A)** The UPJ is excised. **(B)** The ureter is brought either anterior or posterior to the crossing vessel to allow appropriate transposition of the UPJ in relation to those vessels. The proximal ureter is spatulated on its lateral aspect, and corner sutures placed. **(C)** The pyeloplasty is completed in a straightforward manner using fine, absorbable, interrupted sutures as described earlier.

## Ureterocalicostomy: Technique

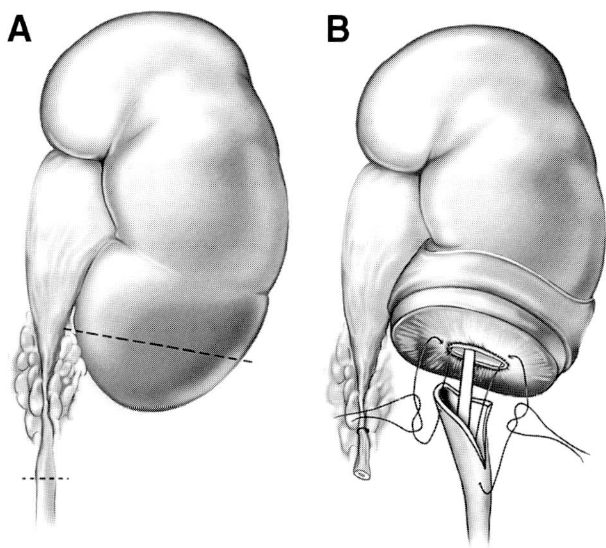


**Fig. 16.13**

The ureter is identified in the retroperitoneum and dissected proximally as far as possible. **(A)** The kidney is mobilized to gain access to the lower pole and to subsequently perform the anastomosis without tension. A lower pole nephrectomy is performed, removing as much parenchyma as necessary to widely expose a dilated lower pole calyx. **(B)** The proximal ureter is spatulated laterally. The anastomosis should subsequently be performed over an internal stent. The initial sutures are placed at the apex of the ureteral spatulation and the lateral wall of the calyx, with a second suture placed 180° from that.

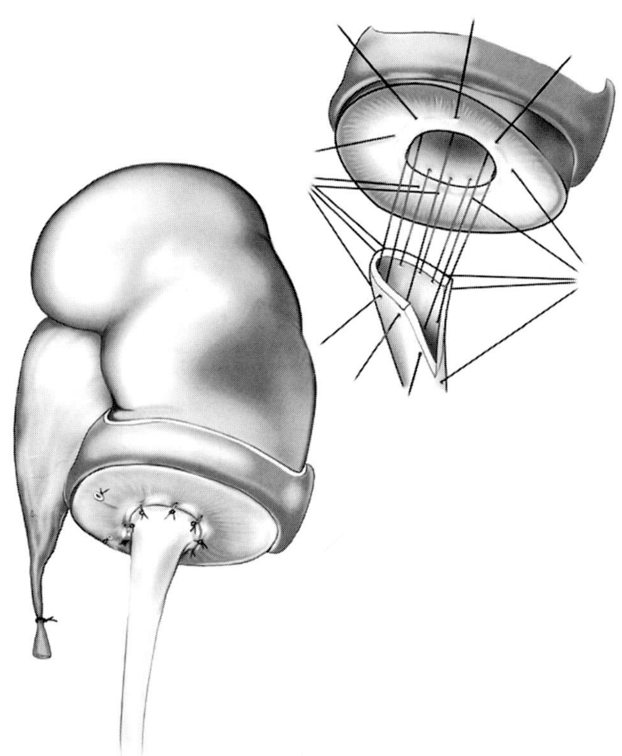

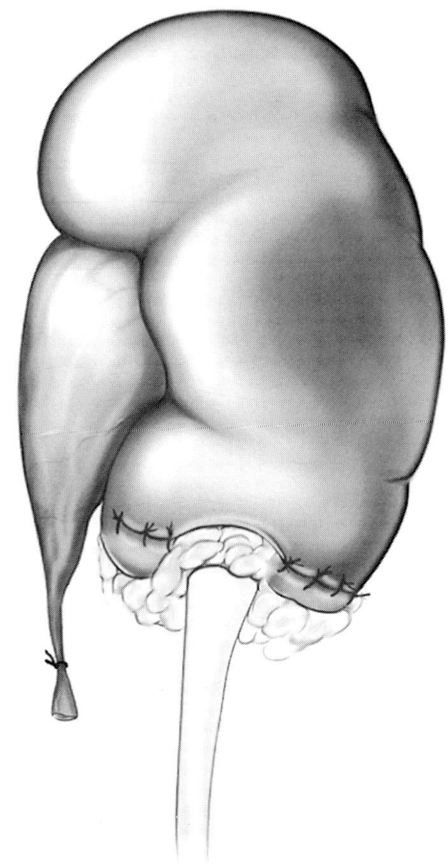

**Fig. 16.15**

The renal capsule may be closed over the cut surface of the parenchyma. However, the capsule should not be closed close to the anastomosis itself, as that may compromise the lumen by extrinsic compression. Instead, the anastomosis should be protected with a graft of perinephric fat or a peritoneal or omental flap.

## POSTOPERATIVE CARE

External drains are advanced and removed when urinary drainage has ceased. This is generally within 48–72 h in uncomplicated cases, especially when internal stents have been placed. It is our preference to remove internal stents on an outpatient basis 4 wk postoperatively. If a nephrostomy tube has been left indwelling, a nephrostogram is generally obtained 7–10 d postoperatively, or even later for particularly complicated repairs. When an antegrade study demonstrates a patent anastomosis

**Fig. 16.14**

The anastomosis is then completed in a "open" fashion, placing each suture circumferentially but not securing them down until the anastomosis is completed.

without extravasation, the nephrostomy tube is removed. Follow-up radiographic studies are generally performed 1 mo following stent extraction.

## Complications

For patients in whom an internal stent had not been left indwelling and urinary drainage persists after 7–10 d, or for such patients in whom urinary drainage recurs after removal of an external drain, retrograde studies are performed and an attempt made to pass an internal stent in a retrograde fashion. Rapid cessation of any external drainage should become evident almost immediately. If an attempt at passing an internal stent is unsuccessful, percutaneous nephrostomy drainage should be instituted, and at times a subsequent attempt is made to pass a stent in an antegrade fashion. Percutaneous nephrostomy drainage is also the next step for patients in whom an internal stent was left indwelling at the time of the procedure, but in whom, again, urinary drainage persists. In some cases urinary extravasation will result in a urinoma despite the appropriate use of stents, drains, or nephrostomy tubes. In those cases the fluid collection is best treated by direct percutaneous drainage using ultrasound or CT guidance. A small drainage tube is left indwelling in the retroperitoneum and removed once the drainage ceases and the urinoma is resolved as proven by ultrasound, or preferably CT, follow-up.

# SPECIAL CONSIDERATIONS IN CHILDREN

## Presentation and Evaluation

Prior to the era of prenatal ultrasound, most children with UPJO presented with symptoms such as pain, urinary tract infection, or hematuria. Since the adoption of nearly universal prenatal ultrasonography, the majority of pediatric UPJOs present as asymptomatic hydronephrosis noted on antenatal ultrasound. Because these UPJOs are incidentally detected, the indications for surgical intervention are unclear. The standard evaluation includes a postnatal ultrasound, a voiding cystourethrogram, and a diuretic renal flow scan. Kidneys that are clearly obstructed on the scan and have decreased function are generally repaired. Those with good function and no apparent obstruction by renal scan criteria should be followed with periodic ultrasound, as approx 20% will ultimately progress. The appropriate management of hydronephrotic kidneys with obstruction by renal scan, but function equal to that of the normal contralateral kidney, is controversial. Natural history studies have shown that 25% of these kidneys followed for several years will ultimately require intervention, most for decreased renal function. Most that lose function on observation will regain normal function following surgical correction of the obstruction. However, approx 5% of all kidneys in this category will lose function irreversibly on an observation protocol. These data have been used to support both close observation and early intervention. When given this information, most parents will elect close observation with intervention if there is deterioration or if no improvement occurs within a year or two. If the renal scan and ultrasound reveal a classic UPJO appearance, then no ureteral imaging is necessary. If there is any question regarding the level of obstruction, a retrograde or antegrade pyelogram is performed just prior to the operation.

## Surgical Intervention

The standard operation for a UPJO in children is a dismembered pyeloplasty. A flank incision in children is generally off the tip of the 12th rib without any rib excision. If the 12th rib is particularly long, a subcostal incision may be employed. Some surgeons employ a dorsal lumbotomy incision. The actual pyeloplasty is performed as described for adults. Crossing vessels are very rare in prenatally detected obstructions. In children the skin is closed with absorbable subcuticular sutures. A Penrose drain is placed in the retroperitoneum. No stent is required for an uneventful pyeloplasty in an infant. In older children a double JJ stent may be employed. Alternatively, a 5 French feeding tube may be placed across the anastomosis. This tube and a nephrostomy tube are brought together through the renal parenchyma and a stab incision in the flank. The feeding tube is tied off so that it serves only as a splint.

Children generally can be discharged from the hospital on postoperative day 1. The feeding tube is removed 7–10 d postoperatively and the nephrostomy tube is clamped. After 1–2 d, if clamping is tolerated, patency of the anastomosis is confirmed by injecting methylene blue diluted in saline through the nephrostomy tube. If the patient voids blue urine, then the nephrostomy tube is removed. If a JJ stent has been used, it is removed 3–4 wk postoperatively under a brief general anesthetic.

Minimally invasive approaches are being applied to children with increasing frequency. Endopyelotomy is not as successful in children as in adults, and the reduction in morbidity is less for children, because children recover from open pyeloplasty very quickly. Endopyelotomy is a very reasonable option in adolescents. Laparoscopic pyeloplasty has been employed in children as young as 6 mo of age. In experienced hands, pediatric laparoscopic pyeloplasty appears to be as successful as the open approach. However, in infants and small children a transperitoneal approach is required and the laparoscopic suturing is more technically challenging.

## SUGGESTED READINGS

1. Anderson JC, Hynes W. Retrocaval ureter: a case diagnosed preoperatively and treated successfully by a plastic operation. Br J Urol 21:209, 1949.
2. Badlani G, Eshghi M, Smith AD. Percutaneous surgery for ureteropelvic junction obstruction (endopyelotomy): technique and early results: J Urol 135:26, 1986.
3. Das S, Amar AD. Ureteropelvic junction obstruction with associated renal anomalies. J Urol 131:872, 1984.
4. Streem SB, Franke J, Smith J. Management of upper urinary tract obstruction. In Campbell's Urology, 8th ed. (Walsh PC, Wein AJ, Vaughan ED Jr., Retik AB, eds). WB Saunders, Philadelphia, 2002.
5. Gerber GS, Lyon ES. Endopyelotomy: patient selection, results, and complications. Urology 43:1, 1994.
6. Inglis JA, Tolley DA. Ureteroscopic pyelolysis for pelviureteric junction obstruction. Br J Urol 58:250, 1986.
7. Kumon H, Tsugawa M, Hashimoto H, et al. Impact of 3-dimensional helical computerized tomography on selection of operative methods for ureteropelvic junction obstruction. J Urol 158:1696, 1997.
8. Matin SF, Yost A, Streem, SB. Ureteroscopic laser endopyelotomy: a 12 year single center experience. J Endourol, in press.
9. Motola JA, Badlani GH, Smith AD. Results of 212 consecutive endopyelotomies: an 8-year follow-up. J Urol 149:453, 1993.
10. Ramsay JW, Miller RA, Kellett MJ, et al. Percutaneous pyelolysis: indications, complications and results. Br J Urol 56:586, 1984.
11. Ransley PG, Dhillon HK, Gordon I, et al. The postnatal management of hydronephrosis diagnosed by prenatal ultrasound. J Urol 144:584, 1990.
12. Ross JH, Streem SB, Novick AC, et al. Ureterocalicostomy for reconstruction of complicated pelviureteric junction obstruction. Br J Urol 65:322, 1990.
13. Sampaio FJB. Vascular anatomy at the ureteropelvic junction. Urol Clin North Am 25:251, 1998.
14. Savage SJ, Streem SB. Simplified approach to percutaneous endopyelotomy. Urology 56:848, 2000.
15. Stephens FD. Ureterovascular hydronephrosis and the "aberrant" renal vessels. J Urol 128:984, 1982.
16. Van Cangh, PI, Wilmart JF, Opsomer RJ, et al. Long-term results and late recurrence after endoureteropyelotomy: a critical analysis of prognostic factors. J Urol 151:934, 1994.

# 17 Laparoscopic Pyeloplasty

*Anup P. Ramani and Inderbir S. Gill*

## INTRODUCTION

Ureteropelvic junction obstruction (UPJO) is one of the most common renal congenital anomalies requiring surgical correction. Despite an array of treatment modalities available, open pyeloplasty remains the gold standard for managing UPJO, with success rates exceeding 90%. Percutaneous antegrade and endoscopic retrograde techniques are effective and have lesser morbidity, but success rates are lower (66–80%). Because it duplicates the technical aspects of open pyeloplasty, laparoscopy has emerged as an attractive option for managing UPJOs at select centers.

Laparoscopic pyeloplasty purports to combine the success rates of open surgery with the decreased morbidity of minimally invasive surgery. Similar to open surgery, laparoscopic pyeloplasty addresses with precision the various anatomical nuances of UPJO, such as redundant pelvis, crossing vessels, and high insertion. The technical goals of excising the strictured segment, relocating the ureter (if necessary), reduction of the renal pelvis (if necessary), ureteral spatulation, and precise mucosa-to-mucosa sutured tension-free approximation is readily achieved laparoscopically, while reducing the postoperative pain, morbidity, and the size relative to the muscle-splitting flank incision of open surgery.

Laparoscopic pyeloplasty, although suitable for the adult patient with UPJO, has also been described in the older child, with good results.

## PREOPERATIVE EVALUATION

The patient undergoes the usual preoperative evaluation to confirm a functionally significant UPJO in an adequately functioning kidney, as well as evaluation for fitness for surgery. Biochemical tests include complete blood count (CBC), metabolic profile, bleeding profile, and urine culture.

Radiological investigations include intravenous pyelography, diuretic isotope renal scan (MAG3/DTPA), and a three-dimensional computed tomography (CT) scan to rule out crossing anomalous vessels. Retrograde pyelography is performed only selectively. These radiological tests evaluate the severity of obstruction, degree of hydronephrosis, renal pelvic size, the anatomical configuration of the UPJ, crossing vessels, and differential renal function.

After general anesthesia, a 4.7 F, 26-cm double-J stent is passed cystoscopically into the renal pelvis. If the patient already has a prior indwelling J-stent *in situ* for more than a month, it is replaced. A Foley catheter is indwelled.

## LAPAROSCOPIC DISMEMBERED PYELOPLASTY

Anderson–Hynes dismembered pyeloplasty is our preferred choice in almost all patients with UPJO. A reductive pyeloplasty can be incorporated as necessary. In addition, anterior or posterior transposition of the dismembered UPJ can be performed when the obstruction is associated with an aberrant lower pole vessel.

In the author's personal tertiary referral experience, a significant proportion of patients are referred with secondary UPJO after having failed previous surgical intervention, such as cutting wire (Acucise) balloon incision, retrograde ureteroscopic endopyelotomy, antegrade percutaneous endopyelotomy, or even failed open pyeloplasty. In these situations, one often encounters dense scarring of the UPJ with peri-ureteral adhesions, edema and inflammation of the full-thickness pelviureteral wall, and subclinical infection. Such altered anatomy increases the technical complexity of the proposed reconstructive surgery of the UPJ. Nevertheless, even in these challenging cases, we have achieved gratifying laparoscopic outcomes by following established surgical principles.

From: *Operative Urology at the Cleveland Clinic*
Edited by: A. Novick et al. © Humana Press Inc., Totowa, NJ

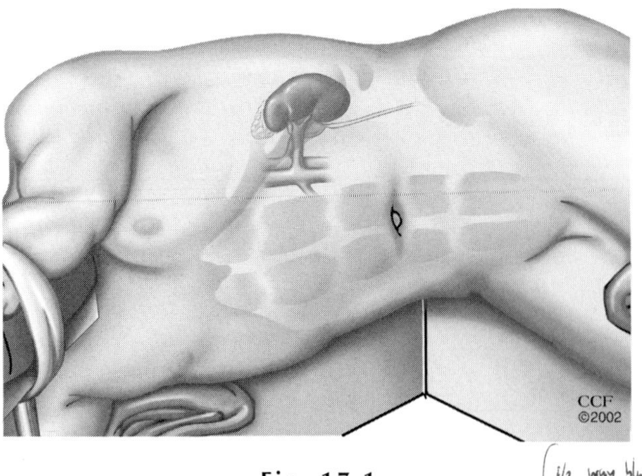


Fig. 17.1

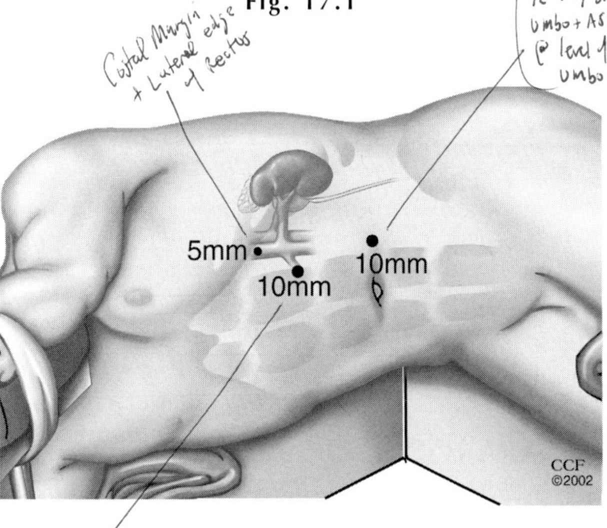


Fig. 17.2

## TRANSPERITONEAL TECHNIQUE

### Patient Position (Fig. 17.1)

The patient is placed in the 45–60° flank position. Extreme care is taken with padding and positioning. The table is flexed somewhat, an axillary roll placed, and the patient is secured to the table with 6-in. cloth tape and safety belt.

### Port Placement (Fig. 17.2)

Peritoneal access is gained using a Veress needle. The abdomen is insufflated with carbon dioxide.

The first port (10 mm) is placed midway between the umbilicus and the anterior superior iliac spine, at the level of the umbilicus. The second port (5 mm) is placed at the angle between the costal margin and the lateral border of the ipsilateral rectus muscle. The third port (10/12 mm) is placed between these two ports, closer to the upper port than the lower one, so as to allow a direct vision of the renal hilum. This port, which houses the 30° laparoscope, may alternatively be placed in the umbilicus.

### Identification of the UPJ Area (Fig. 17.3)

On the right side, the liver is retracted cephaled, and the colon and duodenum are mobilized medially. The colon, spleen, and pancreas are reflected away from the left kidney. On either the left or the right side, the anterior surface of Gerota's fascia is visualized by reflecting the mesocolon in an avascular plane. The psoas muscle is the important landmark that guides the laparoscopic surgeon's orientation and must always be visualized horizontally at the base of

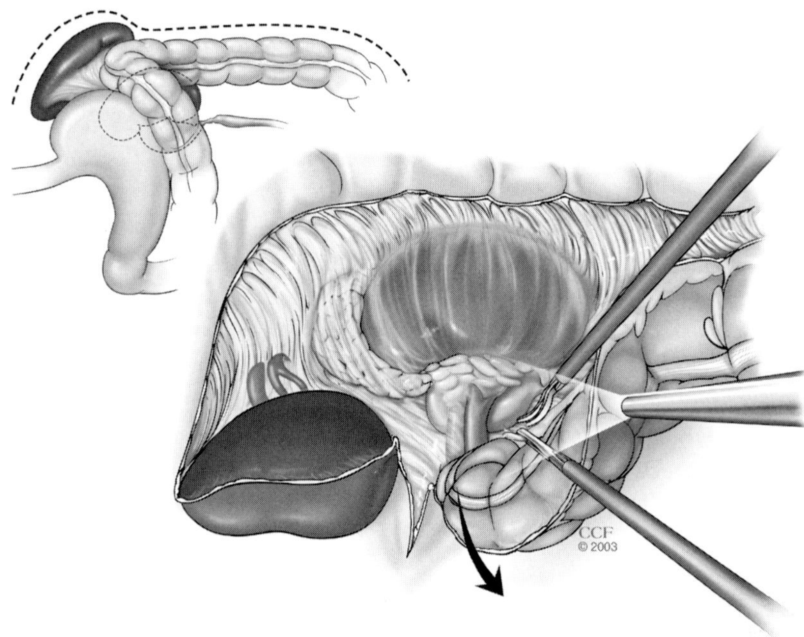


Fig. 17.3

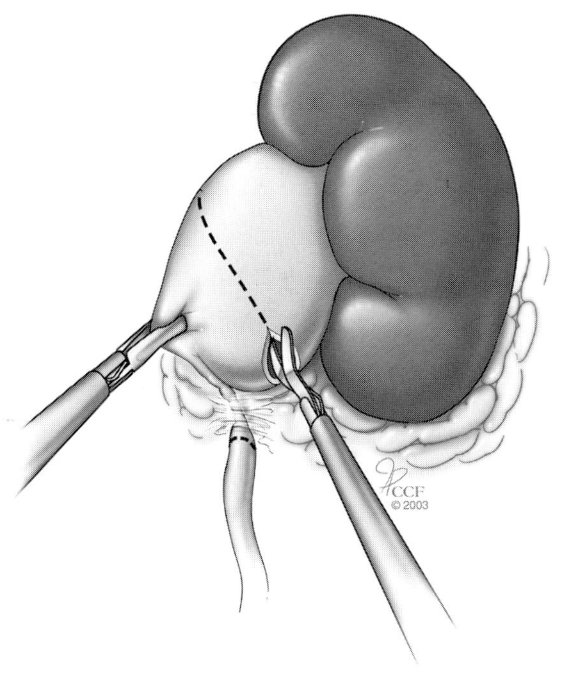


Fig. 17.4

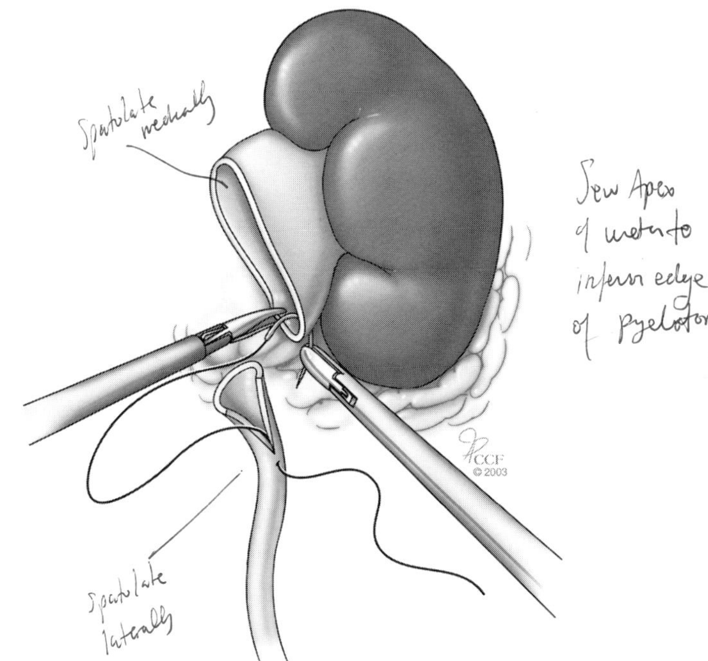


Fig. 17.5

the field. The ureter is identified and dissected toward the renal pelvis. The UPJ area is dissected free from adjacent tissues; this may be technically difficult in case of a secondary UPJ stenosis with significant postsurgical adhesions. Any crossing vessel(s) is/are identified and mobilized. An adequate amount of renal pelvis is also mobilized.

## Excision of the Stenotic UPJ Segment (Fig. 17.4)

The stenotic UPJ is divided obliquely, taking care not to cut the stent. The ureter is spatulated laterally for an adequate length. The stenotic UPJ area may be excised only if excess tissue is available. The renal pelvis is spatulated medially in a generous manner, with or without excision of redundant pelvis. Any excision of pelvic or ureteral tissue should be performed only after careful planning so as not to cause any shortening. The apex of the spatulated ureter is sutured to the inferior edge of the pylotomy with 4-0 Vicryl on RB-1 needle. The knot is kept extraluminal.

## Reconstruction of the UPJ (Figs. 17.5 and 17.6)

Pyeloplasty is performed using two running 4-0 Vicryl sutures, one dyed and the other undyed, on RB-1 needle (suture length 6–8 cm). The anterior wall of the anastomosis is approximated initially across 80% of its length. Anterior traction is placed on this stitch, thus bringing the posterior wall of the anastomosis into view. The second stitch is employed to suture the posterior wall. The cephalad end of the J-stent is reinserted into the renal pelvis. The remainder of the anterior wall is sutured, the two stitches tied, and pelvic suturing completed to secure a watertight anastomosis.

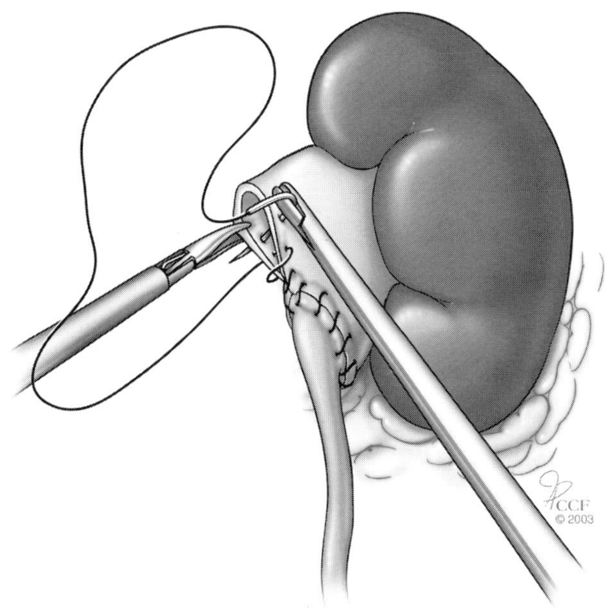


Fig. 17.6

## Aberrant Vasculature (Figs. 17.7–17.9)

When an aberrant lower pole vessel is present, a dismembered pyeloplasty allows proper repositioning of the vessel as necessary. We do not routinely transpose the crossing vessel, performing this maneuver only as dictated by the individual anatomical situation.

## Large Redundant Pelvis (Fig. 17.10)

For a patient with a redundant pelvis, a reductive pyeloplasty avoids stasis and recurrence of obstruction. To perform a reduction pyeloplasty, the entire renal pelvis is

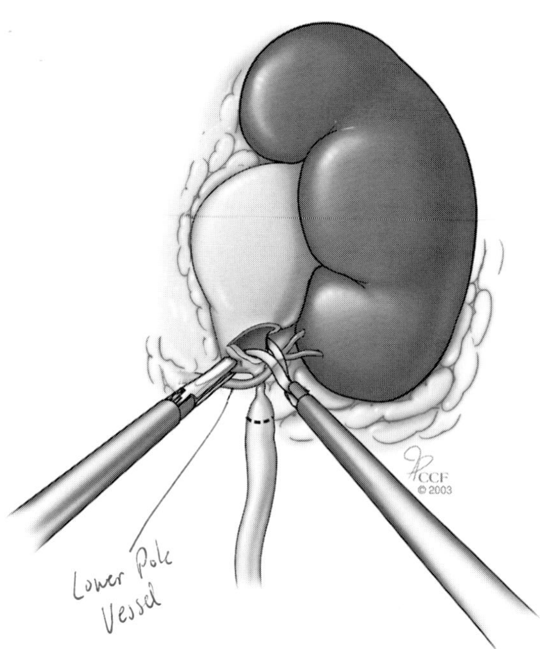


Fig. 17.7

mobilized completely. After dividing the UPJ, the excess, redundant pelvis is excised. Virtually the entire reduction is performed along the medial side of the renal pelvis; the lateral (lower) lip of the pelvis is maintained intact to facilitate adequate funneling of the pelvis. The ureteropelvic junction anastomosis is performed initially as described above. Closure of the large pelvic defect is performed subsequently by running one of the sutures cephalad.

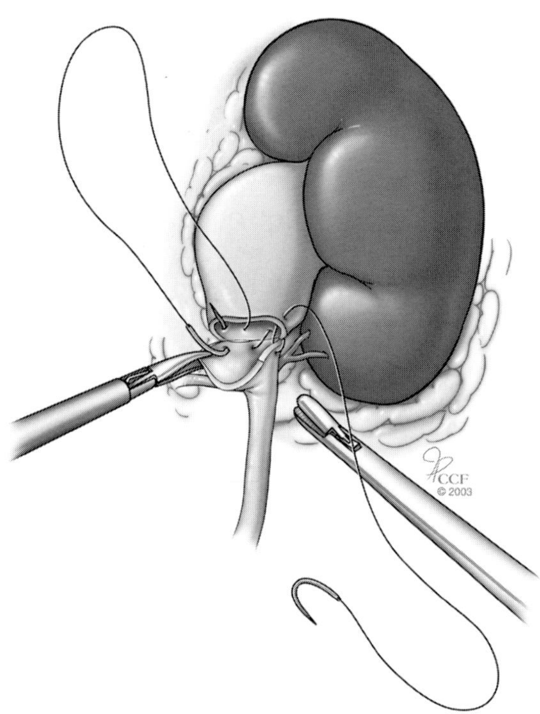


Fig. 17.8

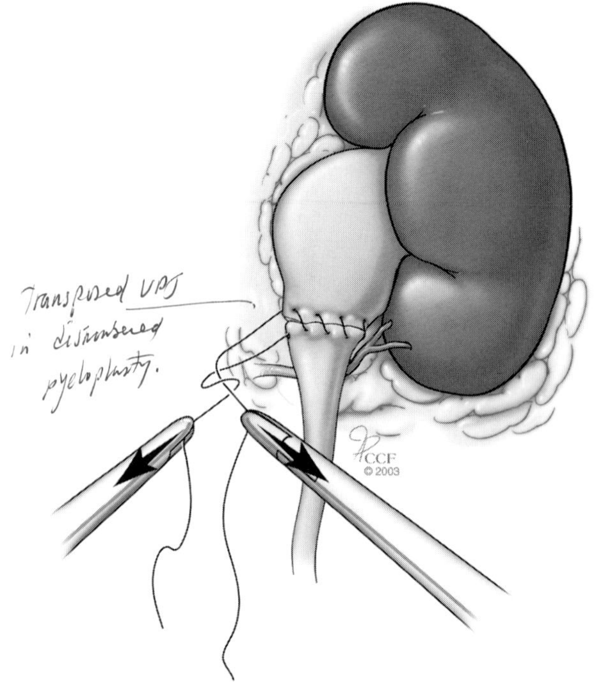


Fig. 17.9

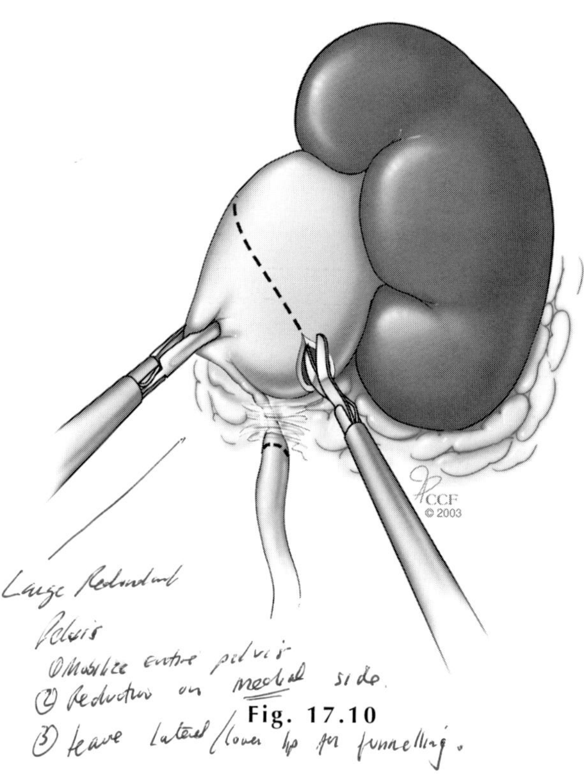


Fig. 17.10

Indigo carmine dye is administered intravenously along with 10-mg lasix to confirm a watertight anastomosis.

If there is any doubt about the integrity of the anastomosis, a Jackson–Pratt (J-P) drain is inserted through one of the ports. Alternatively, a J-P drain may be left routinely. Laparoscopic exit is completed.

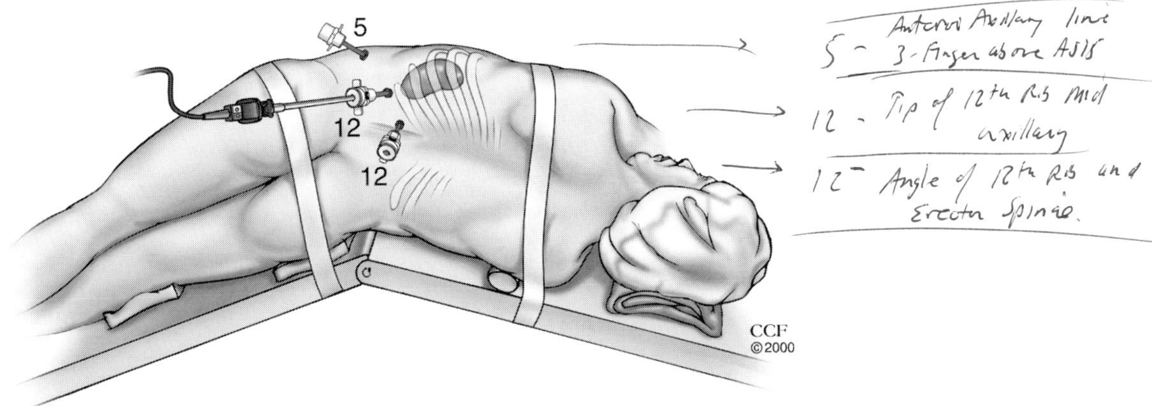


Fig. 17.11

# RETROPERITONEAL TECHNIQUE

## Port Placement (Fig. 17.11)

Our standard three-port retroperitoneal laparoscopic access is achieved. A 1-cm incision is made at the tip of the 12th rib in the mid-axillary line. The incision is deepened up to the dorsolumbar fascia. An incision is made in the dorsolumbar fascia and a finger inserted into the retroperitoneal space. This is confirmed by palpating the psoas muscle and the lower pole of the kidney. A balloon dilator is introduced into the retroperitoneal space and the balloon inflated 50 cc. The balloon is now hitched up against the abdominal wall and inflated an additional 700 cc. This maneuver pushes the peritoneum forward and out of the operative field. The balloon is removed and replaced by a 10/12-mm port. The retroperitoneum is now inspected and correct access confirmed. Insufflation is initiated at 25 mmHg. The second port (5 mm) is placed at the angle of the 12th rib and the paraspinal muscles. The third port (5 mm) is placed in the anterior axillary line, three finger-breadths above the anterior superior iliac spine.

## Mobilization of the Kidney (Fig. 17.12)

The initial step is to identify the ureter below the lower pole of the kidney as it lies above the psoas. The ureter is then dissected cephalad, leaving a good amount of peri-ureteral tissue, until the UPJ is reached. The peri-pelvic fat and the Gerota's fascia are opened and the pelvis exposed.

## Reconstruction

The pyeloplasty is then carried out similar to the transperitoneal technique.

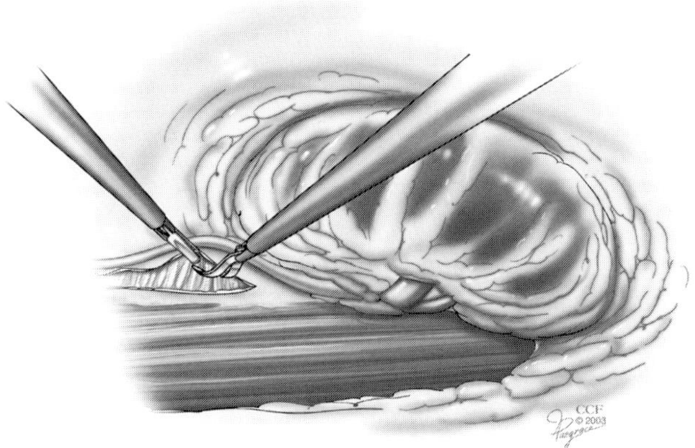


Fig. 17.12

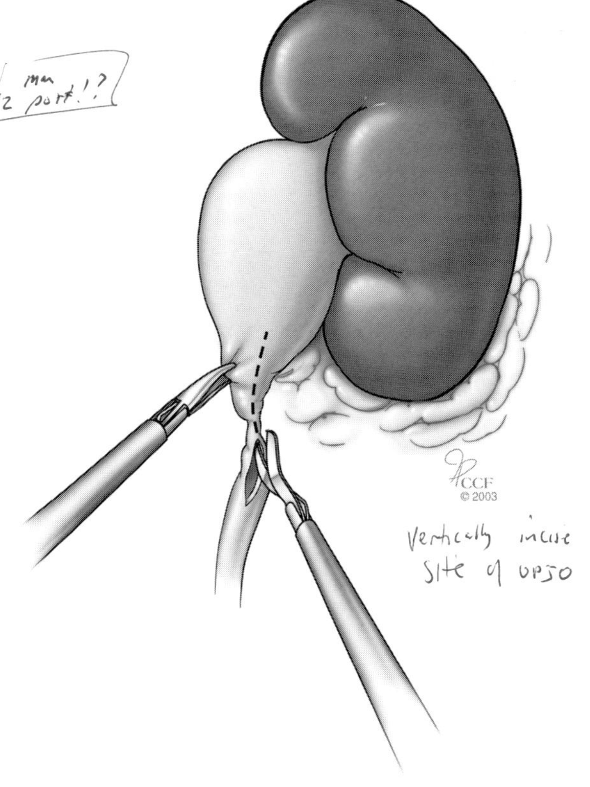


Fig. 17.13

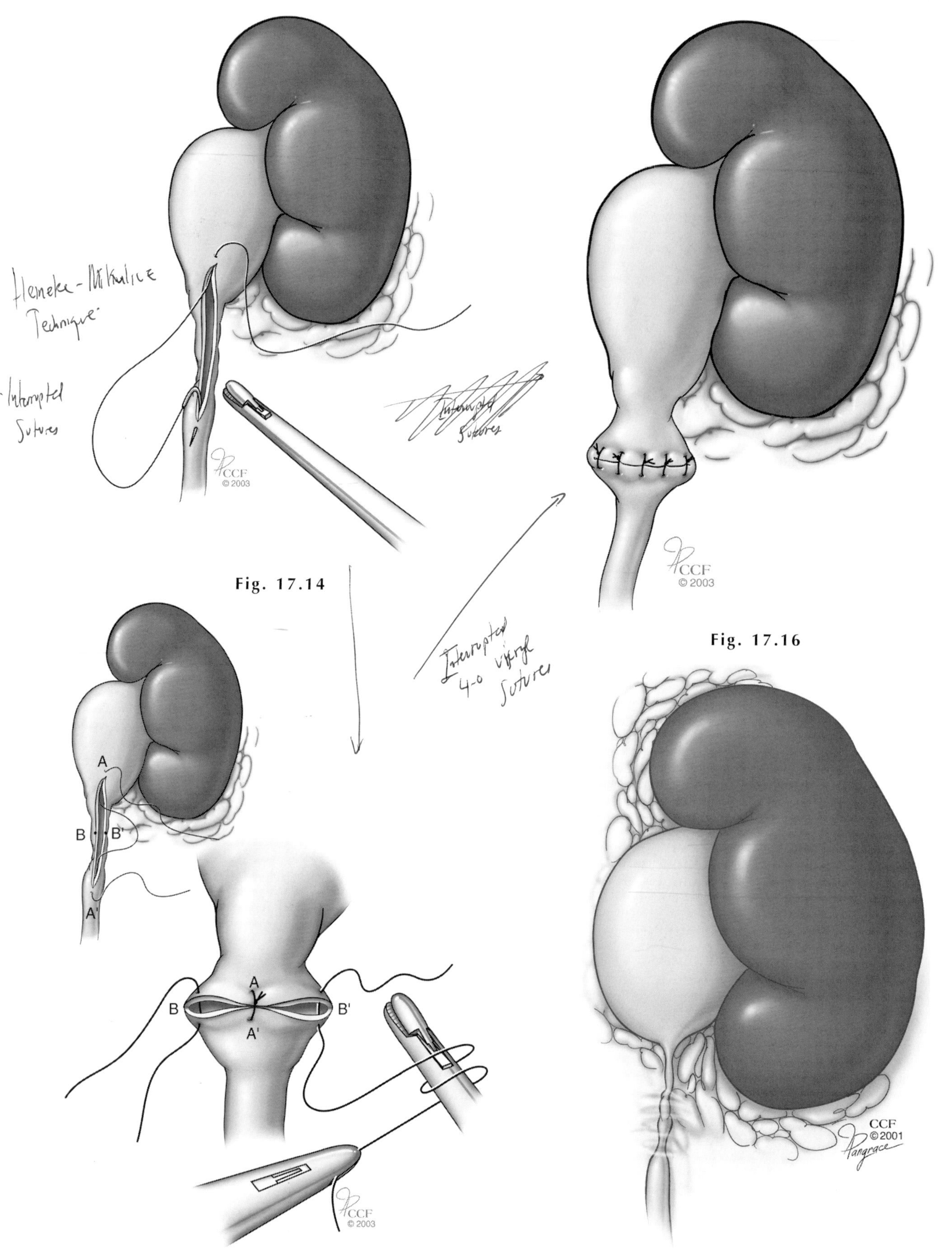


Fig. 17.14

Fig. 17.15

Fig. 17.16

Fig. 17.17

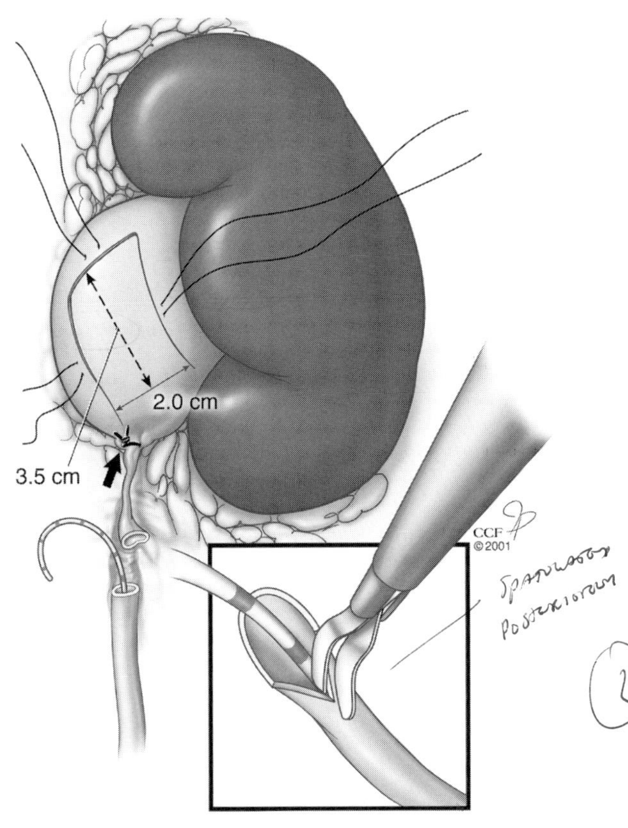


Fig. 17.18

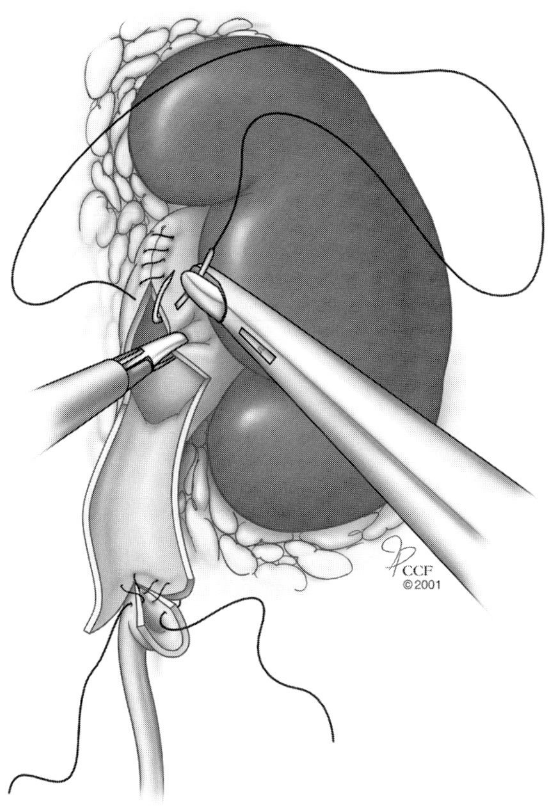


Fig. 17.19

## LAPAROSCOPIC FENGER-PLASTY (HEINEKE–MIKULICZ TYPE) (FIGS. 17.13–17.16)

Laparoscopic endoshears are used to vertically incise the site of the UPJO. A vertical incision is made on the renal pelvis, starting cephalad to the UPJ and continuing across the junction onto the ureter. The upper and the lower angles of the incision are approximated in the midline with 4-0 Vicryl sutures to convert the vertical incision into a horizontal one. Interrupted sutures are now taken to horizontally approximate the rest of the incision. Indigo carmine dye is administered intravenously to confirm no leak from the anastomosis. A J-P drain is inserted, hemostasis confirmed, and laparoscopic exit performed. We have no experience with Fenger-plasty and believe that this procedure is rarely indicated.

## LAPAROSCOPIC DISMEMBERED TUBULARIZED FLAP PYELOPLASTY (FIGS. 17.17–17.20)

Infrequently employed, this technique is indicated for a large, extra-renal pelvis, with dependent, long-segment UPJ or upper ureteral narrowing.

Laparoscopic endoscopic shears are used to excise the strictured area. The renal pelvis is completely transected at the ureteropelvic junction and then closed with a figure-of-eight suture. The strictured upper ureter is excised until healthy ureter is visualized. The cut end of the ureter is spatulated posteriorly. The renal pelvis is completely mobilized and an adequate 3 × 2 cm pelvic flap on a wide inferolaterally directed base is outlined with stay sutures. The flap is created with endoshears and rotated downward to meet the spatulated ureter. Using 4-0 polyglactin suture on RB-1 needle, the most dependent part of the renal pelvis is sutured to the corresponding part of the ureter. Posterior anastomosis is formed in a running manner and the J curl of the ureteral stent positioned in the renal pelvis. The anterior wall of the anastomosis is completed over the stent. Subsequently, the renal pelvis is tubularized by closing it longitudinally in a watertight manner.

Indigo carmine dye is administered intravenously to confirm a watertight anastomosis. A J-P drain is inserted, hemostasis confirmed, and laparoscopic exit performed.

## POSTOPERATIVE CARE

Intravenous antibiotics are continued for 24 h and oral antibiotics for 5 d. Analgesics are administered as required. Oral liquids and ambulation are begun on the evening of surgery.

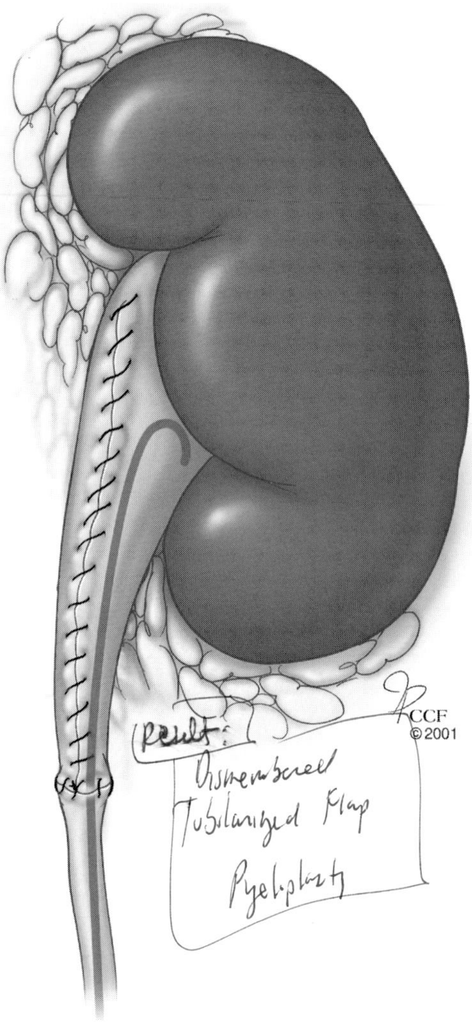


Fig. 17.20

The patient is discharged the next day after removing the Foley catheter. The drain is removed according to the diminution of drainage per the individual patient, normally within 1–3 d. No restrictions are placed on physical activity postoperatively.

## FOLLOW-UP

The J stent is removed at 6 wk. A follow-up isotope diuretic renal scan (MAG3) is performed at 3 mo.

## SUGGESTED READINGS


1. Cassis AN, Brannen GE, Bush WH, et al. Endopyelotomy: review of results and complications. J Urol, 146:1492,1991.
2. Janetshek G, Peschel R, Franscher F. Laparoscopic pyeloplasty. Urol Clin North Am 27:695, 2000.
3. Jarrett TW, Chan DY, Charambura TC, Fugita O, Kavoussi LR. Laparoscopic pyeloplasty: the first 100 cases. J Urol 167:1253–1256, 2002.
4. Kavoussi LR, Peters CA. Laparoscopic pyeloplasty. J Urol 150:1891–1894, 1993.
5. Motola JA, Badlani GH, Smith AD. Results of 221 consecutive endopylotomies: an eight year follow up. J Urol 149:453, 1993.
6. Notely RG, Beaugie JM. The long term follow up of Anderson-Hynes pyeloplasty for hydronephrosis. Br J Urol 45:464, 1973.
7. Persky L, Krause JR, Boltuch RL. Initial complications and late results in dismembered pyeloplasty. J Urol 118:162, 1977.

# 18 Urothelial Tumors of the Renal Pelvis and Ureter

## *Endourological Management*

*Stevan B. Streem*

Standard management of upper tract transitional cell carcinoma (TCC) is a nephroureterectomy. However, there is a distinct subgroup of patients who would be rendered dialysis dependent, or at high risk for functionally significant renal insufficiency, for which a nephron-sparing approach is warranted. With increasing experience, such renal conservative surgery is also being applied to patients with documented low-grade, low-stage disease, even in the setting of a normal, or nearly normal, contralateral kidney.

Historically, the options for nephron-sparing management of upper tract TCC had been limited to variations of open pyelotomy or partial nephrectomy. More recently, endourological techniques have been applied to the management of these difficult patients. For those with relatively small ureteral or pyelocalyceal tumors, definitive treatment may at times be accomplished with a ureteroscopic approach. Although a ureteroscopic approach can be appropriate for patients with small, accessible upper tract lesions, such treatment may be precluded by the size or location of the tumor or by a urinary diversion that makes ureteroscopic access difficult or impossible. Many of these patients can, however, be managed with a percutaneous approach that can provide access to virtually the entire upper tract. The subsequent addition of topical bacille Calmette–Guérin (BCG) as an adjunct to percutaneous upper tract tumor resection may then be beneficial in decreasing the incidence of local recurrence.

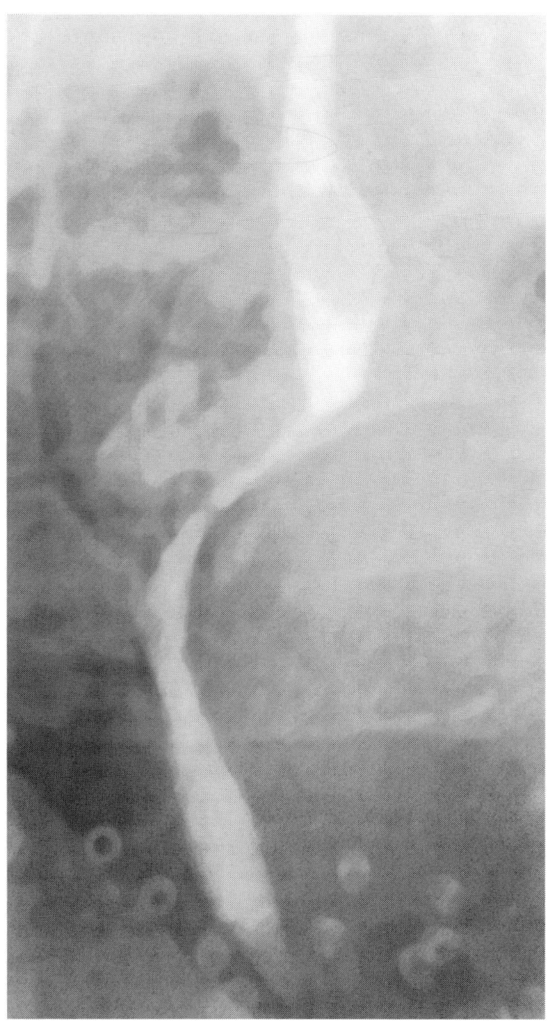

**Fig. 18.1**

A good-quality retrograde pyelogram is performed at the outset of the procedure. For ureteral tumors, a 0.38 guidewire is then passed cystoscopically into the renal pelvis under fluoroscopic control. Most ureteral tumors are approached using a semirigid ureteroscope, though some proximal ureteral tumors in men will require flexible instrumentation.

## URETEROSCOPIC MANAGEMENT

With the introduction of small, semi-rigid ureteroscopes and actively deflectable, flexible ureteroscopes, ureteroscopic treatment of upper tract tumors has become a reasonable alternative to open operative intervention in select patients requiring nephron-sparing management. This treatment is now also being offered to

From: *Operative Urology at the Cleveland Clinic*
Edited by: A. Novick et al. © Humana Press Inc., Totowa, NJ

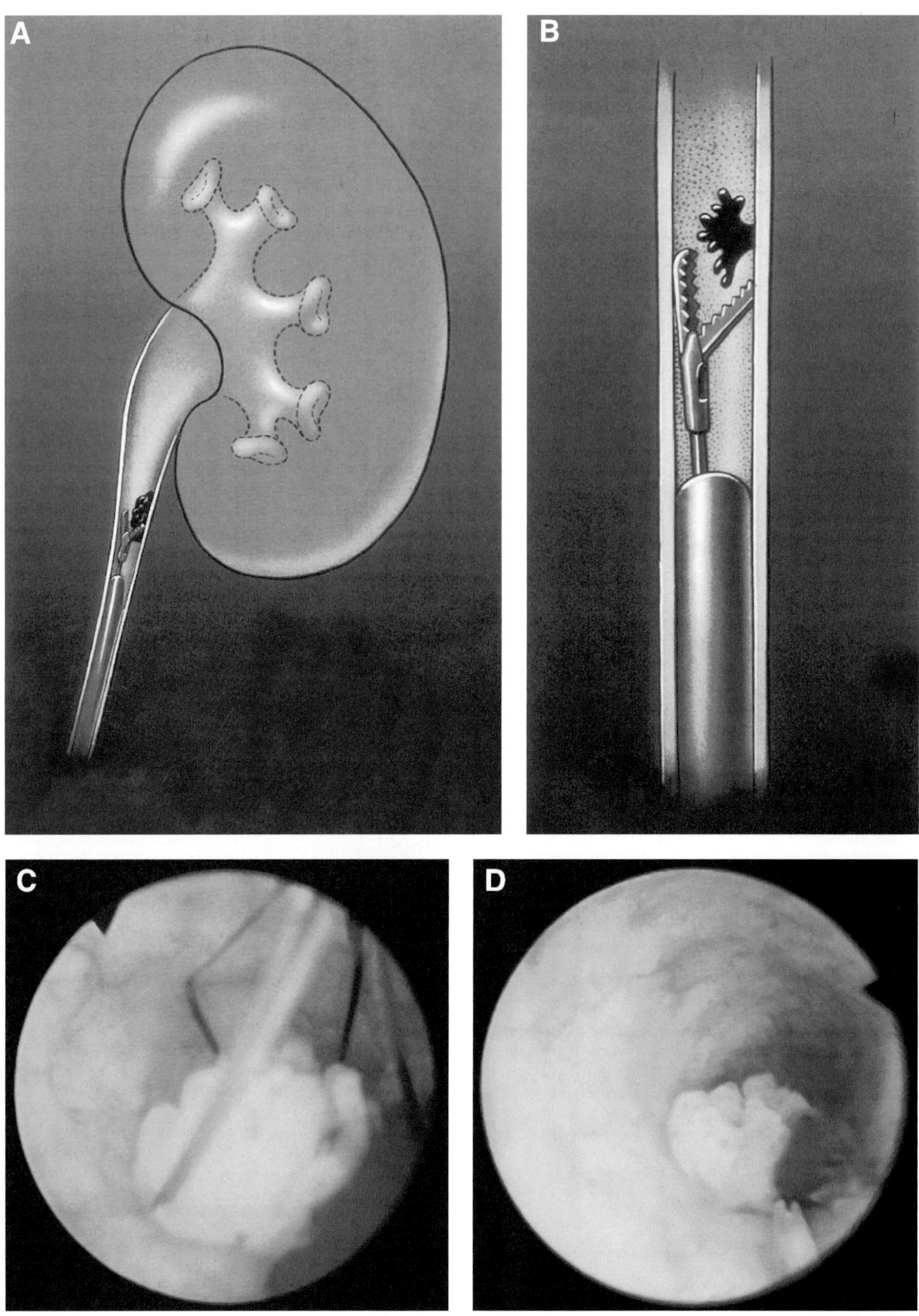


Fig. 18.2

**(A,B)** Papillary tumors may first be debulked using a flexible cup biopsy forceps. **(C,D)** Alternatively, a flat wire basket can be used to snare the base of the tumor. This also provides sufficient tissue for pathological evaluation. **(E,F)** Once the bulk of the tumor has been removed, the base is treated. This can be performed using either electro- or laser fulguration. However, one must be sure not to fulgurate circumferentially in order to prevent ureteral stricture. When using the

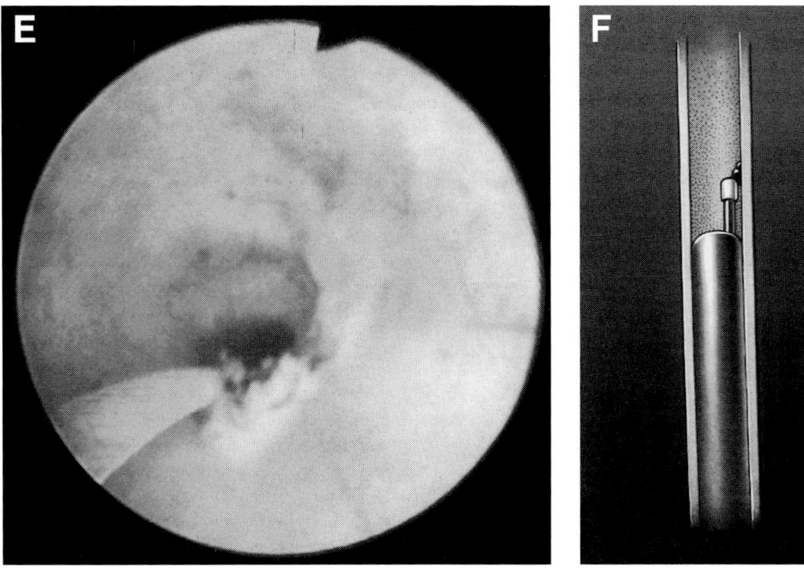

Fig. 18.2 *(Continued)*

Holmium to ablate the tumor, an energy setting of 0.6–1.0 J with a frequency of 10 Hz is recommended. A similar setting may be used for coagulation simply by defocusing the beam.

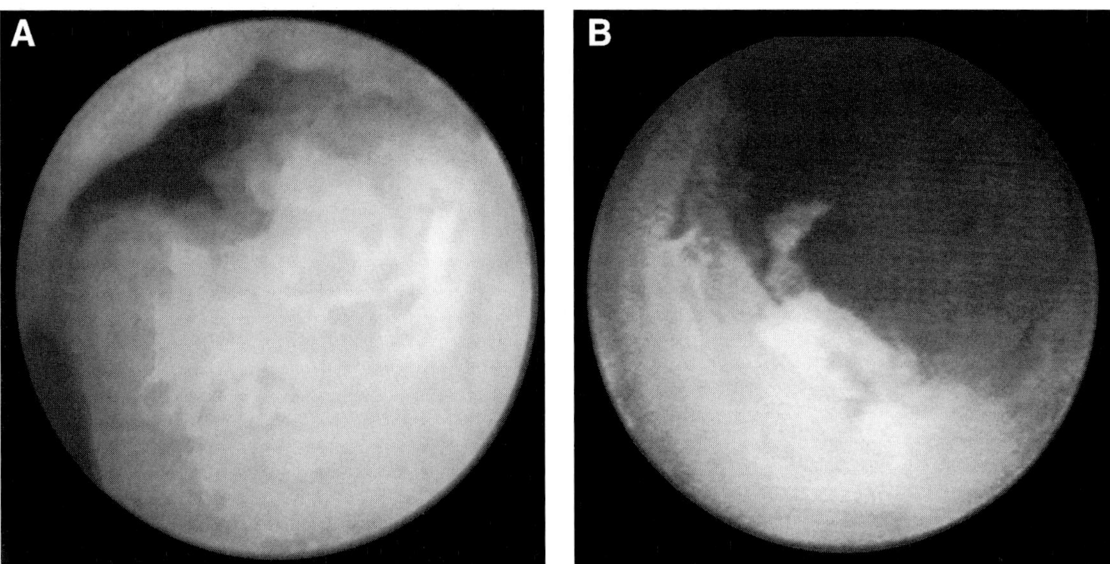

Fig. 18.3

**(A,B)** Larger tumors may be managed with a ureteroresectoscope, as long as the tumors are still of low grade and stage. Because of the large (11 French) diameter of this instrument, prestenting is often a requisite to its use. Care must be taken not to resect too deeply with the resectoscope, as the musculature of the ureter is much thinner than that of the bladder.

some patients with a normal contralateral kidney but with documented low-grade, low-stage disease, who might otherwise undergo nephroureterectomy.

## Equipment

Fluoroscopy table
Hydrophilic guidewires
Pressure irrigation system
Self-dilating semi-rigid ureteroscope (short and long)
Actively deflectable flexible ureteroscope
3 French cup biopsy forceps
3 French flat wire basket
Ureteroscopic Bugbee electrode
Self-retaining ureteral stent

## Optional Equipment

Holmium laser
Rigid ureteroresectoscope

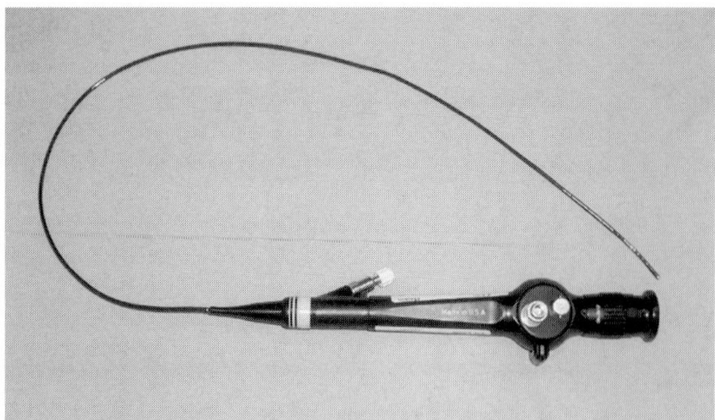

Fig. 18.4

Pyelocalyceal tumors, and some upper ureteral tumors, require actively deflectable, flexible instrumentation. Cystoscopy and retrograde studies are again performed at the outset of the procedure, at which time the first hydrophilic guidewire is passed.

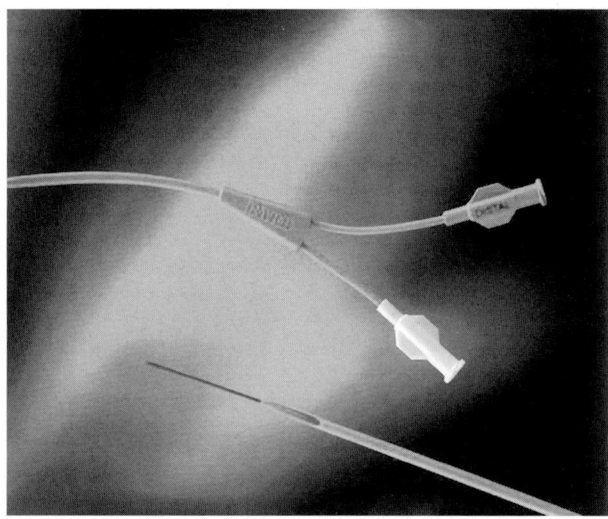

Fig. 18.5

A 10 French dual lumen catheter is passed over the initial guidewire. This acts to both dilate the intramural ureter and to pass a second wire as a "working" wire. Alternatively, the orifice can be dilated with a 5 or 6 French high-pressure balloon, although a second wire still must be passed, leaving both safety and working wires.

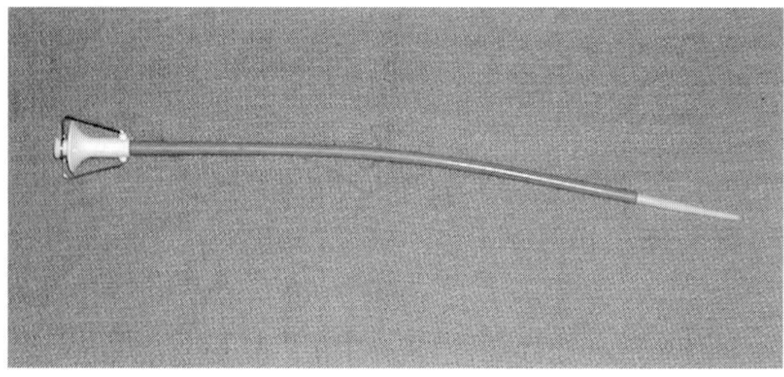

Fig. 18.6

The working wire is used to pass the flexible scope directly, or preferably to place a ureteroscopic working sheath.

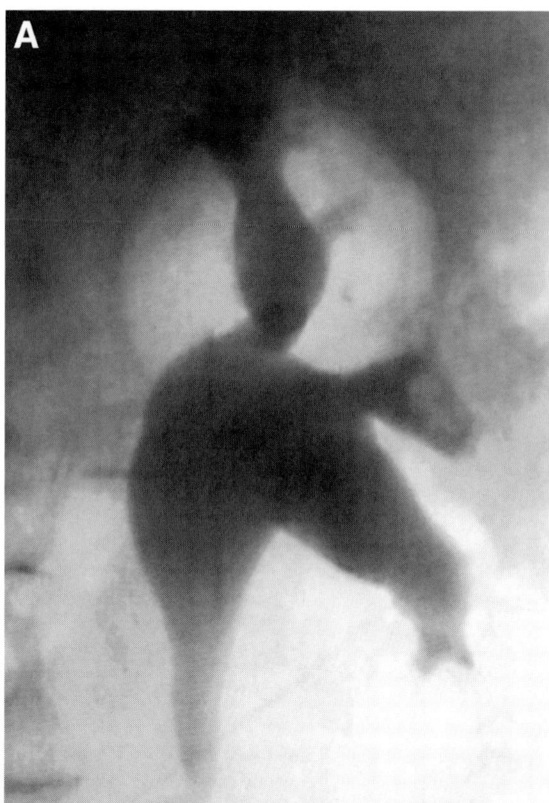


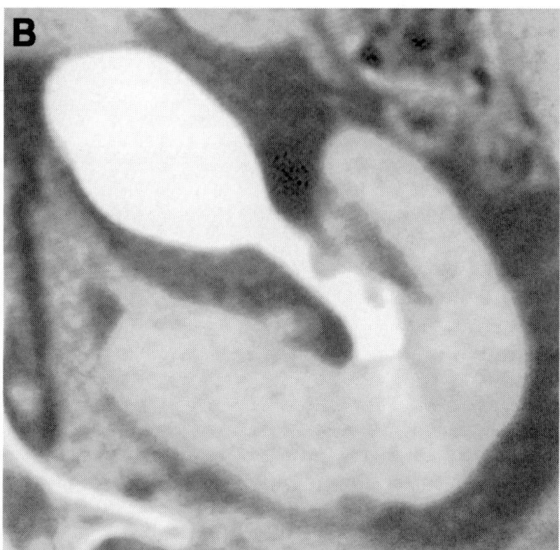


Fig. 18.7

**(A,B)** Retrograde study suggests a filling defect in a mid-lateral calyx on the left. Computed tomography with contrast confirms this.

## Ureteral Tumors: Technique

### Pyelocalyceal Tumors

A standard indwelling ureteral stent is placed for a period of time that depends on the extent of the procedure. For small superficial tumors, the stent can generally be

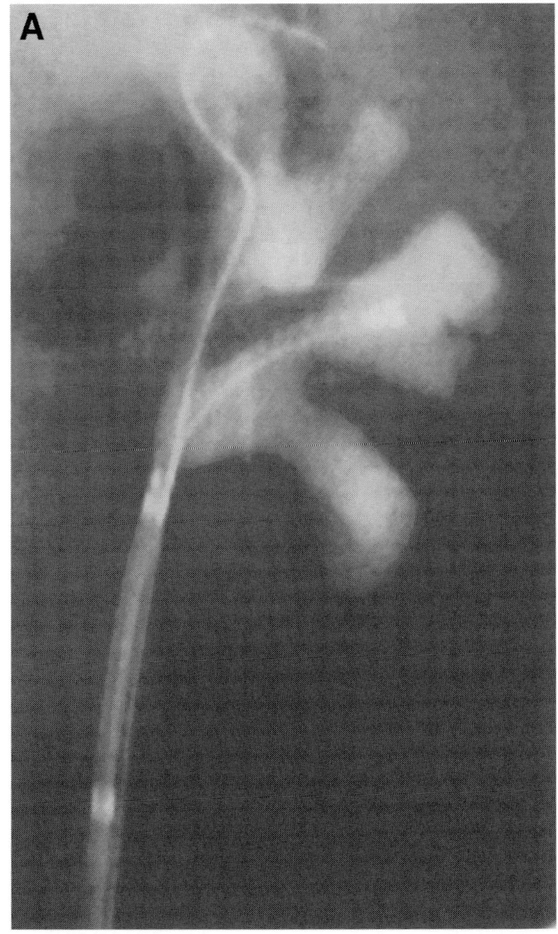


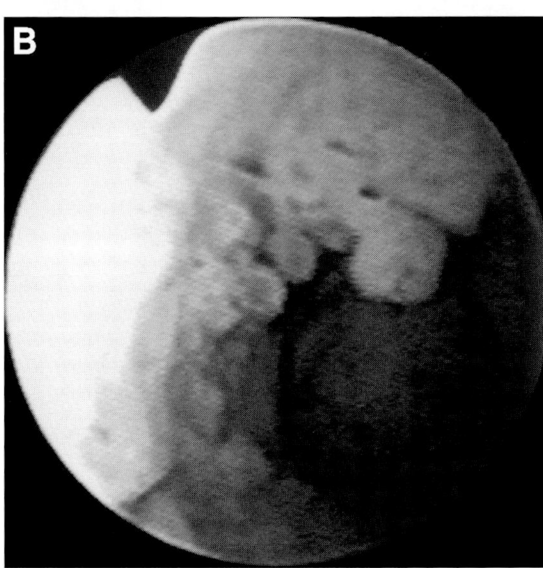


Fig. 18.8

(A,B) The tumor is visualized using a flexible ureteroscope with the aid of fluoroscopic guidance.

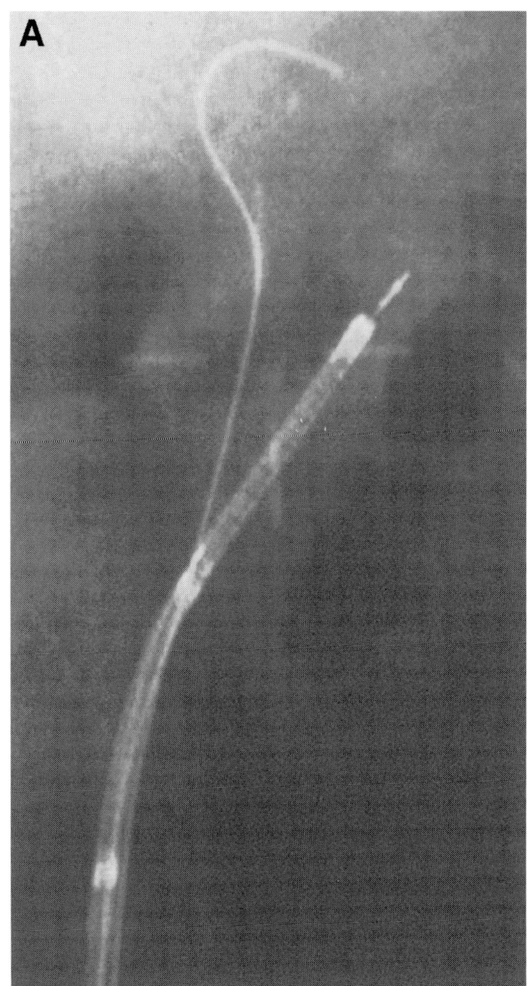


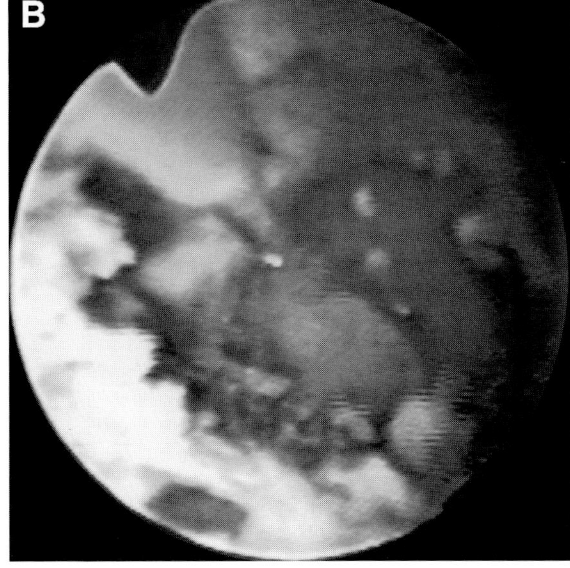


Fig. 18.9

(A,B) Tumor debulking can be accomplished using flexible biopsy forceps or a basket as a snare, and tissue is sent for histological examination. A Holmium laser or small, ureteroscopic Bugbee electrode is used to manage the tumor base.

pulled in 3–4 d with the aid of a retrieval string. For more extensive tumors, a 2- to 4-wk period may be necessary for adequate healing.

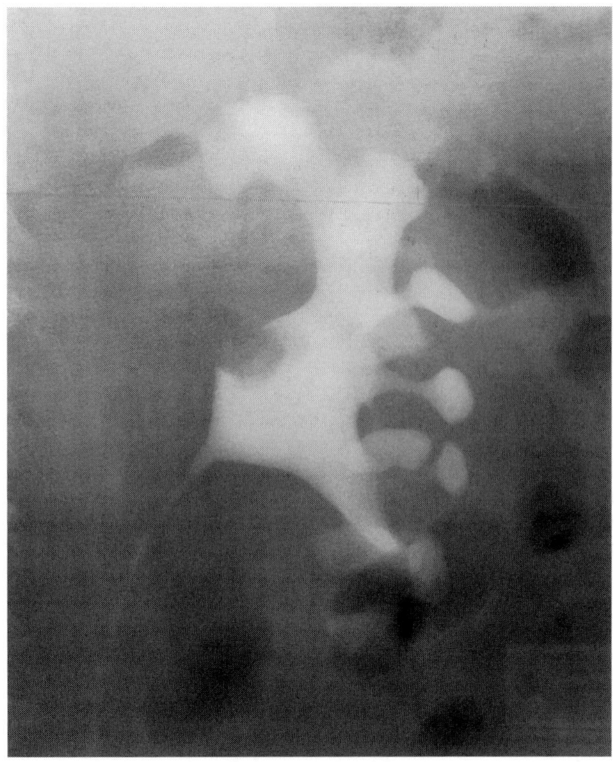

**Fig. 18.10**

The best candidates for percutaneous management are those in whom the tumor is relatively small, low grade, and noninvasive. Such determination is based on cytological and radiographic evaluation, and in some cases, direct ureteropyeloscopic visualization with or without ureteropyeloscopic biopsy. The pyelogram shown here reveals a renal pelvic filling defect on the medial pelvic wall, suggestive of transitional cell carcinoma (TCC). The patient had a TCC of the contralateral ureter as well.

Although the ideal interval has not yet been determined, patients should be followed with periodic cystoscopic and radiographic evaluation, along with interval upper tract endoscopic examination. We maintain a low threshold for nephroureterectomy for patients with recurrent disease and a normal contralateral kidney.

## PERCUTANEOUS MANAGEMENT

Since our first report of percutaneous management of upper tract TCC in 1986, several centers have gained experience managing relatively large numbers of patients who now have been followed for extended time intervals. On the basis of this expanding clinical experience, a logical approach to percutaneous management has been developed. Careful patient selection is a primary consideration when opting for a percutaneous approach. As for any conservative operation for pyelocalyceal TCC, percutaneous management is reserved for those patients in whom nephroureterectomy would result in significant loss of renal function necessitating dialysis or for patients with concurrent medical problems precluding major surgery.

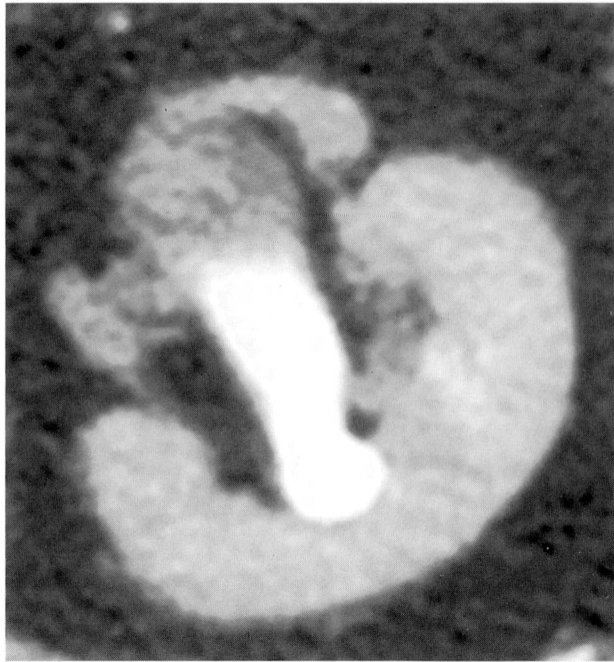

**Fig. 18.11**

A computed tomography scan performed with intravenous contrast confirms this to be an enhancing renal pelvic mass, without evidence of invasion. As such, patient is an excellent candidate for percutaneous management.

### Operative Technique

The site of percutaneous access is chosen in a fashion analogous to that for percutaneous stone removal.

Whenever possible, percutaneous access, tract dilation, and tumor ablation should be accomplished with a single-stage procedure to minimize the risk of potential recurrences along the tract. The optimal technique for tumor ablation depends primarily on the tumor size and location.

At the completion of the procedure, a 24 French nephrostomy tube is left indwelling to drainage. Even in the most experienced hands, visualization of the pelviocalyceal system may be limited at the time of initial access, tract dilation and nephroscopy. As such, "second-look" nephroscopy using rigid and flexible instrumentation is often performed 3–5 d later through a now-mature nephrostomy tract. At that time, the entire pelviocalyceal system can often be easily inspected and any suspicious areas can be biopsied.

Because patients undergoing conservative management of pyelocalyceal tumors are at risk for recurrence, we often utilize the percutaneous tract as access for topical immunotherapy or chemotherapy as an adjunct to definitive resection. With our current protocol, the patient is left with a

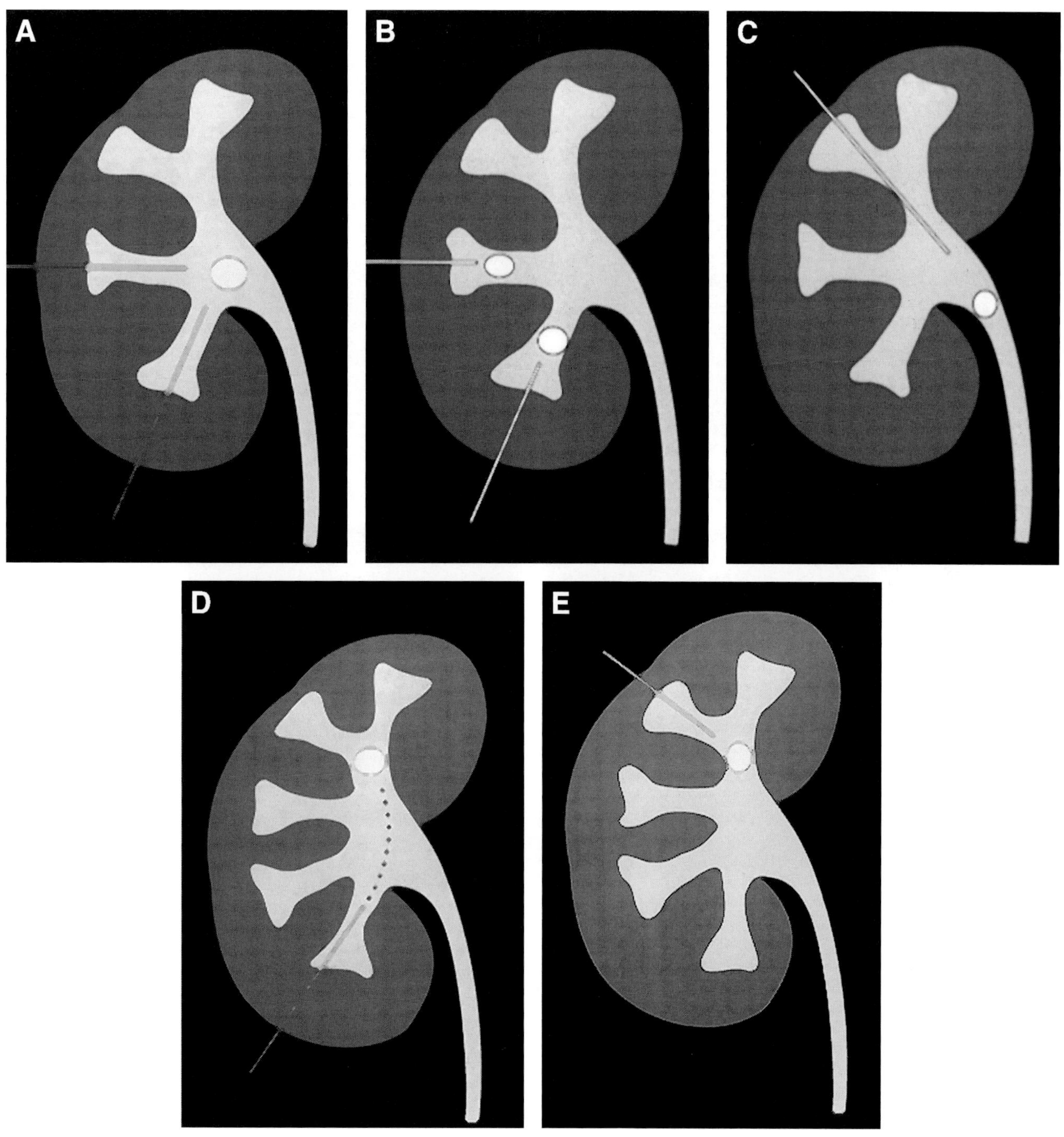


Fig. 18.12

**(A)** Renal pelvic tumors can be accessed via mid or lower pole infundibula. **(B)** Infundibulocalyceal tumors are best approached directly. **(C)** Upper ureteral tumors should be approached via superolateral infundibula. **(D,E)** Upper infundibulocalyceal tumors can be approached indirectly via the lower pole to circumvent the need for supracostal access. However, indirect access to an infundibulocalyceal tumor necessitates tumor ablation with flexible instrumentation. A direct approach is therefore preferable.

22 or 24 French nephrostomy tube indwelling at the time of hospital discharge and returns 2 wk later for a nephrostogram. If there is no obstruction or extravasation on that study, a course of BCG is begun using an ampoule of TICE BCG in 50 cc normal saline infused over 45 min each week for 6 wk. During this 6-wk course, nephrostograms are obtained intermittently to assure a continually nonobstructed system without extravasation. One month after

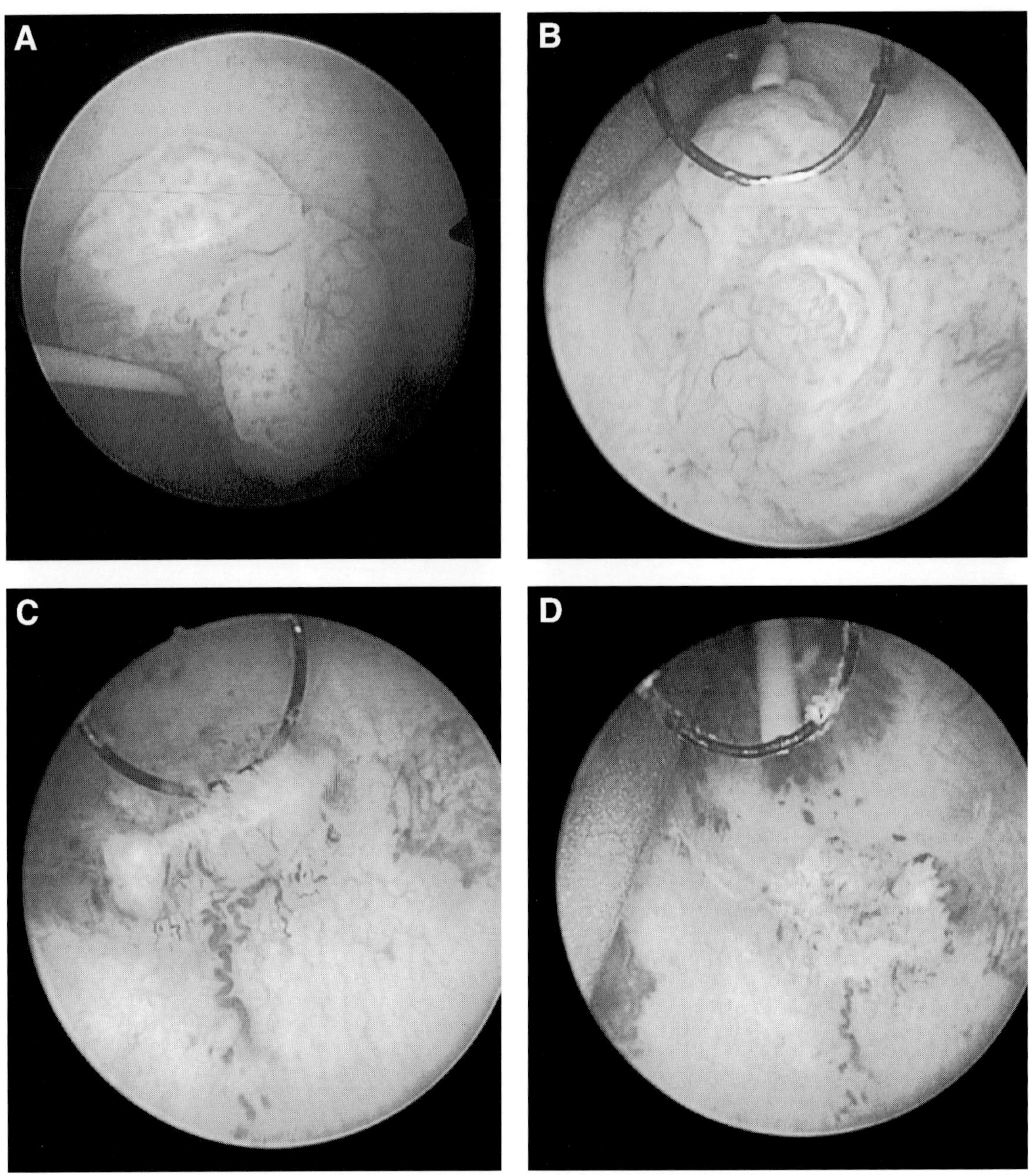


**Fig. 18.13**

**(A–D)** In some cases, the tumor can be managed simply by debulking with an alligator or cup biopsy forceps, following which the base is electrocoagulated with a Bugbee electrode. However, larger tumors are best managed with formal electroresection using a 24 French resectoscope through a working sheath, as seen in these nephroscopic views. In order to obviate the risk of hyponatremia resulting from absorption of fluid, 1.5% glycine is the preferred irrigant at our center whenever electrofulguration or resection is performed.

completion of BCG treatment, i.e., approx 3 mo after initial tumor ablation, a follow-up nephroscopy is often performed with biopsy of any suspicious areas.

## Complications and Results

Complications of percutaneous management of upper tract TCC are analogous to those associated with percutaneous stone management. Immediate complications include bleeding or extravasation, both of which are managed initially with a conservative approach as expectant management will likely result in complete resolution. If bleeding persists, more active intervention is accomplished with selective arterial embolization rather than open operative intervention. Complications specific to management of urothelial tumors include the risk of local tumor seeding along the percutaneous tract or in the peri-renal space, or distantly via the systemic circulation as a result of pyelovenous or pyelolymphatic backflow, although this risk, in properly selected patients, is extremely low. Steps that can be taken to lessen the likelihood of these problems with single-stage percutaneous access, tract dilation and tumor resection, and maintenance of low intrapelvic pressure by resecting through a working sheath and keeping the irrigation bag less than 40 cm above the level of the kidney. Some investigators suggest using sterile water as the irrigant for its osmotic-mediated cytolytic effect. However, our preference is normal saline for nephroscopy and glycine during electroresection or electrocoagulation in order to decrease the possibility of dilutional hyponatremia from absorption.

Others have summarized the long-term results of percutaneous management of upper tract TCC. In a review of patients treated at six different centers, recurrent renal pelvic tumors were reported in 0–45% of patients after follow-up ranging from 4 to 45 mo. At our own center, using a planned, combined approach of percutaneous tumor resection followed routinely with adjuvant topical immuno- or chemotherapy, local recurrence rates remain low, although distant metastatic disease is still a significant problem. However, this is a group of patients at high risk for recurrence. The vast majority had a history of multiple previous tumors elsewhere in the urinary tract, and in those developing metastatic disease, invasive, high-grade disease had already been documented in the bladder at the time of initial presentation.

## SUGGESTED READINGS

1. Blute ML, Segura JW, Patterson DE, Benson RC, Jr, Zincke H. Impact of endourology on diagnosis and management of upper urinary tract urothelial cancer. J Urol 141:1298, 1989.
2. Clark PE, Streem SB, Geisinger MA. 13-year experience with percutaneous management of upper tract transitional cell carcinoma. J Urol 161:772, 1999.
3. Gerber GS, Lyon ES. Endourological management of upper tract urothelial tumors. J Urol 150:2, 1993.
4. Hendin BN, Streem SB, Levin HS, et al. Impact of diagnostic ureteroscopy on long-term survival in patients with upper tract transitional cell carcinoma. J Urol 161:783, 1999.
5. Jarrett T, Sweetser PM, Weiss GH, Smith AD. Percutaneous management of transitional cell carcinoma of the renal collecting system: 9-year experience. J Urol 154:1629, 1995.
6. Keeley FX, Bibbo M, Bagley DH. Ureteroscopic treatment and surveillance of upper urinary TCC. J Urol 157:1560, 1997.
7. Murphy DP, Gill IS, Streem SB. Evolving management of upper-tract TCC at a tertiary-care center. J Endourol 16:483, 2002.
8. Nurse DE, Woodhouse CRJ, Kellett MJ, Dearnley DP. Percutaneous removal of upper tract tumors. World J Urol 7:131, 1989.
9. Savage SJ, Streem SB. Ureteroscopic approach to upper-tract urothelial tumors. J Endourol 14:275, 2000.
10. Shinka T, Uekado Y, Aoshi H, Hirano A, Ohkawa T. Occurrence of uroepithelial tumors of the upper urinary tract after the initial diagnosis of bladder cancer. J Urol 140:745, 1988.
11. Streem SB, Pontes EJ. Percutaneous management of upper tract transitional cell carcinoma. J Urol 135:773, 1986.
12. Studer UE, Casanova G, Kraft R, Zing EJ. Percutaneous bacillus Calmette-Guerin perfusion of the upper urinary tract for carcinoma in situ. J Urol 142:975, 1989.
13. Tasca A, Zattoni F. The case for a percutaneous approach to transitional cell carcinoma of the renal pelvis. J Urol 143:902, 1990.
14. Vasavada SP, Streem SB, Novick AC. Percutaneous BCG as adjunctive therapy to definitive resection in patients with renal pelvic transitional cell carcinoma in solitary kidneys. J Urol 151:258A, 1994.

# 19 Management of the *En Bloc* Distal Ureter and Bladder Cuff During Retroperitoneoscopic Radical Nephroureterectomy

*Osamu Ukimura and Inderbir S. Gill*

## INTRODUCTION

Radical nephroureterectomy with resection of the *en bloc* distal ureter and bladder cuff is the gold standard treatment option for most patients with upper urinary tract transitional cell carcinoma (TCC). Recurrence at the distal ureter and/or peiureteral bladder mucosa in the presence of ipsilateral upper urinary tract urothelial carcinoma has clinical significance. This procedure involves radical nephrectomy and *en bloc* distal ureterectomy with 2- to 3-cm-diameter bladder cuff, with special care to prevent urine spillage. We describe here our pure laparoscopic technique using two suprapubic transvesical ports, with cystoscopic secured detachment and ligation of the *en bloc* bladder cuff and juxtavesical ureter. This laparoscopic technique duplicates established principles of open radical nephroureterectomy.

## PATIENT SELECTION

Patients with upper tract urothelial carcinoma without coexisting active bladder tumor are candidates for this technique. As with all endoscopic methods, our technique is contraindicated in patients with a known urothelial carcinoma in the intramural ureter.

Patients are informed about the general risks of laparoscopy and potential for fluid extravasation/absorption with its associated sequelae, as during transurethral resection of the prostate (TURP). All patients undergo computed tomography (CT) scan for preoperative staging and to identify any abnormal renal vasculature.

## OPERATIVE TECHNIQUE

In the lithotomy position, a 21 Fr 30° cystoscope is inserted transurethrally. The bladder is palpably distended

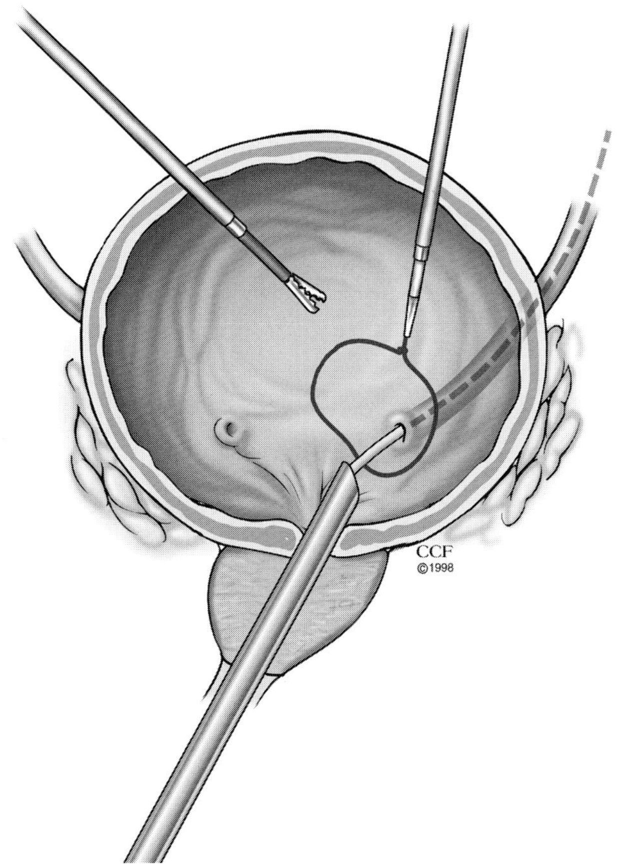


**Fig. 19.1**

A 2-mm endoloop inserted through the needlescopic port on the same side as the targeted ureter is positioned around the targeted ureteral orifice, such that the orifice lies in the center of the open endoloop. A 6 Fr ureteral catheter with a 0.035 guidewire is cystoscopically passed through the endloop up to the renal pelvis. The cystoscope is replaced with a 24 Fr continuous-flow resectoscope mounted with a Collins knife, which is now introduced per urethra alongside the ureteral catheter.

From: *Operative Urology at the Cleveland Clinic*
Edited by: A. Novick et al. © Humana Press Inc., Totowa, NJ

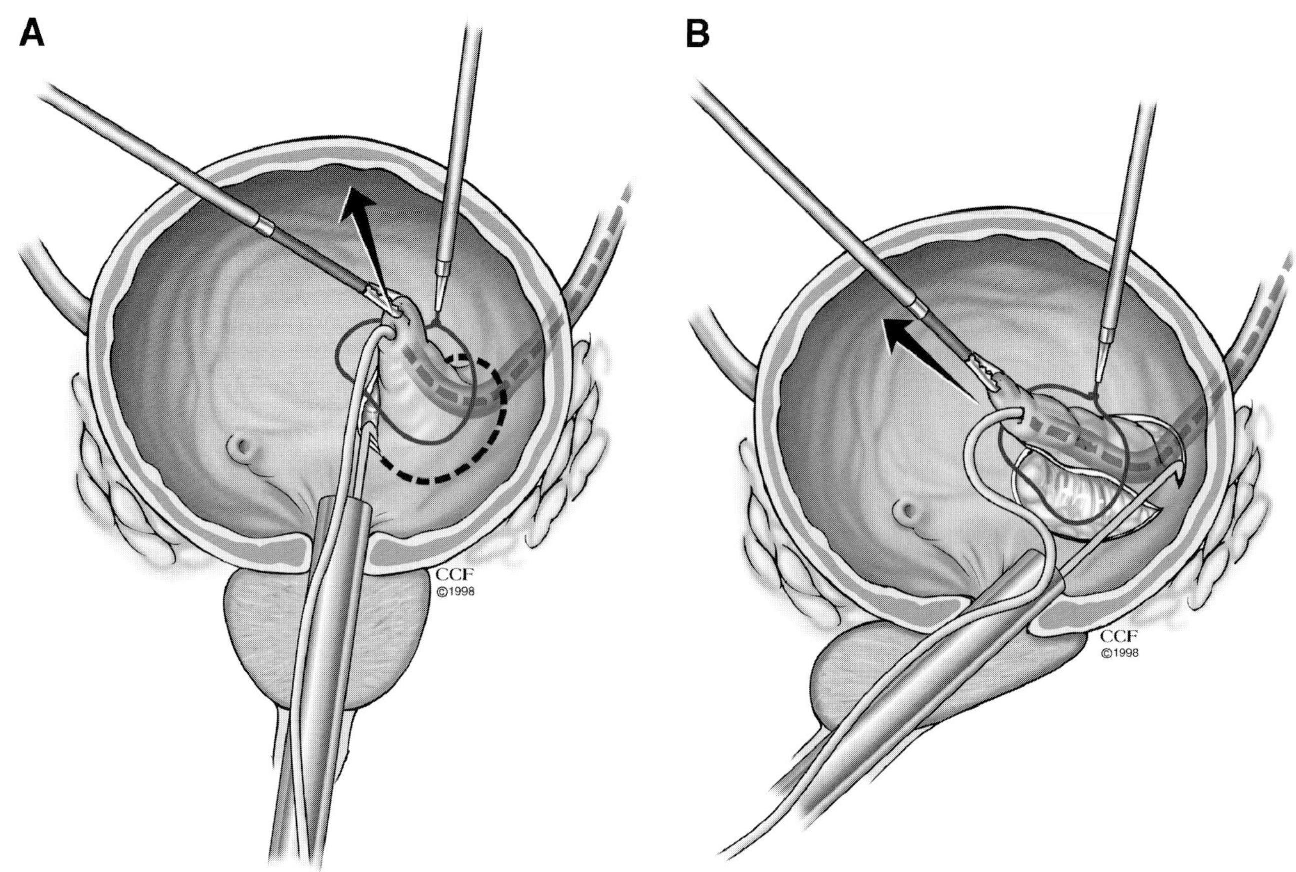


Fig. 19.2

**(A)** A 2-mm needlescopic grasper (arrow) is inserted through the contralateral 2-mm suprapubic port to grasp the targeted ureteral orifice and retract it anteriorly, thus tenting up the adjacent hemitrigone and bladder base. Using an electrocautery Collins knife, the proposed bladder cuff is scored (dotted line), circumferentially around the ureteric orifice and intramural ureter, such that an adequate bladder cuff, 2–3 cm in diameter, is outlined. **(B)** The full-thickness bladder wall is incised with the Collins knife along this scored area. Dissection is carried into the pelvic extraperitoneal perivesical fat until 3–4 cm of the intact extravesical ureter are circumferentially and completely detached *en bloc* and mobilized into the bladder. Arrow denotes direction of traction on the ureter.

with glycine irrigant, and two needlescopic 2-mm suprapubic ports are inserted on either side of the midline, one finger-breadth above the pubic symphysis under direct cystoscopic guidance. When inserting these suprapubic ports, care must be taken to distend the bladder fully and position the port sites close to the pubic symphysis to prevent potential bowel injury. Alternative to 2-mm needlescopic ports, balloon-tipped 5-mm ports (Entec) can be used.

The grasped ureteral catheter acts as a guide to prevent inadvertent entry into the intramural ureter, which must be avoided. Care must be taken not to compromise the contralateral ureteral orifice.

Constant suction is maintained from both suprapubic ports in order to maintain a relatively decompressed bladder with low intravesical pressure in order to minimize extravasation through the created bladder rent.

## POSTOPERATIVE CARE

The 24 Fr Foley catheter is maintained for 1–2 wk. Although the bladder rent is not suture repaired, Foley catheter drainage for 1 wk routinely results in complete bladder healing, which is confirmed with a cystogram. A Jackson–Pratt drain is placed in the pelvis and exteriorized through a 5-mm retroperitoneal port site with no suction on it postoperatively. Because of nonviolation of the peritoneal cavity, paralytic ileus is minimized and any postoperative fluid collections are limited to the retroperitoneum.

## COMMENT

This is the only purely laparoscopic technique that allows formal secured excision of a complete bladder cuff intravesically, with the distal ureter occluded, thus preventing

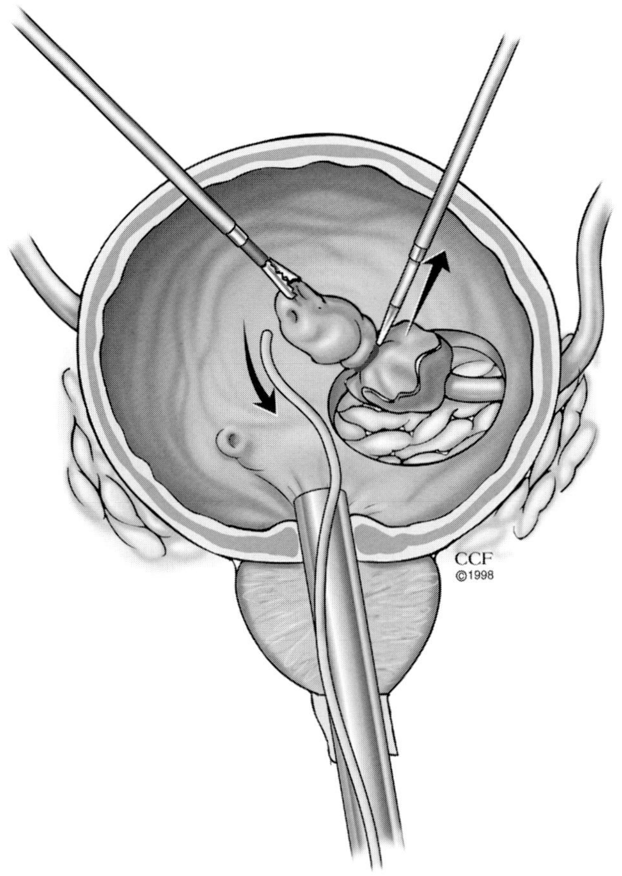


**Fig. 19.3**

Following removal of the ureteral catheter, the previously positioned endoloop is manipulated around the ureter and tightly cinched down to occlude the ureteral lumen. The yellowish pelvic extraperitoneal fat is visible through the bladder rent.
With a rollerball or a resectoscope loop, a 1- to 2-cm margin of the adjacent bladder urothelium is cauterized to ablate the "landing-zone" area. Complete hemostasis is ensured. The suprapubic ports and resectoscope are removed, and a 24 Fr Foley catheter is indwelled. The patient is repositioned in the flank position for the retroperitoneoscopic renal and ureteral dissection. During retroperitoneoscopic mobilization of the distal ureter, visualization of this endoloop tie ensures that the entire ureter with bladder cuff has been removed *en bloc*. As such, the entire nephroureterectomy is performed retroperitoneoscopically, without violation of the peritoneal cavity.

spillage from the upper tract. Further, complete resection of the entire *en bloc* urothelium in the ipsilateral ureter and bladder cuff is confirmed visually intraoperatively. Our recent study suggests that this method of *en bloc* excision of the bladder cuff and distal ureter is oncologically adequate, with adequate overall and recurrence-free survival.

The main disadvantage of this technique is its learning curve. Extravasation may also occur if either the suprapubic port slips out of the bladder or the intravesical pressure is not kept low.

## SUGGESTED READINGS

1. Gill IS, Soble JJ, Miller SD, Sung GT. A novel technique for management of the *en bloc* bladder cuff and distal ureter during laparoscopic nephroureterectomy. J Urol 161:430–434, 1999.
2. Gill IS, Sung GT, Hobart MG, et al. Laparoscopic radical nephroureterectomy for upper tract transitional cell carcinoma: the Cleveland Clinic experience. J Urol 164:1513–1522, 2000.
3. Matin SF, Gill IS. Recurrence and survival following laparoscopic radical nephroureterectomy with various forms of bladder cuff control. J Urol. 173:395–400, 2005.
4. Savage SJ, Gill IS. Laparoscopic radical nephroureterectomy. J Endourol. 14:859–864, 2000.

# 20 Ureteral Disorders in Children

*Jonathan H. Ross and Robert Kay*

## VESICOURETERAL REFLUX

Children with vesicoureteral reflux usually present with a urinary tract infection (UTI), although some cases are diagnosed during the evaluation of prenatally detected hydronephrosis. Approximately 25% of children with a UTI will be found to have reflux. Ultrasound is normal in 75% of children with reflux, and so children with a significant UTI are evaluated with a voiding cystourethrogram (VCUG). Reflux is graded based on the appearance of the VCUG:

Grade 1: Reflux into the ureter only
Grade 2: Reflux into the kidney with no distortion of the collecting system
Grade 3: Reflux into the kidney with blunting of the calyceal angles and/or mild ureterectasis
Grade 4: Reflux into the kidney with hydrouretronephrosis
Grade 5: Reflux into the kidney with marked hydroureteronephrosis and ureteral tortuosity

The grade of reflux is the most important predictor of spontaneous resolution, being approx 90, 80, 50, 30, and 10% for grades 1 through 5, respectively. Most children have mild reflux and are managed expectantly on antibiotic prophylaxis. Treatment of constipation and voiding dysfunction is a critical part of conservative management. Indications for surgery include breakthrough UTI, intolerance of antibiotics and periodic testing, and high-grade reflux. Standard treatment is by ureteral reimplantation, which may be accomplished by an intravesical or extravesical approach. An extravesical approach offers the theoretical advantage of decreased morbidity associated with a bladder incision. However, there is a higher chance of post-operative voiding dysfunction, particularly for bilateral cases. Both approaches have an excellent success rate of greater than 95%. Failures as a result of persistent reflux or ureteral obstruction are rare, except in cases of high-grade reflux requiring ureteral tailoring or tapering, for which reoperation rates are 15–20%.

Injection therapy is an alternative to long-term antibiotic prophylaxis or surgical intervention. Under a brief general anesthetic, cystoscopy is performed and a bulking agent is injected through a needle into the trigone just below the ureteral orifice. This raises a hillock under the intramural ureter discouraging reflux. The complication rate for this procedure is very low, but the reported success rates are less than for open surgical intervention. The bulking agent most frequently used in the United States is Deflux, for which success rates of 65–90% are reported depending on the degree of reflux.

## INTRAVESICAL URETERAL REIMPLANTATION

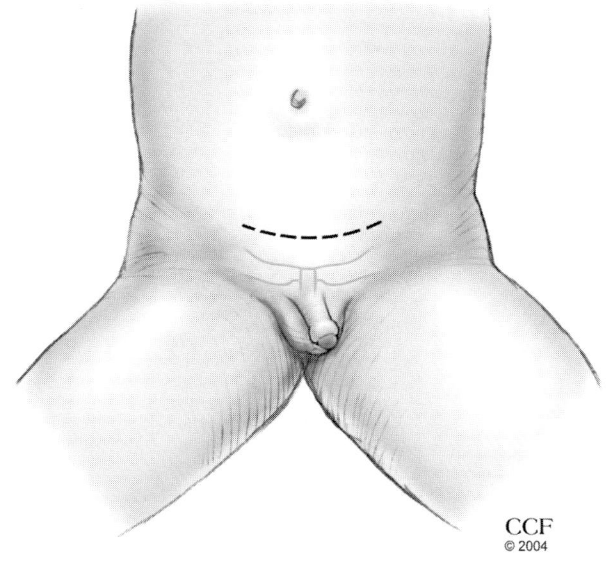


**Fig. 20.1**

A 6- to 7-cm transverse incision (Pfannenstiel) is made one finger-breadth above the pubic symphisis along Langer's lines.

From: *Operative Urology at the Cleveland Clinic*
Edited by: A. Novick et al. © Humana Press Inc., Totowa, NJ

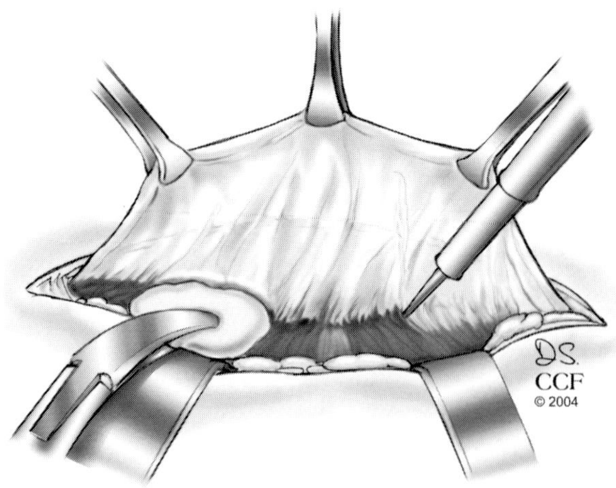


**Fig. 20.2**

Scarpa's fascia is divided, revealing the anterior rectus fascia. This is incised transversely from the edge of one rectus muscle to the other. The fascia is grasped with Kocher clamps, and, with a combination of blunt and cautery dissection, the attachments between the muscle and fascia are divided, elevating the fascia. The superior and inferior leaves of the rectus fascia are elevated from a few centimeters below the umbilicus to the pubic symphisis. The bladder is filled. The rectus muscles are separated in the midline with scissors or cautery exposing the anterior bladder surface. The space of Retzius is bluntly developed on either side of the bladder, and the peritoneum is swept superiorly.

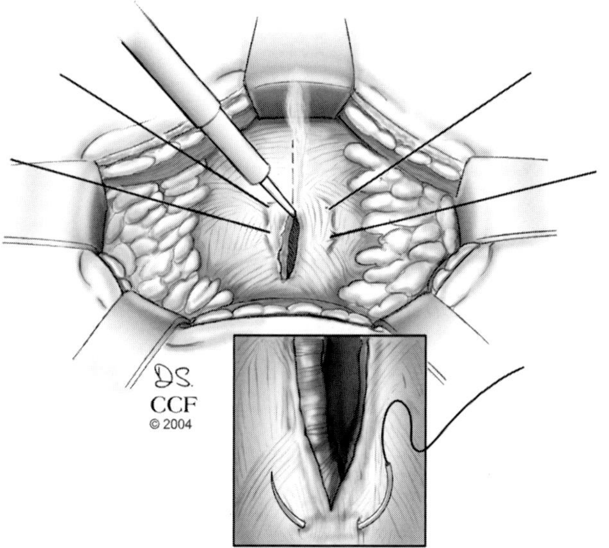


**Fig. 20.3**

The bladder is opened with cautery in the anterior midline from the dome to 1 cm above the bladder neck. A 3-0 chromic suture is placed just distal to the caudal corner of the bladder incision and tied down to prevent tearing of the incision into the bladder neck during subsequent retraction.

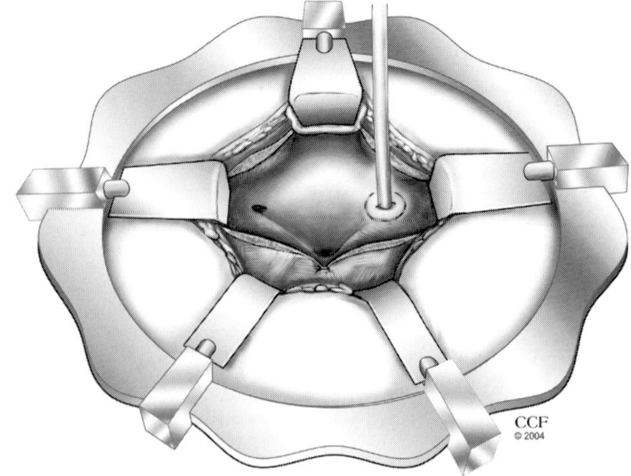


**Fig. 20.4**

Exposure is maintained with a Denis–Browne retractor. One or two moist sponges are placed under the blade in the dome of the bladder. A 5 French feeding tube or 3.5 French umbilical artery catheter is passed up the ureter(s) to be reimplanted and secured with a 4-0 chromic suture.

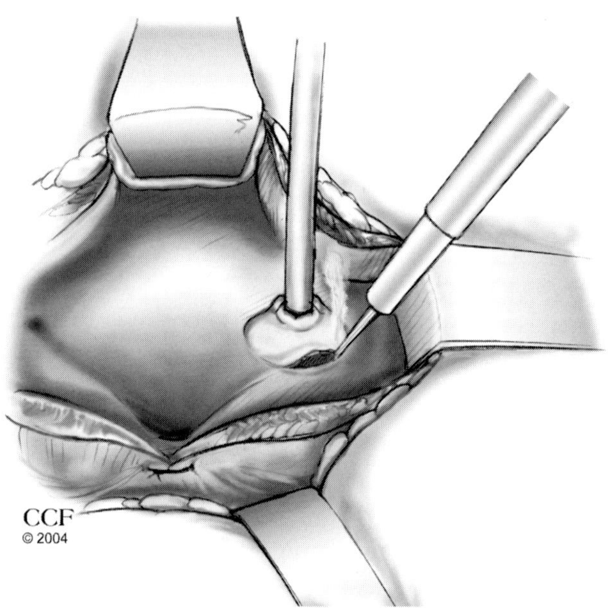


**Fig. 20.5**

Upward traction is placed on the ureter, and the ureteral orifice is circumscribed with pure cutting current, leaving a wide margin to facilitate future reimplantation.

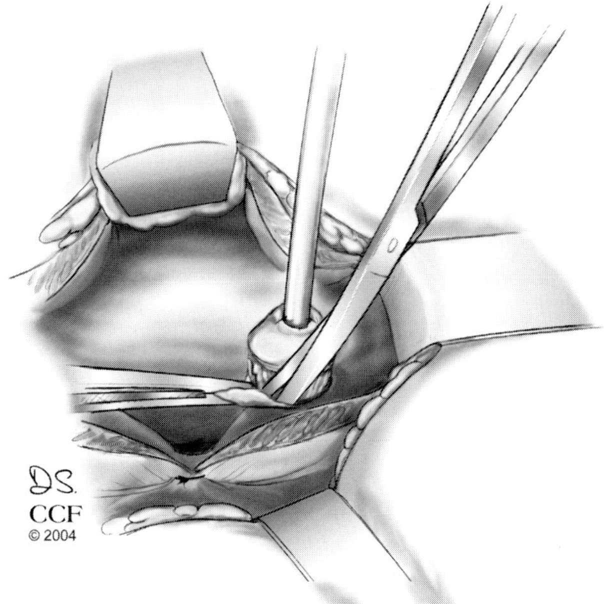


**Fig. 20.6**

The bladder muscle at the caudal aspect of the incision is incised with scissors entering the periureteral plane.

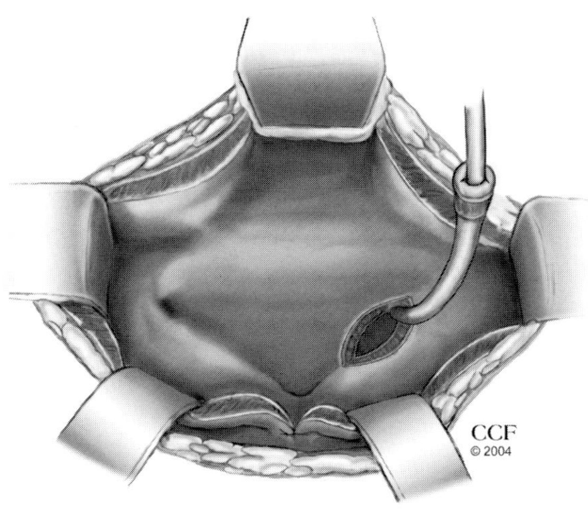


**Fig. 20.7**

With blunt and cautery dissection, the muscular attachments between the bladder and the ureter are divided, hugging the ureter during the dissection. In this way the proper plane is entered. Once free of the trigone, the ureter is easily mobilized from the peritoneum and retroperitoneal attachments with blunt dissection.

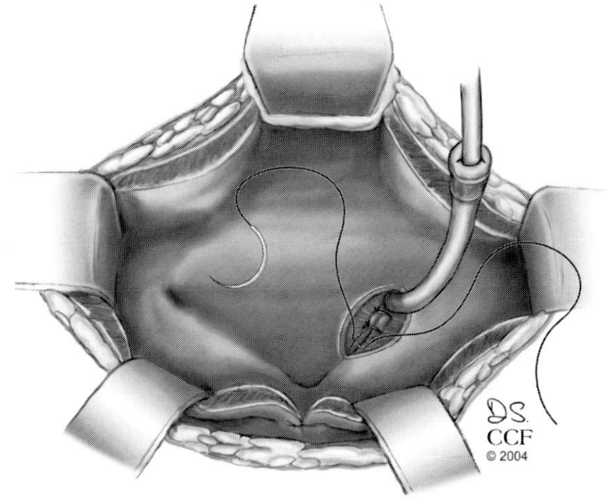


**Fig. 20.8**

The muscular opening at the hiatus is closed with interrupted 3-0 chromic sutures. Care must be taken not to close the opening too snugly against the ureter.

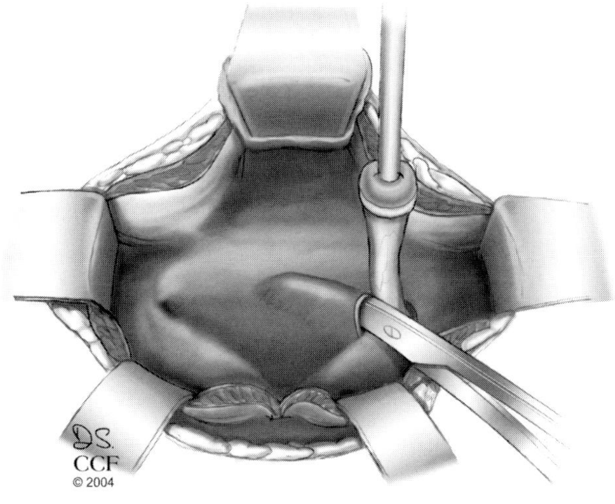


**Fig. 20.9**

A submucosal tunnel in the bladder wall is created. In the Cohen cross-trigonal reimplant, the tunnel extends from the hiatus across the bladder floor to the contralateral side.

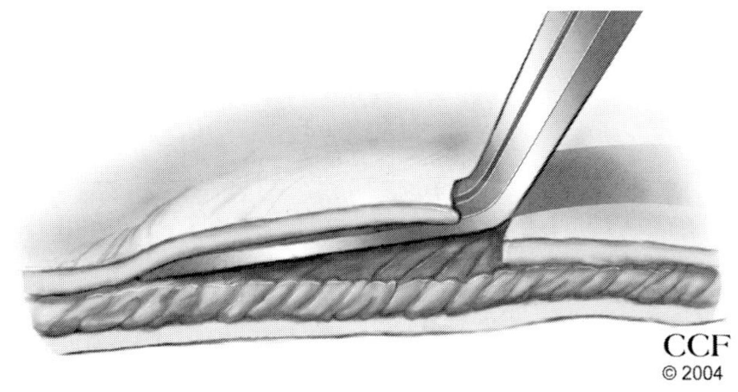


**Fig. 20.10**

The appropriate plane of dissection is between the bladder mucosa and the bladder muscle. If the proper plane is maintained, little bleeding is encountered.

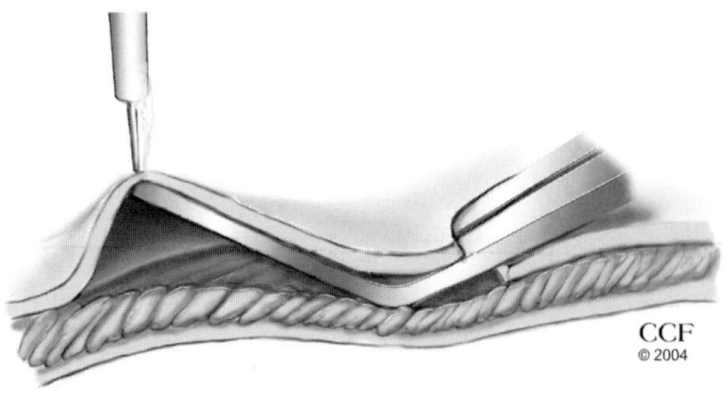


**Fig. 20.11**

Once an adequate tunnel length is dissected a new meatus is created with cautery over the tip of the dissecting instrument.

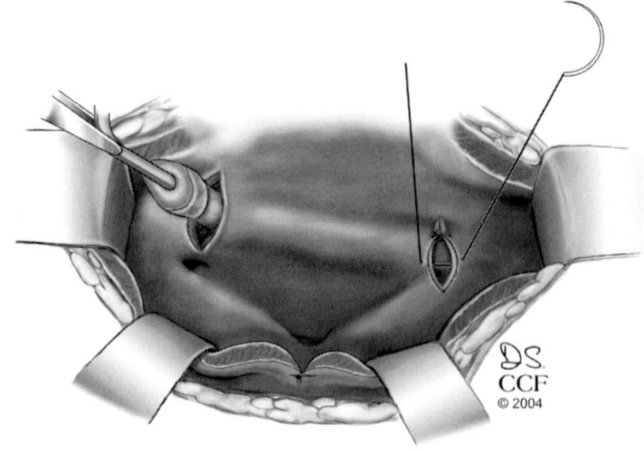


**Fig. 20.12**

The ureter is brought through the new tunnel. The mucosa at the original hiatus is closed with running 5-0 chromic suture. This closure is facilitated by first mobilizing the mucosa off of the muscle circumferentially.

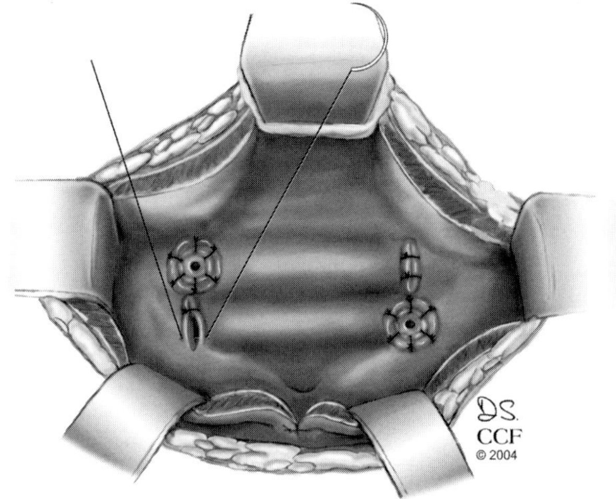


**Fig. 20.13**

The edges of the bladder mucosa cuff on the ureter are secured circumferentially at the new meatus. The three distal-most sutures of 4-0 poliglecapronic-25 extend from the mucosal cuff to the bladder muscle and mucosa, anchoring the neomeatus. The remainder of the approximation is accomplished with mucosa-to-mucosa sutures of 5-0 chromic. The identical procedure is performed on the contralateral ureter when a bilateral reimplantation is undertaken.

A

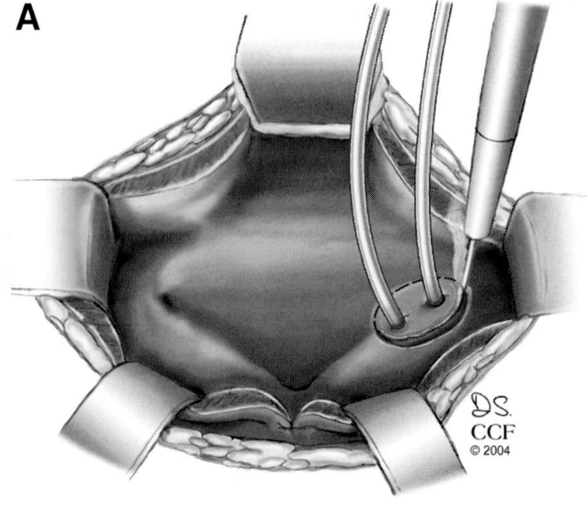


B

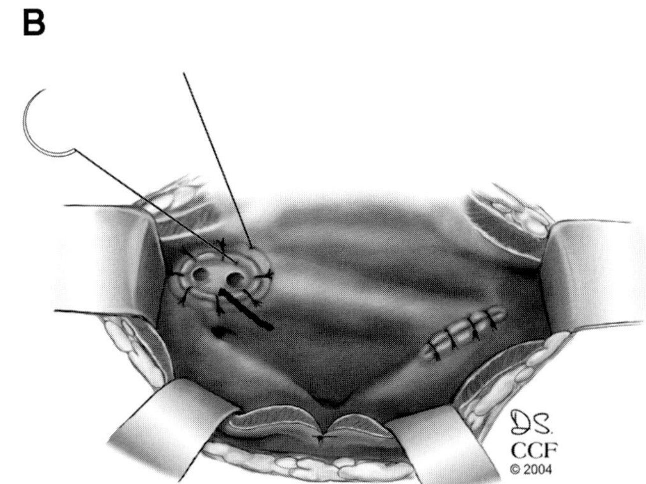


**Fig. 20.14**

**(A,B)** When a duplicated system is present, even if reflux is only present in the lower pole, both ureters should be reimplanted. The ureteral orifices are circumscribed, mobilized, and reimplanted as a unit.

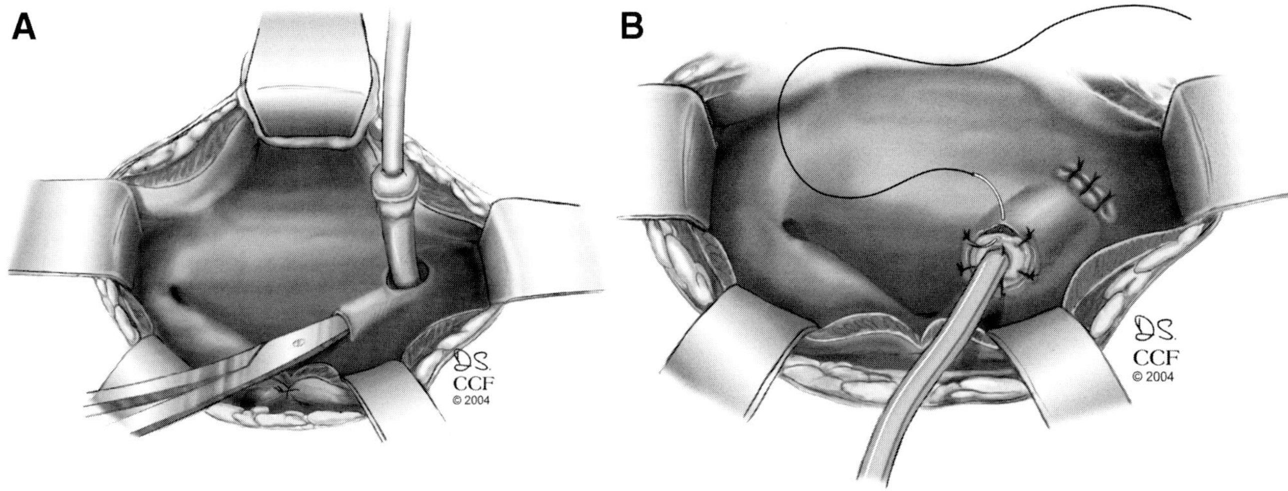


Fig. 20.15

**(A,B)** If the distance from the ureteral meatus to the bladder neck is large, a Glen–Anderson ureteral advancement may be undertaken. The ureter is mobilized and the muscular hiatus repaired as previously described. A submucosal tunnel is then created toward the bladder neck and the ureter reimplanted. The major disadvantage of this approach is the limited tunnel length that can be obtained.

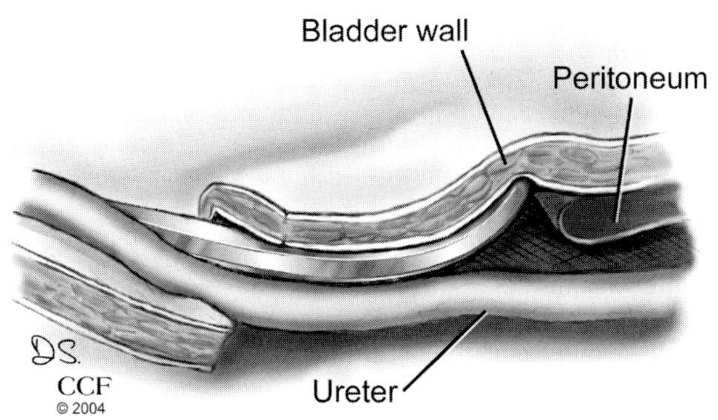


Fig. 20.16

In a Leadbetter–Politano reimplant, the ureteral hiatus is moved cranially to gain tunnel length. Once the ureter has been mobilized, a clamp is passed into the hiatus and is used to bluntly dissect the peritoneum off the back wall of the bladder. A new hiatus is then opened over the tip of the clamp and the ureter drawn up through the new opening.

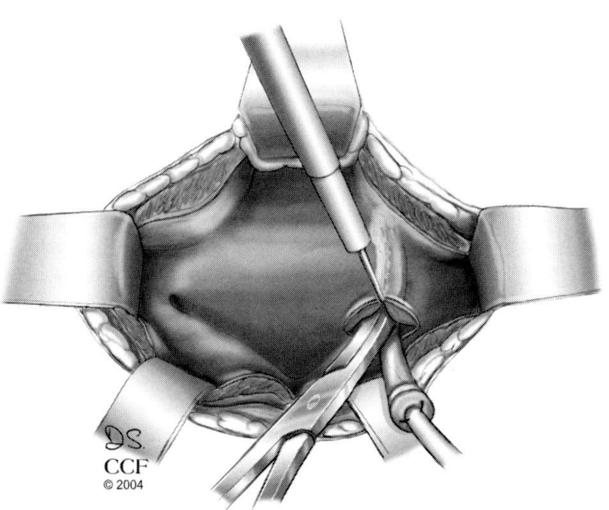


Fig. 20.17

Concern regarding the risk of penetrating the peritoneum during the dissection behind the bladder or kinking the ureter when pulling it through the new hiatus during a Leadbetter–Politano reimplant leads to a modification of the technique. Rather than accomplishing the ureteral transfer blindly, the bladder wall is opened full thickness over the dissecting clamp and the ureter lifted up into the cranial apex of the incision. The bladder muscle is then closed caudal to the neohiatus.

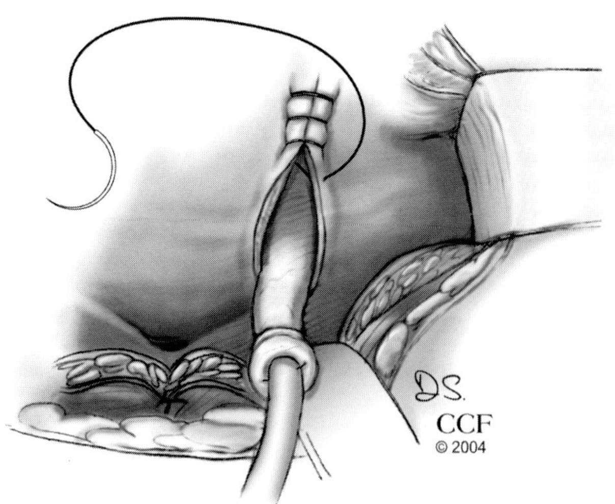


**Fig. 20.18**

The ureter is placed on the closed bladder floor and the mucosa is closed over it with a running 5-0 chromic suture.

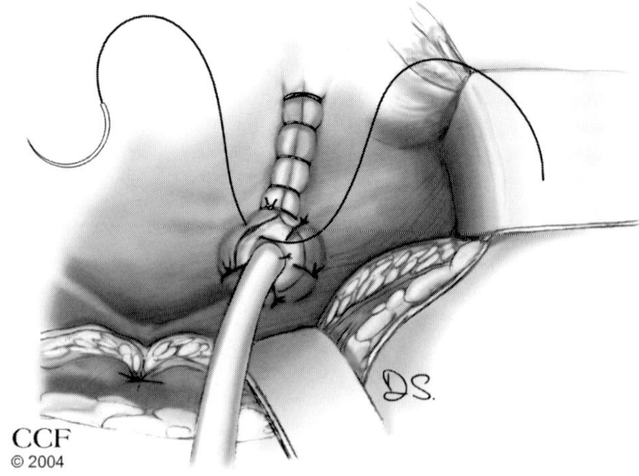


**Fig. 20.19**

The ureter is secured in its neomeatus, which may be at the same site as the original hiatus, or it may be advanced further toward the bladder neck for additional tunnel length.

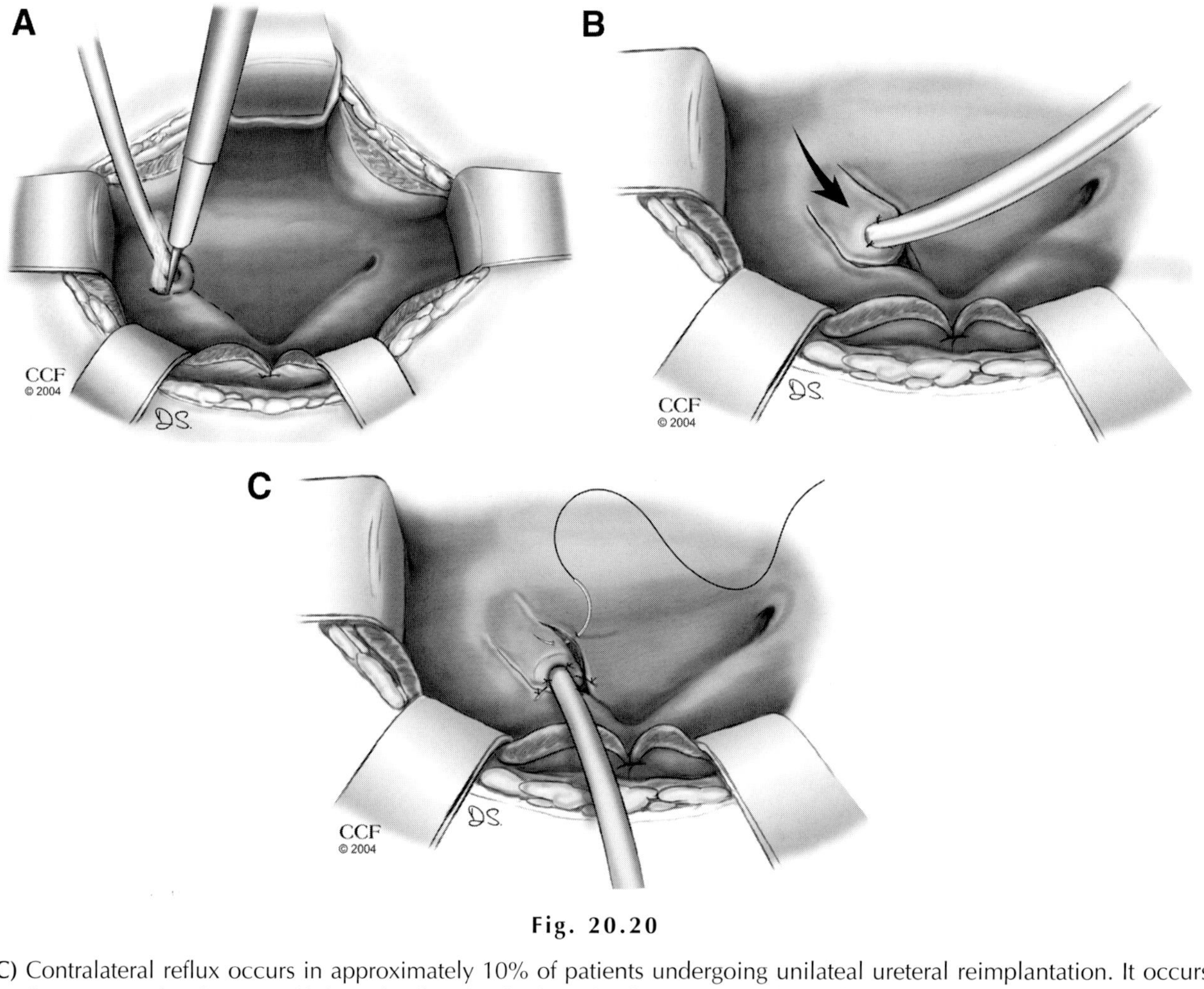

**Fig. 20.20**

**(A–C)** Contralateral reflux occurs in approximately 10% of patients undergoing unilateal ureteral reimplantation. It occurs in 45% of patients with a history of bilateral reflux that had resolved spontaneously on the contralateral side. In such cases, to prevent this complication, bilateral ureteral reimplantation should be undertaken. In cases where the reflux has always been unilateral, the small chance of contralateral reflux may be prevented by a Y-V advancement of the ureteral orifice. A semi-lunar incision is made around the medio-caudal edge of the ureteral orifice and a Y-stem incision from the semilunar incision toward the bladder neck. The ureter is pulled along the stem incision and secured medially with interrupted chromic sutures. While this approach is not routinely employed, it should be considered in cases where the contralateral orifice is laterally ectopic.

# EXTRAVESICAL URETERAL REIMPLANTATION

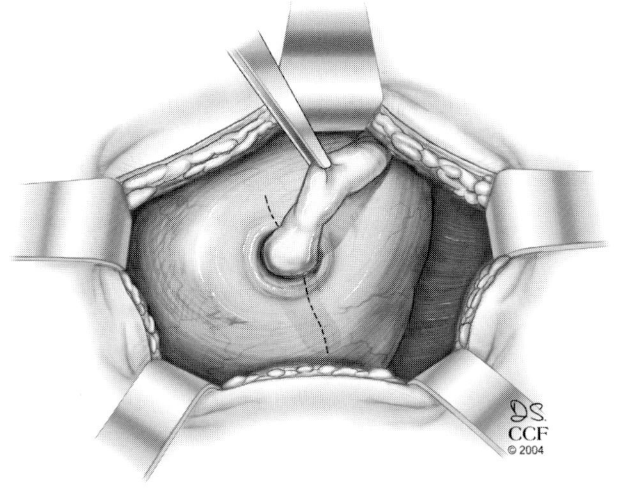


**Fig. 20.21**

A Pfannenstiel incision is made and the space of Retzius developed lateral to the bladder. The olbiterated umbilical artery is divided and the ureter is identified.

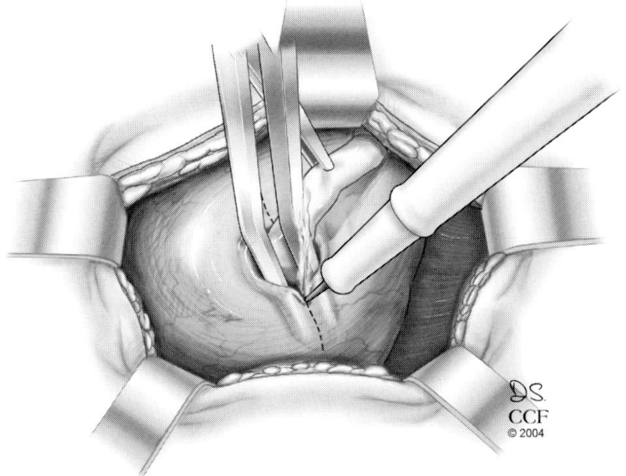


**Fig. 20.22**

The ureter is dissected toward the bladder, and the intramural portion is exposed by dividing the detrussor fibers overlying it. In this way the ureter is dissected until its attachment to the bladder mucosa is exposed.

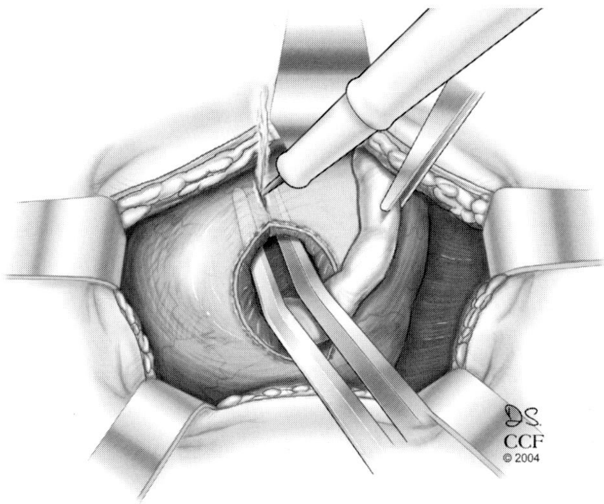


**Fig. 20.23**

The detrussor muscle is dissected off the mucosa cranially and divided up to the peritoneal reflection.

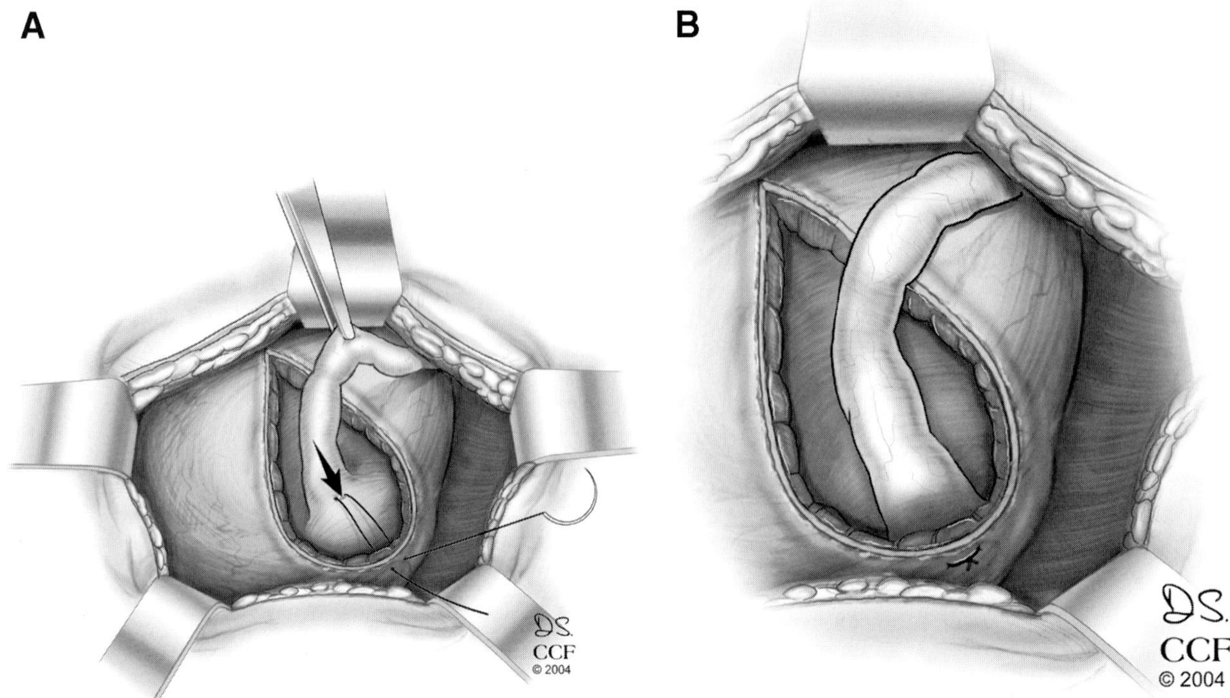


Fig. 20.24

**(A,B)** A U-stitch of 4-0 polyglactin suture is placed advancing the ureteral meatus toward the bladder neck.

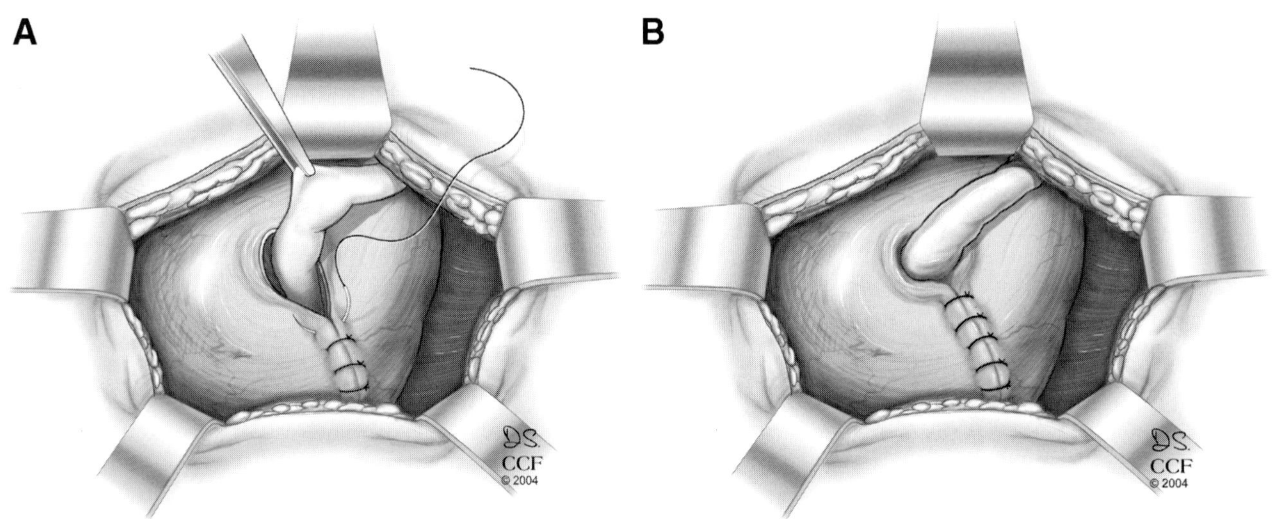


Fig. 20.25

**(A,B)** The ureter is placed on the exposed bladder mucosa, and the previously dissected detrussor muscle is closed over the ureter with interrupted vicryl suture creating a new (and longer) intramural tunnel.

## POSTOPERATIVE CARE

A caudal or epidural block is employed introperatively, but any catheters are removed at the end of the operation. Ketorolac 1.0 mg/kg is administered during wound closure and continued at a dose of 0.5 mg/kg every 6 h until discharge. The urethral catheter is removed on the first postoperative morning, and patients are usually discharged later that day. An ultrasound to rule out iatrogenic obstruction is obtained 4–6 wk postoperatively, and a follow-up ultrasound and VCUG are obtained at 6 mo. Patients are maintained on their antibiotic prophylaxis until the follow-up VCUG confirms a good result.

## MEGAURETERS

Evaluation of obstructed megaureters has traditionally been with intravenous urography and voiding cysto-urethrography. Obstructed megaureters must be distinguished from refluxing megaureters and from nonobstructed, nonrefluxing megaureters, which do not require intervention. Urographic criteria for the diagnosis of obstructed megaureter include moderate or severe hydroureteronephrosis with caliectasis, delayed excretion of contrast on the affected side, decreased density of contrast in the affected ureter, and delayed drainage into the bladder. Reflux should be absent on the voiding cystourethrogram, although, rarely, a ureter may be both obstructed and refluxing. The use of diuretic renography is not established in evaluating washout from dilated ureters, although the analog images may be evaluated with criteria similar to those used for conventional urography. The renal scan has the advantage of offering a more quantitative measurement of relative renal function. In occasional cases, a Whitaker test may be helpful in confirming a significant obstruction.

The widespread use of prenatal ultrasound has raised new questions regarding the management of megaureters. Prior to the use of prenatal ultrasonography, when the vast majority of patients with hydronephrosis presented with a clinical problem, there was little question as to the need for early intervention. However, approx 80% of obstructed megaureters are now detected prenatally. The postnatal detection rate is not significantly different from the preultrasound era, implying that the overall detection rate for these lesions in infants is five times greater than previously. This has stimulated a reassessment of the indications for surgical intervention in what are now primarily asymptomatic neonates with incidentally detected hydroureter. Studies of the natural history of prenatally detected megaureters have shown that most of these megaureters improve spontaneously with little risk of deterioration in renal function. They can be followed with periodic radiographic evaluation. Surgical correction would be reserved for those experiencing a deterioration in renal function or radiographic appearance or those with clinical problems, such as a urinary tract infection. For refluxing megaureters, preemptive reimplantaion may be undertaken at 1 yr of age since the likelihood of resolution is small.

## URETERAL REIMPLANTATION OF MEGAURETERS

The surgical approach to megaureters is similar to that for simple reflux except that additional maneuvers are required to ensure that the submucosal tunnel–to–ureteral diameter ratio is adequate to prevent reflux. These maneuvers include ureteral tapering or tailoring and, when necessary, performance of a psoas hitch or Boari flap.

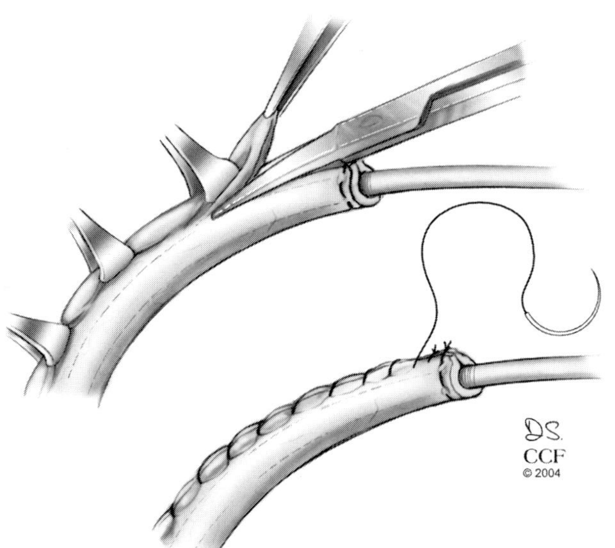


**Fig. 20.26**

Ureteral tapering is performed when the ureteral diameter must be reduced by more than half. After mobilizing the ureter as for any reimplant, an 8 or 10 French catheter is placed in the ureter. Megaureter clamps are placed up against the catheter, taking care not to spiral around the ureter, compromising the blood supply. The redundant ureter is excised and the ureter closed with running 5-0 polydioxanone suture. Interrupted sutures are used at the end in case uereteral trimming or spatulation is required after passing the ureter in to its new submucosal tunnel.

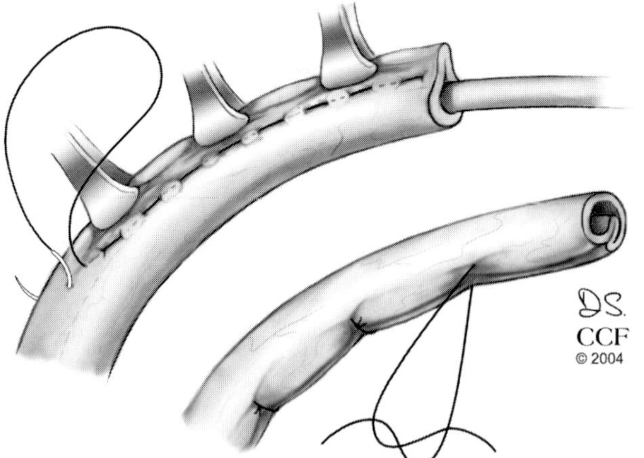


Fig. 20.27

Ureteral tailoring is employed when a more modest decrease in ureteral diameter is required. In theory, this preserves more of the ureteral blood supply than tapering but has the disadvantage of leaving a bulky ureter for reimplantation. Rather than excising the ureter, it is plicated over the catheter with running 5-0 polydioxanone suture and then folded over the ureter and secured in place with interrupted 6-0 polydioxanone suture. Very superficial bites are taken so as not to injure the intrinsic ureteral blood supply.

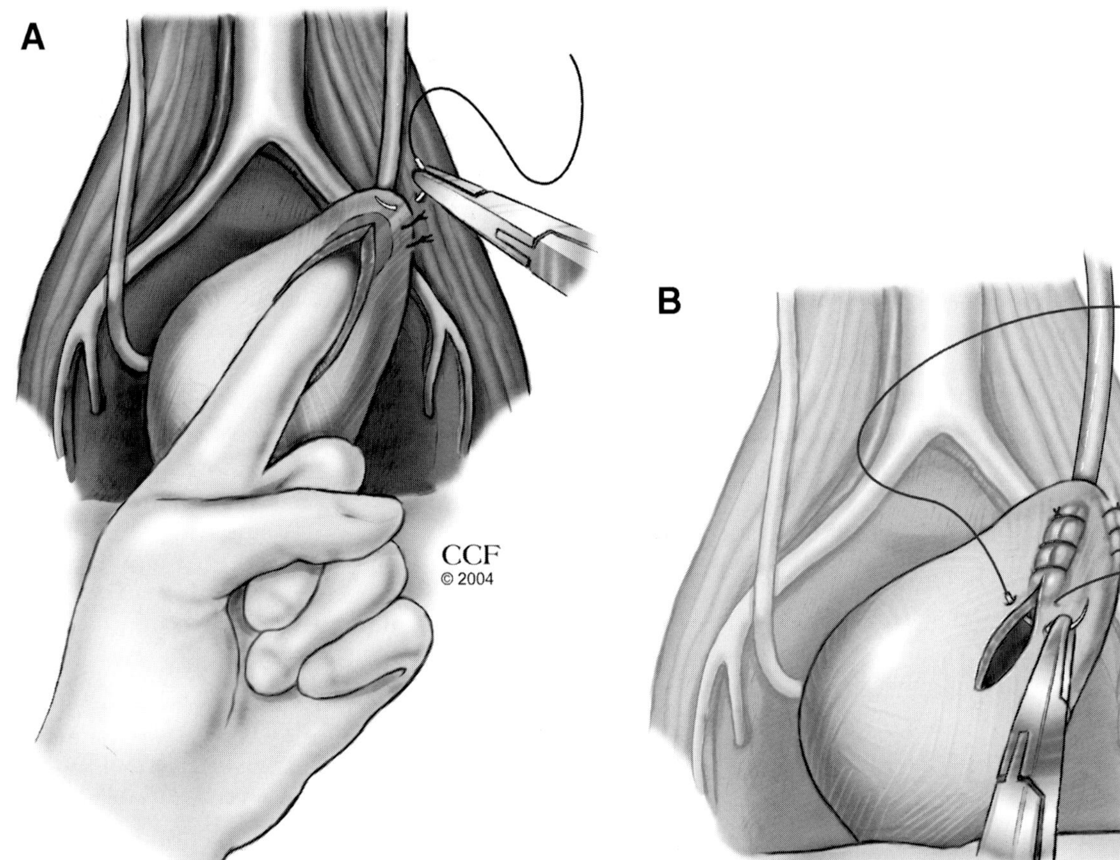


Fig. 20.28

**(A,B)** A psoas hitch can be used to increase tunnel length and/or bridge the gap between a short ureter and the bladder. After mobilizing the ureter, a finger is used to draw the bladder up to the ipsilateral psoas muscle. Prior to sewing the hitch a new hiatus is created near the top of the hitch and a submucosal tunnel is developed. The ureteral catheter is brought through the new hiatus and then the bladder is hitched to the psoas with interrupted 3-0 polydioxanone sutures. The ureter is then drawn through the new submucosal tunnel and reimplanted. The bladder is closed in two layers.

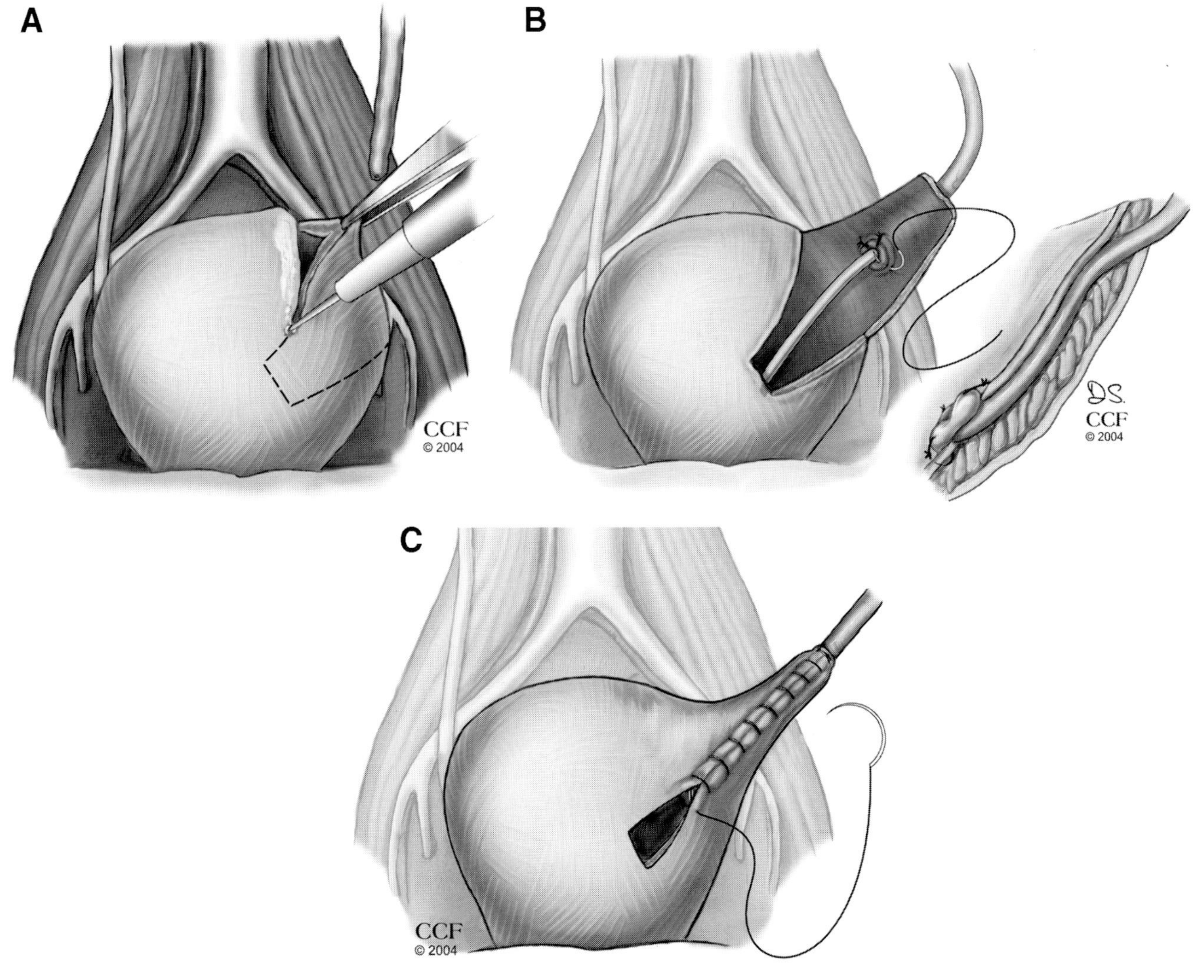


**Fig. 20.29**

**(A–C)** When the ureter cannot be reached adequately with a psoas hitch, a Boari flap is created. A rectangular flap of the bladder wall is created based craniolaterally and flipped toward the ureter along the psoas. A hiatus and tunnel are created in the flap. The flap is hitched to the psoas and closed.

## URETEROCELE AND ECTOPIC URETER

Most ureteroceles and ectopic ureters present as prenatally detected hydronephrosis. However, they may present later in life with UTI or, in a girl, incontinence. The most common prenatal finding is upper pole dilatation in a duplicated system. Lower pole distension may occur due to secondary obstruction by an upper pole ureterocele or to vesicoureteral reflux into the lower pole moiety. Occasionally ectopic ureters and ureteroceles may subtend a single system. These lesions can usually be well characterized by a combination of ultrasound, renal scan, and VCUG. In difficult cases an intravenous urogram and/or cystoscopy with retrograde pyelograms may clarify the anatomy. More recently magnetic resonance urography has been employed. Ectopic ureters in boys usually insert in the posterior urethra or seminal vesicle. In girls, the most common sites of insertion are the urethra, vestibule, and vagina. Ectopic ureters into the urethral sphincter may be obstructed during bladder filling and then reflux when the sphincter relaxes during voiding. This intermittent reflux can be demonstrated by a cyclic VCUG, in which the bladder is imaged during several consecutive cycles of filling and voiding.

Most duplication anomalies are detected on prenatal ultrasonography. Surgical correction during infancy is appropriate. These anomalies may be approached through the flank, the bladder, or both. Because of the technical difficulties encountered in a transvesical approach in the infant, a flank approach is most common. However, 30–50% of patients with ureteroceles will require a bladder operation later in life for persistent

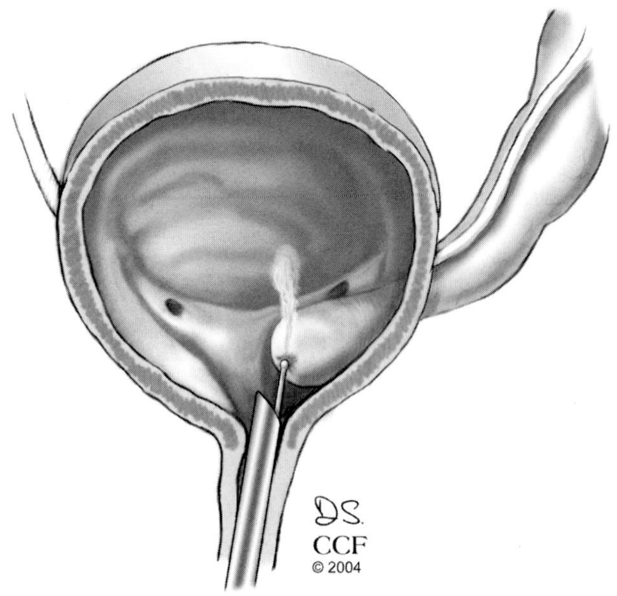


**Fig. 20.30**

A 3 French bugbee is introduced through a pediatric cystoscope. With cutting current the bugbee is pushed through the ureterocele wall with a single puncture. The puncture site should be as caudal as possible just within the bladder neck.

ureterocele, diverticulum at the site of the ureterocele, or persistent lower pole reflux. Therefore, in patients where these complications are felt to be likely, a primary bladder approach may be more appropriate. For ureteroceles, the surgical options include endoscopic puncture, heminephrectomy, upper to lower pole ureteropylostomy, or excision at the bladder level with reconstruction and ureteral reimplantation.

## INCISION OF URETEROCELES

The indications for incising a ureterocele are controversial. It is a well-accepted approach for infected ureteroceles. But its role in the management of asymptomatic ureteroceles is more uncertain. Punctures may be performed under a brief general anesthetic with no skin incision. In some cases the incision is definitive and no further treatment is required. Even when subsequent surgery is needed, it is facilitated by decompression of the dilated ureter. However, particularly in children with associated reflux and ureteroceles that extend beyond the bladder neck, the need for another operation in the future is quite high. In patients without reflux, the inadvertant creation of reflux in the ureterocele may require a bladder operation that could have been avoided if the patient had undergone a heminephrectomy as the original operation. On balance we recommend ureterocele incision in infants diagnosed prenatally unless the ureterocele subtends a nonfunctioning upper pole and there is no associated reflux. In that case, a primary heminephrectomy should be considered, as it is usually curative and precludes the need for future bladder surgery.

## EXCISION OF URETEROCELE

Ureterocele excision with bladder reconstruction (*see* Fig. 20.31) offers definitive management of the obstruction, distortion of the bladder floor, and associated reflux. However, it is the most technically challenging of the surgical options, particularly in young infants. Generally, it is reserved for patients with persistent reflux or bladder outlet obstruction following one of the other treatments. The incision and exposure are the same as for standard ureteral reimplantation.

## HEMINEPHRECTOMY

Heminephrectomy is particularly attractive in the management of ectopic ureters and ureteroceles when there is little or no reflux in the other renal moieties. In this setting it is likely that heminephrectomy will be definitive and no further surgery will be necessary. Heminephrectomy may be performed at 1–2 mo of age. If the patient is doing well and there is no bladder outlet obstruction from the ureterocele, he or she may be maintained on antibiotic prophylaxis and surgery undertaken at 6 mo of age, when the anesthetic risk is slightly lower.

Heminephrectomy is performed through a flank incision. In children this can usually be accomplished off the tip of the 12th rib. It is rare that excision of the rib is required. The muscles are opened in layers preserving the subcostal nerve inferior to the incision between the internal oblique and transversus abdominis muscle. The retroperitoneal space is entered, and Gerota's fascia is opened longitudinally, exposing the surface of the kidney. The kidney is completely mobilized along with the proximal ureters.

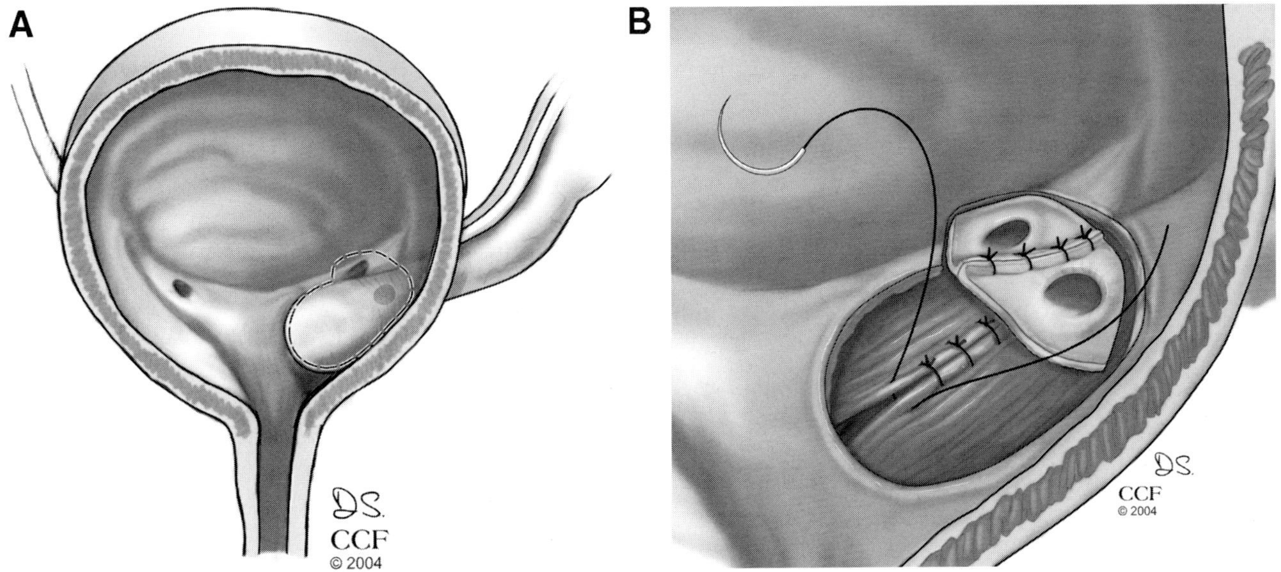


Fig. 20.31

**(A,B)** Once the bladder is opened the ureterocele is unroofed. The epithelial floor of the ureterocele is then excised preserving a cuff of bladder mucosa around the upper-pole and lower-pole ureteral orifices. A double-barrel reimplantation of the ureters is then performed. The bladder muscle is reapproximated in the uretrocele bed and the bladder mucosa closed over the defect. If the ureterocele extends down the bladder neck, then the intravesical portion is excised and the urethral portion may be handled in one of two ways. If it extends a short distance, it may be excised with reconstruction of that portion of the bladder neck. Alternatively, the urethral portion may be left in place and the roof of the urethral portion incised throughout its length to prevent a windsock obstruction during voiding.

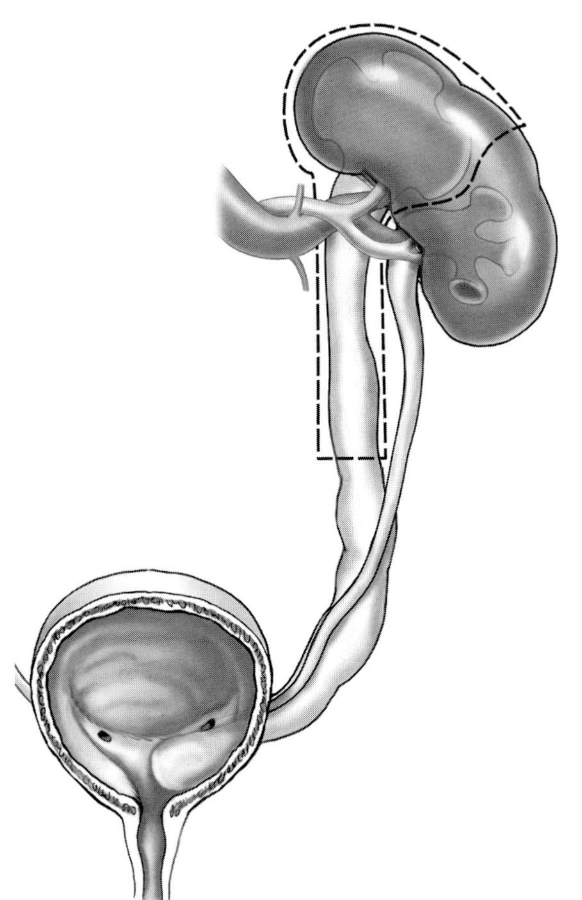

Fig. 20.32

The upper pole ureter is dissected off the lower pole ureter and divided. The cut end of the upper pole ureter may then be grasped as a handle during further mobilization. The upper pole ureter is carefully dissected off of, and passed behind, the hilar vessels. It is dissected up to the renal parenchyma, and the margin between the upper and lower poles of the kidney is delineated. A clamp or catheter may be passed up the upper pole ureter to help define, by palpation, the inferiormost portion of the upper pole collecting system. The parenchyma of the kidney is then divided with electrocautery. If the upper-pole collecting system is entered, it may be peeled off of the lower pole under direct vision. Typically the upper pole is supplied by multiple small arteries, and these may be ligated and divided as they are encountered. Care should be taken to trace all vessels to the upper pole parenchyma before division to avoid ligating accessory vessels to the lower moiety. Bleeding from the cut surface may be controlled with suture ligatures or argon-beam coagulation. Sometimes it is necessary to close the kidney, as after a partial nephrectomy for tumor. The flank incision is closed in layers with absorbable suture, and the skin is closed with subcuticular sutures. A Penrose drain is brought out through a separate stab incision.

## POSTOPERATIVE CARE

A caudal or epidural block is employed intropera-tively, but any catheters are removed at the end of the operation. Ketorolac 1.0 mg/kg is administered during wound closure and continued at a dose of 0.5 mg/kg every 6 h until discharge. The urethral catheter is removed on the first postoperative morning, and patients are usually discharged later that day. The Penrose drain is removed in the office 1 wk later. An ultrasound is obtained at 1 and 6 mo to be sure that no iatrogenic injury to the lower-pole collecting system has occurred.

## URETEROPYELOSTOMY

Ureteropyelostomy may be employed in cases of ureterocele or ectopic ureter in which the upper pole has normal function. However, the upper pole supplies only one-third of the ipsilateral renal function. Therefore, if a ureteropyelostomy is deemed technically difficult (e.g., in the case of marked disproportion in lower and upper ureteral dimensions), then a heminephrectomy should still be performed.

## CUTANEOUS URETEROSTOMY

Cutaneous ureterostomy is occasionally necessary in infants with bladder outlet obstruction or ureterovesical junction obstruction. In small infants this allows immediate relief of obstruction and decompression of the ureter, which may facilitate future reconstruction.

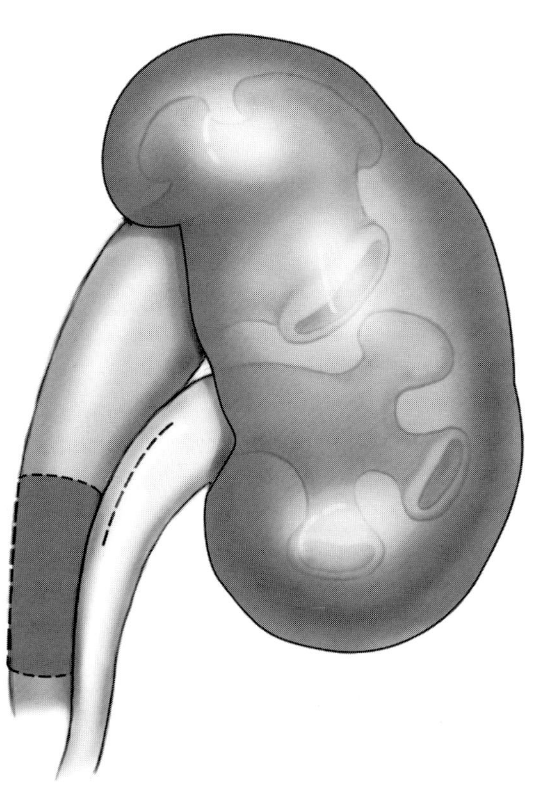

**Fig. 20.33**

The approach is identical to that for a heminephrectomy. Once the kidney is mobilized, the lower-pole ureter is dissected up to the lower-pole renal pelvis. The upper-pole ureter is divided. The lower-pole pelvis/proximal ureter is opened longitudinally to accommodate the dilated upper pole ureter.

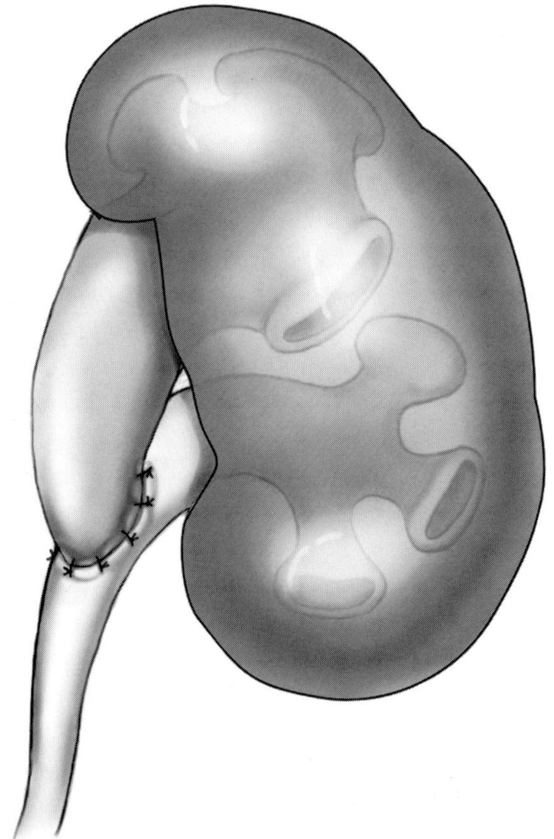

**Fig. 20.34**

The upper-pole ureter is sewn end-to-side to the lower-pole ureter with interrupted absorbable suture. A double pigtail stent may be left traversing the anastamosis. A Penrose drain is brought out through a separate flank stab incision.

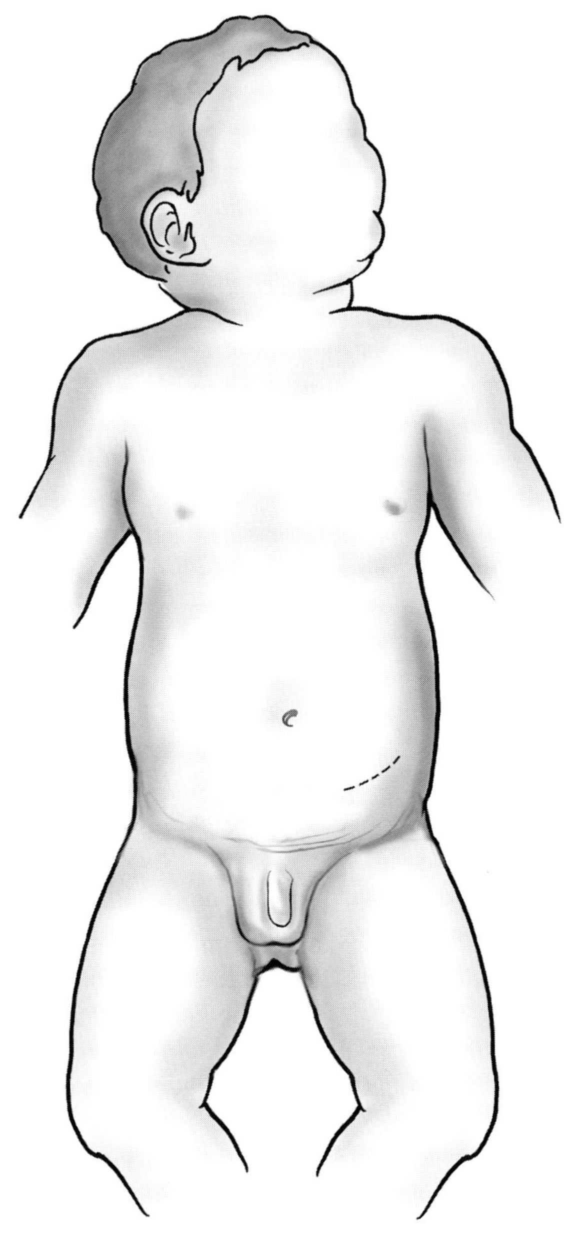

**Fig. 20.35**

A 2-cm Gibson incision is made in a such a way as to allow it to be incorporated in a future Pfannenstiel incision. The muscles are divided with electrocautery, and the retroperitoneum is entered.

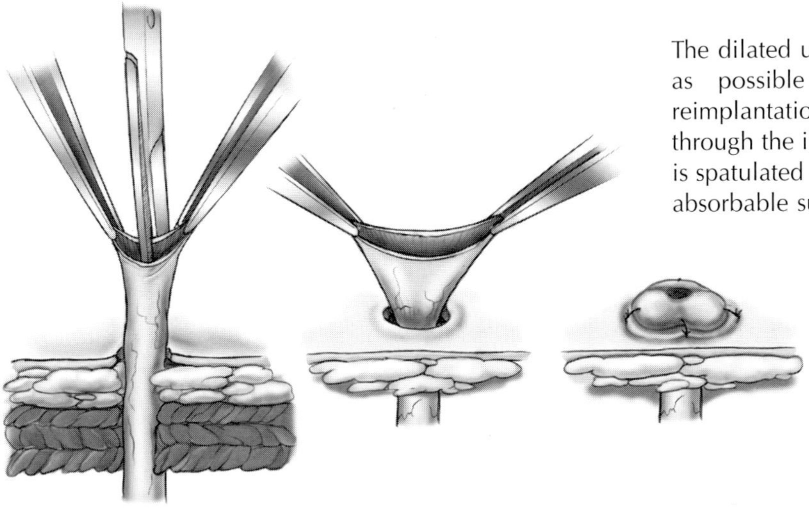

**Fig. 20.36**

The dilated ureter is identified and dissected distally as far as possible to preserve ureteral length for future reimplantation. The ureter is divided and brought out through the incision. If of relatively small caliber, the ureter is spatulated and secured to the skin edges with interrupted absorbable suture.

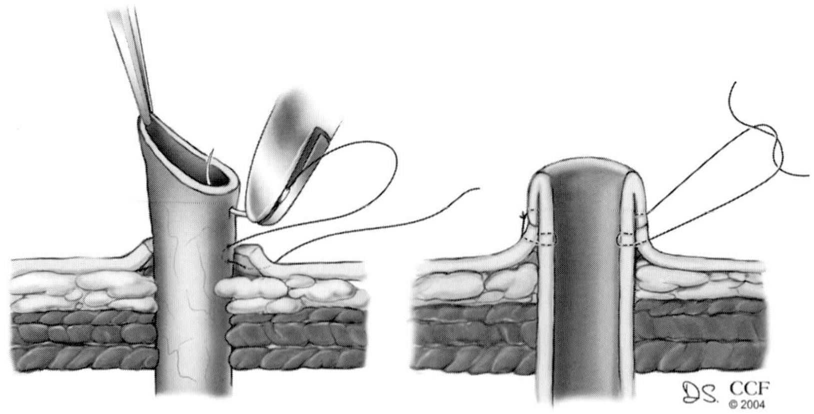


**Fig. 20.37**

For very dilated ureters, the ureter is brought out through the incision and everted. Interrupted absorbable sutures are then passed through the ureteral edge, the ureteral serosa 5–10 mm proximal to the edge, and then through the skin everting the ureter. The ureterostomy may be left intubated for 24–48 h.

## SUGGESTED READINGS


1. Blane CE, DiPietro MA, Zerin JM, Sedman AB, Bloom DA. Renal sonography is not a reliable screening examination for vesicoureteral reflux. J Urol 150:752, 1993.
2. Blyth B, Passerini-Glazel G, Camuffo C, Snyder HM 3rd, Duckett JW. Endoscopic incision of ureteroceles: intravesical versus ectopic. J Urol 149:556, 1993.
3. Capozza N, Caione P. Dextranomer/hyaluronic acid copolymer implantation for vesico-ureteral reflux: a randomized comparison with antibiotic prophylaxis. J Pediatr 140:230–234, 2002.
4. Keating MA, Escala J, Snyder HM 3rd, Heyman S, Duckett JW. Changing concepts in management of primary obstructive megaureter. J Urol 142:636, 1989.
5. Kirsch AJ, Perez-Brayfield MR, Scherz HC. Minimally invasive treatment of vesicoureteral reflux with endoscopic injection of dextranomer/hyaluronic acid copolymer: The Children's Hospitals of Atlanta experience. J Urol 170:211–215, 2003.
6. Koff S. Relationship between dysfunctional voiding and reflux. J. Urol 148:1703, 1992.
7. Peters CA, Mandell J, Lebowitz RL, et al. Congenital obstructed megaureters in early infancy: diagnosis and treatment. J Urol 142:641, 1989.
8. Politano V, Leadbetter W. An operative technique for the correction of vesicoureteral reflux. J Urol 79:932, 1958.
9. Puri P, Chertin B, Velayudham M, et al. Treatment of vesicoureteral reflux by endoscopic injection of dextranomer/hyaluronic acid copolymer: preliminary results. J Urol 170:1541–1544, 2003.
10. Wacksman J, Gilbert A, Sheldon C. Results of the renewed extravesical reimplant for surgical correction of vesicuoreteral reflux. J Urol 148:359, 1992.
11. Weiss R, et al. Results of a randomized clinical trial of medical versus surgical management of infants and children with grades III and IV primary vesicoureteral reflux (United States). J Urol 148:1667, 1992.

# 21 Iatrogenic and Traumatic Ureteral Injury

*Bashir R. Sankari*

Ureteral injuries result from either iatrogenic or external trauma. Iatrogenic ureteral injuries far outnumber traumatic injuries. Ureteroscopy currently accounts for the majority of iatrogenic ureteral injuries. However, most of these injuries are minor and managed with JJ stent. Open pelvic surgery, particularly gynecological procedures, account for the majority of open surgical injuries to the ureter. It is estimated that ureteral injuries occur in 0.5–1% of pelvic surgery. Other abdominal surgical procedures that can result in ureteral injury include colectomy, appendectomy, aorto-iliac bypass, and urological surgeries such as ureteral reimplantation and ureterolithotomy. Many ureteral injuries can be repaired endoscopically with a combination of internal ureteral stenting and percutaneous nephrostomy tube drainage. The rest are amenable to a variety of open surgical techniques depending on the level of injury. Ureteral injuries as a result of external trauma are uncommon, are mostly the result of penetrating gunshot wounds, and are almost always associated with multiple organ injuries.

Operative repair of ureteral injuries requires meticulous techniques. Minimizing ureteral trauma and preservation of adequate blood supply are essential steps for a successful outcome. The ureter should be handled gently to avoid ischemia. The ureter gets its blood supply from multiple sources: renal artery, gonadal artery, aorta, iliac, vesical, uterine, vaginal, and hemorrhoidal arteries. The ureter should be mobilized with a generous periureteral tissue to preserve these collateral circulations. The level of ureteral injury dictates the type of surgical repair feasible for a successful outcome. Whereas a mid-ureteral injury is feasible for ureteroureterostomy, a distal ureteral injury is not, as the distal ureteral stump will be at risk of being devascularized.

## SURGICAL TECHNIQUES

The location of ureteral injury and the length of the defect dictates the type of reconstructive surgery used (Fig. 21.1).

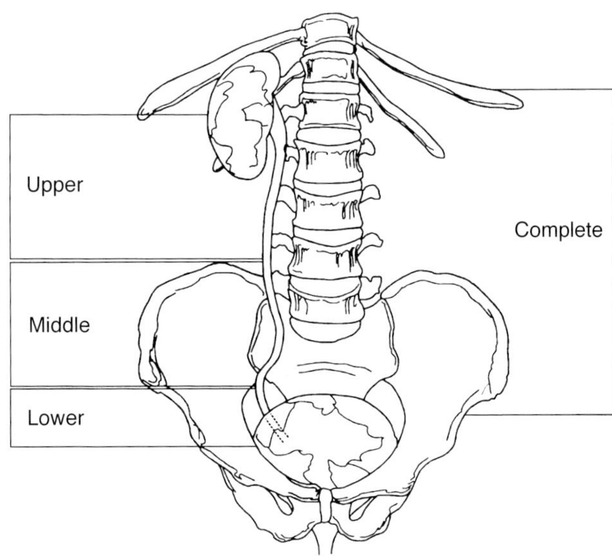


Fig. 21.1

Injuries to the lower ureter can usually be repaired with direct ureteral reimplantation in the bladder alone or with combination of a psoas hitch procedure. Injuries to the mid-ureter may require the addition of a Boari bladder flap or direct ureteroureterostomy if the injured ureteral segment is short. Injuries to the upper ureter may require a transureteroureterostomy. Complete ureteral injury will necessitate an ileal loop ureteral interposition or autotransplantation.

**Table 1**
**Length of Ureteral Defect That Can Be Bridged With Various Surgical Techniques for Ureteral Reconstruction**

| *Procedure* | *Ureteral defect (cm)* |
|---|---|
| Ureteroureterostomy | 2–3 |
| Ureteroneocystotomy | 4–5 |
| Psoas hitch | 6–10 |
| Boari flap | 10–15 |

From: *Operative Urology at the Cleveland Clinic*
Edited by: A. Novick et al. 

Each procedure will allow a certain amount of ureteral gap to be bridged and depending on the length of injury will dictate the appropriate procedure (Table 21.1). Mobilizing the kidney will allow an additional 5–8 cm in length.

## SURGICAL APPROACH

Common surgical approaches to the ureter include subcostal incision for upper ureter, Gibson lower quadrant-type incision for the midureter, and a low midline or Pfannenstiel incision for the lower ureter (Fig. 21.2). A midline intraperitoneal approach allows exposure of the whole ureter and bladder and is useful for complex reconstruction involving possible use of bowel or omentum.

Ureteral injuries identified intraoperatively, whether traumatic or iatrogenic, are usually repaired with the original laparotomy incision.

## URETEROURETEROSTOMY

Primary anastomosis of ureteral injuries is feasible when the defect is short. Injuries to the upper and middle ureter are ideal for primary ureteroureterostomy. In cases of penetrating injuries, the ureter should be debrided to viable tissue. A generous peri-ureteral tissue should be left attached to the ureter during dissection to preserve ureteral blood supply.

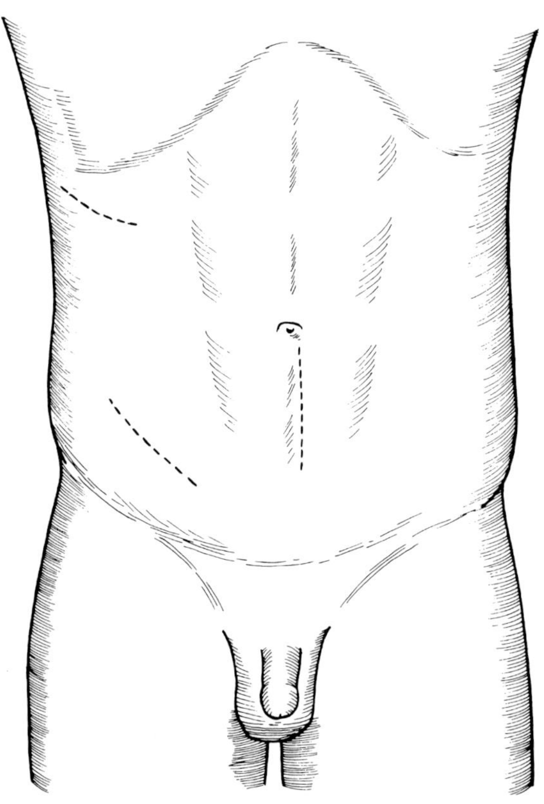

Fig. 21.2

Each end of the transected ureter is spatulated on opposite side for a distance of 5–8 mm. Spatulation may not be necessary in case the ureters are dilated (Fig. 21.3).

Stay sutures of 5:0 or 7:0 polydioxanone (PDS) on a vascular atraumatic needle are inserted from the apex of one ureter to the corner of spatulation of the other ureter (Fig. 21.4).

A watertight anastomosis of the ureteral wall is then performed using either interrupted or continuous sutures of 5:0 or 7:0 PDS (Fig. 21.5). Optical magnification is helpful for accurate suture placement, each bite being taken approximately 1 mm apart and 1–2 mm from the ureteral edge. A JJ stent is inserted after completion of

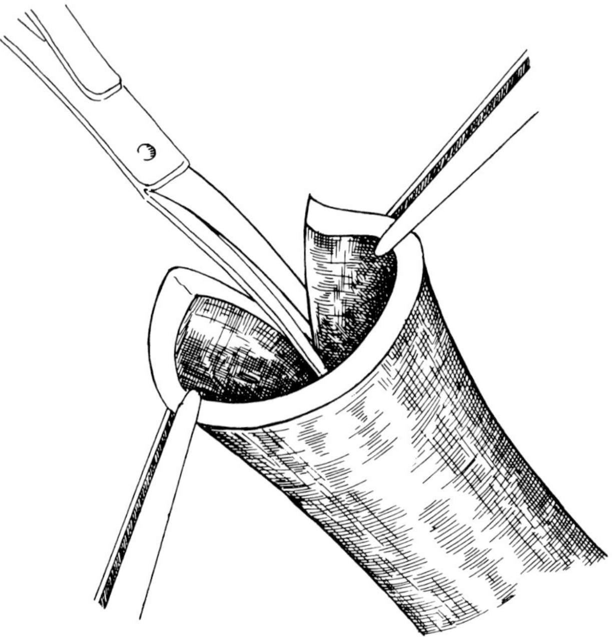

Fig. 21.3

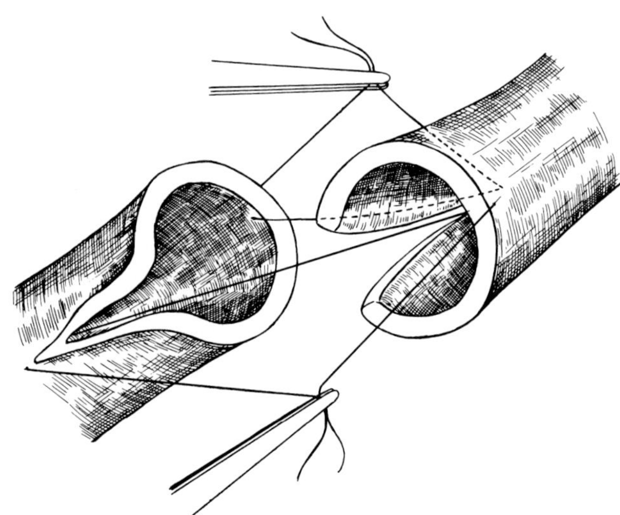

Fig. 21.4

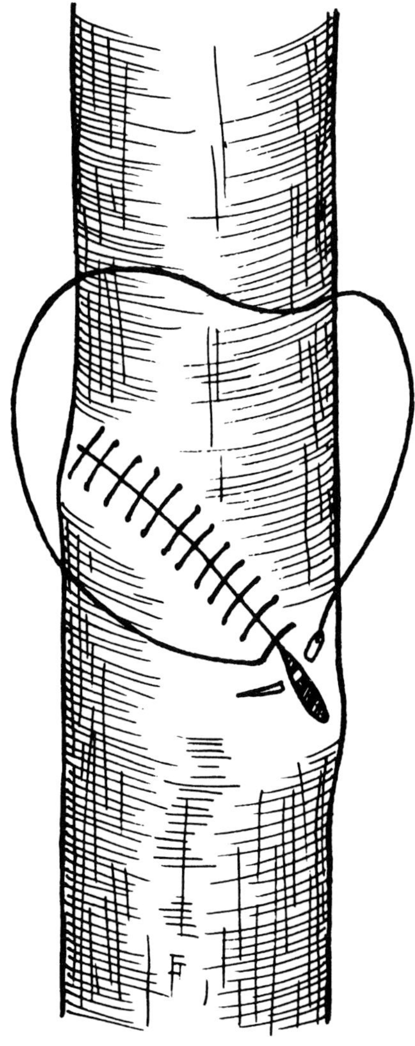

Fig. 21.5

one side of the ureteral anastomosis. In cases of concomitant abdominal surgery, the greater omentum can be mobilized and wrapped around the ureteral anastomosis. This becomes important in cases of abdominal aortic aneurism (AAA) repair, aortoiliac repair, and colectomy. A surgical drain is optional and is removed postoperatively when drainage clears. The JJ stent is removed in 4–8 wk.

## URETERONEOCYSTOTOMY

Ureteroneocystotomy is best indicated for injuries involving the distal 3–4 cm of the ureter. The ureter is mobilized with generous periureteral tissue. The ureter is spatulated and anastomosed to the bladder in an anterior extravesical or intravesical technique. We prefer a modified anterior extravesical approach, as described by Licht, as it avoids a cystotomy incision and decreases the risk of urinary fistula (Fig. 21.6).

Bladder musculature is incised, exposing the bladder mucosa over the entire length of the incision. A buttonhole of bladder mucosa is removed from the distal end of the incision. The ureter is anastomosed to the bladder using continuous or interrupted 5:0 PDS sutures approximating full thickness of the ureteral wall to the bladder mucosa. At the distal aspect of the anastomosis, one or two bites are inserted through the entire wall of the bladder to anchor the ureter and prevent it from pulling out of the tunnel. A JJ stent can be inserted prior to the conclusion of the anastomosis. The bladder muscle is then closed on top of the ureter using interrupted 3:0 chromic sutures to achieve an antireflux mechanism. Care should be taken to avoid tight compression of the ureter.

Alternatively, an intravesical technique can be used. The bladder is opened through an anterior cystotomy.

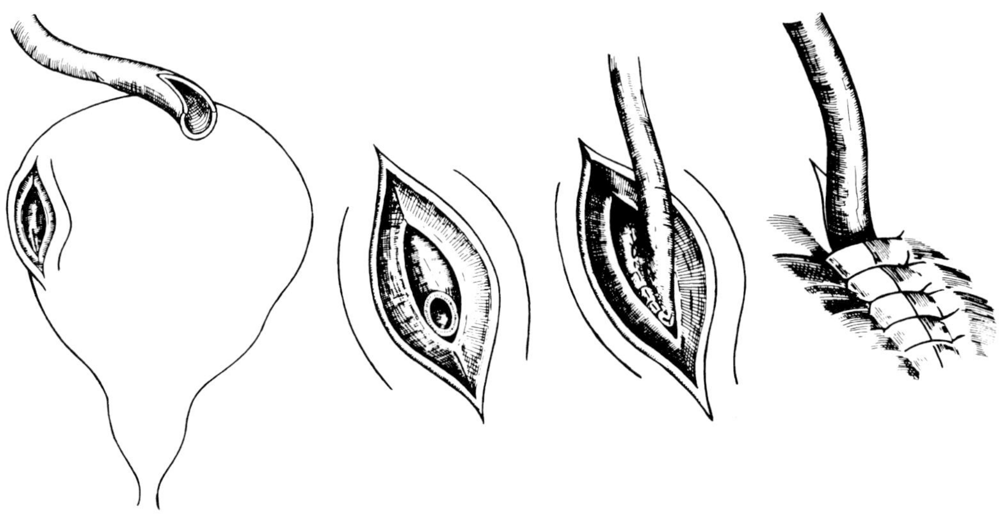

Fig. 21.6

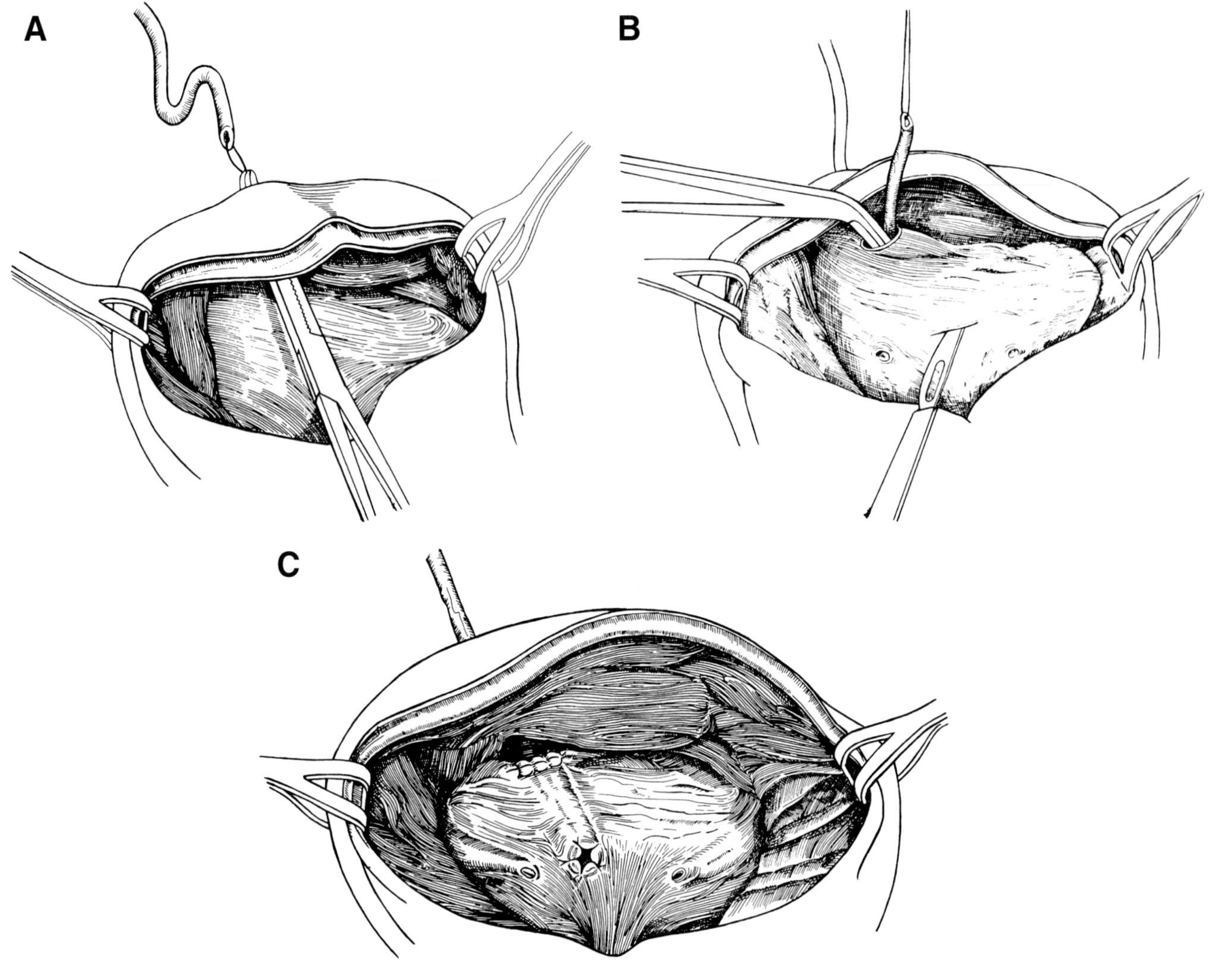


Fig. 21.7

A stab incision is made in the posteriolateral aspect of the bladder (Fig. 21.7A). The ureter is brought through the stab incision and a 2–3 cm submucosal tunnel is fashioned (Fig. 21.7B). The ureter is then brought through the tunnel. The ureter is spatulated and anastomosed to the bladder with interrupted 4:0 or 5:0 chromic sutures. The distal sutures are inserted deeply into the muscularis, and the remaining sutures are placed only through the bladder mucosa. The mucosa overlying the stab incision is closed with a continuous 5:0 chromic suture (Fig. 21.7C). The cystotomy incision is closed in three separate layers.

## PSOAS HITCH

When the distal ureteral injury is more proximal but still below the pelvic brim, a psoas bladder hitch can be used to mobilize the bladder more proximal to allow the performance of a ureteroneocystotomy. A psoas hitch can provide an additional 5 cm of length as compared with ureteroneocystotomy alone. A preoperative cystogram is helpful in assessing bladder anatomy.

The bladder is filled with antibiotic solution. The space of Retzius is entered through a Pfannenstiel or midline incision and the bladder mobilized. The round ligament in the female is divided. The vas deferens in a male may have to be divided. The dome of the ipsilateral bladder should be able to reach superior to the iliac vessels. The contralateral superior vesicle artery can be divided to gain more mobility. The ureter should already have been dissected to normal tissue level and spatulated. The bladder is opened vertically or horizontally. The ureter is anastomosed to the superiolateral aspect of the dome with or without a submucosal tunnel using interrupted suture of 5:0 or 4:0 chromic (Fig. 21.8A). The ipsilateral dome is affixed to the lateral psoas muscle using several interrupted sutures of 2:0 polydiaxonone (Ethicon Inc.) The

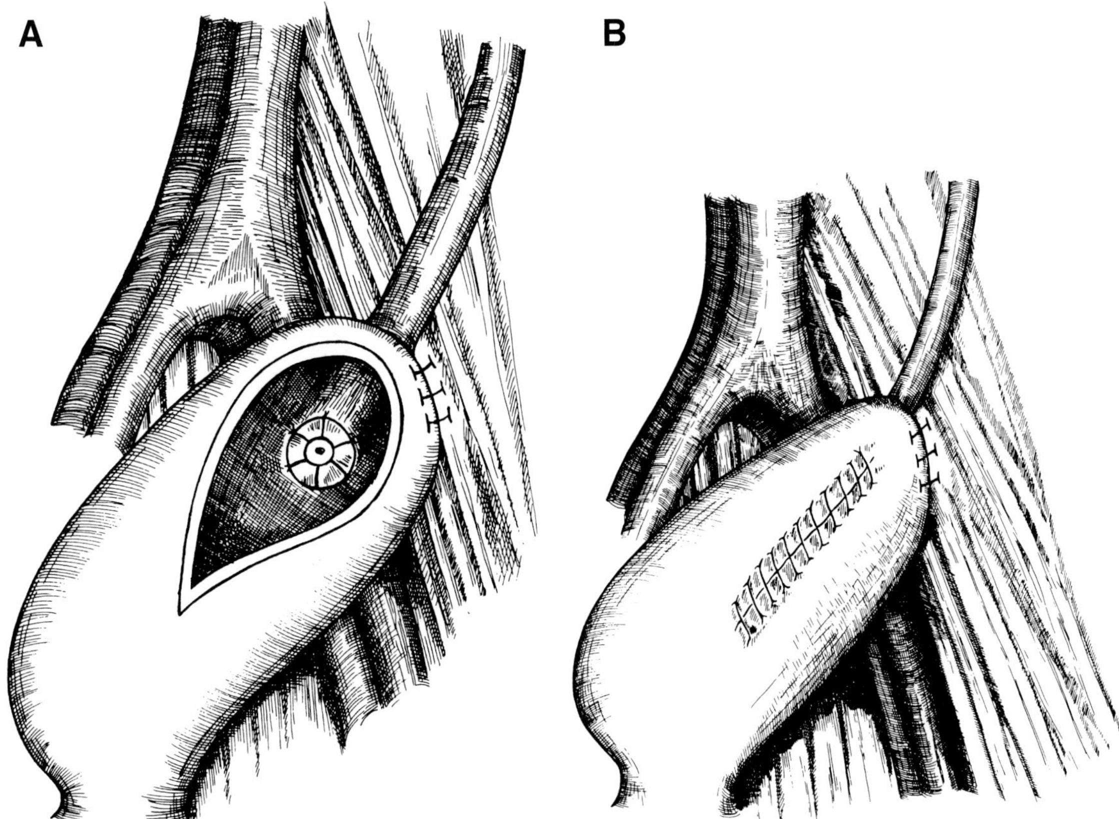


Fig. 21.8

sutures are placed through the full thickness of the posteriolateral bladder wall to the fascia of the psoas muscle. Care should be taken to avoid injury to the genitofemoral nerve. A JJ stent is inserted. The bladder is then closed using three layers (Fig. 21.8B).

## BOARI FLAP

Midureteral injuries with large defects not amenable for primary ureteroureterostomy can be repaired with an anterior bladder wall flap as described by Boari. A ureteral defect 10–15 cm in length can be bridged with this technique, with some spiral flaps reported to reach to the renal pelvis. Generally, Boari flaps are most successful when the injury is below the level of common iliac artery. A small-capacity irradiated bladder is a contraindication for Boari flap. Bladder capacity and anatomy need to be assessed with preoperative cystogram. The operation can be performed retroperitoneally with a modified Pfannenstiel incision, but a midline incision is preferable in order to access the upper ureter and keep other options for reconstruction available. The bladder is filled with antibiotic solution and is mobilized from its peritoneal attachment as in a psoas hitch procedure. The ipsilateral superior vesical artery is identified and a posteriolateral bladder flap based on this artery is outlined (Fig. 21.9A). A U-shaped full-thickness bladder wall flap is usually developed. The length of the flap depends upon the distance between the posterior lateral bladder wall and the distal ureter. If a longer segment is needed, the flap can be fashioned into an L shape by extending the tip laterally at the anterior bladder wall. The base of the flap should be at least 2 cm greater than the apex to ensure good blood supply. The width of the flap should be—three to four times the diameter of the ureter.

The tip of the flap is secured to the psoas muscle with interrupted absorbable sutures. The ureter, which has been spatulated, is then anastomosed to the bladder flap in direct end-to-end fashion or a submucosal tunnel (Fig. 21.9B). A tension-free anastomosis mucosa to mucosa is performed with interrupted absorbable sutures of 4:0 chromic or 5:0 chromic. The flap is closed anteriolaterally and rolled into a tube using two layers of absorbable sutures (Fig. 21.9C). A JJ stent is inserted prior to bladder closure. A drain is inserted. The Foley catheter remains indwelling for 7–10 d. A cystogram is performed prior to removal of the Foley catheter. The JJ stent is removed in 4–8 wk.

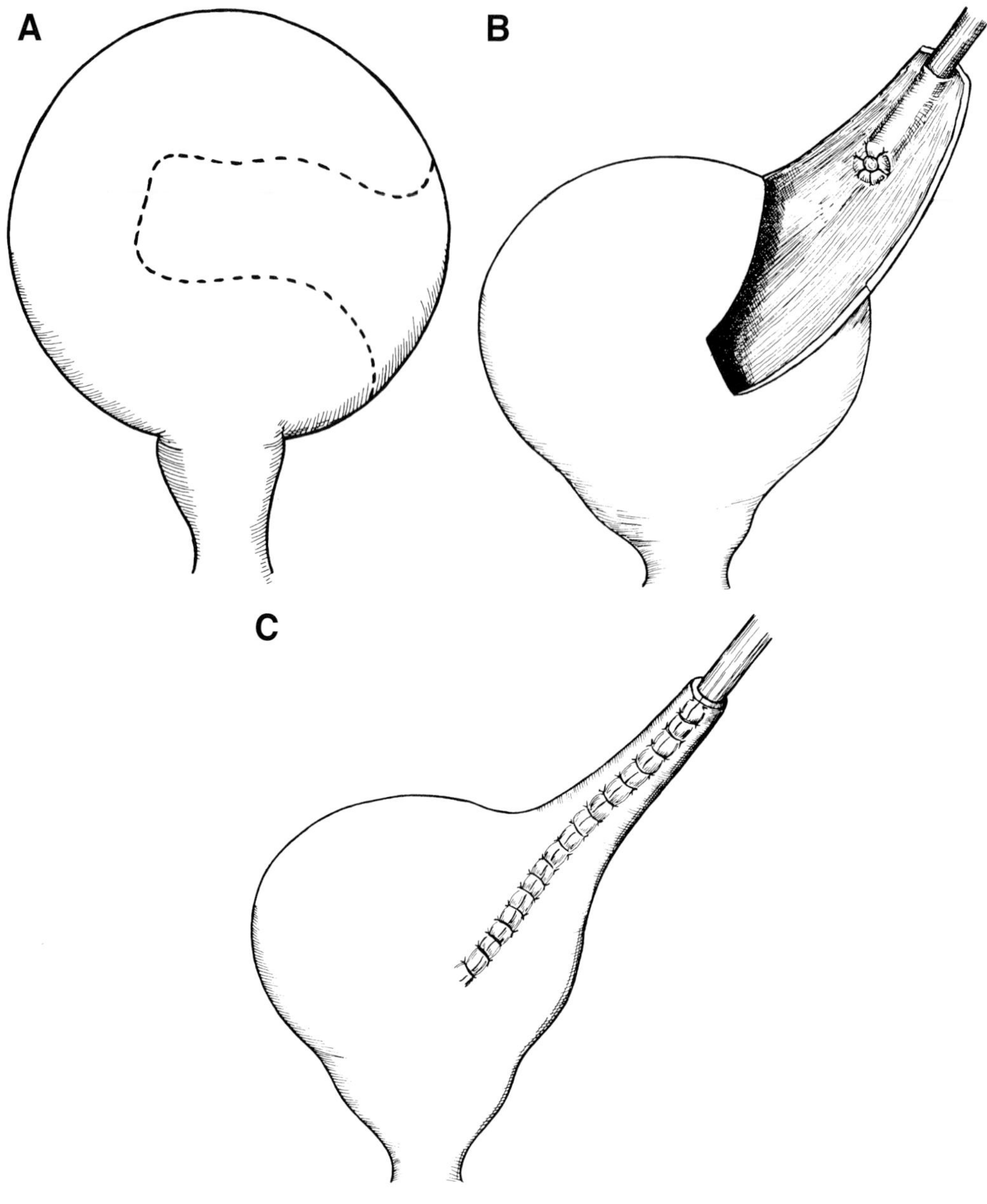


Fig. 21.9

## TRANSURETERO-URETEROSTOMY

Transuretero-ureterostomy is preserved for unilateral ureteral injuries involving the distal half of the ureter with insufficient bladder capacity. Contraindications include a short donor ureter or a diseased recipient ureter.

The procedure is performed through a midline intraperitoneal approach. The colon on the side of the donor ureter is reflected and the ureter dissected out with a generous periureteral tissue that includes the ipsilateral gonadal vessels to ensure viability of the ureter. The donor ureter is mobilized superiorly to gain appropriate length and is passed posterior to the peritoneum above the great vessels. In left-to-right procedures, the ureter is passed above the level of the inferior mesenteric artery to prevent acute angulation at this level (Fig. 21.10A). The posterior peritoneum is then incised over the recipient ureter and the ureter dissected. Excessive periureteral dissection is to be avoided. A ureterotomy is then created in the recipient ureter parallel to its longitudinal axis with an appropriate length to accommodate the donor ureter (Fig. 21.10B). The donor ureter is either spatulated or obliquely transected. Stay sutures of 5:0 PDS are placed in the apex of the recipient ureterotomy and in a corresponding position in the end of the donor ureter. The posterior wall is anastomosed first in a continuous running fashion. It is easier to perform the anastomosis from the inside of the ureter. A JJ stent is inserted at this stage with the proximal end in

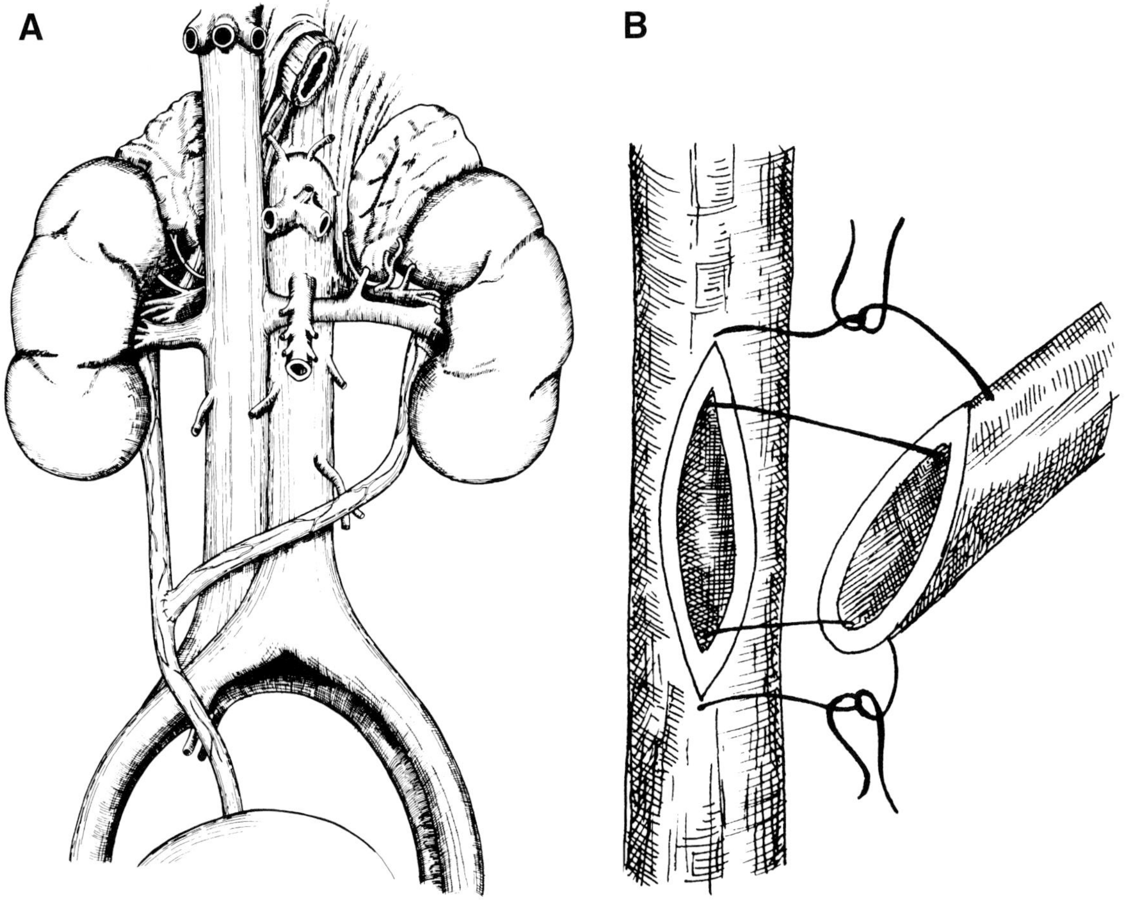


Fig. 21.10

the donor renal pelvis and the distal end going through the recipient ureter to the bladder. The anterior wall anastomosis is then completed with either continuous or interrupted sutures. The opening in the posterior peritoneum is then closed with 3:0 chronic sutures. The colon is repositioned back into its anatomical position.

## ILEAL URETERAL REPLACEMENT

In cases of total ureteral avulsion or when a long segment is diseased or absent, a segment of ileum can be used to reconstruct the urinary system. Candidates for this operation should have relatively normal kidney function with serum creatinine less than 2.5 mg/dL.

The patient is placed on a standard mechanical and antibiotic bowel prep. The operation is performed through a midline intraperitoneal approach. An ileal segment 20–25 cm is mobilized 15–20 cm proximal to the ileocecal valve. Bowel continuity is restored with a stapled end-to-end enteric anastomosis. The isolated ileal segment is then positioned posteriorly in an isoperistaltic fashion. An end-to-end anastomosis between the renal pelvis and the proximal ileal segment is done using running 3:0 chromic suture (Fig. 21.11A). A nephrostomy tube is inserted.

Alternatively, if a proximal ureteral segment is healthy, the anastomosis could be performed between the ureter and the ileal segment in an end-side fashion using interrupted 4:0 chromic suture (Fig. 21.11B). A single J or JJ stent is inserted in the ureter prior to completion of the anastomosis.

Distally the ileal segment is anastomosed to the posterior wall of the bladder. The bladder is mobilized and an anterior cystotomy done. An end-side ileovesical anastomosis is done on the posterior bladder wall. A circular window of the bladder wall is excised. The anastomosis is done in two layers. The inner layer of interrupted or continuous 3:0 chromic sutures inserted through the full thickness of bladder and ileum from within the bladder (Fig. 21.11C).

An outer reinforcing layer of interrupted seromuscular 3:0 chromic sutures is then inserted from outside the bladder (Fig. 21.11D). The cystotomy incision is closed in two layers.

Alternatively, the anastomosis between the distal ileal segment and the bladder can be done in an anterior extravesical fashion direct nontunneled anastomosis. A large 24 Fr

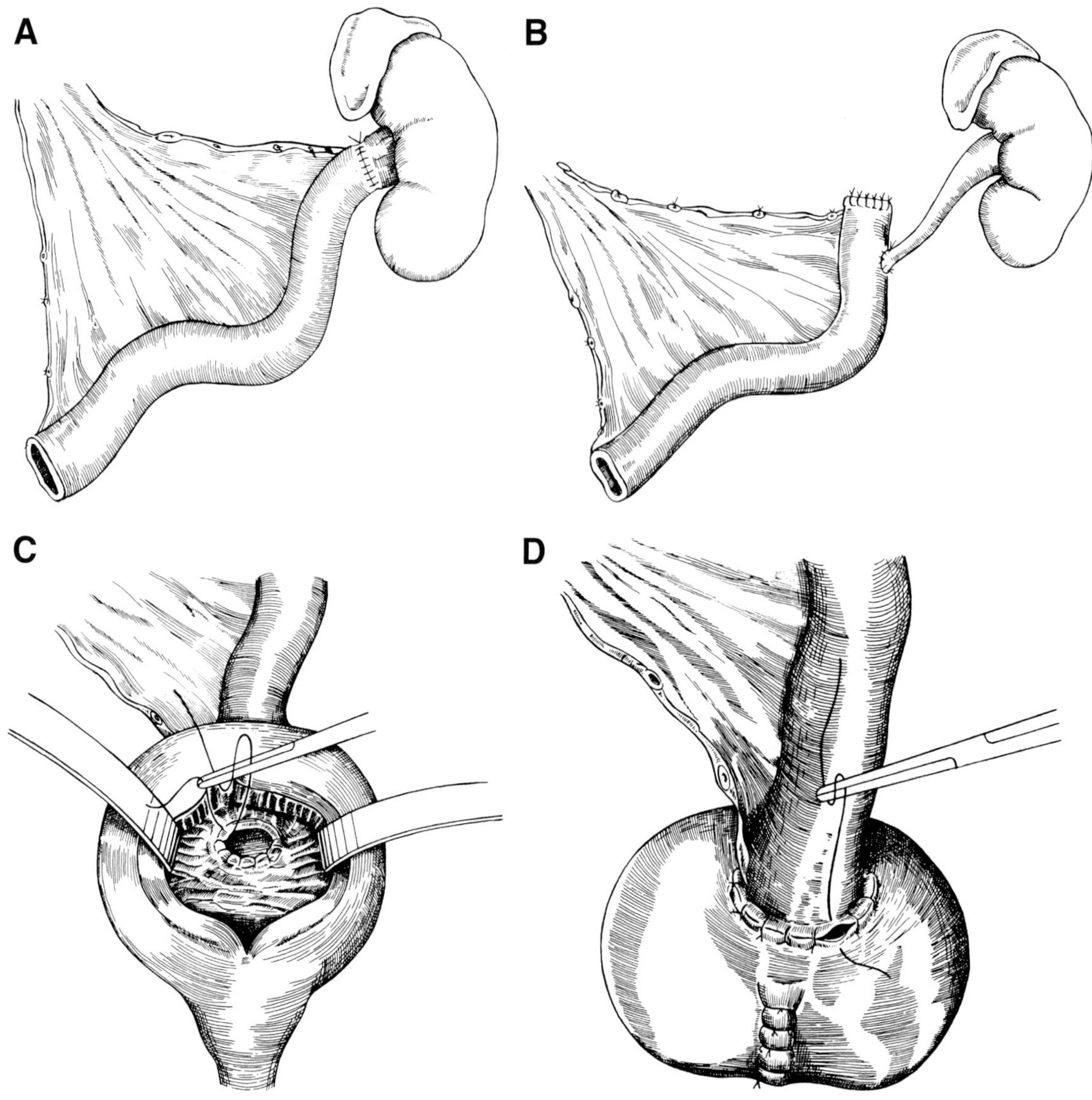


Fig. 21.11

Foley catheter or suprapubic catheter is inserted. Drains are inserted close to all anastomotic sites. The Foley catheter and/or nephrostomy tube are maintained to dependent drainage for at least 1 wk. The bladder catheter may need frequent irrigation. Nephrostogram and cystogram are obtained 1 wk postoperatively to ensure there is no extravasation.

## RENAL AUTOTRANSPLANTATION

Renal autotransplantation is an alternative to ureteral interposition in cases of complete ureteral avulsion or a long diseased ureteral segment. Renal autotransplantation is best reserved for patients with solitary kidney or compromised renal function.

The kidney is best recovered through an intraperitoneal approach. The kidney is usually encased with scar tissue, making retroperitoneal approach hazardous. The kidney is recovered and transplanted in the iliac fossa using standard transplant techniques, as depicted elsewhere in this volume.

## SUGGESTED READINGS

1. Franke JF, Smith JA, Jr. Surgery of the ureter, In: Walsh PC, Retik AB, Vaughan ED, et al., eds. Campbell's Urology, 7th ed., Vol. 1. Philadelphia: Saunders, 1998:3062–3084.
2. Seizman AA, Spirnak JP. Iatrogenic ureteral injuries: a 20 year experience in treating 165 injuries. J Urol 155:878–888, 1996.

# 22 Ureteral Calculi

*Stevan B. Streem*

## URETERAL CALCULI: INDICATIONS FOR INTERVENTION

The indications to intervene for patients with ureteral calculi include pain unresponsive to medical management, progressive obstruction, renal insufficiency associated with the obstruction, infection, socioeconomic factors (travelers, pilots, and others), size judged unlikely to pass spontaneously (>4–5 mm), or failure to progress distally in a reasonable length of time. For those patients with significant renal insufficiency or infection related to the obstructing stone, definitive management should be withheld until the renal failure or infection is controlled with a temporizing stent or percutaneous nephrostomy drainage.

## SHOCK-WAVE LITHOTRIPSY

Stone location is an important determinant of the outcome of shock-wave lithotripsy (SWL). Treatment of upper ureteral stones may result in stone-free rates of 85–92%. For lower ureteral calculi, that is, those below the pelvic brim, stone-free rates of 65–70% can been achieved through various modifications in patient positioning and lithotripter design. With the Storz Modulith SLX, proximal ureteral stones are treated in a supine position modified to place the ipsilateral side slightly down. This ensures that the ureteral stone will project away from the spine. Midureteral stones, that is, those projecting over the sacroiliac, are treated in the prone position in order to circumvent the damping effect that would otherwise occur as the shock wave passes through the bone. Lower ureteral stones, that is, those in the true pelvis, are again treated in a standard supine position, allowing the shock wave to pass unencumbered through the true pelvis.

Despite the fact that SWL can be successful for ureteral calculi, the trend at our center has been to treat almost all mid- and distal ureteral calculi with ureteroscopy. More recently, we are applying this modality with increasing frequency to patients with proximal ureteral stones not only when SWL has failed, but also as primary approach.

## URETEROSCOPY

The advent of ureteroscopy has significantly impacted the management of ureteral calculi. Semi-rigid ureteroscopy can be used in conjunction with pneumatic, laser, and electrohydraulic lithotripsy probes to successfully fragment ureteral calculi, and flexible, actively deflectable ureteropyeloscopes have made access to the upper ureter and intrarenal collecting system a reality of clinical practice. These instruments can be advanced under direct vision or fluoroscopic guidance directly to the level of the stone, which may be fragmented or, when especially small, extracted intact.

Ureteroscopy is a versatile technique that can be used to treat stones throughout the urinary tract. Although the choice of intracorporeal fragmentation technique is frequently based on the location and composition of the stone, the experience of the physician and availability of equipment often dictate this decision. At our center, the Holmium laser is the intracorporeal lithotripter of choice. Most ureteroscopic cases are performed as an ambulatory surgical procedure, with the patient returning to work within 1–2 d.

### Ureteroscopic Visualization: Irrigant Flow

The limited size of the working channels of these smaller ureteropyeloscopes limits the instrumentation that can be utilized. Additionally, this restricts irrigant flow, the result being a negative impact on visualization during the actual procedure. We routinely increase the irrigant pressure by using a large, 1-L inflating pressure bag. One potential drawback to its use is proximal migration of the stone, so that the pressure is used judiciously and only when necessary for visualization. However, placement of most instruments such as baskets, graspers, and even laser fibers through the working channel of any ureteroscope severely

From: *Operative Urology at the Cleveland Clinic*
Edited by: A. Novick et al. © Humana Press Inc., Totowa, NJ

restricts flow. As such, pressure irrigation will almost always be required at some point during the procedure.

## Laser Lithotripsy

The Holmium wavelength is not selectively absorbed and works equally well to fragment stones of varying color and composition. Moreover, the holmium laser has the advantage of being a multipurpose laser system. Not only can it be used for stone fragmentation, it can also be used for its hemostatic and tissue effects, including incision of urinary tract strictures. We now use it almost exclusively as our fragmentation modality of choice with both semi-rigid and flexible ureteroscopes.

## Semi-Rigid Ureteroscopy: Indications

Small-caliber, semi-rigid ureteroscopes are ideally suited for both diagnostic and therapeutic maneuvers performed in any part of the ureter in women and at least the lower third of the ureter in men. The semi-rigid scopes are easy to manipulate in the distal portion of the ureter and allow rapid ureteroscopic stone access in this area. For stones in the upper ureter, especially in men, and in the pyelocalyceal system in any patient, flexible ureteropyeloscopy provides the ideal instrumentation.

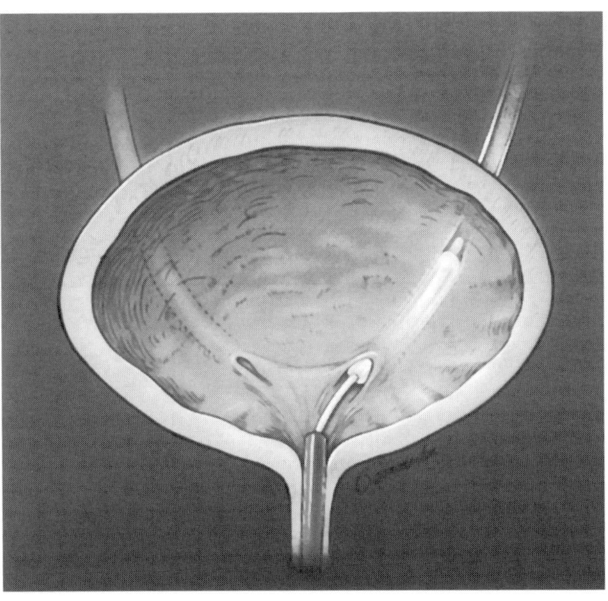

**Fig. 22.1**

If the ureteral orifice will not easily accept the ureteroscope, ureteral dilation is performed with a standard 15–18 French (5–6 mm), 4-cm ureteral dilating balloon. A quick and easy alternative to using a balloon is to use a 9 or 10 French introducing catheter passed over a hydrophilic safety wire.

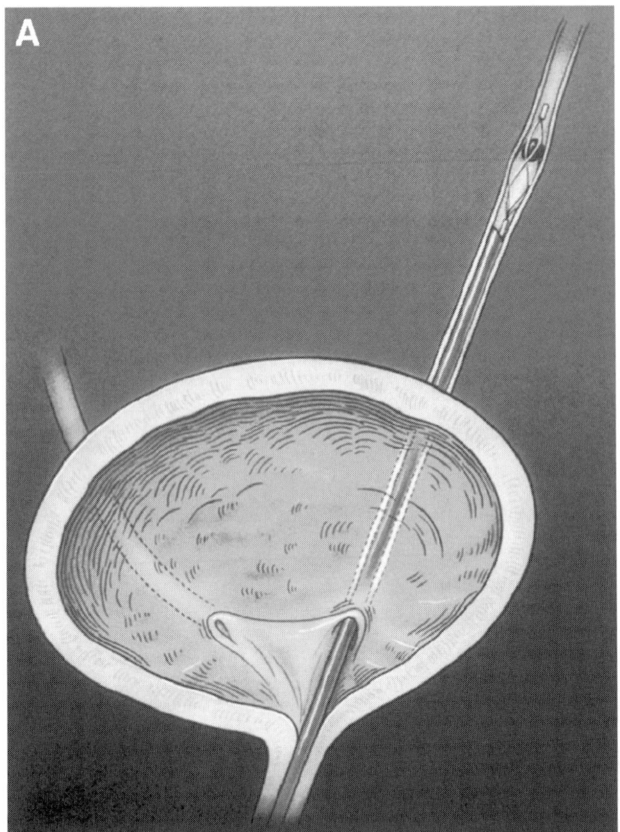


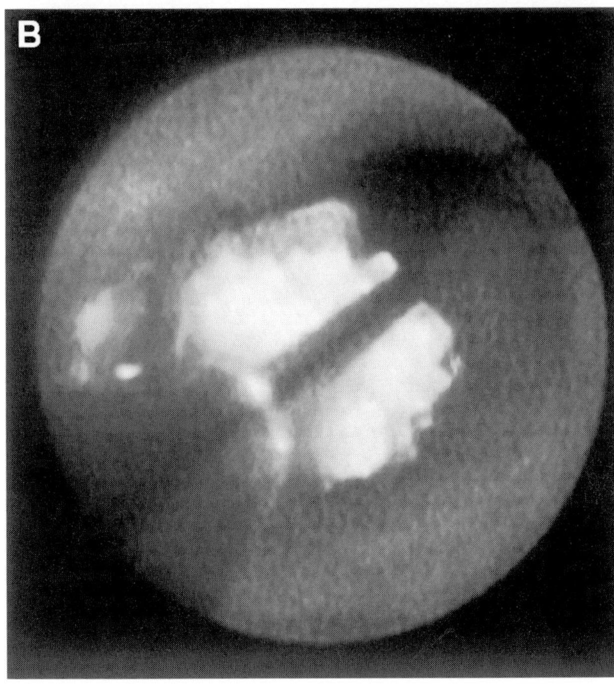


**Fig. 22.2**

**(A,B)** Under direct vision, small stones measuring <5 mm may be trapped within a basket or grasping forceps and simply withdrawn under direct vision.

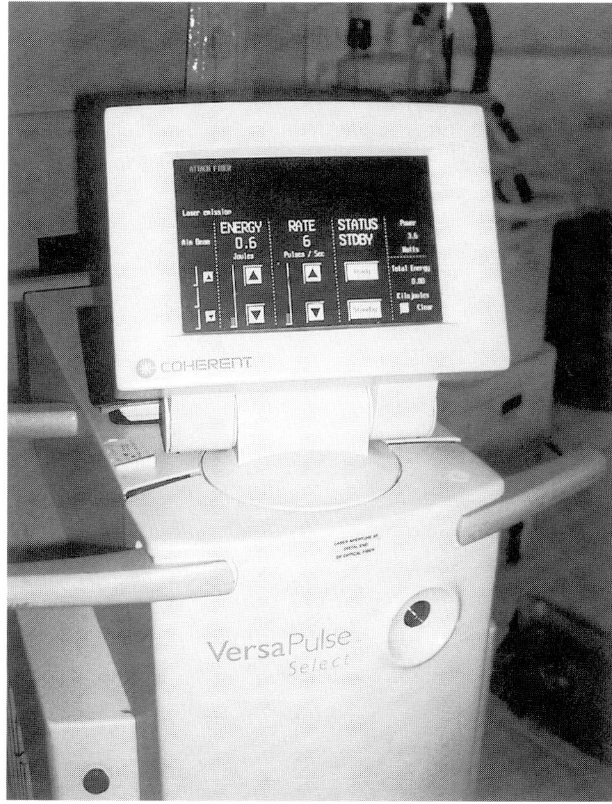


Fig. 22.3

For all but the smallest stones, i.e., those <5–6 mm, fragmentation by intracorporeal lithotripsy begins. With a semi-rigid scope, we prefer a 360-μ fiber. Initially, the power is set at 0.6 J and 6 Hz, although this can be increased as necessary, going as high as 0.8–1.0 J and 8–10 Hz.

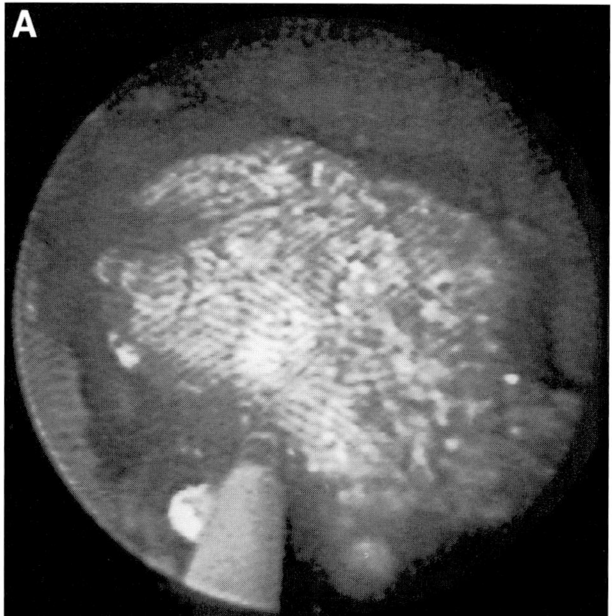


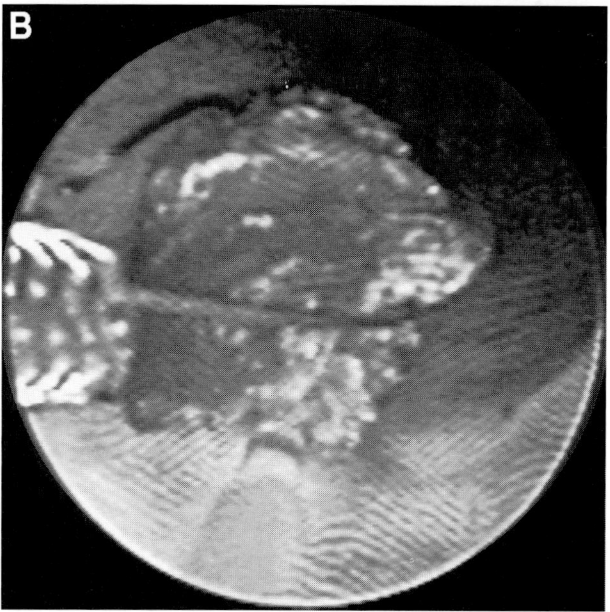


Fig. 22.4

**(A,B)** Fragmentation begins once the stone is well visualized within the ureteral lumen. When the stone is adequately fragmented, larger pieces are withdrawn under direct vision with a basket using a "trolling"-type maneuver, rather than closing the basket down onto the fragments. Smaller fragments are left to pass spontaneously. For uncomplicated cases we do not routinely leave a stent.

## Semi-Rigid Ureteroscopy: Technique

The standard technique involves passage of a 0.038-in. floppy-tipped guidewire under both cystoscopic and fluoroscopic guidance at the outset of the procedure. The semi-rigid ureteroscope is then passed under direct vision alongside the guidewire to the level of the stone.

## Flexible, Deflectable Ureteropyeloscopy: Technique

The flexibility of these small instruments, which allows their manipulation throughout the entire upper tract, may also act as an impediment to their passage. At times the most difficult aspect of flexible ureteropyeloscopy is introduction of the instrument into the distal ureter. Appropriate dilatation of the intramural ureter and introduction of the instrument are integral factors for the performance of flexible ureteropyeloscopy.

## Dilation of the Intramural Ureter

The majority of actively deflectable, flexible ureteropyeloscopes measure between 6.9 and 8.5 French in diameter, thus requiring dilatation of the intramural ureter on occasion.

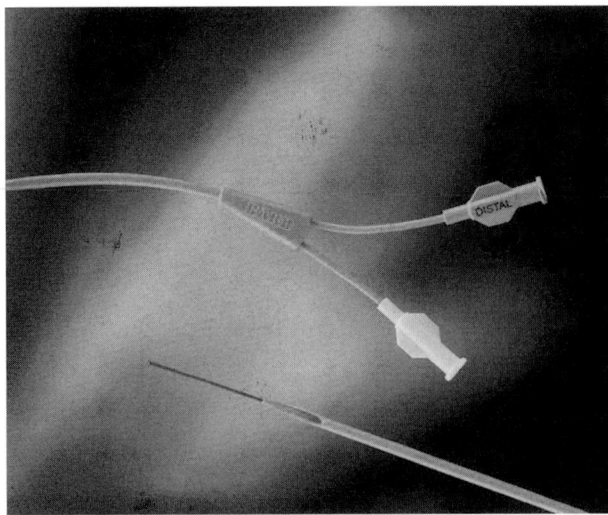


Fig. 22.5

When dilating the ureteral orifice in preparation for flexible ureteroscopy, our preference is to use a dual lumen, 10 French catheter passed over a hydrophilic wire. The second lumen can be used to inject contrast initially if desired and to pass a second "working" wire. The working wire is then used to either pass the flexible ureteroscope directly or to place a working sheath. Alternatively, the intramural ureter can be dilated with a 5-mm balloon passed over a wire under fluoroscopic control, with or without direct cystoscopic visualization. With balloon dilation, a second wire should still be placed, such that both a working and a safety wire are now in the ureter, coiled in the renal pelvis.

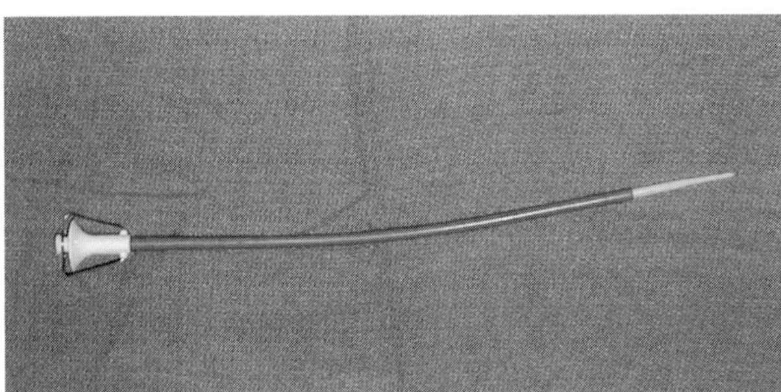

Fig. 22.6

The flexible ureteropyeloscope can be passed directly over a working guidewire. Alternatively, the flexible scope can be passed through a ureteral access sheath, which in fact we use preferentially for larger stones. We generally employ a 12/14 French sheath, although the larger 14/16 French size is often used, especially in prestented patients. The access sheath is passed over a working wire using fluoroscopic monitoring and a safety wire in every case. This allows intermittent monitoring of the procedure and provides access to the renal pelvis should a problem develop, such as proximal stone migration.

## Introduction of the Flexible Ureteropyeloscope

Using both direct vision through the ureteropyeloscope and fluoroscopic monitoring, the flexible ureteropyeloscope is passed up to the stone in the ureter. Once the stone has been reached, the working port is used for passage of

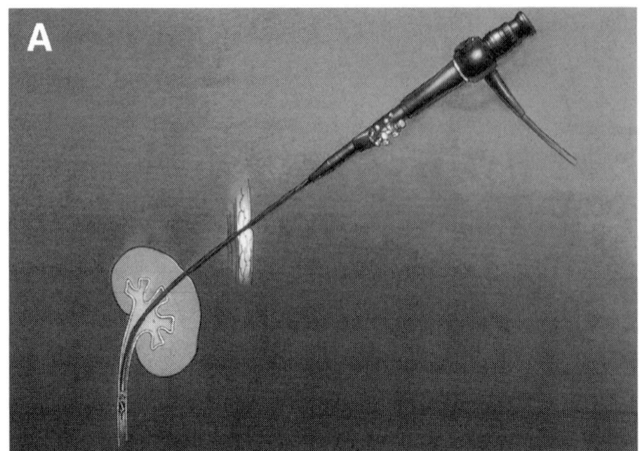


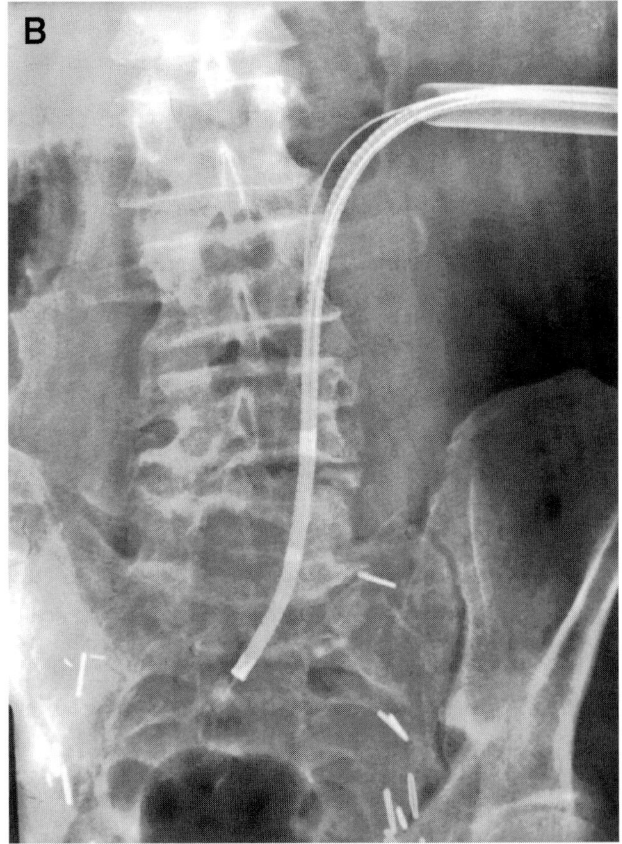


Fig. 22.7

**(A,B)** A mid- or superolateral infundibulocalyceal approach is preferred for better access down the ureter. The flexible scope is then passed through a working sheath. Smaller stones can be basket extracted under vision, while for larger calculi, the Holmium laser is the intracorporeal lithotripter of choice.

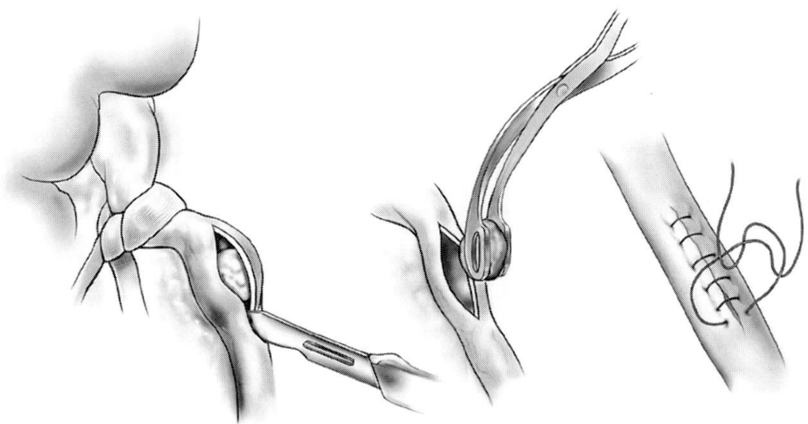

Fig. 22.8

The peritoneum is reflected medially, the ureter is identified, and the stone palpated. Generally, extensive ureteral mobilization is not necessary and should be avoided whenever possible. The ureter proximal to the stone is controlled by placement of a vascular tape. This prevents proximal migration of the stone up into the dilated ureter during the subsequent procedure. A longitudinal ureterotomy is then made directly over the stone utilizing a "banana blade." The stone is extracted with an appropriate-size stone forceps. The ureter is then thoroughly irrigated distally and proximally with a small-caliber red rubber catheter, and distal patency is assured by passage of the catheter all of the way into the bladder. The ureterotomy is closed with interrupted fine absorbable suture and the area drained with a Penrose drain. In the face of extensive ureteral edema or infection, strong consideration should be given to leaving an internal stent placed intraoperatively prior to closure of the ureterotomy.

adjunctive therapeutic instruments. The safety guidewire remains coiled within the renal pelvis at all times. Small stones can be basketed directly under vision. However, almost all stones in the upper two-thirds of the ureter will require intracorporeal lithotripsy. Again, our intracorporeal lithotripter of choice is the Holmium laser. With the flexible scope, our preference is use of the 200-μ fiber, again set at 0.6–0.8 J and 6–8 Hz.

### Antegrade Ureteroscopic Stone Management

When retrograde ureteral access is difficult or has failed for any reason, such as in patients with a urinary diversion, ureteral calculi can be managed with a percutaneous antegrade approach using flexible instrumentation.

### Ureteroscopy: Complications

Complications of ureteroscopy are usually minor and in most cases can be treated with placement of an indwelling ureteral stent. The most common complication is ureteral perforation. Occasionally, stone material may migrate through a ureteral perforation, though several studies have suggested that there are no long-term sequelae if a non-infection-related stone has migrated completely through the wall of the ureter. However, if stone fragments remain within the wall of the ureter, a ureteral granuloma with subsequent stricture formation may result.

The most significant complication of ureteroscopic stone retrieval is ureteral avulsion. This complication is usually a result of basketing a stone that is too large to be extracted intact. When in doubt, intracorporeal stone fragmentation should be performed to obviate the possibility of avulsion. This complication demands open operative reconstruction.

## URETEROLITHOTOMY

Open ureterolithotomy is rarely preformed in contemporary practice. Essentially, the only indication today is a failure of, or a contraindication to, all less-invasive procedures including SWL, retrograde ureteroscopic management, or percutaneous antegrade management. In such cases, an extraperitoneal approach is utilized with the incision positioned at the level of the stone.

## SUGGESTED READINGS

1. Denstedt JD, Wollin TA, Sofer M, et al. A prospective, randomized controlled trial comparing non-stented vs stented ureteroscopic lithotripsy. J Urol 165: 419, 2001.
2. Dretler SP, Cho G. Semirigid ureteroscopy: a new genre. J Urol 141:1314–1316, 1989.
3. Harmon WJ, Sershon PD, Blute ML, Patterson DE, Segura JW. Ureteroscopy: current practice and long-term complications. J Urol 157:28–32, 1997.
4. Huffman JL, Bagley DH. Balloon dilation of the ureter for ureteroscopy. J Urol 140:954–956, 1988.

5. Kourambas J, Byrne RR, Preminger GM. Does a ureteral access sheath facilitate ureteroscopy? J Urol 163(4S):66, 2000.
6. Kramolowsky EV. Ureteral perforation during ureterorenoscopy: treatment and management. J Urol 138:36–38, 1987.
7. Miller OF, Kane CJ. Time to stone passage for observed ureteral calculi: a guide for patient education. J Urol 162:688–691, 1999.
8. Netto R, Ikonomidis J, Zillo C. Routine ureteral stenting after ureteroscopy for ureteral lithiasis: Is it really necessary? J Urol 166:1252, 2001.
9. Peschel R, Janetschek G, Bartsch G. Extracorporeal shock wave lithotripsy versus ureteroscopy for distal ureteral calculi: a prospective randomized study. J Urol 162:1909, 1999.
10. Segura JW, Preminger GM, Assimos DG, et al. Ureteral Stones Clinical Guidelines Panel summary report on the management of ureteral calculi. J Urol 158:1915–1921, 1997.
11. Tawfiek ER, Bagley DH. Management of upper urinary tract calculi with ureteroscopic techniques. Urology 53:25–31, 1999.
12. Wolf JS Jr, Carroll PR, Stoller ML. Cost-effectiveness v patient preference in the choice of treatment for distal ureteral calculi: a literature-based decision analysis. J Endourol 9:243–248, 1995.

# III The Bladder (Malignant)

# 23 Office Procedures

*J. Stephen Jones*

The basics of office-based procedures are easily overlooked in urology training. Mastery of such seemingly simple procedures sometimes eludes the urology resident during times when the spotlight may be on major surgery.

However, the increasing focus on office-based procedures, combined with the fact that large numbers of urologists now function primarily in an ambulatory setting, makes facility with such procedures an increasingly important part of urological specialty care. Although a number of methods to perform cystoscopy, transrectal ultrasound, and prostate biopsy are used, we find that the methods described herein facilitate mastery of these procedures.

## GENERAL PRINCIPLES

Today's typical patient has become an informed medical consumer who justifiably expects minimal pain and to be treated with respect for his or her privacy and modesty.

The examining room layout should minimize the chance that someone opening the door will be able to see the patient in a compromising position. Doors ideally open in a manner that puts the door between someone entering and the patient until completely opened. This increases time delay for the misdirected visitor to stop if errantly entering the room. Curtains in front of the door assist with this as well and undoubtedly make the patient feel less vulnerable. When possible, the examining table should be placed such that the patient in an exposed position is not left in a manner that private body areas are visible from the door. The temperature should accommodate the comfort of the partially clothed patient.

Lubrication for urological instruments is vital. The value of anesthetic-based lubricants has not been definitively demonstrated, but the role of lubrication to minimize the shearing forces of friction against urethral or rectal mucosa is undeniable. We use water-based lubricants such as KY jelly for female cystoscopy and transrectal ultrasound because nothing has been demonstrated to provide better protection from pain. We use lidocaine-based lubricants instilled into the urethra for male cystoscopy despite equivocal demonstration of its value in the peer-reviewed literature. However, we also add water-based lubricant onto the scope because it is a more efficient lubricant than the lidocaine-based lubricant.

The bladder should be evacuated before cystoscopy in order to facilitate visualization. This is especially important if the patient has concentrated urine or has had an excretory urogram on the same day, which can lead to cloudiness in the bladder. In addition, the bladder should be only filled with enough irrigating fluid to see its entirety. Filling beyond that enlarges the surface area that must be examined, increasing the chance of missing a significant finding as well as patient discomfort. (This is also important when obtaining bladder biopsies. The more the bladder is distended, the thinner its wall is and the more likely perforation is and the more the biopsy site expands.)

Finally, it is vital to have a systematic approach to cystoscopy. If the bladder is examined beginning at one point and viewed circumferentially until completely assessed, there is minimal chance of overlooking anything. On the contrary, if the scope is simply moved around in random fashion, the chance that locations have been overlooked is significant and the surgeon cannot be sure when to stop looking.

## RIGID CYSTOSCOPY

Following the advent of flexible cystoscopy, the rigid cystoscope is now primarily used for women unless the patient is under general anesthesia. However, once the scope is placed into the bladder, the technique is basically the same for either gender. Female rigid cystoscopy is used to demonstrate the principles.

Trainees or nursing staff unfamiliar with endoscopic equipment often find a table full of cystoscope parts daunting (Fig. 23.1). This can be simplified in one's mind

From: *Operative Urology at the Cleveland Clinic*
Edited by: A. Novick et al. © Humana Press Inc., Totowa, NJ

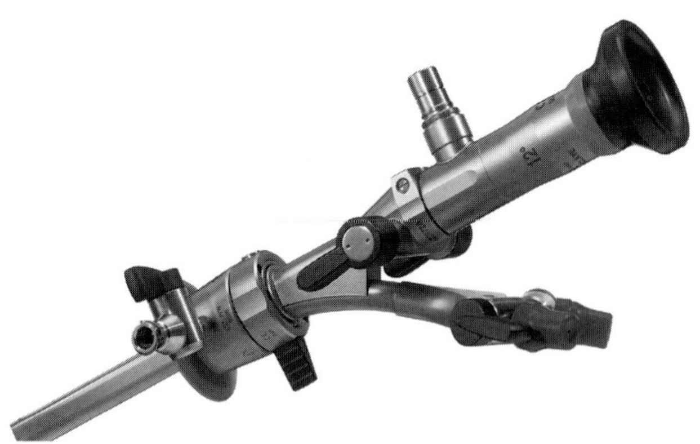

Fig. 23.1

if the "rule of three" is used. Almost all rigid scopes (newer one-piece scopes being the primary exceptions) are comprised of three parts:

1. A lens
2. A sheath
3. A bridge to connect the other two parts

The sheath might be a cystoscope sheath or a resectoscope sheath. The latter can be in one part (traditional resectoscope) or two parts (continuous flow resectoscope). The bridge might be a single- or double-horned bridge (we avoid use of the Albarran bridge because of its sharp edges, which can damage the mucosa) or might be a rigid cold-cup biopsy forcep. Regardless of the bridge, keeping this simple rule in mind helps tame the table full of instruments for the novice.

Modern rod lens systems come in multiple configurations, allowing visualization of fields oriented away from the lens. A 0° lens looks directly away from the eyepiece (it has 0° of deflection from the shaft). It is useful sometimes for urethroscopy, but a 12 or 30° lens is more useful by allowing visualization in front of the lens, but with more angles of freedom if turned. These two lenses are used for working with any instruments, including biopsy forceps, bugbee electrodes, retrograde catheters, and so on. The 70° lens (sometimes inaccurately called a "right-angle lens") allows visualization almost perpendicular to its axis, offering maximal degrees of freedom and the most complete look at the bladder. Thus, we teach that the 30° lens is for working, but the 70° lens is for complete visualization.

The cystoscope should be placed into the non-anesthetized woman's bladder with an obturator in place and the protruding tip pointed rostroventrally (Fig. 23.2). Despite the predominance of a straight urethra depicted in most anatomical texts, the female urethra usually has an upward curvature at the bladder neck. This leads to pain if the cystoscope is placed straight into the bladder. We find that placement is less painful if the cystoscope eyepiece is

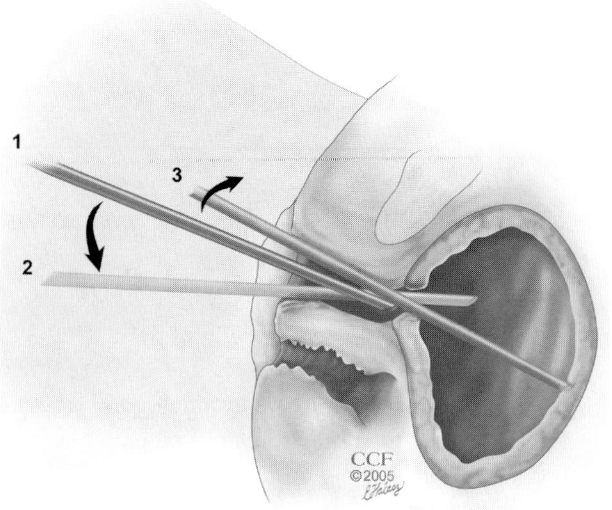


Fig. 23.2

directed slightly downwards (caudally) as it enters the urethra *(1)*. As it approaches the bladder neck, dropping the cystoscope down allows its tip to point up (rostrally) and go over the lip of the bladder neck atraumatically *(2)*.

Once the scope is in the bladder, it is placed gently against the posterior wall above the trigone (the trigone is the most sensitive and friable part of the bladder, so touching it is to be avoided). If done carefully, the obturator can be removed and replaced with the lens that has been placed through a bridge without allowing urine to escape *(3)*.

The obturator is used only in women, as passage is performed under direct visualization in men.

Using the 70° lens for office-based cystoscopy, the bladder is visualized in its entirety by utilizing its angle of deflection (Fig. 23.3). Because the lens visualizes opposite the light cord, the latter is a good reference and serves as a handle to turn the scope. Novices may find it difficult to depend on the angle of deflection to allow complete visualization and often resort to compressing the patient's abdominal wall in order to bring the area of interest into the field of view. This is discouraged, as it is unnecessary if the scope is pointed in the right direction. Moreover, unless the patient is under anesthesia this can be an unpleasant experience. This difficulty is often due to having the axis of the scope pulled in the direction towards the side of interest, which actually pulls the field of view away from the area of interest as shown. (The lens angle is shown without the smooth tip of the cystoscope in order to demonstrate the field of view.)

We prefer to angle the scope eyepiece away from the side of interest in order to allow the field of view to be directed at the contralateral bladder wall (Fig. 23.4).

If the light cord is used to recognize the side away from the field of view, the surgeon's end of the scope ends up

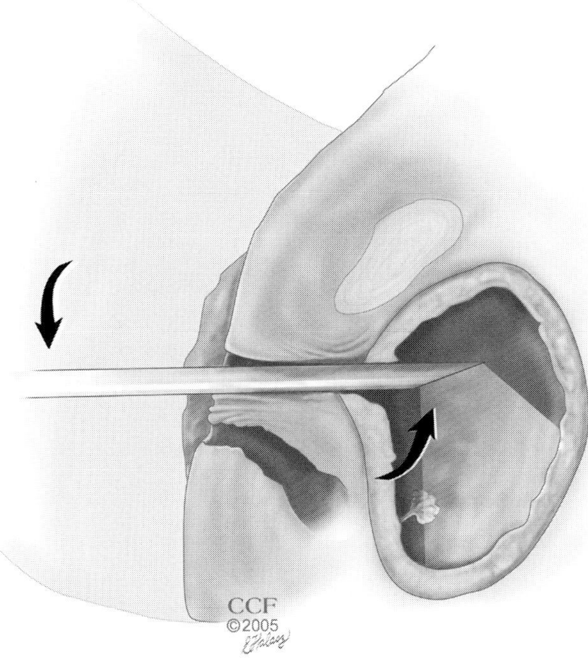


Fig. 23.3

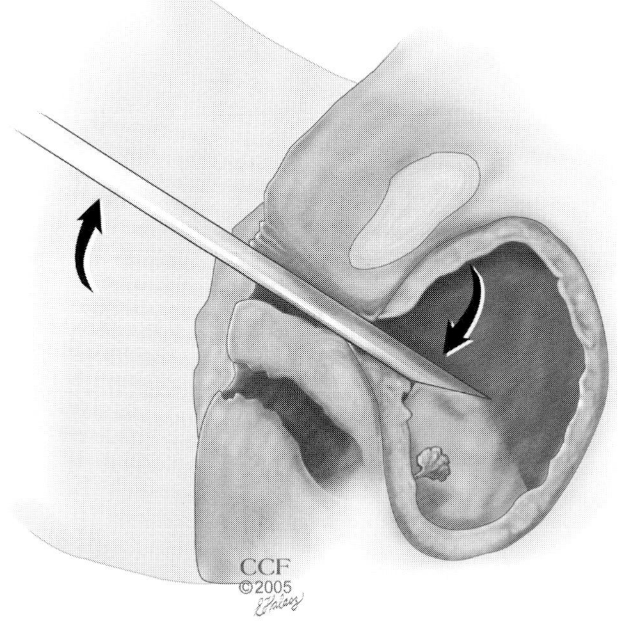


Fig. 23.4

being directed away from the area of interest, bringing the field of view to visualize the bladder wall at that point (Fig. 23.5). If the scope is twisted as it moves around the bladder circumferentially, its arc resembles a cone, as shown. The tip of this imaginary cone is the urethra and bladder neck, whereas the broad base of this cone is the eyepiece. The surgeon's nondominant hand keeps camera orientation upright at all times and ideally never leaves the camera head

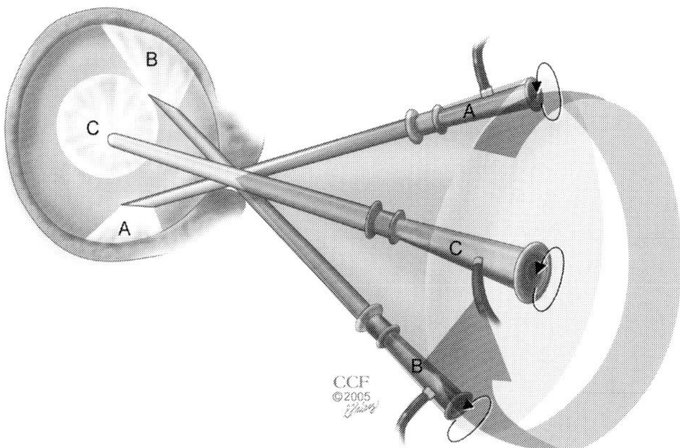


Fig. 23.5

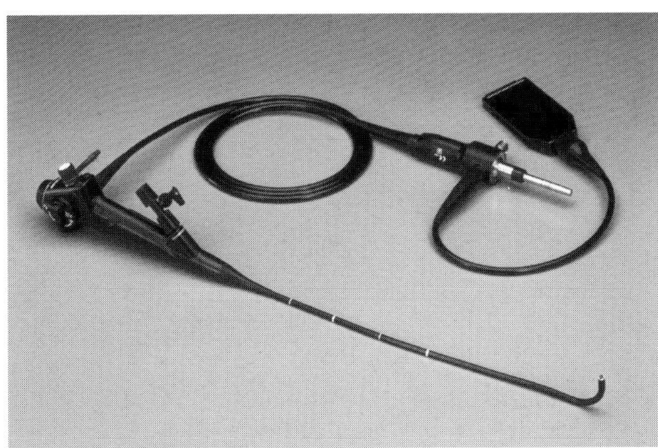

Fig. 23.6

during this arcing maneuver. (Images are shown in schematic form in order to demonstrate the geometric principles.)

## FLEXIBLE CYSTOSCOPY

Until recently, most flexible cystoscopy was performed on men. Curvature of the male urethra made its development a major advance in office-based endoscopy. With the female urethra being shorter and less curved, rigid cystoscopy maintained dominance for women, especially because previous generations of flexible cystoscopes sacrificed visual acuity for flexibility. Finally, most flexible cystoscopes have flat tips that can be difficult and painful for passage through the female urethra.

Newer flexible scopes use digital chip imaging technology that gives a view superior to that of even the best rod lens systems, so the entire bladder can be visualized in seconds. This minimizes the major advantage of rigid cystoscopes for women (Fig. 23.6, courtesy of Olympus, USA).

A thumb-operated control allows the tip of the scope to be placed into any number of degrees of deflection (Fig. 23.7). Moreover, rounded ("bullet") tips on the

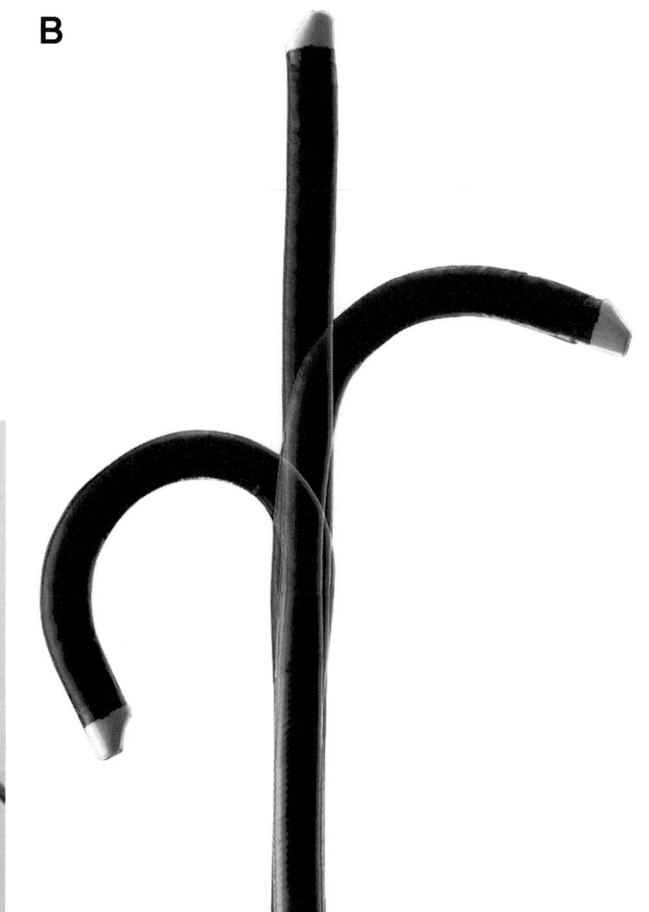


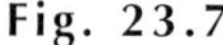

Fig. 23.7

newest generations of digital chip scopes allow relatively atraumatic passage through both the male and female urethra. Their tapered shape also allows gentle dilation of mild or moderate strictures as well (Fig. 23.8, courtesy of Olympus, USA).

Modern tower-holding digital chip cystoscopic processing equipment (Fig. 23.9, courtesy of Olympus, USA) involves light source, processor, photo printer, and digital capture functions. The monitor allows the findings to be recorded digitally, in analog printout, or as video footage.

We perform cystoscopy using video monitors for several reasons. Most important, minimizing exposure to urine enhances safety for the surgeon and staff. Second, photographs or video images can document findings. This is helpful in surveillance, allowing comparison of changes in the bladder. Educating residents is easier and has less of an impact on patients when both can visualize the bladder, whether the attending surgeon or the resident maneuvers the scope. Moreover, we have found that men who observe the video monitor tolerate the procedure with almost 50% less pain, as evidenced by visual analog pain scores compared to men who undergo cystoscopy without being able to see the live images. (This advantage has not been noted in women for unclear reasons.) Finally, printed images or those visualized on the monitor during real-time endoscopy help patients better understand the disease process and help foster a better informed health care consumer.

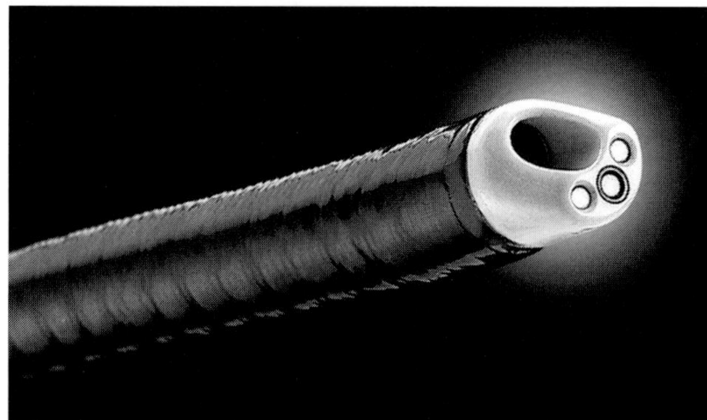

Fig. 23.8

Because flexible cystoscopy offers its greatest advantages in men, its use is demonstrated in a male model (Fig. 23.10). As noted, anesthetic lubricants are popular, and we continue to use them in men (there is no good evidence of their use in women, and they can impair visualization, so we do not recommend them for women).

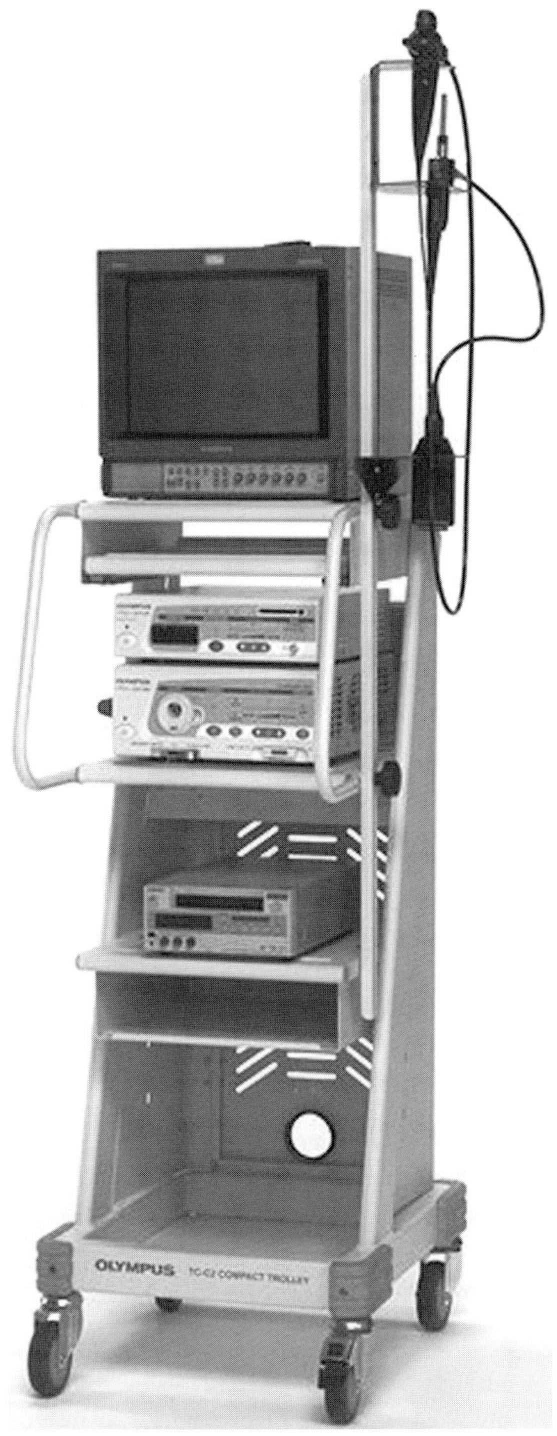


Fig. 23.9

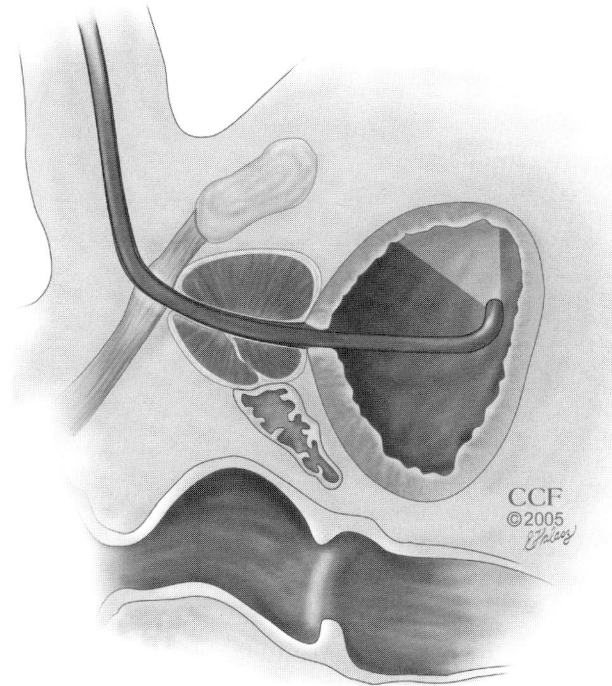


Fig. 23.10

More important, however, is adequate lubrication from addition of a more viscous agent, such as KY jelly. The penis is pulled on stretch by the fourth and fifth fingers of the nondominant hand. They also serve as a tourniquet to keep irrigating fluid in the urethra so it distends well, while spillage of irrigating fluid is minimized. This combination prevents the urethra from buckling like an accordion as the scope advances and is painless. The scope is advanced under direct visualization to the external urethral sphincter, which is readily recognized as a seemingly fixed narrowing. Asking the patient to "relax your bottom" often allows easier passage. Once through the sphincter, the scope is directed upwards (ventrally) in order to pass through the prostatic urethra.

Once the scope reaches the prostatic urethra, it should sit just inside the bladder neck in order to visualize the dome. The magnification afforded by digital chip endoscopy allows this to occur while in that position unless the bladder is overdistended. Keeping the scope handle in the neutral position with respect to the patient's midline helps prevent pulling the scope back into the bladder neck, which can cause trauma and bleeding. Moreover, it allows the surgeon to rotate the handle so that the left and right walls are easily visualized.

Using the thumb control to move the tip, the scope can visualize one side of the bladder if it is rotated towards that side and the tip is deflected in the right direction. Turning it back to the other side and using the thumb-controlled deflection up–down allows it to be visualized similarly. One thing that helps the novice remember how to systematically view the dome is to think of the scope tip tracing the letter H. When the tip goes through that motion, the entire dome and lateral walls will be visible.

After the superior or dome half of the bladder is visualized as above, the scope is advanced toward the dome and posterior wall. Beginning an upwards deflection before reaching mucosa will allow it to come against the back

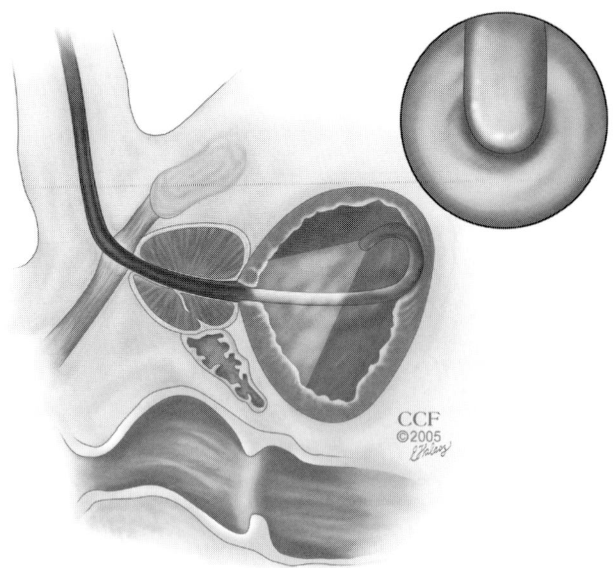


Fig. 23.11

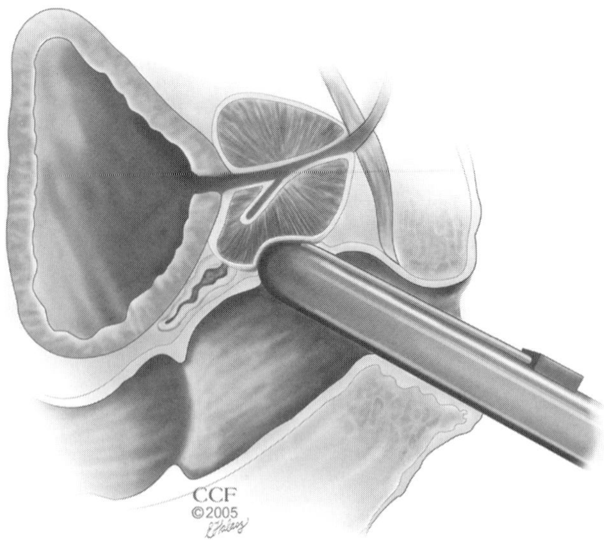


Fig. 23.12

wall in order to retroflex on itself for visualization of the bladder base.

Once the scope reaches the bladder dome, passive deflection allows it to advance into the retroflexed position (Fig. 23.11). While looking back at the bladder neck, its tip can trace another letter H in order to visualize the floor. If performed in systematic fashion, this completely shows the bladder in seconds. The scope can advance toward areas of interest as needed. The inset shows the view of the scope looking back at itself as it exits the bladder neck.

Alternatively, some urologists prefer the multiple-pass approach with either rigid or flexible cystoscopy—most likely the latter. This was necessary when endoscopic equipment lacked the acuity and magnification of today's scopes. The scope is passed beginning at the bladder neck and advancing up the wall at multiple locations (perhaps 12, corresponding to the hours on a clock face). We find these multiple passes to offer a less reliable systematic view and to increase the chance of pain or bleeding from trauma to the bladder neck.

Whichever method is used, surgeons have the greatest control when keeping their elbows at their sides. Movement of the handle by twisting or thumb control of flexion offers all degrees of mobility, so moving the handle in wide arcs only makes control of the tip more difficult. Moreover, if using imaging systems that have a detachable camera head, the surgeon's nondominant hand should maintain camera orientation. Newer integrated digital systems cannot maintain such orientation, which can be disconcerting during the initial attempts at their use. We found that adoption of these up-to-date units took few cases to make the mental adjustment and find their superior optics outweigh any potential disadvantages.

## TRANSRECTAL ULTRASOUND AND PROSTATE BIOPSY

Patient comfort is paramount to successful use of transrectal ultrasound and prostate biopsy. This begins with the room setup. Respect for modesty is medicolegally advisable, but more importantly is the right thing to do. Sheets to cover the legs allow the patient to feel some control over an embarrassing situation.

Modern transrectal ultrasound probe sizes are easily tolerable—some no larger than an examining finger. Adequate (perhaps abundant) lubrication minimizes the coefficient of kinetic friction and shearing forces against the anus. Attempts at anal mucosa and sphincteric anesthesia have yielded mixed results, so lubrication and gentle technique remain the mainstays of comfort measures.

Probe placement should be controlled, applying light but slowly increasing pressure against the probe as its tapered end dilates the sphincter during entry. The anal canal may be oriented slightly in varying anatomical directions, so allowing the probe to find the route of least resistance through this technique minimizes pain.

The physician should remain mindful of the topical anatomy throughout the procedure. Just as the laparoscopic surgeon observes the body during instrument entry and exit, the ultrasonographer should be observant that the probe should point in the direction of the rectal course during probe placement.

After placement, the handle can be pulled dorsally to allow contact with the prostate, the position of which is predictably behind the pubic symphysis (Fig. 23.12). Such firm contact is important for three reasons. First, it allows better sound transmission and so improves image quality.

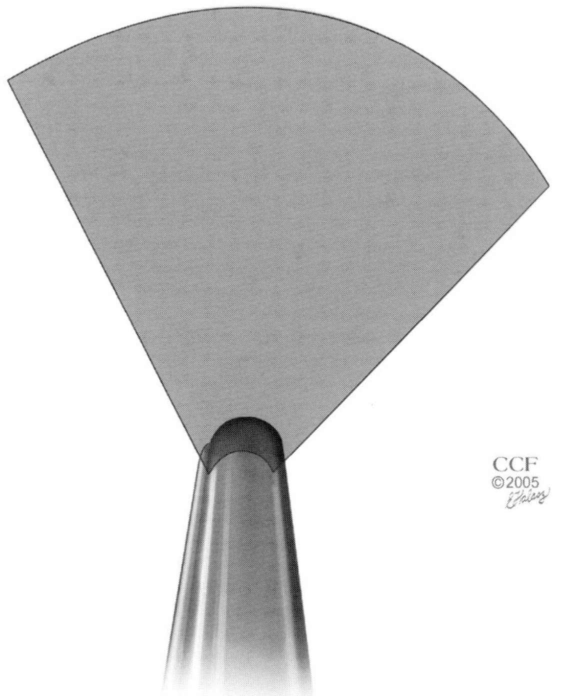


Fig. 23.13

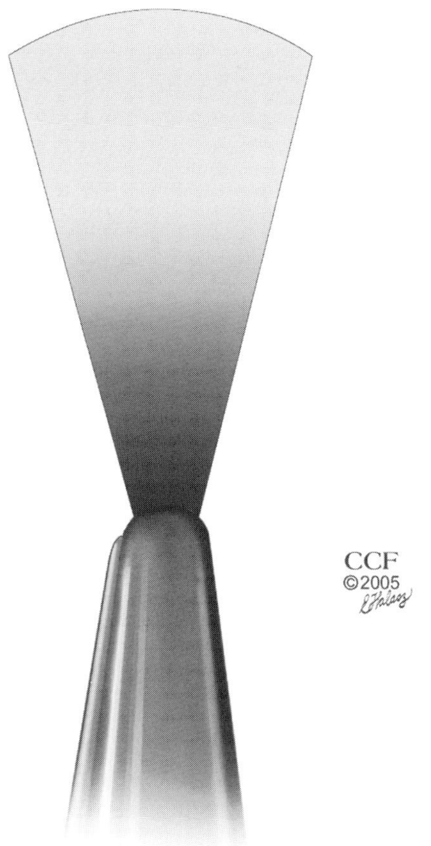


Fig. 23.14

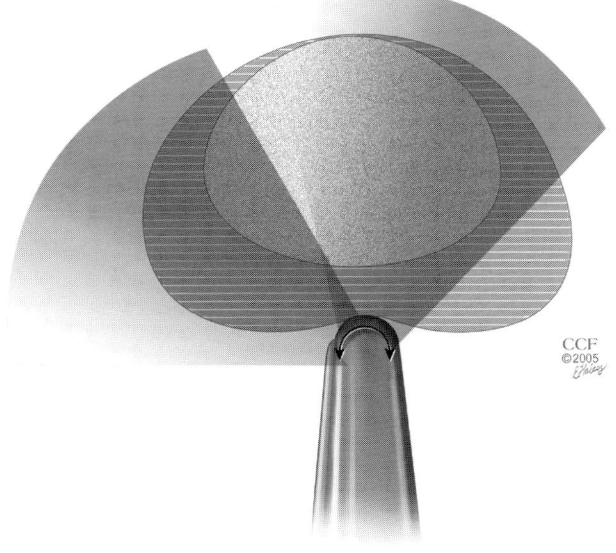


Fig. 23.15

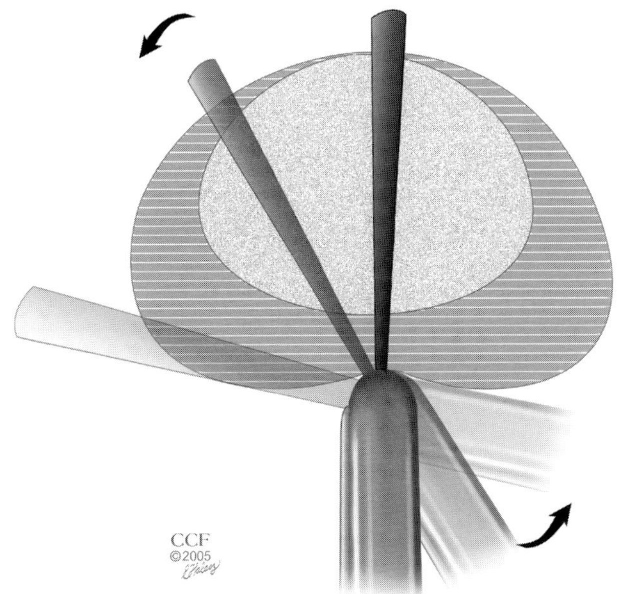


Fig. 23.16

Second, it helps tamponade rectal wall vessels to minimize bleeding. Finally, such pressure helps overcome painful stimuli by its effect on the "gate theory" of pain threshold.

Although it initially seems an unnatural hand position, the surgeon has a greater range of motion to move the probe where needed if holding it between the thumb and forefinger instead of using a "racquet grip."

## PROBE GEOMETRY

There are two types of prostate ultrasound probes: side-fire (Fig. 23.13) and end-fire (Fig. 23.14). Understanding their differences is key to mastery of transrectal ultrasound, since they give an entirely different viewpoint

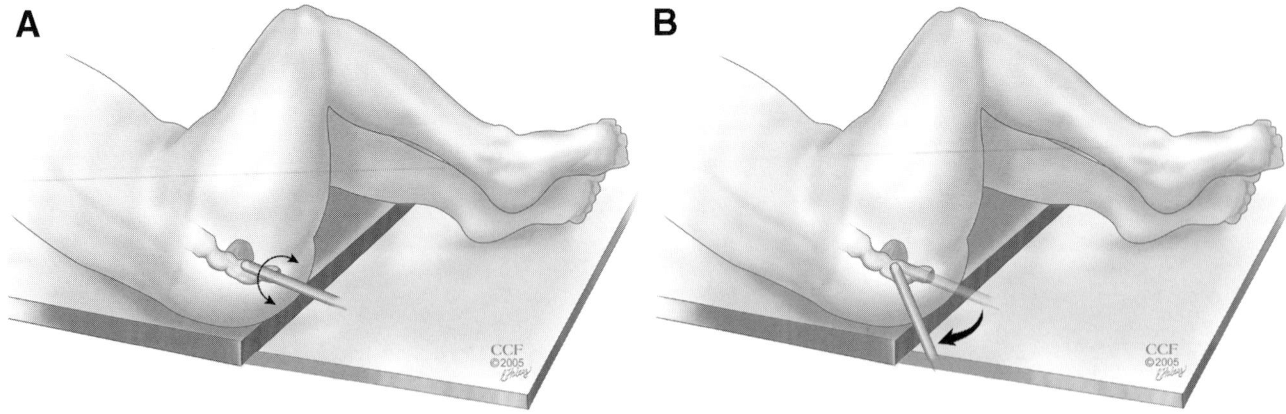


Fig. 23.17

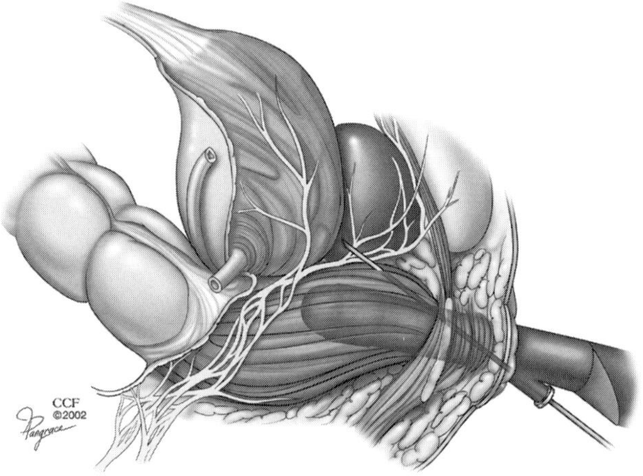


Fig. 23.18

that will create confusion if one uses one in the manner that is appropriate for the other. The direction of imaging should be obvious from their depictions (end- or side-fire), but the implications may not.

Side-fire probes project laterally (Fig. 23.15). For this reason, twisting the probe while keeping its axis neutral with respect to the sagittal plane laterally enables lateral visualization.

In contrast, end-fire probes project an imaging plane either directly or at a slight angle from the end of the probe (Fig. 23.16). This requires that the probe handle be angled away from the side of interest in order to visualize the lateral areas, using the anus as a fulcrum to gain accurate placement (i.e., the handle is moved downward, toward the patient's dependent left side, in order to visualize the right side of the prostate, and vice versa).

The geometric requirements just discussed mean that the male patient undergoing prostatic ultrasound using a side-fire probe should have the probe remain essentially in the midline, twisting to reach the lateral aspects. This makes patient positioning relatively unimportant, as long as the anus is accessible (Fig. 23.17A).

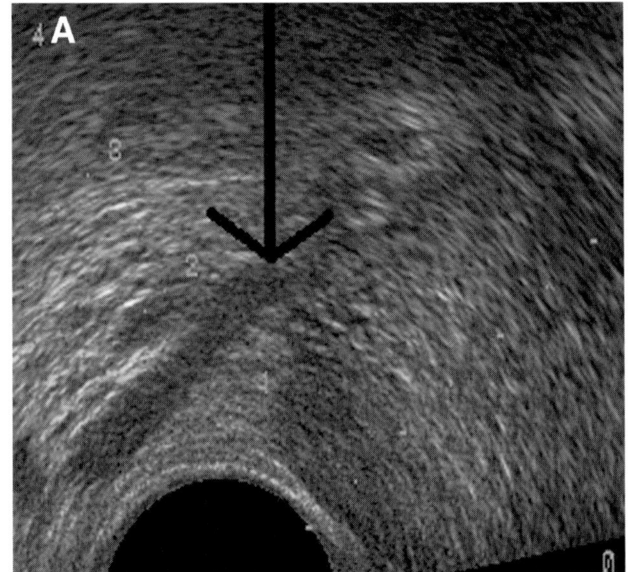


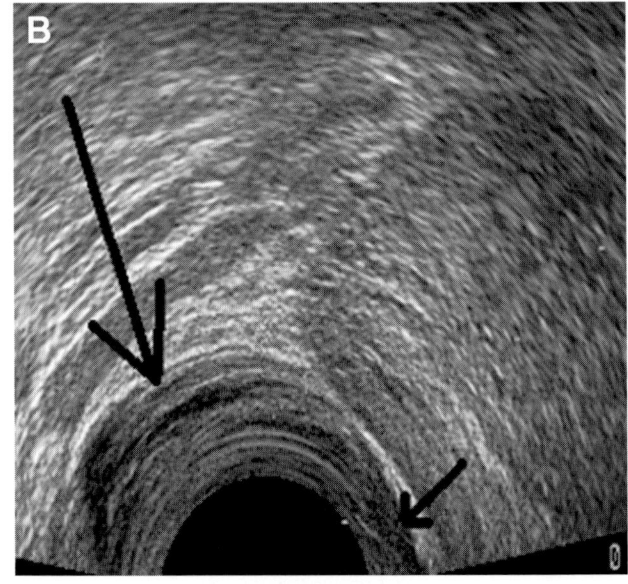


Fig. 23.19

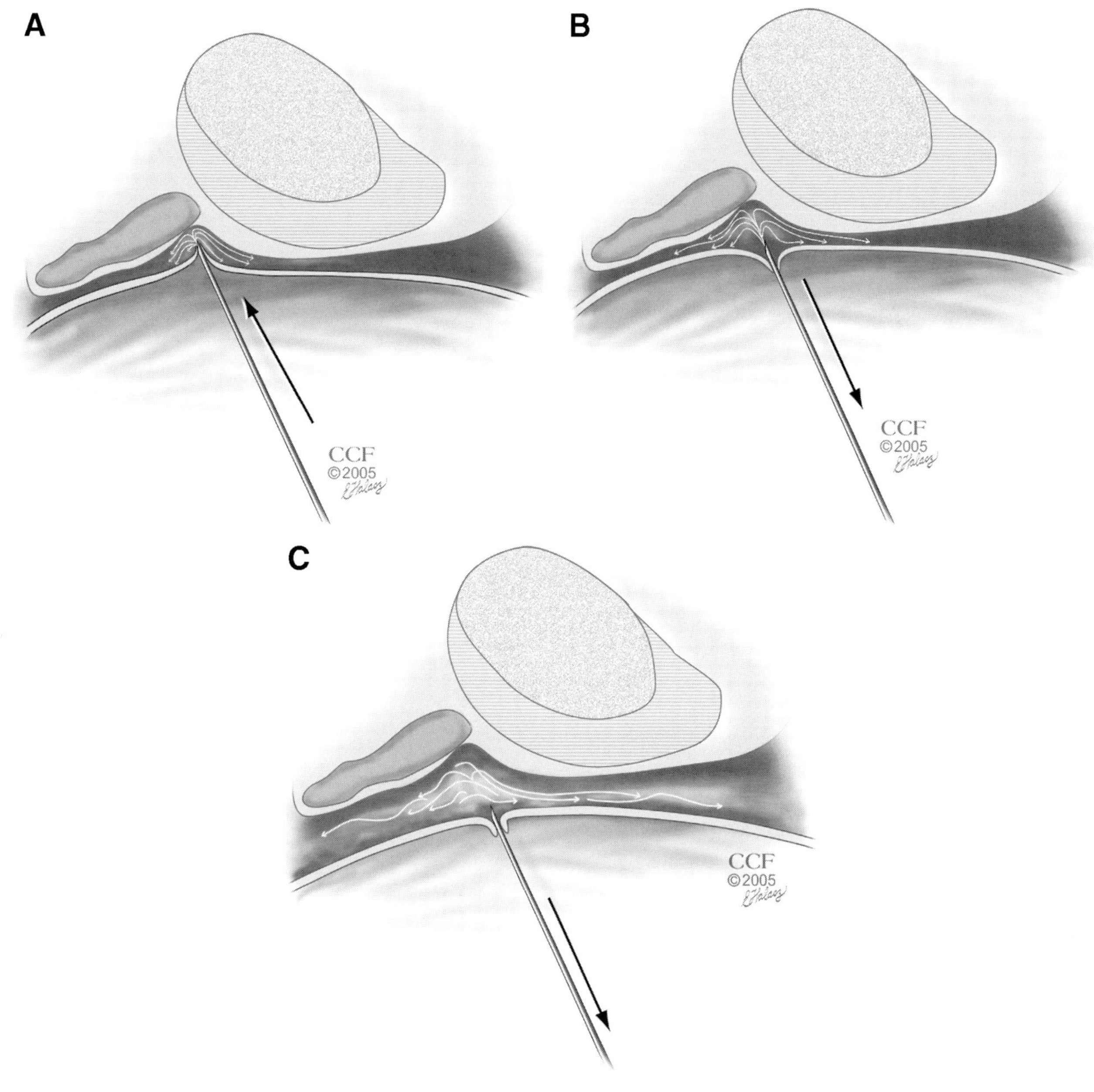


Fig. 23.20

Conversely, the man undergoing ultrasound using an end-fire probe must be positioned as shown in order to allow the ultrasound probe handle to be dropped far enough to reach beneath the plane of the examination table when visualizing the right lateral border of the prostate. This is most readily accomplished if his buttocks are directly over the corner of the table, with his legs flexed toward his chest and held by the table extension (Fig. 23.17B).

Limited visualization of the lateral aspects using either style probe can result in two problems. First, periprostatic block as described here is performed laterally at the junction of the seminal vesicles and prostate. Equally important, the lateral aspects of the peripheral zone are the areas most likely to harbor cancer, so limiting such access risks inadequate and false-negative biopsies. We find that lateral visualization is most readily achieved using an end-fire probe, although we routinely perform biopsies successfully using either.

Another advantage of the end-fire probe is that the needle exits its guide in a trajectory more directly toward the prostate instead of tangentially. This allows easier biopsy of the apex and anterior horn of the peripheral zone, further minimizing the possibility of false-negative biopsy.

## PERIPROSTATIC NERVE BLOCK

Periprostatic block is performed by placing a needle into the notch between the prostate and seminal vesicle laterally (Fig. 23.18).

This is identified ultrasonographically as a white pyramidal area (*see* the arrow in Fig. 23.19A) that we call the "Mount Everest sign." Fat in this location makes its visualization on ultrasound easy. We find that trainees have a tendency to avoid placing the probe deep enough into the rectum to reach the Mount Everest, so named because it is a white (hyperechoic) pyramid that resembles a snowy mountain peak. Difficulty finding this notch immediately upon probe placement is usually either due to inadequate depth of probe placement (easily remediable) or due to inadequate visualization laterally, often because the novice is twisting the end-fire probe or angling the side-fire probe, which leads to loss of bearings and perspective for either, as described previously.

Injection of 5 cc of a local anesthetic agent (either lidocaine or bupivacaine) creates a hypoechoic fluid area (*see* the large arrow in Fig. 23.19B) in the same site as the Mount Everest sign shown in Fig. 23.19A. The "ultrasonic wheal" describes visualization of anesthetic agent reaching the periprostatic nerves. This is demonstrated in the same patient shown above, where the large arrow points to hypoechoic fluid that is replacing the white area previous demonstrated.

Although some authors advocate multiple injections along either side, anesthesia is assured if the hypoechoic agent is visualized dissecting along the nerve bundles between prostate and rectum. The "ultrasonic wheal" doing so confirms that anesthetic has reached the entire neurovascular bundle coursing along each side of the prostate. If it dissects caudally along the neurovascular bundles (small arrow), prostatic anesthesia is assured whether a single or multiple injections are used.

Getting the anesthetic into the proper plane is facilitated by injecting as the needle enters the space in order to expand its distance (Fig. 23.20A), and then pulling back slightly (Fig. 23.20B) in order to open up the potential space until anesthetic is seen dissecting caudally (Fig. 23.20C). Note that the space between rectal wall and prostate widens when this fluid dissects into this plane.

The biopsy needle tract should primarily include peripheral zone tissue owing to the fact that most cancers arise in this location (Fig. 23.21). Parasagittal biopsies will contain some transition zone tissue as they traverse the gland, so this region is biopsied, though not purposefully. Lateral biopsies will include more peripheral zone tissue, as shown. This increases their yield compared to parasagittal biopsies, as does the fact that the lateral areas of the peripheral zone are the most likely areas for cancer to develop.

Measurements on the onscreen needle guide allow the surgeon to judge the depth of the gland. Most spring-loaded biopsy guns have a trajectory length or "throw" of 2–3 cm. If the gland is small enough that this distance as measured on the onscreen needle guide will go beyond the distant border of the prostate, the needle should be pulled back accordingly. A perfect biopsy will involve needle placement that ends with the needle tip against the prostatic capsule on the far side.

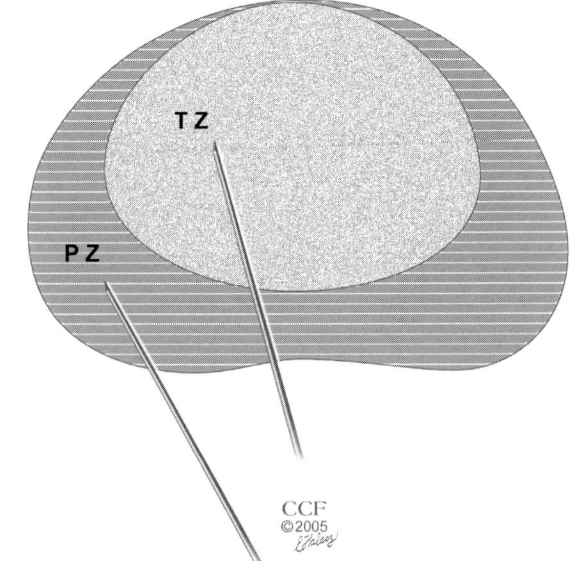


Fig. 23.21

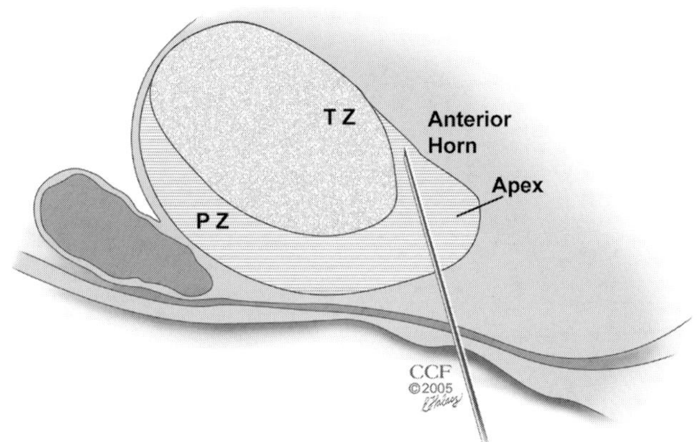


Fig. 23.22

Although many books state that the needle fails to contain tissue from the first 0.5 cm of the "throw,"we have not found this to be the case in bench testing, so do not intentionally pull the needle back this distance away from the tissue prior to firing the gun unless the needle guide measurements indicate that the length from rectal wall to the far side of the prostate is less than the needle's trajectory. If this is the case, the needle should be placed all the way outside its guide and visualized onscreen prior to pulling back in order to assure that overcorrection is avoided.

Apical biopsy is crucial because of the predominance of cancers in this location, especially in the anterior portion of the apex (Fig. 23.22). This area is named the anterior

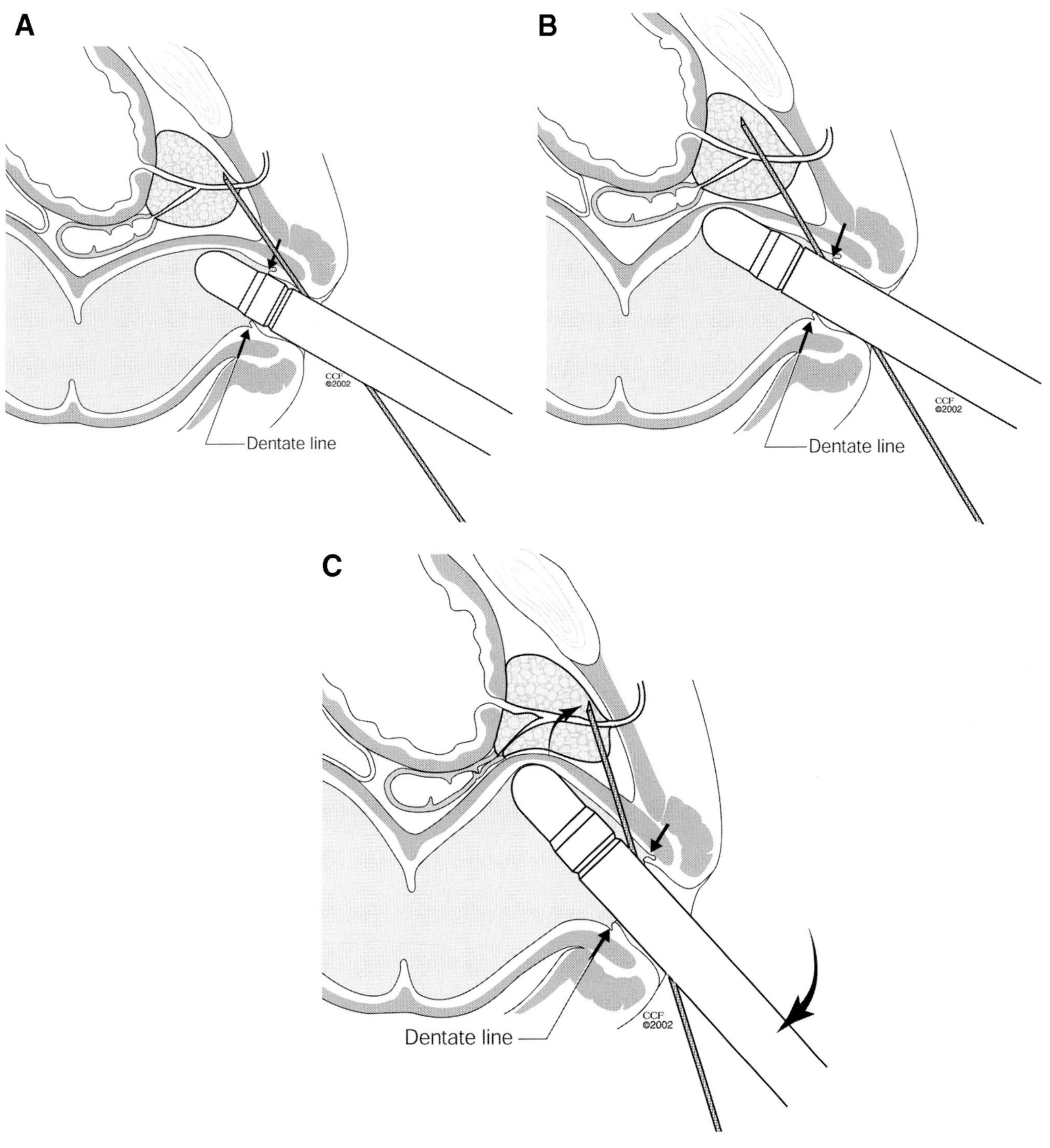


Fig. 23.23

horn because of its beaked appearance as it wraps around the transition zone (where needle is placed). Studies indicate that this is the most likely site of cancer to be missed during a false-negative previous biopsy. We believe this is because of two factors. The first is that it is difficult to reach, especially using side-fire probes because of their tangential needle tract. The second is the perception by urologists that biopsy of the apex is more painful than biopsy of other areas of the prostate.

We have determined that pain of apical biopsy is not prostatic pain; rather, it originates from anal pain fibers below the dentate line of the rectum, which approximately corresponds to the superior limit of such sensory pain fibers *(1)*. As this is often near the level of the prostatic apex, a needle often traverses such areas, resulting in significant anal—not prostatic—pain (Fig. 23.23A). The dentate line, identified by the rectal sensation test, is shown with arrows. During this test the needle is lightly applied against mucosa. It is

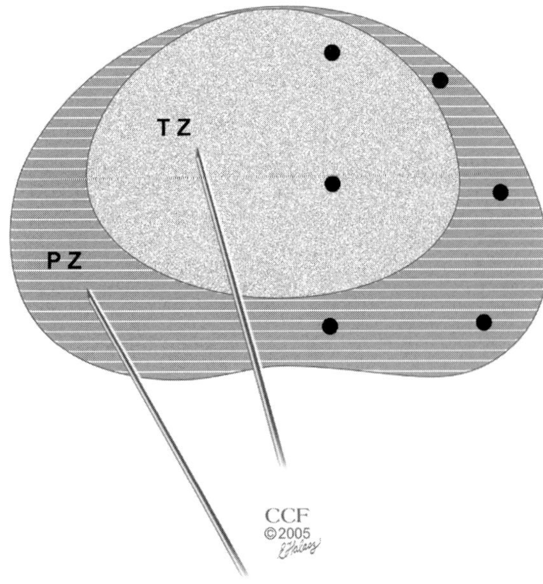


Fig. 23.24

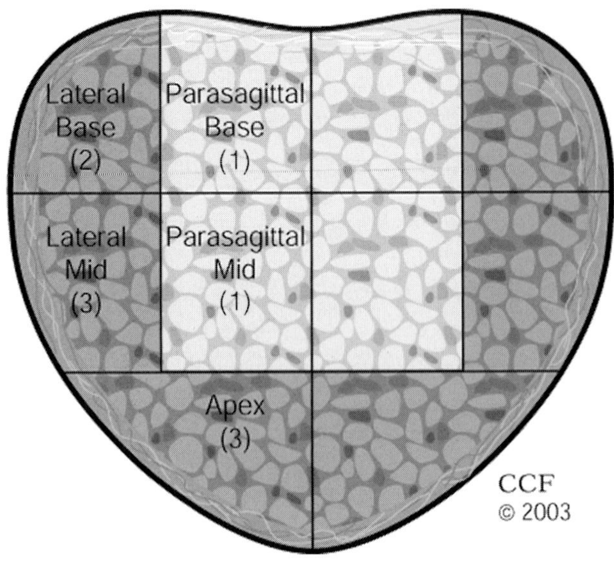


Fig. 23.25

immediately and strikingly obvious upon even light touch whether anal pain fibers are present at the level. If the patient answers affirmatively that he feels sharpness, the needle is repositioned 1–2 mm higher until reaching an asensate area.

When the needle is advanced cranially above dentate line, the trajectory is often towards the midgland, precluding adequate apical biopsy (Fig. 23.23B). This is especially problematic because of the need to biopsy the "anterior horn" or peripheral zone tissue, as described earlier.

Angling the probe handle craniodorsally, as indicated by curved arrows (Fig. 23.23C), allows the needle to pull the rectal mucosa caudally. Painless apical biopsy may then be obtained, bypassing the sensory fibers below the dentate line. This must be performed carefully in order to avoid dragging the needle against hemorrhoidal vessels in the rectum, which could lead to excessive bleeding. Using the needle tip as the fulcrum instead of dragging allows this to occur safely.

We currently recommend 12-core biopsy as an initial biopsy strategy based on our findings that increasing the number of cores beyond that yields no benefit for initial investigation *(2)*. We place six cores parasagittally in the same sites as originally described by Hodge and Stamey (Fig. 23.24). Six additional cores are obtained lateral to those sites, with an emphasis on going as far laterally as will allow full-length cores. The black dots show a typical distribution. Because the needle tract projects toward the base, it is often appropriate to have the entrance site be more towards the apex in order to avoid having most of the tissue be from the superior portion of the gland, which is the area less likely to harbor malignancy.

We have found that patients who have findings suspicious for cancer (abnormal digital rectal examination or persistently elevated prostate-specific antigen [PSA] or depressed free PSA) harbor cancer in almost 30% of biopsies when traditional 6- to 12-core techniques have been used. In this setting we perform office-based saturation biopsy. We have found that biopsies obtaining more than 20 laterally based cores yield minimal additional information, so limit such biopsies to this number. It is rare that parasagittal cores are positive as an isolated finding (i.e., in the absence of positive lateral cores), so the focus of all but two cores on each side is in the lateral regions, with specific attention to the anterior horn of the apex *(3)* (Fig. 23.25).

We do not find general or regional anesthesia to facilitate saturation biopsy as described, so perform all such procedures in the office setting.

## REFERENCES

1. Jones JS, Zippe CD. Rectal sensation test helps avoid pain of apical prostate biopsy. J Urol 170:2316–2318, 2003.
2. Jones JS, Patel A, Rabets JC, Magi-Galluzzi C, Zippe CD. Saturation technique does not improve cancer detection as an initial prostate biopsy strategy, J Urol 2005.
3. Patel A, Jones JS, Rabets J, DeOreo G, Klein E, Zippe CD. Parasaggital biopsies add minimal information in repeat saturation prostate biopsy. Urology 63:87–89, 2004.

# 24 Radical Cystectomy and Orthotopic Diversion in Men and Women

*Eric A. Klein*

Radical cystectomy remains the mainstay of surgical therapy for bladder cancer, both for those with *de novo* invasive tumors and those who fail intravesical therapy or otherwise progress from superficial disease to a higher grade or stage. Cystectomy may be an integrated part of multimodality therapy, as in those treated with neoadjuvant chemotherapy, and for the occasional patient who fails alternative therapies, such as radiation combined with chemotherapy. Cystectomy is also occasionally indicated in patients with benign disease, trauma, or after radiation- or cryotherapy-induced damage to the lower urinary tract. Regardless of the indication, the surgical approach and postoperative care are similar.

Various forms of urinary diversion have been described in the literature. Ample clinical experience in both men and women over the last 20 yr has demonstrated that orthotopic bladder replacement is technically feasible with good functional, cosmetic, and psychological results and should be the procedure of choice in the absence of a clear contraindication. Construction of an orthotopic pouch requires an undiseased segment of bowel of sufficient length for pouch construction, complete detubularization, and a usable urethra with an intact sphincter. Although preoperative parameters may be used to identify those at low risk of urethral involvement by cancer, an intraoperative negative frozen section of the bladder neck in women and the apical prostatic urethra in men is required before proceeding with orthotopic replacement *(1,2)*. A positive biopsy in either instance suggests a risk of leaving residual tumor and is an indication for total urethrectomy and an alternative form of diversion. Voluminous literature attests to the virtues of various forms of orthotopic pouches derived from large bowel, small bowel, or a combination. Smith has convincingly demonstrated, however, that good functional results in terms of preservation of the upper tracts, reasonable voiding intervals, and continence depend more on creating an adequate-capacity, high-compliance pouch, and careful preservation of the sphincter mechanism than on which bowel segment or configuration is used *(3)*. Accordingly, the choice of pouch should be left to the preference of the surgeon, with the best results in terms of expeditious harvest, configuration, and adaptation to variations in patient anatomy accruing from repeated experience with the same technique. Although controversy has existed in the past regarding the need for an antirefluxing ureteral-pouch anastomosis, recent data suggest that sterile reflux in the context of a closed-system, low-pressure reservoir is not detrimental to renal function *(4)*. Furthermore, refluxing anastomoses are less prone to obstruction and may be safely used in adults without contributing to upper tract deterioration. Finally, some controversy exists over whether orthotopic diversion should be used in patients with node-positive or locally advanced tumors for fear of delaying the onset of adjuvant chemotherapy, difficulty in administering chemotherapy, or mechanical interference of the pouch from tumor recurrence. Extended experience has demonstrated the psychological benefit of proceeding with the planned orthotopic diversion and the lack of associated problems with additional therapy or tumor recurrence in this high-risk patient subset *(5,6)*.

## PATIENT SELECTION AND PREOPERATIVE PREPARATION

Older age is not *per se* a contraindication to cystectomy and orthotopic diversion, but it is associated with a higher incidence of cardiopulmonary and other comorbidities, which should be identified and addressed prior to surgery. Consultation with specialists in internal medicine and its subspecialities should be sought when needed for advice on preoperative optimization of medications, pulmonary and cardiac status, and any special postoperative concerns.

From: *Operative Urology at the Cleveland Clinic*
Edited by: A. Novick et al. © Humana Press Inc., Totowa, NJ

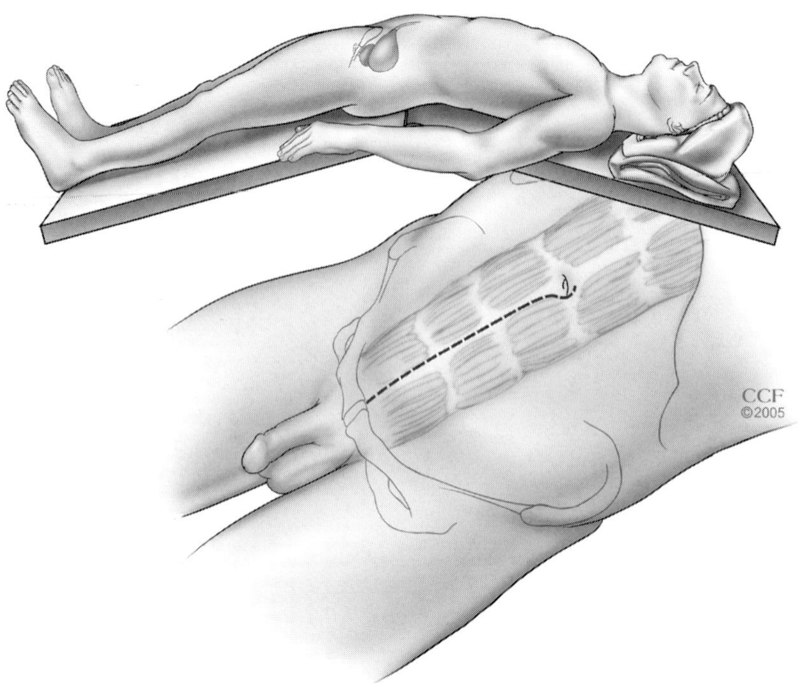


**Fig. 24.1**

The patient is placed in the supine position. Slight hyperextension of the table may be used to facilitate pelvic exposure. A midline infraumbilical incision is used.

Even in the absence of identifiable comorbidities, older patients typically have less physiological reserve and may not tolerate even a minor complication as well as younger patients.

A mechanical bowel preparation of magnesium citrate or GoLytely is administered 1 d prior to surgery. Intravenous ceftizoxime and metronidazole are give on call to the operating room and continued for 48 h postoperatively. Intermittent compression devices are used on the calves for prophylaxis of deep venous thrombosis (DVT). An epidural catheter is placed for use with a patient-controlled analgesia pump postoperatively.

## RADICAL CYSTECTOMY IN MEN

The patient is placed in the supine position, and an 18 F Foley catheter is placed transurethrally. The table may be hyperextended slightly to facilitate intrapelvic exposure. A midline incision is made from the umbilicus to the top of the pubis (Fig. 24.1). The space of Retzius is developed bluntly, and the bladder is mobilized off the pelvic sidewall bilaterally and palpated anteriorly, laterally, and posteriorly to assess resectability. The peritoneum is also mobilized superiorly, exposing the psoas muscles bilaterally. The peritoneum is entered at the level of the umbilicus, and the urachal remnant is identified and divided (Fig. 24.2). A self-retaining retractor is then placed.

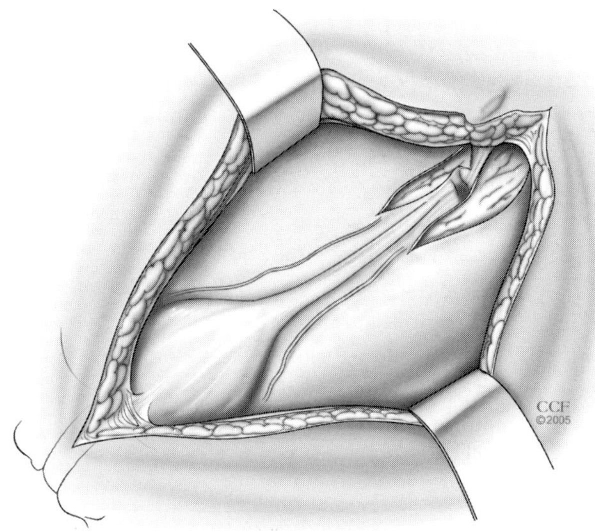


**Fig. 24.2**

The peritoneal cavity is entered and the urachal remnant is identified and divided.

Using the urachus as a handle, the bladder is elevated anteriorly and the peritoneum incised lateral to the lateral umbilical ligaments to the level of the internal inguinal rings (Fig. 24.3). The vas deferens are divided between clips near the pelvic sidewall (Fig. 24.4). The posterior peritoneum is next lifted and divided in a cephalad direction (Fig. 24.5), exposing the ureters as they cross over

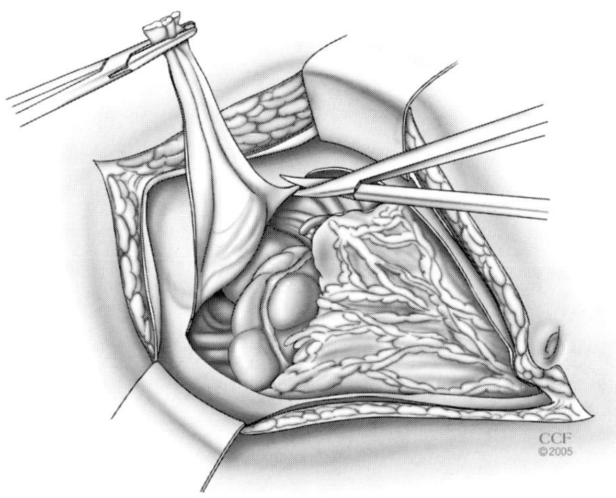


**Fig. 24.3**

The peritoneum lateral to the lateral umbilical ligaments is incised sharply, using the urachus to retract the bladder anteriorly.

the iliac vessels. The ureters are then mobilized proximally with care to preserve the periureteral blood supply for a sufficient length to allow later anastomosis to the neobladder (Fig. 24.6) and distally to the level of the bladder where they are divided. The distal 1–2 cm of ureter are excised and sent for frozen section to rule out the presence of carcinoma *in situ*, and the remaining ureter is packed out of the field superiorly.

Mobilization of the bladder and ureter in this fashion allows excellent exposure of the common, external, and

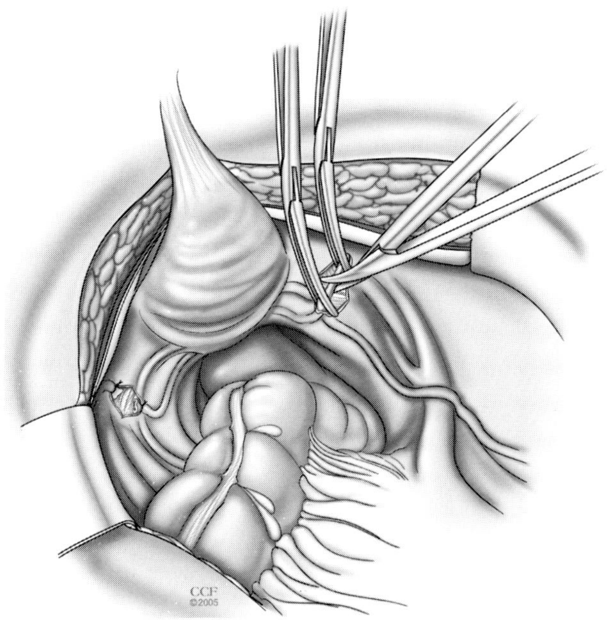


**Fig. 24.4**

The vas deferens are divided between clips.

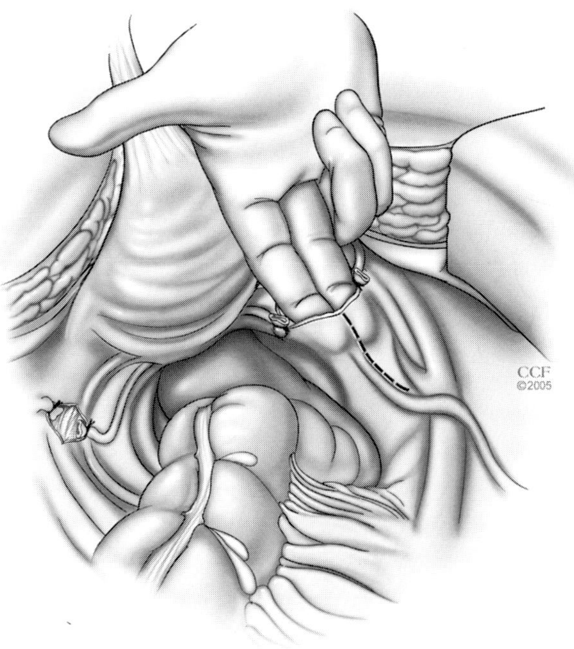


**Fig. 24.5**

The posterior peritoneum is incised to expose the ureters.

internal iliac vessels and the obturator fossa and facilitates completion of a pelvic lymphadenectomy. Alternatively, assuming that cystectomy will be completed even in the face of positive lymph nodes, the lymphadenectomy can

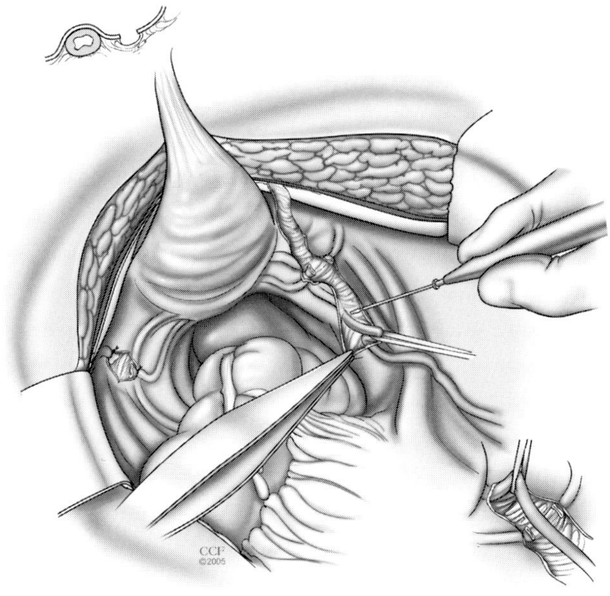


**Fig. 24.6**

The ureters are mobilized proximally and distally and detached from the bladder. The distal 1–2 cm of ureter are sent for frozen section to check for the presence of carcinoma *in situ*.

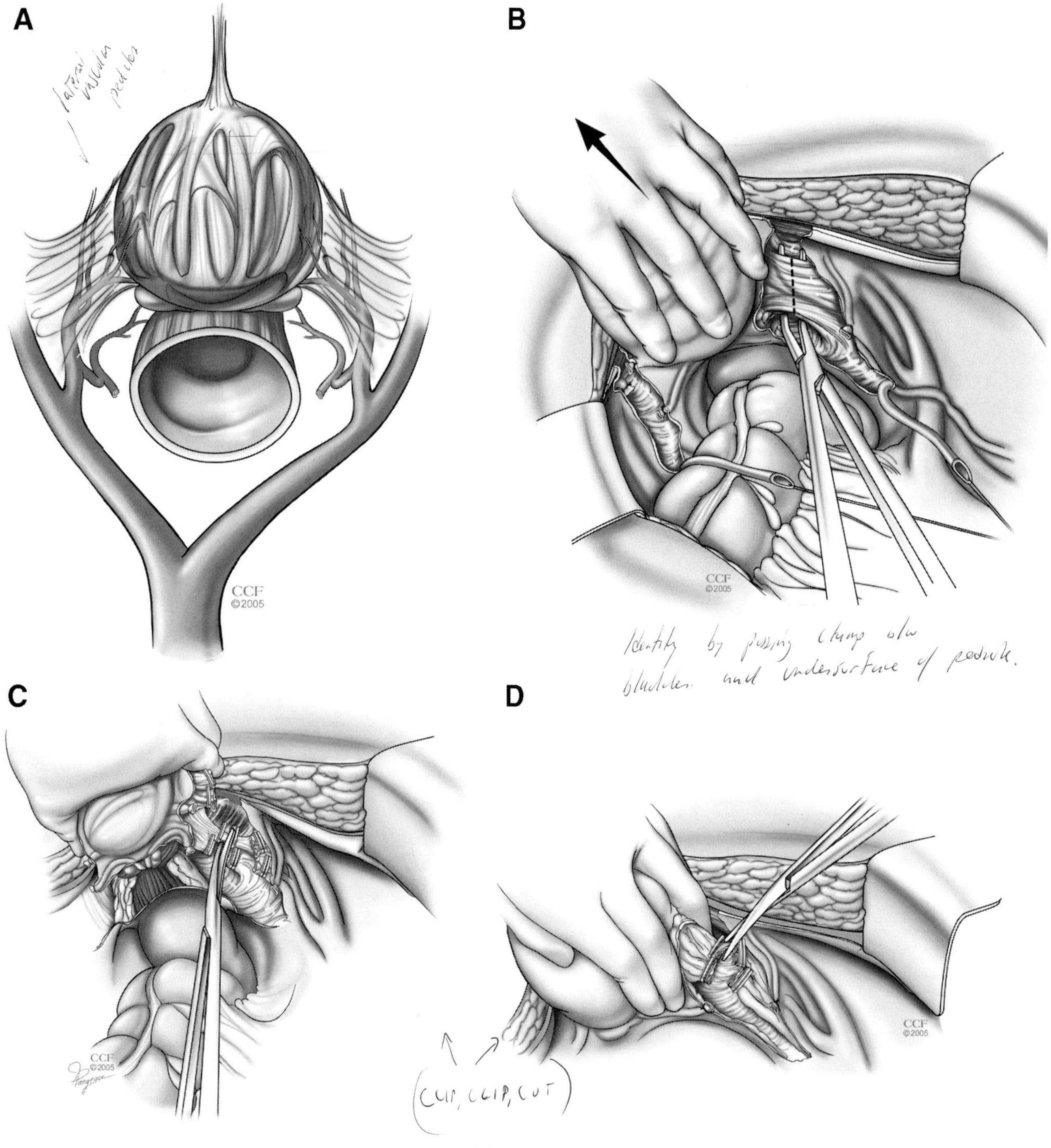

**Fig. 24.7**

**(A)** Skeletonized depiction of the relationship of the lateral vascular pedicles to the bladder, rectum (cut away), and iliac arteries. **(B)** The right lateral vascular pedicle is identified by passage of a clamp between the bladder and undersurface of the pedicle. **(C,D)** The pedicle is sequentially ligated and divided.

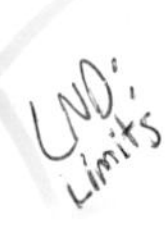


be performed after the bladder is removed (this approach is preferred by the author). The limits of lymphadenectomy include the inguinal ligament distally, the pelvic side wall laterally to the genitofemoral nerve, the anterior surface of the internal iliac vessels, and the aortic bifurcation, based on recent evidence of a therapeutic benefit to an extended dissection *(7)*. All of the fibrofatty tissue surrounding the common and external iliac vessels is removed, ligating the proximal and distal extent of the nodal packets to help prevent lymphoceles.

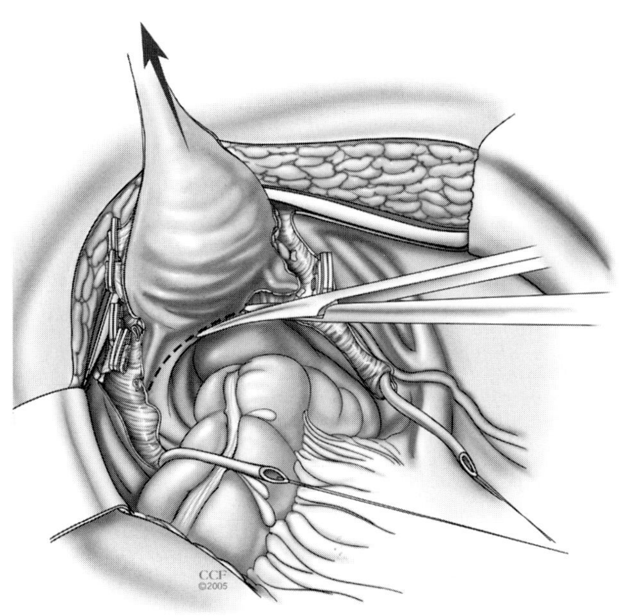


**Fig. 24.8**

The peritoneum in the rectovesical cul-de-sac is incised.

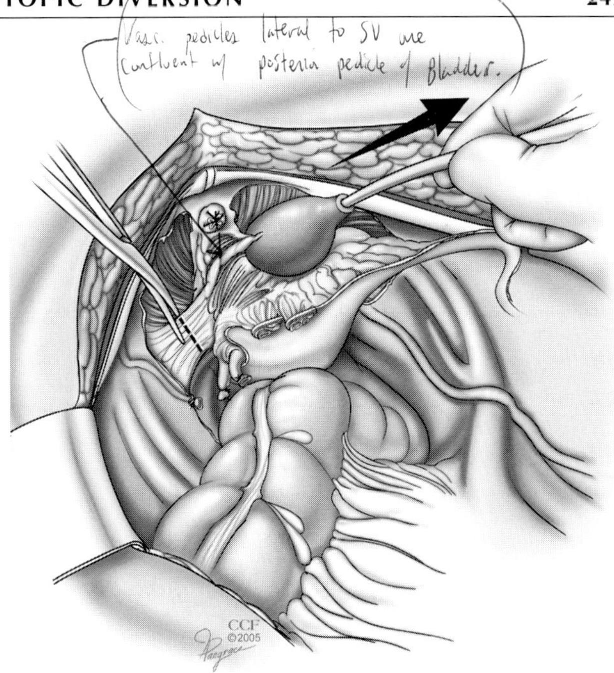


**Fig. 24.9**

Following completion of the apical dissection as performed for radical prostatectomy, the posterior vascular bladder pedicles are ligated, divided, and the specimen is removed.

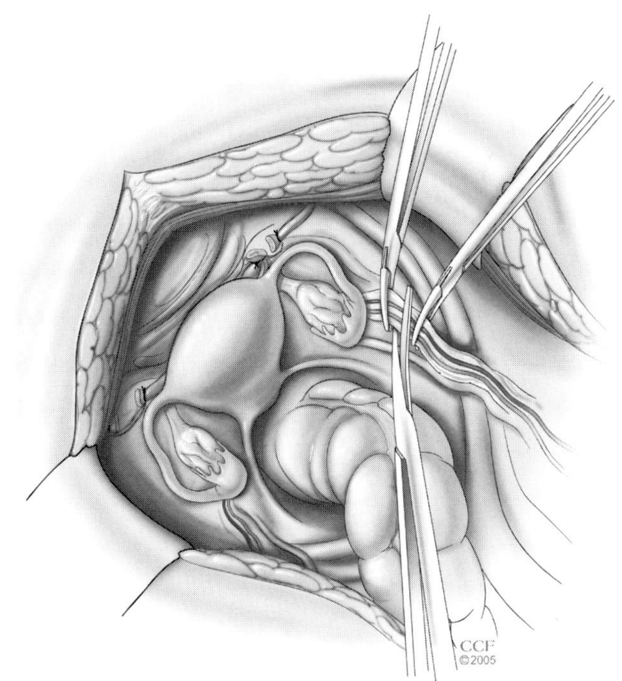


**Fig. 24.10**

The infundibulopelvic ligaments, which contain the ovarian arteries, are ligated and divided.

The endopelvic fascia lateral to the prostate in then cleared of the overlying fat, defining the inferior extent of the lateral vascular bladder pedicles. These pedicles contain the superior vesical arteries, obliterated umbilical arteries, and associated veins and extend at a 45° angle from the bladder to the internal iliac vessels (Fig. 24.7A). The entire pedicle can usually be defined by passing a clamp or finger between its undersurface and the bladder (Fig. 24.7B), facilitating easy ligation and division between clips (Fig. 24.7C,D). The bladder is next retracted anteriorly, and an incision is made in the peritoneal reflection of the rectovesical cul-de-sac (Fig. 24.8). A plane is then established sharply between the posterior bladder wall and the anterior surface of the rectum behind the seminal vesicles and prostate.

Preparation of the urethra for neobladder–urethral anastomosis is identical to that used for radical prostatectomy, and the remainder of the cystectomy is performed identical to that described for radical prostatectomy. The endopelvic and lateral pelvic fascias are incised, and the dorsal vein is ligated proximally and distally and divided. The neurovascular bundles are dissected off the prostate bilaterally, and the urethra is incised anteriorly with placement of the anastomotic sutures. The posterior urethra is divided, and the vascular pedicles lateral to the seminal vesicles, which are confluent with the posterior bladder pedicles, are divided and the specimen removed (Fig. 24.9). The advantage of this approach over the antegrade approach to the posterior bladder pedicles is familiarity with the apical dissection from experience with radical prostatectomy, better preservation of the neurovascular bundles, and a lower risk of rectal injury; its main disadvantage is the need for earlier division of the dorsal vein with its attendant bleeding.

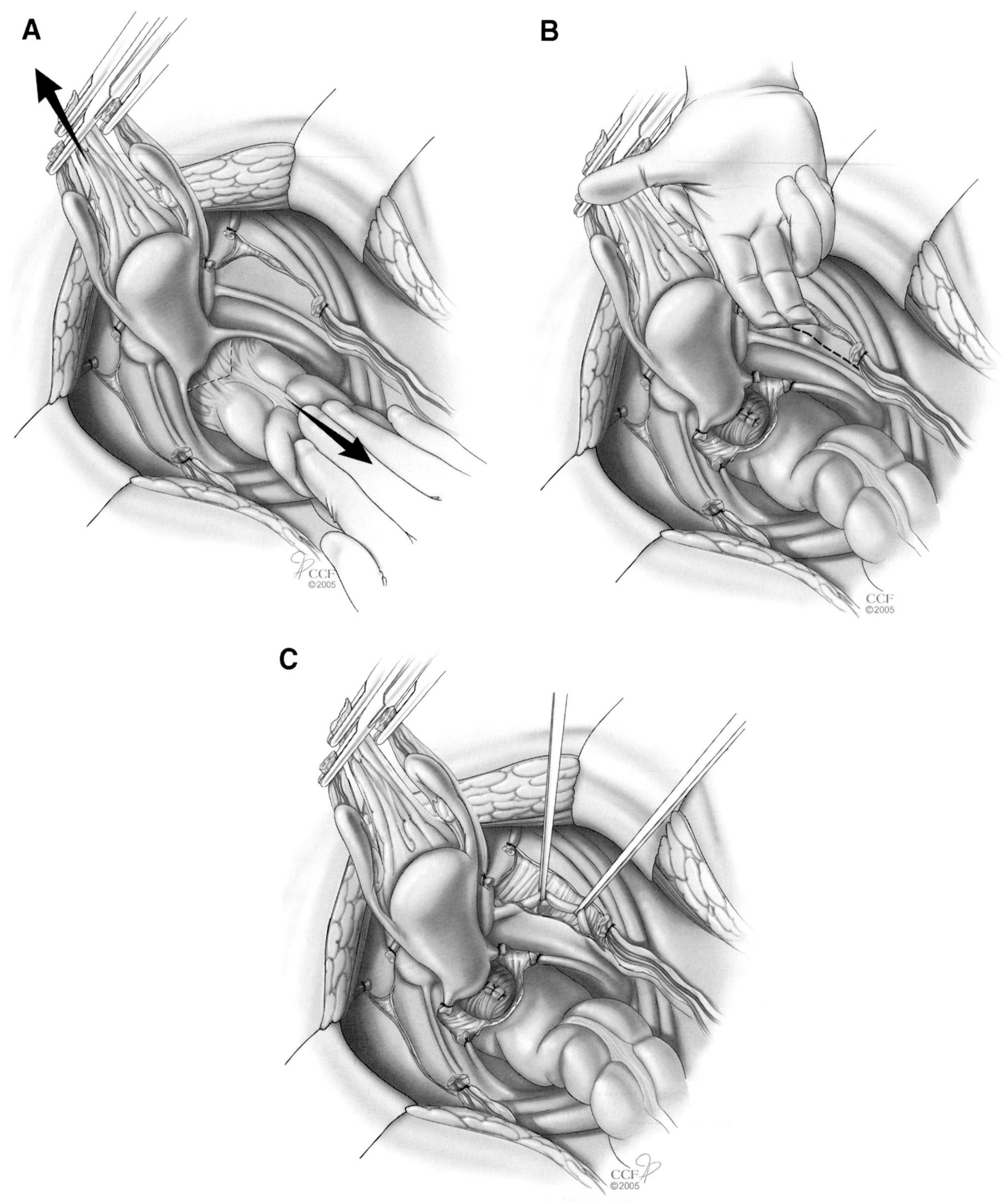


Fig. 24.11

**(A)** The round ligaments are divided. **(B)** The broad ligament is incised and the ureter is identified, mobilized, and detached from the bladder.

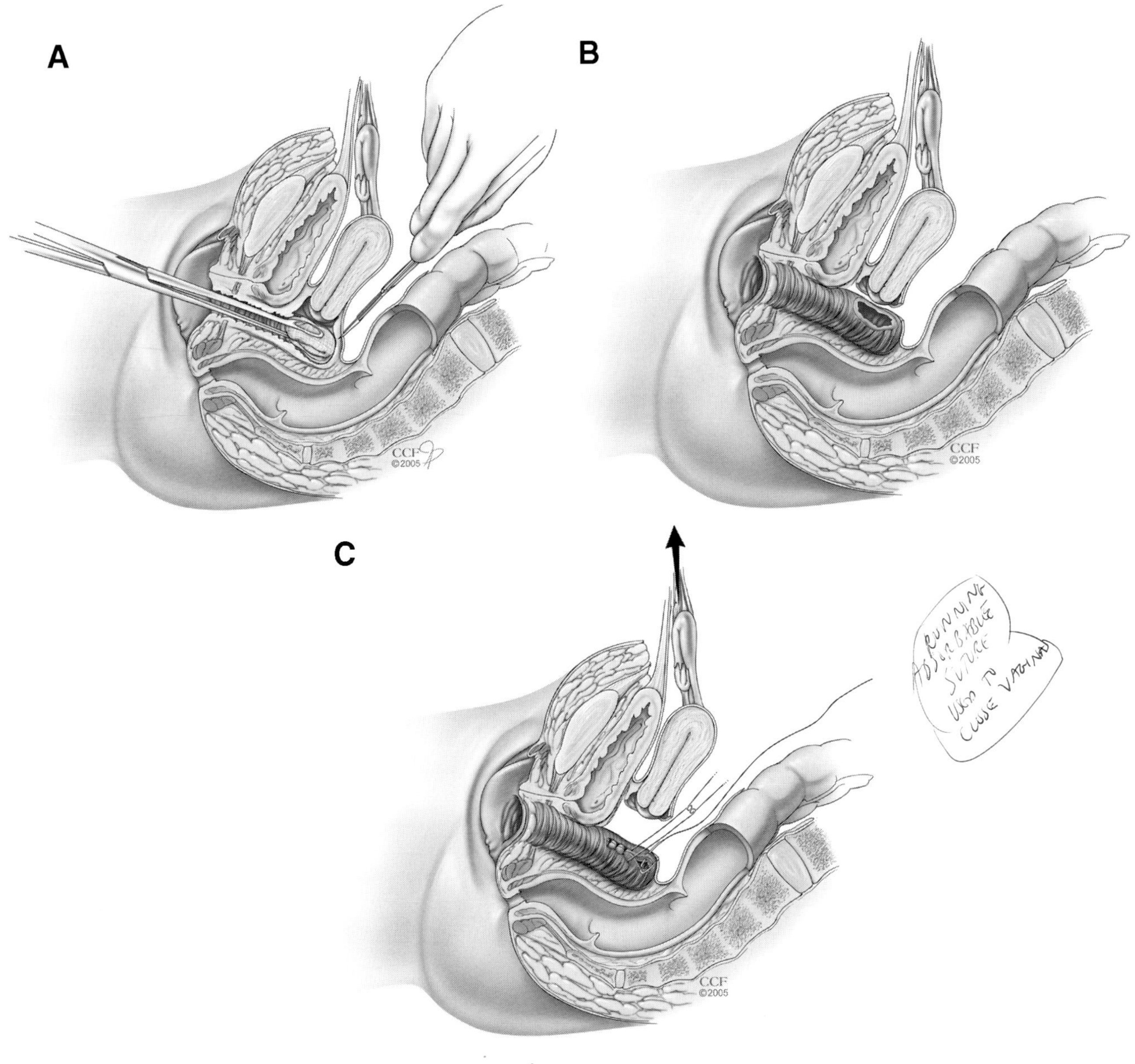


**Fig. 24.12**

**(A)** A sponge stick is placed in the vagina to facilitate dissection of the cervix, which is sharply circumscribed. **(B)** The defect in the vagina after removal of the cervix is shown. **(C)** The vaginal defect is closed with a running absorbable suture.

Following removal of the specimen, hemostasis is obtained and attention is turned to formation of the neobladder (*see* below).

## RADICAL CYSTECTOMY IN WOMEN

Cystectomy in women begins similar to that in men, with supine position, placement of a Foley catheter, and a lower midline incision. Bending the knees and placing the legs slightly frog-legged can facilitate access to the vagina, which is prepped into the field. Depending on age and reproductive desires, the uterus and ovaries may or may not be removed; the technique for anterior pelvic exenteration with vaginal preservation is illustrated here.

The dissection begins with blunt mobilization of the bladder from the pelvic side walls and palpation for resectability. The urachus is identified and divided and used for anterior displacement of the bladder. The infundibulopelvic ligaments, which contain the ovarian artery, are identified, ligated, and divided close to the pelvic side wall (Fig. 24.10). The round ligaments, female anlagen to the vas, are next divided, and the broad

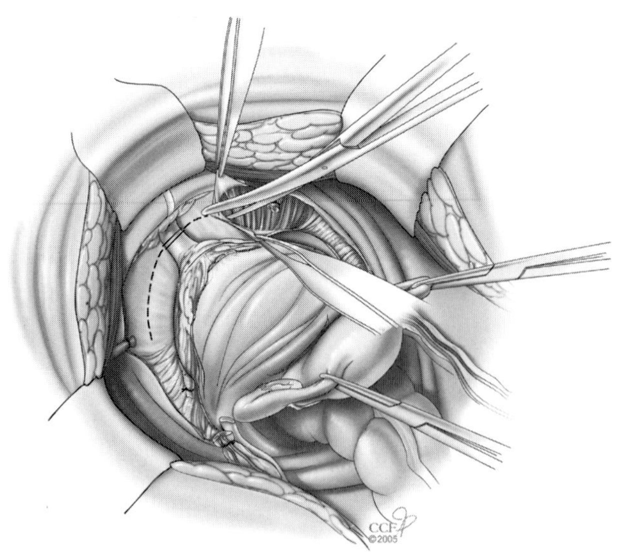


**Fig. 24.13**

The endopelvic fascia is incised. The bladder-neck urethral junction is identified.

ligaments are incised to expose the ureters, which are identified, mobilized, and divided as in the male (Fig. 24.11).

The bladder, uterus, and ovaries are retracted anteriorly and a sponge stick placed in the vagina is pushed up and in against the vaginal apex (Fig. 24.12A). The cervix is circumscribed sharply with a circumferential incision in the anterior vaginal wall (Fig. 24.12B), and the resulting vaginal defect is closed with a running absorbable suture (Fig. 24.12C). Dissection of the plane between the anterior vaginal wall and posterior surface of the bladder is best accomplished in a retrograde fashion, and the remaining dissection proceeds from the apex as for men. The endopelvic fascia is incised, and the urethra and bladder neck are identified by blunt dissection with a sponge stick (Fig. 24.13). Prior to division at its junction with the urethra, the bladder neck is occluded with a clamp or by downward traction on an overfilled Foley balloon to prevent tumor spill. The urethra is divided circumferentially at its junction with the bladder neck (Fig. 24.14A). Traction on the Foley is used to elevate the bladder anteriorly and cephalad, and the bladder is sharply dissected away from the anterior vaginal wall, ligating the posterior vascular pedicles as bleeders are encountered (Fig. 24.14). Care should be taken to avoid buttonholes in the vagina, which may lead to urethro- or neobladder-vaginal fistulae, and to avoid damage to the neural plexus lateral to the vagina, which subserve clitoral sensation and vaginal lubrication *(8)*. Finally, the specimen is removed and five or six anastomotic sutures are placed in the urethral stump (Fig. 24.15). When accomplished easily, an omental flap is brought into the pelvis and sutured posterior to the urethra to help prevent posterior angulation of the neobladder.

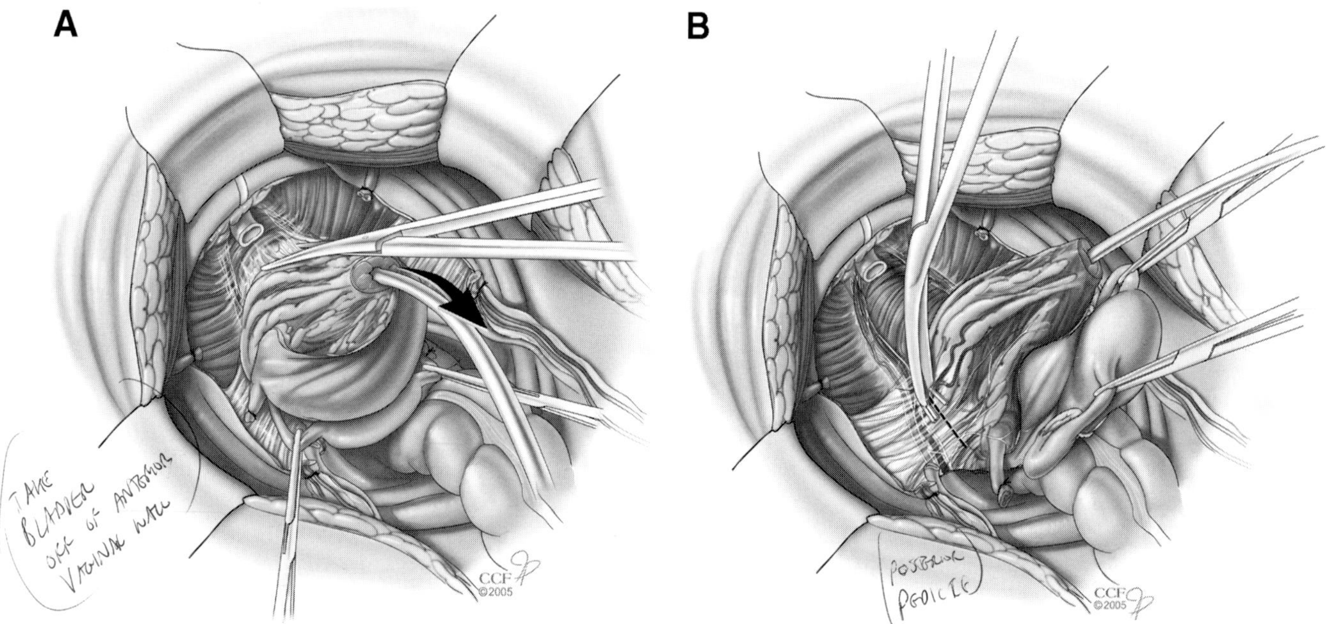


**Fig. 24.14**

**(A)** The urethra is divided and the plane between the anterior vaginal wall and bladder is developed sharply. **(B)** The bladder is dissected sharply away from the vagina and vascular pedicles are ligated. Care should be taken to avoid "buttonholing" the vagina, which can lead to fistula formation.

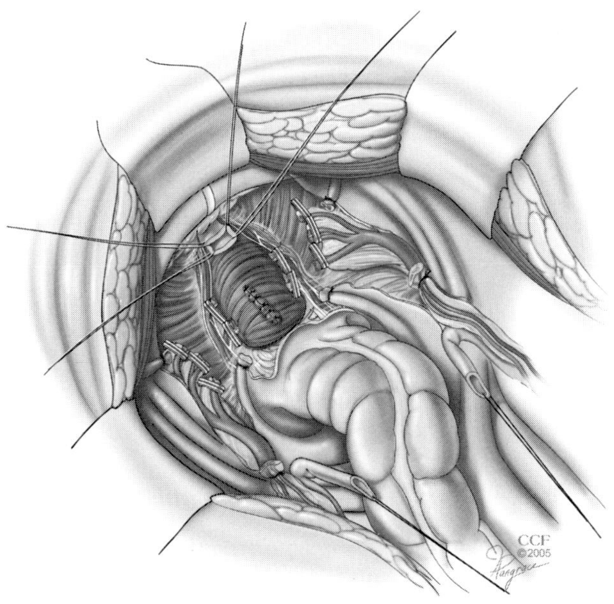

**Fig. 24.15**

Final appearance of the pelvis after removal of the bladder, showing preplaced urethral anastomotic sutures.

## ILEAL NEOBLADDER

As discussed, a variety of bowel segments and configurations for creation of an orthotopic neobladder have been described. Our preference is for the Studer pouch, which easily recapitulates creation of an ileal conduit, is easily manipulated into the pelvis, allows for a proximal limb of whatever length is needed to reach the ureters (especially important in the event of CIS involving the distal ureters), and can be easily converted into an ileal conduit in the event of a urethral recurrence.

Creation of the pouch begins with isolation of a 55-cm segment of ileum, beginning 25 cm proximal to the ileocecal valve (Fig. 24.16A). Starting this proximal to the ileocecal valve will ensure adequate blood supply to the distal most ileum and cecum by preserving the ileocecal artery. The cut in the mesentery closest to the ileocecal valve needs to be made deeper than the more proximal one in order to allow the neobladder to be placed in the pelvis without tension. The bowel is reanastomosed in end-to-end fashion using staplers. The bowel segment is irrigated with *warm* saline (room temperature or colder fluid

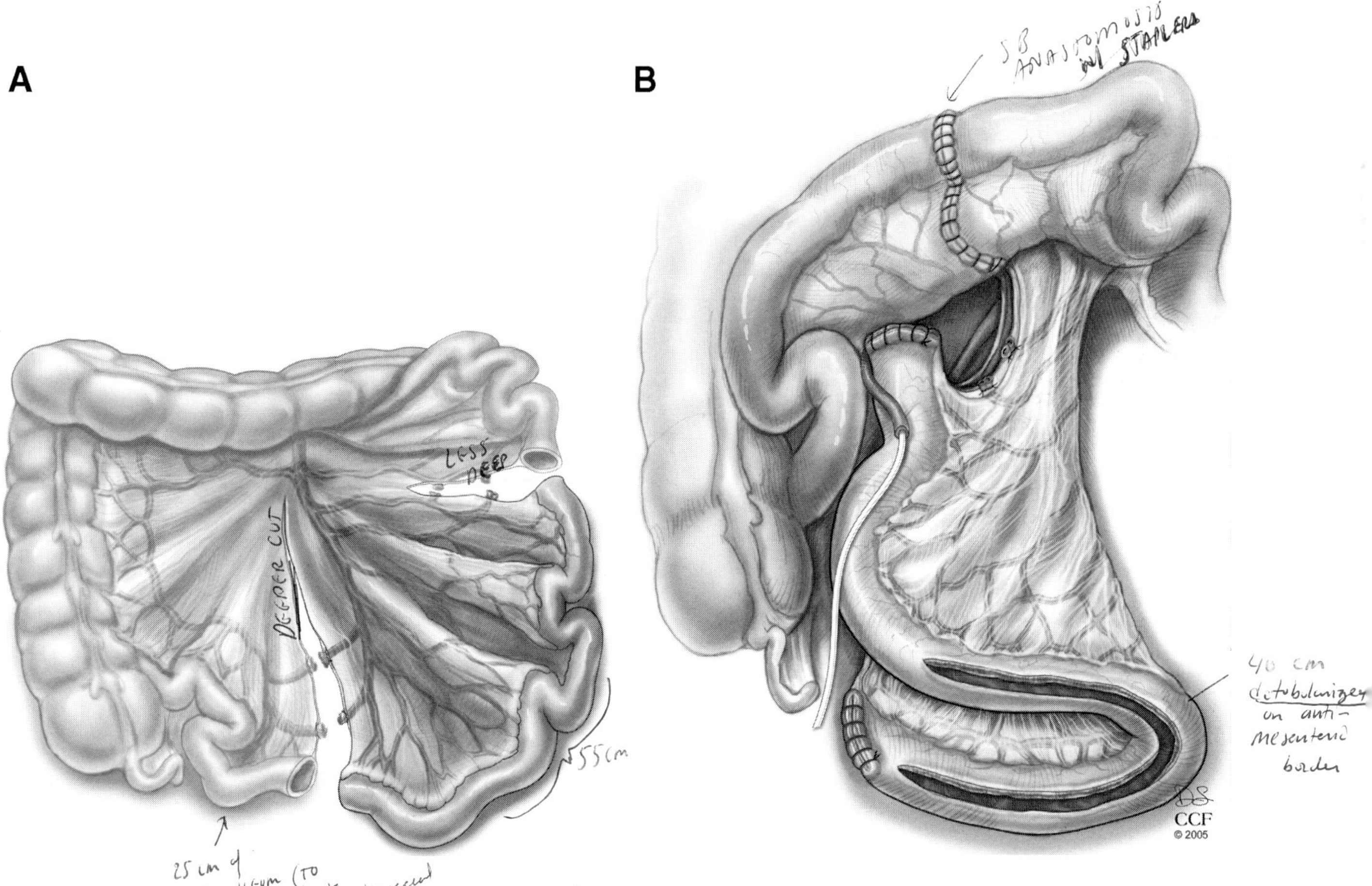

A

B

**Fig. 24.16**

Construction of an ileal neobladder. **(A)** 55 cm of distal ileum is isolated, beginning 25 cm proximal to the ileocecal valve. The distal mesenteric cut is deeper than the more proximal one to permit the neobladder to descend into the pelvis without

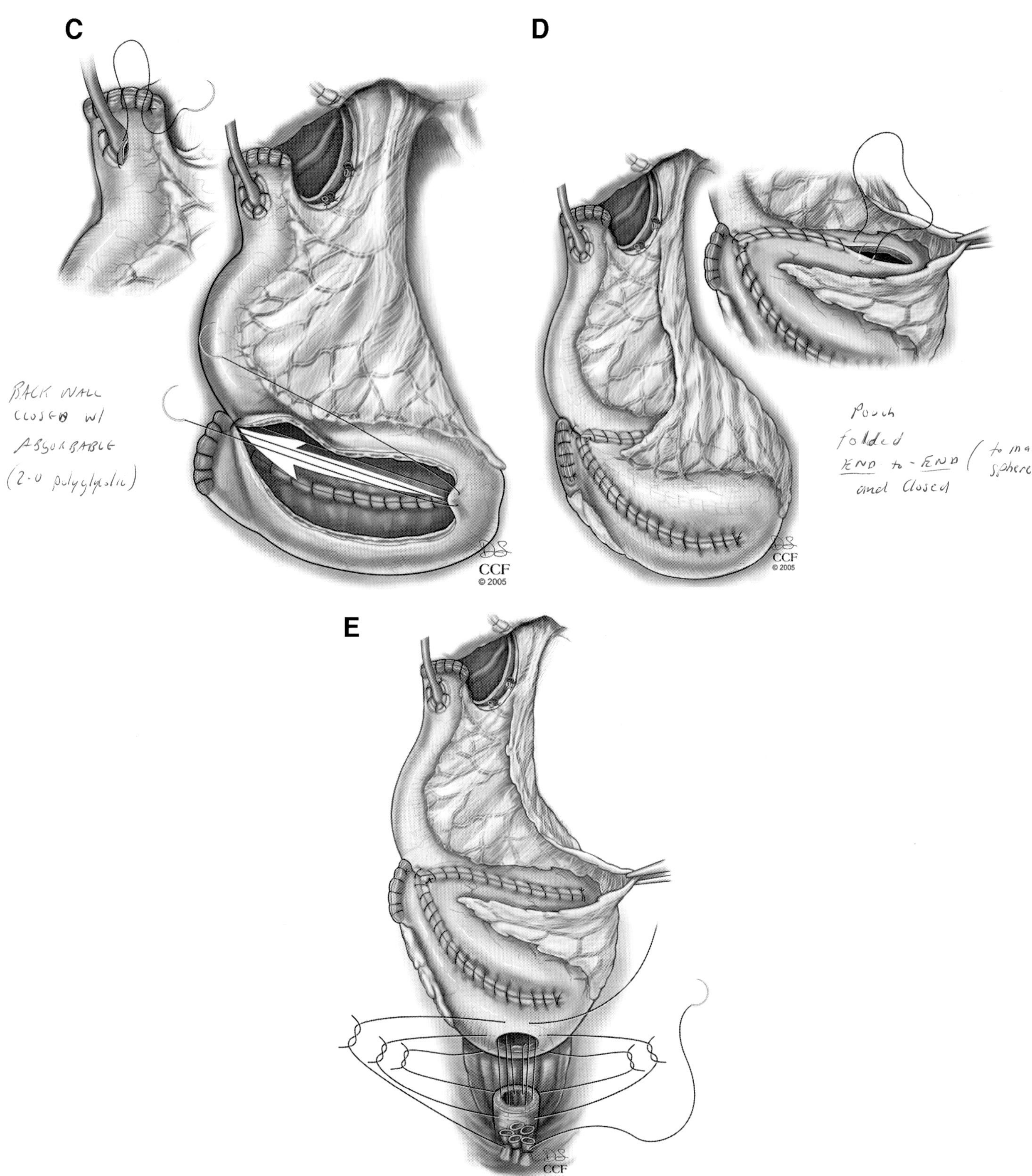


**Fig. 24.16** ***(Continued)***

tension. 10–15 cm of the proximal segment is left intact for attachment to the ureters. **(B)** The small bowel anastomosis is completed with staplers. 40–45 cm of the bowel is detubularized along the antimesenteric border. **(C)** The back wall of the neobladder is closed with running absorbable suture. The neobladder is then folded end-to-end and closed with additional running suture. **(D)** Appearance of the completed neobladder. **(E)** Completion of the neobladder-urethral anastomsis. (After Studer & Zingg Urol Clin North Amer 24:784, 1997.

will cause it to go into spasm and make it hard to work with) until it is free of fecal material. Approximately 40 cm of the pouch is then detubularized on the antimesenteric border, leaving the proximal 10–15 cm intact for later attachment of the ureters (Fig. 24.16B). The adjacent detubularized limbs are folded into a U shape, and the back wall is closed with a running 2-0 polyglycolic suture in a single layer (Fig. 24.16C). The time needed to construct the pouch can be reduced by having two surgeons sew simultaneously in opposite directions. The pouch is then folded over on itself end-to-end (not side-to-side) to form a roughly spherical shape, and additional running sutures are placed to complete the neobladder (Fig. 24.16C,D). The pouch is distended with warm saline to ensure water-tightness, and while full its most dependent portion is identified. An incision of approximately 20F diameter is made in the most dependent portion of the neobladder for anastomosis to the urethra (Fig. 24.16E). The previously placed urethral anastomotic sutures are placed in the corresponding position of the opening of the neobladder and tied over a 20 French Foley catheter (Fig. 24.16E).

The ureters are next anastomosed to the tubularized limb of the pouch over 90-cm single J stents in end-to-side refluxing fashion using running 4-0 chromic suture. Typically the left ureter is passed to the right side of the pelvis through an opening to the sigmoid mesentery. The stents are brought out through a separate stab incision at the base of the tubularized segment and secured there with a pursestring suture of 4-0 chromic. A 22 F mallecot catheter with two of the wings cut off is placed into the uppermost portion of the pouch and secured with a pursestring suture of 2-0 chromic. The ureteral stents and the mallecot catheter are brought out through the skin through separate stab incisions and secured to the skin. The stents serve to keep the pouch decompressed for 5–7 d while the suture line is healing. The mallecot catheter ensures adequate pouch drainage and serves as a conduit for irrigating mucous that might otherwise clog the Foley. A closed suction drain is placed in the pelvis and is also brought through a separate stab incision in the skin. The incision is then closed in a single layer using running 0-PDS, and the skin is approximated with staples.

## POSTOPERATIVE CARE

The nasogastric tube is removed in the recovery room or the following morning. The patients are ambulated on the first postoperative day, and oral intake is begun at 72 h. The ureteral stents, mallecot catheter, and Foley catheter are left to gravity drainage, and the mallecot and Foley are irrigated every 4 h to prevent mucous plugging. The stents are removed when the bowel ileus resolves and the closed suction drain 24 h later. Patients return at 14 d for a pouchogram and removal of the mallecot and Foley if no extravasation is demonstrated.

## REFERENCES

1. Nieder AM, Sved PD, Gomez P, Kim SS, Manoharan M, Soloway MS. Urethral recurrence after cystoprostatectomy: implications for urinary diversion and monitoring. Urology 64:950–954, 2004.
2. Stenzl A, Draxl H, Posch B, Colleselli K, Falk M, Bartsch G. The risk of urethral tumors in female bladder cancer: can the urethra be used for orthotopic reconstruction of the lower urinary tract? J Urol 153:950–955, 1995.
3. Parekh DJ, Gilbert WB, Smith JA, Jr. Functional lower urinary tract voiding outcomes after cystectomy and orthotopic neobladder. J Urol 163:56–58, 2000.
4. Minervini A, Boni G, Salinitri G, Mariani G, Minervini R. Evaluation of renal function and upper urinary tract morphology in the ileal orthotopic neobladder with no antireflux mechanism. J Urol 173:144–147, 2004.
5. Ward AM, Olencki T, Peerboom D, Klein EA. Should continent diversion be performed in patients with locally advanced bladder cancer? Urology 51:232–236, 1998.
6. Hautmann RE, Simon J. Ileal neobladder and local recurrence of bladder cancer: patterns of failure and impact on function in men. J Urol 162:1963–1966, 1999.
7. Bochner BH, Cho D, Herr HW, Donat M, Kattan MW, Dalbagni G. Prospectively packaged lymph node dissections with radical cystectomy: evaluation of node count variability and node mapping. J Urol 172:1286–1290, 2004.
8. Zippe CD, Raina R, Shah AD, et al. Female sexual dysfunction after radical cystectomy: a new outcome measure. Urology 63:1153–1157, 2004.

# 25 Laparoscopic Radical Cystectomy With Intracorporeal Urinary Diversion

*Jihad H. Kaouk and Inderbir S. Gill*

Laparoscopic cystectomy followed by conventional open urinary diversion has been reported by multiple investigators over the past decade *(1–5)*. However, it was not until laparoscopic reconstructive techniques, mainly intracorporeal free-hand suturing experience, matured that laparoscopic radical cystectomy with urinary diversion performed using intracorporeal techniques exclusively was performed *(5–10)*. Surgical steps of the laparoscopic approach follow the already established principles of oncological surgery with an effort to duplicate open conventional technique.

Our laparoscopic technique employs a six-port transperitoneal technique and includes radical cystectomy, extended bilateral pelvic lymphadenectomy, isolation of an ileal segment, restoration of bowel continuity, bilateral ureteral mobilization, and stented uretero-ileal anastomoses. During orthotopic ileal urinary diversion, a Studer-type ileal pouch is constructed, and ileo-urethral anastomoses are completed intracorporeally.

## PATIENT PREPARATION AND POSITIONING

Mechanical bowel preparation includes a clear liquid diet and 4 L of polyethylglycol the day prior to surgery. A stoma site is marked preoperatively for all patients. Broad-spectrum intravenous antibiotics are administered at anesthesia induction. The patient is placed in the low lithotomy position with both arms adducted. All body pressure points are well padded. Sequential compressing stockings are applied. The operation table is placed in the Trendelenburg position. A Foley catheter is inserted after sterile preparation and draping of the patient.

## LAPAROSCOPIC PORT PLACEMENT

A Veress needle is inserted into the abdomen at the inferior umbilical crease and $CO_2$ pneumoperitoneum is achieved at 15 mmHg. A 10-mm primary port is placed at the same umbilical site, and a 10m laparoscope with a 0° camera is introduced. A six-port transperitoneal technique is employed (Fig. 25.1). The surgeon stands on the left side of the patient and the camera holder on the right side.

From: *Operative Urology at the Cleveland Clinic*
Edited by: A. Novick et al. © Humana Press Inc., Totowa, NJ

## RADICAL CYSTECTOMY

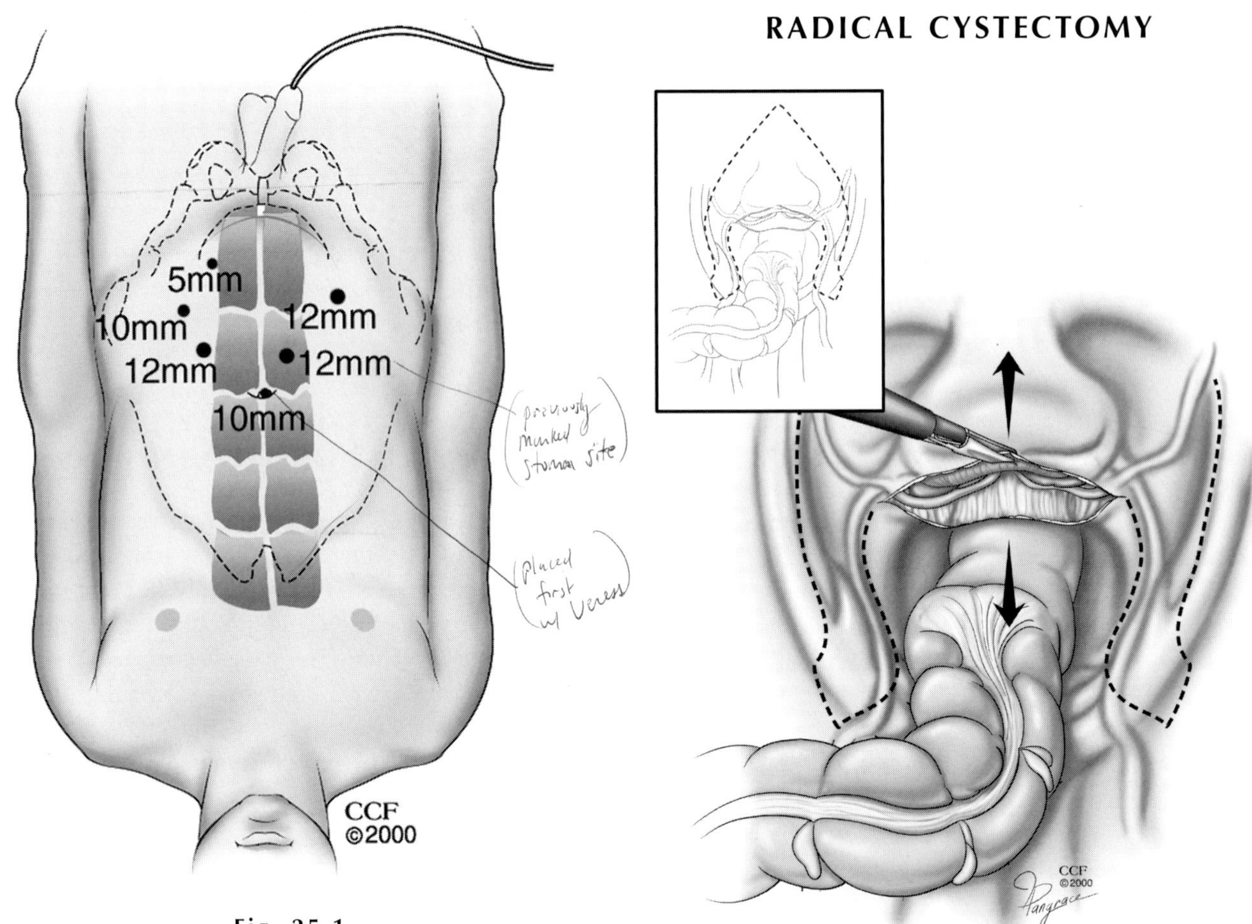


Fig. 25.1

After insertion of the primary port in the umbilicus, five secondary ports are inserted under visualization. A 12-mm right upper port is placed at the previously marked stoma site and is inserted through the belly of the right rectus muscle, carefully avoiding the right inferior epigastric vessels under clear visualization. For ileal conduit diversion, this port is removed and an ileal stoma is constructed at this site. Three other secondary ports are placed: a 1–2mm left upper port at the lateral edge of the left rectus muscle just below the level of the umbilicus, and 10- and 5-mm ports placed medial to the left and right anterior superior iliac spines, respectively. An additional sixth 5-mm port is placed midway between the umbilicus and the symphysis pubis at the time of urinary diversion.

Fig. 25.2

(Inset) The dotted line outlines the initial parietal peritoneal incision. A transverse peritoneotomy is created in the rectovesical cul-de-sac and extended superolaterally toward the ureteral crossing over the common iliac artery bilaterally. The peritoneal incision is continued along the external iliac artery toward the pubic bone. While applying cephalad traction to the base of the bladder, Denonvilliers' fascia is incised horizontally to reveal the perirectal fat, indicating entry into the proper prerectal plane. The seminal vesicles and vasa are not mobilized individually, but are maintained *en bloc* with the bladder specimen.

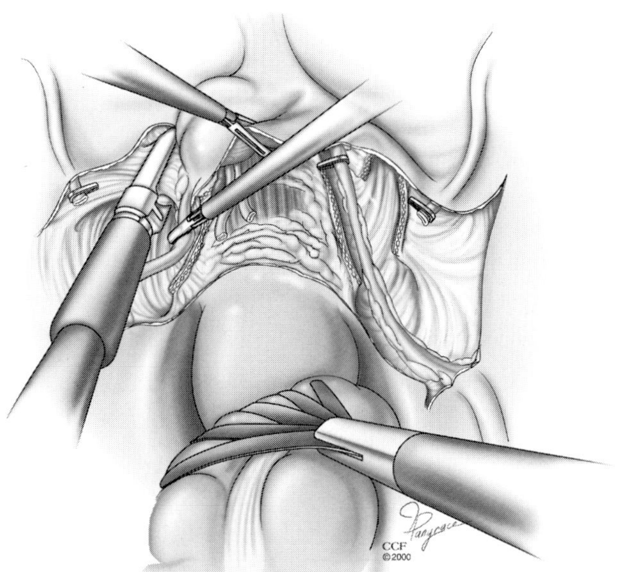


**Fig. 25.3**

The vasa are clipped and divided bilaterally. The distal ureters are traced from their crossing over the common iliac arteries and dissected close to the bladder, where they are clipped and divided. The distal ureteral margins are sent for frozen section evaluation. The lateral and posterior vascular pedicles of the bladder and prostate are controlled and transected with sequential firing of the Endo-GIA stapler. (Courtesy U.S. Surgical, Norwalk, CT.)

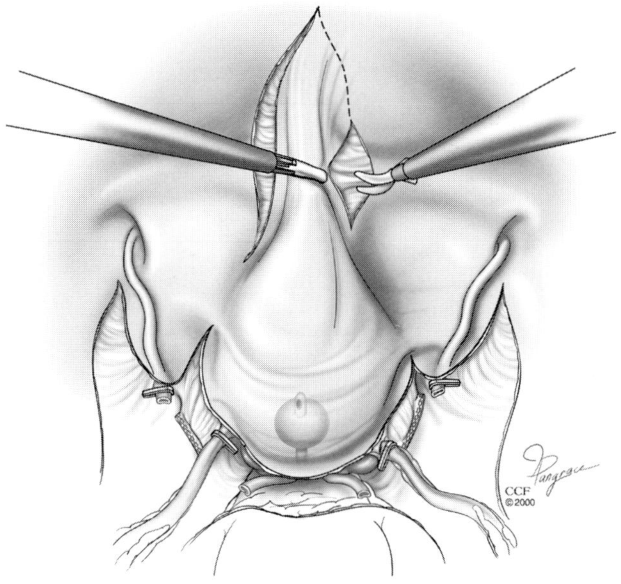


**Fig. 25.4**

The bladder is distended with 200 cc of saline and the Foley is occluded. An inverted U-shaped peritoneotomy is created lateral to the medial umbilical ligament towards the urachus that is transected high near the umbilicus. The antero-lateral bladder surface along with the perivesical fat is mobilized, and the space of Retzius is entered.

## MOBILIZATION OF THE URETERS

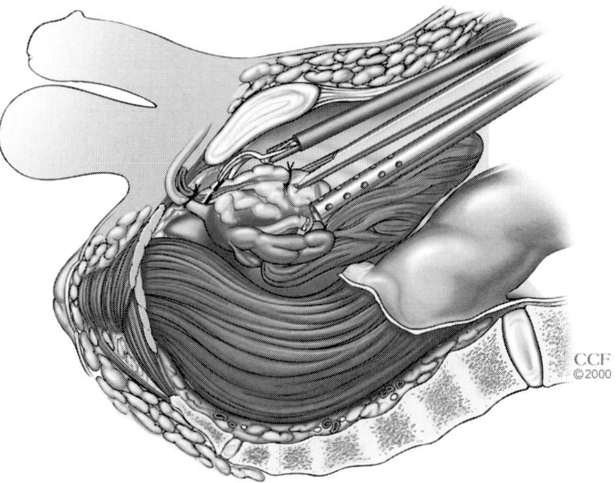


**Fig. 25.5**

The endopelvic fascia is incised and the dorsal vein complex is suture-ligated and then divided. The urethra is divided beyond the prostate apex. In women, a sponge stick inserted into the vagina helps to identify the anterior vaginal wall and subsequent plane of dissection. The anterior vaginal wall along with the uterus is excised. A frozen section evaluation of the urethral margin is performed. The specimen is entrapped in an Endocatch-II bag (U.S. Surgical, Norwalk, CT) for later extraction at the end of the procedure. In women, the specimen could be extracted intact through the already open vaginal vault after which the vaginal wall defect is reconstructed. However, if orthotopic neobladder is planned, we attempt to preserve the integrity of the anterior vaginal wall to guard against subsequent development of a neobladder-vaginal fistula. Bilateral extended pelvic lymph node dissection is then completed, extending from the common iliac artery proximally to the pubic bone distally, and from the genitofemoral nerve laterally to the obturator nerve infero-medially, circumferentially mobilizing both external iliac artery and vein and dissecting clean the pelvic wall.

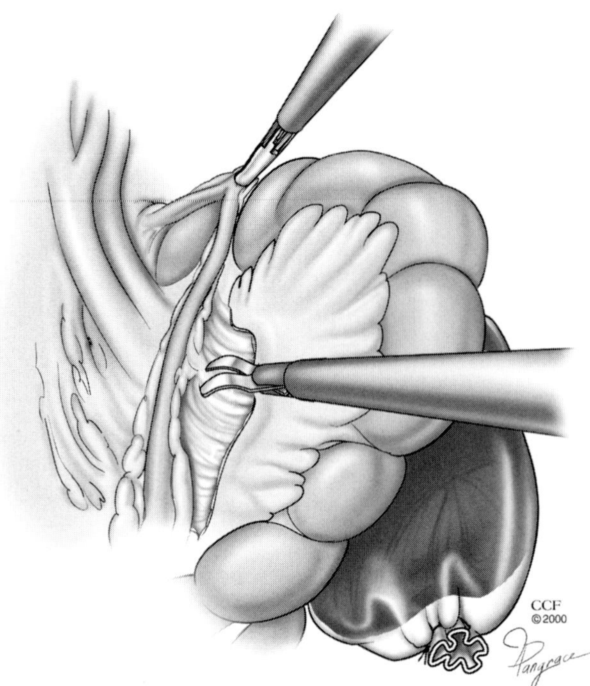


**Fig. 25.6**

Both ureters are mobilized cephalad, with adequate periureteral tissue to avoid ischemic injury to the ureters. Left ureteral dissection is shown.

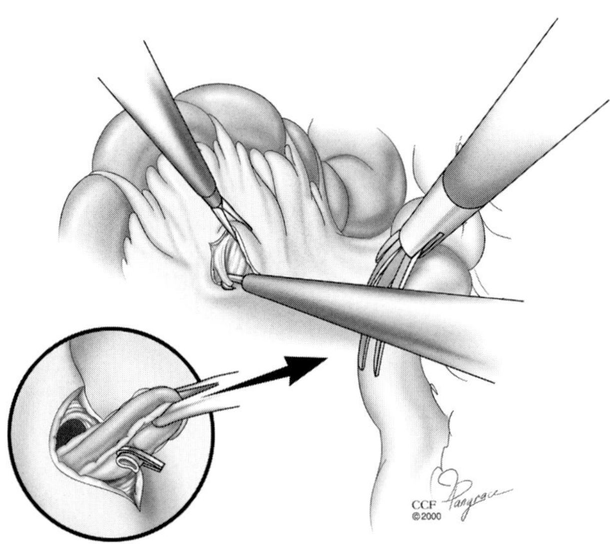


**Fig. 25.7**

Retroperitoneal transfer of the left ureter to the right pelvic side: an adequate opening in the base of the sigmoid mesentery is created just above the sacral promontory. The left ureter (inset) is then transferred through the mesenteric opening to the right side.

## ISOLATION OF ILEAL SEGMENT AND RESTORATION OF BOWEL CONTINUITY

The laparoscope is repositioned in the left lower 10-mm port while the surgeon and the camera holder are at the left side of the patient. Using the 5-mm infraumbilical port for the left hand and the right upper pararectal 12-mm port for the right hand (*see* Fig. 25.1), the surgical field is shifted to the right pelvic and abdominal side (Figs. 25.8–25.10).

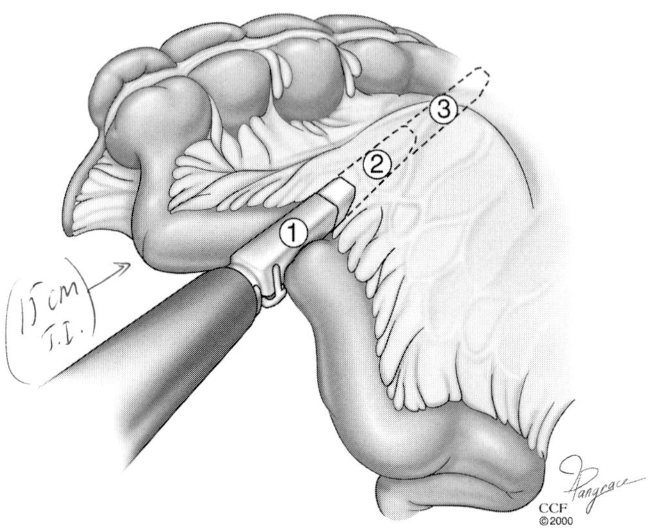


**Fig. 25.8**

An ileal segment is selected (15 cm for an ileal conduit and 60 cm for a Neobladder). Endo-GIA with a 45-mm bowel (1) stapler is used to transect the distal end of the ileal segment 15 cm away from the ileocecal junction. Two sequential firing of 45-mm vascular (2,3) staplers are used to transect the distal mesentery as shown, taking care not to compromise the major arterial arcade.

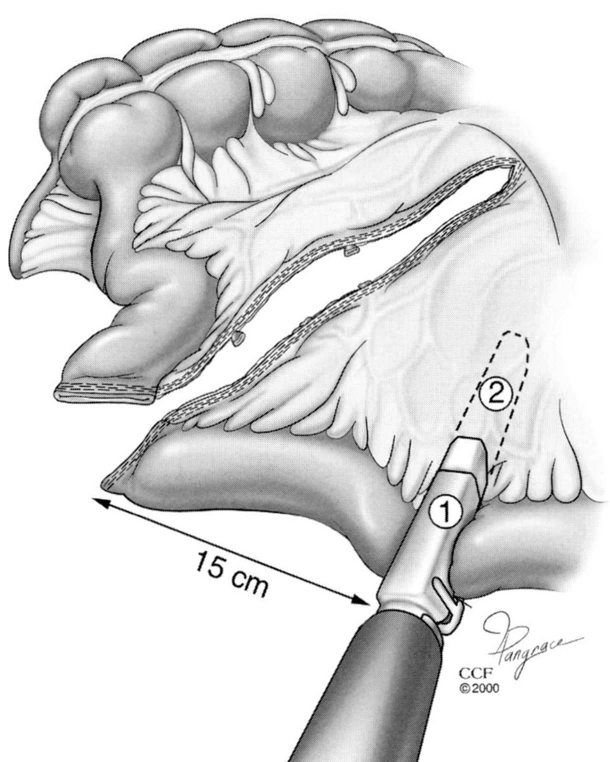


**Fig. 25.9**

The proximal end of the selected ileal segment is transected using an Endo-GIA with a 45-mm bowel (1) stapler. At the same site, one additional 45-mm vascular (2) stapler is used to transect the mesentery. Ileal segment is dropped posteriorly in preparation for restoration of bowel continuity anteriorly.

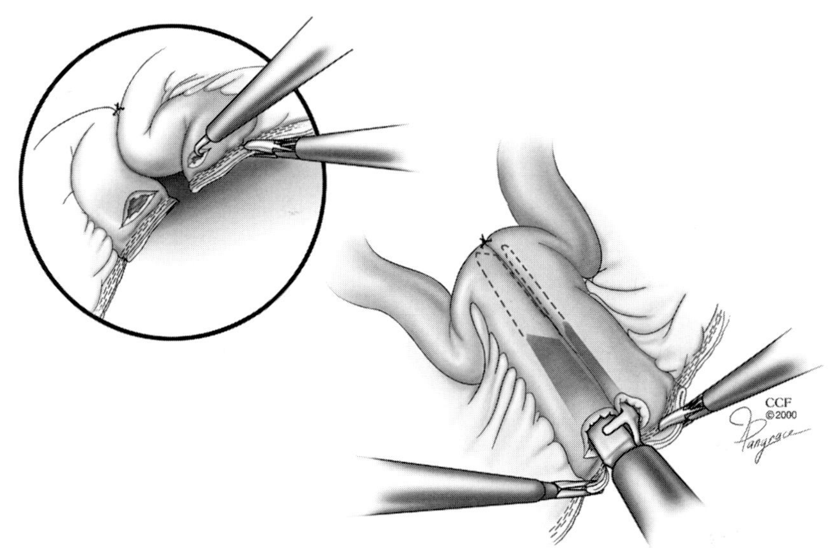


**Fig. 25.10**

Bowel continuity is achieved via side-to-side ileo-ileal anastomoses. The proximal and distal loops of the ileum are approximated and fixed together with a serosal suture along the antimesenteric border. The distal end of each ileal loop is opened (inset) to admit the Endo-GIA stapler, as shown. Two sequential stapler firings achieve adequate ileo-ileal anastomoses. Open ends of the joined ileum are closed with two transverse firings of an additional Endo-GIA followed by a suture reinforcement of the stapled anastomosis line, if felt to be necessary.

## ILEAL CONDUIT URINARY DIVERSION

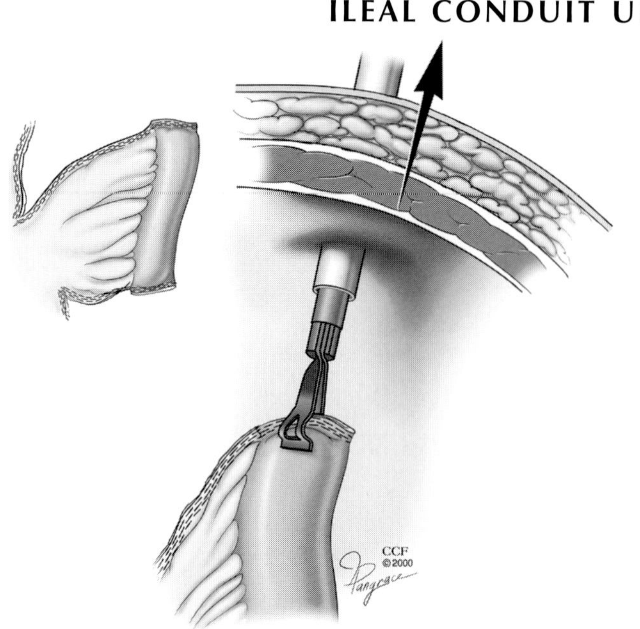


Fig. 25.11

The 12-mm port positioned at the previously marked stoma site is removed. The skin and fascia incisions are extended to admit the ileal conduit. The distal end of the isolated ileal segment is exteriorized, and the stoma is constructed using the conventional surgical technique.

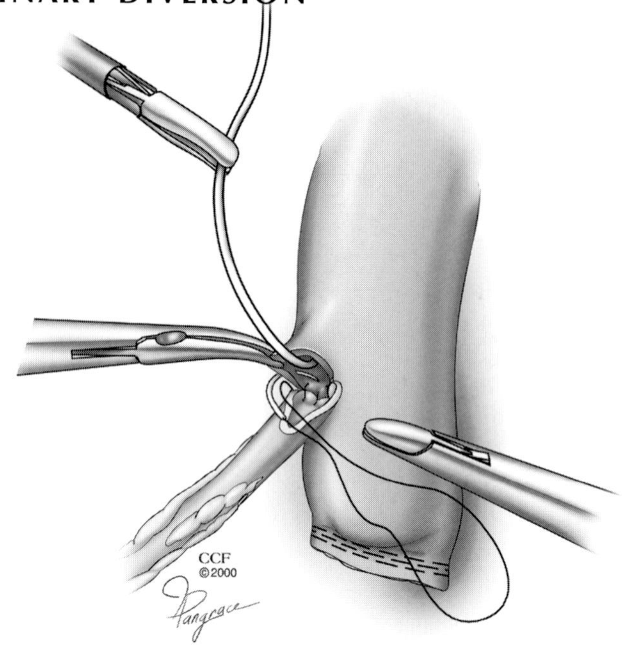


Fig. 25.13

The ureteral edge is refreshed and spatulated. Ureteroileal anastomosis is performed using two sutures of 3-0 vicryl on RB-1 needle. Initially, the apex of the spatulated ureter is fixed at the ileotomy site, as shown, and the stent is passed into the ureter up to the kidney. The anastomosis is then completed in a continuous suturing fashion. The same procedure is repeated for the contralateral ureter.

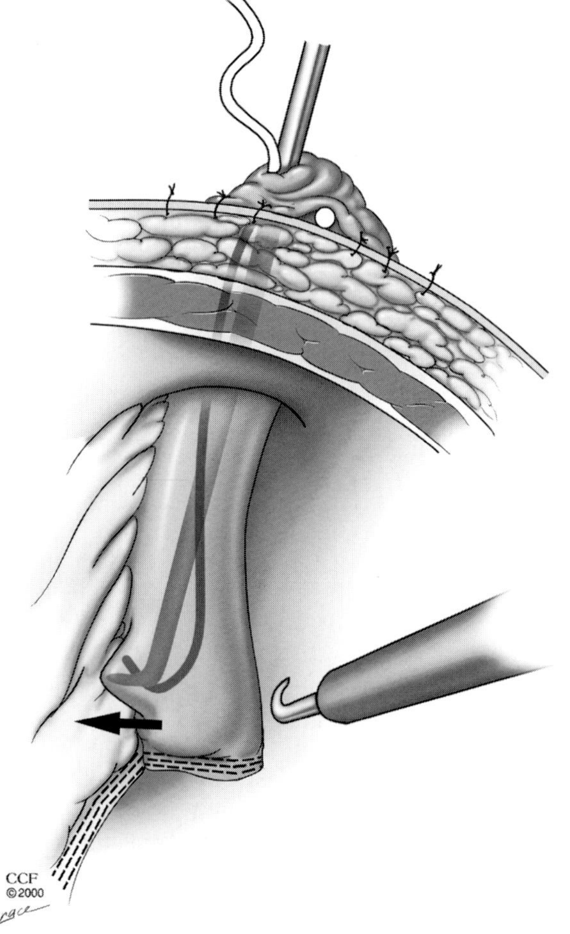


Fig. 25.12

A 5-mm laparoscopic right-angle clamp grasping the tip of a 90-cm single J-stent is inserted through the stoma into the conduit and advanced to a suitable site for uretero-ileal anastomosis under laparoscopic vision. The stent is then passed into the abdominal cavity through a small ileotomy.

# ORTHOTOPIC ILEAL NEOBLADDER URINARY DIVERSION

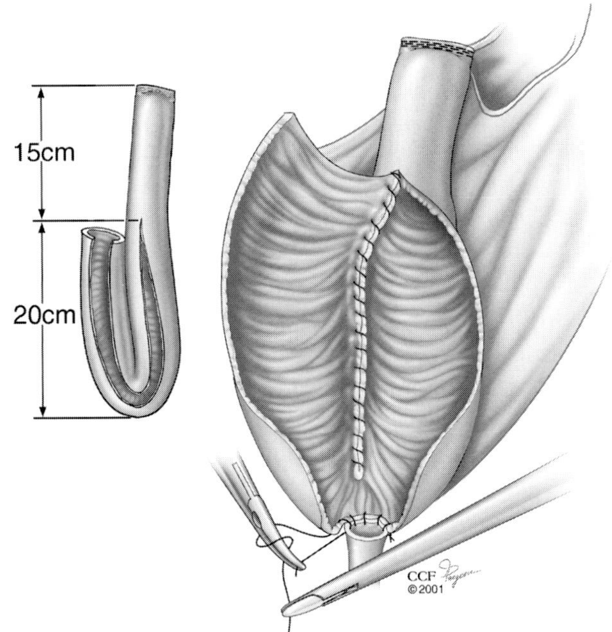


**Fig. 25.14**

The excluded ileal segment is cleaned by inserting the irrigation–suction device into the bowel lumen through a small ileotomy. The ileal segment is detubularized along its antimesenteric border preserving the proximal 15 cm intact as a Studer limb. The remaining 40 cm of detubularized ileum is then folded into a U-shape, and the inner edges of the ileum are sutured together using 2-0 vicryl sutures on CT-1 needles, forming the posterior neobladder plate. The posterior plate is advanced into the pelvis, and the urethroileal anastomosis is performed using two separate sutures of 2-0 vicryl on UR-6 needle.

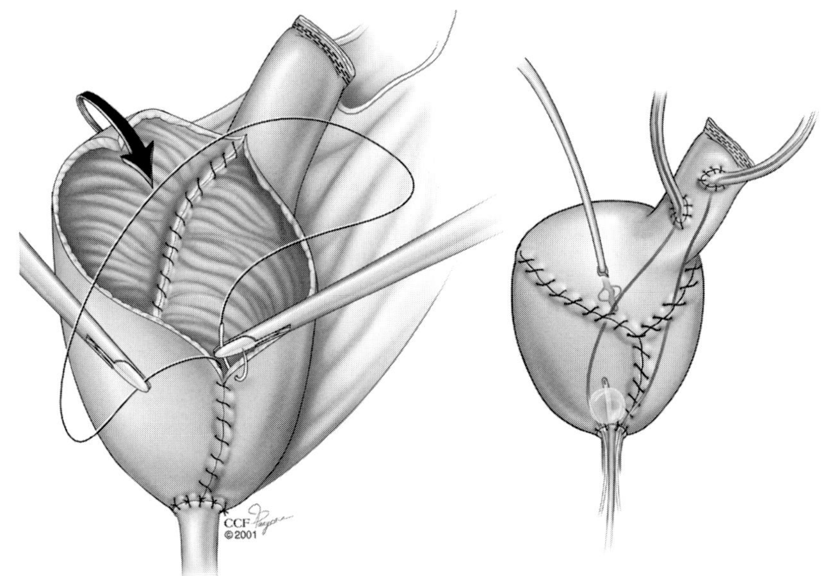


**Fig. 25.15**

The anterior wall of the neobladder is constructed after completion of urethroileal anastomosis over a 22 French Foley catheter. The curved arrow indicates the anteroposterior approximation of ileal plate to develop a spherical shape of the neobladder. Prior to complete construction of the anterior neobladder wall, two 90-cm single J-catheters are delivered through a small ileotomy into the anterior neobladder wall and exteriorized through two small separate ileotomies (1.5 cm each) in the Studer limb at the proposed ureteroileal anastomosis. The J-stents are inserted into each ureter toward the kidneys, and ureteroileal anastomosis is completed using 3-0 vicryl sutures over RB-1 needle. If necessary, a suprapubic catheter is inserted into the neobladder through the midline port site incision.

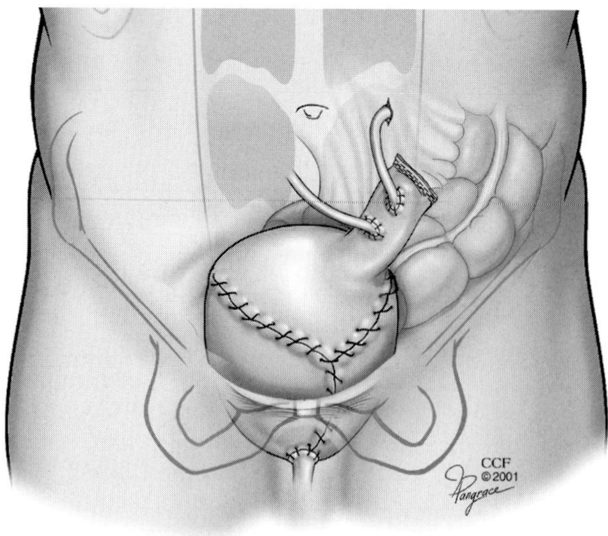


**Fig. 25.16**

The constructed neobladder is irrigated through the Foley catheter, and any obvious leakage from the suture line is repaired by a figure-of-eight stitch.

## SPECIMEN EXTRACTION AND LAPAROSCOPIC EXIT

Two Jackson–Pratt drains are inserted into the pelvis, one through the lower port site on each side. The specimen is extracted intact within the Endocatch bag through circumumbilical extension of the umbilical port site incision. If the specimen is large, a muscle-splitting Pfannenstiel extraction incision can be used. For women, specimen extraction through the vagina obviates the need for an additional incision.

## POSTOPERATIVE CARE

The neobladder is gently irrigated with 50 cc of saline every 4 h to prevent mucus plugging of the Foley catheter. The ileo-ureteral stents are removed 2 wk after a negative intravenous pyelogram. The Jackson-Pratt drains are removed sequentially, as per decrease in their output. The urethral Foley catheter and suprapubic catheter are removed 4 wk after a normal pouchogram.

## SUGGESTED READINGS

1. Denewer A, Kotb S, Hussein O, et al. Laparoscopic assisted cystectomy and lymphadenectomy for bladder cancer: initial experience. World J Surg 33:608, 1999.
2. Fergany AF, Gill IS, Kaouk JH, et al. Laparoscopic intracorporeally constructed ileal conduit after porcine cystoprostatectomy. J Urol 166:285, 2001.
3. Gill IS, Fergany A, Klein EA, et al. Laparoscopic radical cystoprostatectomy with ileal conduit performed completely intracorporeally: the initial 2 cases. Urology 56:26, 2000.
4. Gill IS, Kaouk JH, Meraney AM, et al. Laparoscopic radical cystectomy and continent orthotopic ileal neobladder performed completely intracorporeally: the initial experience. J Urol 168(1):13, 2002.
5. Kaouk JH, Gill IS, Desai MM, et al. Laparoscopic orthotopic ileal neobladder. J Endourol 15:131, 2001.
6. Kozminsky M, Partamian KO. Case report of laparoscopic ileal conduit. J Endourol 6:147, 1992.
7. Parra RO, Andrus CH, Jones JP, et al. Laparoscopic cystectomy: initial report on a new treatment for the retained bladder. J Urol 148:1140, 1992.
8. Puppo P, Perachino M, Ricciotti G, et al. Laparoscopically assisted transvaginal radical cystectomy. Eur Urol 27:80, 1995.
9. Sanchez de Badajoz E, Gallego Perales JL, Reche Rosado A, et al. Laparoscopic cystectomy and ileal conduit: case report. J Endourol 9:59, 1995.
10. Turk I, Deger S, Winkelmann B, et al. Laparoscopic radical cystectomy with continent urinary diversion (rectal sigmoid pouch) performed completely intracorporeally: the initial 5 cases. J Urol 165:1863, 2001.

# IV THE BLADDER (BENIGN)

# 26 Bladder Augmentation With or Without Urinary Diversion

*Raymond R. Rackley, Joseph Abdelmalak, and Jonathan Ross*

## INTRODUCTION

Augmentation cystoplasty (AC) is used as a reconstructive technique for creating a compliant, large-capacity urinary storage unit to protect the upper urinary tract and can provide urinary continence when more conservative management fails. The standard enterocystoplasty involves anastomosing an adequate-sized, well-vascularized patch of bowel with the urinary bladder. This procedure is classically performed through an open laparotomy incision utilizing various segments of the gastrointestinal system: stomach, ileum, cecum, and ascending and sigmoid colon. However, no intestinal segment is a perfect physiological substitute for a native bladder, and all have the potential for a variety of complications, including urinary tract infection, stone formation, small bowel obstruction, metabolic complications, fistula formation, and, rarely, malignancy transformation. The choice of the bowel segment is based on the primary clinical requirements of the patient and the secondary preference of the surgeons. Recently, the laparoscopic approach to bladder augmentation as outlined has become the primary approach for procedures of augmentation enterocystoplasty. As demonstrated below, the technical steps in performing a laparoscopic bladder augmentation are designed to emulate its open surgical counterpart in every aspect, producing similar functional results with an improved recovery.

## INDICATIONS AND PATIENT SELECTION

AC is indicated in chronically contracted bladders caused by tuberculosis, schistosomiasis, interstitial cystitis, neurogenic bladder dysfunction (resulting from spinal cord injuries), multiple sclerosis, myelodysplasia, and detrusor instability. In addition, various congenital conditions can result in a small, poorly compliant bladder that requires augmentation. For patients with physical disabilities who are unable to catheterize themselves via the urethra, a continent catheterizable abdominal stoma may be required in addition to a bladder augmentation.

A few contraindications to AC include bowel disease (Crohn's disease), abnormal or short bowel (especially after radiotherapy), bladder tumors, and severe radiation cystitis. Significant renal impairment may be a relative contraindication for AC in some patients.

## PATIENT PREPARATION

A complete evaluation of the upper and lower urinary tract is required, including blood urea nitrogen, serum creatinine, serum electrolytes, whole blood cell count, urinalysis, urine culture (when appropriate), renal ultrasonography, intravenous pyelography, a urodynamic study, and cystourethroscopy.

A clear liquid diet may be given to the patient for 2 d before the operation, and a bowel preparation is performed 1 d prior to the operation. Prophylactic antibiotics for bowel and urinary tract are required, as is antifungal medication when indicated. Barium enema is necessary to rule out diverticulosis if the sigmoid colon will be used. Many patients with neurological diseases have chronic constipation and may need more time for an adequate bowel preparation.

## SURGICAL TECHNIQUE

The patient is placed in the supine position, and pneumatic compression stockings are applied to both legs. After induction with general anesthesia and endotracheal

From: *Operative Urology at the Cleveland Clinic*
Edited by: A. Novick et al. © Humana Press Inc., Totowa, NJ

intubation, an oral gastric tube is inserted; both arms are tucked and protected along the sides. A 20 French urethral catheter is placed to provide effective intraoperative urine and pelvic fluid drainage. Depending upon an open or laparoscopic approach, either a midline incision or a lower abdominal transverse incision versus laparoscopic port placement is performed.

## BLADDER MOBILIZATION AND CYSTOTOMY

The bladder is distended with saline instillation through the uretheral catheter. The loose areolar tissue surrounding the bladder is bluntly dissected to expose the anterior bladder neck and perivesical spaces. A transverse wide U-shaped cystostomy incision is created, with the apex approaching the anterior bladder neck and the base extending posteriorly past the mid-coronal plane of the bladder dome. This type of cystostomy ensures a large disruption of the bladder musculature to increase the linear length of the bladder wall for bowel anastomosis. Other options may include a midline sagittal or mid-transverse cystotomy.

The surgical technique of enterocystoplasty has the following prerequisites: (1) selection of an optimal segment of bowel based on a broad, well-vascularized mesenteric pedicle, (2) isolation of the bowel segment, (3) reestablishment of bowel continuity and closure of the mesenteric defect, (4) detubularization and reconfiguration of the bowel segment without peritoneal soiling of bowel contents, (5) bladder mobilization with formation of an adequate-sized cystotomy, (6) creation of a tension-free, watertight, full-thickness circumferential anastomosis of the bowel to the bladder, and (7) confirmation of adequate postoperative urinary drainage.

## BOWEL SELECTION AND MOBILIZATION

Various segments of bowel can be used for augmentation depending on the clinical requirements of the patient and the preference of the surgeons. A length of 15–20 cm is usually desirable to attain an adequate augmented bladder capacity.

In ileocystoplasty, the initial step is identification of the ileocecal junction. Then a 20- to 25-cm segment of ileum at least 15 cm proximal to the ileocecal junction is required.

In sigmoidocystoplasty, a loop of sigmoid colon is identified. The sigmoid colon is the preferred segment of bowel for harvesting if the patients can easily perform intermittent catheterization via the urethra and a continent catheterizable stoma formation is not required. In addition, many patients may have a redundant sigmoid segment secondary to neurogenic bowel dysfunction.

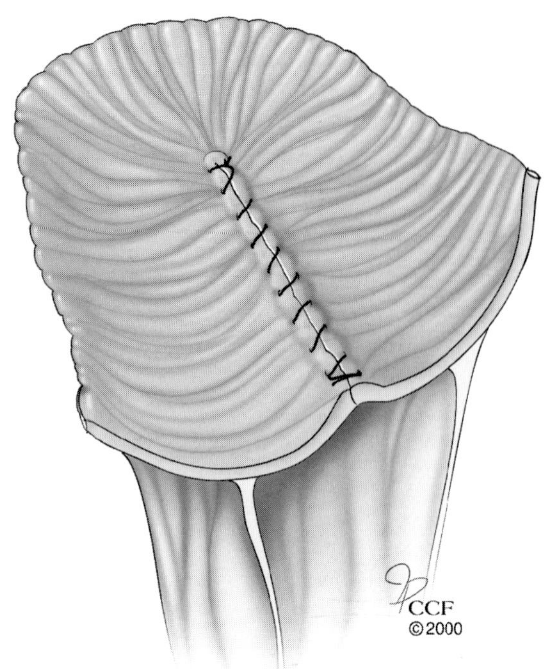


**Fig. 26.1**

Detubularization and reconfiguration of a U-shaped plate of bowel.

In ileocecocystoplasty, the cecum and ascending colon are used for the bladder augmentation, and 10–12 cm of terminal ileum are used to create the catheterizable conduit and stoma at the umbilicus. The peritoneum lateral to the cecum and ascending colon and the peritoneum of the terminal aspect of the Z line are incised, and the entire right colon and terminal ileum are mobilized.

The preselected loop of bowel is isolated with its pedicle between bowel clamps. Care is taken to prevent any twisting of the mesenteric pedicle and to ensure proper proximal-distal orientation of the loop. The excluded bowel segment is draped in moist warm sponges and then irrigated thoroughly with normal saline until the returning irrigation is clear. The antimesenteric border of the bowel is incised using electrocautery. For the small bowel or sigmoid, a U-shaped plate is created by a side-to-side anastomosis with 2-0 vicryl sutures (Fig. 26.1). Bowel continuity is reestablished using a gastrointestinal anastomosis stapling device, and the mesenteric window is closed.

For patients requiring a catheterizable stoma, the right colon and the terminal ileum are utilized and are extracorporealized through the laparoscopic port site for reconstructive purposes. Following detubularization of

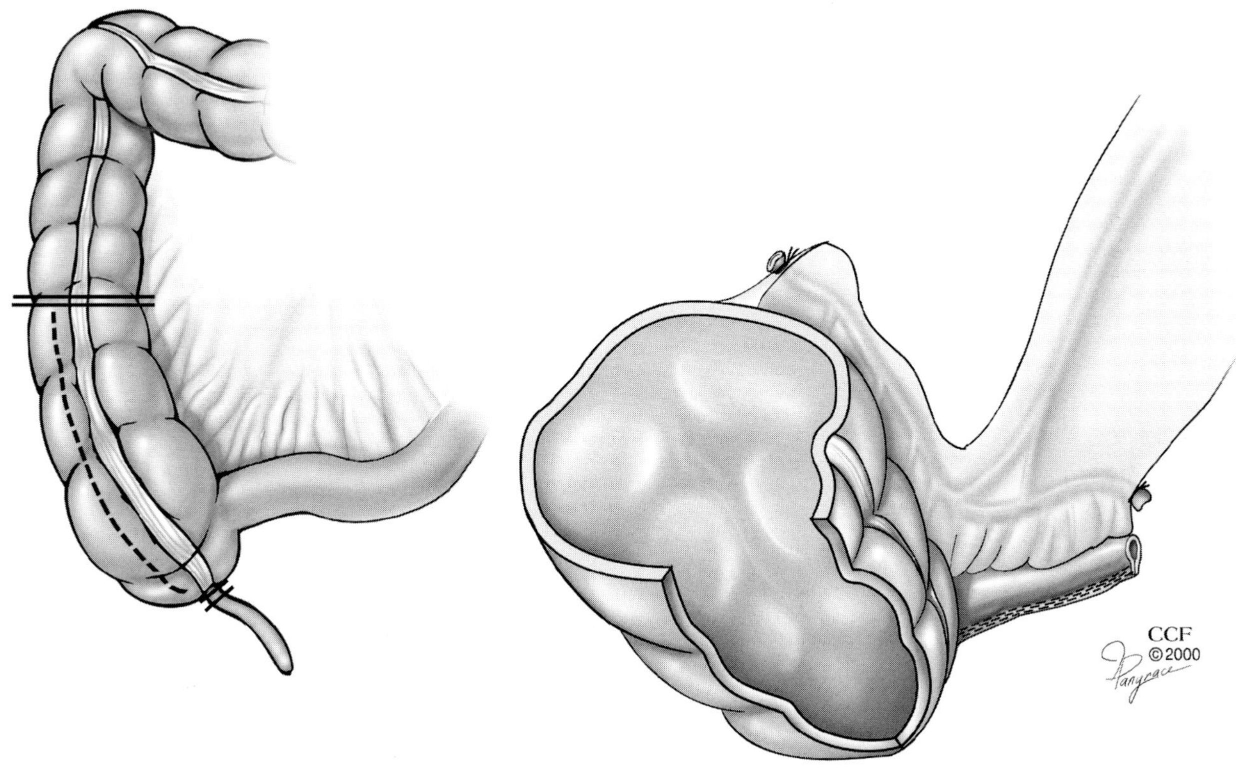


**Fig. 26.2**

Detubularization and reconfiguration of the right colon and ileum for cecocolocystoplasty in preparation for formation of a catheterizeable stoma.

the cecum and proximal colon, an appendectomy is performed (Fig. 26.2). The terminal ileum is narrowed over an 16 French red rubber catheter using a GIA stapler, and the ileocecal junction is imbricated and intussuscepted using 2-0 braided polyester sutures to augment the continence mechanism of the ileocecal valve (Fig. 26.3).

A circumferential, continuous, full-thickness, single-layer anastomosis of the bowel to the bladder is started posteriorly using 2-0 braided absorbable sutures (Fig. 26.4). At the completion of the anastomosis, the bladder is distended to confirm a watertight anastomosis. A drain is inserted into the pelvic cavity. Bladder drainage is maintained with a 24 French urethral catheter in women; a suprapubic tube may be an additional option in men who require a smaller urethral catheter.

In patients who require a catheterizable stoma, the previously refashioned ileal segment is delivered to the umbilicus and secured to the anterior rectus fascia and skin at the level of the umbilicus using 4-0 chromic sutures. A 16 French catheter is placed through the stoma and into the bladder to optimize the bladder drainage and the healing of the newly created catheterizable segment during the early postoperative period.

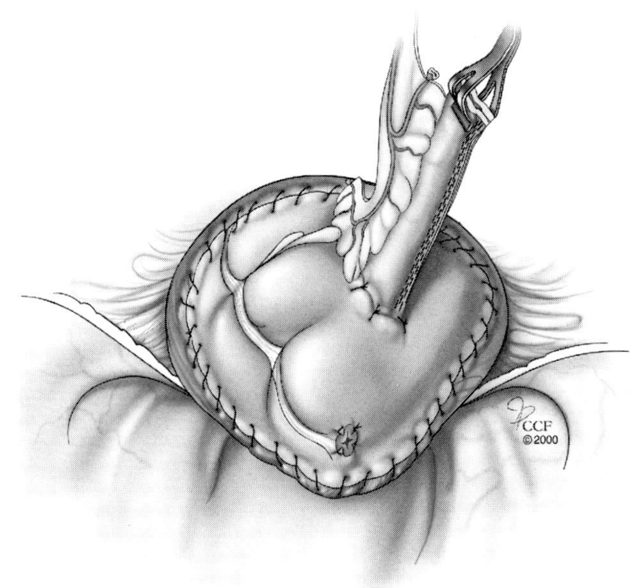


**Fig. 26.3**

The terminal ileum is narrowed over a 16 French red rubber catheter using a stapler and the ileocecal junction is imbricated and intussuscepted to augment the continence mechanism of the ileocecal valve.

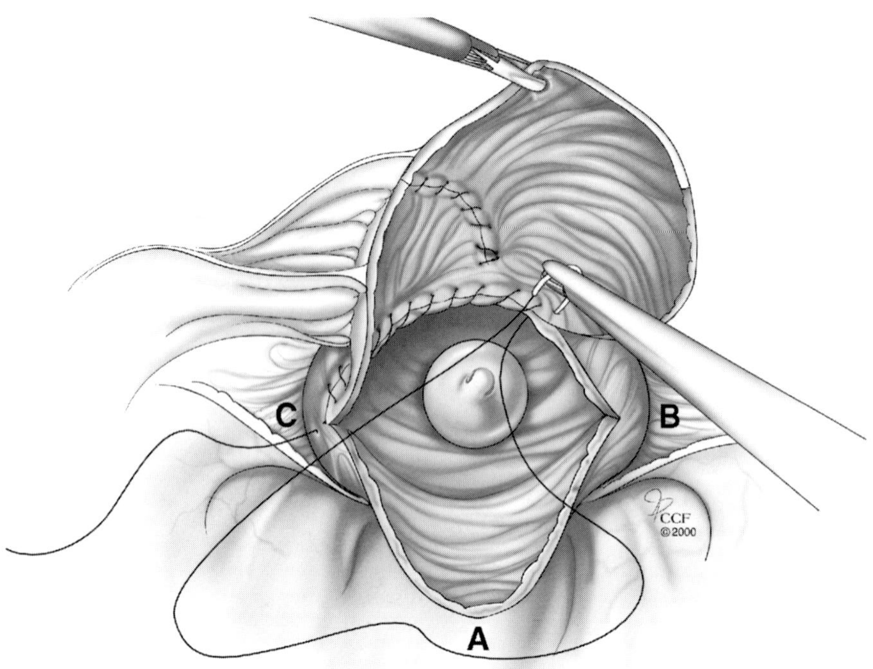


**Fig. 26.4**

Performing the circumferential, continuous, full-thickness, single-layer anastomosis of the bowel to the bladder.

In gastrocystoplasty, either the antrum or a wedge of stomach from the greater curvature can be used. The pyloric antrum of the stomach is excised and is brought down to the pelvis on a pedicle of omentum, along with its blood supply from the left gastroepiploic artery (Fig. 26.5).

When using a wedge of stomach from the greater curvature (Fig. 26.6), the greater omentum is incised along the edge of the greater curvature of the stomach. The gastric wedge is resected using a stapling device. The gastric wedge, with its blood supply from right gastroepiploic artery, is retroperitonealized through the mesentery of the transverse colon and small bowel and brought down into the pelvis. The stable line of the stomach is then removed and the incision is closed using a two-layer closure.

## LAPAROSCOPIC AUGMENTATION CYSTOPLASTY

The patient is placed in the supine position, and pneumatic compression stockings are applied to both legs. After induction with general anesthesia and endotracheal intubation, an oral gastric tube is inserted, and the patient is placed in the low-lithotomy position for the remainder of the operation. Both arms are tucked and protected along the sides so that the surgical team can direct its operative movements deep into the pelvis. Effective intraoperative urine and pelvic fluid drainage can be provided by intermittently opening the 20–24 French urethral catheter to preserve the pneumoperitoneum.

An incision is made at the superior umbilical crease, and a disposable 10- to 12-mm port with occluding balloon and cuff is introduced under direct vision into the peritoneal cavity. A 10-mm, 0-degree laparoscope is introduced, and the subsequent reusable ports are introduced under visual guidance. Ten- or 5-mm ports are inserted bilaterally at the lateral borders of the rectus muscle at the level of the umbilicus (Fig. 26.7). Most of the operative suturing takes place via the two paraumbilical ports. The 10-mm port facilitates the introduction of sutures by the primary surgeon. An additional 5-mm port is inserted at the level of the left anterior superior iliac spine. Other ports may be placed depending on the bowel mobilization required and the surgeon's preference.

## LAPAROSCOPIC BOWEL SELECTION AND MOBILIZATION

As is true in open enterocystoplasty, various segments of bowel can be used for the procedure. depending on the clinical requirements of the patient. A length of 15–20 cm is usually desirable to attain an adequate augmented bladder capacity.

In laparoscopic ileocystoplasty, after identification of the ileocaecal junction, a 25-cm segment of ileum at least 15 cm proximal to the ileocecal junction is identified. A 5-mm laparoscope may be introduced through the lower left port to transilluminate the mesentery and to

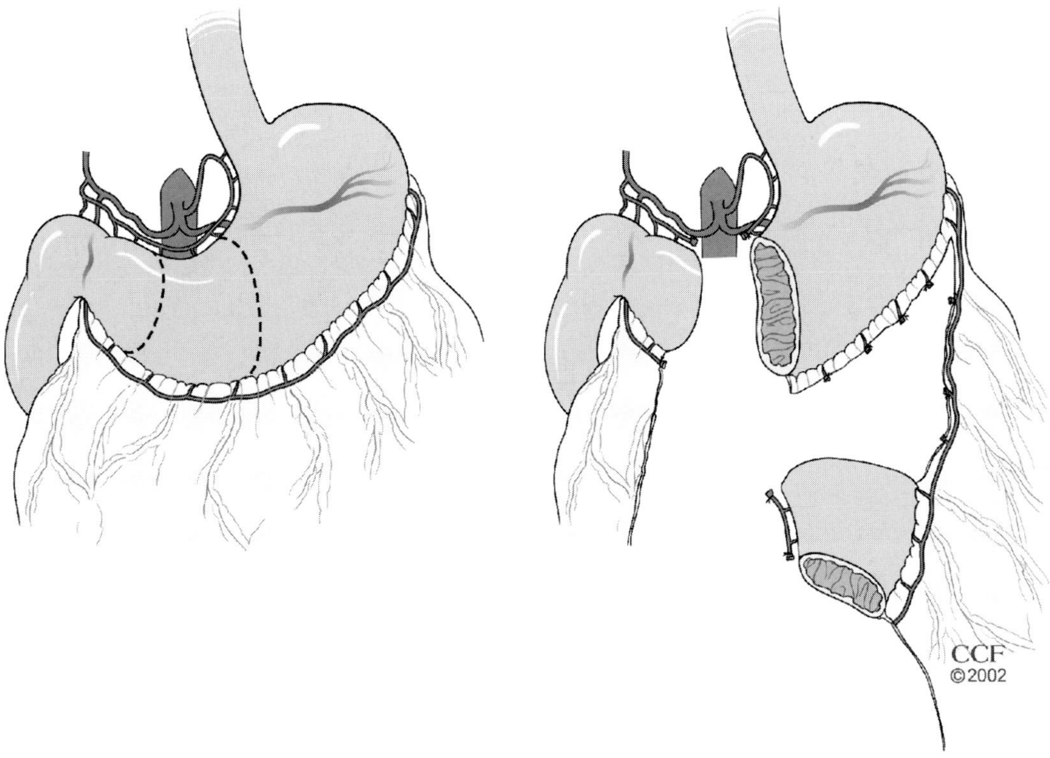


**Fig. 26.5**

Excising the pyloric antrum of the stomach on a pedicle of omentum with its blood supply.

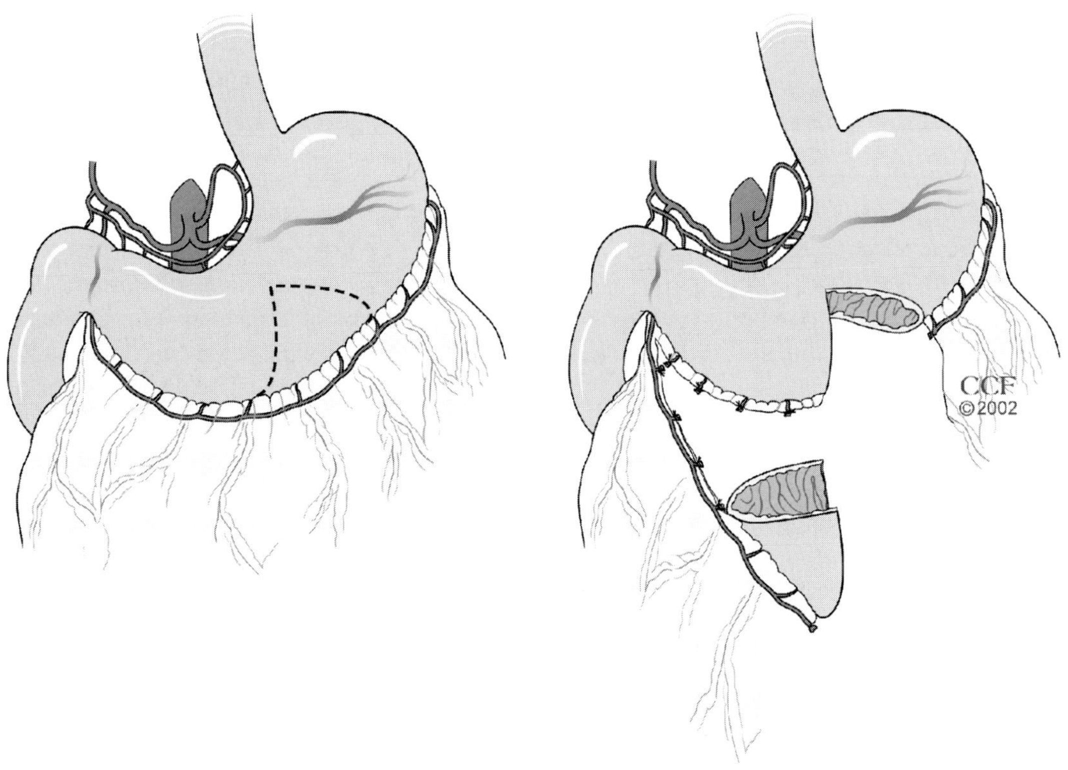


**Fig. 26.6**

Incising the greater omentum along the edge of the greater curvature of the stomach using a stapler.

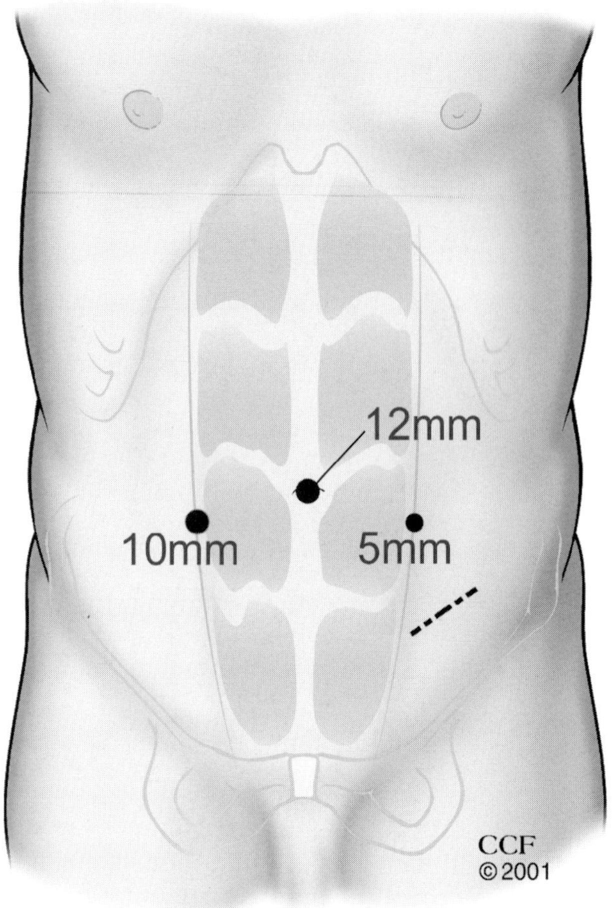


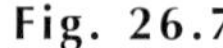
**Fig. 26.7**

Options for selection of port sizes and location in laparoscopic enterocystoplasty procedures.

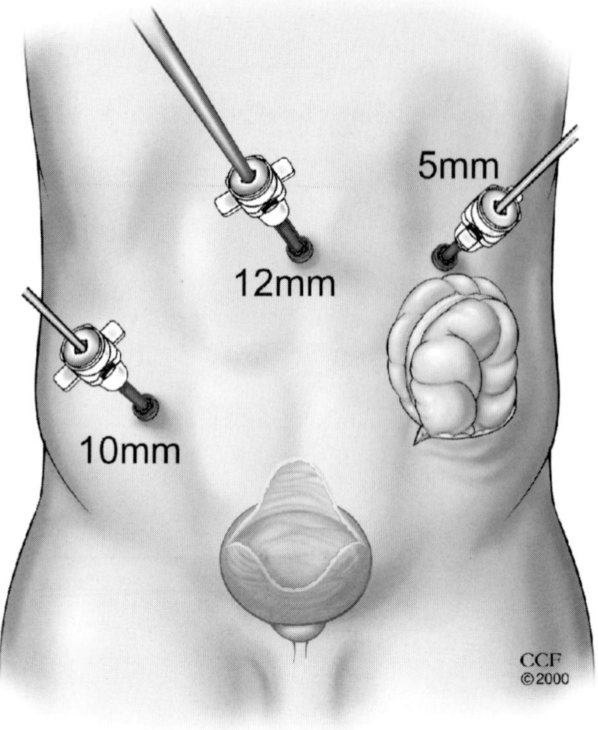


**Fig. 26.8**

Selection of port sizes and location for laparoscopic sigmoidocystoplasty.

identify its vascular pedicle. The mesentery adjacent to the proximal and distal ends of the selected bowel loop is scored with laparoscopic electrosurgical scissors for subsequent extracorporeal identification.

In laparoscopic sigmoidocystoplasty, a loop of sigmoid colon is selected using similar techniques. A 10-mm port is placed medial to the level of the right anterior iliac spine and facilitates sigmoid mobilization for extracorporeal manipulation via extension of the lower left abdominal port defect (Fig. 26.8).

The right colon and terminal ileum are selected in patients who, in addition to bladder augmentation, require a continent catheterizable abdominal stoma using the same traditional open surgical techniques. The entire right colon and terminal ileum are mobilized for extracoporeal manipulation via the extended incision of the umbilical port. Ensuring a low position of the patient's thighs with low lithotomy enables proper manipulation of the laparoscopic instruments through the lower abdominal ports for mobilization of the right colonic flexure.

## LAPAROSCOPIC EXCLUSION AND REANASTOMOSIS OF THE BOWEL

The pneumoperitoneum is then desufflated, and the umbilical port is removed. The umbilical incision is enlarged circumumbilically and extended inferiorly in obese cases for an additional 2 cm. The preselected loop of bowel is delivered extracorporeally through this incision. Care is taken to prevent any twisting of the mesenteric pedicle and to ensure proper proximal-distal orientation of the loop. Using traditional open surgical techniques, the 20 cm of bowel segment with its pedicle is divided between bowel clamps and isolated as performed in ileocystoplasty (Fig. 26.9). Bowel continuity is reestablished using traditional open techniques, and the mesenteric window is closed. The bowel anastomosis is performed cephalad to the excluded segment of bowel, and the reanastomosed bowel is returned to the abdominal cavity before any further manipulations. This step reduces the potential need to enlarge the circumumbilical incision for reintroduction of an edematous combination of both the bowel reanastomosis and the reconfigured bowel segment for augmentation.

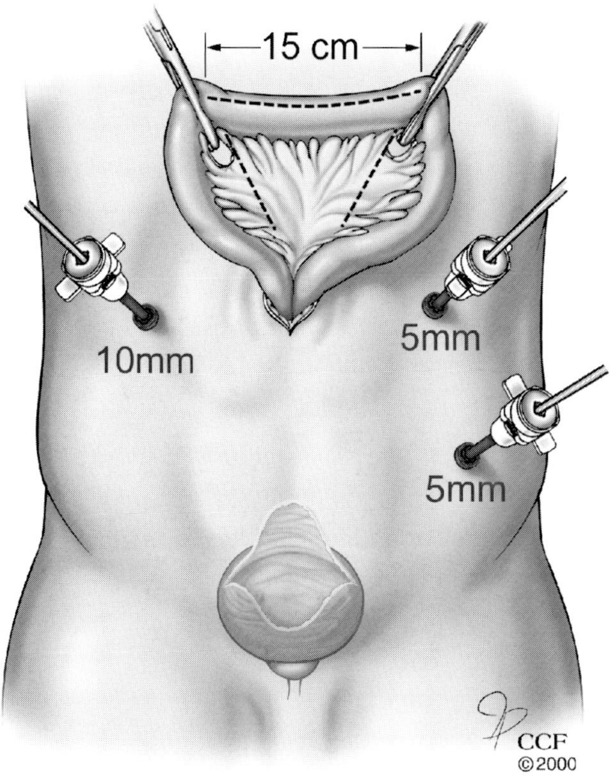


**Fig. 26.9**

Extracorporeal isolation and manipulation of the small bowel via the umbilical port site.

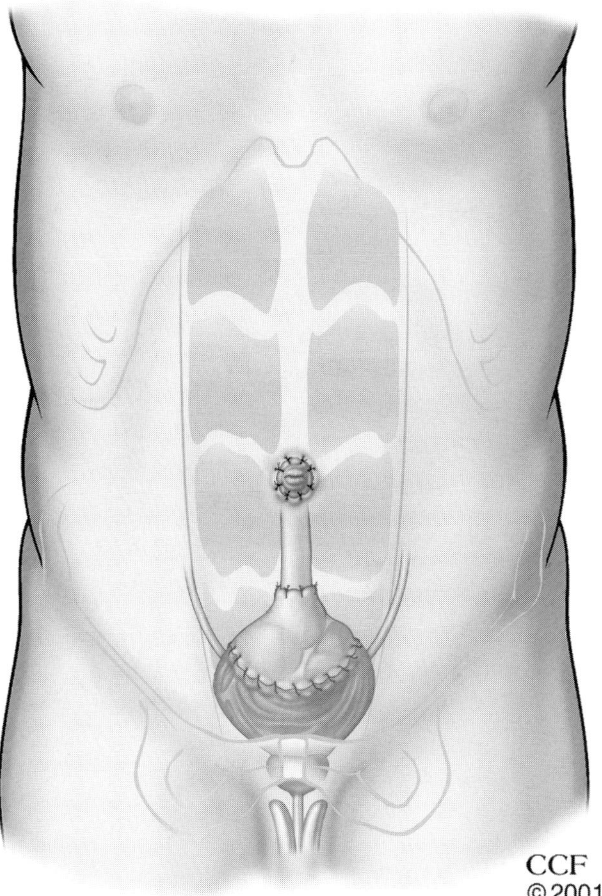


**Fig. 26.10**

View of the completed laparoscopic bowel to bladder anastomosis in preparation for maturation of the catheterizeable stoma to the umbilicus.

## REFASHIONING OF THE ISOLATED BOWEL SEGMENT

The excluded bowel segment is draped in moist warm sponges and then irrigated thoroughly with normal saline until the returning irrigation is clear. The antimesenteric border of the bowel is incised using electrocautery. For the small bowel or sigmoid, a U-shaped plate is created by a side-to-side anastomosis with 2-0 braided absorbable suture, as shown in Fig. 26.1. After the isolated bowel segment for augmentation is reintroduced into the peritoneal cavity, the ports are replaced to reestablish the pneumoperitoneum. In laparoscopic AC, reintroducing a disposable 10- to 12-mm, blunt-tip port with a fascial retention balloon and foam cuff to minimize gas leakage is advantageous.

In sigmoidocystoplasty, the extended lower left abdominal port incision is reduced to accommodate a 10-mm port. The pneumoperitoneum is then reestablished and the laparoscope inserted. The isolated bowel segment is oriented appropriately and inspected to exclude torsion of the pedicle.

For patients requiring a catheterizable stoma, the right colon and terminal ileum are utilized. Following detubularization of the cecum and proximal colon, an appendectomy is performed. The terminal ileum is narrowed over a 16 French red rubber catheter using a gastrointestinal stapling device, and the ileocecal junction is imbricated and intussuscepted to augment the continence mechanism of the ileocecal valve using 2-0 braided polyester sutures (Fig. 26.10). Orientation sutures are placed at the cephalic end and the caudal end of the bowel patch to facilitate intracorporeal laparoscopic identification and manipulation. The 16 French red rubber catheter is secured to the terminal end of the catheterizable segment of ileum with a 2-0 silk suture for atraumatic intracorporeal manipulation and for delivering this terminal segment to the umbilicus for stoma maturation at the end of the procedure. The isolated bowel patch is then returned to the abdominal cavity, and the infraumbilical incision is closed over a 10- to 12-mm blunt-tip port with a fascial retention balloon and foam cuff to minimize gas leakage for the remainder of the operation. After the pneumoperitoneum is reestablished and the laparoscope

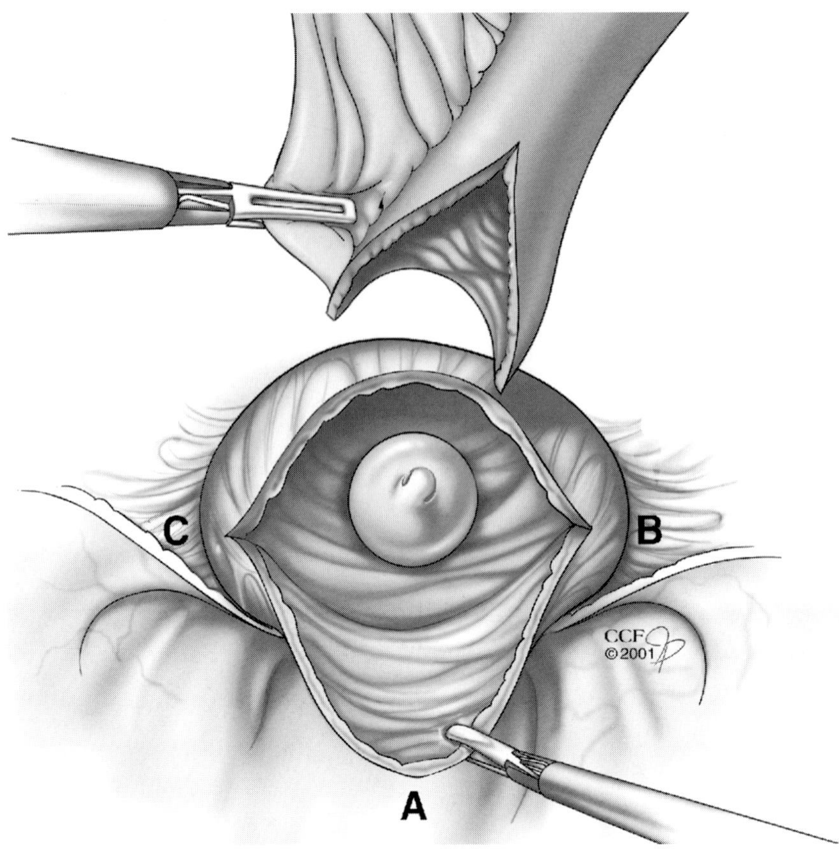


**Fig. 26.11**

An anterior bladder flap cystotomy incision used for performing a laparoscopic ileovesicostomy.

inserted, the isolated bowel segment is oriented appropriately and inspected to rule out torsion of the pedicle.

Exclusion of the bowel segment and subsequent restoration of bowel continuity can be performed intracorporeally using endoscopic staplers. We prefer performing these manipulations extracorporeally by delivering the bowel outside the abdomen through the umbilical or lower abdominal port site, respectively, for several reasons. The bowel segment can be measured precisely, and incision of the mesentery may be performed after ensuring good vascularity. The reanastomosis of the bowel can be performed meticulously using open surgical techniques with increased confidence. The irrigation of the excluded loop can be performed without any peritoneal spillage, thereby eliminating the potential for subsequent pelvic abscess formation. The detubularization and desired modification of the isolated loop can be performed expeditiously by traditional open suturing. If the mesenteric length allows the segment to be delivered outside the anterior abdominal wall comfortably without evidence of bowel ischemia, it is also likely to reach the bladder without tension. The extracorporal approach allows considerable savings in overall operative time and cost.

## LAPAROSCOPIC BLADDER MOBILIZATION AND CYSTOTOMY

Placing the patient in the Trendelenburg position aids in displacement of bowel loops from the pelvic cavity and facilitates the subsequent steps of the procedure. The bladder is distended with saline through the uretheral catheter. The peritoneum overlying the bladder is incised at the medial border of the left medial umbilical ligament and extended to the right in a linear fashion to the right medial umbilical ligament. The median umbilical ligament is taken down during the procedure using the electrosurgical scissors. If needed, the lateral peritoneum incisions are extended down along the medial umbilical ligaments to increase exposure. The loose areolar tissue surrounding the bladder is bluntly dissected for exposure of the anterior bladder neck and perivesical spaces. A large cystostomy is created by making an anterior bladder wall flap through a curvilinear incision that positions the apex approaching the bladder neck and the base extending posteriorly past the mid-coronal plane of the bladder dome as shown for performing a laparoscopic ileovesicostomy urinary diversion (Fig. 26.11). This type of cystostomy ensures a large dysfunctional disruption of the bladder musculature for increasing the linear length of bladder wall for bowel anastomosis. It is most useful in cases where the uterus is present and potentially prevents an adequate cystostomy incision. Furthermore, adequate exposure for enterovesical anastomosis in all of the procedures described previously is preserved by avoiding closure of a deep posterior bladder wall incision in the pelvis that will be obscured by bowel and the isolated bowel segment to be used for the augmentation.

## LAPAROSCOPIC ENTEROVESICAL ANASTOMOSIS

Although different approaches can be used for intracorporeal suturing of the bowel segment to the bladder, we prefer to begin by running the preplaced suture on the posterior wall of the reconfigured bowel patch to the apical aspect of the bladder flap in a medial to lateral direction on each side. Completion of the posterior wall of the reconfigured bowel segment from an intravesical approach beginning medially (point A) and finishing laterally (points B and C, respectively) facilitates the best exposure to ensure a watertight anastomosis (Fig. 26.4). If one attempts to complete the anterior wall of the reconfigured bowel patch to the bladder first, visualization for suturing the posterior wall anastomosis to the bladder may be difficult because of the constraints of the pelvic anatomy.

To complete a circumferential, continuous, full-thickness, single-layer anastomosis of the bowel to the bladder, we run the preplaced sutures of the anterior wall of the reconfigured bowel patch and additional sutures as required. The entire suturing is performed exclusively using freehand laparoscopic suturing and intracorporeal knot-tying techniques. A 5-mm needle holder is used to perform the anastomosis. An assistant follows the sutures with a 5-mm grasper. At the completion of the anastomosis, the bladder is distended to confirm a watertight anastomosis. A drain is inserted into the pelvic cavity through a lower lateral 5- or 10-mm port site. In female patients, bladder drainage is maintained with a 20–24 French urethral catheter. Because a smaller urethral catheter is preferred for postoperative drainage in males, a suprapubic tube is placed through the bladder wall and externalized via the remaining lower port site. The umbilical port and any remaining 10-mm ports are closed in layers.

In patients who require a catheterizable stoma, the previously refashioned ileal segment is located and the attached red rubber catheter is grasped with an endo-clamp via the umbilical port site, as shown in Fig. 26.10. After the pneumoperitoneum is decompressed, the terminal end of the ileal segment is delivered to the umbilicus and secured to the anterior rectus fascia and skin at the level of the umbilicus. A Y-V flap maturation of the stoma to the skin of the umbilicus is performed using 4-0 chromic sutures. In obese patients, use of the umbilicus as the site of stoma formation decreases the amount of ileum needed to mature the stoma to the skin. A 16 French catheter is placed through the stoma and into the bladder to optimize bladder drainage and the healing of the newly created catheterizable segment in the early postoperative period.

## POSTOPERATIVE MANAGEMENT

The oral-gastric decompression tube is removed before extubation. The pelvic drain is removed when the drainage is less than 25 mL or fluid chemistries suggest peritoneal fluid. Discharge criteria are met when the patient is afebrile and able to complete three consecutive meals without abdominal distention or symptoms of nausea and vomiting; the first meal is usually started on the first postoperative day. Patients are discharged with the indwelling urethral catheter used for bladder drainage and daily bladder irrigation with 100 mL of sterile saline. Low-dose antibiotics for prophylaxis are continued during the first 3 postoperative weeks. At that time the urinary catheter is removed and intermittent catheterization is initiated. For patients who have an indwelling catheter via the umbilical stoma, the catheter is usually capped at the time of hospital discharge but may be used to flush the augmented bladder at the time of the daily bladder irrigation.

## SUGGESTED READINGS

1. Gill IS, Rackley RR, Meraney AM, Marcello PW, Sung GT. Laparoscopic enterocystoplasty. Urology 55:178, 2000.
2. Rackley RR, Abdelmalak JB. Laparoscopic augmentation cystoplasty. Surgical technique. Urol Clin North Am 28:663, 2001.
3. Rackley RR, Abdelmalak JB, El-Azab AS, Vasavada SP, Gill I. Laparoscopic bladder augmentation and urinary diversion. In: Kreder K, Stone A, eds. Urinary Diversion: Scientific Foundations and Clinical Practice, 2nd ed. Taylor and Francis, 2004:363–377.

# 27 Vaginal Sling Surgery for Stress Urinary Incontinence

*Sandip P. Vasavada, Raymond R. Rackley, Howard Goldman, and Firouz Daneshgari*

## INDICATIONS

Vaginal sling procedures are indicated in the management of stress urinary incontinence secondary to both intrinsic sphincteric deficiency (ISD) and urethral hypermobility resulting in anatomical incontinence. Although we currently do not attempt to distinguish between these two entities, it remains important that a procedure help both types of incontinence. Several long-term reviews have demonstrated that pubovaginal slings are among the most versatile and durable of the surgical approaches for stress incontinence. Still, the goal remains to create a procedure that supports and compresses the urethra during an increase in intra-abdominal pressure while minimizing the attendant morbidities of the approach. Recent efforts have concentrated on using a variety of materials to help create a hammock of support for the damaged sphincteric unit. These include autologous fascia, anterior vaginal wall, dura mater, bovine pericardium, xenograft tissues, a host of synthetic meshes, and allograft tissues. It is beyond the scope of this chapter to discuss all the pros and cons of each approach because many investigators have their individual preferences.

The latest refinements in technique seem to lead towards the division of the bladder neck and mid-urethral zones in regard to placement of the sling. Our increased understanding and comfort level with synthetics have allowed us to use a synthetic sling under minimal, if any, tension at primarily the mid-urethral location. Its exact mechanism of action is unclear, but European data at 7 yr appears to be quite good, with minimal morbidity. We describe the pubovaginal sling (bladder neck), the mid-urethral synthetic sling, our innovative minimally invasive sling, and new techniques utilizing a transobturator approach.

## DIAGNOSIS

Most patients complain of leakage of urine with stress maneuvers, but those with poor sphincter function secondary to ISD may have gravitational leakage of urine with minimal if any stress. An important phenomenon to consider is that of precipitated micturition. This represents a condition whereby the patient senses urine in the proximal urethra most likely secondary to stress incontinence or lack of proper coaptation of the sphincter. This reflex translates to the sense of urge and frequency to void. Consequently, these patients may necessitate correction of the stress component to help the urge-related symptoms.

The diagnostic evaluation includes a history and physical exam and in certain circumstances may include cystoscopy and radiographic imaging. All cases of stress incontinence do not require urodynamic evaluation, yet in cases of mixed incontinence urodynamics may be quite valuable. Cystourethroscopy may demonstrate rigidity and scarring of the bladder neck and proximal urethra in cases of ISD, while in anatomical incontinence, the urethra will open and funnel with straining maneuvers. Similar findings may be evident with radiographic studies, including voiding cystourethrograms, videourodynamics, or even magnetic resonance imaging. Measurements of valsalva leak point pressure (VLPP) may be less than 60 cm$H_2O$ in cases of ISD, whereas higher values are typical of anatomical stress incontinence.

The decision to perform a bladder neck sling vs a mid-urethral tension-free sling is based on the history (prior operations), the degree of urethral mobility, and in some cases urodynamic findings. In cases with primarily ISD where the urethra is relatively fixed (minimal mobility) or a very low VLPP is noted, we have found less than satisfactory results with mid-urethral

From: *Operative Urology at the Cleveland Clinic*
Edited by: A. Novick et al. © Humana Press Inc., Totowa, NJ

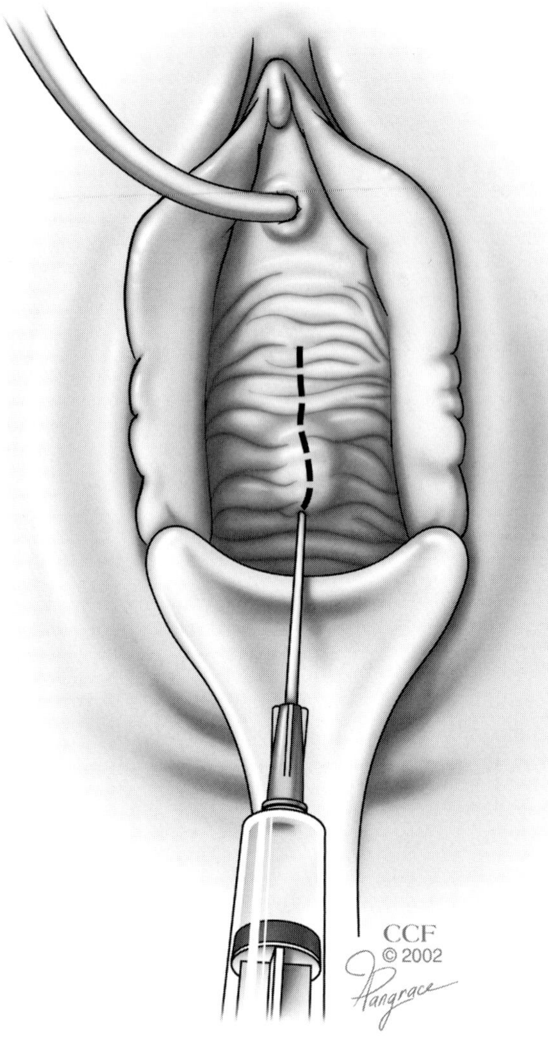


Fig. 27.1

slings and, accordingly, will recommend a formal pubovaginal (bladder neck) sling. This point is certainly debatable, and some proponents advocate mid-urethral slings for all patients. The majority of slings we currently perform are mid-urethral synthetic slings.

However, cases of severe, recurrent incontinence tend to require a more classic approach, and we will, therefore, place a bladder neck sling in those instances.

## BLADDER NECK SLING

The patient is prepped and draped in the usual sterile fashion in the dorsal lithotomy position (Fig. 27.1). After a Foley catheter and/or suprapubic catheter is inserted, an Allis clamp applies upward traction to the anterior vaginal wall. Two oblique incisions or a midline incision is made in the anterior vaginal wall after it is infiltrated with normal saline or vasoactive substances.

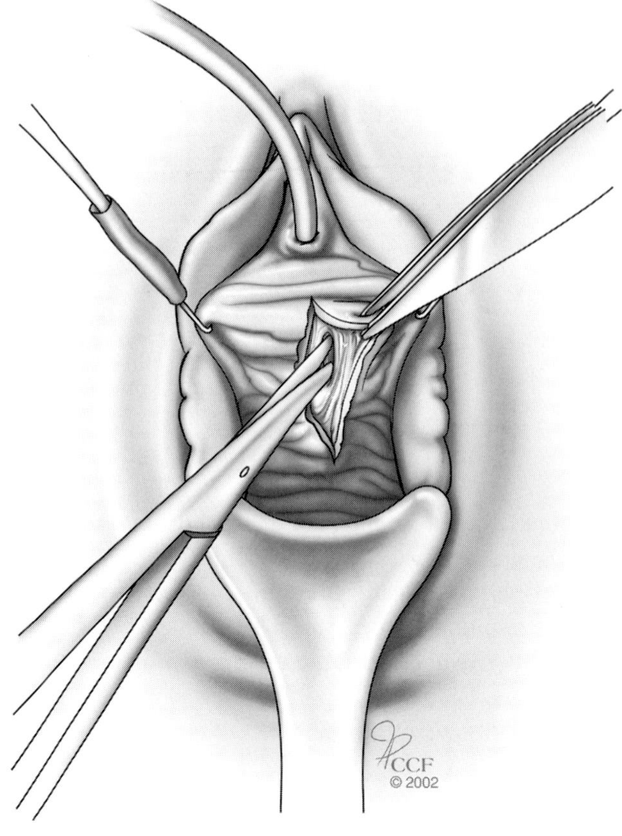


Fig. 27.2

The dissection is carried out laterally over the periurethral fascia toward the ipsilateral shoulder (Fig 27.2). A curved Mayo scissors is used to enter the retropubic space at thc level of the bladder neck. It is important to enter the space at the bladder neck level rather than near the bladder base to avoid perforation into the bladder. The urethropelvic ligament is detached from the arcus tendineus. The adhesions are freed either bluntly or sharply.

A segment of autologous, xenograft or allograft fascia is isolated and placed on the back table for suture placement (Fig. 27.3). Typically, a 2 × 6 to 2 × 12 cm sling is used. Two separate O-polypropylene sutures are placed in the corners of the sling for transfer into the suprapubic incision.

Two small incisions for use of a stamey device or a single stab incision is made just above the pubic symphysis to allow placement of the Raz-Peyrera ligature carrier and allow it to be delivered under complete fingertip guidance into the vaginal incision (Fig. 27.4). The ends of the polypropylene sutures are passed into the ligature carrier and brought back up to the abdominal incision. Cystoscopy is performed to exclude the possibility of

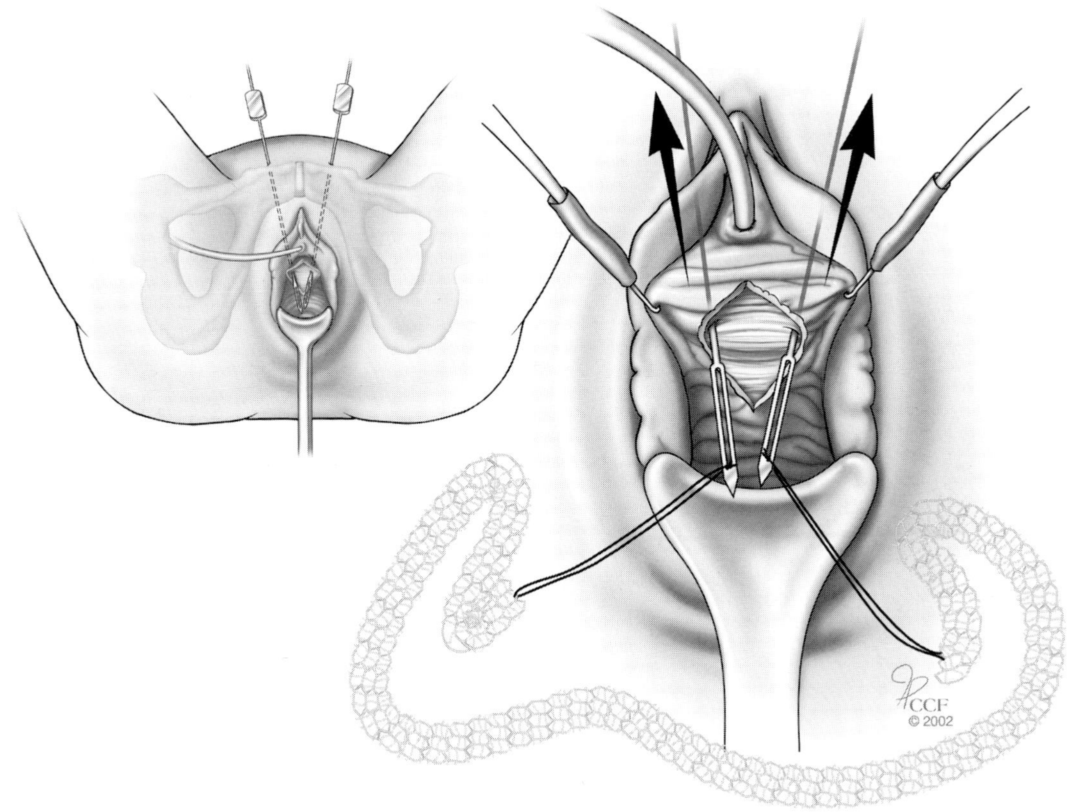


Fig. 27.3 and 4

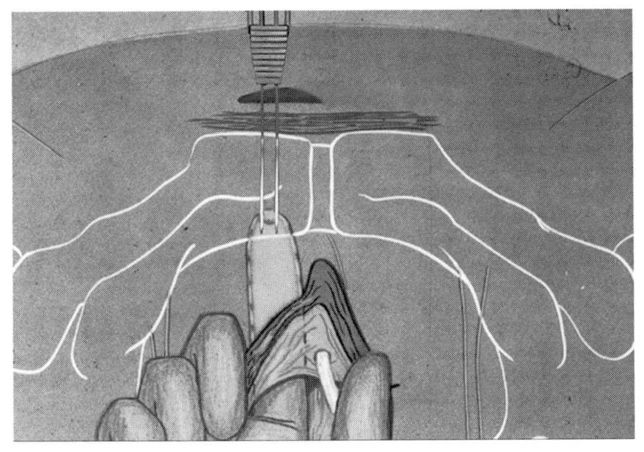

Fig. 27.5

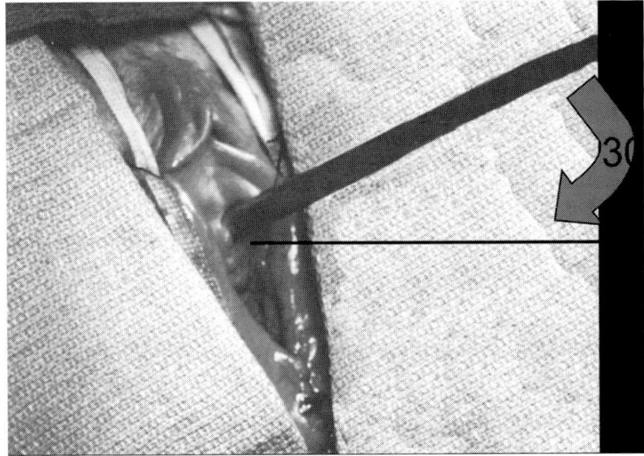

Fig. 27.6

intravesical suture transfer or bladder perforation and to confirm proper position to the suprapubic tube if placed.

The suspension sutures are brought into the suprapubic incision prior to tying (Fig. 27.5).

Proper tying of the sutures to avoid oversuspension of the bladder neck is performed with use of a cystoscope sheath (Fig. 27.6). It is placed in the urethra and bladder neck and not allowed to have greater than a 30º deflection from the horizontal after the sutures are tied. This is similar to the normal urethrovesical angle as seen in voiding cystourethrography. Alternatively, an open Kelly clamp may be placed under the sling itself while the sutures are tied in order to prevent excess tension. The vaginal incisions and suprapubic incision are closed with absorbable sutures. A vaginal pack is placed for hemostasis.

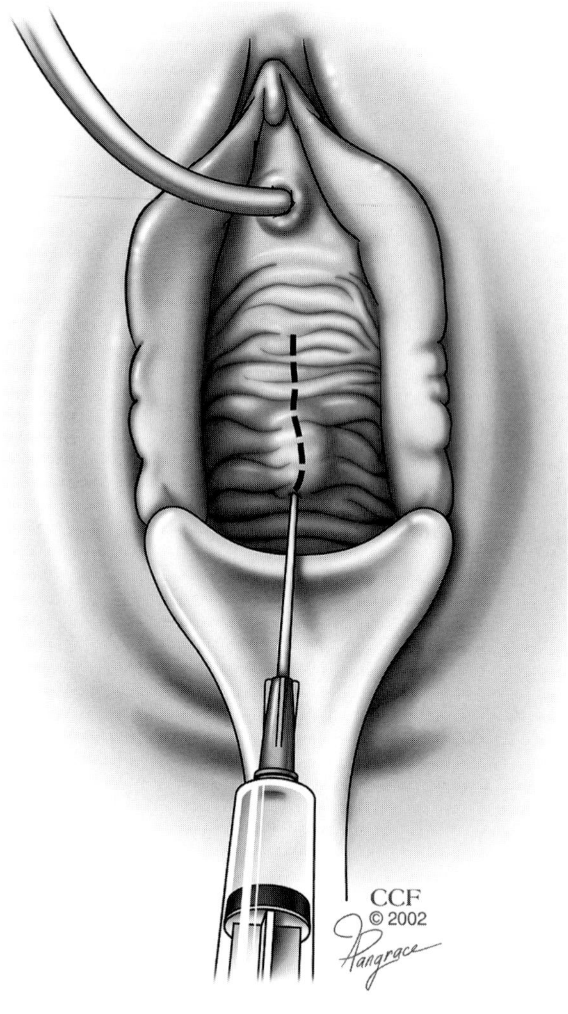


Fig. 27.7

## MID-URETHRAL SLING (PERCUTANEOUS VAGINAL TAPE [PVT])

Obtain vaginal exposure via the dorsal lithotomy position (Fig. 27.7). Use a marking pen to draw the abdominal percutaneous puncture and mid-urethral vaginal wall incision sites. Place an 18 French urethral catheter into the bladder, and then place the catheter guide into the catheter and lift the catheter guide handle to bring the anterior vaginal wall closer to the surgical field for making the mid-urethral vaginal incision.

### Vaginal Incision

Use a scalpel to make a midline anterior vaginal wall incision at the level of the mid-urethra (Figs. 27.8 and 27.9). Develop a pocket at the level of the mid-urethra between the vaginal wall and underlying urethral and paraurethral tissue by dissecting the vaginal wall tissue off laterally with the

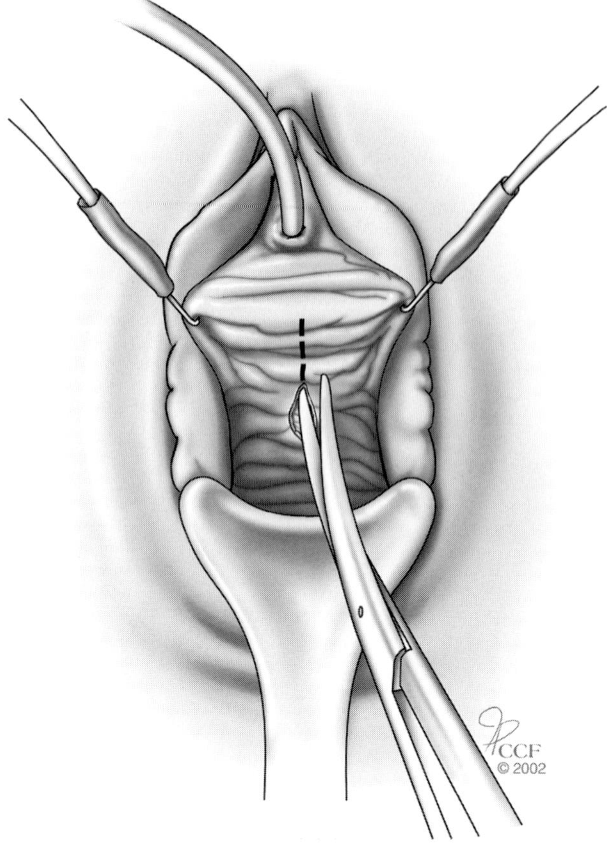


Fig. 27.8

curved Mayo scissors from the 1.5- to 2.0-cm midline incision to the lateral anterior vaginal sulcus.

When the pocket is completed laterally to the junction of the inferior aspect of the pubic ramus and the urethropelvic complex, one can proceed with passage of the needle carrier in either an antegrade or a retrograde fashion. This may be facilitated by use of a catheter guide through the urethal Foley catheter and displacement of the bladder neck away from the side of the carrier passage to decrease the likelihood of bladder perforation. Stabilize the urethral catheter by moving the catheter with guide to the side of interest (right side to start) to open up the mid-paraurethral space for passing through the percutaneous ligature carrier or vaginal trocar in the retropubic space (Fig. 27.10).

Whether passing the percutaneous ligature carrier antegrade or the vaginal trocars retrograde through the retropubic space, several issues are worth discussing. The bladder should be emptied of all fluid. The handle of the catheter with guide should be aligned on the same side of retropubic interest in order to move the bladder and urethra away from where the ligature carrier or trocar will pass. The patient's position on the operating table should result in placement of the symphysis pubis in a near-vertical

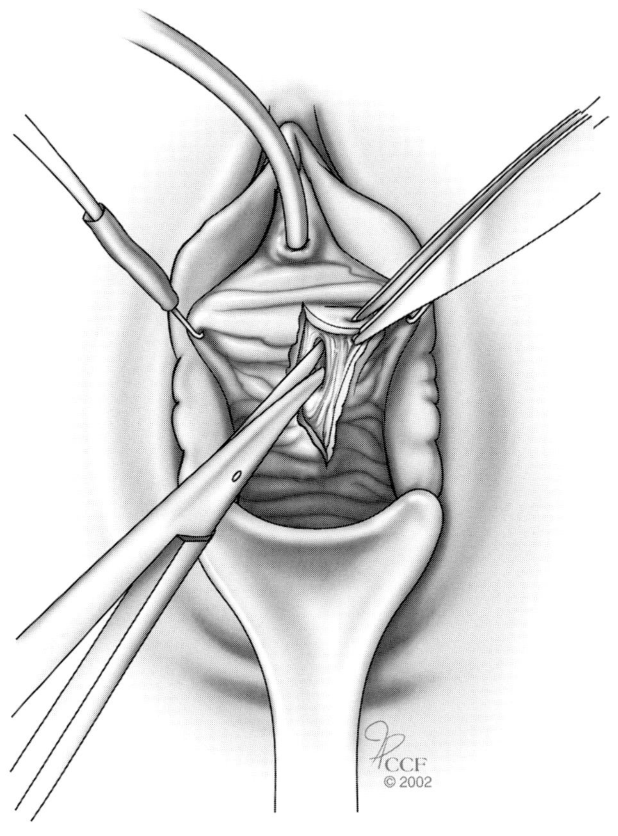


Fig. 27.9

plane; this usually means keeping the patient's torso and head in a level horizontal position or slightly up in a reverse Trendelenburg position.

Small 5-mm stab incisions are made through the abdominal skin overlying the top of the symphysis approx 2.5 cm from the midline on either side. This maneuver allows easier manipulation of the ligature carrier for the antegrade approach or vaginal trocars for the retrograde approach by avoiding any resistance at the skin level. It also provides a visual location for avoiding the perforation of the skin and rectus fascia too laterally because that may lead to the reported complication of ilioinguinal nerve or inferior epigastric vascular damage.

For the tension-free vaginal tape (TVT) procedure, place the vaginal trocars in the anterior vaginal wall pocket. After it is "seated" in the pocket (~2–3 cm), turn the trochar tip toward the ipsilateral shoulder and guide it under the pubis with the nondominant hand. By cradling the trochar with the nondominant hand and holding the handle with the dominant hand, the trochar is gently advanced in an upward fashion behind the posterior aspect of the symphysis and out through the abdominal stab wounds. Attention to staying on the

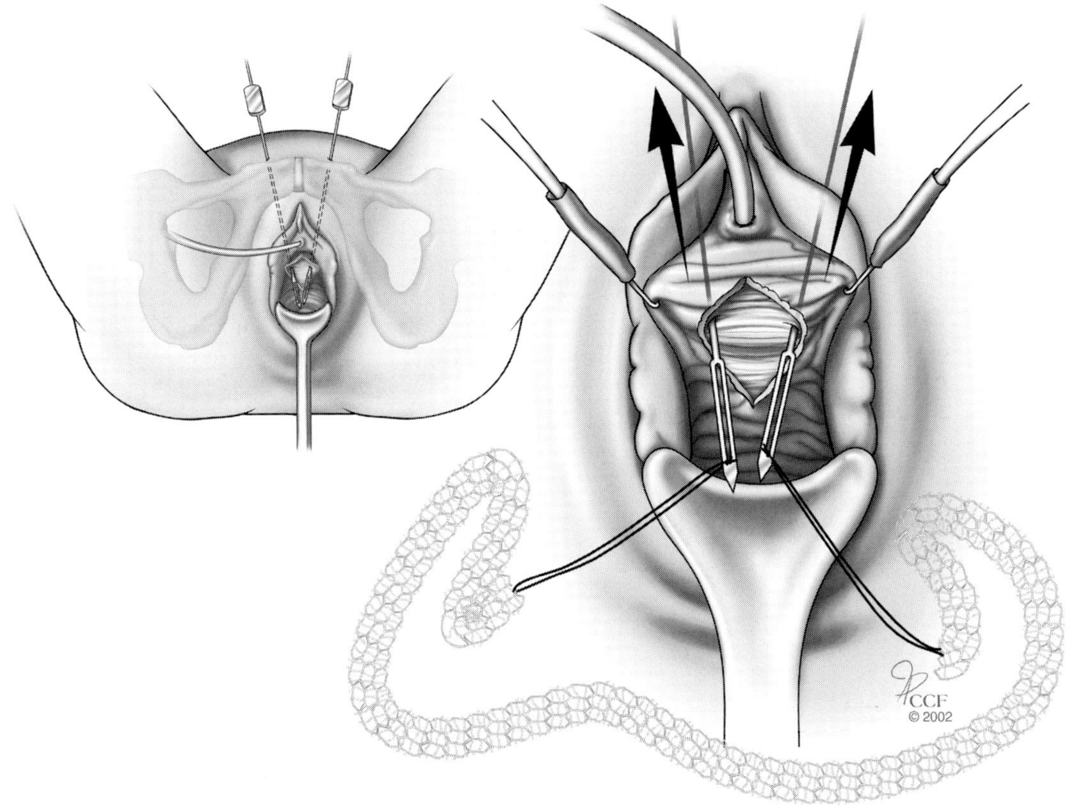


Fig. 27.10

posterior or back side of the symphysis is required to prevent entering the rectus muscle and fascia too far cephalad from its insertion on the symphysis. Removal of the weighted speculum from the vagina and cradling the curve of the trocar in the nondominant hand ensures total control of the device and helps to guide the device in a straight upward direction as pressure is applied with both hands.

When using the percutaneous ligature carrier, we fashion the free sling from a large sheet of polypropylene mesh (PML, Ethicon, Somerville, NJ) to approximately the same size as supplied in the TVT kit (1.2 cm wide × 30 cm long) (Fig. 27.4A). Using 0-Ethibond suture, we simply weave suspending sutures into each end of the prolene sling for placement into the ligature carrier. For passing the ligature carrier in an antegrade fashion, begin by placement of the carrier through the previously marked skin sites. Be sure to stay in contact with the symphysis as the ligature carrier is passed down in an antegrade fashion to the urethropelvic complex at the location described above for locating the insertion of the vaginal trocars for the TVT procedure. To guide the ligature carrier into the vagina, the periurethral pocket must be developed further toward the arcus tendineus to allow entrance of one's finger to guide the carrier out and into the vagina. The suspending sutures of the tape are then threaded into the carrier and retrieved at the abdominal skin site (Fig. 27.4B).

Cystoscopy is performed to inspect for foreign body material within the urinary tract, and it is best to do this inspection when the ligature carrier for PVT or vaginal trocar for TVT is still within the retropubic space. Inspection must take place with a full bladder and use of the 70° lens. A clue that a perforation of the bladder has taken place is the finding of cystoscopic fluid extravasation around the trochar or the sling material at the level of the abdominal skin. If the ligature carrier or vaginal trocar device has been placed through the bladder, simply extract the device and try again. Most surgeons would leave a urethral catheter for several extra days to ensure bladder healing of the injury in hopes of avoiding any chance that postoperative urinary retention would lead to urinary extravasation. Unlike bladder perforations, trocar injury of the urethra rarely occurs. If urethral perforation does occur, terminate the procedure and return at a later date to repeat the surgery. Leave a Foley catheter in for at least 10 d.

## Positioning the Sling

Having completed the procedure on both sides, the next part of the procedure is to set the mid-urethral sling to stabilize, not suspend, the urethra (Figs. 27.11 and 27.12). For a TVT, the trocars are cut from the attached tape covered by a plastic sheath. The plastic sheath theoretically protects the sling material from potential intraoperative contamination and provides for a smooth movement of the sling through the surrounding tissues. The plastic sheath is separated at the midpoint of the sling so that it can be removed once the sling is in the correct position, as described below. Even after removal of the plastic sheath, the TVT tape can be moved, albeit with a fair degree of resistance.

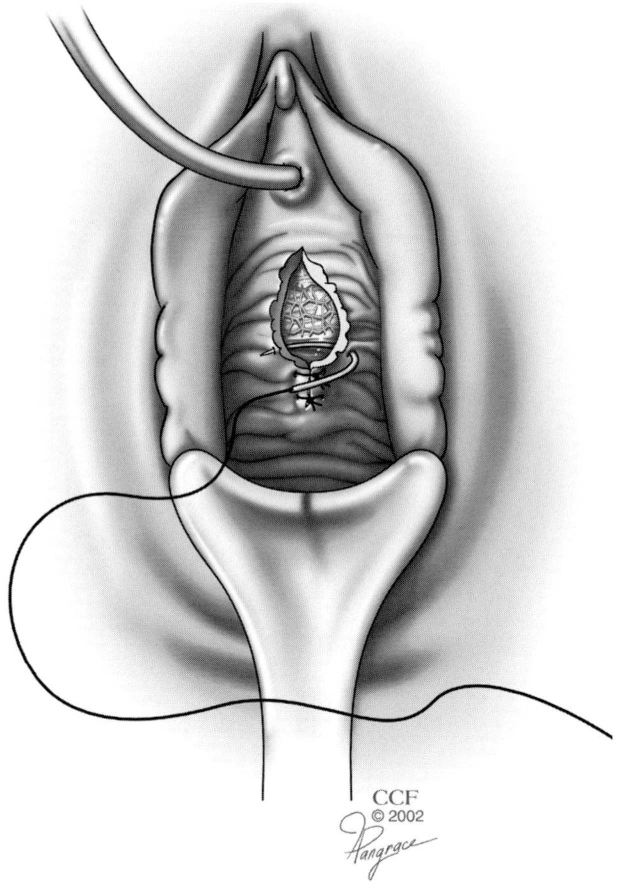


Fig. 27.11

Sling stabilization of the urethra should ensure that at least 30–45° of urethra hypermobility exists as tested by urethral manipulation with the cystoscopic sheath or catheter with guide. We prefer to place the tips of a curved Mayo scissor or a 10 French Heger dilator between the urethra and the sling to ensure ample looseness of the sling. For procedures performed under local anesthesia and sedation or spinal anesthesia, some surgeons prefer to ask the patient to cough or valsalva in order to witness a urinary leak with the sling in place to ensure that the urethra is not obstructed before closing the vaginal incision. This intraoperative cough/stress test for all patients undergoing the

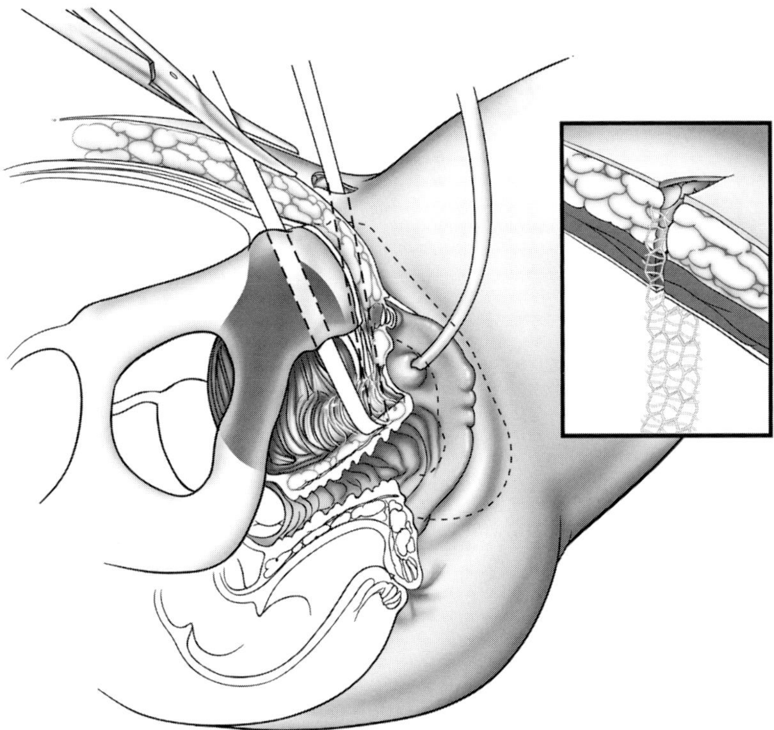

Fig. 27.12

procedure does not make physiological sense because many patients with documented stress urinary incontinence never leak in the supine or lithotomy position.

Once proper positioning of the sling is achieved, the plastic sheath around the TVT tape is removed. Slight countertraction should be applied to the instrument between the mesh and urethra to avoid unwanted tensioning as the sheath is pulled off. The remaining excess sling material at the abdominal skin site for both TVT and PVT is cut below the level of the skin. The vaginal incision site is irrigated with copious amounts of an antibiotic or iodine solution and the incision closed with a running absorbable suture. The skin edges of the abdominal puncture site are approximated with skin adhesive closures. A vaginal pack and urethral catheter are placed for patients remaining in the hospital overnight; otherwise, the bladder is drained, and a urethral catheter and vaginal pack are not usually placed in patients planned for same-day discharge from the recovery room.

## TRANSOBTURATOR SLING PLACEMENT

Recently, transobturator passage of synthetic slings using specially designed instruments has been introduced. Theoretically, this may be a safer approach in that it should avoid the possibility of bowel and other intra-abdominal organ injury. Early outcome data seem to match that reported for the other mid-urethral slings. Two techniques — in-out (passing the device from the vagina out) and out-in (passing the device from the thigh area inward to the vagina) — will be described here. A number of commercial devices are available for the out-in approach. Currently, only one kit is available for the in–out approach (Gynecare, Sommerville, NJ), although several more are in development.

### Technique

As with other sling procedures, the patient is placed in the dorsolithotomy position. Access to the obturator foramen is easier with the thighs at a right angle to the pelvis. The area is prepped and draped, taking care to include the inner thighs in the area prepped.

A 1- to 2-cm incision is made in the vaginal wall over the mid-urethra about 1 cm proximal to the meatus (Figs. 27.13 and 27.14). Sites are marked on the inner thighs approx 2 cm lateral to the thigh crease and 2 cm anterior to the level of the urethral meatus. Stab wounds are made at these thigh sites.

#### Out–In Technique

A pocket is developed periurethrally to the level of the internal obturator membrane (Fig. 27.15). The medial rim

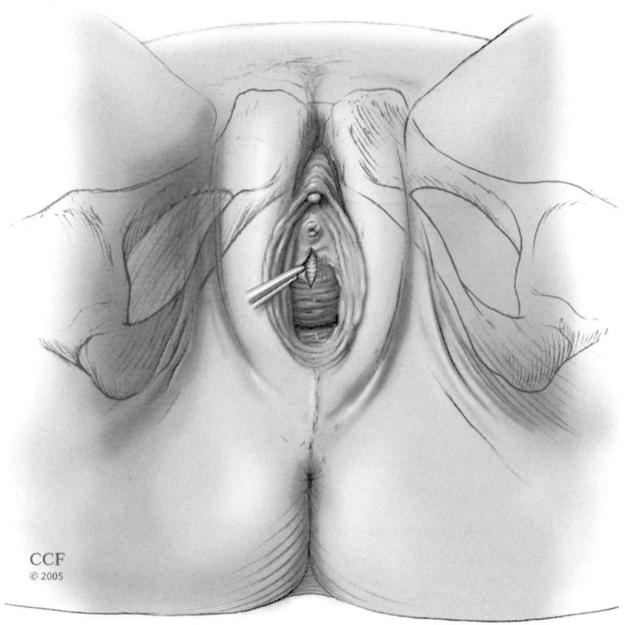


Fig. 27.13

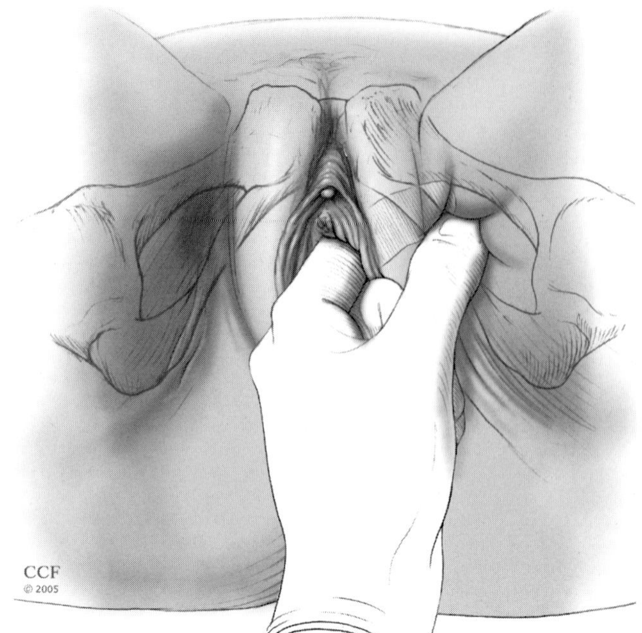


Fig. 27.15

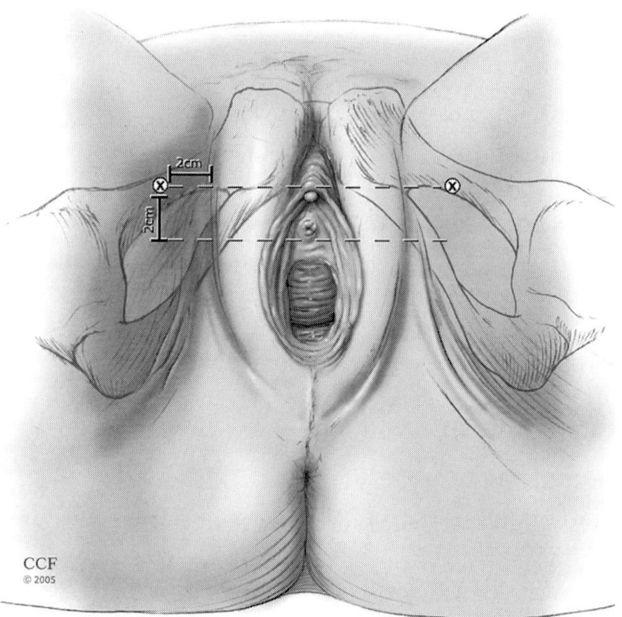


Fig. 27.14

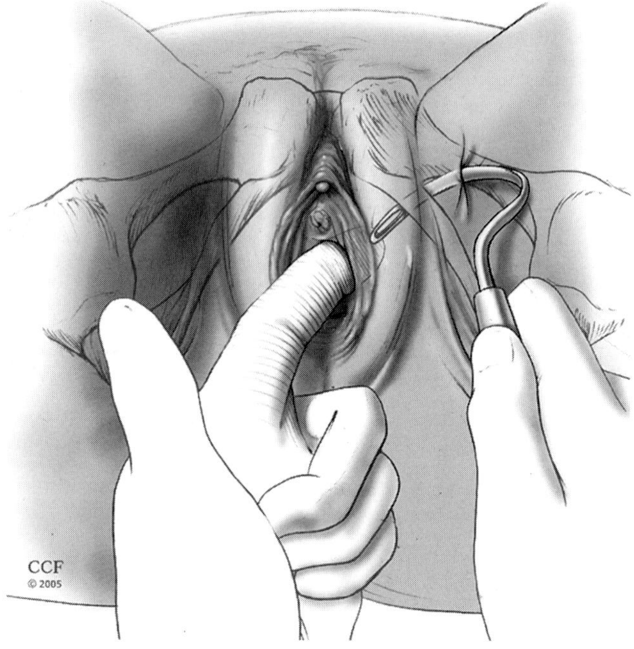


Fig. 27.16

of the obturator foramen is pinched between a vaginal finger and one on the inner thigh near the stab wound at the premarked site.

A curved device is passed from the inner thigh site, through skin, muscle, and fascia onto the vaginal finger and then rotated into the vagina (Fig. 27.16). Cystoscopy should be done at this point to exclude any bladder or urethral perforation.

The sling material is attached to the curved instrument and brought out to the thigh area (Fig. 27.17). This is then repeated on the contralateral side.

### In–Out Technique

Using fine scissors, a tunnel is developed under the vaginal wall to the level of the internal obturator fascia by dissecting at a 45° angle to the vertical plane

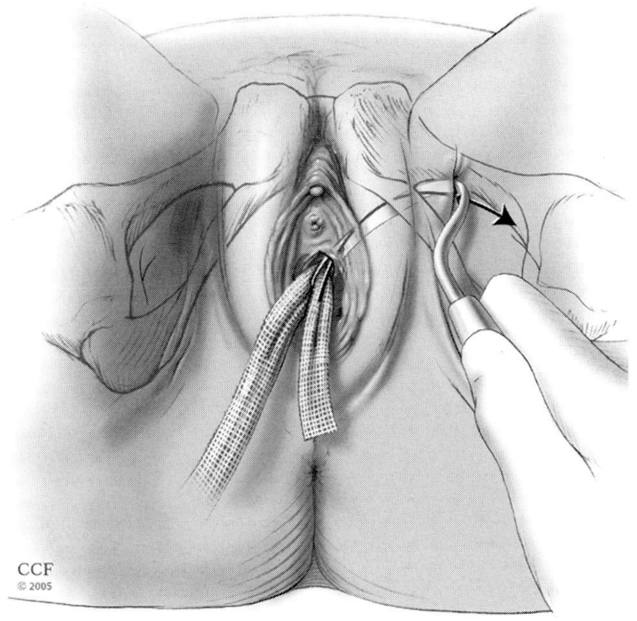


Fig. 27.17

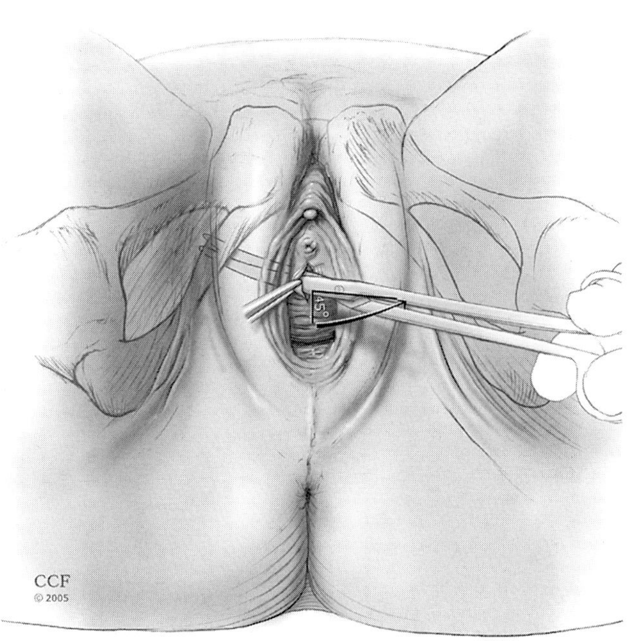


Fig. 27.18

aiming slightly upward (Fig. 27.18). The fascia is then perforated.

A specialized guide is placed in the tunnel and carefully passed through the fascia at the site of perforation (Fig. 27.19).

A specialized spiral instrument with sling attached is passed via the groove of the guide through the foramen and rotated while bringing the handle of the device into a

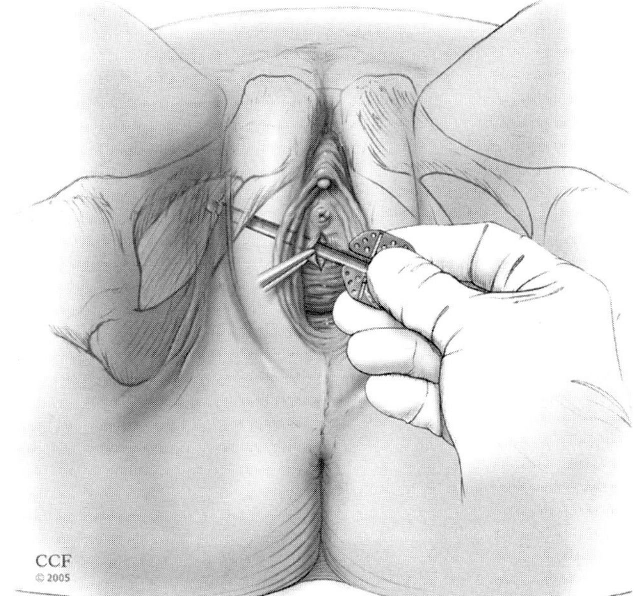


Fig. 27.19

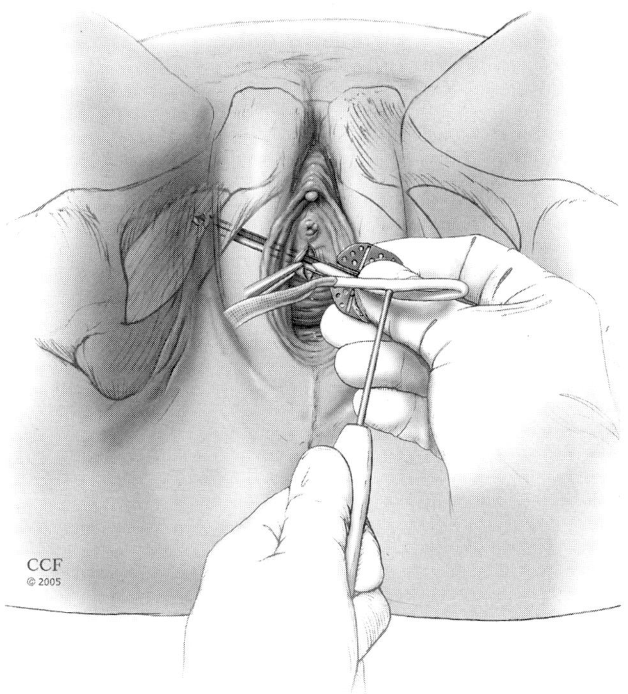


Fig. 27.20

vertical position and the tip out through the premade inner thigh stab wound (Figs. 27.20–27.22).

The sling is pulled through the thigh incision while the spiral device is backed out (Fig. 27.23). This is all repeated on the contralateral side. Because one is always aiming away from the urethra and bladder, many feel cystocopy is unnecessary in the in–out approach.

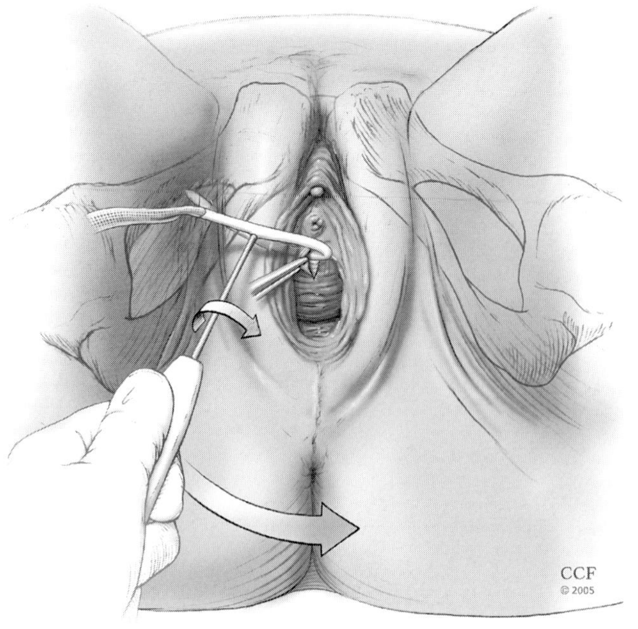


Fig. 27.21

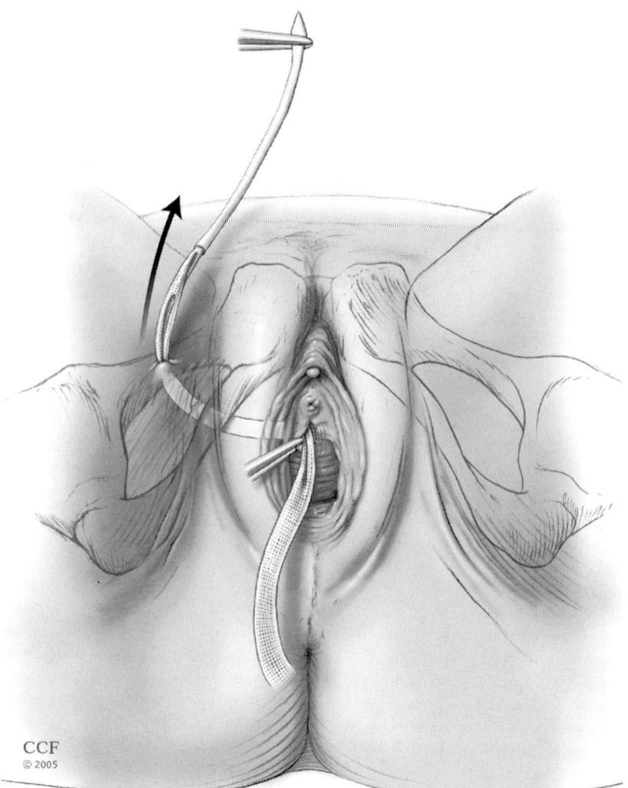


Fig. 27.23

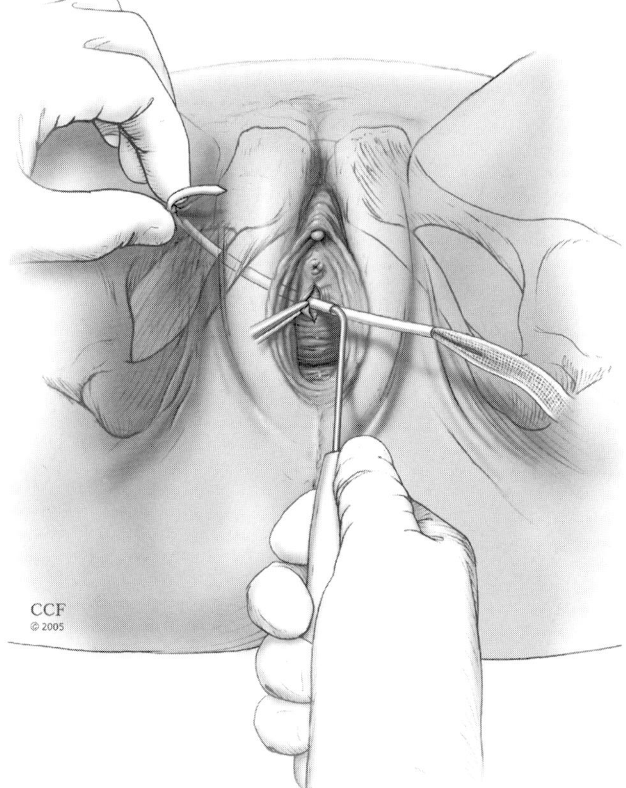


Fig. 27.22

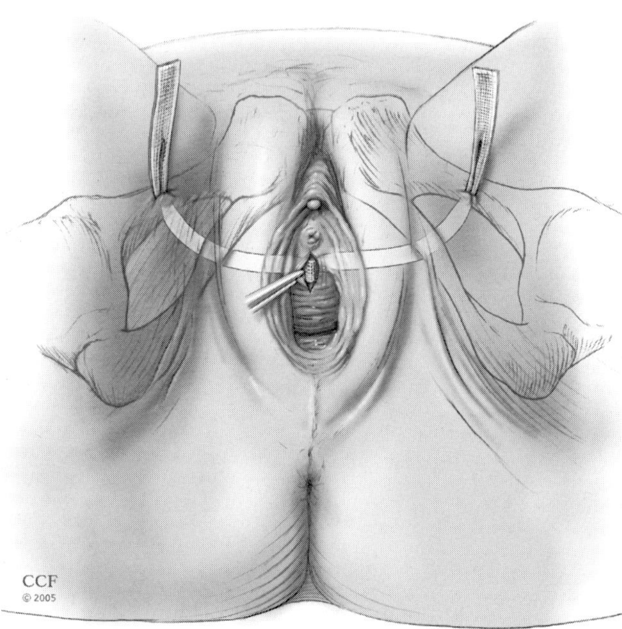


Fig. 27.24

If a plastic sheath is present, it is pulled off, making sure to leave an instrument between the mesh and urethra such that a small air loop is present — the urethra should not be under any tension (Fig. 27.24). All incisions are irrigated, the vaginal wall incision is closed with absorbable suture, excess mesh in the thigh is excised, and the thigh incisions can be closed with a simple chromic stitch or a skin sealant.

### Postoperative Care

Many surgeons who perform the TVT or PVT procedure under local anesthesia with sedation without concomitant prolapse repairs send patients home the same day without a catheter if a voiding trial is successfully completed. If a patient cannot void immediately after the procedure in the recovery room or the bladder was perforated during the procedure, catheter drainage for a brief period of 1–2 d may be required and a voiding trial completed as an outpatient.

## POSTOPERATIVE COMPLICATIONS

Bleeding, either intraoperatively or postoperatively, can be dealt with using a few simple maneuvers. Most mild bleeding will stop once the sling material is pulled into place. If there is still mild bleeding at the end of the case, it will often subside simply with bed rest and the prolonged use of a vaginal pack. In cases of more severe bleeding, one may require placement of a Foley catheter with 60–80 mL in the balloon and inflate it posterior to the packing to assist in hemostasis. Persistent bleeding may require surgical exploration, but this is a rare occurrence and has not happened in our experience.

Postoperative pain may occur in the suture sites where the suspension sutures are located either suprapubically in anterior vaginal wall sling cases or in the area of the pubic bone in bone-anchor techniques. The suspending prolene sutures must not be tied over a mobile portion of the rectus muscle so as to prevent the possibility of nerve entrapment.

Urinary retention can be problematic to deal with. Most patients will void shortly after the catheters are removed or, in the case of suprapubic tube use, with low residuals. It is the experience of the authors that the degree of postoperative bladder dysfunction (urge-type symptoms or period of urinary retention after voiding) is longer with patients undergoing bladder neck slings as they are placed with some degree of tension/support. The majority of patients undergoing mid-urethral tension-free slings void spontaneously in the recovery room and may be discharged home without catheter drainage. Some patients may develop prolonged bouts of retention or carry excessively high residuals. They may complain of irritative and obstructive voiding symptoms, and these should be addressed, as they may or may not be secondary to retention of urine. There exists no clear-cut method of determining outlet obstruction as the cause for these symptoms, but the temporal relation between surgery and the onset of these irritative or obstructive symptoms is a good clue that iatrogenic obstruction has occurred. We have divided the management of obstructive symptoms into the two surgical categories (after bladder neck or mid-urethral sling placements). Because mid-urethral sling placements are typically done with synthetic materials, we prefer to simply incise the sling early in the postoperative period (within several days to weeks) to avoid prolonged voiding problems. Bladder neck sling patients may take a longer time to achieve normal voiding and, accordingly, are given a longer period of time before intervention is contemplated. Voiding cystourethrography and physical exam may confirm a hypersuspended urethra and pressure flow analyses may demonstrate high pressures and low flow rates, but this is variable. Management consists of early institution of intermittent self-catheterization with a prudent trial of waiting. If spontaneous voiding does not resume within 3 mo, one may proceed with transection of the sling, and most will void after this maneuver. Only rarely is formal transvaginal urethrolysis required.

# 28 Transvaginal Closure of the Bladder Neck

*Sandip P. Vasavada, Raymond R. Rackley, Howard Goldman, and Firouz Daneshgari*

## INTRODUCTION

Transvaginal closure of the bladder neck represents an uncommon surgical procedure, as its main indication is in patients who have urethral destruction secondary to prolonged catheter drainage of a neurogenic bladder. The resultant effect of the catheter and Foley balloon on the urethra is erosion and pressure necrosis as well as spontaneous urethral extrusion from severe bladder spasms. The usual course of events is progressive worsening of leakage around the catheter, necessitating larger catheters and more fluid placement in the balloon. These sequential increases in catheter size, along with the concomitant urethral destruction, results in a wide, patulous, and severely damaged urethra. Accordingly, proper management of these patients requires transvaginal closure of the bladder neck and simultaneous urinary diversion with a continent catheterizable augmentation, incontinent ileovesicostomy, or suprapubic catheter.

Although most patients who would be candidates for transvaginal closure of the bladder neck suffer from a neurogenic bladder and have urethral destruction secondary to long-term catheter drainage, other indications include refractory urethrovaginal fistula, severely shortened urethra, and severe refractory intrinsic sphincteric deficiency.

## DIAGNOSIS

Visual inspection of the urethra demonstrates a large, patulous urethra that is shortened and may even permit visualization of the bladder neck or bladder itself (Fig. 28.1). Cystoscopy is performed to confirm the absence of other pathology in the bladder such as stones, neoplasms, or diverticuli that may accompany long-term catheter drainage. Simultaneous study of the upper urinary tracts may be indicated to evaluate for hydronephrosis or ureteric obstruction. The patient should also be evaluated for manual dexterity or have an adequate caregiver to facilitate catheterization of the augmented segment. If this is not feasible, one must plan for an incontinent augmentation (ileovesicostomy) and subsequent stomal drainage or suprapubic catheter drainage. Urine cultures should be routinely assessed preoperatively because these patients are prone to infections. Broad-spectrum antibiotics are essential prior to surgery.

## SURGICAL TECHNIQUE

Initial preparatory steps include placement of the patient in the dorsal lithotomy position and prepping and draping the lower abdomen and vagina in the usual sterile fashion. If a suprapubic tube placement is necessary, it is placed at this time, typically with use of a Lowsley retractor elevating the bladder to the anterior abdominal wall.

Normal saline or vasoactive substances are injected into the vaginal wall to develop a subepithelial plane around the urethra (Fig. 28.2). A circumscribing incision is made around the urethra and an inverted U incision is made inferior to this in the anterior vaginal wall. A vaginal flap is created by sharp dissection in the anterior vaginal wall separating the epithelium from the underlying vesicopelvic fascia. This dissection is carried laterally around the open bladder neck.

The dissection is continued toward the bladder neck, freeing the bladder from its attachments to the symphysis pubis and lateral pelvic sidewall (Fig. 28.3). This necessitates entering the retropubic space by detaching the urethropelvic ligaments on either side of the bladder neck and transecting the pubourethral ligaments above the urethra. Typically, the attenuated urethra requires some degree of excision; however, we often

From: *Operative Urology at the Cleveland Clinic*
Edited by: A. Novick et al. © Humana Press Inc., Totowa, NJ

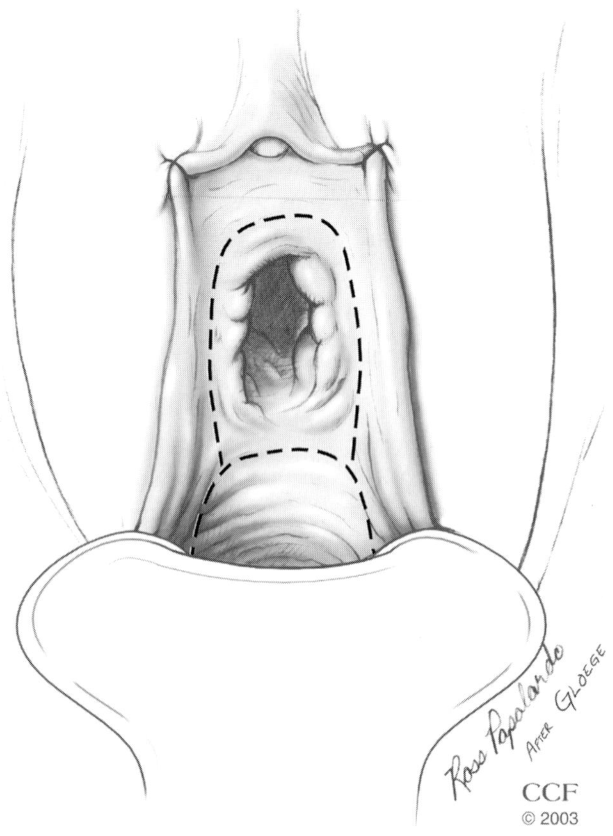


Fig. 28.1

use it to create an additional layer of closure. Indigo carmine is administered intravenously to facilitate identification of the ureteral orifices to prevent injury during bladder neck closure.

The bladder neck is closed using a vertical closure of 2-0 polyglycolic acid suture in an interlocking fashion (Fig. 28.4).

A second layer of interrupted 2-0 polyglycolic acid suture incorporates the bladder neck and anterior bladder wall in order to prevent overlapping suture lines and transfer the closed bladder neck into the retropubic space, high behind the pubic symphysis (Fig. 28.5). After this second layer, placement of the attenuated posterior urethral plate allows a third layer of support of the closure. If necessary, a Martius flap may be placed at this time in order to advance yet another layer over the repair. When no simultaneous continent urinary augmentation is planned, a separate penrose drain is advanced through a suprapubic incision.

The anterior vaginal wall flap is advanced as the final layer of closure and covers the original urethral opening (Fig. 28.6).

## POSTOPERATIVE CARE

A vaginal pack is placed in the vagina to prevent bleeding. The suprapubic tube is irrigated and confirmed to function properly to allow for adequate drainage and

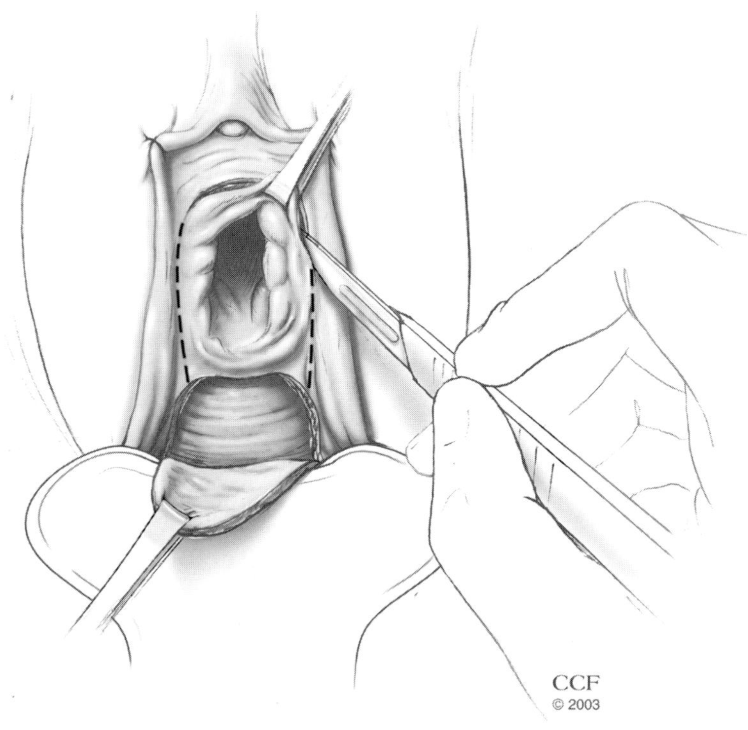


Fig. 28.2

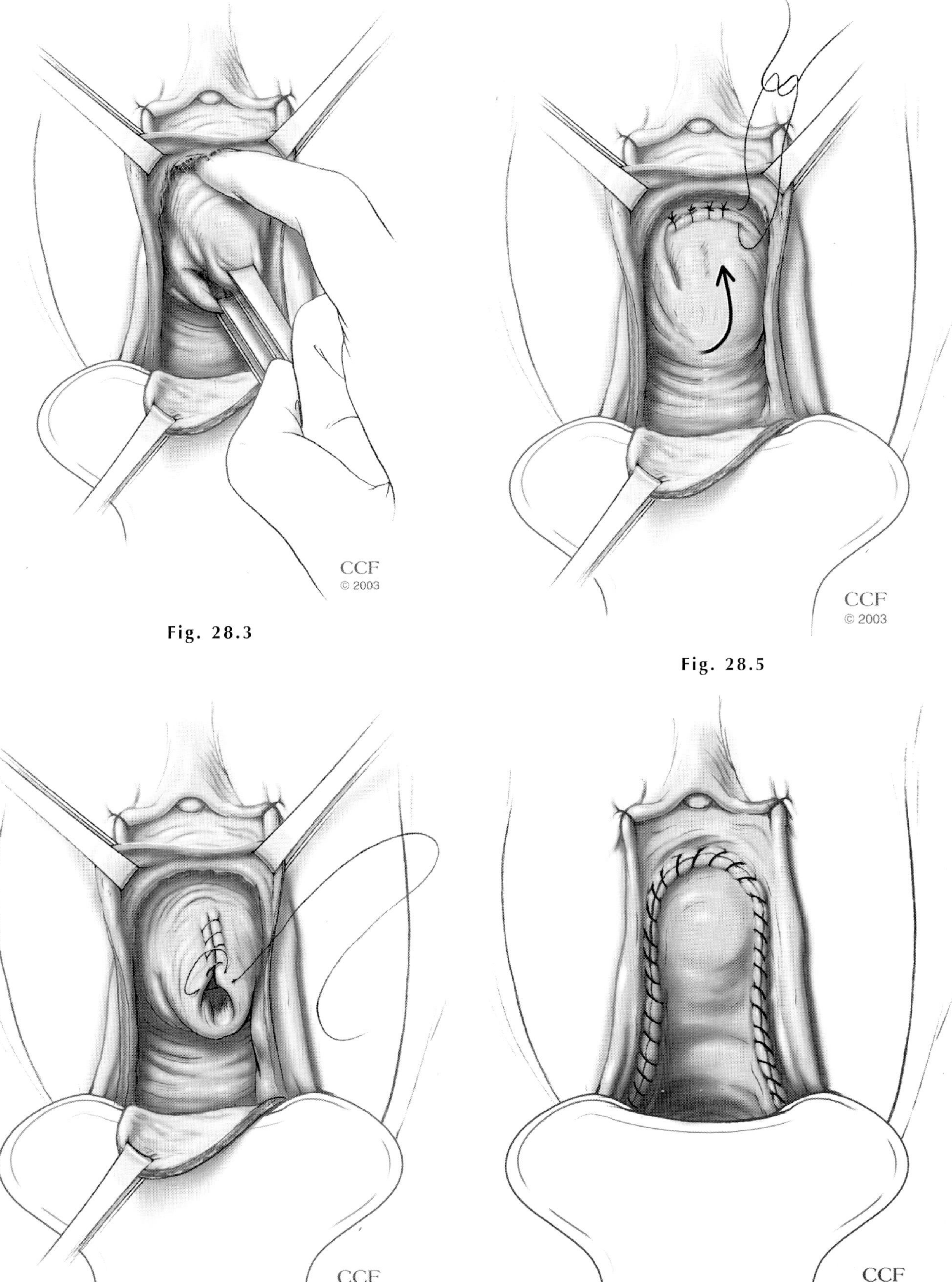


Fig. 28.3

Fig. 28.5

Fig. 28.4

Fig. 28.6

healing of the incisions. Antibiotics are used postoperatively for 2 wk during the healing period. Depending on whether or not a continent catheterizable augment is performed, a cystogram may be performed to ensure proper healing, and the suprapubic tube may be allowed to remain or be removed at that time.

## POSTOPERATIVE COMPLICATIONS

The most significant complication of transvaginal bladder neck closure is postoperative vesicovaginal fistula. This may occur early or late in the healing period. Steps one can perform to prevent the development of fistulas include (1) use of several layers of closure, (2) watertight closure, (3) positioning the bladder neck high in the retropubic space, (4) avoidance of postoperative bladder spasms with anticholinergics, (5) use of a Penrose drain, and (6) use of a Martius flap when necessary. Bleeding and infection may require surgical drainage. If fistula formation occurs, secondary repair may be performed after a prudent period of observation. Often a rotational flap may be required to assist in the closure. Alternatively, an abdominal approach may be utilized with interposition of an omental flap to cover the repair.

# 29 Urethral Diverticula

*Sandip P. Vasavada, Raymond R. Rackley, Howard Goldman, and Firouz Daneshgari*

## INTRODUCTION

A urethral diverticulum remains an elusive diagnosis in the female patient presenting with a constellation of irritative voiding symptoms. Many changes in the standard evaluation of suspected urethral diverticula have been realized over the last few years to the point that often an exact diagnosis can be obtained with a combination of physical exam and appropriate radiographic imaging. We present our method of evaluation for female urethral diverticulum and describe some of the salient technical points to accomplish a successful reconstruction and avoid complications in this setting.

## ETIOLOGY

In most cases, a urethral diverticulum results from repeated infection and obstruction of the periurethral glands. Initially, a suburethral cyst is formed both by the irritative process of infection and by the high pressures created within an obstructed periurethral gland. These cysts subsequently rupture into the urethral lumen. The resulting draining abscess cavity is eventually epithelialized, and a urethral diverticulum is formed. Other less common causes of urethral diverticula involve congenital and posttraumatic factors.

## DIAGNOSIS

A history of dyspareunia, dysuria, postmicturition dribbling, and recurrent urinary tract infections is highly suggestive of a urethral diverticulum. Urgency, frequency, and hematuria may also be seen with this condition. On occasion, the diverticulum may be complicated by stones, bladder outlet obstruction, and, rarely, malignancy. Romanzi et al. recently reviewed their experience with diverse presentations of urethral diverticula and concluded that when symptoms that mimic other disorders do not respond to standard therapy, one should entertain the possibility of a urethral diverticulum *(1)*. In their experience, 48% presented with urethral/pelvic pain, incontinence (35%), dyspareunia (24%), and frequency/urgency (22%). Therefore, one must have a high index of suspicion for this process, as many patients may not be overtly symptomatic upon initial evaluation. In general, one should entertain the possibility of a urethral diverticulum in any case of persistent lower urinary tract symptoms unresponsive to therapy.

On physical examination, the urethra may be tender, and often a suburethral mass is palpable. Manual compression may cause the drainage of purulent material or urine from the external meatus. In rare instances, the patient may present with signs of sepsis and acute inflammation from a tense, infected diverticulum. Significant manual compression should be avoided, and more definitive therapy should be planned.

The presence of urethral hypermobility and stress incontinence should be documented during the initial visit. Q-tip testing and/or provocative testing with a bedside cystometrogram and subsequent Valsalva maneuvers may confirm the presence or absence of leakage. Evidence of urethral hypermobility and stress incontinence may require follow-up urodynamic assessment to determine any need for a simultaneous sling with excision of the diverticulum.

## RADIOGRAPHIC EVALUATION

In the past, evaluation and confirmation of the presence of a diverticulum often involved both voiding cystourethrography (VCUG) and positive pressure urethrography (PPUG) with a double balloon catheter. While these studies are specific in defining the location, size, and number of diverticula, their sensitivity is questionable. Wang et al. reviewed a 3-yr experience using standard VCUG vs PPUG in the evaluation of urethral diverticula and found

From: *Operative Urology at the Cleveland Clinic*
Edited by: A. Novick et al. © Humana Press Inc., Totowa, NJ

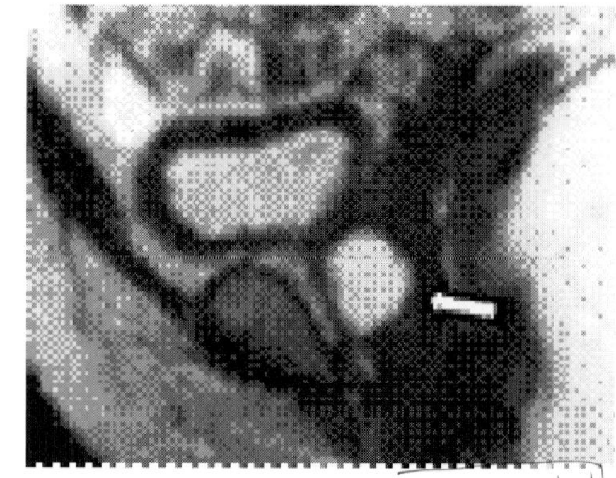

Fig. 29.1

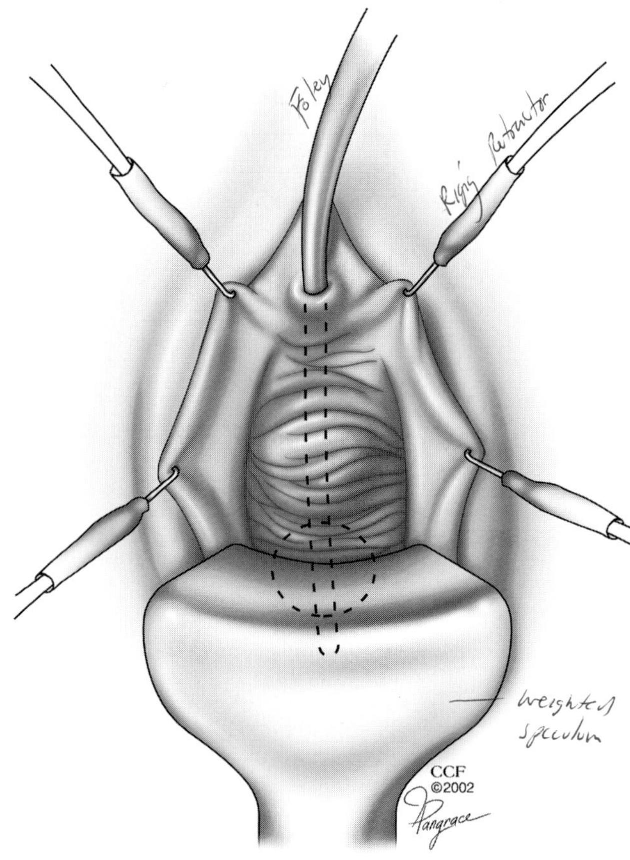


Fig. 29.2

that the positive predictive value of VCUG after PPUG was only 60% *(2)*. While this indicates some benefit over VCUG alone, there is some hesitation about recommending a PPUG in all patients with suspected diverticula because of the discomfort involved in the procedure and its invasiveness. More recently, magnetic resonance imaging (MRI) has proved to have a higher sensitivity in detecting urethral diverticula when compared to PPUG *(2–4)*. Neitlich et al., in a series of 13 patients being evaluated for urethral diverticula, found 6 patients with urethral diverticula *(3)*. Four of these patients were diagnosed by MRI only and two by MRI and PPU. A number of other recent studies have also demonstrated the superiority of MRI over other imaging exams. Therefore, at the present time it appears that MRI has become the procedure of choice for evaluation of a suspected urethral diverticulum.

## INDICATIONS FOR SURGERY

Patients who have significant symptoms related to the urethral diverticulum are best treated with surgery. In acute situations where there is a significant amount of inflammation and an abscess is suspected, incision and drainage may be required prior to performing definitive surgery. Stress urinary incontinence and urethral hypermobility may coexist with urethral diverticula and, if suspected, should be evaluated prior to surgery with formal urodynamic assessment.

## TREATMENT

Some patients who do not have significant symptoms from a diverticulum may be followed and treated with conservative measures, including antibiotics and anticholinergics. In general, however, most patients desire definitive repair. There exist three surgical options for urethral diverticulum repair: (1) transurethral incision of the diverticula communication, transforming a narrow-mouthed into a wide-mouthed diverticulum, (2) marsupialization of the diverticula sac into the vagina by incision of the urethrovaginal septum, and (3) excision of the diverticulum. In acute sepsis situations, the diverticulum may also be transvaginally drained and fixed at a later time.

## SURGICAL PROCEDURE

At our institution complete excision of the diverticulum is performed if at all possible. After the patient is prepped and draped, a 12 French urethral Foley catheter is inserted, and the bladder is filled with 200 cc of normal saline. A suprapubic tube may then be placed with a Lowsley retractor. The urethral foley catheter is replaced and a ring retractor and weighted vaginal speculum are used for retraction. A marking pen is used to outline an inverted U incision up to the distal aspect of the urethra just proximal to the urethral meatus. Occasionally if a diverticulum is quite eccentric, a laterally based flap — with the base over the ostial side of the diverticulum — is utilized.

A mid-sagittal MRI view of the pelvis shows an arrow pointing toward the mid-urethra with prominent diverticulum on T2-weighted sequence (Fig. 29.1).

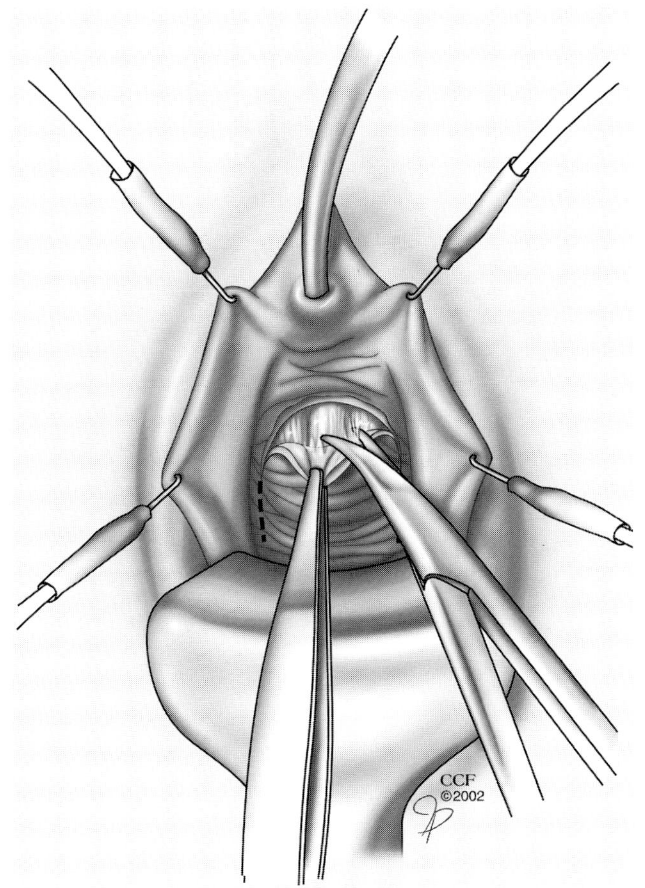


Fig. 29.3

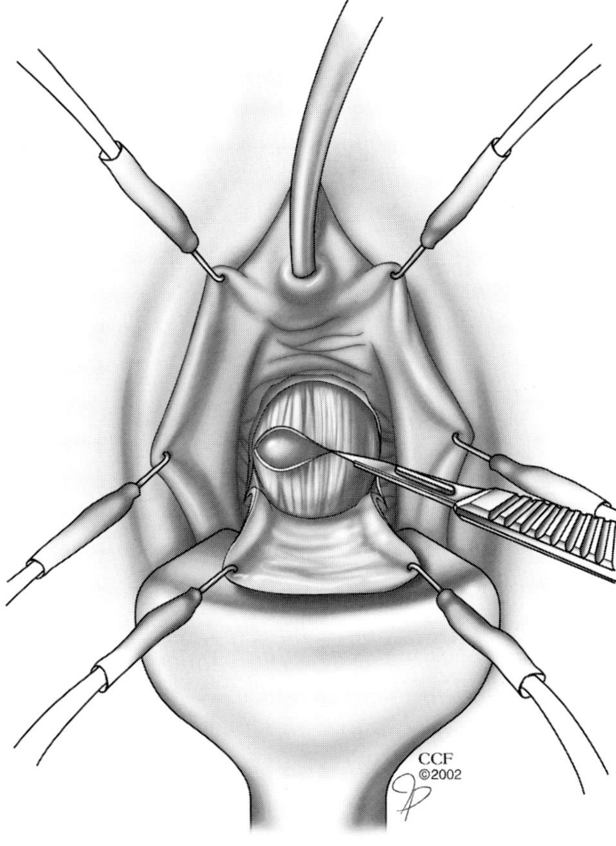


Fig. 29.4

Initially, both urethral and suprapubic catheters are placed to assure maximum postoperative drainage (Figs. 29.2 and 29.3). A 10–12 French urethral Foley catheter is inserted to facilitate identification of the urethral wall during the subsequent dissection. Normal saline or lidocaine with epinephrine solution is administered just beneath the vaginal wall to create a plane for dissection. Following this, an inverted U incision is created in the anterior vaginal wall with the tip of the U just proximal to the urethral meatus. The vaginal wall flap is dissected posteriorly, thus exposing the periurethral fascia. It is important to not enter the fascia or the diverticulum at this point so as to facilitate later dissection and reconstruction. Exposed periurethral fascia flaps are created above and below, thereby exposing the diverticulum only (Fig. 29.4). The periurethral fascia is then incised in a transverse direction over the diverticulum. This layer may be quite thin, and again, care must be taken to avoid entry into the diverticulum.

The superior and inferior flaps are created, leaving only the submucosal layer of the urethral wall and the diverticula sac (Fig. 29.5).

The diverticula sac is sharply freed from the surrounding structures, and the communication and neck of the diverticulum is then excised flush with the wall of the urethra (Figs. 29.6 and 29.7). If the patient had a prior infected diverticulum or has severe inflammatory changes, the diverticulum may be adherent to the other layers, necessitating entry into the sac in order to excise it. The entire diverticula sac should be excised, including extensions laterally and anteriorly. The mucosal defect may be quite large, and the urethral Foley catheter may be identified. The urethral wall is reconstructed using longitudinal closure of the urethral defect using a 3-0 absorbable suture. This must be closed in a watertight fashion without any tension. Moreover, the defect in the periurethral fascia should be closed in order to prevent the chance of recurrent diverticula formation. One must take care to not incorporate the underlying urethral catheter into the closure.

The periurethral fascia is trimmed back to healthy tissue edges and closed horizontally with an absorbable 3-0 suture (Fig. 29.8). This layer of closure is perpendicular to the urethral closure to avoid overlapping suture

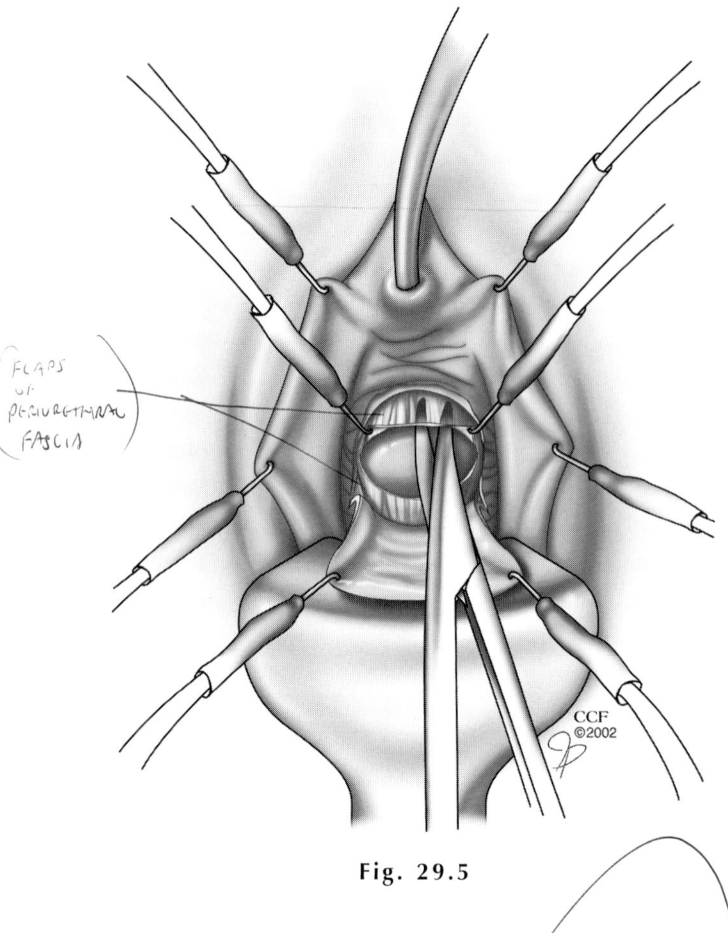


Fig. 29.5

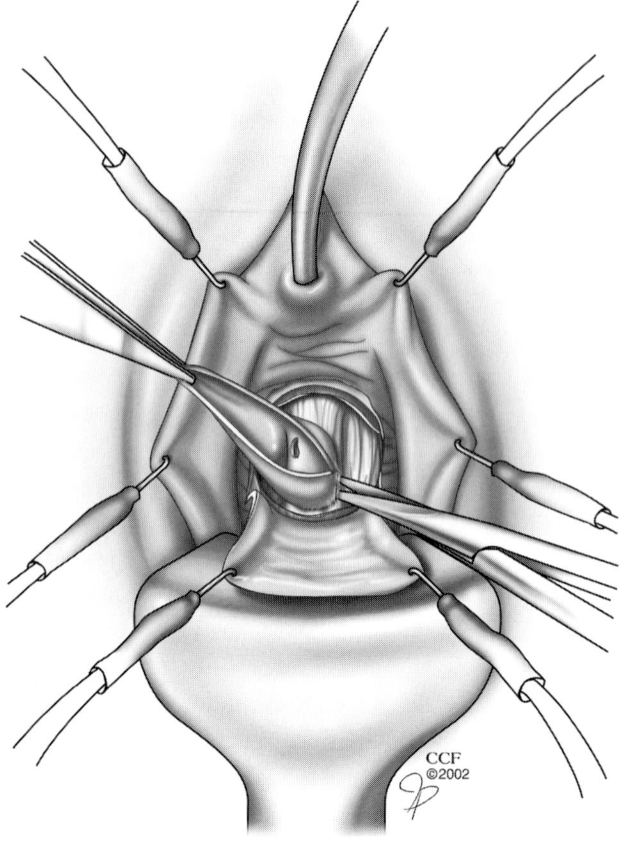


Fig. 29.6

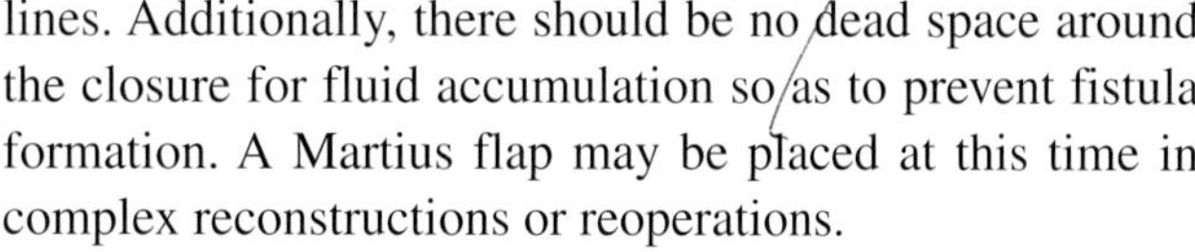

lines. Additionally, there should be no dead space around the closure for fluid accumulation so as to prevent fistula formation. A Martius flap may be placed at this time in complex reconstructions or reoperations.

The anterior vaginal wall flap is advanced over the periurethral fascia suture lines to again avoid overlapping suture lines (Fig. 29.9). A vaginal pack is placed, and the urethral and suprapubic catheters are placed on gravity drainage.

## POSTOPERATIVE CARE

Patients are discharged either the same day or within 23 h with both the urethral Foley catheter and suprapubic tubes to gravity drainage. Patients are treated with oral antibiotics for 2 wk after surgery. Anticholinergic therapy is begun in the immediate postoperative period to prevent bladder spasms. A voiding cystourethrogram is performed 2 wk postoperatively to rule out extravasation. If a small amount of extravasation is present, the suprapubic tube alone is allowed to remain in place and to gravity drainage while the urethral Foley catheter is removed. A repeat study may be performed in 1 wk to demonstrate resolution of the extravasation. The suprapubic tube may then be capped and voiding trials carried out until the patient can void with low residual urine volumes.

## COMPLICATIONS

### Intraoperative Complications

Excessive bleeding occurs rarely, and it is usually controlled well with judicious use of electrocautery and, ultimately, vaginal packing.

Difficulty in closing the urethral mucosa may be encountered as the result of a large defect created during the excision of the diverticulum. In this situation it may be necessary to expose the urethral wall further and to close the urethral mucosa over a 5–8 French feeding tube.

In patients with severely inflamed or poor quality tissue, a fibrofatty labial (Martius) flap can be used between the periurethral fascia and the vaginal wall. This flap will add an extra protective layer, thereby helping to prevent formation of a urethrovaginal fistula *(7)*.

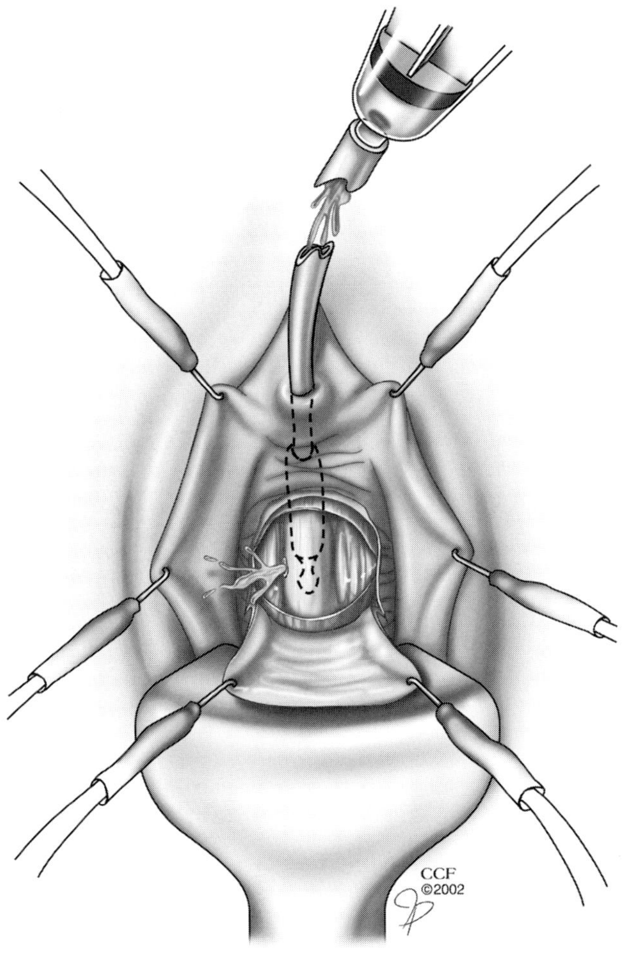


Fig. 29.7

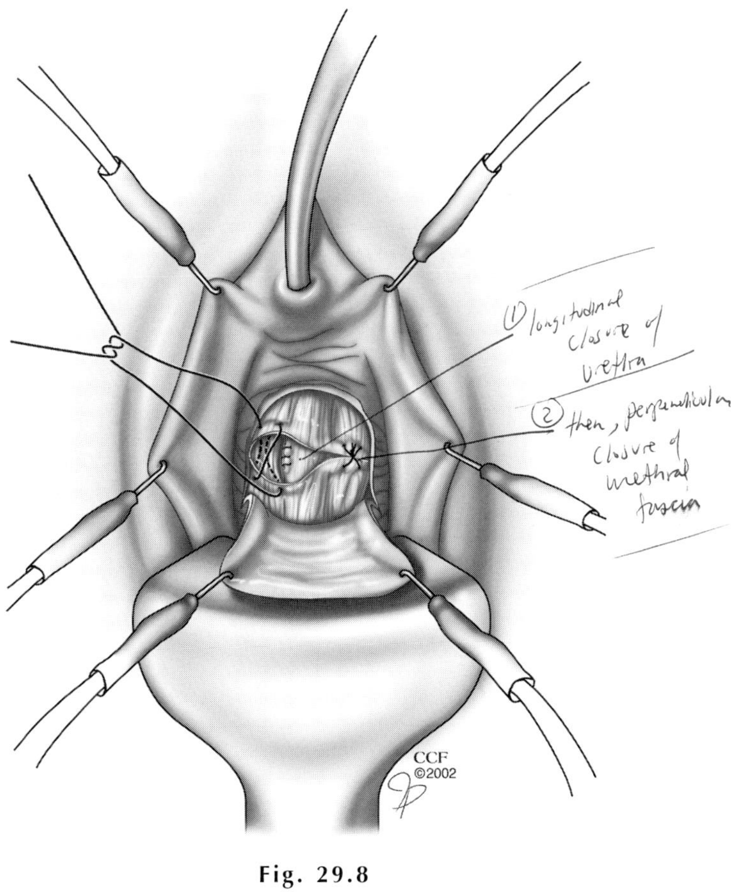


Fig. 29.8

The finding of a large periurethral abscess may require a staged procedure in which the abscess is drained and excision of the diverticulum is performed as a secondary procedure.

A large proximal urethral diverticulum may extend into the trigone and bladder. Instillation of indigo carmine into the bladder will assure bladder integrity, and cystoscopy after intravenous injection of indigo carmine may be performed in select cases to rule out ureteric injury *(8,9)*.

## Postoperative Complications

Urethrovaginal fistula formation is the most difficult complication of diverticula surgery and should be treated after a reasonable period of healing. This may require at least 3 mo of maturation to allow the inflammatory response after surgery to subside in order to optimize the subsequent surgical repair. Often, a Martius flap is placed over the repair to improve the chances of success. If an abscess forms, surgical drainage is required despite the potential damage to the repair.

Risk factors for diverticula recurrence include active urethral infection, difficult dissection, and excessive suture-line tension. Secondary urinary stress incontinence not present before surgery is rare but may develop in patients with prior anatomical defects because of dissection of the urethral support mechanisms. Severe incontinence caused by a nonfunctional sphincter may result from extensive dissection of the urethral wall. Surgical therapy for this condition may require a sling procedure or periurethral injection.

## CONCLUSIONS

The evaluation of the female urethral diverticulum has evolved greatly over the past several years. Still, its ultimate diagnosis may be difficult. However, once the appropriate diagnosis is made, the management scheme is fairly straightforward. Strict adherence to principles of surgical reconstruction allows one to eradicate the diverticulum while simultaneously preventing recurrence and complications.

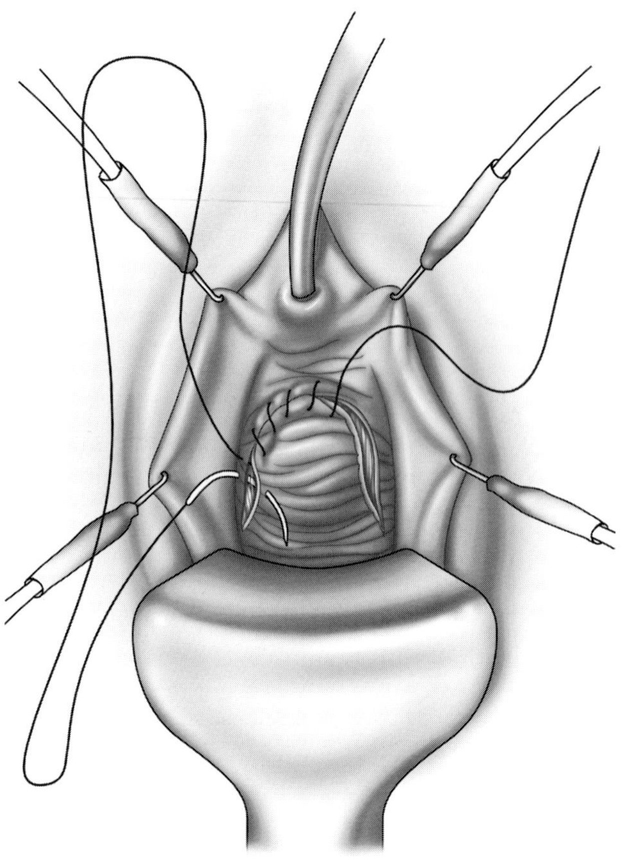

Fig. 29.9

## REFERENCES


1. Romanzi LJ, Groutz A, Blaivas JG. Urethral diverticulum in women: diverse presentations resulting in diagnostic delay and mismanagement. J Urol 164: 428–433, 2000.
2. Wang AC, Wang CR. Radiologic diagnosis and surgical treatment of urethral diverticulum in women: a reappraisal of voiding cystourethrography and positive pressure prethrography. J Reprod Med 45(5): 377–382, 2000.
3. Neitlich JD, Foster HE, Glickman GG, Smith RC. Detection of urethral diverticula in women: comparison of a high resolution fast spin echo technique with double balloon urethrography. J Urol 159:408–410, 1998.
4. Gousse AE, Barbaric ZL, Safir MH, Madjar S, Marumotot AK, Raz S. Dynamic half Fourier acquisition, single shot turbo spin-echo magnetic resonance imaging for evaluating the female pelvis. J Urol 164(5): 1606–1613, 2000.
5. Leng WW, McGuire EJ. Management of female urethral diverticula: a new classification. J Urol 160: 1297–1300, 1998.
6. Faerber GJ. Urethral diverticulectomy and pubovaginal sling for simultaneous treatment of urethral diverticulum and intrinsic sphincteric deficiency. Tech Urol 4(4):192–197, 1998.
7. Leach GE. Urethrovaginal fistula repair with Martius labial fat pad graft. Urol Clin North Am 18:409–413, 1991.
8. Pallapattu G, Vasavada SP, Comiter CV, Raz S. Repair of urethral diverticulum. In: Raz s,ed. Atlas of the Urologic Clinics of North America — Vaginal Surgery, Vol. 8. Baltimore: Williams and Wilkins, 2000:61–70.
9. Vasavada SP, Comiter CV, Rovner ES, Raz S: How to prevent complications in vaginal surgery. J Bras Urol. 25(2):152–160, 1999.

# 30 Repair of Anterior Vaginal Wall Prolapse

*Sandip P. Vasavada, Raymond R. Rackley, Howard Goldman, and Firouz Daneshgari*

## INTRODUCTION

A grade IV cystocele represents prolapse of the anterior vaginal wall outside of the introitus at rest. The etiology of this severe form of prolapse is secondary to defects in several areas of pelvic support, including (1) the attenuation of the vesicopelvic fascia, (2) loss of lateral attachments from the bladder to the pelvic sidewall resulting in lateral/sliding cystoceles, (3) loss of bladder neck support, and (4) separation of the cardinal ligaments. These four defects often accompany most grade IV cystoceles and must be corrected in order to achieve good support and elevation of the bladder base and a solid repair.

A central defect cystocele is manifest by loss of the support of the vesicopelvic fascia and results in central herniation of the bladder base into the introitus. The lateral support may be retained, and clinically on examination, the lateral sulcus may retain its H shape. If, however, there is loss of lateral support and a sliding herniation of the bladder, loss of the H shape may result. Additionally, as central and lateral support structures are weakened, the cardinal ligaments become lax and separate. Paramount to the management of high-grade cystoceles is the fact that many patients have associated urethral hypermobility and would develop significant stress incontinence if support to the urethra were not given at the same setting. Thus, a preoperative urodynamics study with vaginal packing is important. Proper repair of the grade IV cystocele requires isolation and fixation of all defects.

## DIAGNOSIS

Clinical examination demonstrates prolapse of the anterior vaginal wall outside the introitus at rest. One must delineate the nature of the prolapse accurately, as appearance may be difficult to differentiate from an enterocele or a large rectocele. We have used single-shot turbo fast spin echo dynamic magnetic resonance imaging (MRI) sequences to further define the nature of the prolapse and evaluate for potential enteroceles, rectoceles, or uterine prolapse. Many patients with severe anterior vaginal wall prolapse have defects in pelvic floor relaxation such that they are predisposed to formation of these other forms of prolapse. The MRI also allows simultaneous viewing of the distal ureters in order to demonstrate ureteral dilation that may accompany high-grade cystoceles with kinking of the trigone. This information is invaluable as a preoperative tool because it allows one to properly define the exact nature of the prolapse. In the office setting, we have also found it useful to use a light test to more accurately differentiate a cystocele from other types of vaginal prolapse. This is performed during cystoscopy with the tip of the cystoscope aimed downward. Although this test is quite simple, it can yield important information as well.

## TECHNIQUE

A midline incision is created in the anterior vaginal wall as in other grade IV cystocele approaches (Fig. 30.1). The dissection is carried laterally to remove the vaginal epithelium from the perivesical fascia up to the lateral sulcus. The retropubic space is entered sharply with the curved Mayo scissors to allow palpation of the pubic bone if simultaneous pubovaginal sling is required. Alternatively, it can be preserved if a tension-free or other mid-urethral sling is to be performed.

The cardinal ligaments are isolated and plicated with 2-0 polyglycolic acid sutures in order to correct their separation and laxity (Fig. 30.2). This forms the basis for the repair of one of the important defects in cystoceles.

From: *Operative Urology at the Cleveland Clinic*
Edited by: A. Novick et al. © Humana Press Inc., Totowa, NJ

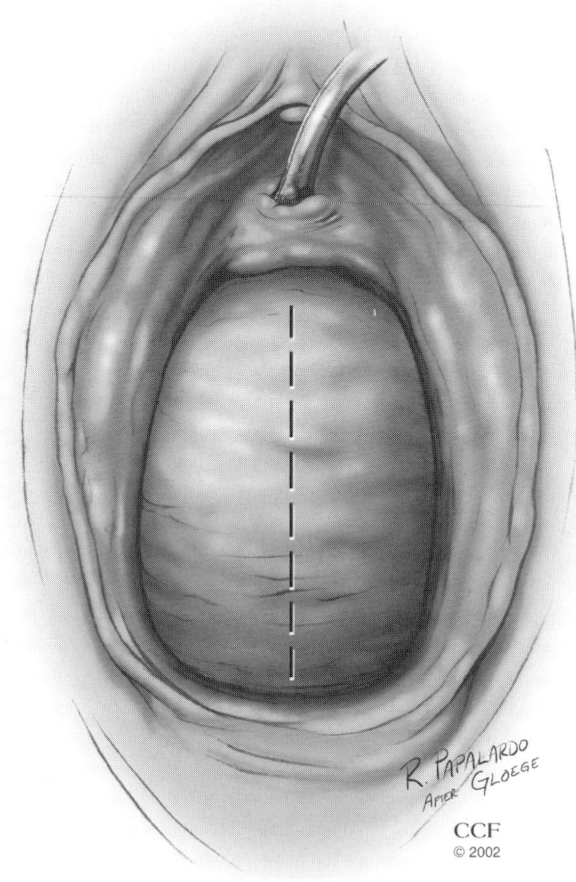


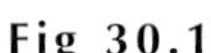

Fig 30.1

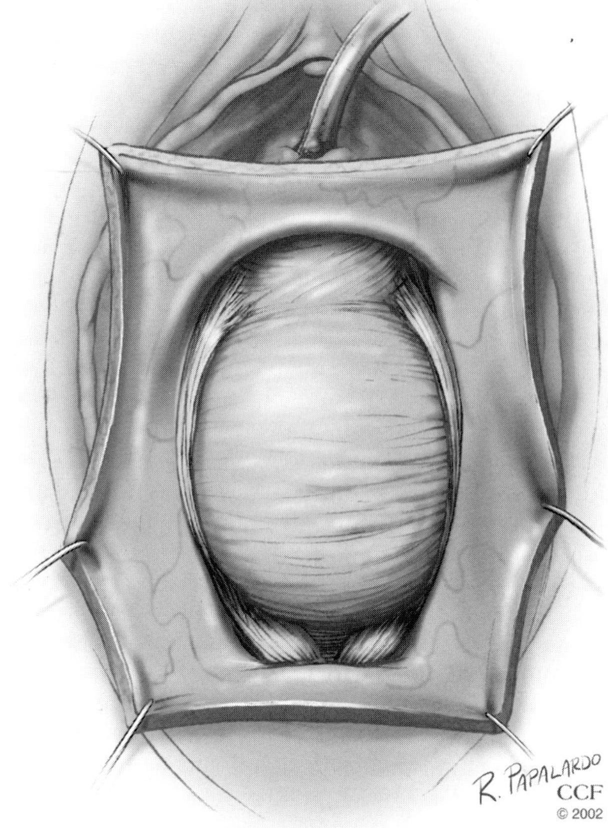


Fig 30.2

The sutures are placed into the levator fascia on each side, thereby preventing the sliding defect herniation of the bladder base. Additionally, the cardinal ligaments form the base of the cystocele repair and anchor the posterior portion of the patch if used.

The perivesical fascia is plicated after the central defect cystocele is reduced with use of an optional absorbable mesh (Fig. 30.3). The fascia is reapproximated with horizontal mattress sutures of 0-polyglycolic acid sutures in order to avoid ureteric injury. The tissue is brought to the midline over the mesh to facilitate reapproximation without tension, and this maneuver also helps reduce the incidence of ureteric injury. Prior to this, intravenous indigo carmine dye is administered to ensure patency of the ureters. A separate set of polyglycolic acid sutures is placed into the levator fascia distally at the level of the bladder neck to support the distal portion of the patch if used.

A segment of allograft, xenograft or synthetic mesh is then fashioned such that the width spans from levator fascia or even obturator fascia to the contralateral side (Fig. 30.4). The sutures are placed in the corners of the patch 5 mm from the edge. The length of the fascial segment is dependent on the size of the cystocele and the distance between the pubic bone and the cardinal ligaments. We routinely trim a 5- to 7-cm segment to fit this distance appropriately. The lower set of sutures (through the cardinal ligaments) is placed through the patch segment in a similar fashion.

The excess vaginal epithelium is then trimmed and the incision is closed with use of a 2-O polyglycolic acid suture incorporating the underlying mesh in order to prevent any dead space for fluid accumulation. An antibiotic-impregnated vaginal pack is then placed for postoperative hemostasis.

## INTRAOPERATIVE COMPLICATIONS

There exists a wide spectrum of potential complications that may occur during the repair of a high-grade cystocele. Clearly, the most common intraoperative complications would include excessive bleeding and urethral or bladder injuries as well as ureteric injury. Because in most instances high-grade prolapse leads to thinning and attenuation of the perivesical fascia, it can be easy to enter the bladder during dissection. In order to prevent this, one must stay very lateral in the initial dissection and immediately

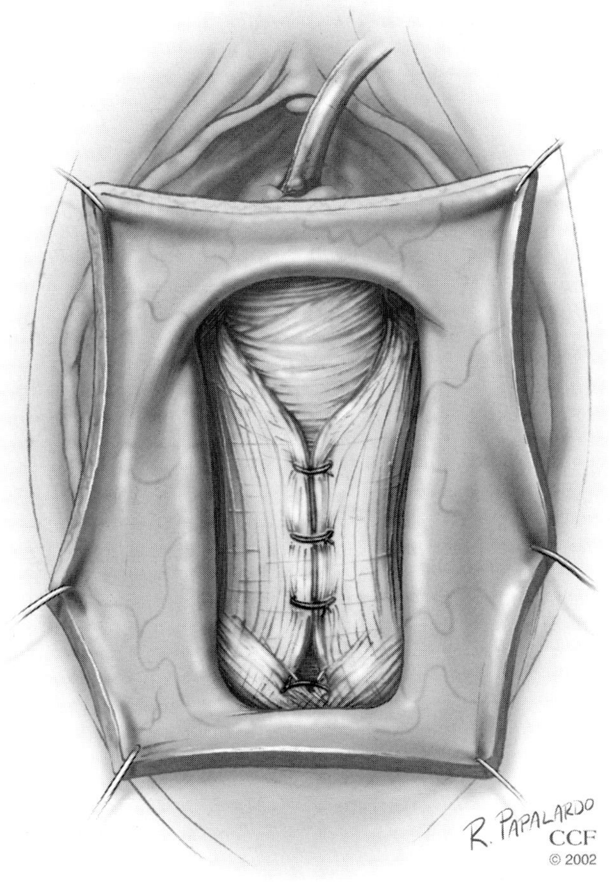


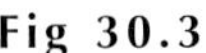
Fig 30.3

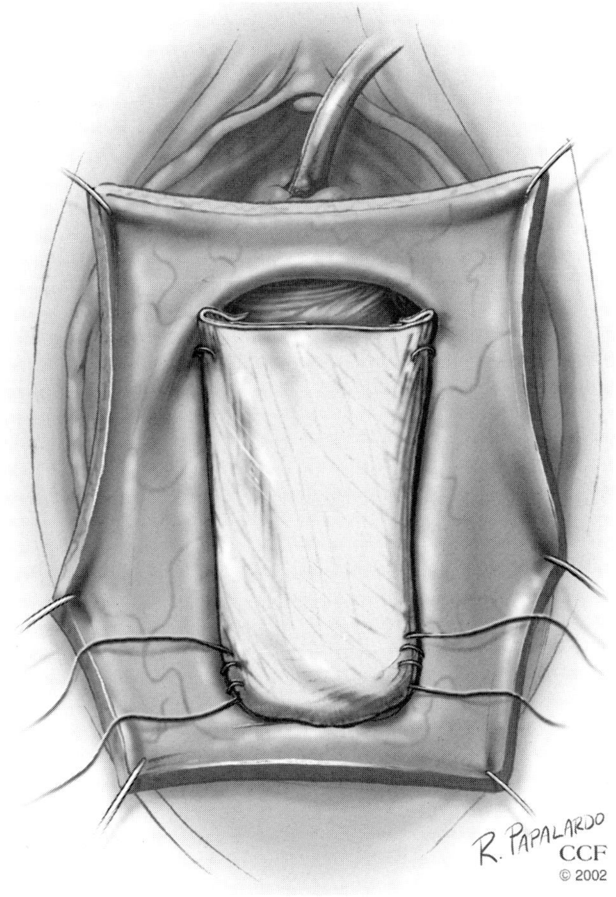


Fig 30.4

below the level of the vaginal epithelium, with care to preserve what little perivesical fascia there is to facilitate reconstruction. In the event of bladder entry, one must perform a multilayer repair with absorbable sutures and prolonged bladder drainage.

Ureteric injury can be prevented with several simple maneuvers. This includes placement of an absorbable mesh over the central defect or upward retraction with use of a Haney retractor to mobilize the trigone away from the sutures. Subsequent suture placement should be lateral to the midline in a horizontal mattress fashion, and the perivesical fascia should be brought over to the midline in the repair. Finally, indigo carmine dye is administered intravenously, and cystoscopy is performed to ensure patency of the ureteric orifices. If doubt exists concerning the patency of the ureters, either a stent may be passed or the sutures removed and replaced.

## POSTOPERATIVE CARE

A vaginal pack is placed and allowed to remain either for 2 h postoperatively (outpatient surgery) or overnight if the patient remains in the hospital. The drainage catheter is removed either at hospital discharge or 48 h postop for those done as outpatient surgery. A voiding trial is performed to ensure reasonable voiding prior to discharge.

## POSTOPERATIVE COMPLICATIONS

Postoperative complications in grade IV cystocele repair are not unlike those of other vaginal reconstructive procedures. These may include prolonged urinary retention, *de novo* urinary urge or stress incontinence, recurrent prolapse, vaginal shortening, or ureteric obstruction.

Urinary retention is usually a transient phenomenon and often resolves on its own. Rarely, one may require a prolonged course of catheter drainage or intermittent catheterization until satisfactory spontaneous voiding occurs.

*De novo* urinary incontinence (urge or stress) may occur in a small portion of patients. Urge incontinence may subside with time but often requires behavioral therapeutic modifications as well as anticholinergic therapy to assist in controlling symptoms. New-onset stress incontinence may result from inadequate bladder neck and urethral support or due to intrinsic sphincteric dysfunction. In order to minimize the occurrence of postoperative stress incontinence, we almost always support the urethra and bladder neck in the course of high-grade cystocele repairs, as they almost always have poor support.

In our experience, patients with grade IV cystoceles often require concomitant surgical procedures to correct severe pelvic floor relaxation in the form of enterocele, rectocele, or uterine prolapse. Simply repairing the cystocele without addressing these other potential defects in pelvic support may lead to recurrent vaginal bulges and require secondary procedures. As the anterior vaginal wall is transferred superiorly, this may allow a weakened cul-de-sac and posterior vaginal wall to prolapse in the form of an enterocele or rectocele.

Vaginal shortening can be avoided by minimizing the amount of anterior vaginal wall tissue that is excised; thus this should be a rare complication.

Ureteric obstruction may occur postoperatively, despite patency being demonstrated on cystoscopic examination, as kinking of the ureters results from the support sutures. If this occurs, one must address the obstruction by placement of either a stent or a percutaneous nephrostomy tube and passage of a glide wire down the narrowed channel. After a period of observation, if no patency ensues, one may proceed with ureteric reimplantation. Our preference is to not disturb the repair site, avoiding transvaginal exploration.

## SUGGESTED READINGS

1. Comiter CV, Vasavada SP, Raz S. Dynamic MRI grading of pelvic floor prolapse. Urology 54(3): 454–457, 1999.
2. Comiter CV, Vasavada SP, Raz S: Transvaginal culdosuspension technique for vaginal prolapse. Urology 54(5):819–822, 1999.
3. Vasavada SP, Comiter CV, Raz S. Cystoscopic light test to aid in the differentiation of high-grade pelvic organ prolapse. Urology 54(6):1085–1087, 1999.
4. Vasavada SP, Comiter CV, Raz S. Repair of anterior vaginal wall prolapse. In: Raz S, ed. Atlas of the Urologic Clinics of North America—Vaginal Surgery, Voil. 8. Baltimore: Williams and Wilkins, 2000: 109–132.
5. Vasavada SP, Comiter CV, Rovner ES, Raz S. How to prevent complications in vaginal surgery. J Bras Urol 25(2):152–160, 1999.

# 31 Repair of Bladder Fistulae

*Mark J. Noble, Sandip Vasavada, and Ian C. Lavery*

## VESICOGENITAL FISTULAE

### Vesicovaginal Fistula

Leakage of urine through an abnormal communication between the bladder and the vagina, or vesicovaginal fistula, can be one of the more troubling disorders faced by women so afflicted. In some cultures, uncontrolled leakage of urine from the vagina results in social ostracism *(1,2)*. In others, women may simply be embarrassed and may view the condition as quite incapacitating. There is little doubt that patients are quite grateful when this condition is corrected.

Most vesicovaginal fistulae were historically caused by child birth injuries, but improvements in management of labor and delivery have resulted in this condition becoming much rarer after childbirth. Currently, these types of fistulae most often result from complications of hysterectomy or other pelvic operations *(3)*. Cancer- or radiation-induced tissue necrosis can also cause vesicovaginal fistula, and such fistulae are generally more difficult to treat successfully *(3)*.

Historically, the first successful repair of vesicovaginal fistula is credited to Marion Sims *(4)*. He failed in more than 100 attempts before succeeding in May 1849, when he performed curative surgery in a slave who herself had already suffered 29 unsuccessful operations. Interestingly, other surgeons reported cures prior to Sims, so it is unclear why history credits him with the first success. For example, Hayward reported two successes, the first in 1839 and the second in 1847, while Gosset related a cure in 1834 *(4)*.

Current methodology for repair of vesicovaginal fistula emphasizes a number of important principles. These include (1) total separation of the tissues comprising the wall of the vagina and the wall of the bladder, (2) closure of the defects with nonoverlapping suture lines, (3) where possible, interposition of alternative tissue between the two suture lines, (4) control of urinary infection, (5) avoidance of postoperative bladder distension, and (6) attention to proper hemostasis throughout *(4,5)*. It is still controversial as to the optimum timing of repair of traumatic vesicovaginal fistula. Some believe in repair within a few weeks *(6,7)*, whereas others recommend the more traditional allowance of a 3-mo delay in order to permit subsidence of edema, inflammation, and the catabolic state that ordinarily persists for a period of time following the initial (causative) surgery. In general, transvaginal repair may be performed sooner after an abdominal causative surgery as the lack of intra-abdominal adhesions via the vaginal route permit earlier repair. There exists no evidence that one cannot successfully operate earlier in the post-event period, assuming there is absence of infection, severe inflammation, or other adverse factors that may preclude a successful repair. Thus, one should try to ensure that the first attempt is performed under the best of conditions.

One debatable advantage to waiting 3 mo before surgery is that a few fistulae may close spontaneously, especially small ones, thus saving the patient an operation *(8)*. Furthermore, although intraversial, very small fistulae can sometimes be cured with simple fulguration and continuous bladder drainage *(9)*. This may certainly be worth trying before performing an open surgical procedure.

Fistulae resulting from radiation therapy or cancer represent more difficult problems than do traumatic fistulae resulting from pelvic surgery or birth injury. These have a higher recurrence rate and are usually best treated with a transabdominal or suprapubic, transvesical approach (discussed later) *(10–12)*. In most such cases, this facilitates interposition of fresh tissue, such as omentum, between the bladder and the vagina, and has been shown to maximize the success rate of reparative surgery.

### Transvaginal Repair

Repair of vesicovaginal fistulae can be successfully performed through either a transvaginal or a suprapubic approach. In this section, transvaginal repair will be discussed first and its advantages described. First and

From: *Operative Urology at the Cleveland Clinic*
Edited by: A. Novick et al. © Humana Press Inc., Totowa, NJ

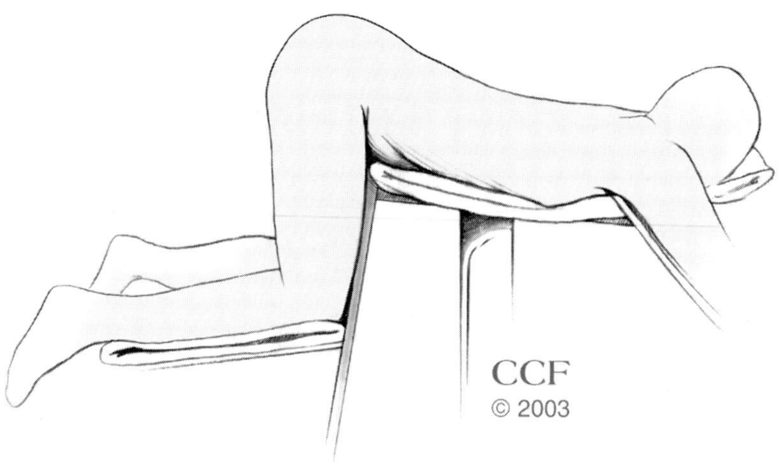


Fig. 31.1

foremost, a transvaginal repair tends to be lower risk and much less painful than an abdominal repair. This type of repair can often be performed on an outpatient basis or at least with 23-h observation (minimal hospital time). Recovery from surgery also tends to be quicker than for an abdominal operation. The basic principles listed earlier should be followed, and in addition, patient selection for this approach is a key to success. If the fistula is located anatomically in a particular patient such that surgical exposure will be compromised by the vaginal approach, then a suprapubic approach is preferable.

#### Exposure

A vaginal approach may be performed in either the lithotomy or the Kraske (jackknife) position (Fig. 31.1). The latter has the advantage of permitting the surgeon to work in a normal, comfortable position and is preferred by some authors for that reason. (Repair from the perspective of the Kraske position is illustrated herein; by simply turning the figures upside down, one can obtain the perspective for a surgical approach from the lithotomy position.) One begins by utilizing wide adhesive tape to spread the upper thighs and buttocks laterally. Redundant labia majora may be sewn apart with temporary stay sutures of 2-0 silk clipped to the drapes. A Sims retractor or equivalent is used to retract the posterior vaginal wall upward.

One next inserts a Foley catheter through the fistulous tract into the bladder, and the balloon is then inflated (Fig. 31.2). If one has chosen to use a urethral catheter rather than a suprapubic catheter (for bladder drainage), then this should be kept well out of the way from the dissection; leading it down in a dependent fashion is straightforward if the patient is in the Kraske position. If the fistulous tract is too small to permit insertion of a small catheter (8 or 10 French), the tract can be dilated with a hemostat, lacrimal probes, or Hagar dilators first. If cystoscopy has not been performed recently, or if there is some doubt about location of the fistula (and catheter) within the bladder, then a cystoscopy may be performed at this time. The catheter will help to stabilize the bladder wall during excision of the fistulous tract.

#### Dissection and Hemostasis

The vaginal mucosa is first injected with 1% xylocaine with epinephrine to facilitate hemostasis and create a plane of dissection in the vaginal wall (Fig. 31.3). Furthermore, there should be minimal bleeding, and thus, no extensive electrocautery or suturing should be needed during the fistulous exposure to minimize potential devascularization. A circumferential incision around the fistula (and catheter) is created through the vaginal mucosa, including an adequate margin of normal tissue, while the catheter is placed on gentle traction to allow the fistula to be brought into the operative field. An inverted J incision is made around the fistula to permit exposure of the flaps prior to fistula closure. The vaginal mucosa is opened by means of sharp dissection with either Metzebaum scissors or curved thoracic scissors.

The issue of fistula tract exision is controversial, but the advantage of leaving it intact is that it allows a strong epithelialized layer to permit closure sutures to be anchored securely (Fig. 31.4). Fistula tract excision may enlarge the fistula, increase bleeding (i.e., one may need to use electrocautery and risk further devascularization injury), or create poor tissue for anchoring closure sutures. The fistula should be closed in at least two and preferably three layers in a tension-free fashion. There should be at least one layer for the bladder and separate layers for the pubocervical fascia and vaginal mucosa.

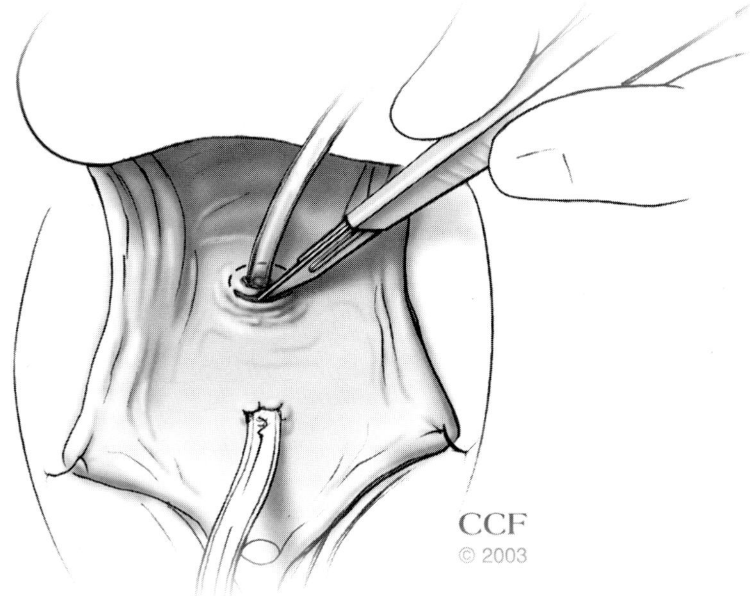


Fig. 31.2

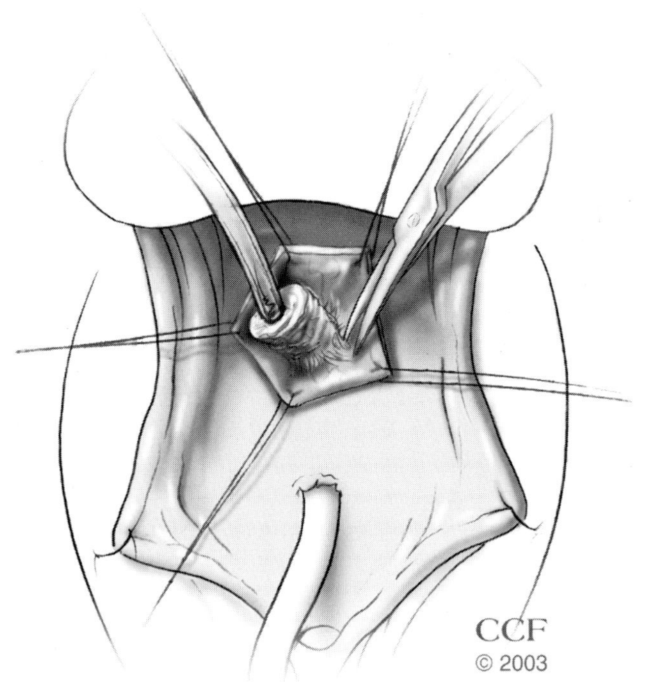


Fig. 31.3

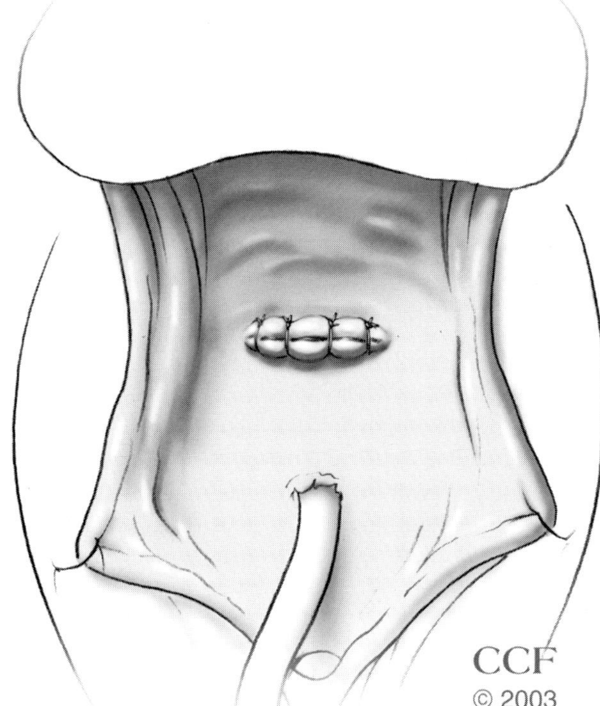


Fig. 31.4

The use of nonopposing suture lines is prudent. In special circumstances, a Martius, peritoneal, or labial fat pad flap may be placed between the vagina and bladder to reinforce the repair (not shown). We prefer 3-O polyglycolic acid (PGA) absorbable suture for each layer. It is important to try to invert the bladder mucosa to prevent it from becoming trapped in the vaginal closure suture line; if trapped in this way, it could lead to recurrence of the fistula. It is helpful to pressure test the integrity of the repair with distention of the bladder using saline instilled through a urethral Foley catheter; a proper repair should show no leakage. The final steps allow the vaginal flap to be trimmed and mobilized over the entire closure to

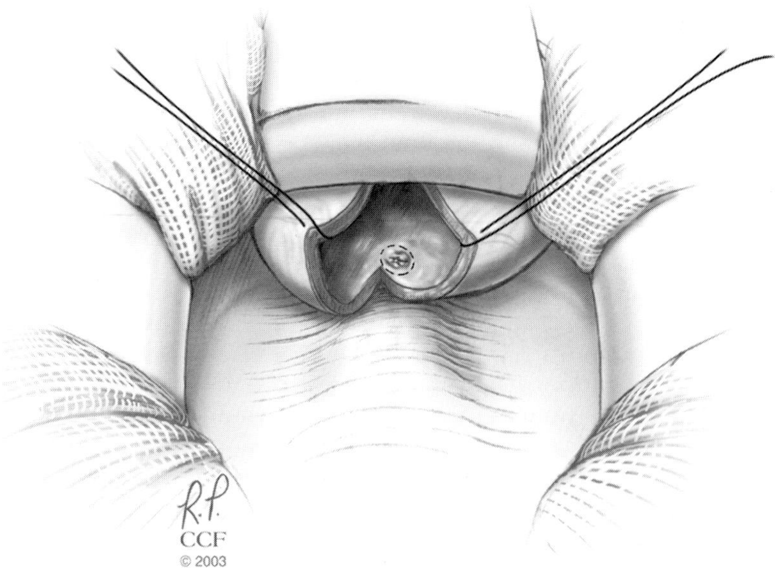


Fig. 31.5

ensure, again, no overlapping suture lines. A vaginal pack should be placed overnight to help with hemostasis and to eliminate dead space between tissue layers.

### Postoperative Care

If the repair site is close to the bladder neck, a urethral Foley might induce breakdown of the suture line owing to pressure of the balloon on the tissues. For these cases some authors prefer a suprapubic catheter over a long-term urethral catheter. If such is to be utilized, it is best placed and secured *before* the patient is positioned prone in the Kraske position. Sterilization of the urine prior to surgery is also important, and antibiotics utilized preoperatively should be continued well into the postoperative period. It is very important that the catheter not become clogged or kinked during the postoperative healing phase. Otherwise, distention of the bladder might contribute to breakdown of the suture line and to recurrence of the fistula. Furthermore, use of antispasmodic agents postoperatively may decrease troublesome bladder spasms. While the patient is encouraged to walk and may climb stairs or perform light duties, she should be advised to avoid straining, performance of heavy lifting (more than 10 lb), or sexual intercourse sooner than 6 wk following surgery. A stool softener can help prevent constipation and thus avoid straining at stool. Although the time for catheter drainage can vary, we prefer 2–3 wk of catheter drainage to ensure the best result. A speculum examination may be performed at 3 wk, and if healing appears normal, the patient can be given a voiding trial in the office. For difficult repairs or if there is lingering doubt regarding the success of the repair, a gravity cystogram can be obtained to ensure that there is no leak from the bladder (prior to removal of the catheter). The patient should be cautioned that her bladder capacity will be small at first, and she will need to void frequently as a result of bladder shrinkage over several months while the fistula was draining. She should be reassured that normal bladder capacity is usually achieved in 2–4 mo.

## Suprapubic Transvesical Repair

In those cases where a fistula is large, it is situated very high in the vaginal vault, or there is scarring that prevents adequate vaginal exposure to the fistula, a suprapubic approach becomes the preferred one for surgical repair. One should create an incision that permits exposure of the pouch of Douglas, the vaginal apex, and the entire bladder. Furthermore, if there is likelihood that omentum would be employed to further protect the repair (e.g., tissues that were previously irradiated with marginal blood supply), the incision should permit dissection and mobilization of the omentum as well. A vertical (midline) lower abdominal incision permits all options in this type of repair, as it is easily extended in a cephalad direction when necessary. A Pfannenstiel incision is more cosmetic but makes omental mobilization more difficult (but not impossible if the patient is fairly slender and there are no bowel adhesions).

### Exposure

The retropubic space is opened through a suitable incision, as described above (Fig. 31.5). The bladder is mobilized anteriorly and laterally, and care is taken to preserve the blood supply to the bladder and vagina. If possible,

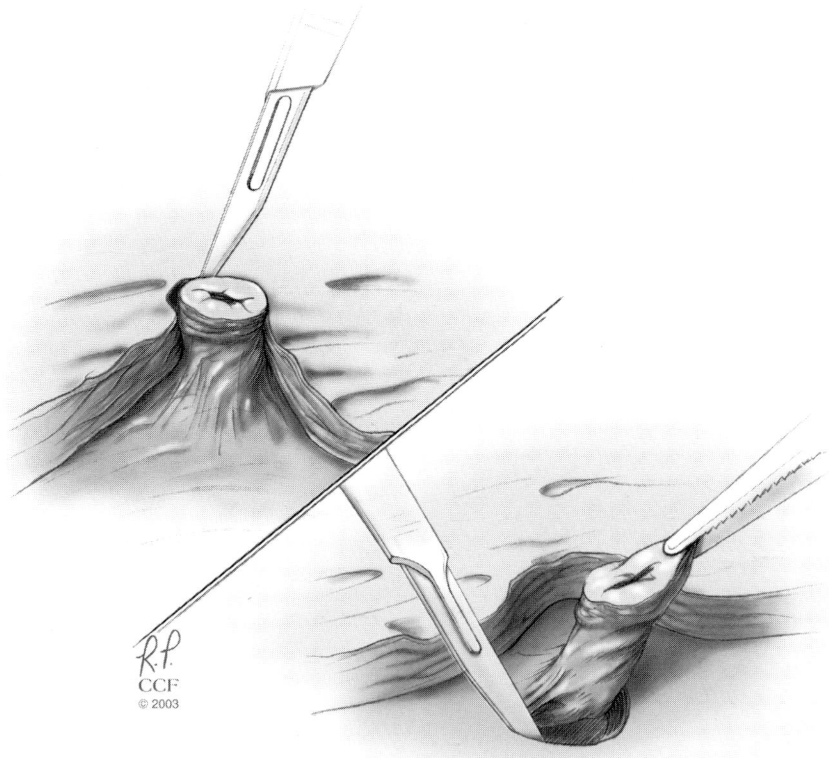


Fig. 31.6

the peritoneal cavity should not be entered at this time, but if the peritoneum is opened, then bowel must be packed away to keep it out of the operative field. If the fistula is extremely close to one or both ureteral orifices, then it may become necessary to reimplant one or both ureters after the fistula is excised. Placement of double J stents enables one to judge the proximity of the fistula to the submucosal ureteral tunnels. Although open-ended ureteral catheters can be placed cystoscopically prior to the abdominal incision and anchored to a Foley catheter, they are less easily manipulated in the event of ureteral reimplantation. A midline cystotomy should be carried posteriorly down to the fistula, as shown.

### Dissection and Repair

The fistulous tract is excised by circumscribing its bladder portion (Fig. 31.6a), dissecting it down to the vaginal wall, and removing it by a circumscribing incision in the vagina (Fig. 31.6b). Sufficient margin should be removed to ensure normal, well-vascularized tissue will remain for closure of bladder and vagina.

The edges of the vaginal wall are freed up by sharp dissection to permit adequate mobilization for closure without tension (Fig 31.7). Interrupted 2-0 or 3-0 PGA sutures are used to close the vagina, inverting the mucosa to avoid its entrapment in the closure (which might recreate the fistula). The bladder incision is only closed posteriorly (approximately half of the total cystotomy) at this stage, enough to repair the area formerly involved with the fistula. Running 4-0 PGA or chromic suture is used to close the bladder mucosa, and interrupted 2-0 or 3-0 PGA suture is used to close the outer bladder wall (muscle and serosa). If a ureteral reimplantation is required, it can easily be accomplished by one of several techniques, but with the anterior bladder still open, a modified Ledbetter-Politano reimplant is facilitated. Double J stent(s), if utilized, can be placed or adjusted at this time as well.

The remainder of the cystotomy can now be closed in the accustomed fashion (Fig. 31.8a). If a suprapubic tube is desired, it can be placed and secured at the time of anterior cystotomy closure and brought through a separate stab wound in the abdominal wall in the usual manner. If omentum is to be interposed between the bladder and vaginal wall, it should now be mobilized with careful preservation of its blood supply. If the peritoneal cavity was not previously entered, it must now be opened for this step. An omental flap should then be brought down without tension and secured in place with a few 3-0 or 4-0 chromic catgut sutures distal to the repair (Fig. 31.8b).

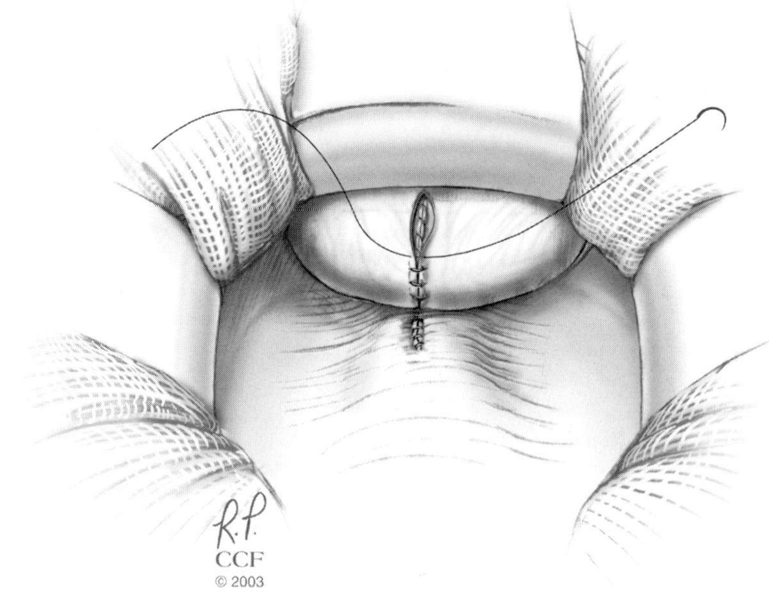


Fig. 31.7

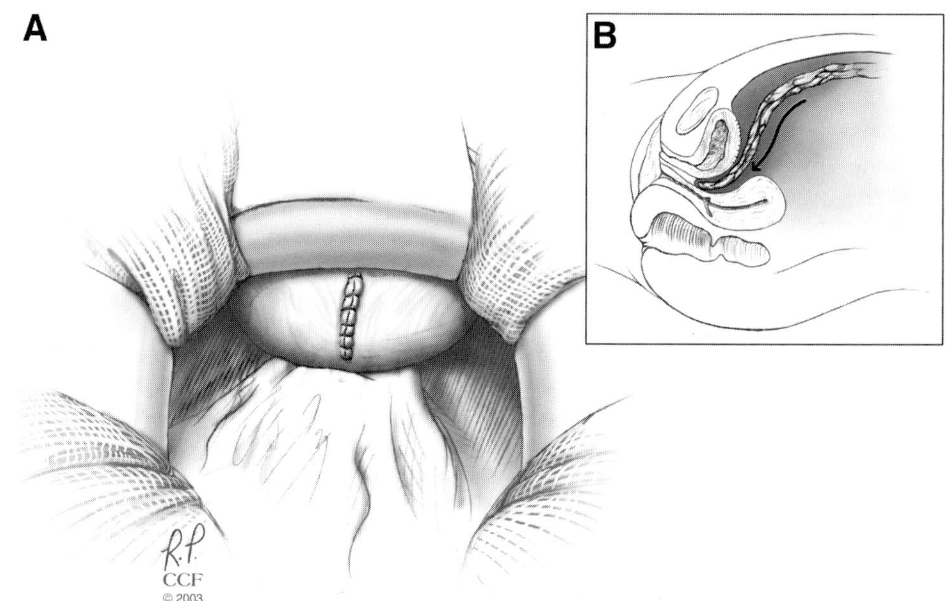


Fig. 31.8

A drain placed near but not directly on the suture line(s) of the fistula repair site is brought out through a separate stab wound in the lower abdomen and secured to skin. The wound is closed in layers in the standard manner.

### Postoperative Care

Preoperative antibiotics should be maintained well into the postoperative period. Foley and/or suprapubic catheter drainage should be continued for a minimum of 2 wk. This should be extended if there are other factors that might slow healing (diabetes, heart disease, prior radiation, etc.). A gravity cystogram should be performed to confirm no extravasation, and then a voiding trial may be performed. It was once customary to keep patients at bed rest for prolonged periods of time, just as was historically done after hernia repairs and other abdominal operations. But there is no scientific evidence that prolonged bed rest improves the fistula cure rate, and there is much evidence that it will increase morbidity from a variety of complications, including deep venous thrombosis. We believe in early ambulation but recommend avoidance of heavy lifting (>10 lb) for 6 wk, as with any abdominal surgical procedure. Sexual intercourse is prohibited for 6 wk and until a pelvic examination reveals complete vaginal healing. Routine use of stool softeners to help prevent constipation (and straining at stool) is recommended as well.

#### Concluding Comments

A very high success rate can be expected with the suprapubic transvesical approach to vesicovaginal fistula repair *(10,11,13)*. Success rates vary from 70 to 90% depending on the patient mix (previously radiated patients have a lower rate of success). This repair is ideal for patients in whom previous transvaginal repair has failed, as it permits exposure via a previously nonoperated plane as well as use of omentum to bolster the repair. In patients where omentum is not available, a peritoneal flap interposition, a Martius fat pad interposition, or a gracilis or rectus muscle flap interposition can often be substituted *(7,14)*.

### Urethrovaginal Fistulae

Urethrovaginal fistulae can be caused by injury from childbirth, poor healing following vaginal or urethral surgery (e.g., failed urethral diverticulum repair), tissue breakdown from pessaries or pelvic radiotherapy, or direct blunt or penetrating trauma. If the fistula is small and involves the distal urethra, the continence mechanism may often remain fully functional, and the patient will be asymptomatic and will not require surgery. However, if the fistula involves the continence mechanism at the bladder neck, then the patient's incontinence may vary from mild (from a small fistula) to severe or total incontinence (from a large one). Because no single methodology serves for repair of urethrovaginal fistulae, detailed operative techniques will not be presented in this treatise. If there is extensive tissue loss, reconstruction must be highly individualized and would depend on available tissue flaps, history of previous radiation exposure, and a variety of other factors, some possibly complex *(15–19)*. Most reports suggest that successful fistula repair can be performed in the majority of cases, but restoration of continence may not be successful, even with bladder neck and urethral reconstruction utilizing flaps from the bladder itself or from other viable tissue sites. In such cases supravesical urinary diversion may be the best solution for restoration of urinary control.

### Vesicouterine and Vesicocervical Fistulae

This type of fistula is becoming more common due to the increase in cesarian section for delivery *(20–22)*. It is felt to occur when there is injury to the bladder as well as to the uterus (or cervix), and these injuries are in close proximity. Some believe that the behavior is similar to external endometriosis. Patients may present with cyclic urinary bleeding at the time of menses, with passage of lochia in their urine, or with passage of urine vaginally (through the cervical os). Diagnosis is sometimes difficult and demands a high index of suspicion, careful examination, computed tomography (CT) or magnetic resonance imaging, differential pad testing (to localize the source of urine if incontinence is part of the presentation), and sometimes other tests as well. Surgical repair is usually straightforward, but some believe that hormonal management may be successful and can avoid surgery *(21)*. Hormonal blockade with luteinizing hormone-releasing hormone agonist-antagonist medication, as with conventional endometriosis, can permit endometrial epithelium in the fistulous tract to involute and die, resulting in spontaneous closure of the fistula. In rare cases, however, the damage is too severe, and hysterectomy is necessary during reparative surgery on the bladder *(22)*.

## ENTEROVESICAL FISTULAE

Enterovesical fistulae most commonly originate from sigmoid diverticulitis, cancer of the sigmoid colon, Crohn's disease of the terminal ileum, and radiation injury to the bladder, small intestine, or sigmoid colon and rectum *(23–27)*. Less common causes are carcinoma of the bladder, trauma, and other miscellaneous conditions *(28–33)*.

Enterovesical fistulae are most common in males. They are less common in the female patient, usually occurring in patients who have had a hysterectomy. The most common symptoms are those of cystitis, i.e., frequency, urgency, dysuria, and sometimes gross hematuria. Frequently, there are no symptoms referable to organs other than the bladder. Recurrent urinary tract infections or persistent pyuria are common modes of presentation. The classical symptom of an enterovesical fistula is pneumaturia. There are often only minimal symptoms with apparently clear urine in an established fistula. Feces are rarely seen in the urine, and the urine is sometimes sterile.

### Diagnosis

The development of urinary symptoms in a patient with one of the known causes of an enterovesical fistula heralds the onset of an incipient fistula or an already established fistula. The demonstration of pneumaturia or fecaluria is diagnostic. Sigmoidoscopy rarely demonstrates a fistulous opening. Examination of the sigmoid colon with a rigid sigmoidoscope is usually unsuccessful due to tethering of the sigmoid colon to the bladder. With the flexible sigmoidoscope an area of inflammation and edema is seen but the fistulous opening is rarely seen. Sigmoidoscopy, however, allows installation of air into the bladder to make pneumaturia more obvious.

Barium enema or small bowel roentgenographic contrast studies will demonstrate pathology in the intestine but will only occasionally demonstrate a fistula. However, after one of these studies barium may be passed in the urine. Cystoscopy is not useful in demonstrating a fistulous opening in most cases, but an area of cystitis may be seen and is a clue to the site of the fistula, and focal bullous edema may commonly be seen. Pelvic ultrasound may sometimes reveal inflammatory pathology associated with a fistula *(34)*. CT can be helpful in diagnosing an enterovesical fistula, as it can show the extraluminal disease process as a walled-off mass encompassing the borders of bladder and intestine *(33,35)*.

For the patient whose symptoms suggest the diagnosis of an enterovesical fistula but in whom there is difficulty in establishing a diagnosis by the above methods, the diagnosis may be confirmed by taking charcoal by mouth. The appearance of charcoal in the urine confirms the presence of a fistula. A cystogram may rarely demonstrate a fistula but usually proves nondiagnostic *(25)*.

## Treatment

An enterovesical fistula will not heal without resection of the diseased segment of bowel *(36)*. The presence of a large inflammatory mass or abscess in association with a fistula may dictate that a preliminary diversionary procedure be performed (ileostomy or colostomy) *(37)*. In otherwise uncomplicated elective bowel resections, it is usually unnecessary to make a preliminary diversion. The difficulty of bowel resection with an anastomosis is often less than anticipated, and the decision for concomitant proximal colonic diversion is made at the conclusion of the procedure based on local conditions, such as the extent of the residual inflammatory process, quality of bowel preparation, and medical condition of the patient *(37)*.

## Preoperative Bowel Preparation

### Mechanical Bowel Preparation

GoLYTELY or Fleet phosphasoda is given over a 2-h period on the day before surgery (4 PM).

### Dietary Preparation

The patient is given a clear liquid diet on the day before surgery.

### Antibiotics

We use intravenous preoperative antibiotics in the presence of an inflammatory mass. Metronidazole 1 g and ciprofloxacin 400 mg are given with premedication and continued for 24 h postoperatively.

### Irrigation of the Rectum Immediately Preoperatively

A 32 French mushroom (dePezzar) catheter is inserted in the rectum, and the rectum is irrigated with normal saline until the return of fluid is clear.

### Preoperative Cystoscopy

This may demonstrate edema and cystitis in the dome of the bladder. Infrequently, the fistulous opening is seen. The main purpose for cystoscopy is to eliminate other pathological conditions in the bladder as a cause of the fistula (i.e., bladder cancer). If the fistula is caused by carcinoma of the sigmoid colon, this may be confirmed by endoscopic biopsy. After cystoscopy, an 18 French Foley catheter is left indwelling in the bladder, where it remains for the operative procedure.

## Repair for Diverticulitis

The patient is placed in the lithotomy Trendelenburg position using Lloyd-Davies stirrups that permit a conventional hand-sewn anastomosis or the use of stapling instruments (Fig. 31.9). The abdomen is opened through a midline incision extending from the symphysis pubis to the mid-epigastrium. The small intestine is displaced to the upper abdomen, and the pelvic viscera are inspected.

In diverticulitis, the sigmoid colon and upper rectum are usually mobile above and below the fistulous opening into the dome of the bladder (Fig. 31.10). Even if a large mass is present, uninvolved bowel can be isolated proximally and distally to help isolate the fistula.

The fistulous tract is defined and divided by pinching between the thumb and index finger (Fig. 31.11). This leaves an area of granulation tissue through which the fistula enters the bladder.

The descending colon is occluded with a 1/2-in. linen tape to prevent contamination from the proximal bowel during the procedure (Fig. 31.12). A sigmoid colectomy is then performed. Extensive resection of the mesentary is not necessary, but it is essential that the entire sigmoid colon be resected, proximally and distally. Where a concomitant carcinoma of the sigmoid colon cannot be excluded, as is occasionally the case, the procedure should be as described for a fistula due to a carcinoma of the sigmoid colon. The rectum is identified as that part of the bowel that has no teniae and corresponds approximately to the level of the sacral promontory or 4–5 cm above the

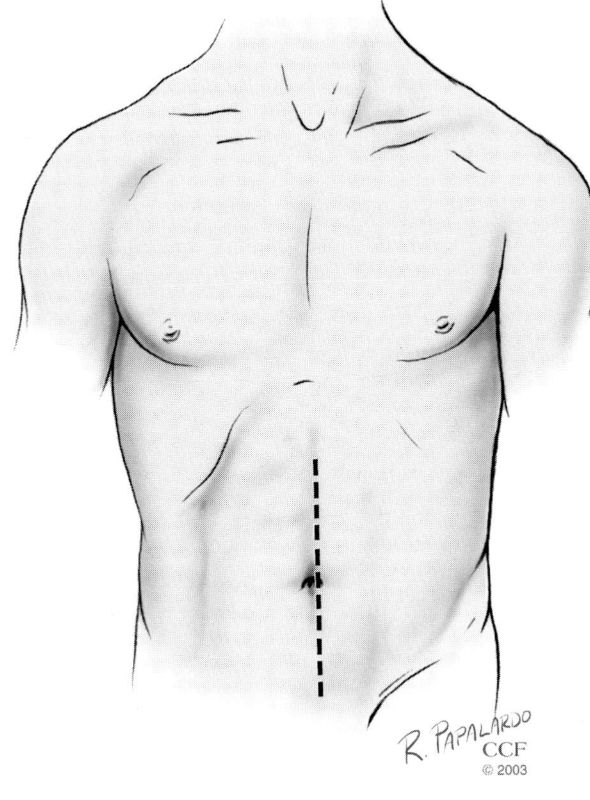


Fig. 31.9

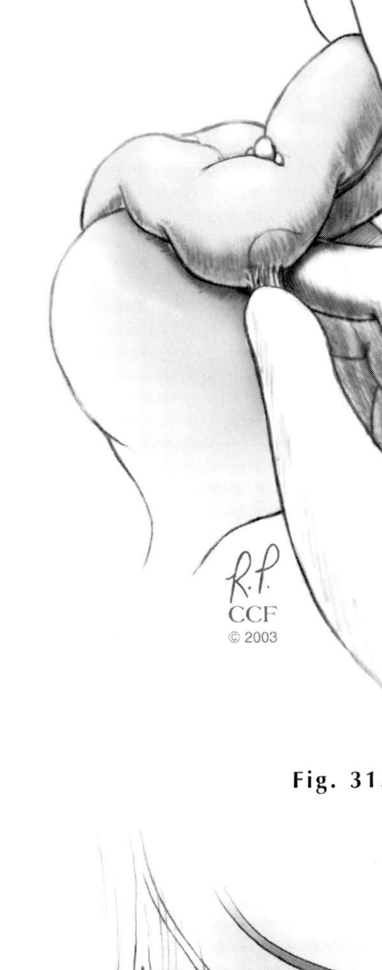


Fig. 31.11

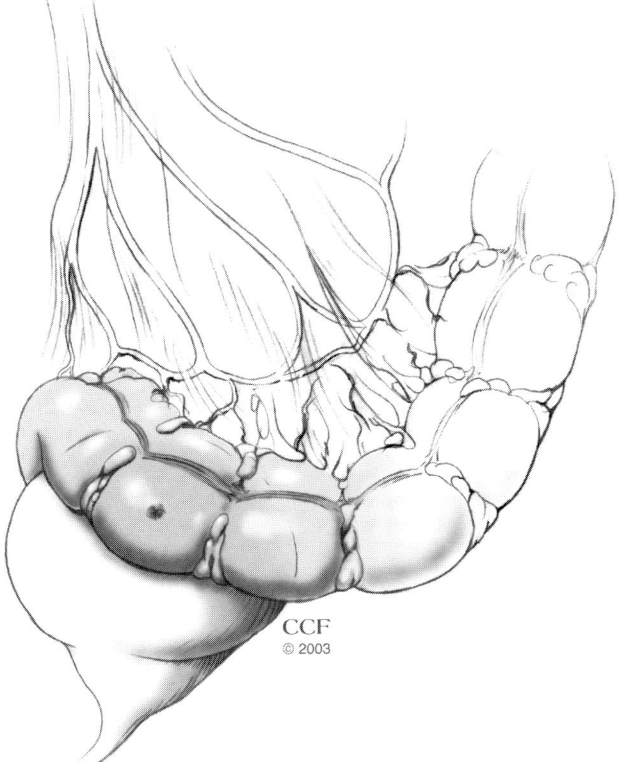


Fig. 31.10

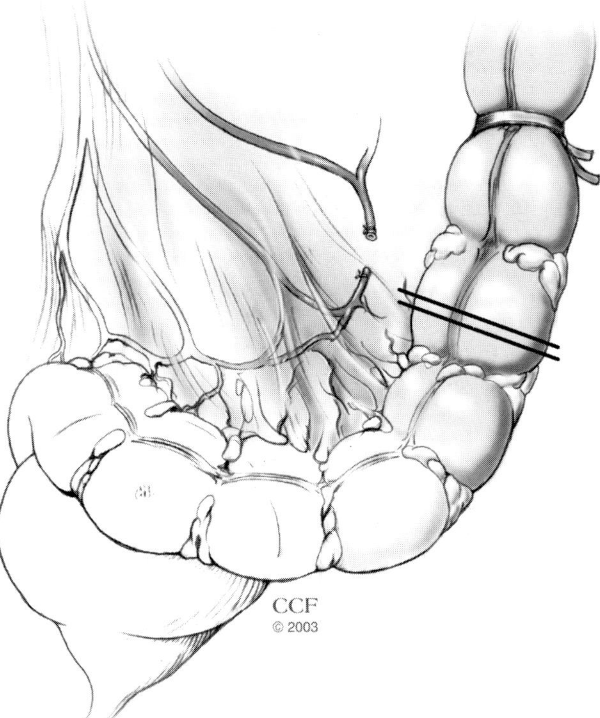


Fig. 31.12

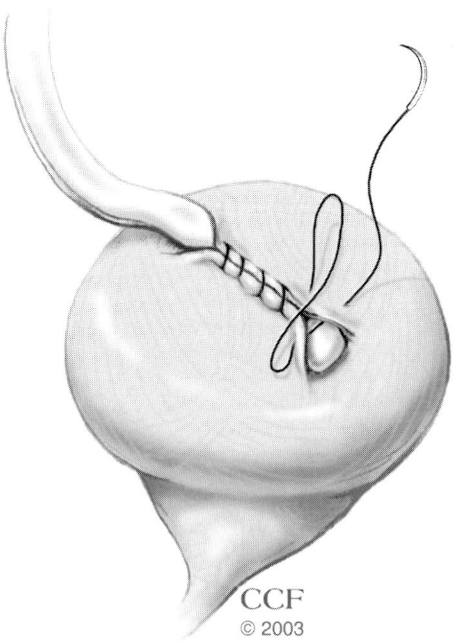


Fig. 31.13

peritoneal reflection. There is no need—and, in fact, it is contraindicated—to enter the presacral space when performing resection of the upper rectum.

The granulation tissue of the pyogenic membrane is curetted from the fistulous opening in the bladder wall and from the dome of the bladder (Fig. 31.13). This prevents further suppuration that will occur if this infected material is not removed. No attempt is made to close the bladder opening. If the area of granulation tissue is large or the hole is more than a few millimeters in size, a double layer of 7/8-in. Penrose drain is placed over the opening and invaginated into the bladder, approximating the serosal surface of the dome of the bladder using 0-chromic catgut. Invaginating the drain presents a serosal surface to lie adjacent to the colorectal anastomosis rather than the raw surface at the site of the fistulous opening.

An anastomosis is performed between the descending colon and the rectum approx 3 cm above the peritoneal reflection (Fig. 31.14a). The anastomosis is performed using an end-to-end stapling instrument introduced through the anus.

The anastomosis may also be performed by hand using an inner layer of interrupted vertical mattress sutures of 3-0 chromic catgut and an outer layer of seromuscular sutures of 3-0 Ethibond (Fig. 31.14b).

If the greater omentum is long enough, it is sutured into the pelvis, separating the colorectal anastomosis from the bladder (Fig. 31.15). If there is insufficient length in the omentum, a pedicle of omentum based on the left gastroepiploic vessel is created by detaching the omentum from the greater curvature of the stomach.

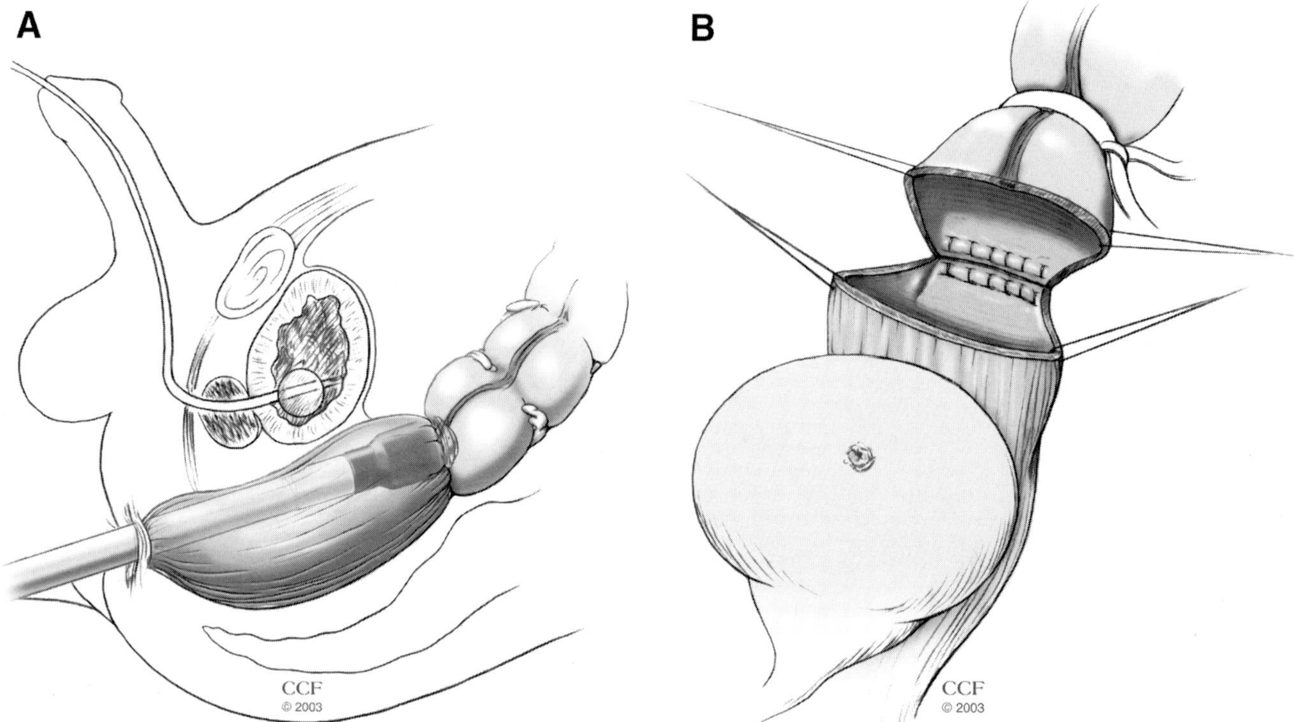


Fig. 31.14

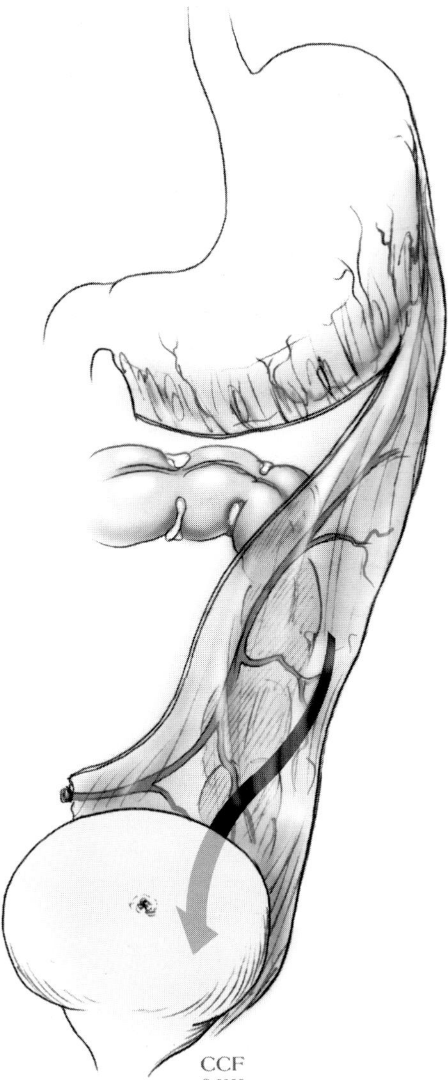


Fig. 31.15

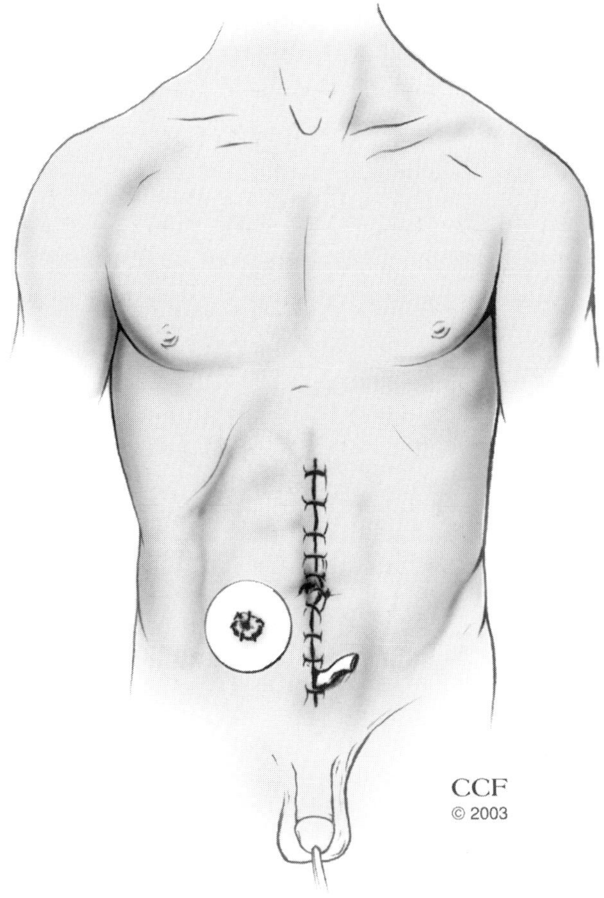


Fig. 31.16

The abdomen is closed in a routine fashion and the 7/8-in. Penrose drain from the bladder is brought out through the lower end of the wound (Fig. 31.16). This effectively exteriorizes the hole in the bladder and allows urine to drain to the exterior, should the urine not drain out the indwelling catheter for any reason. A proximal loop ileostomy is created if a chronic inflammatory nest remains in the pelvis or if bowel preparation is inadequate.

## Postoperative Care

The Foley catheter remains indwelling in the bladder for 7 d. On the seventh postoperative day, a cystogram is performed with postevacuation films to ascertain that there is no extravasation from the bladder. When this has been ascertained, the catheter is removed. The Penrose drain is removed 1 d later. Urinary antiseptics (Bactrim DS), one tablet daily, are given for 3 wk from the time of the operative procedure. Urine cultures are performed at the 6-wk follow-up visit. Ileostomy closure is performed in 3 mo, after radiographic demonstration of anastomotic integrity.

## Carcinoma of the Sigmoid Colon

Involvement of the bladder by a carcinoma of the sigmoid colon is managed differently from that of a fistula due to diverticulitis (Fig. 31.17). A wider resection of the sigmoid mesentery is performed using the preliminary lympho-vascular isolation technique to ligate the inferior mesenteric artery at its origin. The left colic artery is ligated and divided proximal to its bifurcation into ascending and descending colic branches, and the marginal artery is divided at the junction of the sigmoid and descending colon where the bowel is transected. The distal line of resection is in the rectum at least 5 cm distal to the lower border of the cancer.

No attempt must be made to pinch the bladder from the bowel (Fig. 31.18). This only causes seeding of the

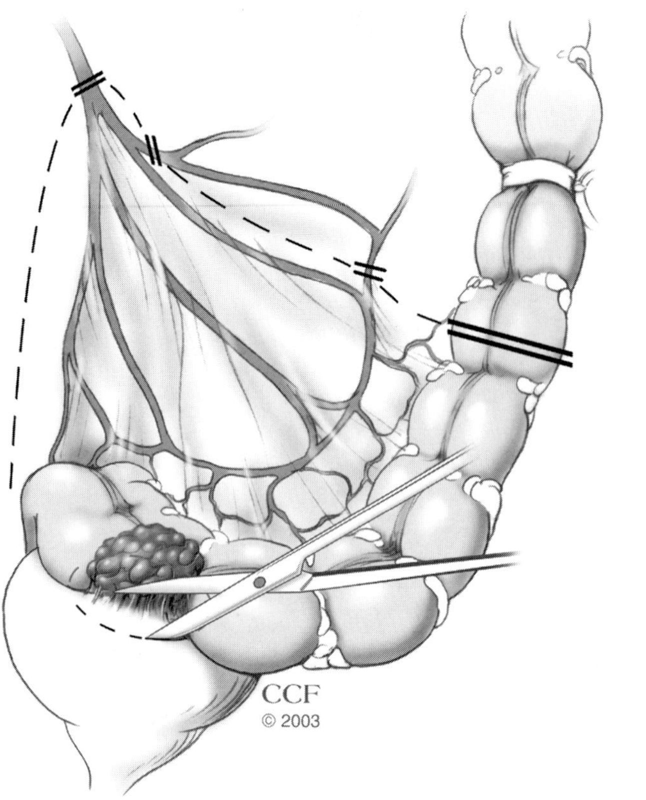


Fig. 31.17

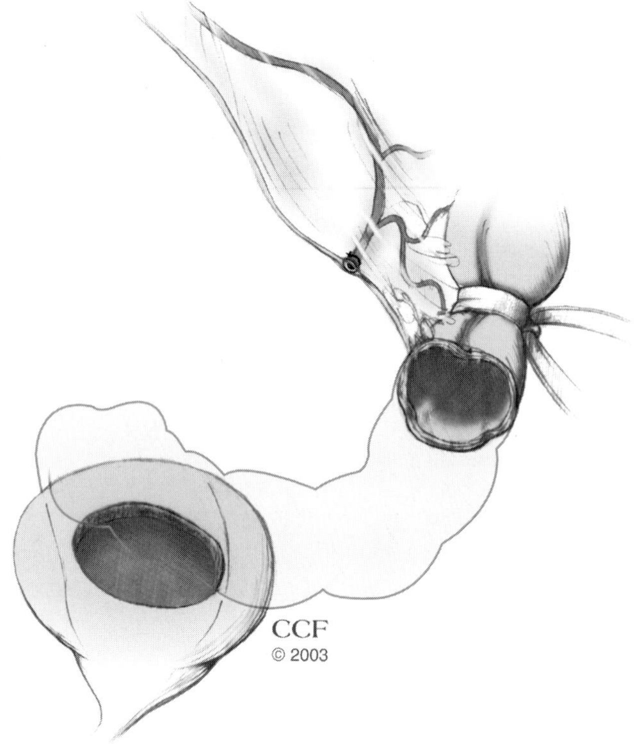


Fig. 31.18

peritoneal cavity with malignant cells. A wedge of bladder with a 1.5-cm margin from the site of attachment is excised *en bloc* with the tumor. Where the bladder is involved with an adjacent bowel malignancy, there is no associated inflammatory process. The bladder is closed in two layers using inverting sutures of O-chromic catgut.

## ILEOVESICAL FISTULAE FROM CROHN'S DISEASE

Being an inflammatory process with a propensity to fistulize, Crohn's disease of the ileum often will fistulize into adjacent organs such as the bladder and sigmoid colon (Fig. 31.19). Ileosigmoid and ileovesical fistulae are commonly encountered in the same patient in whom the primary condition is Crohn's disease. Recognition of this is important because failure to repair the ileo sigmoid fistula leads to severe pelvic sepsis with its resultant complications. The bladder, ileum, and sigmoid colon are separated by pinching apart with thumb and forefinger. This leaves an area of granulation tissue on the bladder through which the fistulous opening passes into the bladder.

The lines of resection are in macroscopically normal bowel (Fig. 31.20). The proximal line is determined by the absence of fat encroachment over the ileum from the mesenteric border. At this point, the mesenteric border of the bowel is visible with a definite angle between the bowel and the mesentery. The distal line of resection is in the ascending colon when the bowel is of normal dimensions without stenosis, thickening, serositis, or abnormal blood vessels. Termination of involvement is abrupt, and a 5-cm margin of macroscopically normal bowel proximally and distally is sufficient. Early involvement at the line of resection can be identified by aphthoid ulcers in the mucosa on the mesenteric border of the bowel. Further conservative resection is performed to remove the disease unless the early involvement is over a long segment. If there is extensive involvement of the small intestine, the anastomosis is performed in diseased bowel rather than resecting a long segment of minimally involved intestine.

An end-to-side ileocolic anastomosis is made using a circular stapling instrument (Fig. 31.21). The exposed shaft is introduced through the open end of the ascending colon and through a stab incision in the wall. After the anvil has been reapplied, the ileum is placed over it with a pursestring suture, and the anastomosis is performed (Fig. 31.21a). After removal of the instrument, the open end of the colon is closed with a linear stapler (Fig. 31.21b).

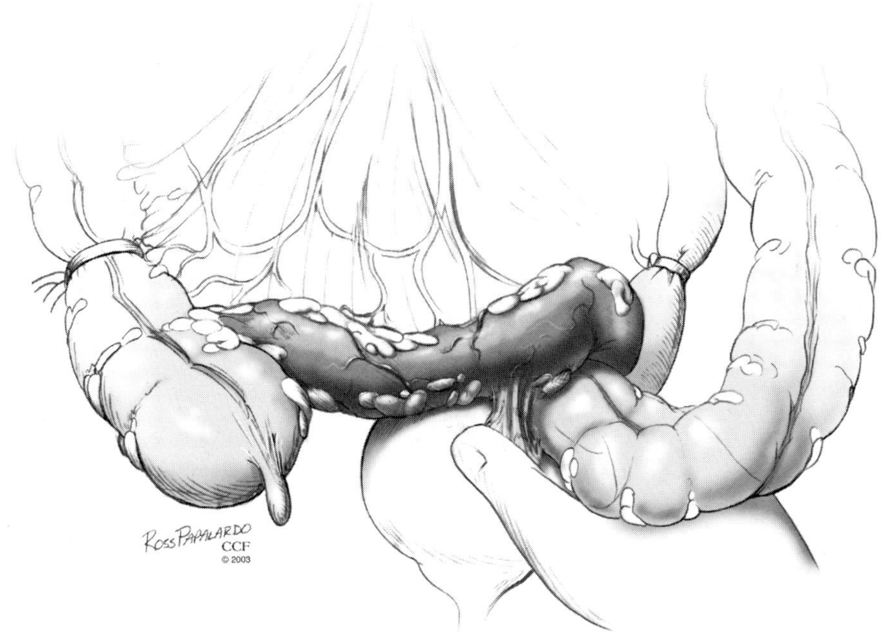


Fig. 31.19

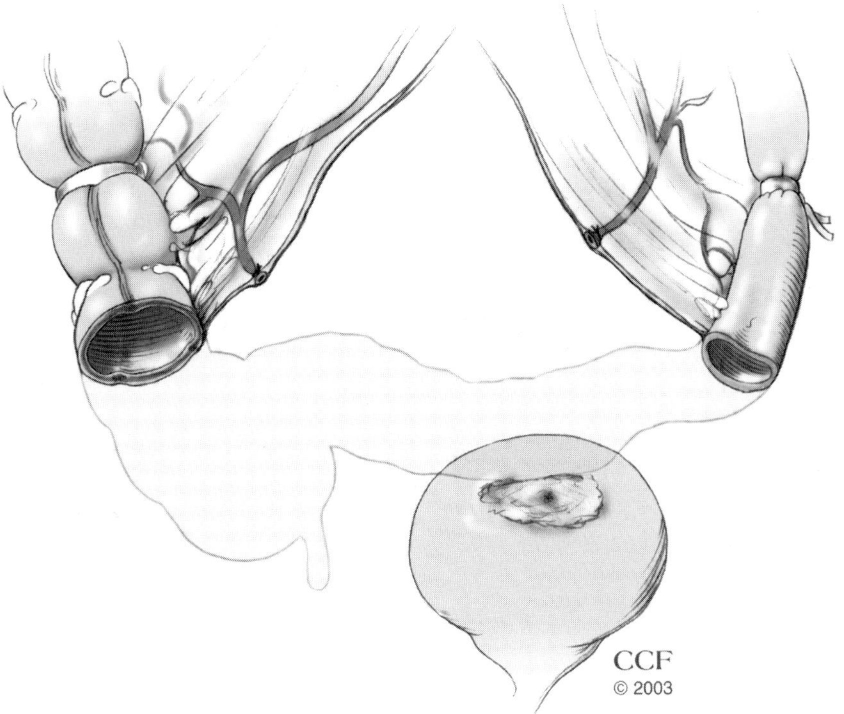


Fig. 31.20

The anastomosis may also be made meticulously in two layers by hand. An inner layer of interrupted vertical mattress sutures of 4-0 chromic catgut and an outer layer of seromuscular sutures of nonabsorbable material (Ethibond 4-0). A Cheatle slit is performed on the antimesenteric side of the ileum to make the two circumferences to be sutured equal in size. This maneuver eliminates puckering on the large colonic side of the anastomosis, minimizing the chance of leakage. In the presence of an inflammatory nest, particularly if the anastomosis has been performed in the right colon and the sigmoid colon, it may be prudent to perform a proximal diverting

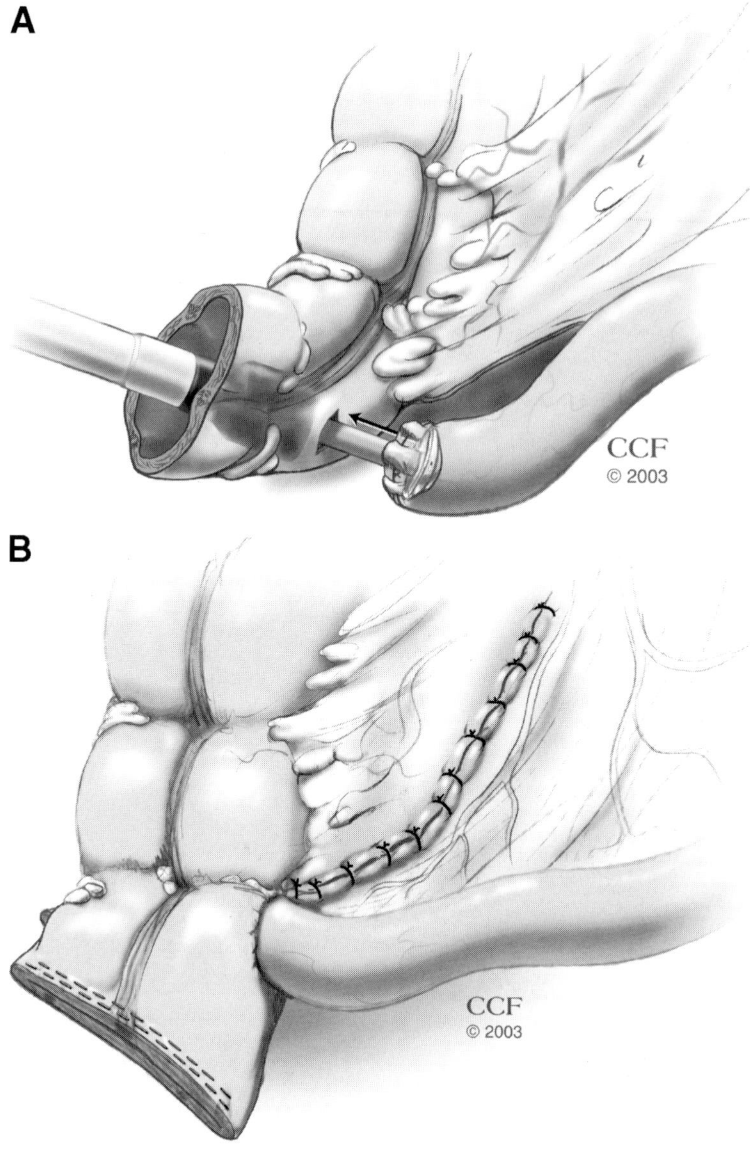


Fig. 31.21

ileostomy. The bladder is managed as illustrated for diverticulitis, and the postoperative care is the same. If an ileostomy is constructed, it is closed in 3 mo after demonstration of anastomotic integrity.

## REFERENCES

1. Elkins TE, Drescher C, Martey JO, et al. Vesicovaginal fistula revisited. Obstet Gynecol 72:307, 1988.
2. Falandry L. [Treatment of post-partum urogenital fistulas in Africa. 261 cases observed in 10 years]. Prog Urol 2:861, 1992.
3. Langkilde NC, Pless TK, Lundbeck F, et al. Surgical repair of vesicovaginal fistulae—a ten-year retrospective study. Scand J Urol Nephrol 33:100, 1999.
4. Krieger J. Repair of bladder fistulae. In: Pontes ACN, ed. Stewart's Operative Urology, Vol. 2, 2nd ed. Baltimore: Williams & Wilkins, 1989:539–551.
5. Vitale L, Revelli G, Kiss A, et al. [Vesico-vaginal fistula after abdominal hysterectomy. Use of the Legueu technique]. Minerva Chir 49:977, 1994.
6. Fourie T. Early surgical repair of post-hysterectomy vesicovaginal fistulas. S Afr Med J 63:889, 1983.
7. Raz S, Bregg KJ, Nitti VW, et al. Transvaginal repair of vesicovaginal fistula using a peritoneal flap. J Urol 150:56, 1993.
8. Frang D, Jilling A. Techniques for surgical repair of vesicovaginal fistulae. Int Urol Nephrol 15:161, 1983.

9. Stovsky MD, Ignatoff JM, Blum MD, et al. Use of electrocoagulation in the treatment of vesicovaginal fistulas. J Urol 152:1443, 1994.
10. Huang WC, Zinman LN, Bihrle W, 3rd. Surgical repair of vesicovaginal fistulas. Urol Clin North Am 29:709, 2002.
11. Kristensen JK, Lose G. Vesicovaginal fistulas: the transperitoneal repair revisited. Scand J Urol Nephrol Suppl 157:101, 1994.
12. Diaz Calleja E, Calatrava Gadea S, Caldentey Garcia M, et al. [Surgical repair of vesico-vaginal fistulae with abdominal-transvesical approach. Comments on this technique and long-term results]. Arch Esp Urol 50:55, 1997.
13. Weyrauch HM, Rous SN. Transvaginal-transvesical approach for surgical repair of vesicovaginal fistula. Surg Gynecol Obstet 123:121, 1966.
14. Patil U, Waterhouse K, Laungani G. Management of 18 difficult vesicovaginal and urethrovaginal fistulas with modified Ingelman-Sundberg and Martius operations. J Urol 123:653, 1980.
15. Bissada NK, McDonald D. Management of giant vesicovaginal and vesicourethrovaginal fistulas. J Urol 130:1073, 1983.
16. Koraitim M. A new retropubic retrourethral approach for large vesico-urethrovaginal fistulas. J Urol 134:1122, 1985.
17. Khanna S. Posterior bladder flap plasty for repair of vesicourethrovaginal fistula. J Urol 147:656, 1992.
18. Hedlund H, Lindstedt E. Urovaginal fistulas: 20 years of experience with 45 cases. J Urol 137:926, 1987.
19. Rangnekar NP, Imdad Ali N, Kaul SA, et al. Role of the martius procedure in the management of urinary-vaginal fistulas. J Am Coll Surg 191:259, 2000.
20. Jozwik M. [Hormonal dependence of vesicouterine fistulas]. Ginekol Pol 69:717, 1998.
21. al-Rifaei M, el-Salmy S, al-Rifaei A, et al. Vesicouterine fistula—variable clinical presentation. Scand J Urol Nephrol 30:287, 1996.
22. Kottasz S, Gergely I. Successful pregnancy after surgical repair of vesico-uterine fistula. Int Urol Nephrol 18:289, 1986.
23. Paul AB, Thomas JS. Enterovesical fistula caused by small bowel lymphoma. Br J Urol 71:101, 1993.
24. Miyashita M, Hao K, Matsuda T, et al. Enterovesical fistula caused by inflammatory bowel diseases. Nippon Ika Daigaku Zasshi 59:467, 1992.
25. Lubbers EJ. Bladder fistulae in Crohn's disease. Arch Chir Neerl 31:93, 1979.
26. Levenback C, Gershenson DM., McGehee R, et al. Enterovesical fistula following radiotherapy for gynecologic cancer. Gynecol Oncol 52:296, 1994.
27. Daniels IR, Bekdash B, Scott HJ, et al. Diagnostic lessons learnt from a series of enterovesical fistulae. Colorectal Dis 4:459, 2002.
28. Wyczolkowski M, Klima W, Labza H, et al. Vesicoileal fistula caused by a foreign body. Urol Int 66:164, 2001.
29. Urdiales Viedma M, Martos Padilla S, Navarrete Gonzalez P, et al. [Enterovesical fistula secondary to leiomyosarcoma]. Arch Esp Urol 45:474, 1992.
30. Vidal Sans J, Pradell Teigell J, Palou Redorta J, et al. Review of 31 vesicointestinal fistulas: diagnosis and management. Eur Urol 12:21, 1986.
31. McBeath RB, Schiff M, Jr., Allen V, et al. A 12-year experience with enterovesical fistulas. Urology 44:661, 1994.
32. Liu CH, Chuang CK, Chu SH, et al. Enterovesical fistula: experiences with 41 cases in 12 years. Changgeng Yi Xue Za Zhi 22:598, 1999.
33. Fraley EE, Reinberg Y, Holt T, et al. Computerized tomography in the diagnosis of appendicovesical fistula. J Urol 149:830, 1993.
34. Di Nardo R, Capanna G, Iannicelli E, et al. [Diagnostic imaging in the evaluation of pelvic complications in intestinal diseases]. Radiol Med (Torino) 88:49, 1994.
35. Goldman SM, Fishman EK, Gatewood OM, et al. CT in the diagnosis of enterovesical fistulae. AJR Am J Roentgenol 144:1229, 1985.
36. Nishimori H, Hirata K, Fukui R, et al. Vesico-ileosigmoidal fistula caused by diverticulitis: report of a case and literature review in Japan. J Korean Med Sci 18:433, 2003.
37. Moss RL, Ryan JA, Jr. Management of enterovesical fistulas. Am J Surg 159:514, 1990.

# V THE PROSTATE

# 32 Open Benign Prostatectomy

*Charles Modlin*

Open prostatectomy for the treatment of bladder outlet obstruction is rarely performed today because of the advances in technique of transurethral prostatectomy and anesthesia and α-blocker medical therapy for benign prostatic hyperplasia (BPH). Nevertheless, the urological surgeon must be familiar with the indications and techniques for performing open prostatectomy. The main techniques for performing open prostatectomy consist of the transvesical suprapubic prostatectomy and simple retropubic prostatectomy. Today, indications for open prostatectomy consist mainly of situations of failed medical therapy for BPH as well as situations in which the urologist considers transurethral surgery to be of increased risk to the patient compared with open prostatectomy (Table 32.1).

## OPEN PROSTATECTOMY

### Preparation

The patient should be given informed consent and counseled regarding the risk for blood loss, infection, incontinence, and erectile dysfunction. Blood should be available during the surgery. Preexisting azotemia, urinary tract infection, and dehydration should be corrected if present preoperatively. Open prostatectomy, as an elective procedure, should proceed only after the patient has been screened for cardiovascular, pulmonary, and coagulation disorders as indicated. Spinal anesthesia is the preferred method of anesthesia unless contraindicated. The suprapubic transvesical approach is preferred over the simple retropubic approach in situations where concomitant intravesical or bladder procedures are planned or anticipated and where a large intravesical prostatic component is present. Patients on anticoagulation medications present a special challenge and should have anticoagulation discontinued 5–7 d preoperatively following consultation with the medical physician and/or cardiologist.

**Table 1**
**Indications for Open Prostatectomy**

| |
|---|
| Enormous prostate gland size (>100 g) |
| Coagulopathy |
| Contraindication to transurethral resection fluid absorption |
| Congestive heart failure |
| Cardiomyopathy |
| Orthopedic contraindication to dorsolithotomy position |
| Need for concomitant bladder surgery: |
| Bladder diverticulectomy |
| Cystolithotomy |
| Reconstruction of bladder neck |
| Ureteral reimplantation |
| Prior urethral stricture reconstruction surgery |

### Instrumentation

The operating room should have available a basic laparotomy set along with self-retaining retractors with bladder blades, ureteral catheters, indigo carmine or methaline blue, vaginal packs, sponge sticks, hooked 11 or 15 blade scalpel, large-bore three-way urethral catheter with 30-cc or greater balloon, two-way urethral catheter with 5-cc balloon, and continuous bladder normal saline irrigation.

## SUPRAPUBIC PROSTATECTOMY

### Positioning of the Patient

The patient is most commonly placed supine on the operating table, or alternatively may be positioned in the low litotomy position to allow placement of a third assistant or nurse. A lumbar role may aid exposure to the retropubic area, and additional exposure may be obtained with gentle breakage of the table. The right-handed surgeon should stand on the left side of the patient. Following anesthesia, the abdomen and penis are prepped and draped, and the bladder is catheterized with a urethral

From: *Operative Urology at the Cleveland Clinic*
Edited by: A. Novick et al. © Humana Press Inc., Totowa, NJ

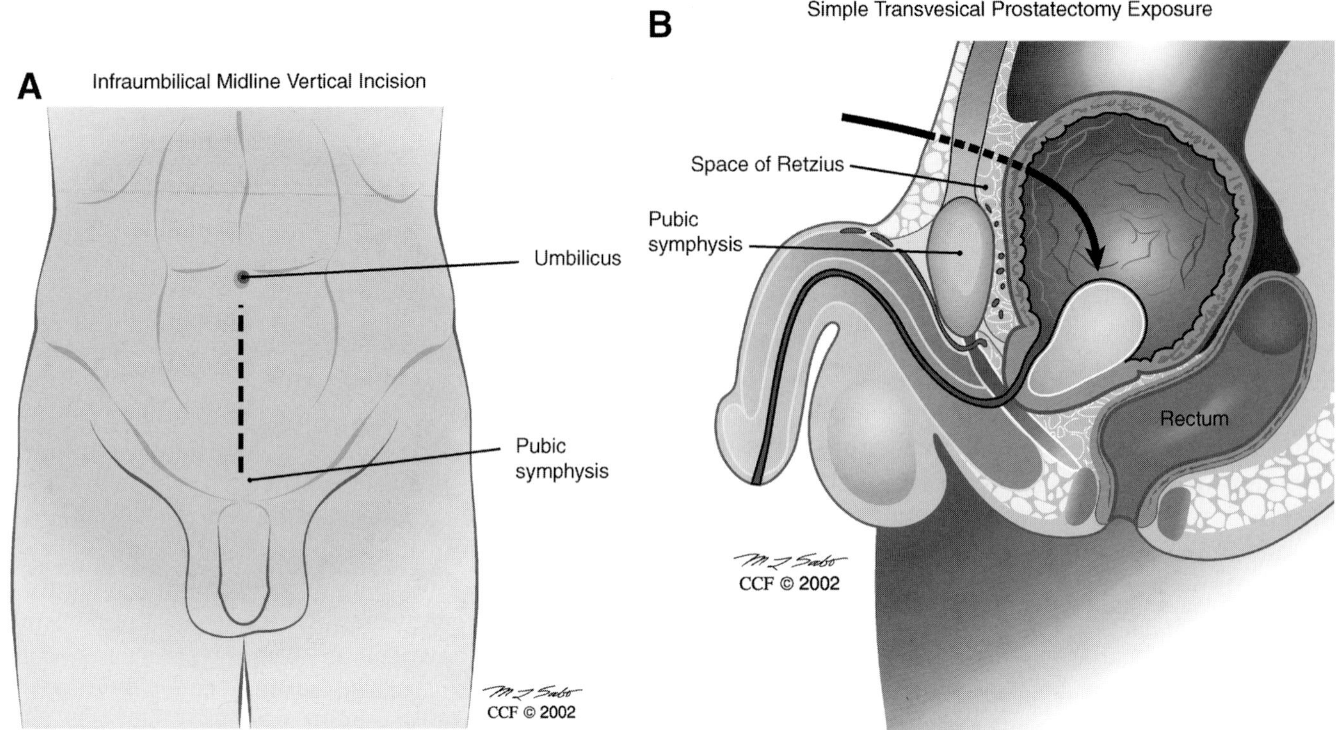


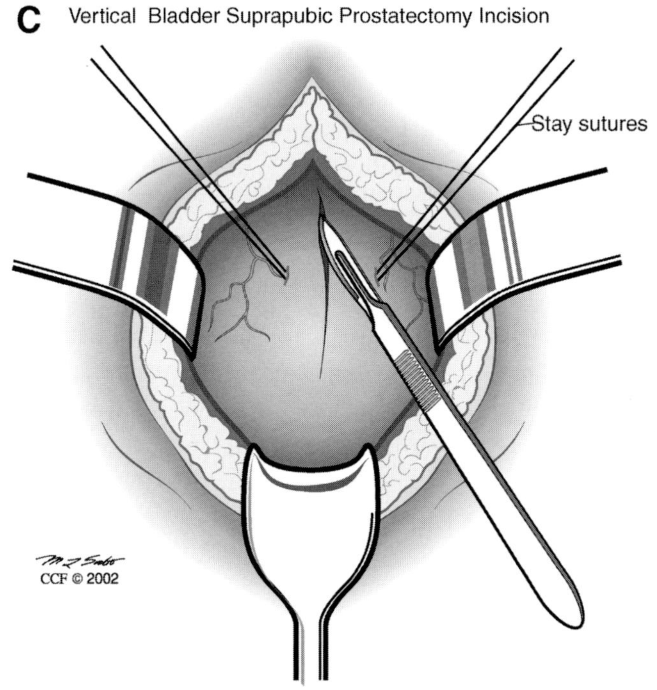


Fig. 32.1

catheter using sterile technique (16–22 French) and the urine sent for culture and sensitivity. The bladder is then distended with antibiotic irrigation to capacity and the urethral catheter clamped.

## Incision

Most urologists utilize a vertical midline incision (Fig. 32.1A), but a transverse incision works as well. Using the vertical midline approach, the skin is incised with a knife from just below the umbilicus to the pubic symphysis (Fig. 32.1A) over the distended palpable bladder (Fig. 32.1B). The rectus fascia is opened in the midline with electrocautery to expose the perivesical fat, space of Retzius, and detrussor muscle. A self-retaining retractor is then positioned to facilitate exposure of the distended bladder. At this point, O-chromic

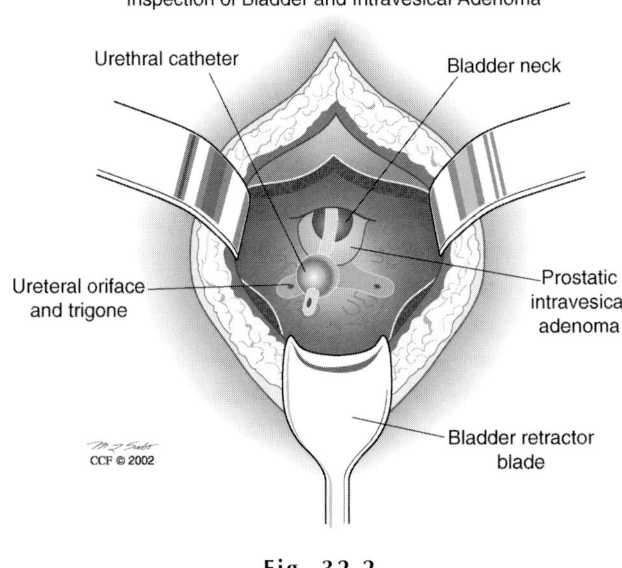


Fig. 32.2

catgut stay sutures are posited at 3 and 9 o'clock positions. With a knife and/or electrocautery the bladder is open vertically in the midline between the stay sutures and the bladder fluid aspirated (Fig. 32.1C). At the caudal end of the bladder incision, a figure-of-8 2-0 chromic suture is positioned and tied to prevent caudal tearing of the bladder incision during manual retrieval of the prostate adenoma. At this point, the location of both ureteral orificies is identified (Fig. 32.2). Intravenous dye may be given to facilitate identification. Some urologists cannuate ureters with ureteral catheters to mark the location of the orifices during the intravesical operation. At this point, concomitant bladder surgery, if required, such as bladder diverticulectomy, cystolithotomy, ureteral reimplanation, etc., is performed prior to prostatic enucleation; otherwise bleeding may ensue and complicate the concomitant procedure. The urethral catheter can now be removed. The scrub nurse should be ready with a vaginal packing following enucleation and the anesthesiologist comfortable with fluid resusitation and patient stability prior to proceeding with prostatic enucleation.

## Prostatic Enucleation

The initial step of enucleation consists of incision of the bladder neck mucosa only from the 5- to 7-o'clock position with the aid of a curved scalpel blade (Fig. 32.3A). The urologist should then advance the index finger (pointed up) of his dominant hand into the bladder down through the bladder neck and into the prostatic urethra down to the apex of the prostate. Once at the apex, the index finger firmly sweeps anteriorly to fracture the anterior commissure of the prostate, from apex to bladder neck (Fig. 32.3B). Then, the with the finger back at the apex, the entire hand of the surgeon should be rotated clockwise or counterclockwise with a firm index finger effectively separating the adenoma from the compresed surgical capsule of the prostate, the portion of the prostate that will remain *in situ*. Additionally, movement of the index finger will assist in enucleation of the adenoma. Both lobes of the adenoma are separated in this fashion up the area of the bladder neck (Fig. 32.3C). The last step of the enucleation consists of removing both lobes from the region of the bladder neck by pinching the adenoma to remove it. Often sharp incision with scissors is needed at this final stage to remove the adenoma from the bladder neck to prevent laceration and tearing of the bladder neck and injury to the trigone. Following removal of the adenoma, the urologist should inspect the prostatic fossa again with the finger to determine completeness of enucleation.

## Hemostasis

The prostatic fossa is then tightly packed with vaginal packing and held tightly in the fossa with a sponge stick to ensure hemostatis for 5–10 min (Fig. 32.4). The packing is then removed, and hemostatic figure-of-8 chromic catgut sutures are positioned at 5 and 7 o'clock at the bladder neck for additional hemostasis (Fig. 32.4). Electrocautery may be utilized sparingly, taking care to avoid coagulating the ureteral orifice and avoiding ischemic damage to the bladder neck. In rare instances of uncontrolled hemorrhage, the packing may be left *in situ* and brought out through the bladder incision and separate suprapubic stab incision. The use of a hemostatic bladder neck suture with or without a bladder pack may be also necessary in very rare instances (Fig. 32.5). In situations where a pack is utilized, a suprapubic cystotomy tube should be positioned through a separate stab bladder incision and suprapubic incision.

## Closure

Following adequate hemostasis, a large-bore three-way or multichannel urethral catheter 22–28 French should be positioned. Many urologists routinely also leave a 20–26 French suprapubic cystotomy catheter, although this is left at the discretion of the surgeon (Fig. 32.6). A rationale for leaving a suprapubic tube is situations of anticipated continued or delayed bleeding to facilitate irrigation and situations where it is believed that the patient may have detrussor hypocontractility, resulting in urinary retention following urethral catheter removal. The bladder is closed using a running chromic

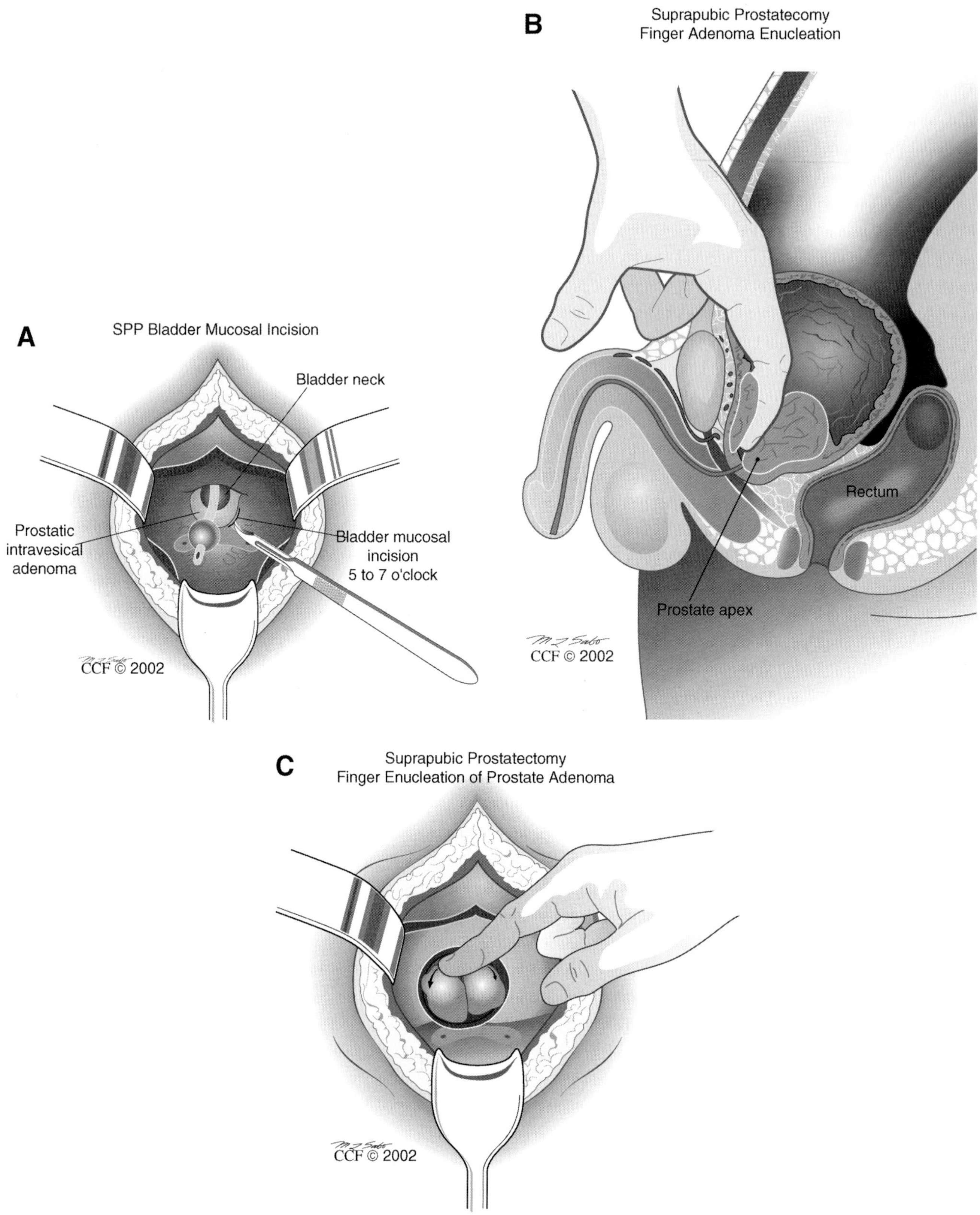

A
SPP Bladder Mucosal Incision
Bladder neck
Prostatic intravesical adenoma
Bladder mucosal incision 5 to 7 o'clock
CCF © 2002
B
Suprapubic Prostatecomy
Finger Adenoma Enucleation
Rectum
Prostate apex
CCF © 2002
C
Suprapubic Prostatectomy
Finger Enucleation of Prostate Adenoma
CCF © 2002

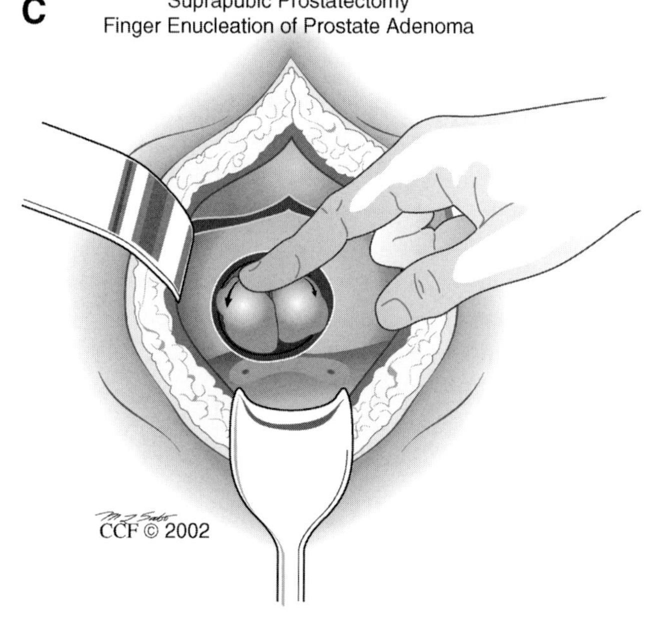

Fig. 32.3

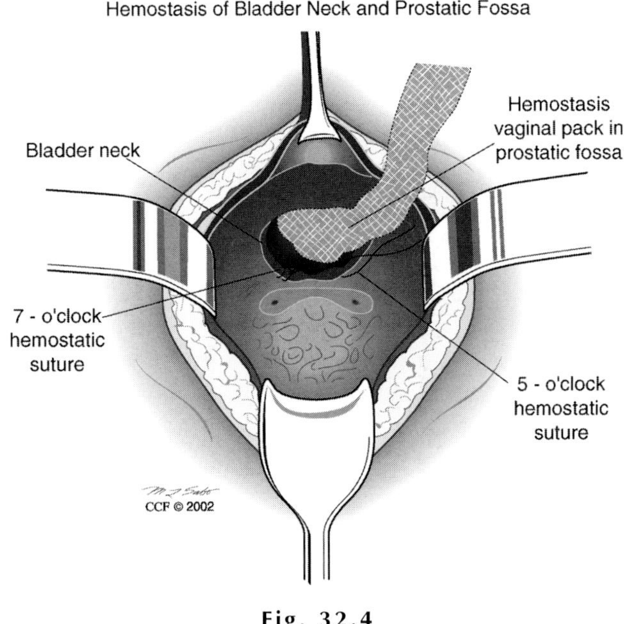


Fig. 32.4

catgut suture in one or two layers. If two layers are used, the first layer closes the bladder mucosa with a 2-0 chromic suture and the second layer an O-chromic catgut suture closing the detrussor muscle. A large Penrose drain is placed anterior to the bladder in the space of Retzius (Fig. 32.6) and brought out through a separate skin incision and secured to the skin with a drain stitch. The fascia is closed with a running absorbable suture and the skin closed using skin staples. The urethral catheter is connected to a drainage bag and/or three-way irrigation. In situations where a suprapubic tube is used, continuous bladder irrigation fluid is instilled via the suprapubic tube (SPT) and drained out the urethral catheter. For additional hemostasis, the urethral catheter balloon is distended with 30–60 mL of sterile water and placed on gentle traction and secured to the anterior thigh. Traction is removed after several hours to avoid ischemic necrosis of the glans penis, which has been reported secondary to prolonged heavy traction.

## Postoperative Management

The duration of urethral catheterization is operator dependent but has traditionally been 3–7 d, after which a voiding trial is performed with clamping of the SPT when present. Electrolytes and complete blood counts should be monitored while the patient is in the recovery room and as needed thereafter. In patients with preexisting uncorrected obstructive uropathy, monitor fluid status closely and watch for possible postobstructive diuresis syndrome. Empirical intravenous antibiotics are often administered for 24 h postoperative and discontinued if the intraoperative cultures are negative. In patients who were on preoperative anticoagulants, it is advisable to avoid reexposure to anticoagulants for several days until the urethral catheter has been removed and the patient is voiding well.

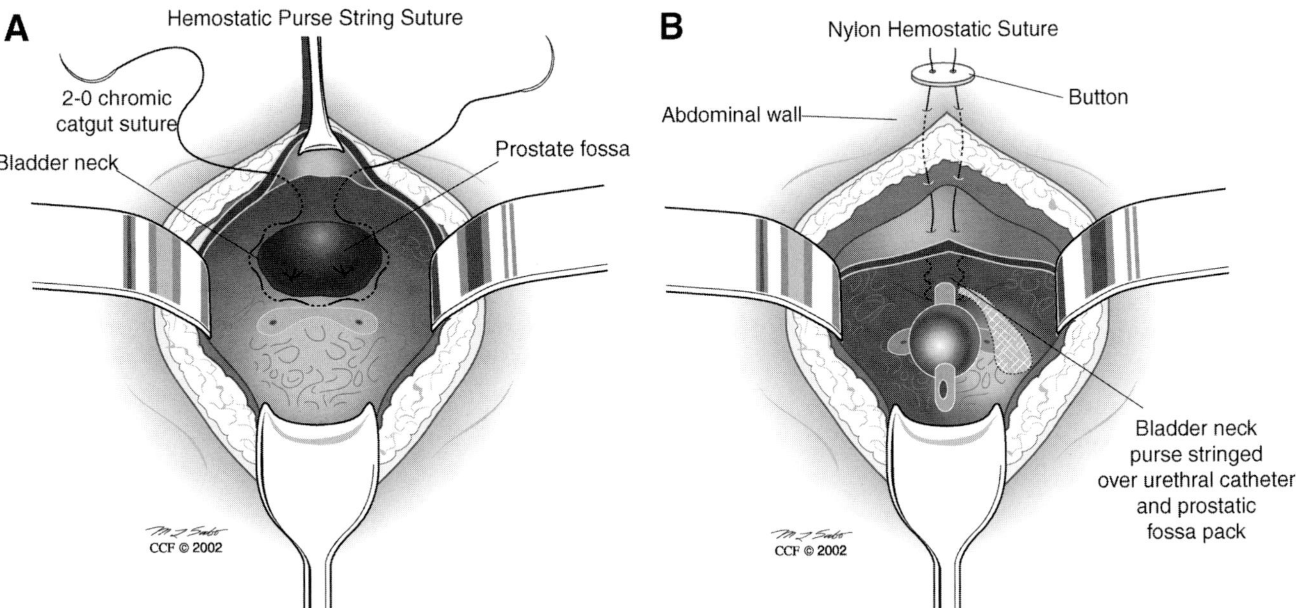


Fig. 32.5

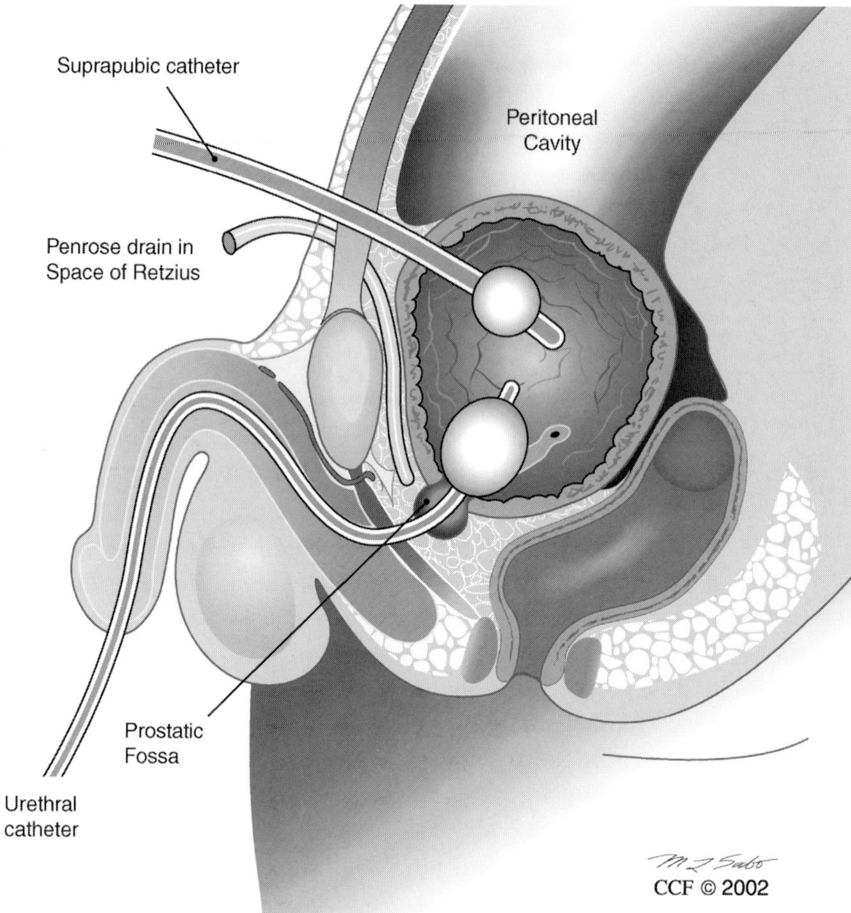


Fig. 32.6

## SIMPLE RETROPUBIC PROSTATECTOMY

Indications for simple retropubic prostatectomy parallel those of suprapubic transvesical prostatectomy except in situations where access to the interior of the bladder is desired ( intravesical prostatic median lobe, need for bladder diverticulectomy, etc.).

The advantages of simple retropubic prostatectomy over the transvesical approach are improved visualization and hemostasis of the prostatic fossa and avoidance of bladder or ureteral trauma and bladder hemorrhage. The patient is positioned as described above, and a urethral catheter is inserted. There is no need to distend the bladder. A vertical midline incision is made (Fig. 32.1) through the rectus fascia to expose the space of Retzius. The self-retaining retractor is positioned to keep the rectus muscles separated. Fat on the surface of the prostate is removed with electrocautery. Figure-of-8 chromic catgut sutures and electrocautery are used to achieve hemostasis of blood vessels overlying the anterior surface of the prostatic capsule (Fig. 32.7). Care is taken to avoid bleeding by avoidance of the lateral prostatic pedicles. A horizontal incision is made with a knife blade or cautery through the prostatic capsule (Fig. 32.8), and the index finger is inserted through this incision and the adenoma enucleated with a sweeping and pinching motion (Fig. 32.9). Following removal of the adenoma, the fossa is packed with vaginal packing and held with a sponge stick for 5–10 min. The packing is removed, and under direct vision cautery is used to achieve hemostasis. With the capsule open, the urethral catheter is inserted via the penis and guided with the finger into the bladder and balloon inflated and placed on gentle traction. The prostatic fossa is closed with running chromic catgut, and a Penrose drain is placed over the capsular closure in the space of Retzius and brought out via a separate fascial and skin incision. The fascia and skin are closed as described above.

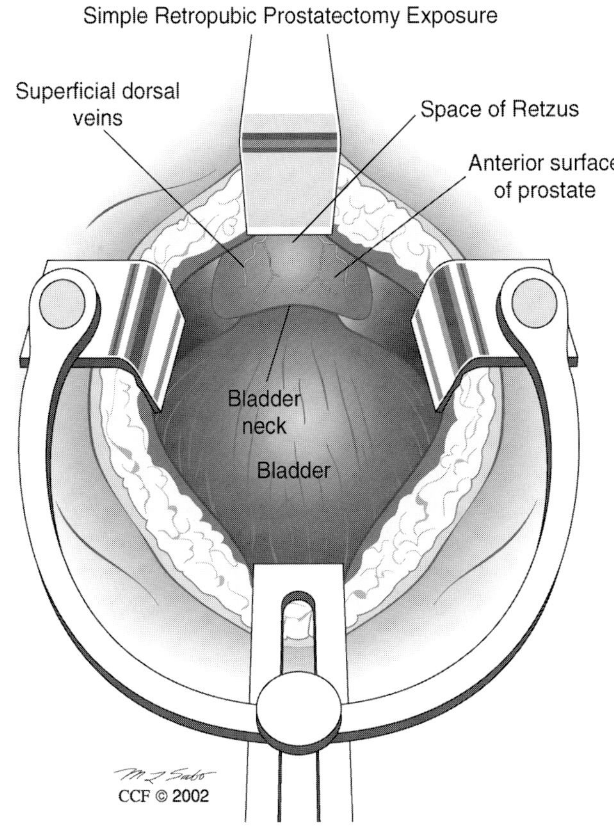


Fig. 32.7

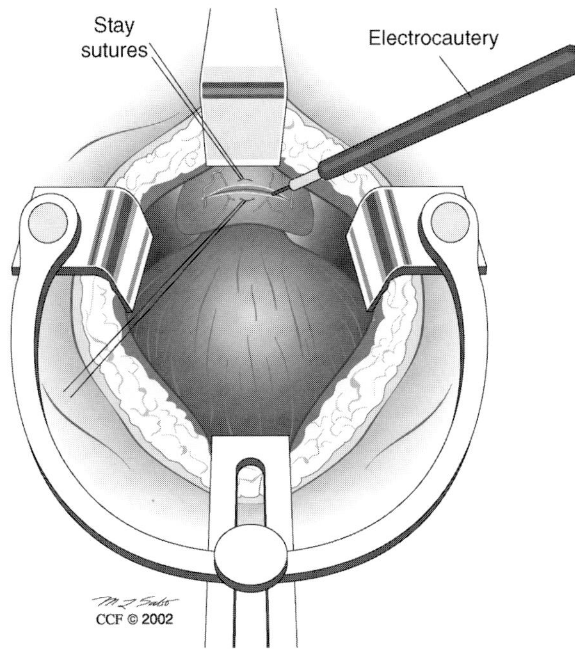


Fig. 32.8

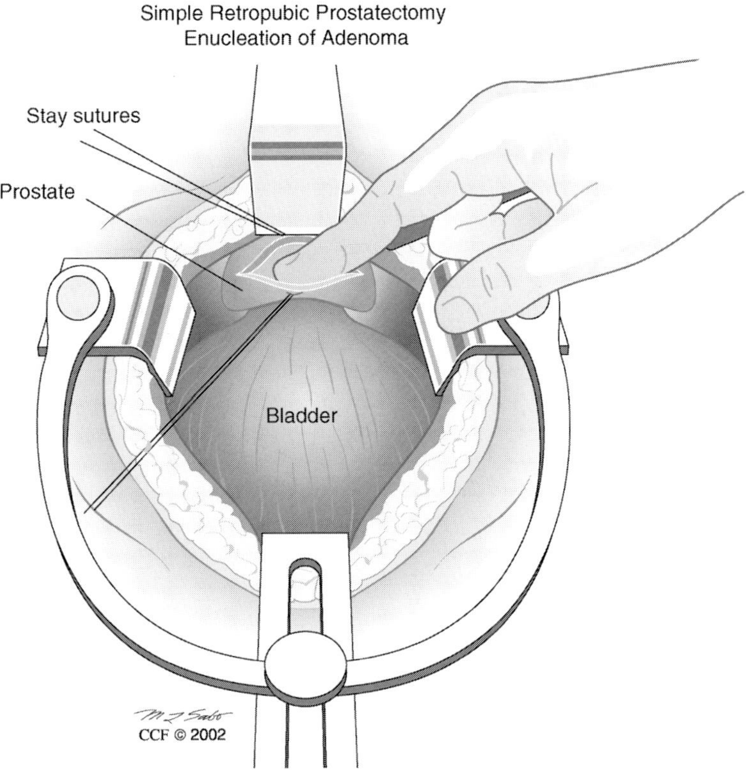


Fig. 32.9

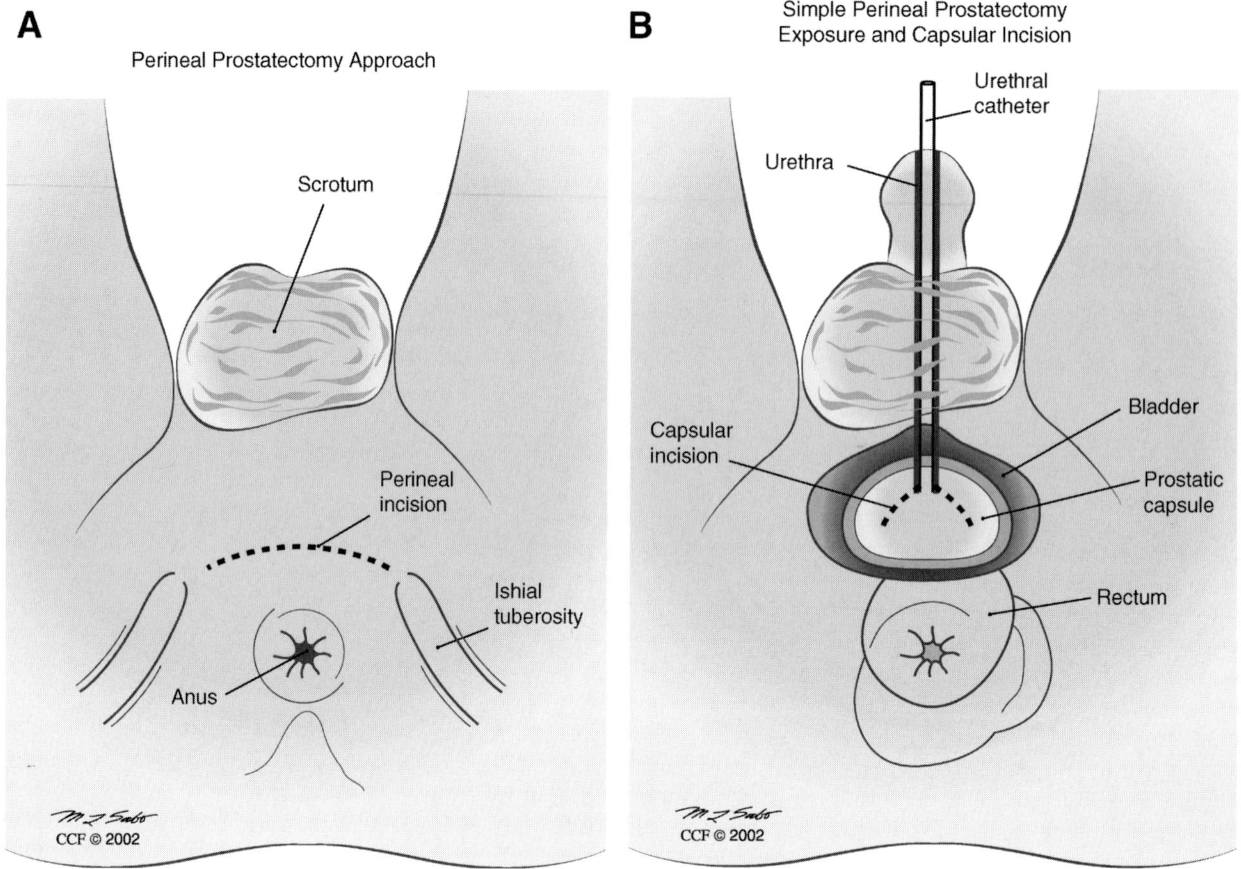


Fig. 32.10

## OTHER ROUTES FOR OPEN SIMPLE PROSTATECTOMY

Other approaches for simple prostatectomy are rarely used as there are few indications. Simple perineal prostatectomy (Fig. 32.10) is an approach indicated in the patient in whom transurethral surgery is either contraindicated or ill-advised and in whom a suprapubic incision is contraindicated (such as in a patient with a femoral–femoral bypass graft *in situ*). The approach is the same as that described for radical perineal prostatectomy (described elsewhere) with the exception of when the prostatic capsule is approached, in which case a horizontal or vertical capsular incision is made and the adenoma enucleated from the perineal approach.

Another approach is the transsacral approach, which is largely of historical reference and has not been utilized by the author.

# 33 Benign Prostatic Hyperplasia

## *Minimally Invasive and Endoscopic Management*

*James C. Ulchaker and Elroy D. Kursh*

Transurethral resection of the prostate is performed under intermittent or continuous irrigation using a nonconducting iso-osmotic irrigant solution (e.g., glycine). Resection is accomplished by a low power current, with the active electrode connected to the resectoscope and the neutral electrode fixed to the skin. The urethra is calibrated using urethral sounds prior to inserting the resectoscope. Cystoscopic examination of the urethra, external sphincter, verumontanum, prostate, bladder neck, and bladder is then performed (Fig. 33.1). Once other intravesical pathology has been ruled out, the resection may then commence.

With the resection loop, successive fragments of adenomatous tissue are systematically resected and hemostasis maintained. Glycine is normally used as the irrigation fluid in an effort to limit electrolyte disturbances. However, technological advances have led to the development of a bipolar electrode that allows saline to be used as the irrigant. One must maintain the proper three-dimensional perspectives throughout the dissection with constant knowledge of the whereabouts of the bladder neck and verumontanum.

The resection begins with the removal of any middle lobe and/or intravesical extension of prostatic tissue (Fig. 33.2). The bladder neck is next resected in a 360° fashion until exposure of bladder neck muscular fibers are visualized (Fig. 33.3). An anterior grove is created at the 12-o'clock position. This is a vascular area with the dorsal venous complex just above, and hemostasis is essential to

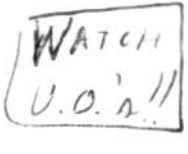

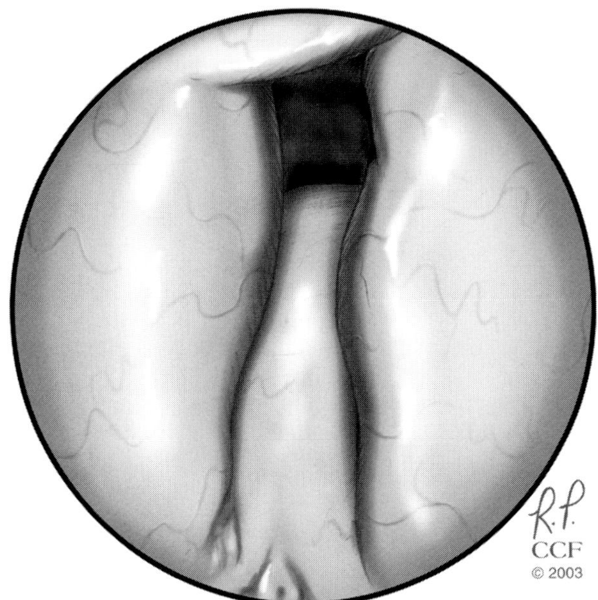


Fig. 33.1

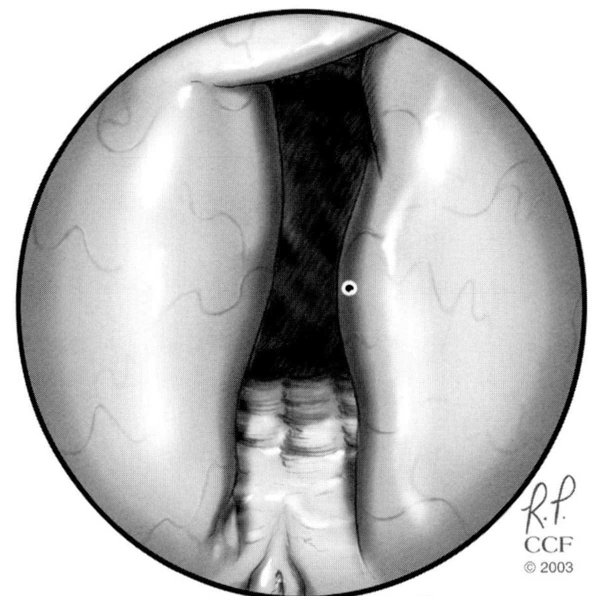


Fig. 33.2

From: *Operative Urology at the Cleveland Clinic*
Edited by: A. Novick et al. © Humana Press Inc., Totowa, NJ

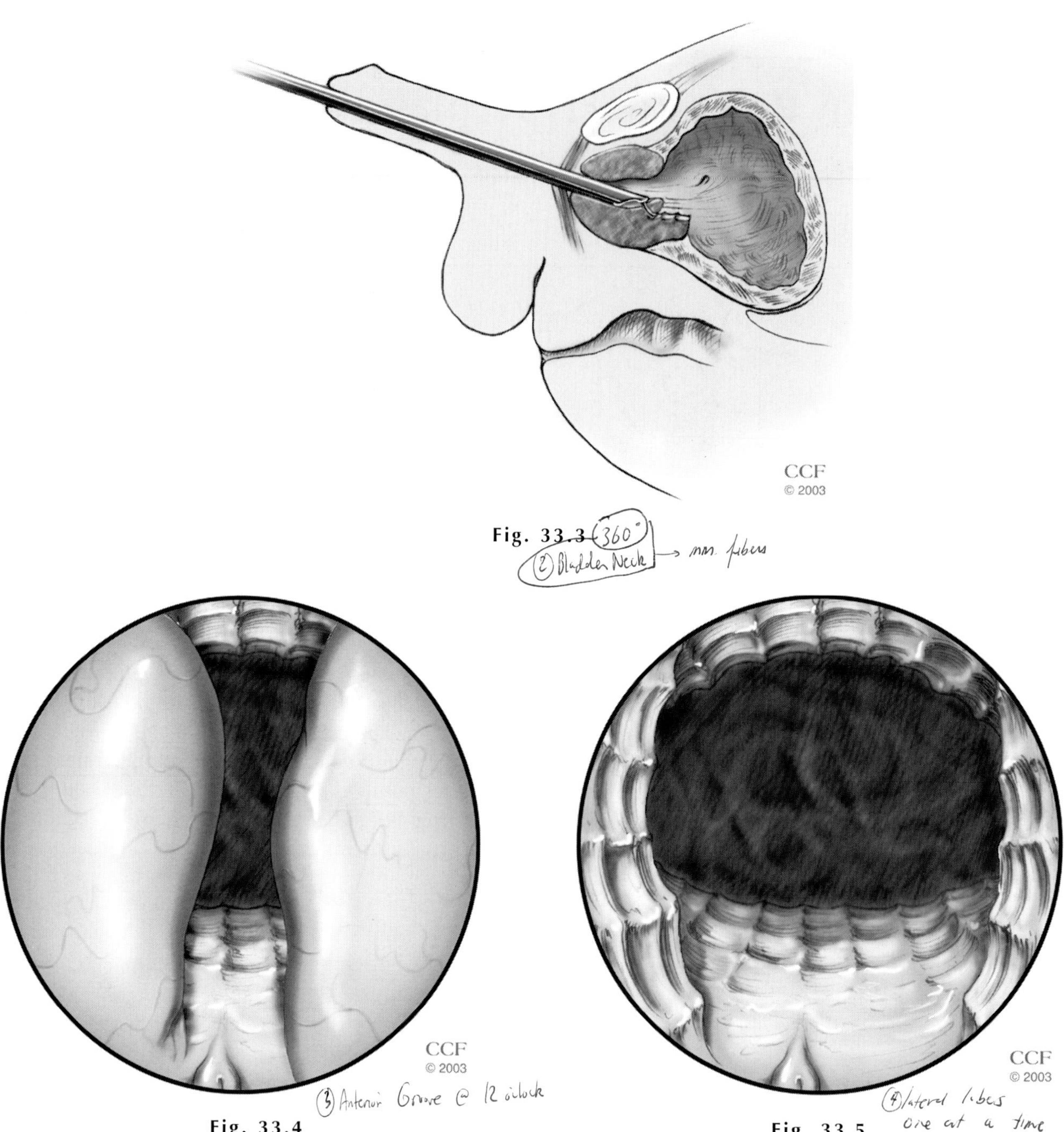


Fig. 33.3

Fig. 33.4

Fig. 33.5

allow proper visualization for the remainder of the resection (Fig. 33.4). Resection of each lateral lobe is then performed. The complete removal of tissue from the first side is recommended prior to working on the contralateral side to aid in visualization and decrease potential blood loss and fluid absorption. Resection is performed using long smooth strokes from the bladder neck to the verumontanum until the capsular fibers are visible (Fig. 33.5). Intermittently, these prostatic chips are irrigated from the bladder and hemostasis obtained.

Point cautery is used to control arterial and venous bleeding. The remaining prostatic floor and apical tissue is then resected including tissue adjacent and just distal to the verumontanum (Fig. 33.6). This dissection must be done with great care to avoid damage to the external sphincter. Visual confirmation of all chips removed from the bladder is performed, and hemostasis once again is performed, the final time with the irrigation off. A 24 French three-way catheter is placed with 40 cc of sterile $H_2O$ in the balloon. The catheter is placed on traction. The following morning the irrigation and traction are discontinued, and if the urine remains fairly clear the catheter is removed.

Over the years, and especially recently, a variety of minimally invasive procedures for benign prostatic

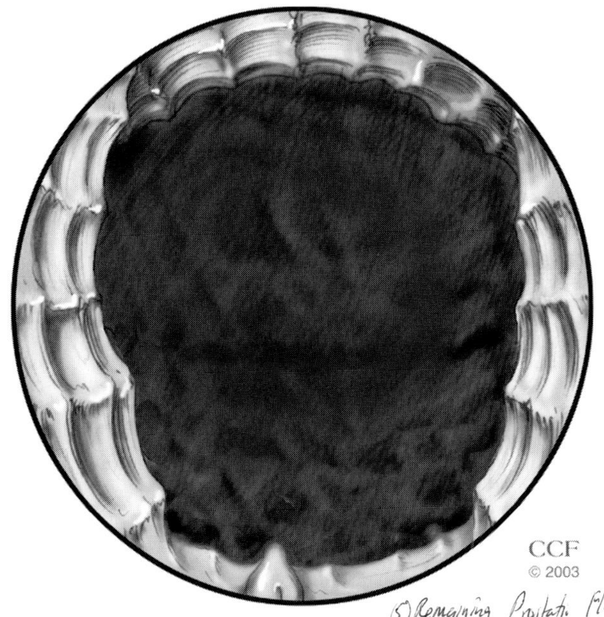


Fig. 33.6

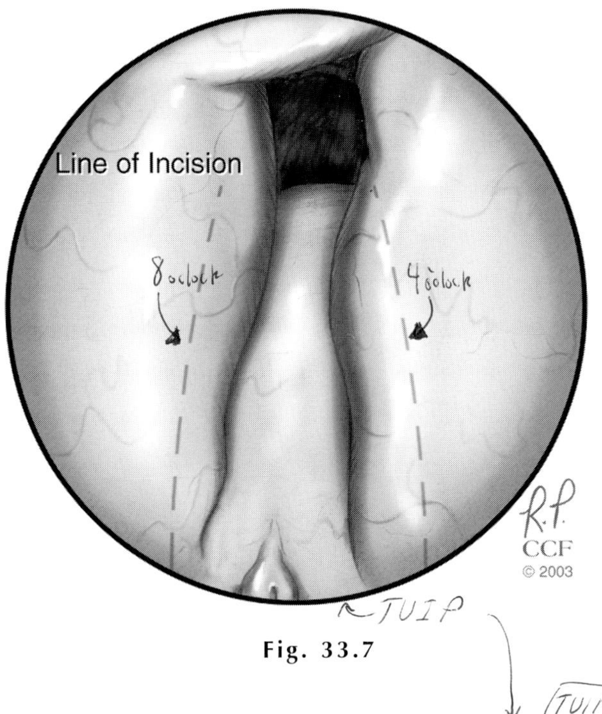


Fig. 33.7

hyperplasia have been developed. The first is transurethral incision of the prostate. This is most useful in prostate glands that are short in length as well as ones that have a high bladder neck. It is not useful when a significant middle lobe is present. When performing a transurethral incision of the prostate, a pair of incisions using a Collins knife or laser are performed at the 4- and 8-o'clock positions of the prostate and carried from the bladder neck to the verumontanum. This is designed to "spring open" the bladder neck and prostatic tissue (Fig. 33.7).

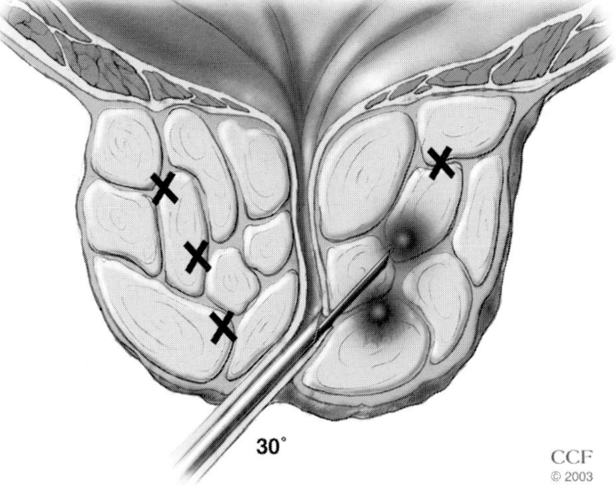


Fig. 33.8

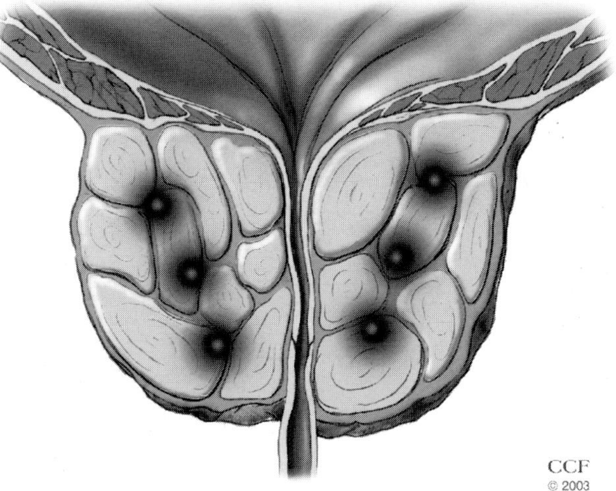


Fig. 33.9

Microwave devices, laser probes, and radiofrequency antennae are also currently part of our benign prostatic hyperplasia armamentarium in the early 21st century. Currently there is a variety of microwave devices in which a microwave heat applicator (antenna) embedded in a transurethral catheter delivers energy to the prostate to produce coagulation necrosis. Some of these systems combine heating with conductive cooling in an attempt to limit urethral morbidity. Other technologies use either a diode laser or radiofrequency to deliver energy to the prostate. These latter two technologies use probes passed deep into the obstructing prostatic tissue and subsequently heat the prostatic adenoma for various lengths of time in an effort to produce coagulation necrosis and subsequent reabsorption. When performing interstitial laser coagulation (shown) or transurethral needle ablation (not shown), we try to achieve a 30–45° angle of entry on each puncture to create the most optimal thermal defect (Figs. 33.8 and 33.9). A Foley catheter is left

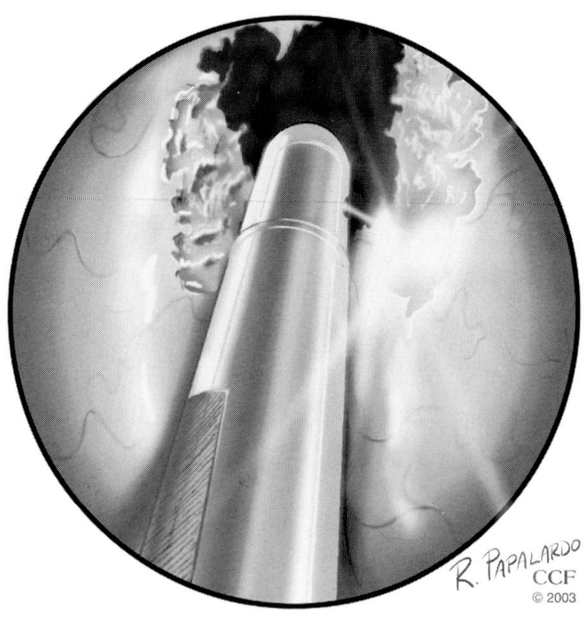


Fig. 33.10

for at least a week secondary to the tissue edema that develops from the heat treatment. Modest results in flow rate improvement and symptom score have been achieved using this technique.

Finally, photoselective vaporization of the prostate has most recently been added to our benign prostatic hyperplasia treatment armamentarium using the Greenlight PVP™ laser. The prostate is slowly vaporized in a near-bloodless fashion using a continuous-flow cystoscope. Saline serves as the irrigant of choice (Fig. 33.10). Care is taken to rotate the fiber between the fingers in a pendulum-type fashion. This allows for optimal vaporization with little charring and a significant depth of penetration of the energy. Following this procedure a catheter may or may not be placed, depending on the individual circumstance.

# 34 Radical Retropubic Prostatectomy

*Eric A. Klein*

## PREOPERATIVE PREPARATION

All patients undergo face-to-face preoperative counseling, preferably including partners, for discussion of the general nature of the procedure, potential complications, including incontinence, impotence, and the potential need for transfusion, and the postoperative routine. Specific emphasis is placed on the use of epidural anesthesia, whether or not lymphadenectomy is to be performed, whether or not a nerve-sparing procedure is contemplated, and planned hospital length of stay. Patients donate one or two units of autologous blood at their option. A preoperative urinalysis should demonstrate no active infection. The diet is restricted to clear liquids on the day prior to surgery, and no bowel preparation is used. Patients are admitted to the operating room (OR) on the day of surgery. A second-generation cephalosporin is given intravenously on call to the OR and for two doses postoperatively. Intermittent compression stockings are used for prophylaxis against deep venous thrombosis.

## ANESTHETIC CONSIDERATIONS

Epidural anesthesia alone is the preferred technique for all patients. The epidural catheter is placed in low thoracic position preoperatively and dosed with 0.1% bupivacaine and morphine sulfate 0.05 mg/mL upon arrival in the OR. This combination of position and drugs has been demonstrated to promote early return of intestinal function by sympathetic blockade and results in less postoperative pain by induction of pre-emptive analgesia *(1)*. Analgesia is maintained intra- and postoperatively with morphine sulfate or fentanyl, and low doses of anxiolytics are given parenterally throughout the procedure as needed. Epidural anesthesia avoids the need for ventilatory support and eliminates pulmonary and laryngeal complications, causes less sedation, results in less narcotic use, requires fewer transfusions, and is less expensive than general anesthesia *(2)*.

## PATIENT POSITIONING

The patient is placed in the supine position with the table in mild reverse Trendelenburg position to facilitate exposure of the apex. Once the apical dissection is completed, the table is placed in mild Trendelenburg position to facilitate visualization and dissection of the bladder neck.

## INCISION, EXPOSURE, AND RETRACTOR PLACEMENT

An 18 French Foley catheter is placed transurethrally, and the balloon is inflated with 10 cc of water prior to incision. A midline incision is made from below the umbilicus to the top of the pubis (Fig. 34.1), usually 4–6 in. in length depending on individual patient anatomy. The space of Retzius is developed bluntly, and the bladder is mobilized off the pelvic sidewall bilaterally. The peritoneum is also mobilized superiorly, exposing the psoas muscles bilaterally. The vas deferens is not routinely divided. A Bookwalter retractor with blades specifically modified for the performance of radical prostatectomy is placed *(3)* (Fig. 34.2). When pelvic lymphadenectomy is performed, a malleable blade is secured to the ring for lateral retraction of the bladder, permitting full visualization of the obturator fossa (Fig. 34.3).

## PELVIC LYMPHADENECTOMY

Based on published nomograms and our own experience, pelvic lymphadenectomy is omitted in selected patients at low risk for lymph node metastases based on preoperative serum prostate-specific antigen (PSA), tumor grade, and palpable tumor extent. Specifically,

From: *Operative Urology at the Cleveland Clinic*
Edited by: A. Novick et al. © Humana Press Inc., Totowa, NJ

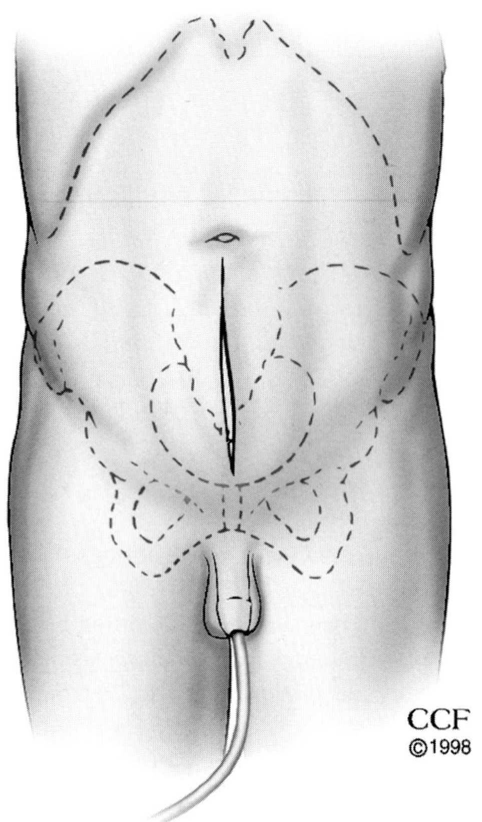


**Fig. 34.1**

An 18 French Foley catheter is placed transurethrally, and an extraperitoneal incision is made in the lower midline.

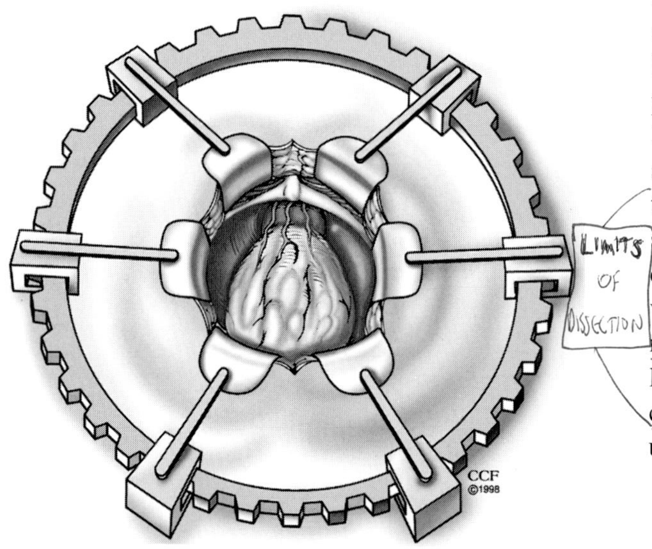


**Fig. 34.2**

A self-retaining, table-fixed ring retractor is placed. The two cephalad blades pull the bladder out of the pelvis and obviate the need to overinflate the Foley balloon. The prostatic apex is to the top.

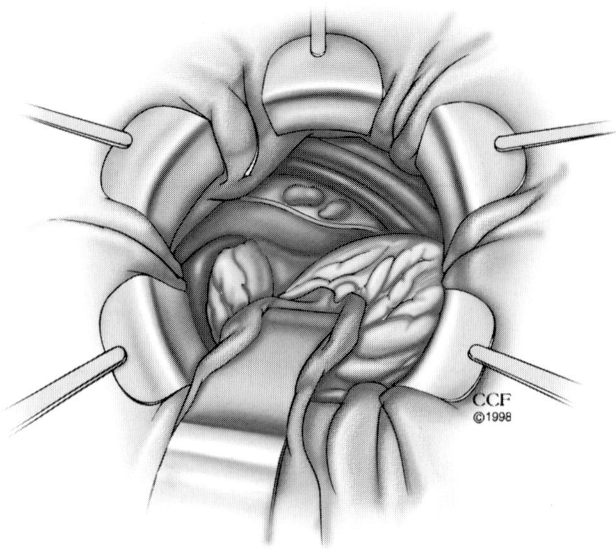


**Fig. 34.3**

A malleable blade is used for exposure of the obturator fossa when pelvic lymphadenectomy is performed.

lymphadenectomy is omitted in patients with all three of the following criteria: preop PSA of 10 ng/mL or less, biopsy Gleason sum of 6 or less, and clinical stage T1c (nonpalpable) or T2a (nodule involving less than one-half of one lobe). Such patients have only a 0.3% likelihood of positive nodes, much less than the estimated 1% chance of a complication resulting from lymphadenectomy. Furthermore, omission of lymphadenectomy in men with these characteristics does not increase the likelihood of biochemical failure *(4)*. Pelvic lymphadenectomy is routinely performed in any patient with preop PSA greater than 10 ng/mL, any Gleason sum of 7 or more, and for clinical stage of T2b or higher. When performed, lymphadenectomy is limited to the obturator fossa bilaterally and is considered prognostic but not therapeutic. The limits of dissection include the undersurface of the external iliac vein superiorly, the pelvic sidewall laterally, the obturator nerve deep, the bifurcation of the common iliac vein cephalad, and the origin of the superficial circumflex iliac vein caudally. Frozen section analysis is not routinely performed unless the nodes are grossly suspicious.

## ENDOPELVIC AND LATERAL PELVIC FASCIA, SANTORINI'S PLEXUS, AND DORSAL VEIN COMPLEX

The apical dissection begins with vertical incisions of the endopelvic fascia at the apex bilaterally (Fig. 34.4). The attachments of the levator muscles to the lateral

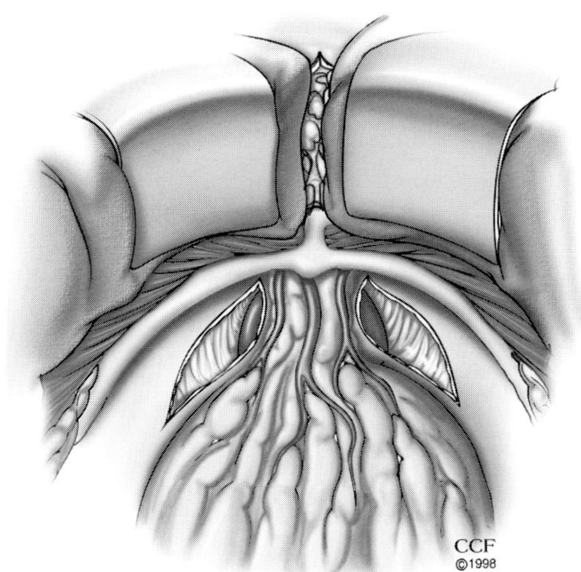


**Fig. 34.4**

The endopelvic fascia is incised bilaterally just lateral to the prostatic apex. The attachments of the levator muscles to the lateral surface of the prostate are taken down sharply with scissors. The puboprostatic ligaments are left intact. The apex is to the top.

surface of the prostate are taken down sharply with scissors. Blunt dissection of these attachments should be avoided to prevent shearing of small blood vessels, which may be difficult to control. The puboprostatic ligaments are left intact. The urethral catheter will be easily be palpable beyond the prostatic apex when all of the muscular attachments have been released.

Next, the lateral pelvic fascia (the visceral portion of the endopelvic fascia) covering the prostate is incised bilaterally beginning from the initial incision in the apical endopelvic fascia and extending to the base of the prostate (Fig. 34.5). The incision is performed high on the lateral surface of the prostate to avoid injuring the neurovascular bundles (NVBs). When completed, this maneuver allows clear visualization of the prostatourethral junction and location of the NVBs and facilitates bunching of the ramifications of the dorsal vein over the prostate. The cut edges of the lateral fascia are then grasped with Turner-Babcock clamps, incorporating the branches of the venous plexus on the dorsolateral surface of the prostate (Fig. 34.6A). The plexus is suture-ligated with two individual figure-of-8 0-chromic ligatures (Fig, 34.6B and C). This technique prevents back-bleeding when the dorsal vein is divided and helps identify the plane between the dorsal vein and urethra.

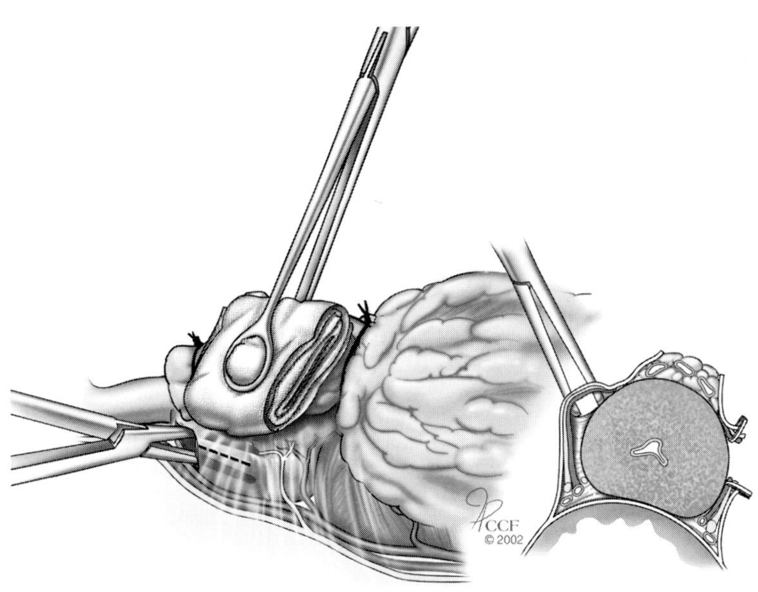


**Fig. 34.5**

The lateral pelvic fascia (the visceral layer of the endopelvic fascia covering the prostate) is elevated with a right-angled clamp and incised sharply with a knife (along the dotted line) from the apex to base of the prostate. This maneuver exposes the anterior prostatourethral junction and the position of the neurovascular bundles and facilitates control of the ramifications of the dorsal vein over the prostate. The maneuver is then repeated on the opposite side (not shown). The apex is to the left.

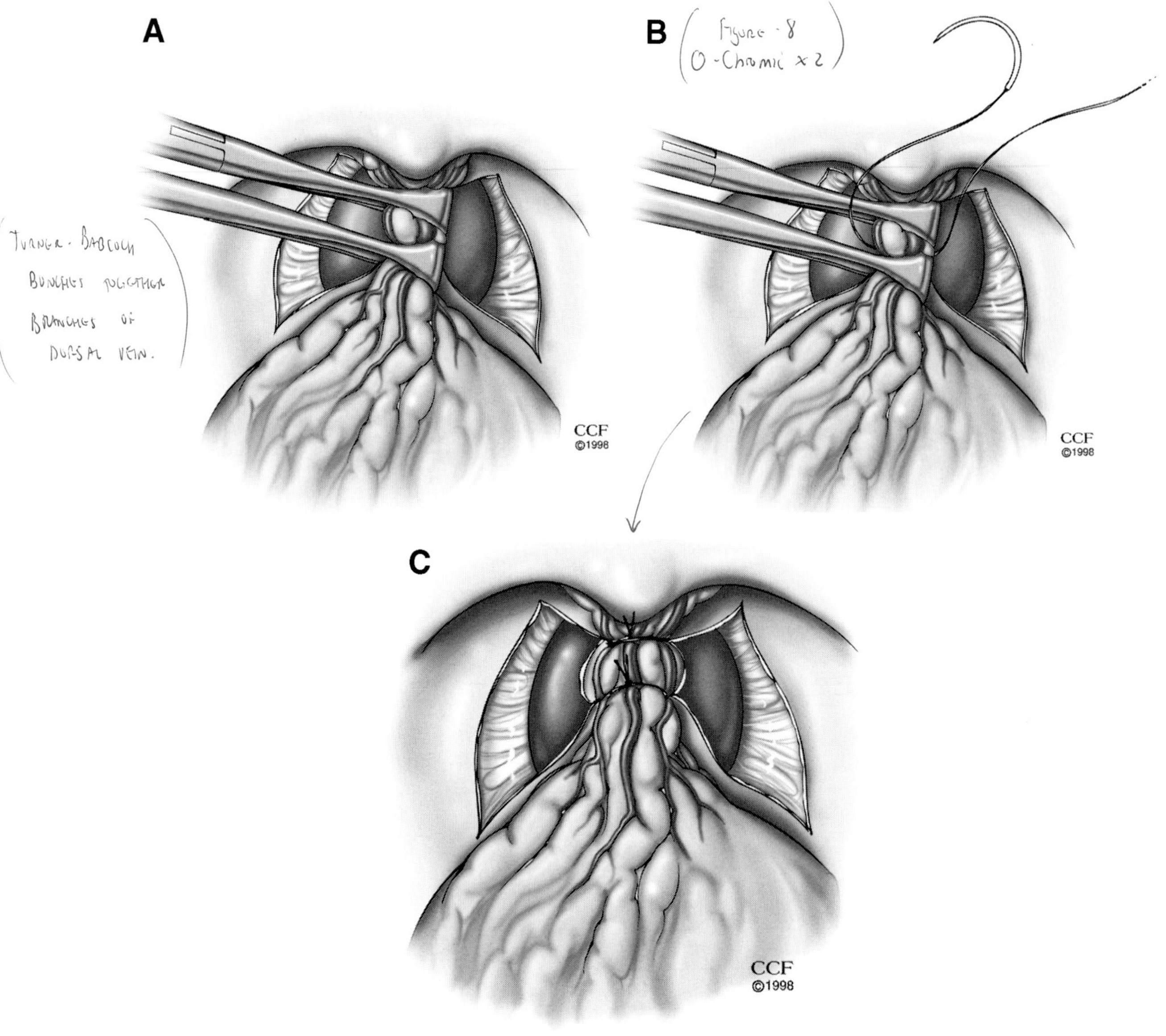


**Fig. 34.6**

Bunching technique for control of the dorsal venous complex. **(A)** Turner-Babcock clamps are used to bunch together the branches of the dorsal vein covering the dorsal surface of the prostate. **(B)** Two figure-of-8 sutures are used to ligate these branches, incorporating the cut edges of the endopelvic fascia. **(C)** Appearance after both sutures have been placed. The apex is to the top.

Incision and control of the dorsal vein varies by individual patient anatomy. In patients in whom a clear separation or notch is palpable between the posterior surface of the dorsal vein and anterior surface of the urethra, a right-angled clamp is passed between them (Fig. 34.7A). Identification of this plane is facilitated by finger palpation of the prostatic apex and urethral catheter, and in many patients this maneuver can be performed under direct vision. Precise placement behind the fascial sheath of the dorsal vein complex will also permit it to retract fully and help minimize bleeding. The dorsal vein is divided sharply between the sutures (Fig. 34.7B). A figure-of-8 0-chromic suture is placed for additional hemostasis (Fig. 34.7C). When correctly performed this technique does not compromise the anterior prostatic margin and results in excellent visualization of the urethra (Fig. 34.7D). In some patients the dorsal vein and urethra are closely approximated and

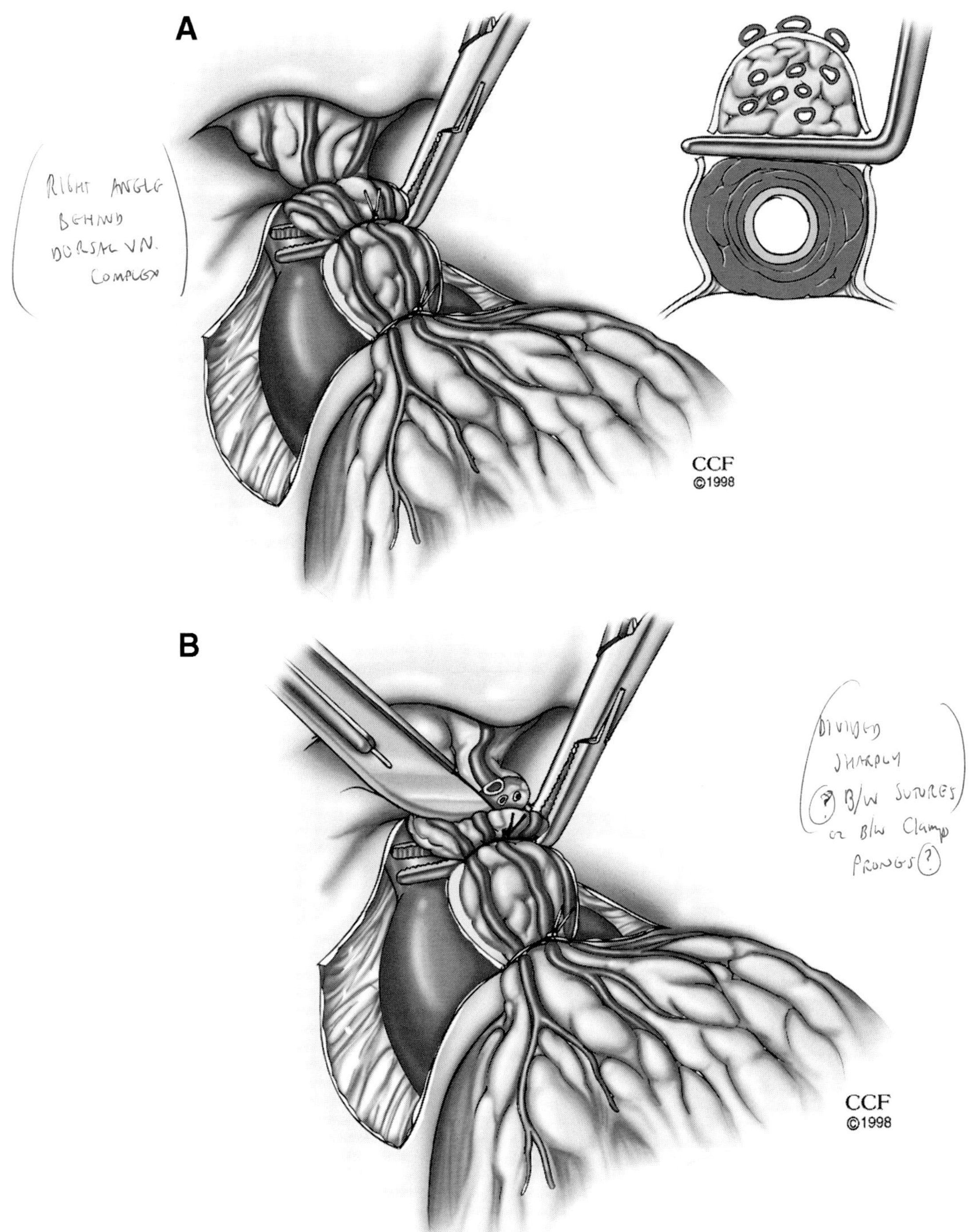


Fig. 34.7

passage of an instrument between them carries the risk of damaging the anterior striated sphincter. In such patients the dorsal vein is divided with scissors. This technique is usually associated with more bleeding than with passage of a clamp between the dorsal vein and urethra but, with experience, does not compromise the anterior prostatic margin and is safer in some patients.

## RELEASE OF NVBS

For nerve-sparing procedures, the NVBs are next released from the prostate from the apex to the level of the vascular pedicle lateral to the seminal vesicles. The dissection is performed with fine-tipped scissors and begins at the mid-prostate with identification of the most

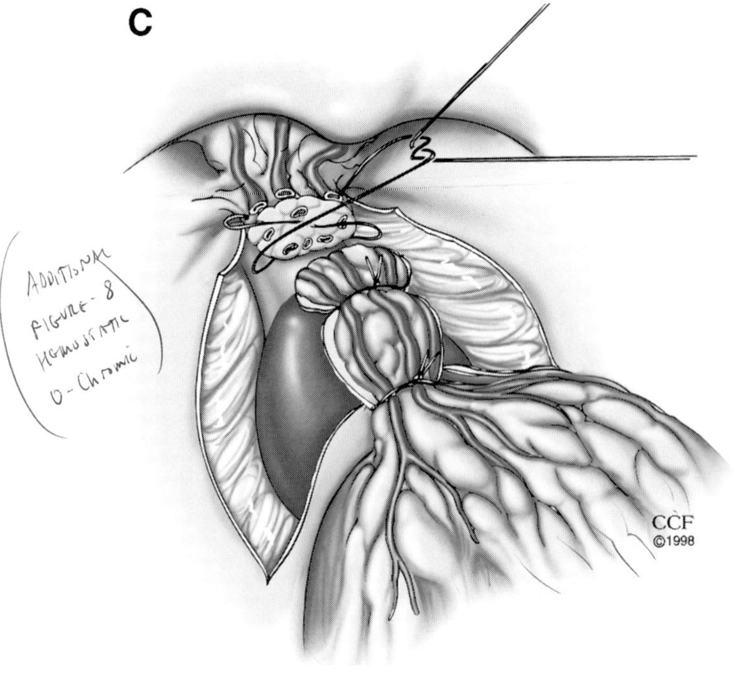


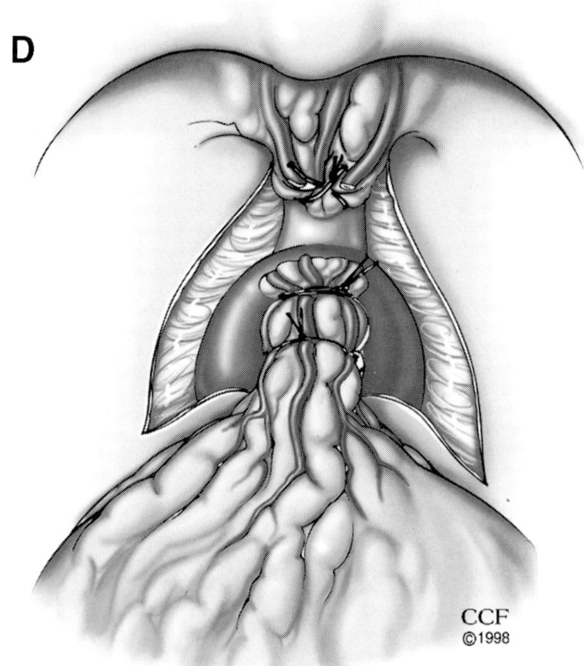


**Fig. 34.7** ***(Continued)***

Division and control of the dorsal vein. The prostatic apex is to the left. **(A)** A right-angled clamp is placed between the anterior surface of the urethra and posterior surface of the dorsal vein distal to the figure-of-8 sutures. The inset shows the correct plane between the dorsal vein and urethra. **(B)** The dorsal vein is divided sharply with a knife. **(C)** The cut surface of the dorsal vein is suture-ligated for hemostasis. **(D)** Appearance of the urethra after division and ligation of the dorsal vein.

superior peri-prostatic vein, which marks the upper extent of the bundle. The dissection is carried sharply around the edge of the prostate bilaterally, entering the plane posterior to Denonvilliers' fascia and anterior to the rectum (Fig. 34.8). This plane is fully developed by sharp dissection, using a sponge stick for gentle rotation of the prostate (Fig. 34.8A); blunt dissection with an instrument or finger runs the risk of fracturing the neurovascular bundle and should be avoided. When this plane is fully developed, the prostate can be lifted off the rectal surface (Fig. 34.8B). This maneuver yields excellent visualization of the prostatourethral junction both anteriorly and posteriorly and allows precise transection of the urethra without risk of incision into the prostatic apex. For a non-nerve-sparing procedure, the incision in the lateral pelvic fascia is made lateral to the bundles to permit wide excision of all periprostatic tissue (Fig. 34.8C). The plane between the prostate and rectum is developed similarly.

There are several advantages to the described approach. Initial release of the lateral pelvic fascia allows superior visualization of the junction between the rectum and prostate, with precise definition of the plane of dissection between these organs leaving all layers of Denonvilliers' fascia on the prostate. This reduces the likelihood of a positive margin along the posterior aspect of this fascia. Lifting the prostate off the rectum early in the dissection also permits precise delineation of the anatomy of the prostatic apex, especially posterior to the urethra, and prevents leaving small amounts of prostatic tissue attached to the urethra. Improved visualization of the apex using this technique also incorporates one of the main advantages of the perineal approach while still permitting adequate visualization and resection of the bladder neck and seminal vesicles. This technique also fully preserves the posterior fascial attachments of the urethra. Finally, dissection of the neurovascular bundles away from the prostate prior to transection of the urethra lowers the risk of traction injury when the apex is elevated.

## DIVISION OF THE URETHRA AND PLACEMENT OF URETHROVESICAL SUTURES

Following division of the dorsal vein complex and release of the lateral fascia and NVBs, the prostate remains attached at the apex only by the urethra. Division of the urethra begins with an incision of the anterior surface between 3- and 9-o'clock (Fig. 34.9A), exposing the Foley

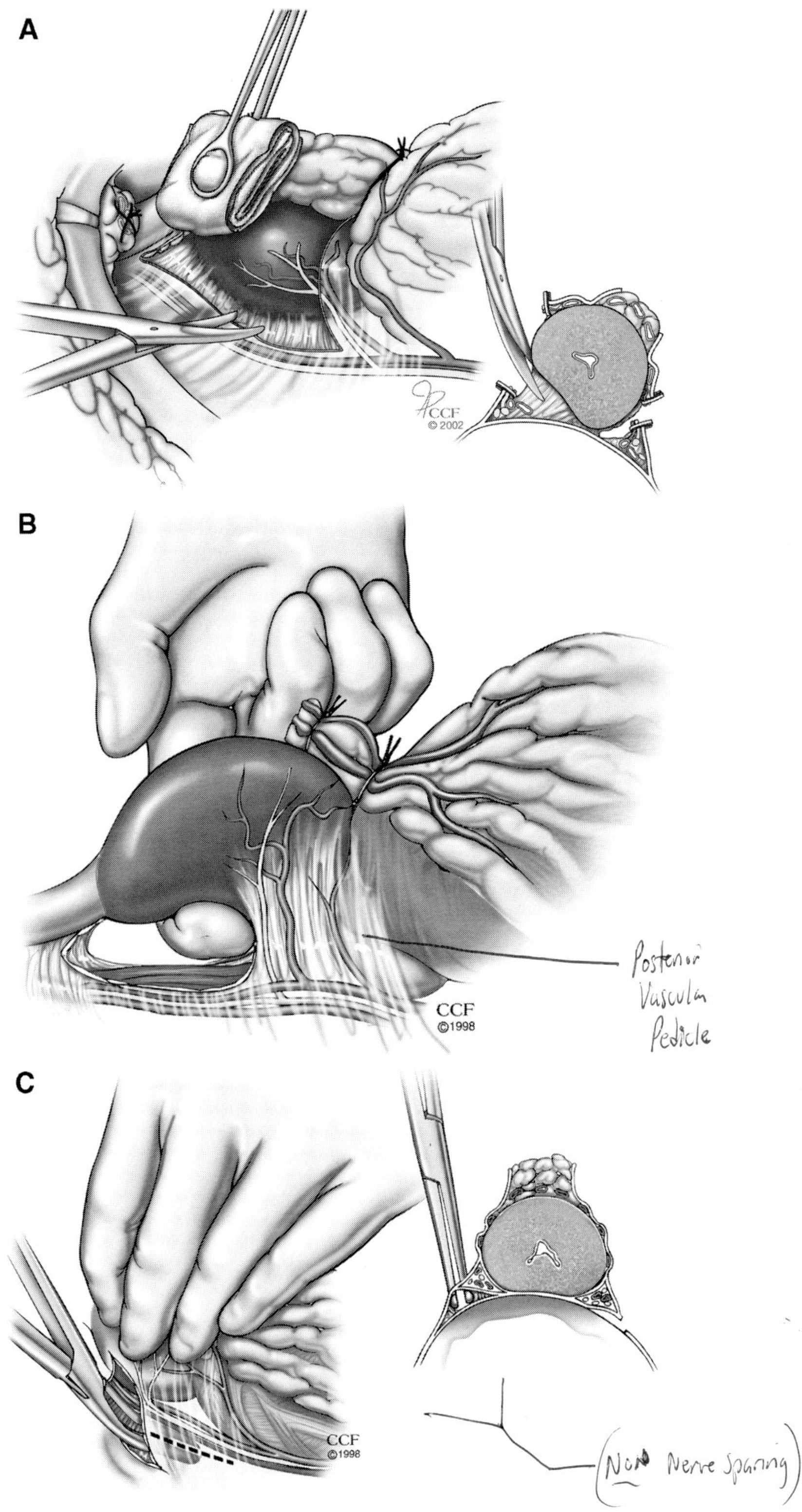


**Fig. 34.8**

Release of the neurovascular bundles. The prostatic apex is to the left. **(A)** The left neurovascular bundle is exposed by rotating the prostate medially with a sponge stick and released from the prostate by sharp dissection from the apex to the posterior vascular pedicle. The inset shows the plane of dissection medial to the bundle and posterior to Denonvilliers' fascia. A similar dissection is performed on the other side. **(B)** When the dissection is complete, the prostate can be lifted off the anterior surface of the rectum. The urethra remains intact at this point of the dissection. **(C)** The dissection is similar for non-nerve-sparing procedures, except that the lateral fascia is incised lateral to the neurovascular bundles. The plane between the prostate and rectum is developed similarly to the nerve-sparing technique.

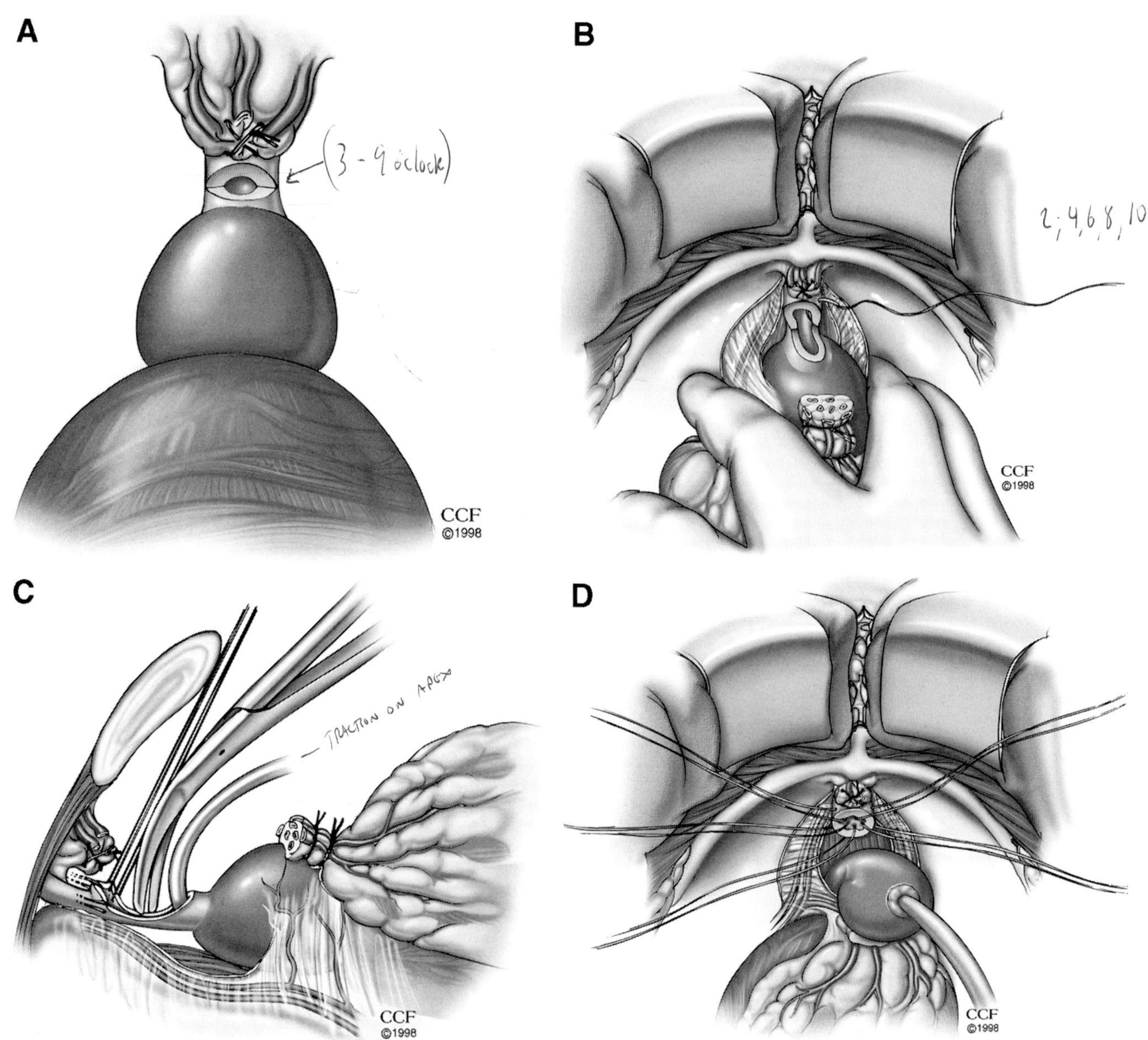


**Fig. 34.9**

Urethral division and placement of urethral sutures. **(A)** The anterior urethra is incised sharply from the 3- to 9-o'clock position, exposing the Foley catheter. **(B)** The Foley catheter is removed, and two anterior and three posterior anastomotic sutures are placed at the 2-, 4-, 6-, 8, and 10-o'clock positions. Leaving the posterior urethra attached facilitates suture placement by preventing urethral retraction. **(C)** The posterior urethra is divided sharply under direct vision, using gentle traction on the apex of the prostate for exposure. **(D)** Final appearance of the divided urethra with anastomotic sutures in place.

catheter. The catheter is next removed to allow placement of the vesicourethral anastomotic sutures. Placement of these sutures is facilitated by leaving the posterior urethra attached to the prostate in order to prevent urethral retraction (Fig. 34.9B). Five sutures of absorbable material are used for the anastomosis, placed at the 2-, 4-, 6-, 8-, and 10-o'clock positions, taking care to avoid the NVBs lying posterolaterally. The NVBs may be gently pushed out of the way with a finger to facilitate suture placement. With experience placement of these sutures can usually be easily accomplished from outside to inside without the need for double-armed sutures or a urethral sound. The sutures with needles still attached are held with hemostats labeled with the corresponding clock face position to avoid entanglement until the anastomosis is completed. Urethral transection, including the underlying layers of Denonvilliers'

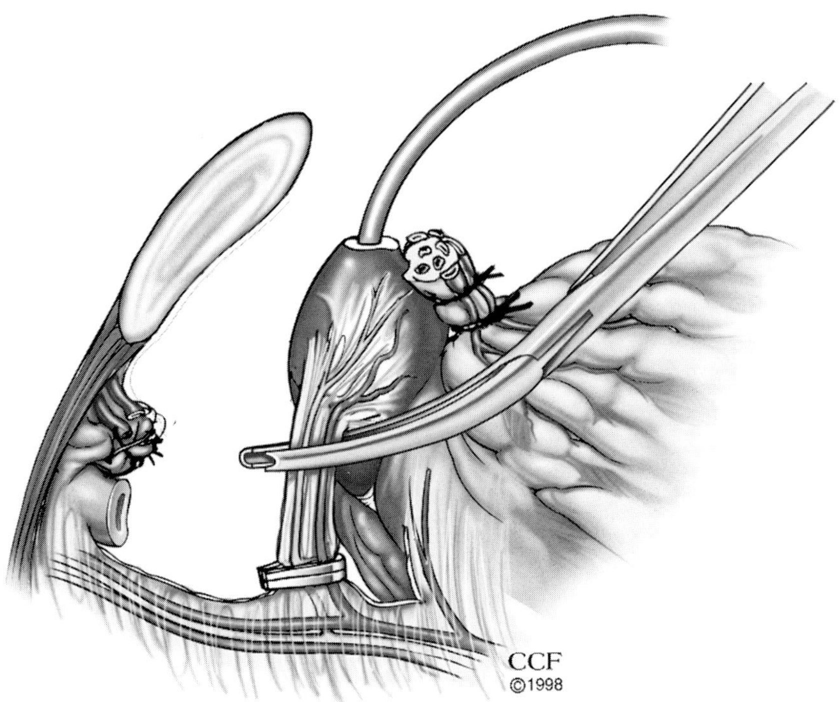


**Fig. 34.10**

The posterior vascular pedicles are divided bilaterally between clips. This exposes the junction of the bladder and prostate.

fascia, is next completed under direct vision using scissors and gentle traction on the prostatic apex for exposure (Fig. 34.9C and D). To minimize traction injury, the Foley catheter is not replaced into the prostate until the NVBs are fully released by division of the posterolateral pedicles.

## POSTERIOR VASCULAR PEDICLES, BLADDER NECK, AND SEMINAL VESICLES

Dissection of the posterior vascular pedicles is easily accomplished after completion of the apical dissection. Placing the table in mild Trendelenburg position and gentle traction on the prostate facilitates visualization for this portion of the procedure. It has generally been our approach to perform the bladder neck dissection prior to dissection of the seminal vesicles to permit leaving as much fascia as possible on both sides of these glands, although the "posterior peel" technique of seminal vesicle dissection prior to bladder neck dissection is occasionally used for glands with large median lobes.

Dissection of the prostate base begins with complete release of the NVB lateral to the posterolateral pedicle. In this area the NVB is typically tethered to the prostate by a single branch, which is divided between small hemostatic clips. Next a right-angled clamp is used to develop the plane between the posterolateral pedicle and the lateral surface of the seminal vesicle (Fig. 34.10). The pedicle should be ligated high to avoid damage to the NVB and pelvic plexus, which lie just lateral to the tips of the seminal vesicles. Ligation of these pedicles allows good exposure of the junction of the prostate and bladder neck and facilitates passage of a right-angled clamp between the posterior bladder neck and anterior surface of the seminal vesicles (Fig. 34.11A). The bladder neck is then incised sharply in a direction that preserves its anatomical integrity as much as possible and avoids cutting into the trigone near the ureteral orifices (Fig. 34.11B). In cases of high-grade or large-volume tumor at the prostate base, a larger cuff of bladder neck is removed to ensure an adequate margin of normal tissue. Release of the prostate from the bladder neck exposes the posterior surface of the vas deferens and seminal vesicles (Fig. 34.11C). The vas are individually ligated with clips and divided; the remaining attachments of the seminal vesicles are then dissected sharply (Fig. 34.11D), ligating the small arterial branch at the tips of the glands, and the specimen is removed.

## COMPLETION OF THE ANASTOMOSIS

The final step is completion of the vesicourethral anastomosis. When necessary, the bladder neck is

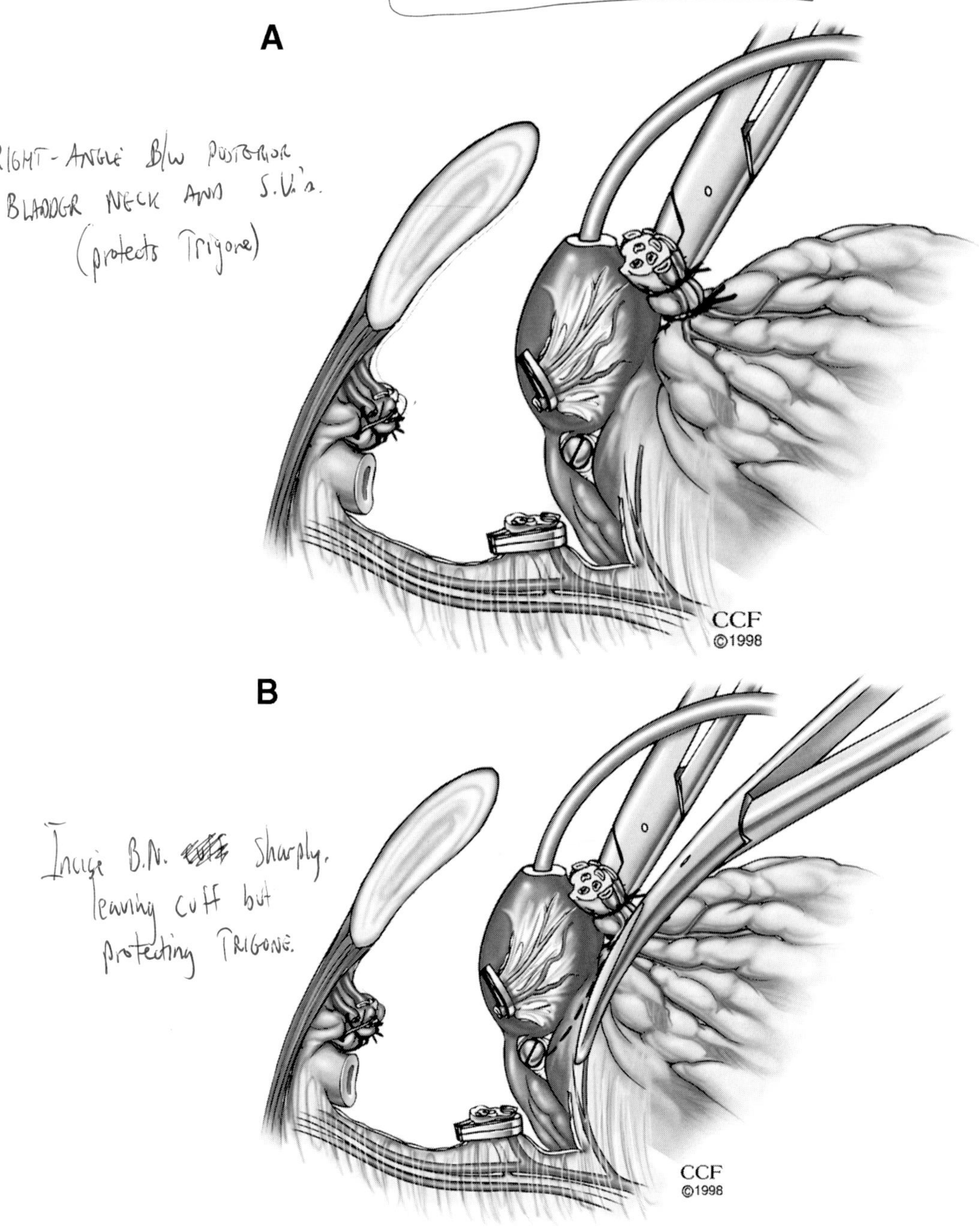


Fig. 34.11

reconstructed using 3-0 chromic suture. The anastomotic sutures previously placed in the urethra are placed in corresponding positions in the bladder neck (Fig. 34.12A). The cephalad two retractor blades (Fig. 34.2) are removed, releasing the bladder into the pelvis. The needles are removed from the sutures and the sutures are tied sequentially, beginning with the posterior row and without a Foley catheter in place. The 4- or 8-o'clock suture is tied first, followed by the 6-o'clock suture, followed by the remaining posterior suture. Omitting the Foley catheter while tying the anastomotic sutures allows the surgeons' hands to descend fully into the pelvis to ensure full approximation of the urethra and bladder neck. A 20 French Foley catheter is next placed per urethra and guided into the bladder with a finger placed over the bladder neck opening. The two anterior sutures are then tied to complete the anastomosis (Fig. 34.12B), and the Foley

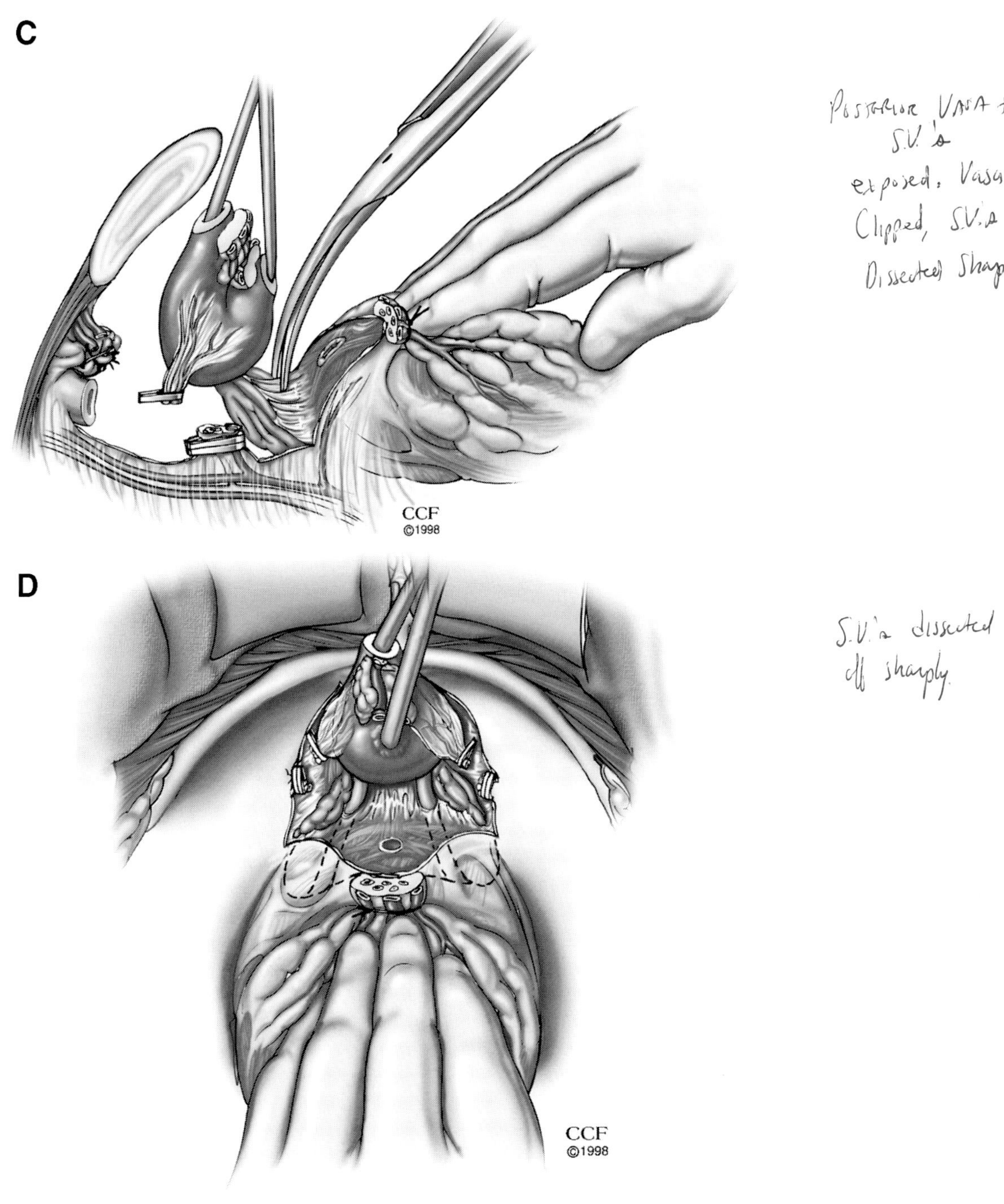


**Fig. 34.11** ***(Continued)***

Bladder neck dissection. **(A)** A right-angled clamp is inserted in the plane between the posterior bladder neck and the seminal vesicles. This maneuver helps identify the correct plane for bladder neck dissection without injury to the trigone. **(B)** The bladder neck is incised sharply, leaving an adequate cuff of bladder neck on the prostate while preserving the anatomical integrity of the bladder neck muscle fibers. **(C)** Release of the prostate from the bladder neck exposes the posterior surface of the vas deferens and seminal vesicles. The vasa are ligated with clips and divided. **(D)** The attachments to the seminal vesicles are divided, and the specimen is removed.

balloon is inflated with 10 cc of water. Use of a Foley with an overinflated balloon and traction on the bladder neck prior to tying the sutures is avoided, as the balloon simply fills up the already small space of the pelvis and may prevent good approximation of the bladder neck and urethra. The anastomosis is checked for

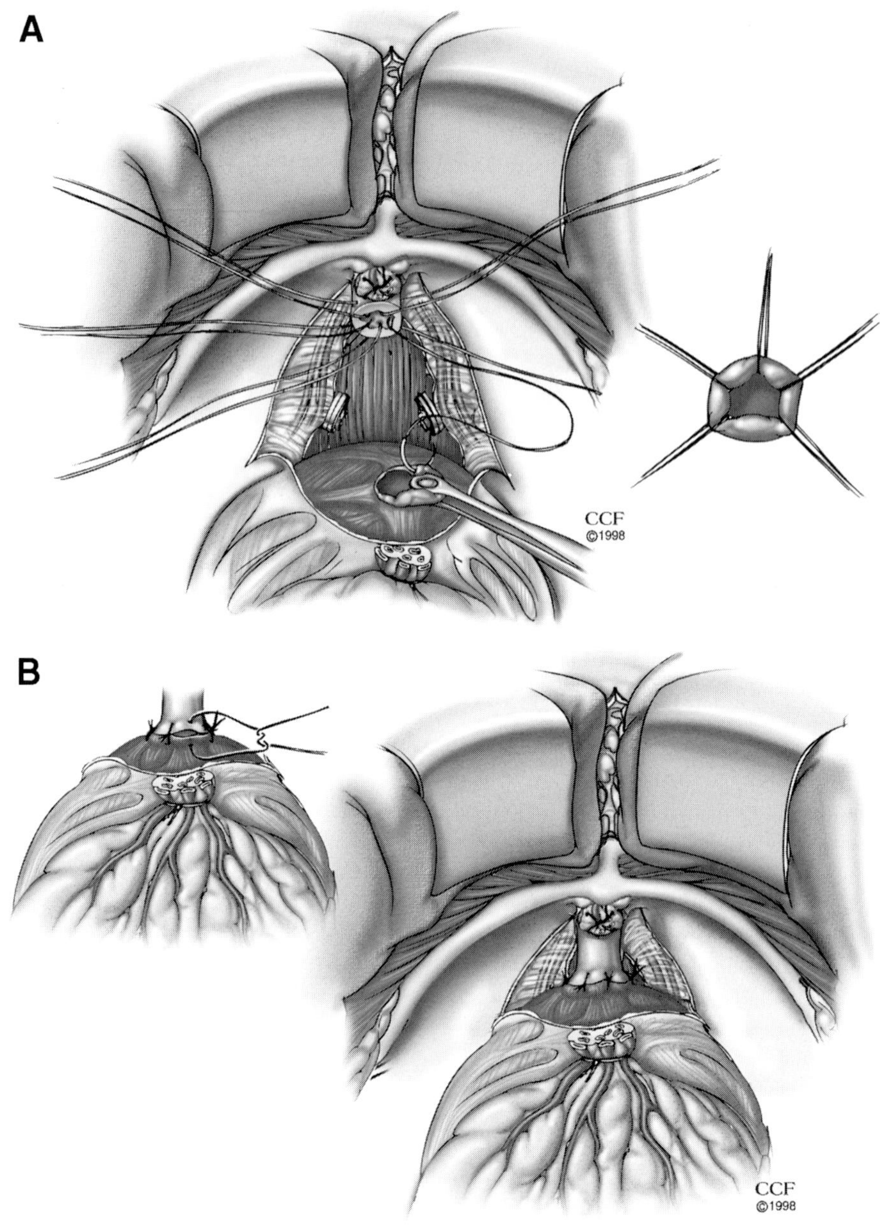


**Fig. 34.12**

Vesicourethral anastomosis. **(A)** The five urethral sutures are placed into the bladder neck at the corresponding positions after eversion of the bladder neck mucosa. The inset shows detail of bladder neck suture placement after mucosal eversion. **(B)** The vesicourethral sutures are tied circumferentially over a 22 French Foley catheter (left). The final appearance of the completed anastomosis is illustrated (right).

watertightness by irrigation via the Foley, and additional sutures are placed if necessary.

Closed suction drains are placed through separate incisions through the body of the rectus muscle and left in the obturator fossa. Only a single drain is used in patients in whom no pelvic lymphadenectomy is performed. The incision is closed in a single layer with running nonabsorbable suture, and the skin is approximated with clips.

## POSTOP ROUTINE

A detailed description of our postoperative regimen has been published elsewhere *(5)*. Briefly, patients are ambulated on the evening of or morning following surgery. A clear liquid diet is begun on postoperative day 1 and advanced as tolerated. Analgesia is maintained with continuous and on-demand morphine sulfate plus bupivacaine via epidural catheter for 24 h, followed by iv/po ketorolac and ibuprofen as needed. The drains are removed after 48 h unless there is clinical suspicion of a urine leak. Ninety-nine percent of patients are discharged after two nights of hospitalization. Patients return 7 d after discharge for incisional staple and catheter removal. Cystograms are not routinely performed. In cases where the vesicourethral anastomosis is not tension-free and in cases of documented urine leak, the Foley is left in longer and a cystogram may be performed before catheter removal.

## REFERENCES

1. Scheinen B, Asantila R, Orko R. The effect of bupivacaine and morphine on pain and bowel function after colonic surgery. Acta Anaesthesiol Scand 31:61–164, 1987.
2. Klein EA. Contemporary technique of radical prostatectomy. In: Klein EA, ed. Management of Prostate Cancer, 2nd ed. Totowa, NJ: Humana, 2004:217–242.
3. Klein EA. Modification of the Bookwalter retractor for radical prostatectomy. Contemp Urol 10:65–69, 1998.
4. Bhatta-Dhar N, Reuther AM, Zippe C, Klein EA. No difference in six-year biochemical failure rates with or without pelvic lymph node dissection during radical prostatectomy in low-risk patients with localized prostate cancer. Urology 63: 528–531, 2004.
5. Klein EA, Grass JA, Calabrese DA, Kay RA, Sargeant MBA, O'Hara JF. Maintaining quality of care and patient satisfaction with radical prostatectomy in the era of cost containment. Urology 48:269, 1996.

# 35 Laparoscopic Radical Prostatectomy

*Massimiliano Spaliviero and Inderbir S. Gill*

## INTRODUCTION

Prostate cancer is the most frequently diagnosed solid organ tumor among men in the United States. Radical prostatectomy is widely considered as the gold standard definitive treatment option for localized prostatic cancer, with excellent long-term (15-yr) cure rates. Therapeutic goals of radical prostatectomy are cancer cure, early return of continence, and preservation of sexual function. The anatomical radical retropubic prostatectomy described by Walsh *(1)* has gained acceptance as the standard open surgical technique.

Laparoscopy has recently been incorporated into the urological armamentarium for the treatment of localized prostate cancer with the goal of combining the advantages of open retropubic prostatectomy with the advantages of minimally invasive surgery. Oncological control and continence and potency maintenance are coupled with reduced peri-operative morbidity, ultimately enhancing global quality of life. After Schuessler et al.'s pioneering report *(2)*, the ultimate credit goes to the French team of Guillonneau and Vallancien, who developed, refined, standardized, and popularized the procedure *(3)*. Subsequently, multiple other reports were forthcoming in short order *(4,5)*. Laparoscopic radical prostatectomy (LRP) represents a paradigm advance in the evolution of urological laparoscopy.

The transperitoneal approach is the most popular technique of LRP. Bollens et al. *(6)* have standardized the extraperitoneal approach to LRP. Reproducible functional outcome data regarding continence and potency from multiple centers are beginning to emerge *(7)*. Using either the transperitoneal or the extraperitoneal approach *(8)*, the senior author has performed more than 600 LRPs at our institution since 1999.

## SELECTION OF PATIENTS

Akin to conventional open surgery, LRP is indicated for appropriate patients with organ-confined prostate cancer and a life expectancy of 10 yr or more. Absolute contraindications for general laparoscopy include abdominal wall infection, active peritoneal inflammatory process, bowel obstruction, uncorrected coagulopathy, and significant cardiopulmonary comorbidity. Relative contraindications are largely determined by the individual surgeon's experience and the patient's local anatomy. In one's early experience, LRP should be reserved for nonobese patients with a medium-sized prostate without a history of periprostatic inflammatory reaction, such as prostatitis or luteinizing hormone-releasing hormone (LHRH) agonist therapy. Similarly, morbidly obese patients and large-sized prostate glands should be avoided initially. Although periprostatic fibrosis increases the difficulty of dissecting the prostate, particularly its posterior wall, with increasing experience we have performed LRP in patients with a prior history of prostatitis, repeated transrectal biopsies, transurethral prostatic resection, open adenomectomy, LHRH agonist hormonal therapy, and $I^{131}$ seed implants. Furthermore, we have performed LRP for prostate size up to 222 g, in obese patients weighing in excess of 430 lb, and in many patients with history of prior inguinal mesh herniorraphy, appendectomy, or aorto-bifemoral grafting. Although laparoscopic salvage prostatectomy following external radiotherapy failure has been reported *(9)*, in our opinion prior history of open retropubic prostate surgery or definitive external beam radiation remain current contraindications to LRP.

## PREOPERATIVE CARE

For bowel preparation, two bottles of magnesium citrate are self-administered by the patient at home on the afternoon before surgery. After overnight fasting, the

From: *Operative Urology at the Cleveland Clinic*
Edited by: A. Novick et al. © Humana Press Inc., Totowa, NJ

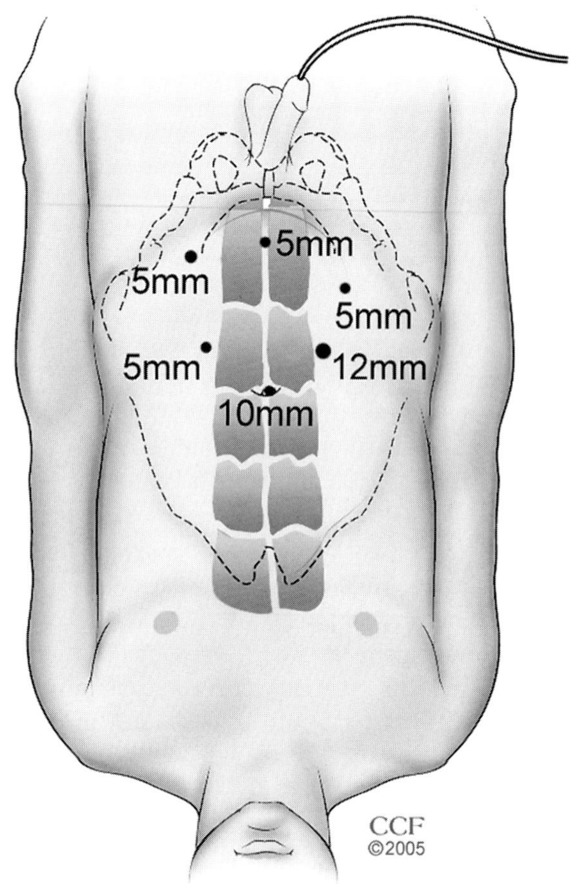


Fig. 35.1

patient is admitted to the hospital on the morning of the procedure and given broad-spectrum intravenous antibiotics and low-molecular-weight subcutaneous heparin (2500 U).

Bilateral sequential compression devices are applied to both legs. To facilitate simultaneous abdominal and perineal access, the patient is placed in a supine, modified lithotomy (abducted thighs) position with the arms adducted by the patient's side. The patient is secured with a safety belt placed across the chest. The anterior abdominal wall, perineal area, and upper thighs are sterilely prepared and draped. A Foley catheter is inserted from the sterile field and the bladder drained. The table is set in a 15–30° Trendelenburg position.

The operative team includes the surgeon standing on the left side of the patient, a first assistant on the right side of the patient, and a second assistant standing next to the surgeon.

We employ a six-port anterior transperitoneal approach (Fig. 35.1). Five ports are placed initially in a fan-array. The initial 10/12-mm port (port 1) is placed at the inferior umbilical crease for the laparoscope (10 mm, 0°). Ports 2 (12 mm; right side for a right-handed surgeon) and 3 (5 mm; left side) are placed at the lateral border of the right and left rectus muscle, respectively, approx 2 fingerbreadths below the umbilicus. *Note*: Caution must be taken regarding injury to the inferior epigastric vessels during placement of the two pararectal ports. Ports 4 (5 mm) and 5 (5 mm) are placed 1–2 fingerbreadths medial to each anterior superior iliac spine and used for retraction and suction purposes. The sixth port (5 mm, suprapubic) is inserted suprapubically during the midpoint of the operation at the time of bladder neck transection.

The patient is placed in a 15–30° Trendelenburg position. Bowel loops are gently retracted out of the pelvic cavity. An inverted U-shaped peritoneotomy with both limbs of the U-incision located medial to the ipsilateral medial umbilical ligament is made. To prevent inadvertent bladder injury, the horizontal part of the incision is cephalad to the dome of the bladder, high on the undersurface of the anterior abdominal wall. The bladder is actively deflated using a bulb syringe (Fig. 35.2). Once entry into the retropubic space is gained, dissection in the prevesical space of Retzius is performed in a deliberate manner, maintaining hemostasis at all times. The superficial dorsal vein, included in the small fatty area in the midline in the vicinity of the puboprostatic ligaments, is coagulated with bipolar electrocautery. Subsequently, the endopelvic fascia is cleaned bilaterally.

The right endopelvic fascia has already been incised (Fig. 35.3). The left side of the endopelvic fascia is being incised along the dotted line. The prostate is retracted to the right, placing the left endopelvic fascia on stretch. The endopelvic fascia is incised using a J-hook electrocautery or cold endoshears. The fascial incision is carried distally up to the lateral-most puboprostatic ligament. Visualization of the prostate apex is the endpoint of this dissection.

The completed incision of the endopelvic fascia bilaterally, exposing the convex contours of the prostatic lobes (Fig. 35.4). The apex of the prostate is defined bilaterally. The lateral puboprostatic ligaments are divided as necessary.

The Foley catheter is replaced with a metallic urethral dilator. This enhances needle orientation during dorsal vein ligation by displacing the urethra posteriorly (allowing better visualization of the precise site for stitch placement). Further, the dilator can be "palpated" with the needle tip. The stitch (CT-1 needle, 2-0 Vicryl) is placed in a right-hand backhanded manner from right-to-left side distal to the apex of the prostate, between the dorsal vein complex and the urethra (Fig. 35.5). Deep placement of

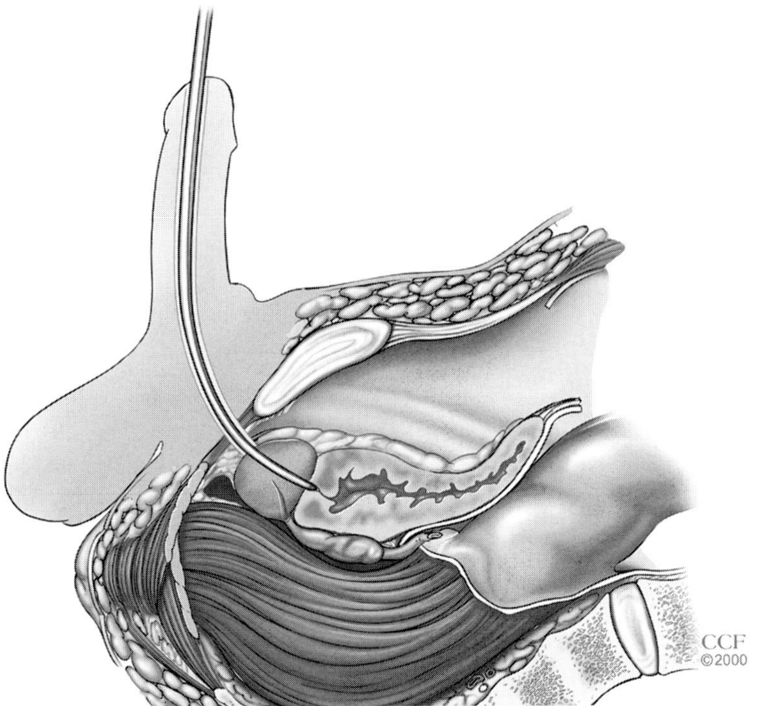


Fig. 35.2

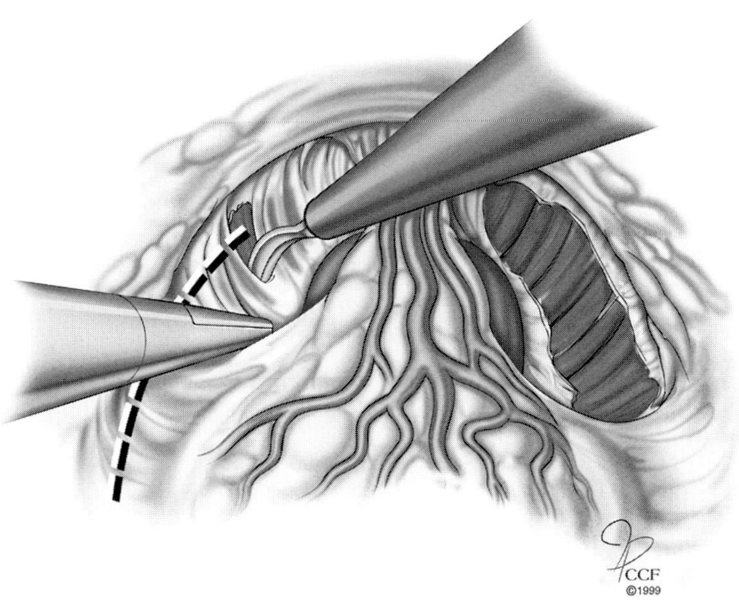


Fig. 35.3

this stitch allows the entire dorsal vein complex to be encompassed. Two sutures provide secure ligation. We incorporate a retropubic urethropexy in the dorsal vein complex ligature by anchoring the stitch to the undersurface of the symphysis pubis.

A back-bleeding stitch (CT-1 needle, 2-0 Vicryl) is placed across the anterior surface of the base of the prostate (Fig. 35.6). The tails of this stitch are cut long to allow anterior traction on the stitch.

The pelvic fascia enveloping the lateral surface of the prostate is incised transversely with cold endoshears in an attempt to drop the neurovascular bundles (NVBs) bilaterally (Fig. 35.7). Laparoscopic visualization of the precise anatomical location of the junction between the prostate

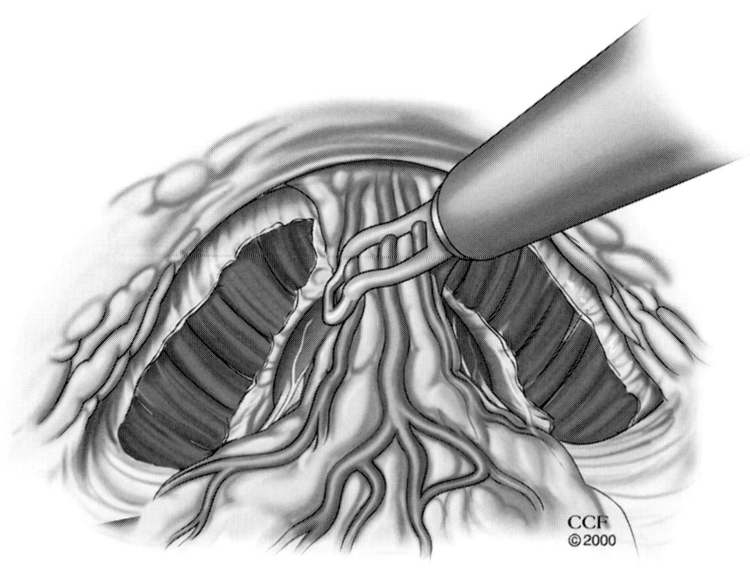


Fig. 35.4

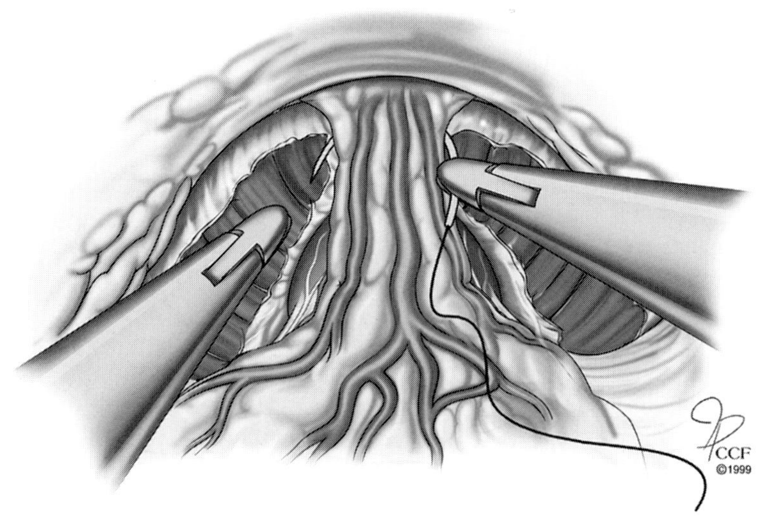


Fig. 35.5

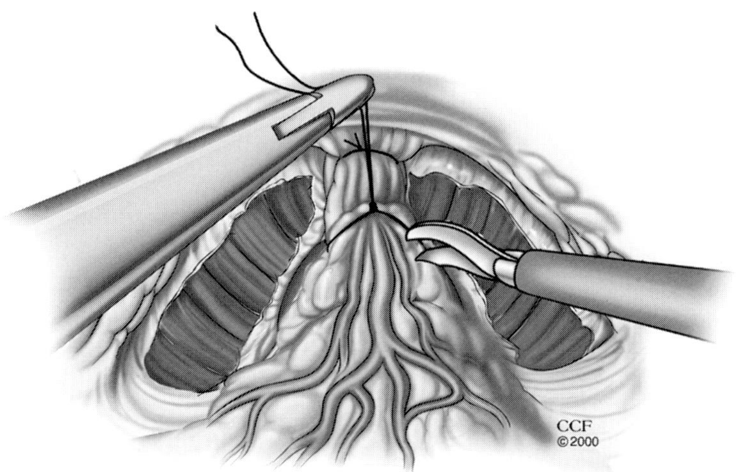


Fig. 35.6

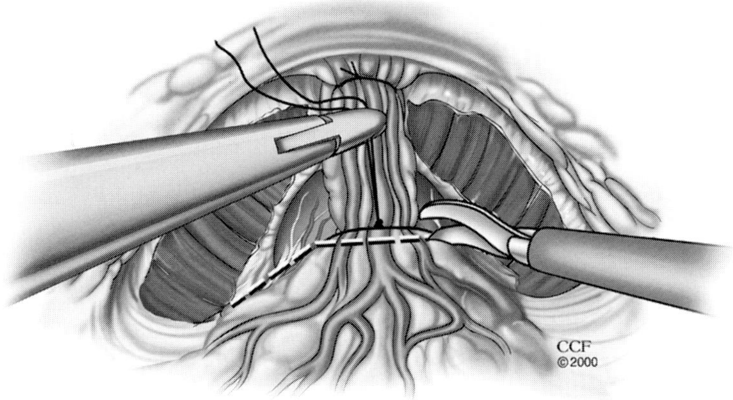


Fig. 35.7

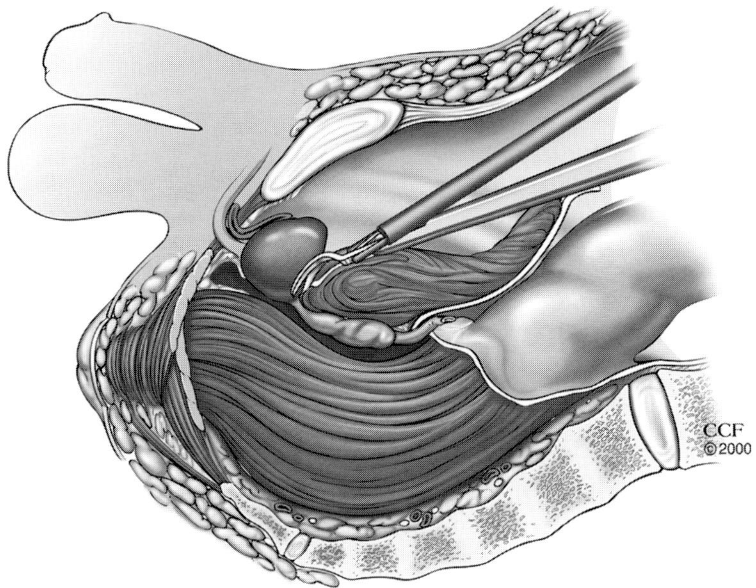


Fig. 35.8

and the anterior bladder neck (transverse dotted line) is difficult. Typically, the bladder neck is located approx 1–2 cm cephalad to the above-mentioned horizontal back-bleeding stitch. Also, the area where the prevesical fat ends roughly represents the prostatovesical junction. Finally, repeated in-and-out movements of the anteriorly pointing, curved tip of the metallic urethral sound may also help to localize the prostate-vesical junction. A horizontal incision is created at this location, and the anterior bladder neck is divided. Anterior retraction on the prostate allows visualization of the posterior bladder neck.

The posterior bladder neck is deeply scored with J-hook electrocautery at the proposed line of transection at a safe distance from the ureteric orifices. As this incision is developed, the posterior lip of the bladder neck is grasped in the midline with a laparoscopic Allis forceps and retracted anteriorly (Fig. 35.8).

This plane is further developed with a J-hook electrocautery until the posterior bladder neck and the prostate are completely separated. The anterior layer of Denonvilliers' fascia is incised. The vas deferens and seminal vesicles are visualized by dividing the few remaining attachments between the bladder and the prostate. The lateral pedicle of the prostate on each side is the lateral endpoint of this dissection. Care must be taken to prevent "buttonholing" of the bladder neck or inadvertent entry into the prostate. Also, the need for bladder neck reconstruction can be minimized by careful mobilization of the bladder neck. Following posterior bladder neck transection, the space between the prostate and the bladder neck is enlarged by retracting these two structures anteriorly and cephalad, respectively, allowing access to the seminal vesicles and vas deferens (Fig. 35.9).

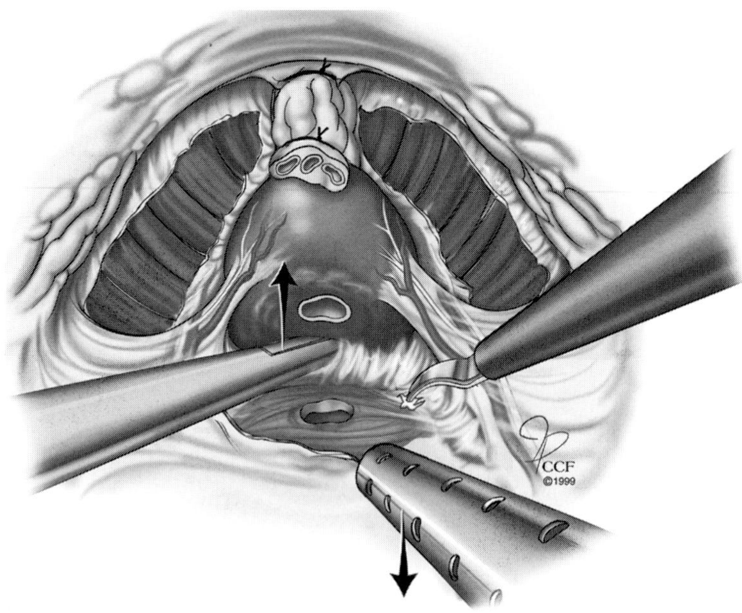


Fig. 35.9

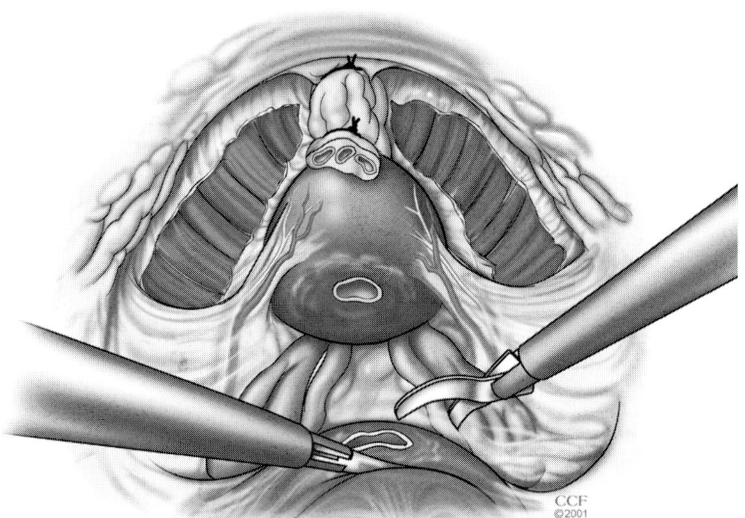


Fig. 35.10

The anterior layer of Denonvilliers' fascia is incised, and vasa deferentia are identified, grasped with an Allis forceps, and retracted anteriorly (Fig. 35.10).

The vas deferens is clipped with a hem-o-lock clip and divided. Blunt dissection is carried laterally to identify the ipsilateral seminal vesicle. After circumferential mobilization of the seminal vesicle, multiple small vesicular vessels (e.g., the seminal vesicle artery entering the tip of the seminal vesicle) are secured using a combination of hem-o-lock clip and harmonic scalpel (Fig. 35.11). Since the tip of the seminal vesicle is in close proximity to the NVBs, we recommend complete avoidance of electrocautery in this area.

Dissection of the seminal vesicles is carried distally up to their junction with the prostate (Fig. 35.12).

Denonvilliers' fascia is transected, and the prerectal plane is developed along the horizontal dotted line (Fig. 35.13). This retro-prostatic dissection is not pursued aggressively at this point for fear of rectal injury.

Preoperative measurements of the prostate and NVB are obtained using a transrectal ultrasound (TRUS) probe (Probe types 8808, Type 2102 Hawk, B-K

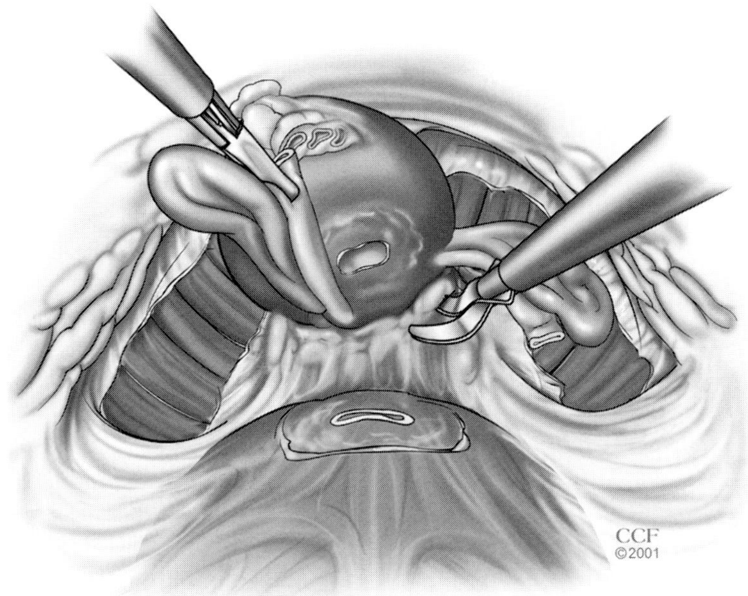


Fig. 35.11

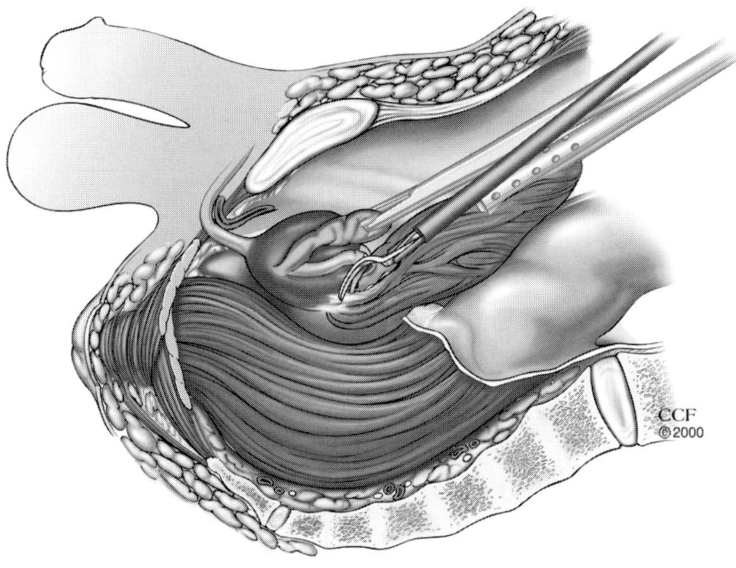


Fig. 35.12

Medical, Copenhagen, Denmark) inserted into the rectum *(10)*. The artery to the seminal vesicle is clipped with a hem-o-lock clip (Weck Closure Systems, Research Triangle Park, NC) and then transected with cold scissors. The right lateral pedicle and NVB are addressed initially. Antero-lateral to the left, taut retraction of bilateral seminal vesicles and vas deferens grasped by an atraumatic bowel clamp introduced through the 5-mm suprapubic port places the right lateral pedicle of the prostate on gentle stretch. A 25-mm, straight, atraumatic bulldog clamp (Fig. 35.14) (CEV565, MicroFrance™ Medtronic Xomed, Inc., Jacksonville, FL) is placed obliquely at a 45° angle across the right lateral pedicle close to the bladder neck, at some distance from the right postero-lateral edge of the prostate *(11)*. A bulldog clamp is placed on the lateral pedicle to obtain temporary vascular control. The lateral pedicle is carefully divided in small tissue bites using cold endoshears. An approx 1- to 2-mm edge of pedicle tissue is left protruding from the jaws of the

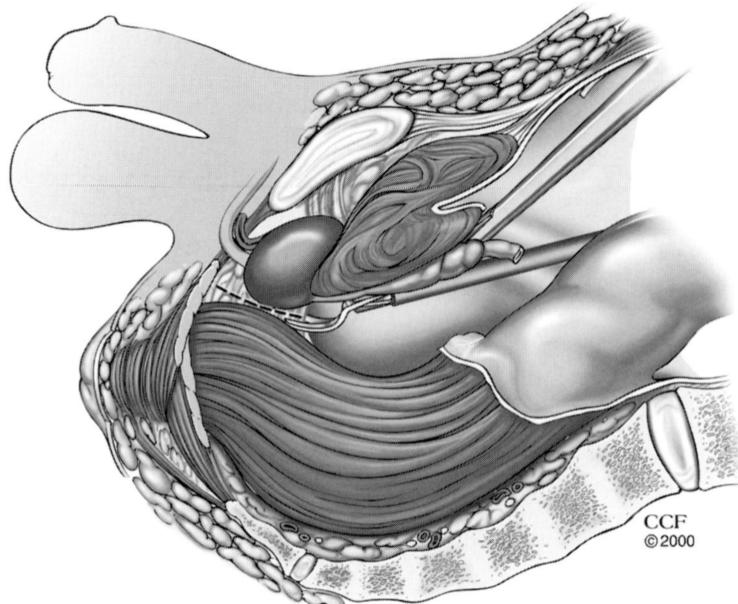


Fig. 35.13

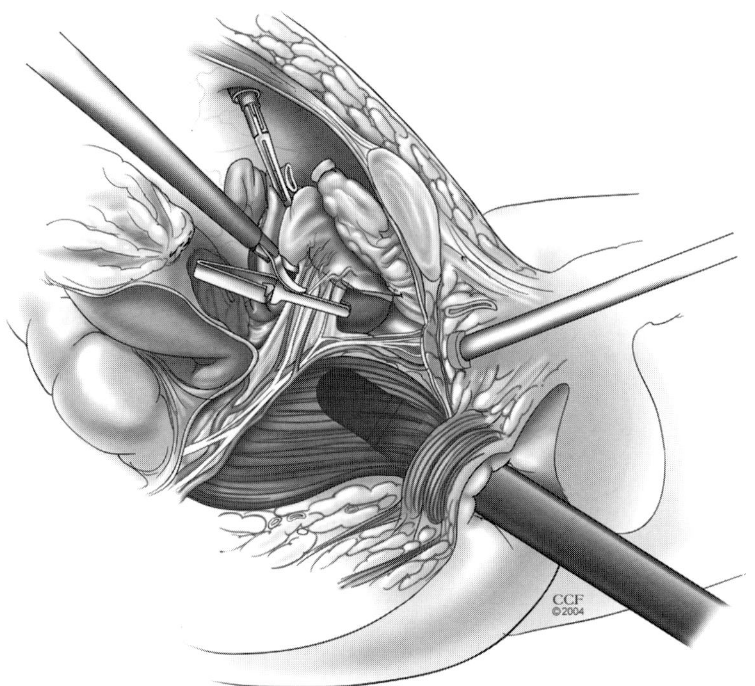


Fig. 35.14

bulldog clamp. Inadvertent compromise of the prostate capsule is minimized using real-time TRUS guidance along the posterolateral edge of the prostate. The NVB begins to be visualized after the division of the last few remaining attachments of the lateral pedicle. The NVB is released in an antegrade manner along the convexity of the prostate toward the apex using a combination of minute sharp scissor cuts and gentle blunt teasing with a soft laparoscopic Kittner. The prostate capsule must be maintained intact along the posterolateral and lateral edge of the prostate. Lateral pedicle hemostasis is achieved with precise superficial suturing of transected blood, and the bulldog clamp is released. The transected lateral pedicle is superficially sutured using a 4-0 Vicryl

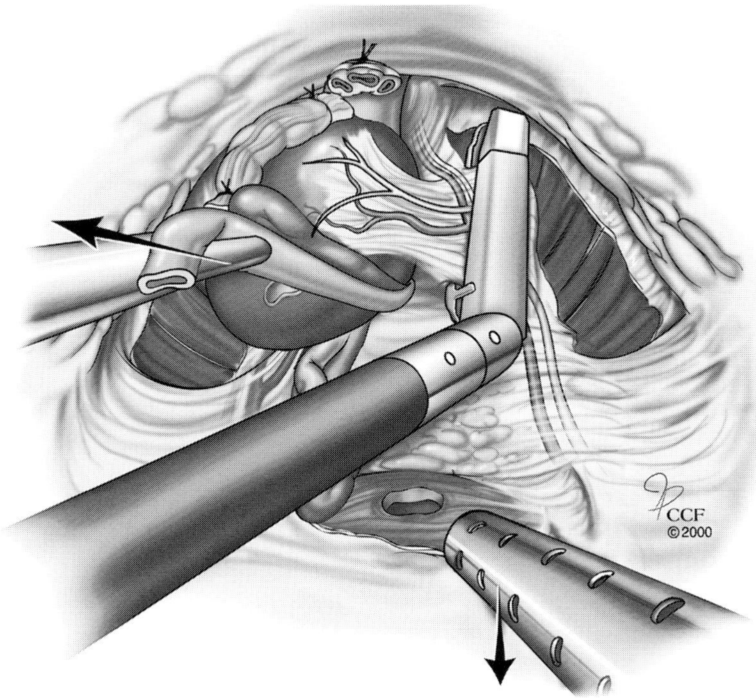


Fig. 35.15

suture on RB-1 needle (suture length 6–8 cm). The initial stitch is placed at the proximal cut end of the lateral pedicle close to the bladder neck. In order to anchor the stitch, one to two additional small suture bites are taken superficial to the jaws of the closed bulldog clamp. After bulldog clamp removal, any bleeding vessel is meticulously sutured for hemostasis. Typically, four to six running suture bites are necessary. The left lateral pedicle is transected and the NVB released in similar manner.

In the non-nerve-sparing technique, the seminal vesicle and vas deferens are retracted to the contralateral side, and each on-traction pedicle is transected with an articulating Endo-GIA stapler (vascular cartridge) (Fig. 35.15). The Endo-GIA stapler must be deployed cephalad to the base of the prostate, with the rectum in constant and clear view. The lateral prostatic edge and the NVB are completely detached from the perirectal fat. The second assistant is asked to insert a finger into the patient's rectum to provide digital guidance. After repetition of this maneuver on the contralateral side, the prostate remains attached only near its apex.

Using laparoscopic graspers, the urethra and the dorsal vein complex are placed on stretch by placing cephalad traction on the transected base of the prostate (Fig. 35.16). The dorsal vein complex is divided using the harmonic scalpel along the curvature of the prostate apex. Meticulous hemostasis is mandatory during this step. The dorsal venous complex is divided, and the anterior urethral wall is visualized. Under clear visualization and hemostasis, the urethra is transected at the prostate apex. The anterior urethral wall is divided close to the concave notch of the prostate with cold scissors, thereby achieving the three goals of maximal urethral length preservation, maintenance of prostate apex integrity, and preservation of the NVBs at the prostato-urethral junction. The tip of the urethral metallic sound is delivered into the retropubic space through the opening in the divided anterior urethral wall. Alternate prostate retraction to the left and right side allows the NVBs to be dissected off the prostate apex. The posterior urethral wall and the recto-urethralis muscles are divided. Inadvertent entry into the prostatic apex and rectum must be avoided using gentle and careful maneuvers under clear visualization and complete hemostasis. The completely detached prostate is entrapped in a 10-mm Endocatch bag and left within the abdomen until extraction at the end of the case.

Figure 35.17 shows a bladder neck stitch at 3 o'clock (outside in, right hand, forehand). To confirm absence of cancer, a posterior bladder neck biopsy is examined by frozen section. The bladder neck is evaluated for size and any inadvertent buttonholing. Both ureteric orifices are identified, and in case of suspicion, intravenous indigo carmine is administered. Prior to performing urethrovesical anastomosis, bladder neck reconstruction

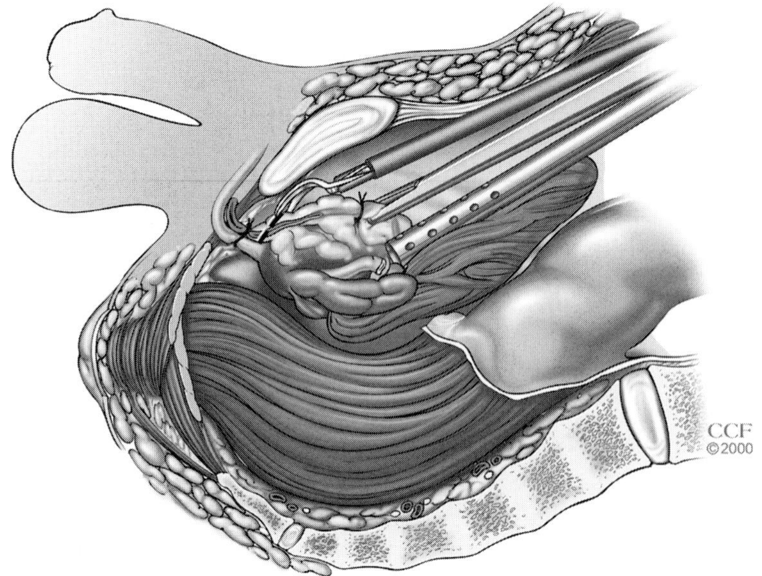


Fig. 35.16

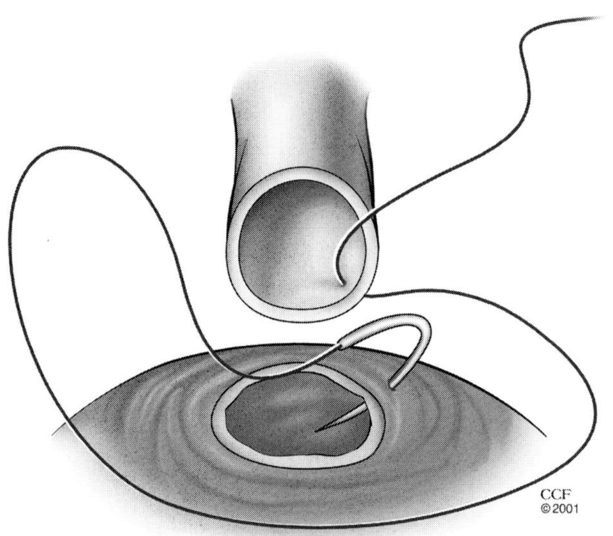


Fig. 35.17

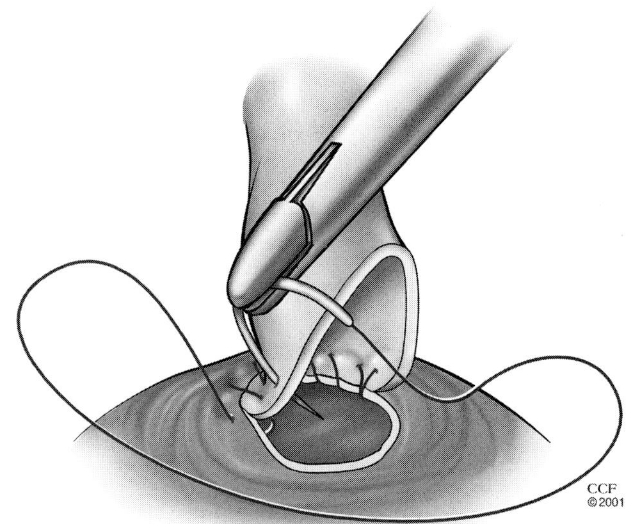


Fig. 35.18

(necessary in only 10–15% of cases) can be performed by placing two to four running stitches (UR-6 needle, 3-0 Vycril) posteriorly in a tennis racket fashion, similar to open surgery. To facilitate urethrovesical anastomosis, the diameter of the reconstructed bladder neck should be somewhat larger than the urethral diameter.

A double-needled suture is created on the back table by tying two UR-6 needled sutures together. Each 11–in. suture is 2-0 monocryl of a different color—one blue and one pale yellow—to facilitate intraoperative identification. The initial stitch is placed at the 6-o'clock position of the bladder neck and the urethral stump. At least three to four needle passes are necessary in a clockwise direction to create an adequate posterior plate. The metallic dilator guides the placement of the needles into the urethra.

Figure 35.18 shows a urethral stitch at 9 o'clock. The two needles are both placed outside in through the bladder neck at 6 o'clock. The left half of the anastomosis is created by running the blue stitch in a clockwise direction from 6-o'clock to the 11-o'clock position. The right half of the anastamosis is created by running the pale yellow stitch in a counterclockwise direction from the 5-o'clock to the 1-o'clock position. These two full-thickness mucosa-to-mucosa hemicircumferential running sutures are placed

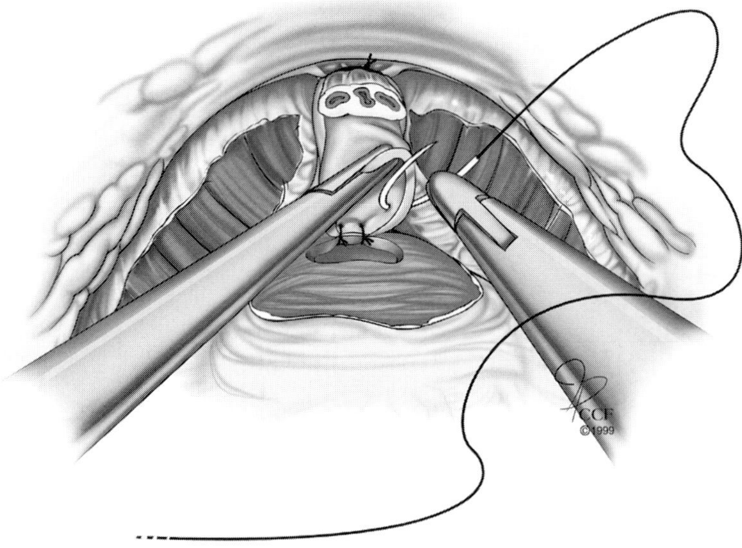


Fig. 35.19

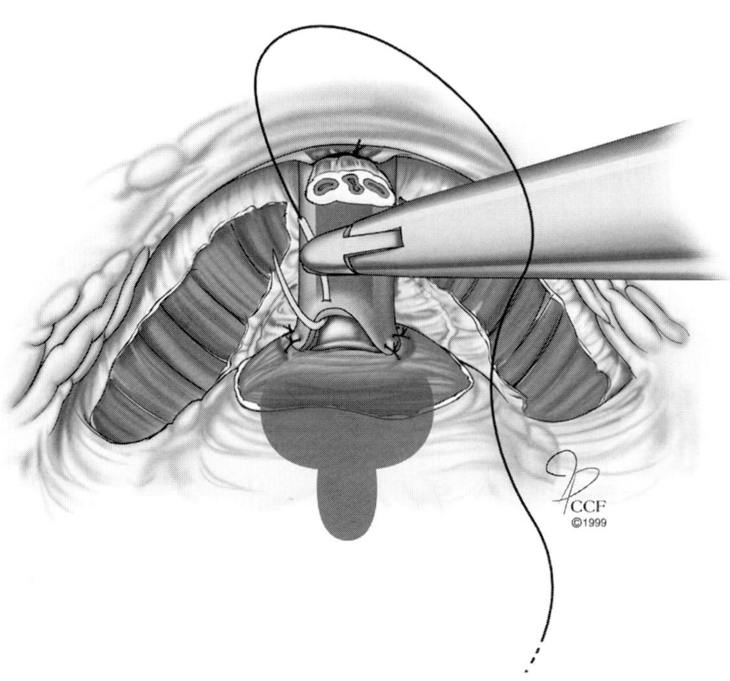


Fig. 35.20

in a preplanned choreographed sequence using two needle holders.

Once the 11 o'clock position is reached, the blue suture is pulled towards the symphisis pubis and maintained under traction by an assistant (Fig. 35.19). The second stitch (pale yellow color) is run along the contralateral edge of the urethral stump and bladder neck in a counter-clockwise direction from 6 o'clock to 12 o'clock.

Alternatively, interrupted sutures can be placed (Fig. 35.20). A 20 # French urethral Foley catheter is inserted into the bladder.

Figure 35.21 shows the completed running urethrovesical anastomosis. A Jackson-Pratt drain is placed in the pelvis. Laparoscopic exit is completed.

## EXTRAPERITONEAL APPROACH

A midline infraumbilical 1.5 cm incision is made through the anterior rectus fascia (Fig. 35.22). A trocar-mounted balloon dissection device is gently inserted along the undersurface of the anterior rectus fascia towards the pelvis for atraumatic creation of working space in the

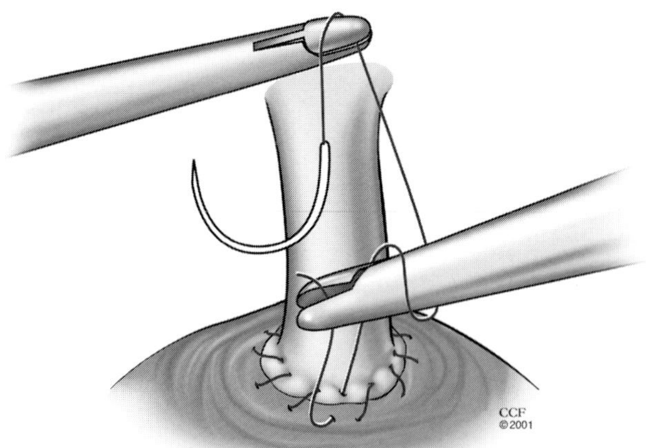


Fig. 35.21

extraperitoneum. The balloon is advanced towards the pelvis until the pubic bone is reached. The tip of trocar is then pushed underneath the pubic bone, the transversalis fascia is breached, and the prevescical space entered. The balloon is inflated with only 200–300 mL of air to develop the extraperitoneal space of Retzius. Insertion of the laparoscope within the balloon confirms adequate positioning of the balloon. The balloon is deflated and removed, and a 10-mm Bluntip trocar is inserted, in preference to the Hasson cannula, for creation of an airtight seal of the primary port.

The inflated manta-ray shaped dilator (200–300 cc) is shown in Fig. 35.23. Pneumoextraperitoneum is created (15 mmHg) and four secondary ports are placed in a fan array similar to the transperitoneal technique. Alternatively, a Hasson cannula instead of the balloon dilator may be inserted, and lateral by-expanding circular

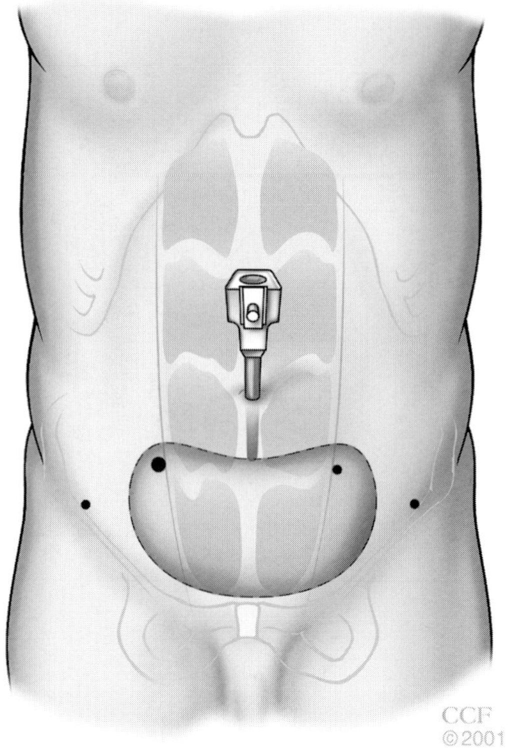


Fig. 35.23

movements of the laparoscope are performed to develop and progressively enlarge the extraperitoneal space further, without any balloon dilation. The remainder of the procedure is generally performed in a similar manner as the transperitoneal approach.

Using laparoscopic graspers, the seminal vesicle is grasped with upward traction, exposing the prostatovesical

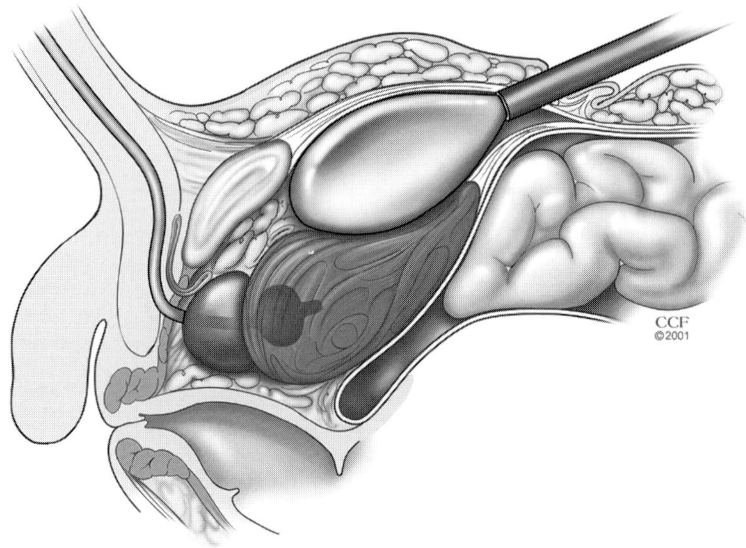


Fig. 35.22

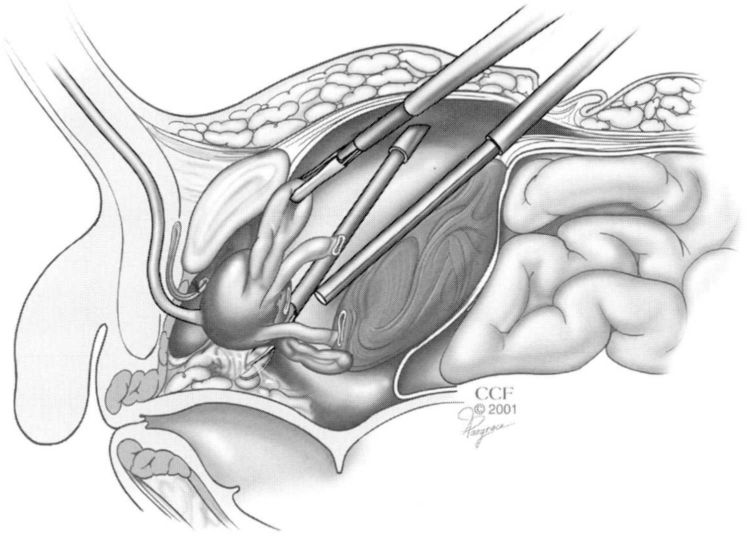


Fig. 35.24

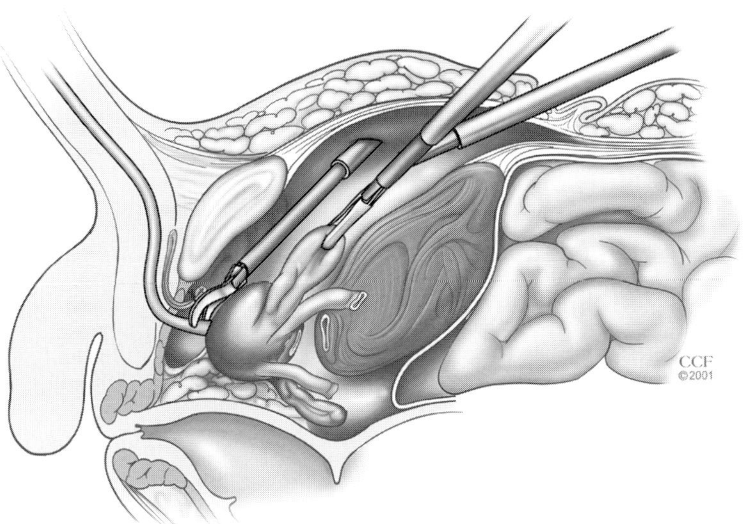


Fig. 35.25

junction (Fig. 35.24). The anterior aspect of the bladder neck is incised. Subsequently, the removal of the Foley catheter exposes the posterior aspect of the bladder neck, and the bladder neck transaction is completed.

After the incision of the anterior urethral wall, the Foley catheter is retracted, exposing the posterior urethral wall, which is transected (Fig. 35.25).

## POSTOPERATIVE CARE

The patient may begin to ambulate the same evening. A liquid diet is resumed the following morning. Depending on the individual recovery, the patient is usually discharged on postoperative d 1 or 2. The catheter is discontinued if no leaks from the anastomotic site are detected on a cystogram performed at 1 wk. The Jackson-Pratt drain is removed after 3 consecutive days of less than 50 cc/d drainage. Follow-up begins with prostate-specific antigen measurement at 3 mo.

## RESULTS

Mean operative time is 4.1 h (range 3.5–4.5 h), and open conversion rate is 1.5% (range 0–4.4%). Owing to improved control of the dorsal vein complex combined with the tamponading effect of pneumoperitoneum (15 mmHg of $CO_2$),

**Table 35.1.**
**Complication Rates After Laparoscopic Radical Prostatectomy**

| | *Mean (%)* | *Range (%)* |
|---|---|---|
| Total complications | 12.5 | (7.7–17) |
| Reoperation | 3.7 | — |
| Conversion to open | 1.2 | — |
| Deep vein thrombosis | 1.35 | (0.3–2.4) |
| Ureteral injury | 0.75 | (0.7–0.8) |
| Bladder injury | 1.38 | — |
| Anastomosis leakage | 10 | — |
| Rectal injury | 1.9 | (1.4–2.4) |
| Urinary retention | 4.6 | — |
| Ileocolonic injury | 0.8 | (0.8–0.9) |
| Postoperative ileus | 2.3 | (1–3.2) |
| Epigastric artery injury | 0.5 | — |
| Incision dehiscence | 0.6 | (0.5–0.7) |
| Anastomosis stricture | 2.5 | (1.6–3.3) |
| Rectourethral fistula | 0.9 | (0.8–1.1) |
| Iliac vein injury | 0.8 | — |

the average blood loss reported is 514 mL (range 185–1230 mL), with an average transfusion rate of 8.4% (range 0–31%). Mean catheter duration is 6.5 d (range 4–10 d).

The laparoscopic technique has the potential to enhance postoperative continence rates because of the superior length of urethral stump, watertight running urethrovesical anastomosis performed under optimal visualization, and meticulous tissue handling and dissection. Published reports demonstrate a continence rate easily comparable to open surgery (75–90% at 6 mo). Continence outcomes depend on surgeon experience, surgical technique, patient age, and method of data collection.

Laparoscopy allows excellent identification and precise handling of the NVBs. Reported 2- to 12-mo follow-up data range between 40 and 87.5% of erections in patients with bilateral nerve sparing and between 22.2 and 51% in patients with unilateral nerve-sparing procedure.

With an average follow-up of 9.9 mo (range 6.8–12 mo), overall positive surgical margin rate reported in the literature is 19.8% (range 16–26.4%); positive surgical margins occurred in 12.1% (range 2.3–16.8%) of pT2 patients and in 32.5% (range 23–48.8%) of pT3 patients; and biochemical failure was detected in 5.1% of cases (range 0–11.4%) *(7)*.

Meta-analysis of complication rates from large laparoscopic radical prostatectomy series is shown in Table 35.1 *(12)*.

## REFERENCES


1. Walsh PC. Anatomic radical prostatectomy: evolution of the surgical technique. J Urol 160:2418, 1998.
2. Schuessler WW, Schulam PG, Clayman RV, et al. Laparoscopic radical prostatectomy: initial short-term experience. Urology 50:854, 1997.
3. Guillonneau B, Vallancien G. Laparoscopic radical prostatectomy: initial experience and preliminary assessment after 65 operations. Prostate 39:71, 1999.
4. Abbou CC, Salomon L, Hoznek A, et al. Laparoscopic radical prostatectomy: preliminary results. Urology 55:630, 2000.
5. Guillonneau B, Vallancien G. Laparoscopic radical prostatectomy: the Montsouris technique. J Urol 163:1643, 2000.
6. Bollens R, Vanden Bossche M, Roumeguere T, et al. Extraperitoneal laparoscopic radical prostatectomy. Results after 50 cases. Eur Urol 40:65, 2001.
7. Guillonneau B, el-Fettouh H, Baumert H, et al. Laparoscopic radical prostatectomy: oncological evaluation after 1,000 cases a Montsouris Institute. J Urol 169:1261, 2003.
8. Gill IS, Zippe CD. Laparoscopic radical prostatectomy: technique. Urol Clin North Am 28:423, 2001.
9. Vallancien G, Gupta R, Cathelineau X, et al. Initial results of salvage laparoscopic radical prostatectomy after radiation failure. J Urol 170:1838, 2003.
10. Ukimura O, Gill IS, Desai MM, et al. Real-time transrectal ultrasonography during laparoscopic radical prostatectomy. J Urol 172:112, 2004.
11. Gill IS, Ukimura O, Rubinstein M, et al. Lateral pedicle control during laparoscopic radical prostatectomy: refined technique. Urology 65:23, 2005.
12. Guillonneau B, Gupta R, El Fettouh H, et al. Laparoscopic [correction of laproscopic] management of rectal injury during laparoscopic [correction of laproscopic] radical prostatectomy. J Urol 169:1694, 2003.

# 36 Laparoscopic Robotic-Assisted Prostatectomy

*Sidney C. Abreu and Inderbir S. Gill*

## INTRODUCTION

Conventional laparoscopy has technical limitations that include two-dimensional visualization, reduced tactile feedback, ergonomic restriction, and counterintuitive movements. For the novice laparoscopist, these limitations constitute a daunting challenge. Incorporation of robotic technology has the potential to correct these impediments *(1)*, enhancing human skills in challenging procedures such as laparoscopic radical prostatectomy.

The Zeus Robotic System (Computer Motion) comprises three essential components *(2)* (Fig. 36.1). The first component is an ergonomically enhanced surgeon console. In this mobile unit, the surgeon sits comfortably in front of a high-resolution video monitor. Two robotic handles are attached to the console. The surgeon manipulates the robotic arms using the handles in a master–slave fashion. Manipulation of the robotic handles around a pivot point allows movements of the instrument tips in three different planes. Force feedback is available during the grasping maneuvers, but not during the actual movements of the instruments. To activate the handles, the surgeon must step on a built-in foot paddle, designed to prevent inadvertent movements of the instruments. The handles' movements are then appropriately scaled, filtered to remove natural human-hand tremor, and transmitted in real time to the instruments tips, which precisely execute the steps of the operation. The second component consists of three interactive robotic arms that are attached to the operating table. The AESOP arm is designated to hold and move a 0°, 10-mm laparoscope under the surgeon's voice control. The other robotic arms manipulate a variety of instruments (scissors, forceps, needle driver). Similar to "conventional" laparoscopy, the surgeon can see the rest of the operation room in addition to the endoscopic view while simultaneously controlling the three robotic arms by voice command and by means of a joystick. The third component is a delicate computer controller, which is responsible for the eletromechanical interface between the surgeon's hands and the robotic arms and instruments. Through an accessory monitor, the surgeon can modify robotic computer parameters such as the translation and rotation movement scale. To increase the degree of fine control of movements at the operative site, a scale of 3.5:1 can be employed. Under this mode, a movement of 3.5 in. of the robotic handles would generate a movement of 1 in. at the tip of the instrument. On the other hand, during rough dissections, an ergonomic economy of robotic handle movements can be achieved using a 1:3 or a 1:2 scale *(3)*.

The da Vinci Robotic Surgical System (Intuitive Surgical) represents another master–slave type of surgical robot (Fig. 36.2). The slave or work unit consists of three telemanipulator arms attached to a main column or surgical cart. The central arm is used for the camera, and the others lateral two arms are used for the 8-mm instruments. The kinematic structure of the robotic arms mimics the "pitch" (up/down) and the "yaw" (side-to-side) flexibility of the human joints. Each arm has a set-up joint release button and a clutch button that are used to achieve optimal position of the articulations; thus, the surgeon can enjoy their maximum range of motion.

In the da Vinci surgical console (master unit), the surgeon rests his or her forehead in a natural relaxed position looking down at the visual stereo display (Fig. 36.3). Completely immersed in the endoscopic operative field, without any external visual interference, the surgeon reaches superb hand–eye coordination and depth of perception. The two finger-controlled handles are linked electronically to the motor-driven arms. Each

From: *Operative Urology at the Cleveland Clinic*
Edited by: A. Novick et al. © Humana Press Inc., Totowa, NJ

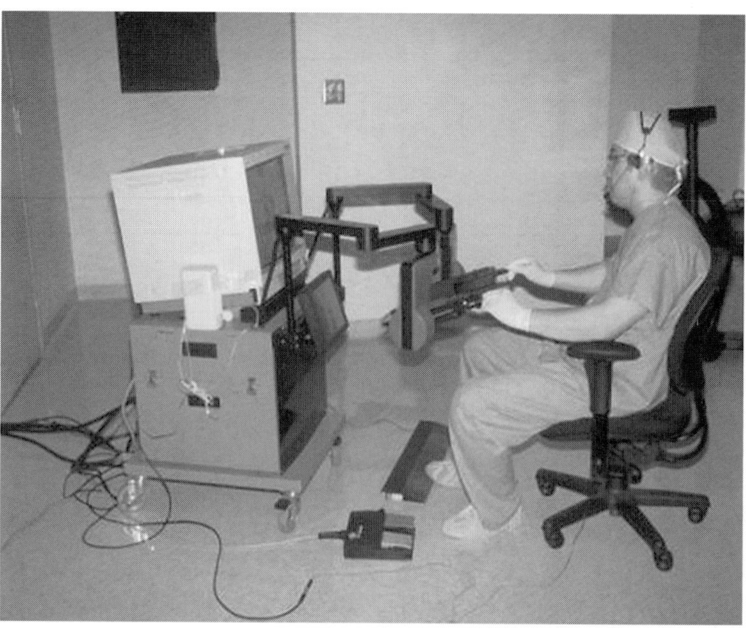

Fig. 36.1

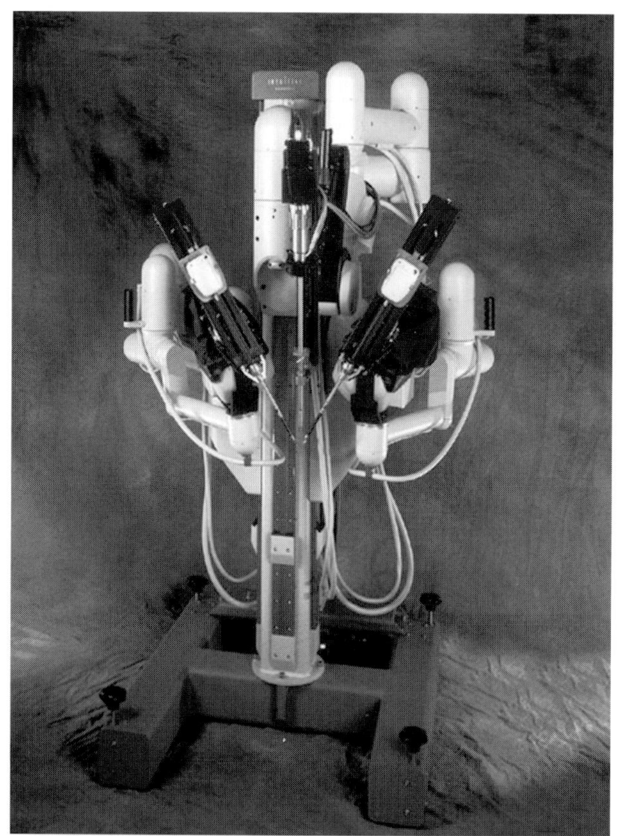

Fig. 36.2

motion of the handles is sensed, filtered, scaled, and transferred to the lateral arms, where they are translated into precise and smooth surgical moves. There are no natural hand tremors or unintended movements owing to fatigue of holding instruments for a prolonged period of time. There is no measurable time delay between the master-handles and the instruments tips because transition is performed using coaxial cables over a short distance. Using the footswitch control, the surgeon can navigate the endoscope without assistance. In this mode, the master manipulators command only the central arm and the surgeon can drive the camera to obtain a new steady view. The clutch pedal is another feature in the footswitch control that allows the surgeon to read just the masters into an optimal position while the instruments remain frozen.

The da Vinci system has unique visual capabilities that provide a high-quality, three-dimensional (3D) view (Fig. 36.4). Two three-chip couple device cameras are mounted on a 3D endoscope (0° and 30°) with two separate optical channels. The images from the operative site are independently acquired and fused into a single, 10× magnified, high-resolution view that appears at the binocular display. The stereoscopic 3D vision enhances the depth of the surgical view simulating the open approach.

The da Vinci instruments incorporate an Endowrist technology that allows a full 7° range of motion at the instrument tips: pitch, yaw, in and out, horizontal, vertical, rotational, and grasping *(1)* (Fig. 36.5). This freedom of movement allows the surgeon to deliver the dexterity of his or her hand and wrist to the operative site, incorporating open surgical maneuvers into laparoscopy without spatial restriction of the movements. Thus, maneuvers such as needle positioning can be facilitated and optimized since the surgeons' fingers intuitively act as

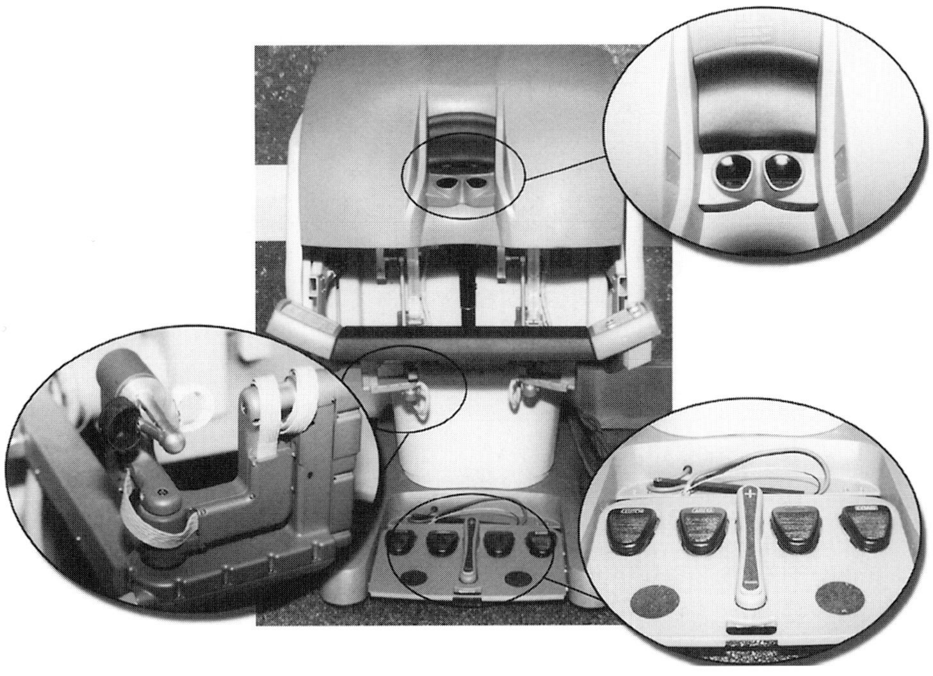

Fig. 36.3

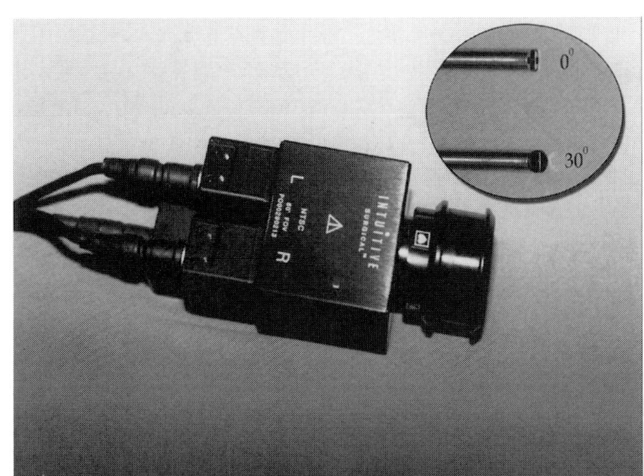


Fig. 36.4

the jaws of the needle holder. Nevertheless, the lack of tactile feedback is a drawback of this currently available robotic technology, especially when judging tension of the suturing material.

The patient is placed in a modified lithotomy position (tights abducted) with the arms adducted by his or her side, and the table is set in a Trendelenburg (Fig. 36.6). The abdomen and perineal region are prepared with iodine-based disinfectant and draped. A Foley catheter is inserted, and bladder is drained. The robotic arms are also draped with sterile plastic coverings and prepared for later docking. Through a peri-umbilical puncture, a 15 mmHg $CO_2$ pneumoperitoneum is created with a Verres needle. Five ports are placed in a fan array. A 12-mm port is introduced at the umbilicus as the camera port. Under visual control of a regular endoscope, the 8-mm robotic ports are inserted respectively in the right and left lateral border of the rectus muscle, approximately two fingerbreadths below the umbilicus. The remote center of the da Vinci instrument arm canulas (marked with a wide black band) must be carefully placed within the abdominal wall for proper function of the instruments. Additionally, two regular ports (5/12 mm on the right side and 5 mm on the left side) are placed two fingerbreadths medial to the anterior superior iliac spine and are used by the right and left patient-side assistants for retraction and suction purpose. Alternatively, a six-port transperitoneal approach can be employed. For this purpose, the camera port is shifted slightly to the left side of the umbilicus, and an additional 5-mm port is inserted in the right side. After port placement, the robotic surgical cart is moved toward the patient's feet, and the main column is properly aligned with the primary (camera) port. The patient-side assistants precisely control and dock the robotic arms, taking care to avoid patient injury by inadvertent compression. The remote surgeon sits in the master unit located in the corner of the operating room.

The initial dissection targets bladder mobilization to gain immediate access to the space of Retzius

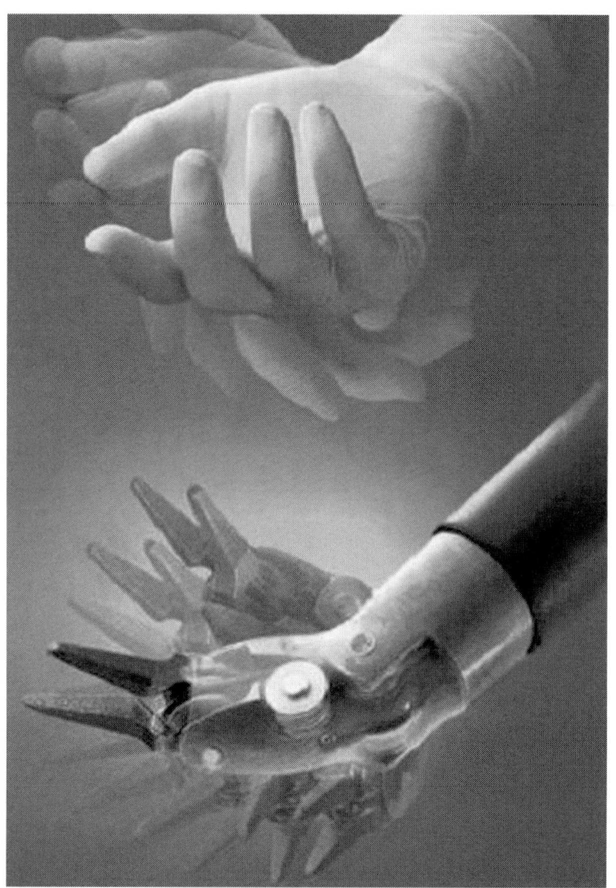

Fig. 36.5

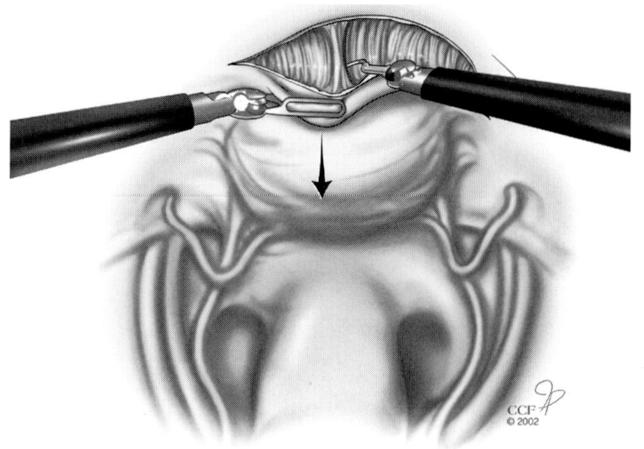


Fig. 36.7

(Fig. 36.7). For this purpose the bladder is distended with 200 mL of saline through the Foley catheter, and an inverted U-shaped peritoneotomy is made. Using a 30° lens looking upwards, the peritoneum is widely incised with the both limbs of the U incision located medial to the ipsilateral medial umbilical ligament. The horizontal part of the U incision is located high on the undersurface of the anterior abdominal wall to prevent an inadvertent bladder injury. Circumferentially, dissection of the bladder is performed in a virtually avascular plane of loose areolar tissue. Although this "modified" transperitoneal route does not completely avoid the peritoneal cavity as in the "pure" extraperitoneal approach, the bowel manipulation is minimal, and a suitable working

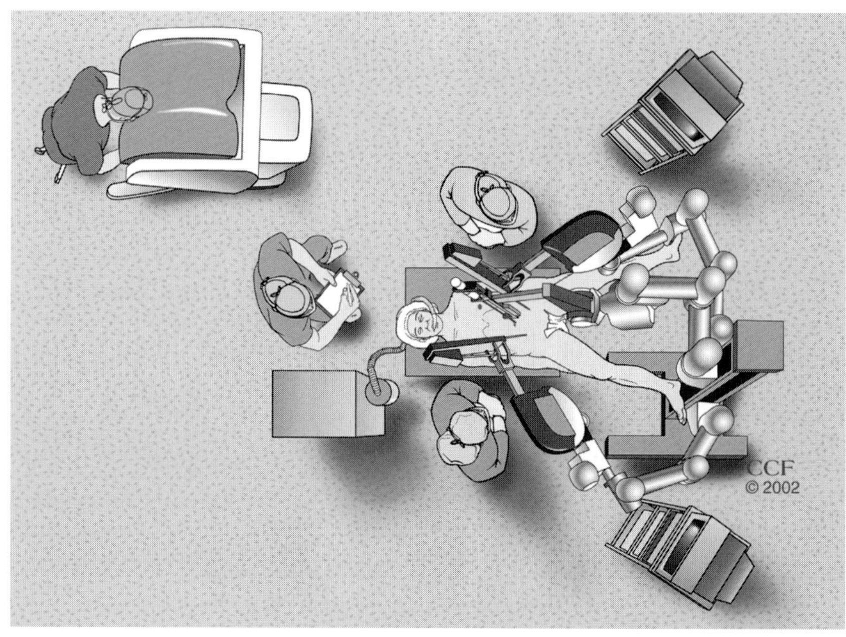


Fig. 36.6

space is achieved, which is critical for the success of this operation.

Under 0° lens visualization, the elbow of the J-hook is used to sweep the fatty tissue from the pubic symphysis espousing the endopelvic fascia and the puboprostatic ligaments (Fig. 36.8). The endopelvic fascia is then incised, and the prostate is mobilized off the levator fibers. Visualization of the prostate apex is the endpoint of this dissection. A laparoscopic Küttner may be used to complete the dissection atraumatically. Dissection distal to the prostate apex should be minimized in order to better preserve this nerve-rich, sphincter-active zone.

Using the index finger and thumb as the jaws of the needle holder, the surgeon intuitively places a CT-1, 2-0 polyglactin stitch distal to the apex of the prostate, from the right to left side, between the dorsal vein complex and the urethra (Fig. 36.9). Routinely, two sutures are placed at the dorsal vein complex to achieve appropriate venous control. Using the clutch pedal, the surgeon can readjust the master handles to tie these stitches snugly enough. Furthermore, in order to enhance the continence outcomes, the dorsal vein stitches are also secured to the puboprostatic ligaments. A back-bleeding stitch is also placed across the anterior surface of the prostate, midway between apex and base.

Since precise anatomical landmarks are not present, the exact identification of the junction between the prostate and the bladder neck is a relatively challenging task (Fig. 36.10). However, close endoscopic 3D visualization with a 30°

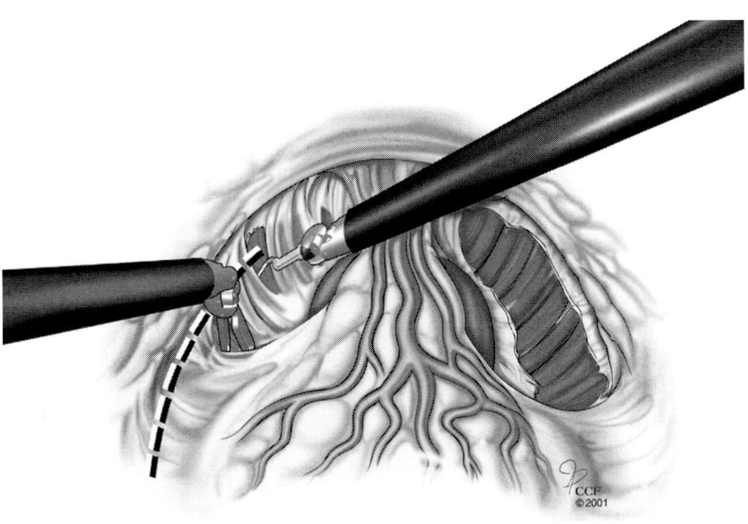


Fig. 36.8

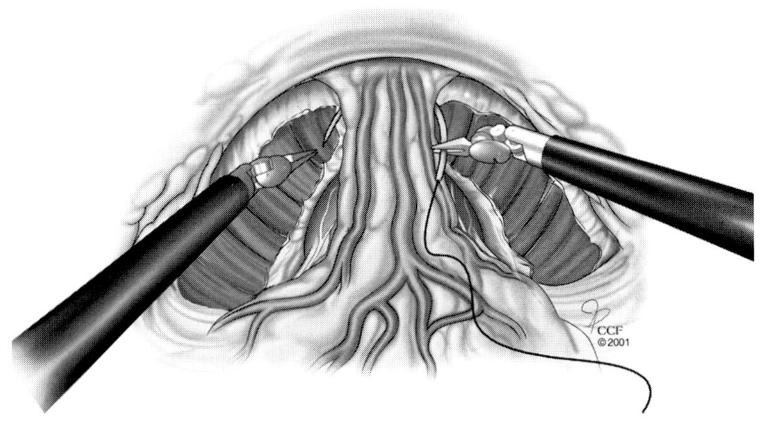


Fig. 36.9

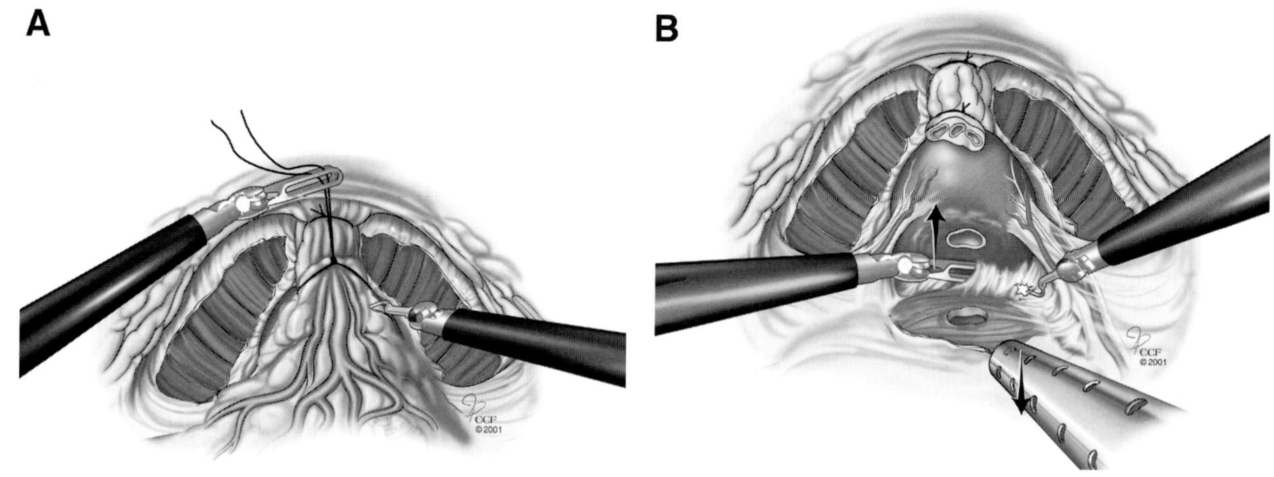


Fig. 36.10

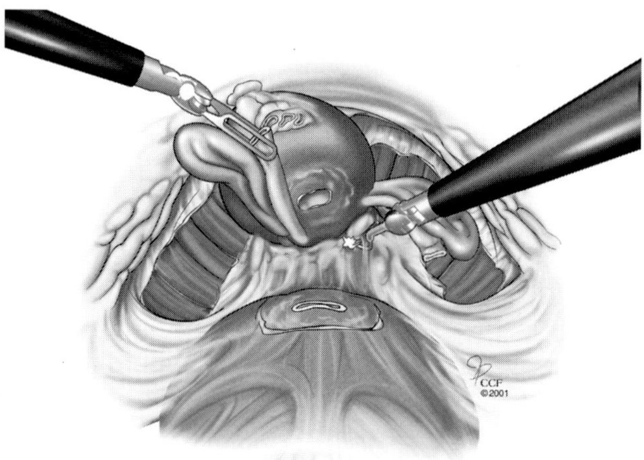


Fig. 36.11

lens looking down usually identifies the area where the prevesical fat ends. At this point a shallow groove between the prostate and the bladder can be identified. Furthermore, repeated in-and-out movements of the metallic urethral dilator, with its curved tip pointing anteriorly, provide an accurate idea of where the bladder ends and where the prostate begins. Using the J-hook electrocautery, the anterior bladder neck is transected while the bleeders are coagulated. No attempts to spare the bladder neck are performed. However, if one can obtain a bladder neck that is not too wide, an extra reconstructive step of the operation can be avoided. Moreover, incising the bladder neck unevenly so that the posterior lip becomes slightly longer than the anterior provides better visualization of the posterior suture line later on during the urethrovesical anastomosis. The posterior bladder neck is then gradually dissected away from the prostate.

Using the da Vinci J-hook, the anterior layer of the Denonvilliers' fascia is incised, exposing the vas and seminal vesicles. The vas deferens is subsequently grasped and transected (Fig. 36.11). Dissection is carried along its lateral border to identify the ipsilateral seminal vesicle, which is circumferentially mobilized using the harmonic scalpel and the hem-o-lock clips (Weck Systems). Subsequently, the bilateral prior mobilized vas deferens and seminal vesicles are retracted anteriorly, which place the posterior layer of Denonvilliers' fascia under traction. The posterior layer of Denonvilliers' fascia is incised 2–3 mm posterior to the junction of the seminal vesicles with the prostate. This allows proper entry into the plane between the prostate and the rectum. Visualization of a yellow perirectal fat confirms the correct plane.

In a non-nerve-sparing procedure, the ipsilateral seminal vesicle and the vas deferens are retracted, thus placing in traction the adjacent lateral pedicle (Fig. 36.12). An Endo-GIA stapler with an articulated vascular cartridge (gray color, 2.5 mm) is fired across the lateral pedicles, away from and cephalad to the base of the prostate. A second articulating vascular cartridge is employed to detach completely the lateral border of the prostate and the neurovascular bundle from the perirectal fat. In a nerve-sparing procedure, a combination of hem-o-lock clips (Weck Systems) and harmonic scalpel is employed.

Using 0° lens, a J-hook eletrocautery is utilized to incise slowly and with meticulous hemostasis the previous ligated dorsal vein complex, exposing the under laying urethra (Fig. 36.13). To minimize the possibility of positive apical margin, the anterior wall of the urethra is transected a few millimeters distal to the concave

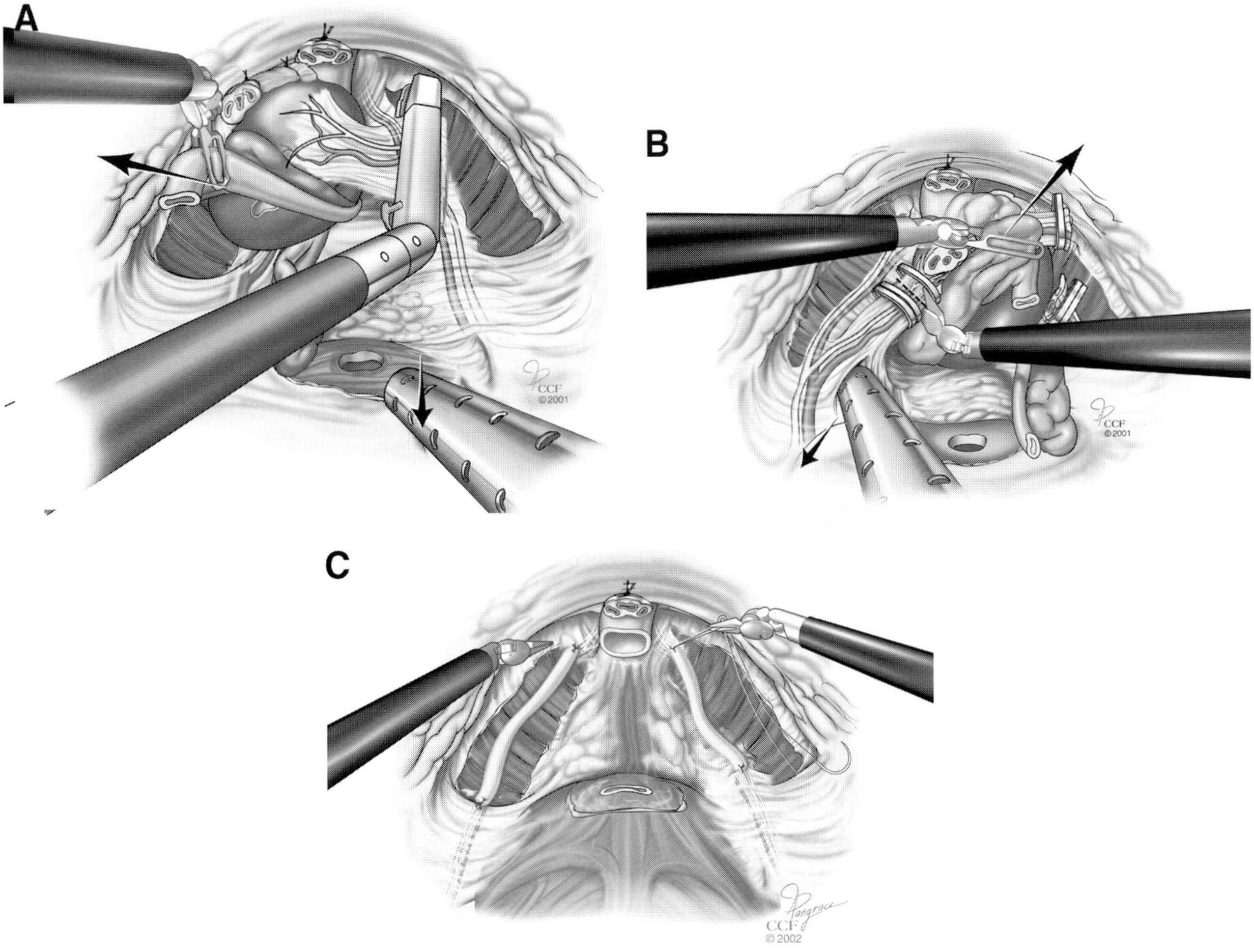

Fig. 36.12

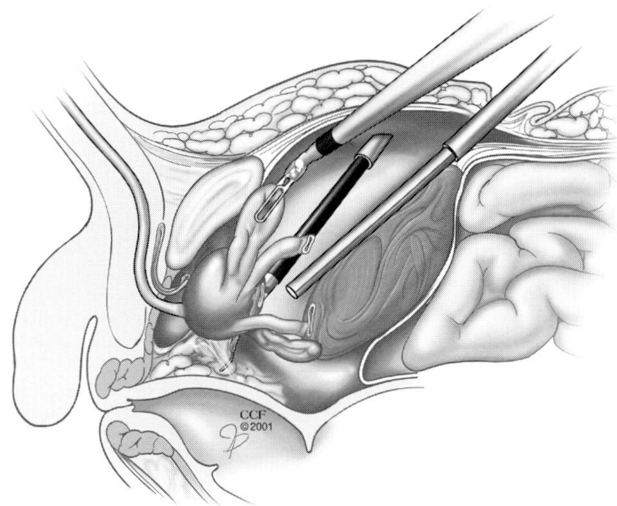


Fig. 36.13

notch of the prostate apex. The tip of the intraurethral metallic sound is delivered into the space of Retzius, and the posterior urethral wall is transected sharply.

During urethrovesical anastomosis, the Endo-wrist technology helps significantly because the sutures can be placed at almost any angle (Fig. 36.14). Using an RB1 needle in a 2-0 polyglactin suture, two full-thickness mucosa-to-mucosa hemicircumferential running sutures are placed. Although no tactile feedback is available with the da Vinci system, the superb 3D view capabilities allow the surgeon to correctly judge the amount of tension that he or she is applying to the thread; thus, the 2-0 polyglactin suture is unlike to be torn during the suturing. The initial suture is placed inside the urethral lumen and outside the bladder at the 5-o'clock position, bringing and anchoring them together. The right hand is used for the urethral stump needle pass and the left hand for the bladder neck needle pass. At least four-needle passes are necessary to create an adequate posterior plate. A 22 French

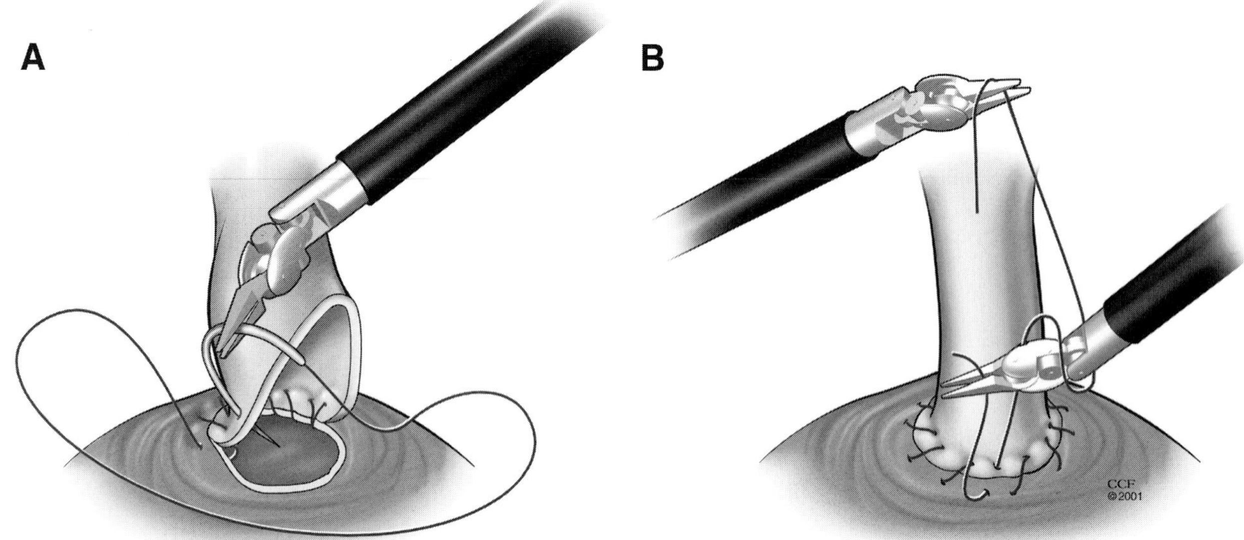


Fig. 36.14

urethral Foley catheter, mounted in an insertion guide, is easily pushed into the bladder. A second stitch begins at 5 o'clock and runs counterclockwise to 11 o'clock, where it is tied to the previous placed stitch. The bladder is filled with 200 cc of saline, and the integrity of the anastomosis is tested.

## REFERENCES

1. Sung GT, Gill IS. Robotic laparoscopic surgery: a comparison of the da Vinci and Zeus system. Urology 58:893–898, 2001.
2. Gill IS, Sung GT, Hsu TH, et al. Robotic remote laparoscopic nephrectomy and adrenalectomy: the initial experience. J Urol 164:2082–2085, 2000.
3. Sung GT, Gill IS, Hsu TH. Robotic-assisted laparoscopic pyeloplasty: a pilot study. Urology 53: 1099–1103, 1999.
4. Hoznek A, Zaki SK, Samadi DB, et al. Robotic-assisted kidney transplantation: an initial experience. J Urol 167:1604–1606, 2002.
5. Abbou CC, Hoznek A, Salomon L, et al. Laparoscopic radical prostatectomy with a remote controlled robot. J Urol 165:1964–1966, 2001.
6. Menon M, Tewari A, Peabody J. Vattikuti institute prostatectomy: technique and contemporary results using the da Vinci surgical system. In press.
7. Kaouk J, Desai M, Abreu SC, Papay F, Gill I. Robotic-assisted sural nerve grafting during laparoscopic radical prostatectomy: the initial experience.

# 37 Radical Perineal Prostatectomy

*Craig D. Zippe*

## INTRODUCTION

Radical prostatectomy can be performed either by a retropubic, a laparoscopic, a robotic or a perineal approach. The radical perineal prostatecomy is a minimally invasive approach that in skilled hands may take no longer than 60 min. Patients have minimal postoperative pain, requiring minimal analgesics, are ambulatory immediately, and are routinely discharged from the hospital on the first or second postoperative day. The three important surgical endpoints of cure, continence, and potency are comparable to the other two approaches. With experienced derived surgeons, the surgical margin status on low-volume prostate cancers is less than 20%, full continence returns in 80–90% of patients, and 1-yr potency rates have been reported as high as 70%. Whether these results can be universally reproduced throughout the urological community remains to be seen. With the recent stage migration in the diagnosis of lower-volume prostate cancers, especially in the younger patient, the necessity of a laparoscopic lymph node dissection has been eliminated, but the emphasis on nerve-sparing techniques has increased. Similar to the evolution of radical laparoscopic and robotic surgery, the ultimate role of radical perineal prostatectomy will depend on the ability to consistently perform successful bilateral nerve-sparing radical prostatectomy.

Fundamental anatomy that facilitates but does not preclude the perineal approach includes (1) sufficient width of the ischial tuberosities, (2) a thin perineum with the apex of the prostate palpably close to the anal verge, and (3) a relatively small to average size prostate that has not previously been operated on. One should consider the size of the prostate with respect to the size of the incision before selecting the perineal route. Pre-existent inflammatory adherence from a prior transurethral resection of the prostate, multiple biopsies, and a history of recurrent prostatitis complicate but do not preclude the perineal approach.

## SURGICAL POSITION AND INCISION

The patient is placed in an exaggerated lithotomy position with the head down (Trendelenburg position). While the full exaggerated lithotomy position is often utilized, making the perineal horizontal to the floor, this degree of lithotomy can produce transitory if not permanent neuropraxia in legs. Consequently, a modified lithotomy as shown is Fig. 37.1 is preferred. In this position, either Allen stirrups or candy cane stirrups are used to elevate the legs such that the perineum is roughly perpendicular to the floor. A role placed under the sacrum may facilitate exposure. The knees and feet are well padded in the stirrups to prevent peroneal nerve compression. A curved Lowsley is placed in the urethra and passed into the bladder to aid in the dissection.

The incision is an inverted U with the top of the incison approx 2 cm anterior to the mucocutaneous anal junction. This top of this incision lies directly above the subcutaneous anal sphincter (Fig. 37.2). Classically, the ends of the incision curve laterally and posteriorly toward, and stop medial to, each ischial tuberosity. However, extending the incision further posteriorly on either side of the anus will facilitate posterior anal retraction and rectal mobilization. The subsequent achievement of the correct plane along the anterior rectal wall beneath the external sphincter is then achieved easier. The ischiorectal fossae are developed by blunt dissection with either a scalpel handle or electrocautery. The central tendon is exposed by passing a finger behind it and connecting the two ischiorectal fossae by digital dissection. The tendon is then divided by electrocautery.

## APPROACHES TO THE PROSTATE

Positioning the Lowsley retractor cephalad towards the abdomen directs the prostate toward the wound and

From: *Operative Urology at the Cleveland Clinic*
Edited by: A. Novick et al. © Humana Press Inc., Totowa, NJ

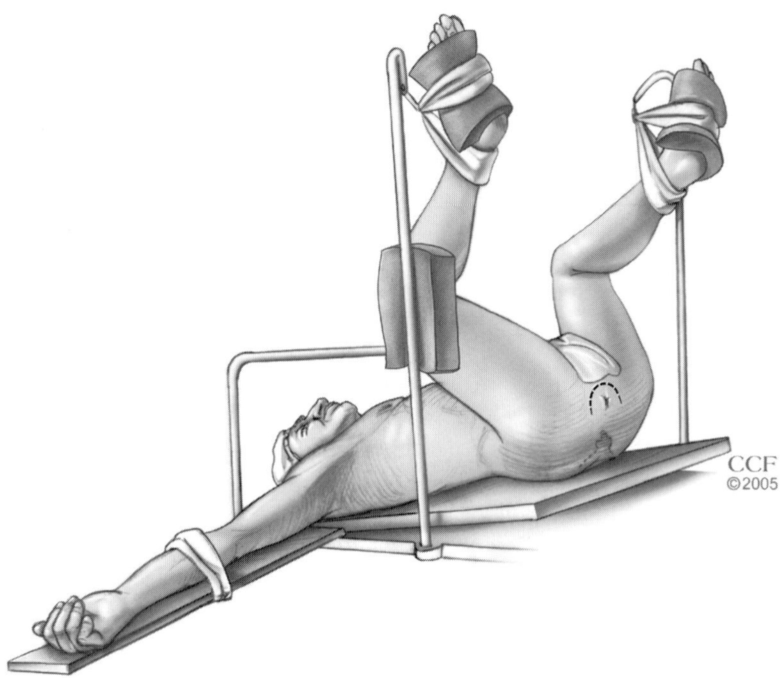


Fig. 37.1

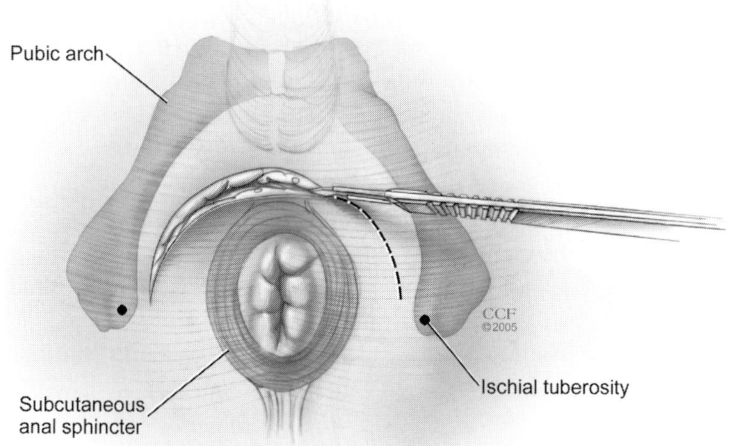


Fig. 37.2

elevates the external anal sphincter. Dissecting initially just above the subcutaneous anal sphincter, the external anal sphincter is dissected off the rectum with sharp dissection with a scissors (line C, Fig. 37.3). Placing a finger in the rectum to feel the space between the dissection and the rectal wall is helpful. Some prefer to use a moist sponge between a finger and the lower aspect of the wound to draw the rectum taut and then dissect the external anal sphincter anteriorly. Line B represents the Hudson approach, such that the subcutaneous anal sphincter is preserved to maximize anal blood supply and sphincter control (Fig. 37.4). Line A represents the classic Young approach, incising the central tendon and rectourethralis muscle, without visualization of the rectum. The classic Young approach produced a significant number of rectal injuries and is not utilized very often today. Line C represents the Belt's approach, which does not preserve the subcutaneous anal sphincter, compromising blood flow to the anus, resulting in a higher incidence of necrotic anal flaps and prolonged healing time. Complete rectal continence is less likely with this approach.

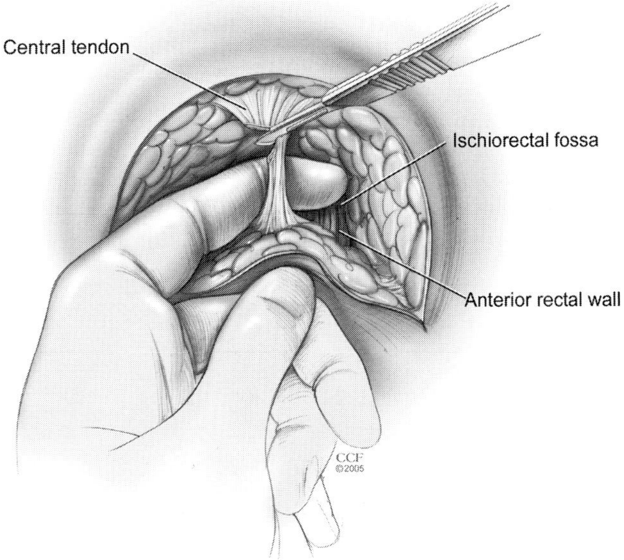


Fig. 37.3

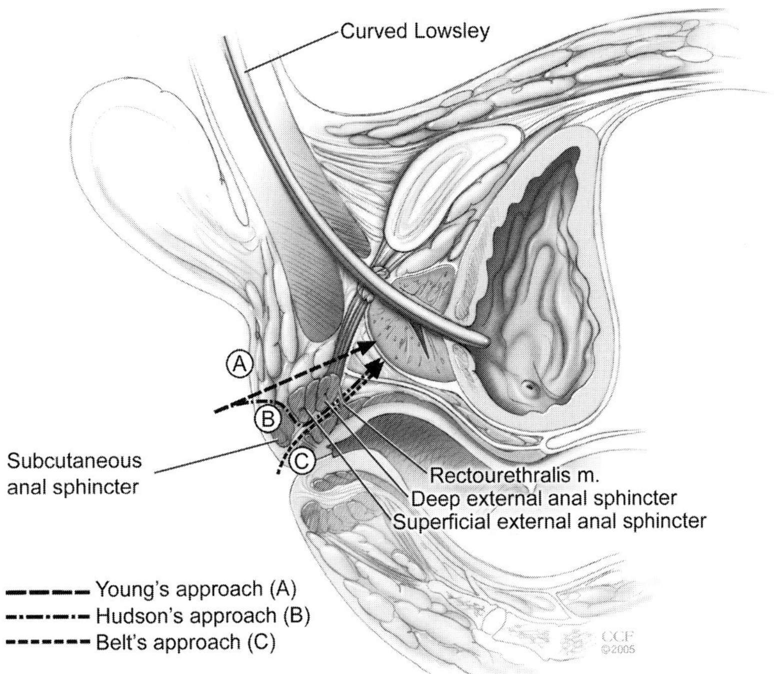


Fig. 37.4

After elevating the superficial and deep external anal sphincters, a condensation of levator muscle fibers are seen in the midline, referred to as the rectourethralis muscle. This muscle lies just in front of the posterior Denonvilliers' fascia of the prostate and needs to be excised (Fig. 37.5). This particular maneuver has the highest incidence of producing a rectal injury, so placement of a finger into the rectum is recommended to check the safety of this maneuver. Using the manual lateral retractors or the self-retaining system (Omni retractor), the remaining levator ani muscles—the right and left leafs of the levator ani—are retracted laterally, exposing the posterior layer of Denonvilliers' fascia (Fig. 37.6). Care must be taken at this point to limit the lateral retraction to avoid injury to the neurovascular bundles.

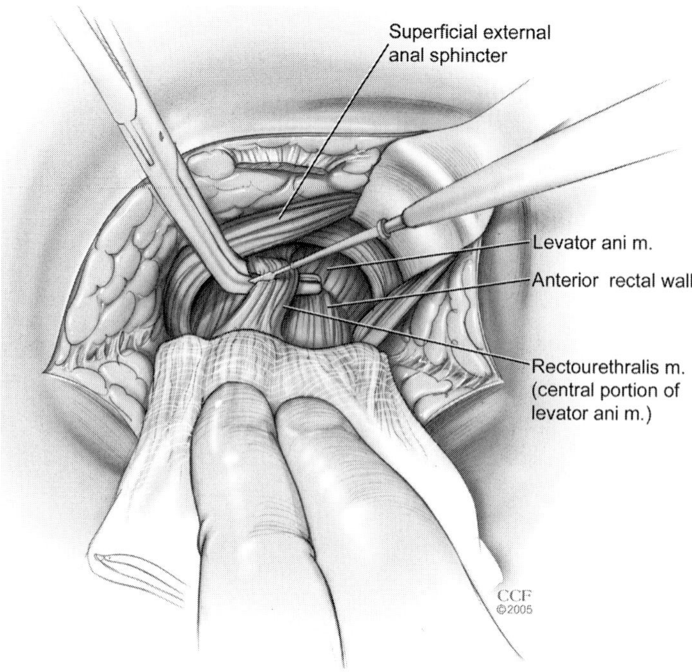


Fig. 37.5

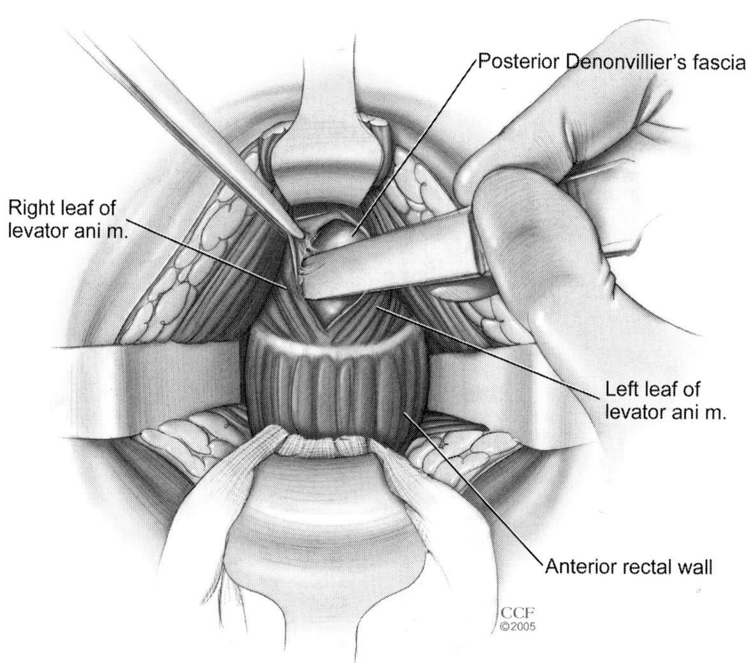


Fig. 37.6

## PRESERVATION OF THE NEUROVASCULAR BUNDLES

The neurovascular bundles anatomically lie in the lateral pelvic fascia, which lies deep, lateral, and cephalad to Denonvilliers' fascia. Thus, a midline, vertical incision is made into Denonvilliers' fascia—along the entire gland extending up the urethra—and the fascia is sharply retracted to the right and left to expose the posterior prostatic capsule (Fig. 37.7). This incision must fully release the neurovascular bundles to allow proper resetting of the retractor blades and thus to avoid a traction injury to the neurovascular bundles. Blunt or sharp dissection is often required to release the bundles far enough laterally to

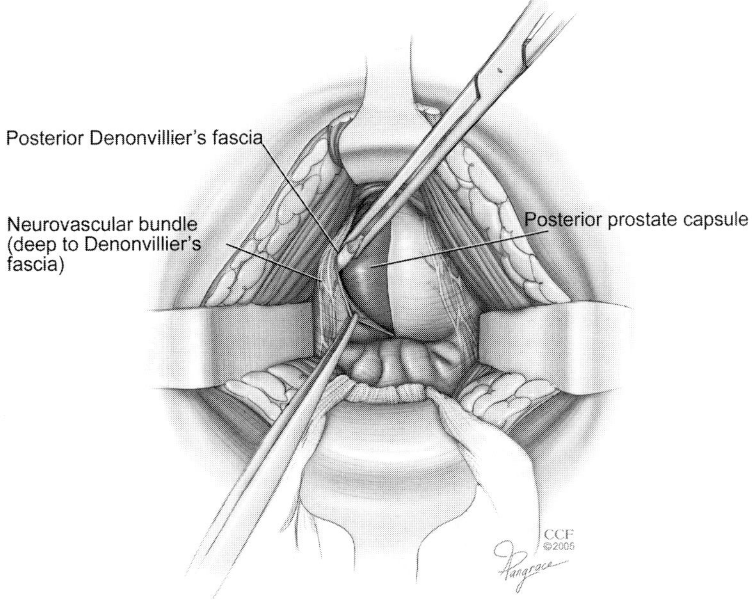


Fig. 37.7

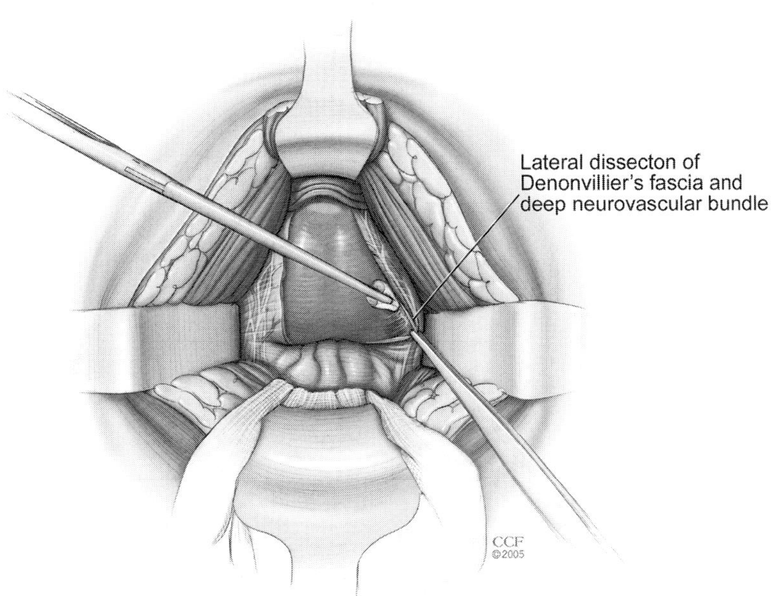


Fig. 37.8

achieve adequate exposure to the posterior prostate base (Fig. 37.8).

## LIGATION OF THE LATERAL VASCULAR PEDICLES

With use of the posterior retractor over a moist sponge to retract the rectum inferiorly, and with anterior pressure on the curved Lowsley, the prostate is gland is visualized more completely and the lateral pedicles can be visualized and ligated (Fig. 37.9). To achieve this exposure, posterior Denonvilliers' is further dissected posteriorly to expose the seminal vesicles and the vas deferens. The seminal vesicles and vas are not ligated at this point in the operation.

## URETHRA AND ANTERIOR PROSTATE DISSECTION

The urethra is then mobilized, and an umbilical tape is passed anterior to the urethra at the prostatic apex. Care is

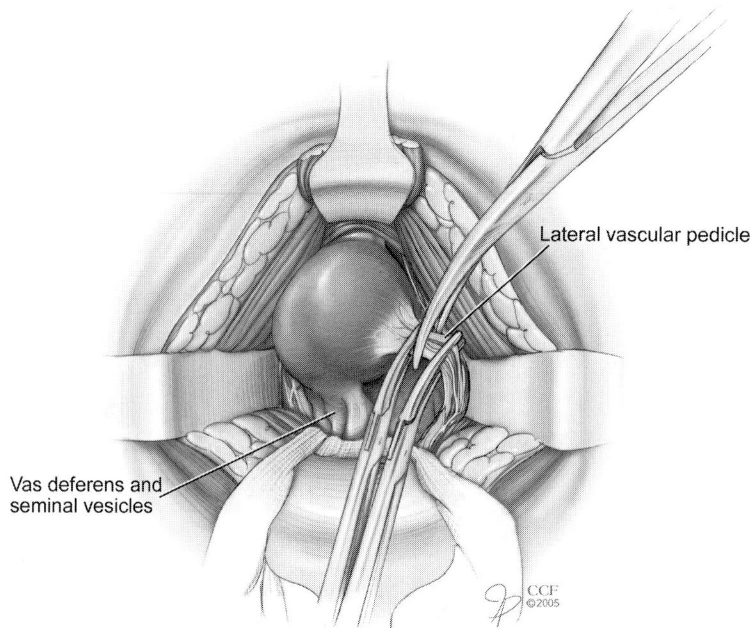


Fig. 37.9

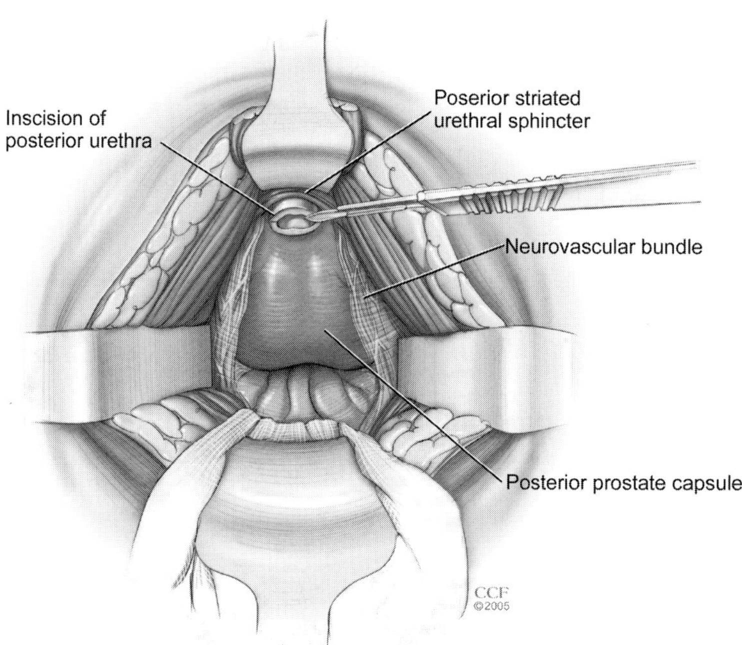


Fig. 37.10

exercised in preserving the periurethral tissue so as not to injure the associated nerves in this region. The posterior surface of the urethra is then incised with the scalpel (Fig. 37.10). This exposes the curved Lowsley retractor, and it is removed and replaced with a straight Lowsley retractor. Retraction on the straight Lowsley retractor toward the incision facilitates the remaining urethra transection and the dissection of the anterior prostate off of the dorsal vein attachments. The anterior prostate dissection is carried out beneath the puboprostatic ligaments and its associated dorsal vein branches, thereby diminishing the potential for significant bleeding.

## BLADDER NECK DISSECTION

After dissection and release of the anterior prostate capsule, the bladder neck vasculature is then is encountered and can be controlled with several interrupted ligatures

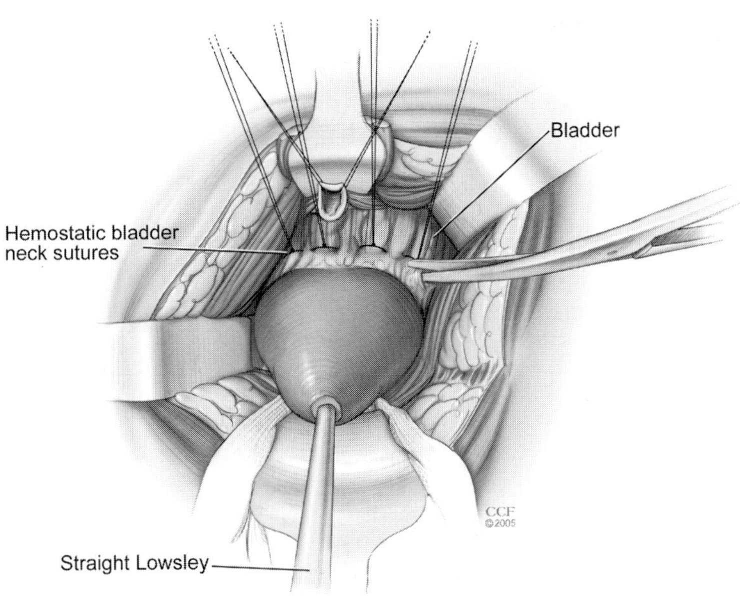


Fig. 37.11

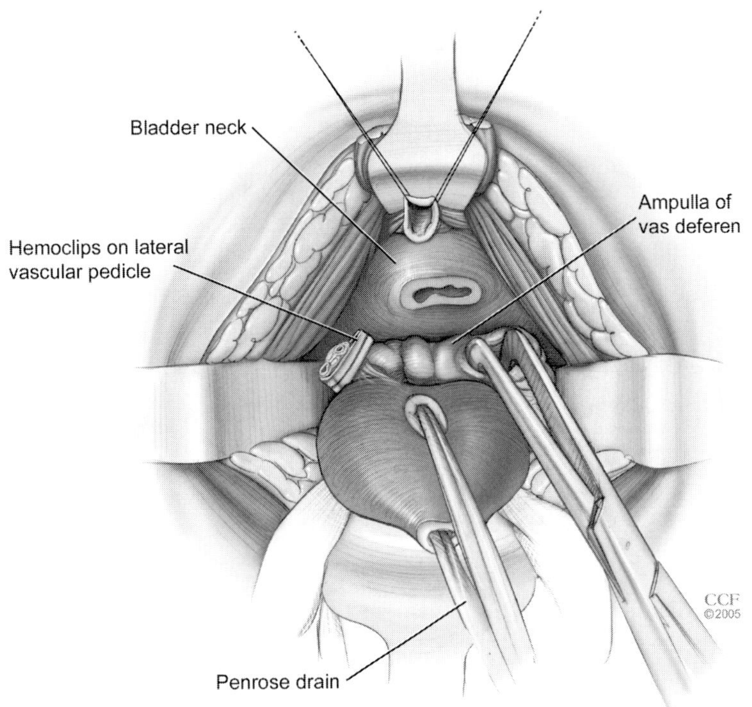


Fig. 37.12

(Fig. 37.11). The blades of the straight Lowsley retractor can be palpated at this point to direct the entry into the bladder and complete the prostate enucleation from the bladder neck. Alternatively, the Lowsley can be removed and a right-angle clamp can be placed through the prostatic urethra and pierced anteriorly through the junction of the prostate and bladder neck. A Penrose drain is grasped with the clamp and pulled back through the urethra to use as traction.

## LIGATION OF THE VAS DEFERENS AND SEMINAL VESICLES

Posterior division of the bladder neck with downward and outward traction on the prostate gland exposes the seminal vesicles and vas deferens (Fig. 37.12). The ampullae of the vasa deferentia are identified and divided with hemoclips or electrocautery.

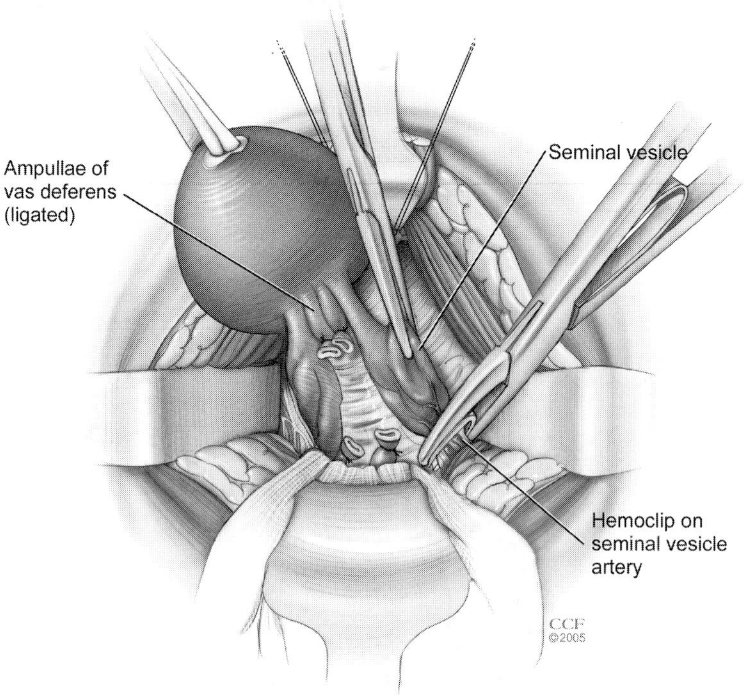


Fig. 37.13

Ligation of the vas deferens facilitates lifting the prostate anteriorly to expose the seminal vesicles. The seminal vesicles are ligated as far distally as possible, with no significant effort made to reach the tip of the seminal vesicle (Fig. 37.13). Once the tips of the seminal vesicle are reached, hemoclips are applied. The specimen is free and can be removed and inspected for surgical margin status.

## VESICOURETHRAL ANASTOMOSIS

The bladder neck is inspected and reconstructed, if necessary, with interrupted 2-0 polyglycolic acid sutures, leaving an opening that will accommodate the tip of the fifth finger. Mucosal eversion sutures of 4-0 chromic can be placed but often are unnecessary.

The anterior row of the vesicourethral anastomosis is then completed with interrupted 2-0 or 3-0 polyglycolic sutures. Approximately three to four anterior sutures are placed—beginning inside the urethra and brought inside the bladder neck, with the knots tied on the inside. A 22 or 24 French Foley catheter (30-cc balloon) is then passed retrograde through the urethral stump into the bladder. The remaining five to six posterior vesicourethral sutures are then placed outside the urethra to outside the bladder neck with the knots tied outside. The posterior wall is most important because of the additional tension of bringing the bladder neck down, and often the 6-o'clock suture is done in a figure-of-8 configuration with the knot tied on the outside of the bladder neck (Fig. 37.14). The Foley is then irrigated with saline, and the vesicourethral anastomosis is inspected for extravasation. Additional sutures are placed as necessary. The typical secure, watertight anasotomosis will easily accommodate eight to nine vesicourethral sutures.

## CLOSURE AND POSTOPERATIVE COURSE

Closure of the surgical wound involves placement of a 1/2-in. Penrose drain at the anastomosis, bringing it out on the skin through a separate stab incision. After inspecting the rectal wall for any inadvertent enterotomy, the levator muscles are reapproximated in the midline with interrupted 2-0 chromic gut sutures (Fig. 37.15).

The central tendon and the subcutaneous tissues are then reapproximated with 3-0 chromic sutures. Vertical mattress sutures of 3-0 nylon are preferred for the skin closure (Fig. 37.16).

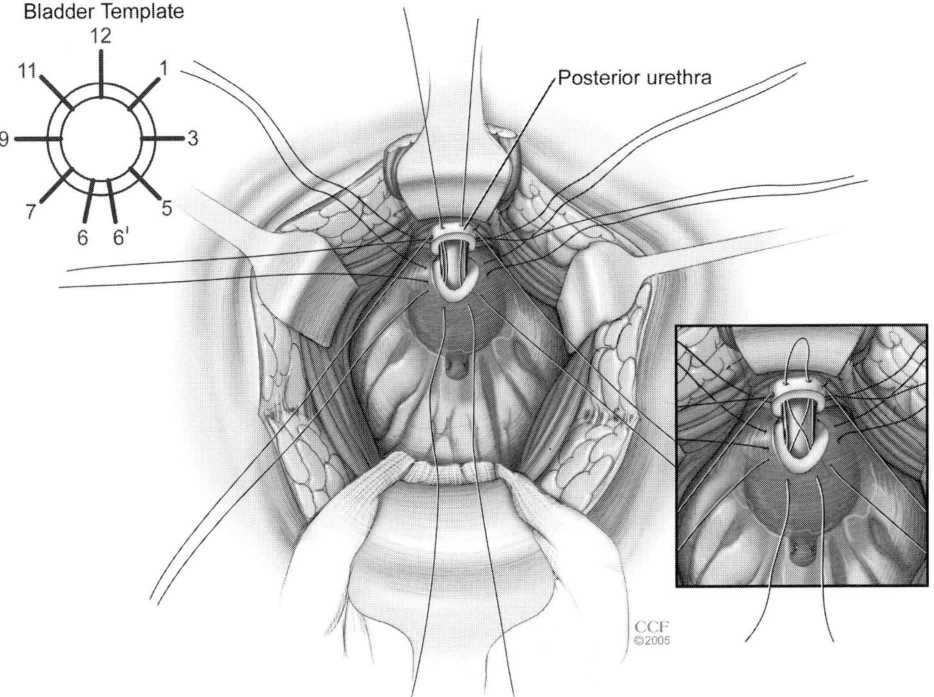


Fig. 37.14

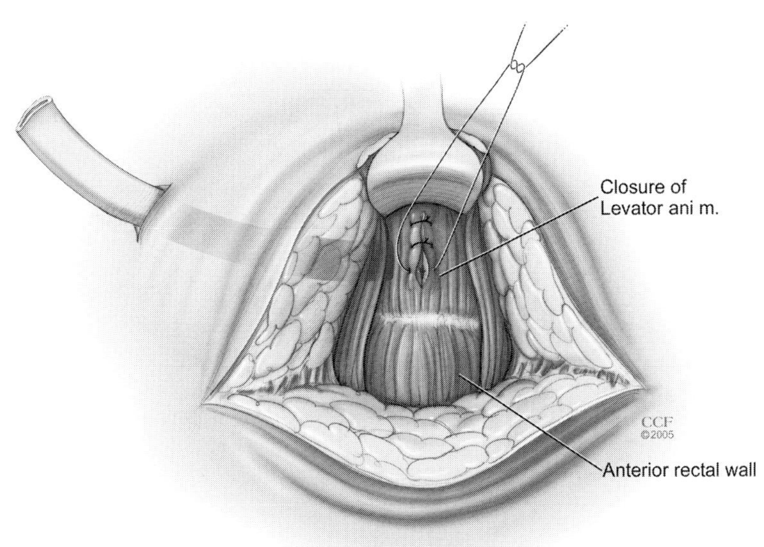


Fig. 37.15

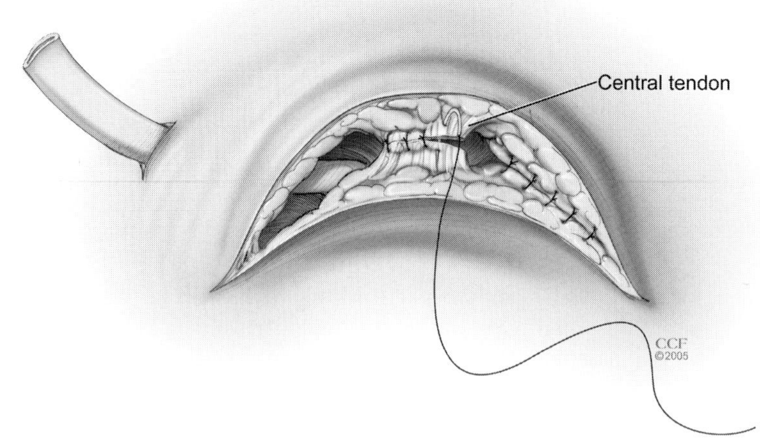


Fig. 37.16

The postoperative course following radical perineal prostatectomy is generally excellent due to the lack of pain, with minimal analgesic requirements. Ambulation begins on the first day, with a typical hospital discharge being on the first or second postoperative day. The Penrose drain remains until drainage stops, usually on the third day. The Foley catheter on a nonleaking anastomosis can be removed 7–10 d after surgery.

## SUGGESTED READINGS

1. Resnick MI, Bernsley CN. Technique of nerve-sparing radical perineal prostatectomy. Atlas Urol Clin North Am 2(2):95–106, 1994.
2. Weldon VE, FR Tavel. Potency-sparing radical perineal prostatectomy: anatomy, surgical technique and initial results. J Urol 140:559–562, 1988.

# 38 Prostate Cancer

## *Brachytherapy*

*James C. Ulchaker and Jay P. Ciezki*

Prostate brachytherapy has been performed since the 1970s, when brachytherapy was administered in a retropubic fashion. Using this approach needles are passed in an anterior to posterior fashion using digital pressure to ensure no perforation of the rectum (Fig. 38.1). This method, over time, has been abandoned secondary to its poor assurance that all areas of the prostate gland are adequately covered by appropriate doses of radiation. As a result, the treatment fell out of favor.

Brachytherapy is rapidly regaining popularity in the United States as a method of treating organ-confined prostate cancer because of the institution of the more accurate perineal approach. In our initial prostate cancer patients, using this approach we used a preplanned dosemetric method for implantation. However, we have now refined our technique and use an intraoperative treatment plan. In this chapter we will describe our current methods for real-time intraoperative treatment planning and radiation seed placement.

There are many potential disadvantages of the preplan method:

1. Alterations in the prostate volume and shape can occur between the time of the preplan and the actual brachytherapy surgery date, especially when hormonal downsizing of the prostate gland has been initiated.
2. Patient positioning, setup, and actual images acquired during the implant may not completely match the preplan.
3. The preplan method requires a separate transrectal ultrasound study, which may be difficult to schedule and is inconvenient for the patient.

The patient is brought to the operating room, and a general anesthetic is administered. This form of anesthesia is strongly recommended to avoid unwanted patient movement during the procedure. The patient is placed in the exaggerated dorsal lithotomy position and sterilely prepped and draped. An adhesive tape or drape is used to hold both the penis and scrotum anteriorly out of the perineal surgical field. The brachytherapy stand is then firmly attached to the operating room table. The transrectal ultrasound probe is the securely fashioned to its cradle, and the ultrasound probe is inserted transrectally. Using cross-sectional images, the most cranial aspect of the prostate is identified, and serial 5-mm step sections of the prostate are then performed in a cranial to caudal fashion (Fig. 38.2). The surgeon must also ensure that the entire prostate and base of the bladder can be visualized on the sagittal image, as this will be an import landmark during seed implantation. The prostatic volume is measured and the number of saved cross-sectional images and the urethral length should appropriately match up, serving as a double-check for accuracy (example.g., a 4.5-cm-long gland requires at least nine cross-sectional images). If the two measurements do not correspond correctly, the images and measurements should be reobtained before proceeding to the next step of the procedure.

Each of the cross-sectional images is then entered into a treatment-planning computer program, which recreates a three-dimensional model of the gland. This specialized computer software allows interactive virtual placement of the seeds within the prostate, instantly superimposing the resultant isodose curves over the images of the cross sections. Extreme care must be taken to ensure adequate coverage of the target volume while limiting the radiation dose to other key structures of the pelvis such as the bladder, rectum, and prostatic urethra (Fig. 38.3). Our common practice is to place vycril stranded seeds in the majority of the gland and loose seeds near the prostatic urethra in a peripherally loaded fashion.

Once the physicist has completed the above, the needle guide template is attached to the ultrasound cradle. A stabilization needle is placed in the midline approx 5–10 mm above the posterior aspect of the prostate.

From: *Operative Urology at the Cleveland Clinic*
Edited by: A. Novick et al. © Humana Press Inc., Totowa, NJ

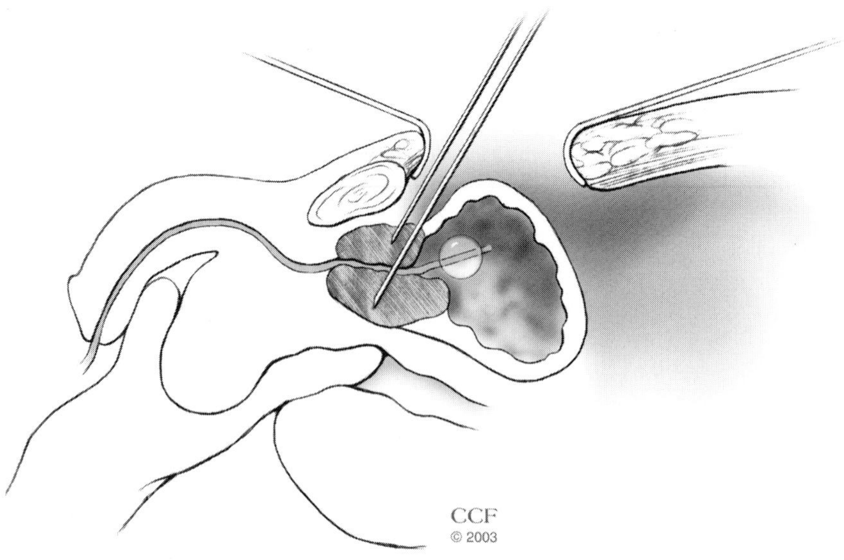


**Fig. 38.1**

Sagittal section of the pelvis during an open anterior permanent prostate brachytherapy procedure. Note the lack of prostatic visualization and reliance on tactile feedback.

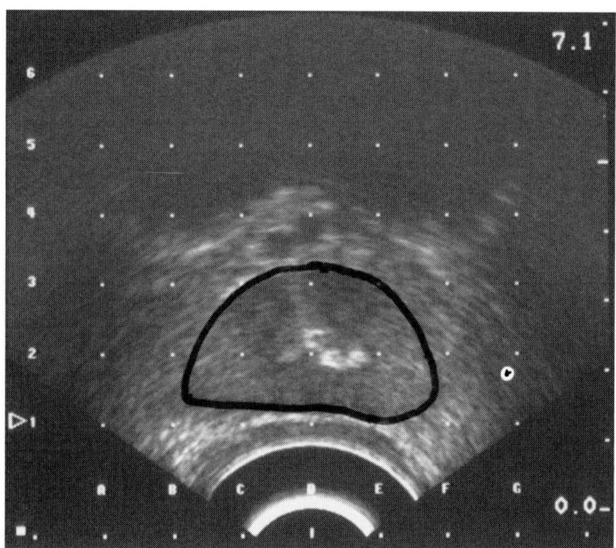

**Fig. 38.2**

Contouring of an axial section of a prostate visualized during the planning phase with a transrectal ultrasound. The gland is oriented symmetrically relative to the center of the probe.

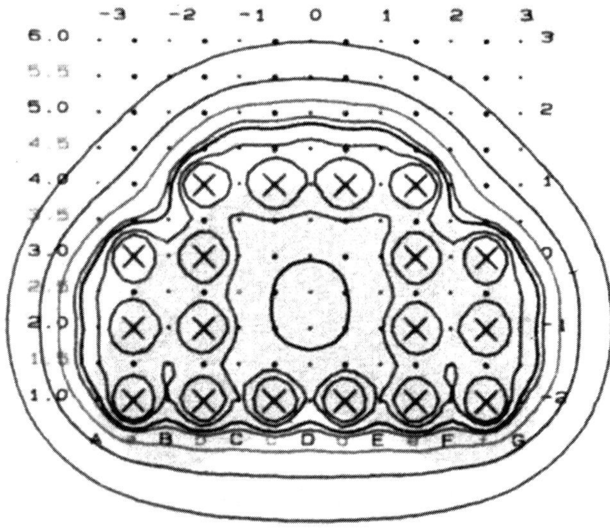

**Fig. 38.3**

Dose distribution computed during the planning phase, which is then superimposed on the prostate images in Fig. 38.2.

Next, using both the cross-sectional and sagittal views of the prostate, the needles are inserted one tier at a time, beginning with the most anterior row. The seeds are then systematically placed following the needle map generated by the treatment-planning computer program (Fig. 38.4).

It is essential to pass each needle up to the level of the prostatic base/ bladder neck to allow accurate deposition of the seeds.

Once all of the needles have been appropriately placed, the stabilization needle is removed. The urethra is milked, and the meatus is inspected for the presence of blood. The presence of blood at the meatus or, if the surgeon feels that significant perforation of the bladder has occurred during seed placement, a cystoscopic evaluation is warranted. All seeds and spacers identified should be carefully removed using an Ellik irrigator or an alligator forceps (Fig. 38.5).

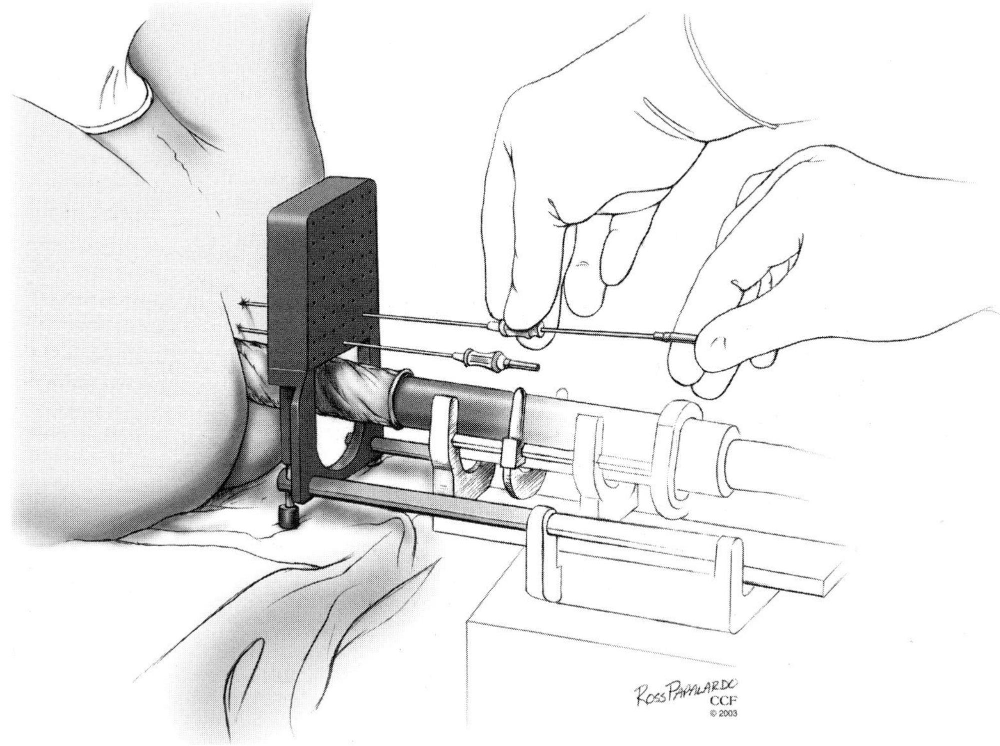


**Fig. 38.4**

Setup of transrectal ultrasound, template, and needles. The grid is from the planning session in Fig. 38.3.

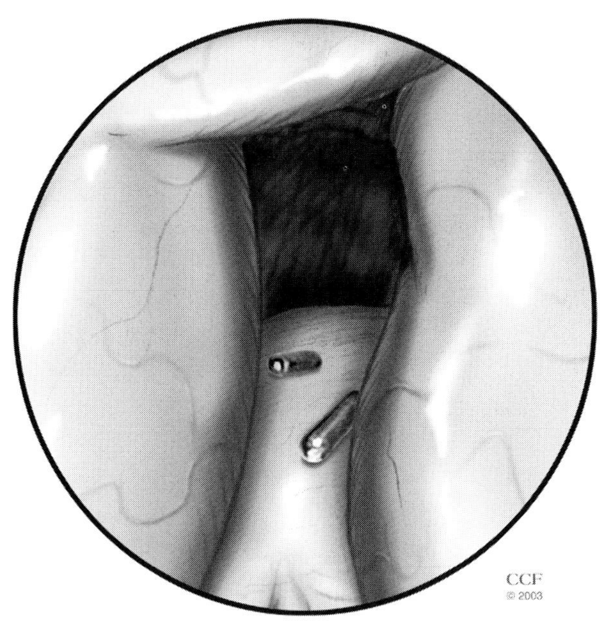


**Fig. 38.5**

Cystoscopic visualization of loose seeds in bladder and prostatic urethra after completion of implant.

All foreign material should be removed before a Foley catheter is placed. The patient's anesthesia is then reversed, and the patient is taken to the recovery room. Patients are generally discharged home from the ambulatory surgery center in a few hours. Postoperative medications often include $\alpha$ blockers, antibiotics, and analgesics. Approximately 30 d following the procedure, a dosemetric evaluation of the implant is performed using a three-dimensional computed tomography scan. We strive to achieve at least 90% of the prescribed dose in 90% of the prostate gland.

## SUGGESTED READINGS

1. Intraoperative planning and evaluation of permanent prostate brachytherapy: Report of the American Brachytherapy Society. Int J Radiation Oncol Biol Phys 51(5):1422–1430, 2001.
2. Herr HW. Radioactive seed implantation for carcinoma of the prostate. In modern technics in surgery: Urologic surgery, Futura Publishing, Chapter 7, 1980.
3. Urology, 4th ed. Radioactive Seed Implantation for Carcinoma of the Prostate. 1986:461–466.

# VI THE PENIS AND URETHRA

# 39 Surgical Anatomy of the Penis

*Kenneth W. Angermeier*

The bulk of the penis is made up of three erectile bodies: two corpora cavernosa and the single corpus spongiosum (Fig. 39.1). The dorsally located corpora cavernosa contain erectile tissue within a compliant sheath of connective tissue, the tunica albuginea. Within the shaft of the penis, there is free communication between the corpora cavernosa through an incomplete midline septum. This septum is composed of multiple strands of connective tissue, similar to that of the tunica albuginea. The septum becomes more complete at the tip of the penis and toward the penile hilum, where the corpora cavernosa become independent and form separate crura.

The erectile bodies are surrounded by the deep penile fascia (Buck's fascia), the superficial penile fascia (dartos fascia), and the skin. Buck's fascia is the sturdy layer immediately surrounding and loosely attached to all three corpora. On the superior aspect of the corpora cavernosa, the deep dorsal vein, dorsal arteries, and dorsal nerves lie within Buck's fascia above the tunica albuginea. Ventrally, Buck's fascia splits to surround the corpus spongiosum. Consolidations of the fascia lateral to the corpus spongiosum fix this structure firmly to the tunica albuginea of the corpora cavernosa. Buck's fascia is attached distally to the undersurface of the glans penis at the corona. Beyond the base of the penis, it extends into the perineum encompassing the crura of the corpora cavernosa and the bulb of the corpus spongiosum.

The dartos fascia of the penis consists of loosely arranged areolar tissue that is typically devoid of fat. It separates the two layers of the preputial fold and continues proximally beneath the penile skin, loosely attached to the skin and to Buck's fascia. The dartos fascia contains the superficial arteries, veins, and nerves of the penis. At the base of the penis, it fuses with the tunica dartos of the scrotum and extends into the perineum, where it is continuous with the layers of the superficial perineal fascia. The penile skin is attached distally to the glans penis at the corona and folds upon itself to form the prepuce or foreskin overlying the glans. The inner layer of the prepuce is confluent with the glabrous skin covering the glans, which in turn is continuous with the mucous membrane of the urethra at the external meatus. The skin covering the penis is very thin and mobile due to the supple nature of the underlying dartos fascia.

The tunica albuginea consists primarily of collagen and elastic fibers, which are oriented into an inner circular layer and an outer longitudinal layer encompassing the majority of the corporal bodies (Fig. 39.2). The only exception is that there are no outer layer fibers between the 5- and 7-o'clock positions adjacent to the corpus spongiosum. At their attachment in the midline dorsally and ventrally, the fibers of the septal strands are interwoven with the fibers of the inner circular layer of the tunica albuginea. The inner space of the corpora cavernosa is filled with erectile tissue consisting of arteries, sinusoids lined with endothelial cells, veins, nerves, smooth muscle fibers, and trabeculae arising from the tunica albuginea. Between this tissue and the tunica albuginea, there is a very thin layer of areolar connective tissue containing a number of vessels.

Proximally, the suspensory ligaments of the penis are located at its base (Fig. 39.3). The outer fundiform ligament is continuous with the lower end of the linea alba and splits into laminae that completely surround the body of the penis. The inner, triangular-shaped suspensory ligament is attached to the anterior aspect of the symphysis pubis and blends with the fascia of the penis below it. Posterior to these ligamentous attachments, the corpus spongiosum enlarges between the crura of the corpora cavernosa to form the penile bulb.

The corpus spongiosum lies within the ventral groove between the two corpora cavernosa. The tunica albuginea surrounding this structure is much thinner than that of the corpora cavernosa, and less erectile tissue is present. The

From: *Operative Urology at the Cleveland Clinic*
Edited by: A. Novick et al. © Humana Press Inc., Totowa, NJ

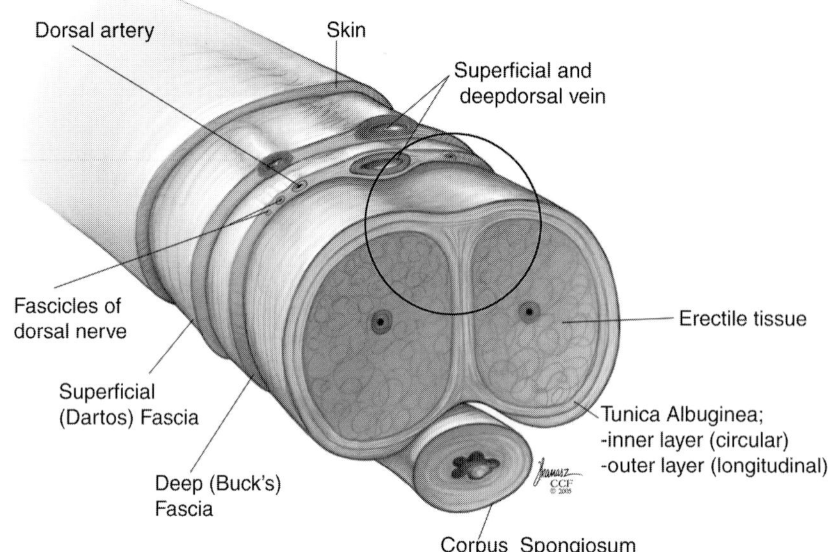


Fig. 39.1

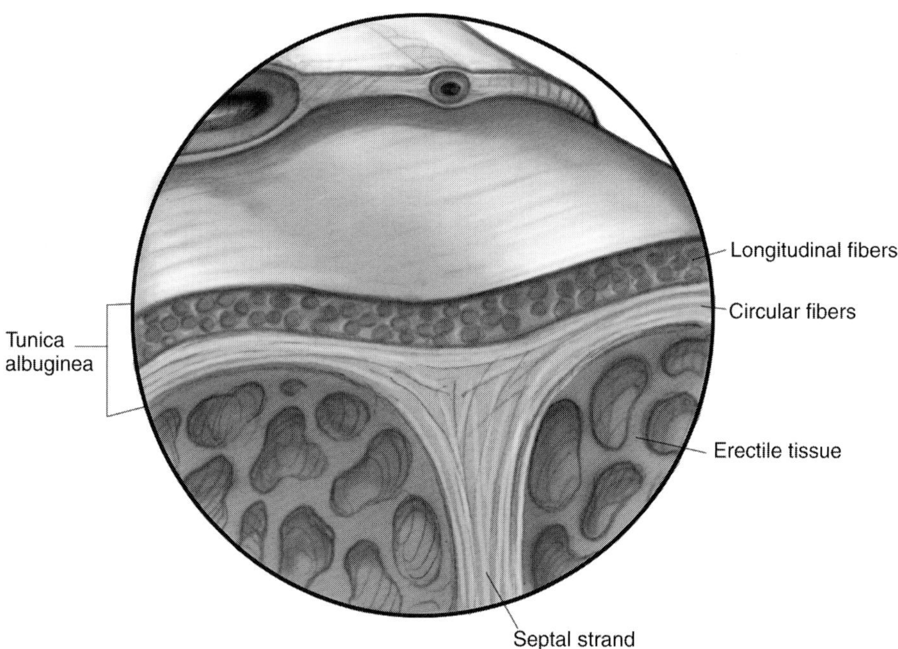


Fig. 39.2

urethra runs the length of the penis within the corpus spongiosum. The corpus spongiosum expands distally to form a broad cap of erectile tissue called the glans penis, which covers the tips of the corpora cavernosa. The urethral meatus lies on the ventral aspect of the tip of the glans penis with its long axis in a vertical direction. The edge of the glans penis overhangs the penile shaft forming a rim called the corona, with the coronal sulcus just proximal to this. The frenulum is a fold of skin attached at the most ventral point of the glans penis, where the corona forms a distally pointing V.

The divisions of the urethra are as follows: (1) glanular, (2) pendulous or penile, (3) bulbous, (4) membranous, and (5) prostatic (Fig. 39.4). The glanular urethra is lined with stratified squamous epithelium. Within the pendulous portion, the epithelium is primarily stratified or pseudostratified columnar with areas of stratified squamous epithelium. It maintains a lumen of constant size roughly centered within the corpus spongiosum. Within the bulb, the urethra widens and lies closer to the dorsal aspect of the corpus spongiosum. The urethra does not traverse the full extent of the bulb, but exits from its dorsal surface

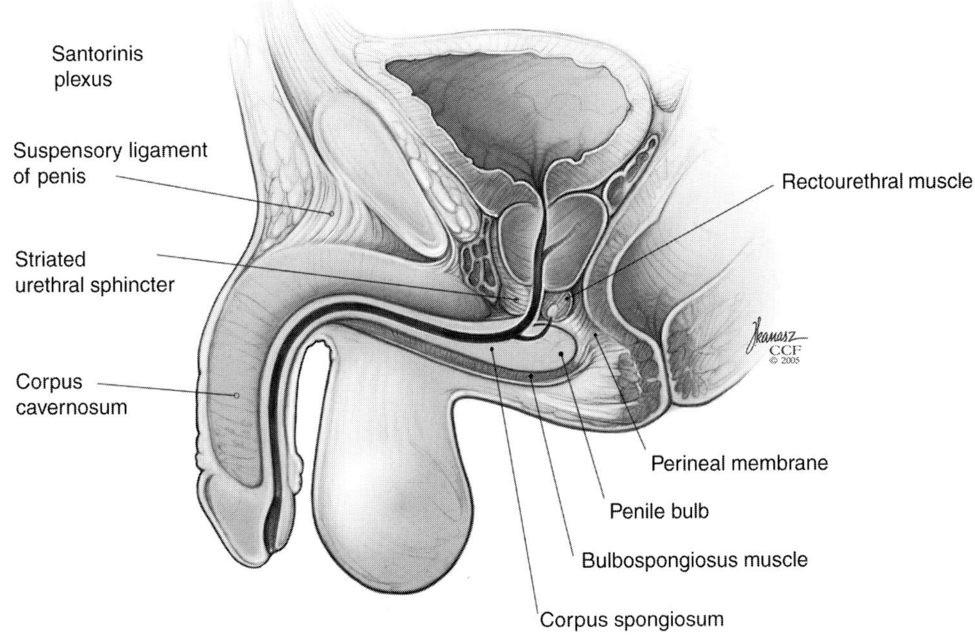


Fig. 39.3

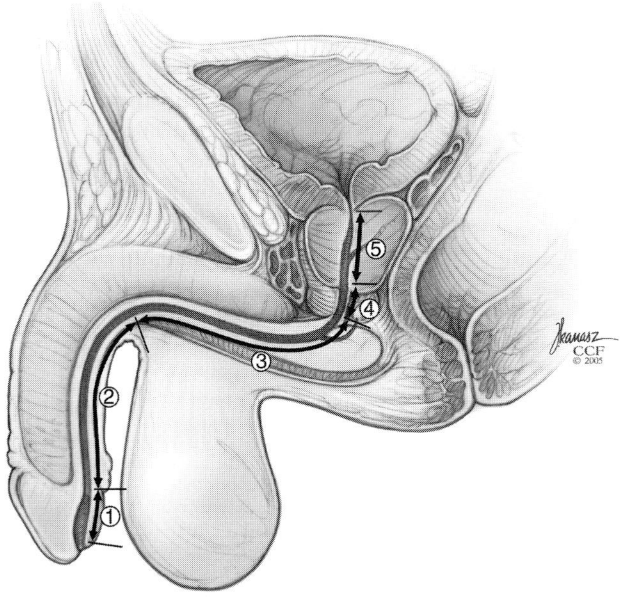


Fig. 39.4

prior to the posterior attachment of the bulb to the perineal body. The bulbous urethra is lined with stratified or pseudostratified columnar epithelium, which continues proximally as the urethra progresses upward into the membranous portion. In this area, there is a gradual change to a transitional epithelium that lines the prostatic urethra. The periurethral (Littre's) glands open into the pendulous and bulbous portions of the urethra along its dorsal surface. Often there is a larger lacuna magna in the dorsal will of the fossa navicularis. The ducts of the bulbourethral (Cowper's) glands open into the urethra within the bulb. More superiorly these ducts are posterolateral to the membranous urethra, extending to the glands located within the striated urethral sphincter.

The superficial arterial supply to the penile skin and dartos is derived from the left and right inferior external pudendal arteries (Fig. 39.5). These vessels arise from the first portion of the femoral artery and cross the upper medial aspect of the femoral triangle to eventually divide into two main branches. These branches run dorsolaterally and ventrolaterally within the dartos fascia on the shaft of the penis, with extensive collateralization across the midline. Fine branches supplying the skin are given off at intervals to form a rich subdermal vascular plexus. Superficial venous drainage is provided by a number of vessels that run in the dartos fascia on the dorsolateral aspect of the penis. These veins unite at the base of the penis to form a superficial dorsal vein, which usually drains into the left saphenous vein. At times there is a communication between a superficial vein and the deep dorsal vein of the penis.

The blood supply to the deep structures of the penis originates from the common penile artery, which is the continuation of the common penile artery distal to the perineal artery (Figs. 39.6 and 39.7). The common penile artery travels along the medial margin of the inferior pubic ramus before dividing into its terminal branches near the urethral bulb. Occasionally one or more of the terminal penile vessels may be derived from an accessory pudendal artery arising within the pelvis, most commonly from the obturator artery or the internal pudendal artery

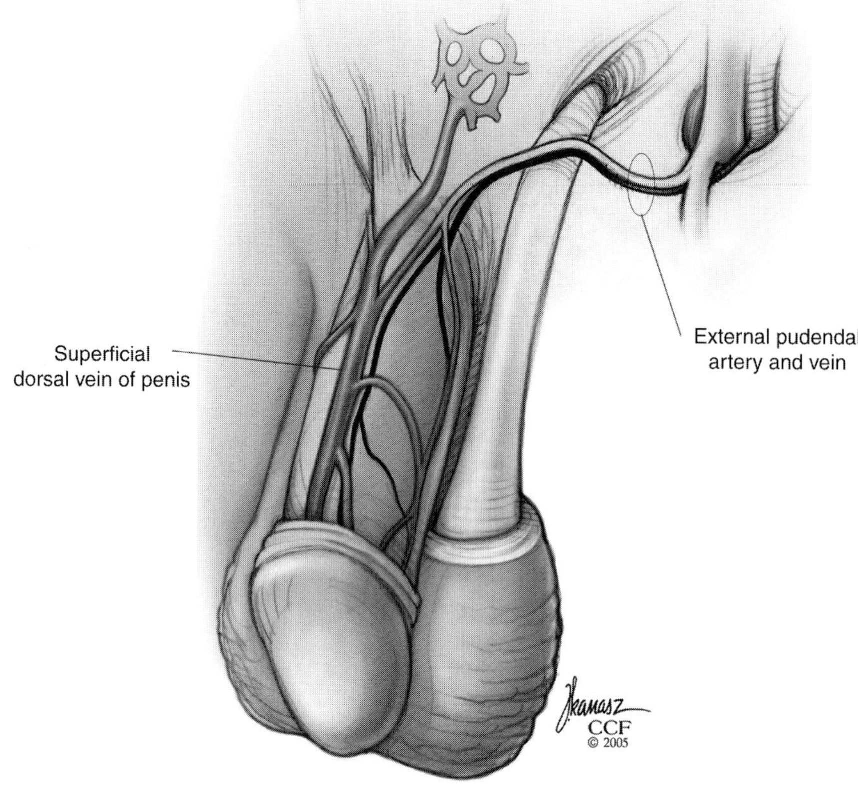


Fig. 39.5

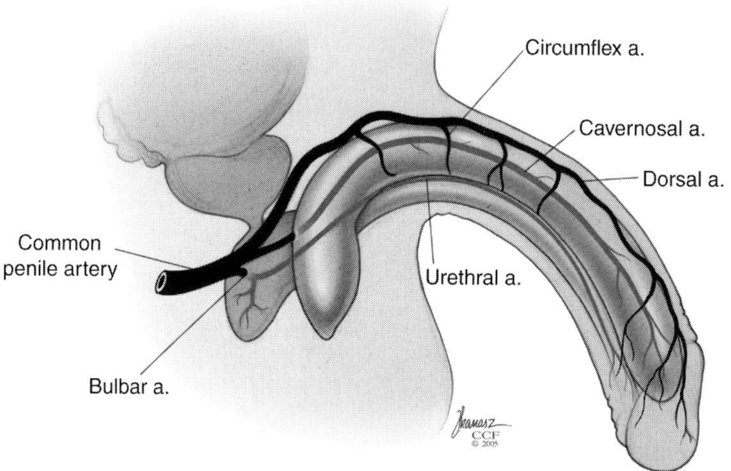


Fig. 39.6

before its entrance into the greater sciatic foramen. The accessory pudendal artery travels along the lower part of the bladder and the anterolateral surface of the prostate to reach the root of the penis.

The first branch of the common penile artery is the bulbo-urethral artery, which traverses the perineal membrane to enter the bulb of the penis. It may also arise as a branch of the dorsal or cavernosal arteries. The urethral artery, which may emerge as a separate branch of the common penile artery, travels within the corpus spongiosum ventrolateral to the urethra and terminates in the glans penis. The dorsal artery of the penis is the continuation of the common penile artery and generally has a constant course. It proceeds along the dorsum of the penis between the deep dorsal vein medially and the dorsal nerves laterally and has a coiled configuration in the flaccid state. It gives off 3–10 circumflex branches that accompany the circumflex veins around the lateral surface of the corporal bodies. The proximal

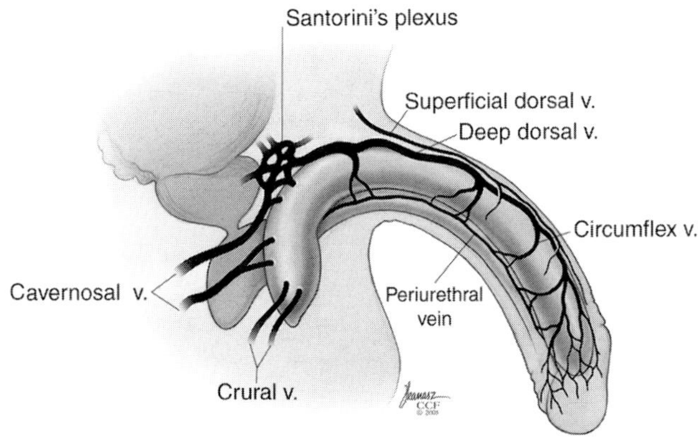


Fig. 39.7

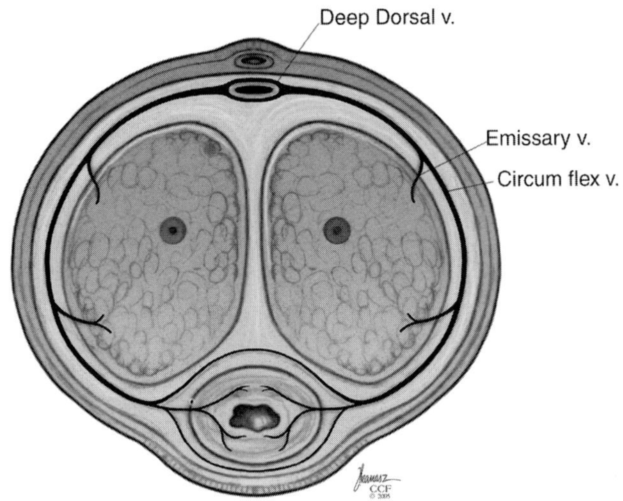


Fig. 39.8

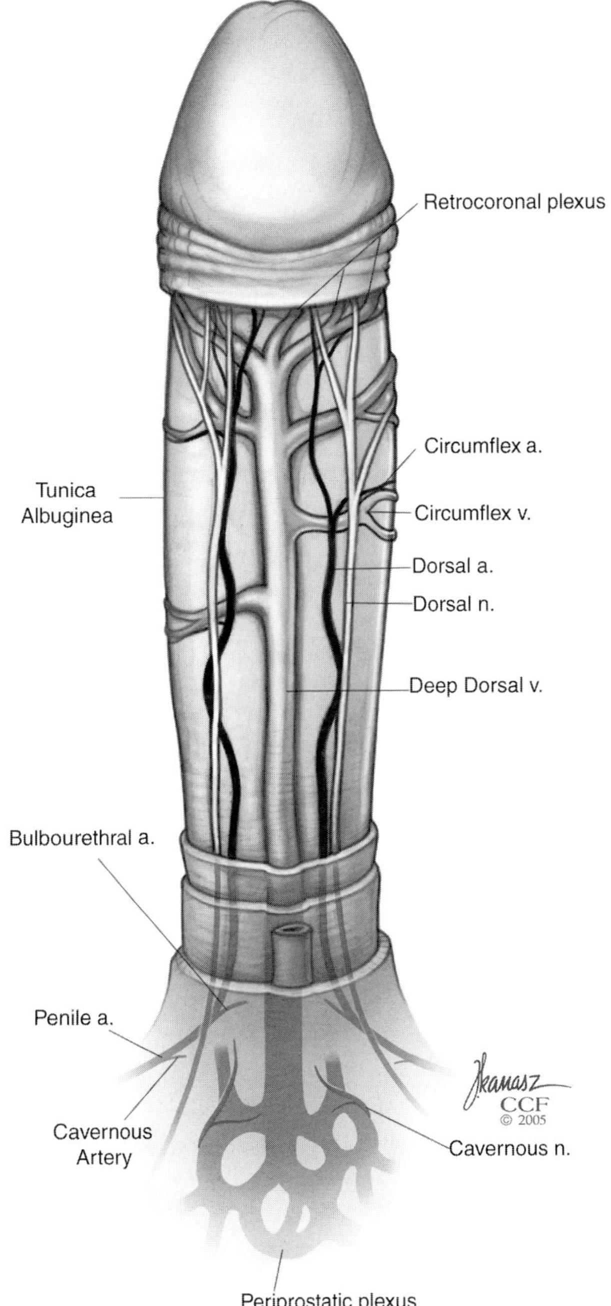


Fig. 39.9

circumflex arteries may also contribute to the blood supply of the corpus spongiosum and urethra. Occasionally a branch of the dorsal artery penetrates the tunica albuginea to supply the erectile tissue. The dorsal artery terminates in the glans penis, contributing to the dual blood supply of the corpus spongiosum, which is important in urethral reconstructive surgery. The final branch of the common penile artery is the cavernosal artery. It enters the corpus cavernosum at the hilum and runs the length of the penile shaft, giving off the many helicine arteries that comprise the arterial inflow portion of the erectile apparatus. The cavernosal artery may arise from an accessory pudendal artery, and variation may occur in the number of arteries and their configuration. There may be a communication between the cavernosal arteries in the midline prior to entering the corporal bodies or a branch from one may enter the corporal body on the opposite side. Occasionally a single artery will branch in the penile shaft to supply both sides.

Veins emerging from the glans penis form a retrocoronal plexus that drains through three to five larger veins into the deep dorsal vein, which lies within Buck's fascia in the midline superior to the corporal bodies (Fig 39.8). The deep dorsal vein proximally passes deep to the suspensory ligaments and then beneath the symphysis pubis to join the prostatic (Santorini's) plexus. Along the penile shaft, the dorsal vein receives drainage from the erectile tissue as well. Small venules drain the blood from the lacunar spaces into a subtunical venous network. Emissary veins arising from this network follow a perpendicular or oblique course through the tunica albuginea. They emerge on the lateral or dorsal surface of the corpora cavernosa and empty into the circumflex

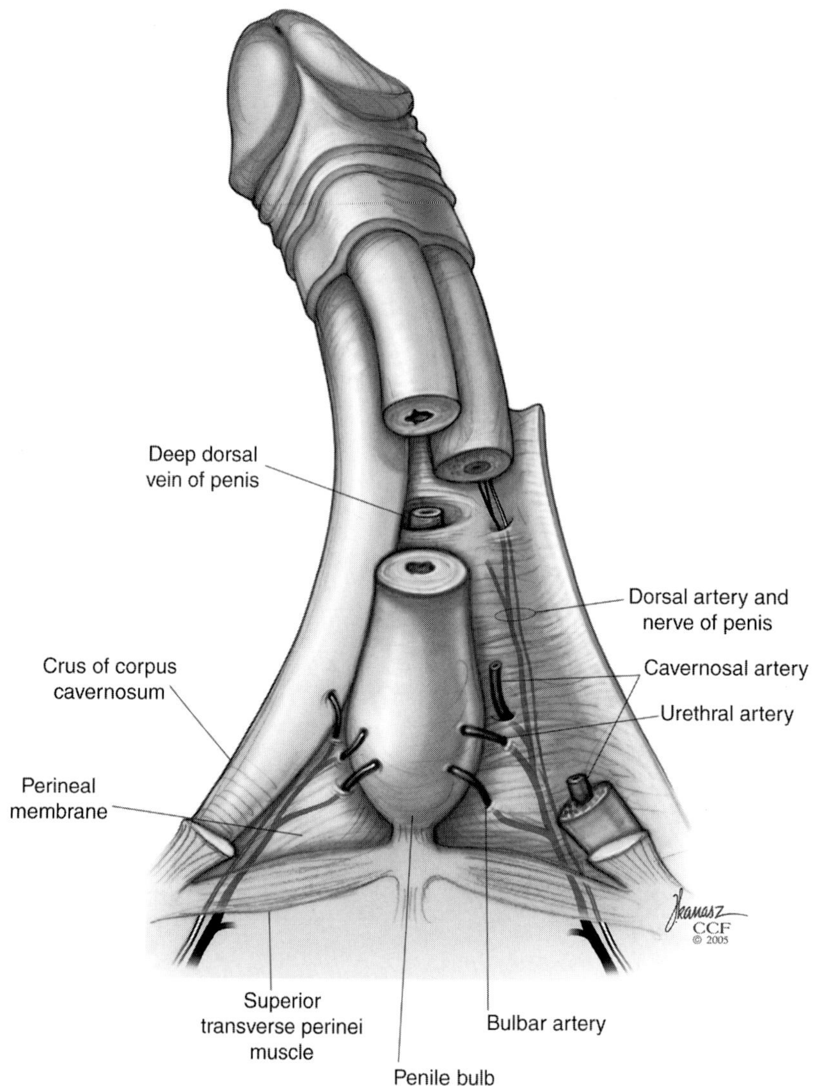


Fig. 39.10

veins or directly into the deep dorsal vein. The circumflex veins are present in the distal two-thirds of the penis. They arise from the corpus spongiosum and traverse the lateral aspect of the corporal bodies, passing beneath the dorsal arteries and nerves to empty into the deep dorsal vein. Confluences at the origins of the circumflex veins may form periurethral veins that run parallel to the corpus spongiosum on each side of the penis.

Emissary veins in the proximal third of the corporal bodies join to from several venous trunks on the dorsomedial surface of each crus. These consolidate into one or more cavernosal veins on each side, coursing deep and medial to the cavernosal arteries and nerves in the penile hilum. These veins drain into the prostatic plexus or run laterally between the penile bulb and the crus for about 2–3 cm before joining with the internal pudendal veins. Three to four small crural veins emerge from the dorsolateral surface of each crus and drain into the ipsilateral internal pudendal vein. The internal pudendal veins run together with the internal pudendal artery and pudendal nerve within Alcock's canal and empty into the internal iliac vein.

The pudendal nerves provide somatic motor and sensory innervation to the penis (Fig. 39.10). These nerves enter the perineum with the internal pudendal vessels through the lesser sciatic foramen at the posterior aspect of the ischiorectal fossa. They travel within Alcock's canal to the posterior border of the perineal membrane. On each side the dorsal nerve arises as the first branch of the pudendal nerve within Alcock's canal. Distally these nerves continue along the dorsal aspect of the corporal bodies, assuming a position lateral to the dorsal artery. Multiple fascicles fan out from the dorsal nerve along the penile shaft, supplying the surface of the tunica albuginea as well as the skin and glans penis.

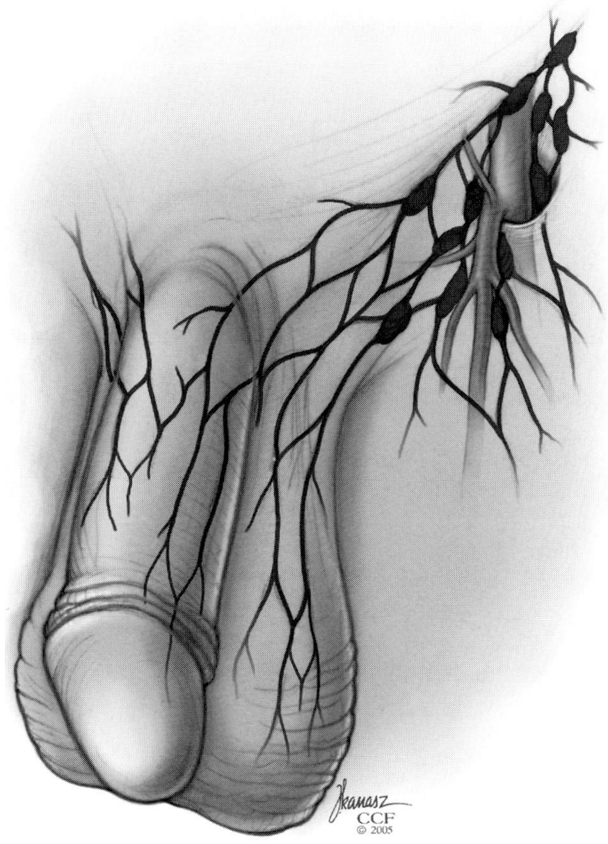

Fig. 39.11

The autonomic innervation of the external genitalia is derived from the pelvic plexus. This plexus is rectangular in configuration and located on either side of the rectum, with its midpoint at the tips of the seminal vesicles. The cavernous nerves emanate from this plexus and distal to the prostate are located posterolateral and lateral to the membranous urethra just outside of the striated urethral sphincter. As they traverse this area, they send fibers to the bulbourethral glands before entering the corpora cavernosa dorsomedial to the cavernosal arteries. The cavernous nerves provide the autonomic innervation to the erectile tissues of the penis.

Lymphatic vessels draining the prepuce and skin of the penile shaft converge dorsally and then divide at the base of the penis to drain into the right and left superficial inguinal nodes (Fig. 39.11). Drainage from the glans penis is toward the frenulum, where large trunks are formed and encircle the corona to unite with those from the other side on the dorsum. They traverse the penis to the base within Buck's fascia, draining via presymphyseal lymphatics into the superficial inguinal nodes and the deep inguinal nodes of the femoral triangle.

## SUGGESTED READINGS

1. Breza J, Aboseif SR, Orvis BR, Lue TF, Tanagho EA. Detailed anatomy of penile neurovascular structures: surgical significance. J Urol 141: 437–443, 1989.
2. Brock G, Hsu GL, Nunes L, von Heyden B, Lue TF. The anatomy of the tunica albuginea in the normal penis and Peyronie's disease. J Urol 157:276–281, 1997.
3. Devine CJ, Jr., Angermeier KW. Anatomy of the penis and male perineum, part 1. AUA Update Series, Volume 13, Lesson 2, 1994.
4. Devine PC, Horton CE. Strictures of the male urethra. In: Converse JM, ed. Reconstructive Plastic Surgery, Vol. 7, 2nd ed. Philadelphia:WB Saunders, 1977: 3883–3895.
5. Dewire D, Lepor H. Anatomic considerations of the penis and its lymphatic drainage. Urol Clin North Am 19:211–219, 1992.
6. Goldstein AM, Padma-Nathan H. The microarchitecture of the intracavernosal smooth muscle and the cavernosal fibrous skeleton. J Urol 244:1144, 1990.
7. Gosling JA, Dixon JS, Humpherson JR. Functional Anatomy of the Urinary Tract–an Integrated and Color Atlas. Baltimore:University Park Press, 1982.
8. Juskiewenski S, Vaysee PH, Moscovici J, Hammoudi S, Bouissou E. A study of the arterial blood supply of the penis. Anat Clin 4:101–107, 1982.
9. Lue TF, Zeineh SJ, Schmidt RA, Tanagho EA. Neuroanatomy of penile erection: its relevance to iatrogenic impotence. J Urol 131:273–280, 1984.
10. Rouviere H (Tobias, MJ, trans.). Anatomy of the Human Lymphatic System. Ann Arbor, MI:Edwards Bros., 1938.
11. Schlegel PN, Walsh PC. Neuroanatomical approach to radical cystoprostatectomy with preservation of sexual function. J Urol 138:1402–1406, 1987.
12. Tobin CE, Benjamin JA. Anatomical study and clinical consideration of the fasciae limiting urinary extravasation from the penile urethra. Surg Gyn Obstet 79:95–204, 1944.

# 40 Anterior Urethral Reconstruction

*Kenneth W. Angermeier*

## INTRODUCTION

A urethral stricture is a scar that occurs as a result of tissue injury. As the scar heals, circumferential contraction may occur, leading to luminal narrowing. In the past, the most common etiology of urethral stricture disease was inflammatory urethritis. With the advent of more effective antibiotic therapy, external trauma and urethral instrumentation have emerged as the most frequent causes today.

### Urethral Anatomy (*see* Chapter 39)

The glanular portion of the adult male urethra lies within the glans penis. The pendulous or penile urethra extends from the corona of the glans to the level of the suspensory ligaments of the penis. It maintains a lumen of relatively constant size, centered within the corpus spongiosum. From the suspensory ligaments proximally to the level of the perineal membrane, the bulbous urethra widens and lies closer to the dorsal than to the ventral aspect of the corpus spongiosum. The urethra exits from the dorsal surface of the bulb just prior to its attachment to the perineal body. The membranous urethra lies between the perineal membrane and the verumontanum and is the sphincter-active portion of the urethra. The prostatic urethra is the remaining component of the adult male urethra, extending to the bladder neck.

The anterior urethra, consisting of the glanular, pendulous, and bulbous regions, is encompassed by the corpus spongiosum, as described above. There is a dual blood supply to the corpus spongiosum that is of significance when planning urethral reconstructive surgery. After giving off its perineal branch, the internal pudendal artery becomes the common penile artery. On each side, this artery gives rise to several branches, the largest of which is the bulbourethral artery, which directly enters the bulb and represents the majority of the posterior vasculature of the corpus spongiosum. The urethral artery, which may also arise as a separate branch of the common penile artery, travels within the corpus spongiosum ventrolateral to the urethra. It terminates in the glans penis, where it anastomoses with branches of the dorsal artery. The dorsal artery of the penis also arises from the common penile artery and travels along the dorsum of the penis between the deep dorsal vein medially and the dorsal nerves laterally. Its terminal branches supply the glans penis. This dual blood supply to the corpus spongiosum, consisting of anastomoses between branches of the urethral artery and dorsal artery in the glans, allows the urethra to be divided surgically with its vascularity coming in retrograde fashion from the glans unless inflammation or trauma has occluded these vessels.

### Symptoms

Most patients with urethral stricture disease present with obstructive voiding symptoms, which often have an insidious onset. The inciting trauma may be unrecognized or forgotten, with the patient presenting years later with symptoms. Some patients will present with an episode of prostatitis, epididymitis, or hematuria. The infections may be severe, resulting from chronic high-pressure voiding with dilation of the prostatic ducts and stasis of urine. Postvoid urethral bleeding and terminal hematuria are usually the result of acute dilation of the urethra proximal to the stricture during voiding with cracking of the mucosa and subsequent hemorrhage. Spraying of the urinary stream or a split stream has often been considered to be a hallmark of a urethral stricture. However, this occurs most commonly as a consequence of a decreased urinary stream, which can be present for a variety of reasons. This symptom does not seem to be specific for a urethral stricture. Urinary retention may infrequently occur and is usually preceded by a period of gradually increasing symptoms. Alternatively, acute trauma may result in urethral injury or disruption leading to a dense or obliterative stricture shortly thereafter.

From: *Operative Urology at the Cleveland Clinic*
Edited by: A. Novick et al. © Humana Press Inc., Totowa, NJ

### Evaluation

In evaluating the patient with urethral stricture disease, it is important to determine the location and extent of the stricture and to estimate the depth of associated spongiofibrosis. Dynamic retrograde urethrography, voiding urethrography, and endoscopy are the primary means of assessing these parameters. Endoscopy is used to confirm the radiographic findings and to examine the urethral mucosa and associated scar visually. Although advocated by some, we have not found that ultrasound or magnetic resonance imaging adds significant information to the above. Direct palpation of the urethra may be helpful in assessing spongiofibrosis. A thorough examination of the genital skin is important to identify areas with adequate vascularity that may serve as a skin island for substitution urethroplasty.

Based on the above information, an anatomical classification of anterior urethral stricture disease was proposed in 1983, ranging from minimal disease in the form of a urethral mucosal fold or scar without spongiofibrosis to severe scarring with full thickness spongiofibrosis and associated infection or fistula. Based on this classification, an anatomical approach to the treatment of urethral stricture disease has been adopted in which the stricture is treated initially with what is deemed to be the most appropriate procedure. This is in contrast to the so-called reconstructive ladder approach, in which management of virtually all strictures begins with the simplest procedure (dilation) and proceeds sequentially to more involved forms of treatment (direct vision internal urethrotomy [DVIU] and then open urethroplasty). With use of an anatomical approach initially for the treatment of anterior urethral stricture disease, as well as recent advances in tissue transfer techniques, significantly improved success rates have been realized.

### DVIU

Internal urethrotomy consists of endoscopic incision of a urethral stricture, allowing the underlying soft elastic tissue to expand the urethral lumen. To be effective, the incision must extend through the entire depth of the spongiofibrosis. Although the most common location for the incision in the past has been at the 12-o'clock position, it should be realized that there is little corpus spongiosum dorsally there in the area of the bulbous urethra. Therefore, incisions at 10 o'clock and 2 o'clock (± 6 o'clock) or some minor variation thereof have been described as a means of ensuring that the incision extends through the depth of the scar into healthy spongy tissue. A catheter is left indwelling for 3–7 d, depending on the density of the stricture and the extent of the incision. Internal urethrotomy may be curative for relatively short strictures consisting of a mucosal fold or scar with no spongiofibrosis or for those with an iris configuration and minimal spongiofibrosis. When successful, the final result is often a stable, wide-caliber urethral scar. Two recent long-term studies of men undergoing primary DVIU have demonstrated a recurrence rate of 34–58% for bulbous urethral strictures. Factors leading to an increased incidence of recurrence include: stricture length greater than 1 cm, penile or penoscrotal location, multiple strictures, and prior DVIU.

If the initial attempt at internal urethrotomy fails, then the patient should be reassessed radiographically and endoscopically. If these studies show improvement, then the procedure may be repeated. However, two or three times should be the limit. When there is significant scarring of the urethral mucosa and deep spongiofibrosis, re-epithelialization will not occur and open urethroplasty may be necessary. In patients who are not good medical candidates for open surgery, internal urethrotomy followed by self-dilation may help maintain patency of the urethra. This is done two or three times a day initially and usually can be tapered to once or twice a week. If self-dilation is discontinued in patients with significant urethral scarring, however, the stricture will almost certainly recur at about the same rate as it would have without self-dilation.

## URETHRAL RECONSTRUCTION

Open urethral reconstruction is the procedure of choice for urethral strictures associated with dense spongiofibrosis or other factors, suggesting that DVIU will not be effective. It is also indicated when more conservative forms of treatment have failed. It is important to have the urethra be free of instrumentation for 3 mo prior to radiographic evaluation and urethral reconstruction in order to allow the stricture to fully declare itself and be at its worst at the time of repair and not underestimated. If a patient cannot make it for 3 mo, a suprapubic catheter is required. A number of surgical techniques are available to the reconstructive surgeon depending on stricture length, location, and density. Currently, the overwhelming majority of open procedures consist of excision of the stricture with a primary urethral anastomosis or reconstruction using buccal mucosa in some fashion. Therefore, I focus primarily on these approaches in the remainder of this chapter.

### Excision with Primary Urethral Anastomosis (EPA)

EPA is the optimal method of urethral reconstruction when feasible (Fig. 40.1). It is limited to patients with strictures in the bulbous urethra that are 2.5–3 cm in

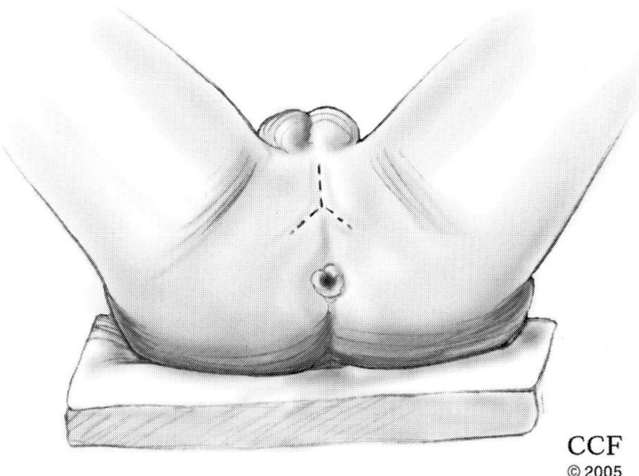


Fig. 40.1

length. A stricture can be reconstructed at the upper end of that range if it is in the proximal bulbous urethra as opposed to the distal bulbous urethra, where mobilization does not result in as much gain in extensibility. Excisional procedures cannot be done in the penile urethra because urethral mobilization would result in penile curvature or undue tension on the repair. The patient is placed in the exaggerated lithotomy position using boot-type stirrups. The buttocks are elevated on a specially made solid gel pad for support and exposure. I do not use compression stockings while the patient is in exaggerated lithotomy in order to maximize lower extremity perfusion, but all patients are given subcutaneous heparin preoperatively. We ensure that there are no undue pressure points and that the buttocks and thighs are soft and comfortable.

A modified lambda incision is made in the perineum, and dissection proceeds to the level of the bulbospongiosus muscle using electrocautery and scissors (Fig. 40.2A). The corpus spongiosum is identified just distal to the muscle, and the muscle is divided in the midline to fully expose the bulb of the corpus spongiosum (Fig. 40.2B). A modified Denis-Browne retractor is used for exposure. The corpus spongiosum is dissected circumferentially off of the underlying corporal bodies (Fig. 40.2C). Distally this is limited in potent patients to the level of the suspensory ligament of the penis to avoid ventral erectile curvature. Proximally the dissection is done close to the level of the departure of the urethra from the bulb. Posterior and lateral to the proximal bulb, attachments are taken down to help mobilize it. In the posterior midline, these are attachments to the inferior-most aspect of the central tendon. One should take care not to divide the posterior blood supply to the bulb (the bulbar arteries [Fig. 40.2I]). A bougie or flexible cystoscope is passed distally to identify the distal end of the stricture, and the urethra is divided with scissors right through the area of the stricture (Fig. 40.2D). Proximally, if the lumen is evident, I start with a dorsal urethrotomy through the stricture until one enters healthy urethra and corpus spongiosum. This often needs to be carried to the level of the bulbomembranous junction. The scarred urethra is excised, and the healthy segment is spatulated so that it accommodates a 30 French bougie. If there is no identifiable lumen, the proximal scar is excised until the lumen is identified. This is often aided by passing a sound or flexible cystoscope antegrade into the urethra through the suprapubic tract. Retrograde flexible cystoscopy is performed to confirm that there is no additional stricture. If needed, the intracrural space can be developed sharply using a knife and then scissors to incise between the corporal bodies down to the level of the dorsal vein of the penis. This can aid proximal exposure and decrease tension on the urethral anastomosis by straightening the pathway from the proximal to the distal end of the urethra. The distal urethra is then spatulated ventrally into healthy tissue, and the scar is excised (Fig. 40.2E). Buck's fascia is then meticulously dissected off of the distal corpus spongiosum to aid its extensibility. The anastomosis is then done using interrupted sutures of 4-0 polydioxanone (PDS) along the back wall to the lateral edge of the closure (Fig. 40.2F,G). I then convert it to a two-layer closure by suturing the urethral mucosa using interrupted 5-0 PDS and the corpus spongiosum with running 4-0 PDS (Fig. 40.2H). This helps to prevent a full-thickness scar. The proximal urethral segment is then tacked to the adjacent tunical albuginea of the corporal bodies to fix the urethra in place and take further tension off of the anastomosis. A 16 or 18 French soft silicone catheter is passed and placed to drainage. A small suction drain is placed in the periurethral region, and the bulbospongiosus muscle is closed in the midline using interrupted 3-0 vicryl sutures. A 7-mm suction drain is placed in the perineum overlying the muscle, and Colles' fascia is closed using running 3-0 vicryl, followed by skin closure with running 4-0 chromic. A clear adhesive dressing is placed, and the patient is placed supine. In most cases I do not place a suprapubic catheter for an EPA, but we will continue with suprapubic drainage in a patient with a pre-existing catheter. The catheter is taped upward onto the lower abdomen without tension.

## Ventral Buccal Mucosa Onlay Graft

Strictures that cannot be reconstructed by EPA require substitution urethroplasty (Fig. 40.3). In this technique, a urethrotomy incision is made through the stricture and into healthy urethra proximally and distally. Tissue in the form of a graft or a flap is then transferred into the urethral defect and sutured to the existing urethral plate to re-establish urethral patency. Buccal mucosa has emerged as the most effective material for substitution

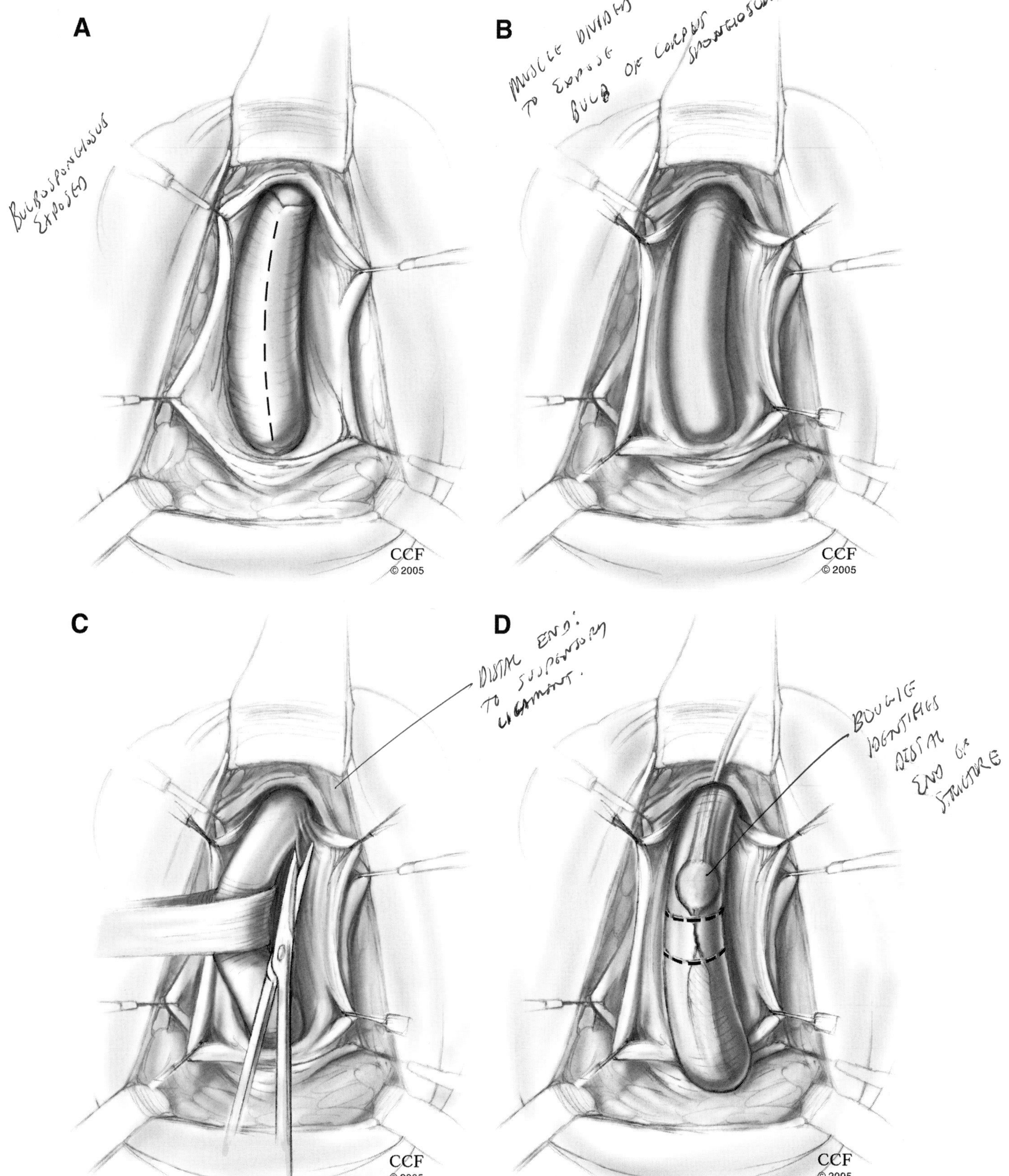


Fig. 40.2

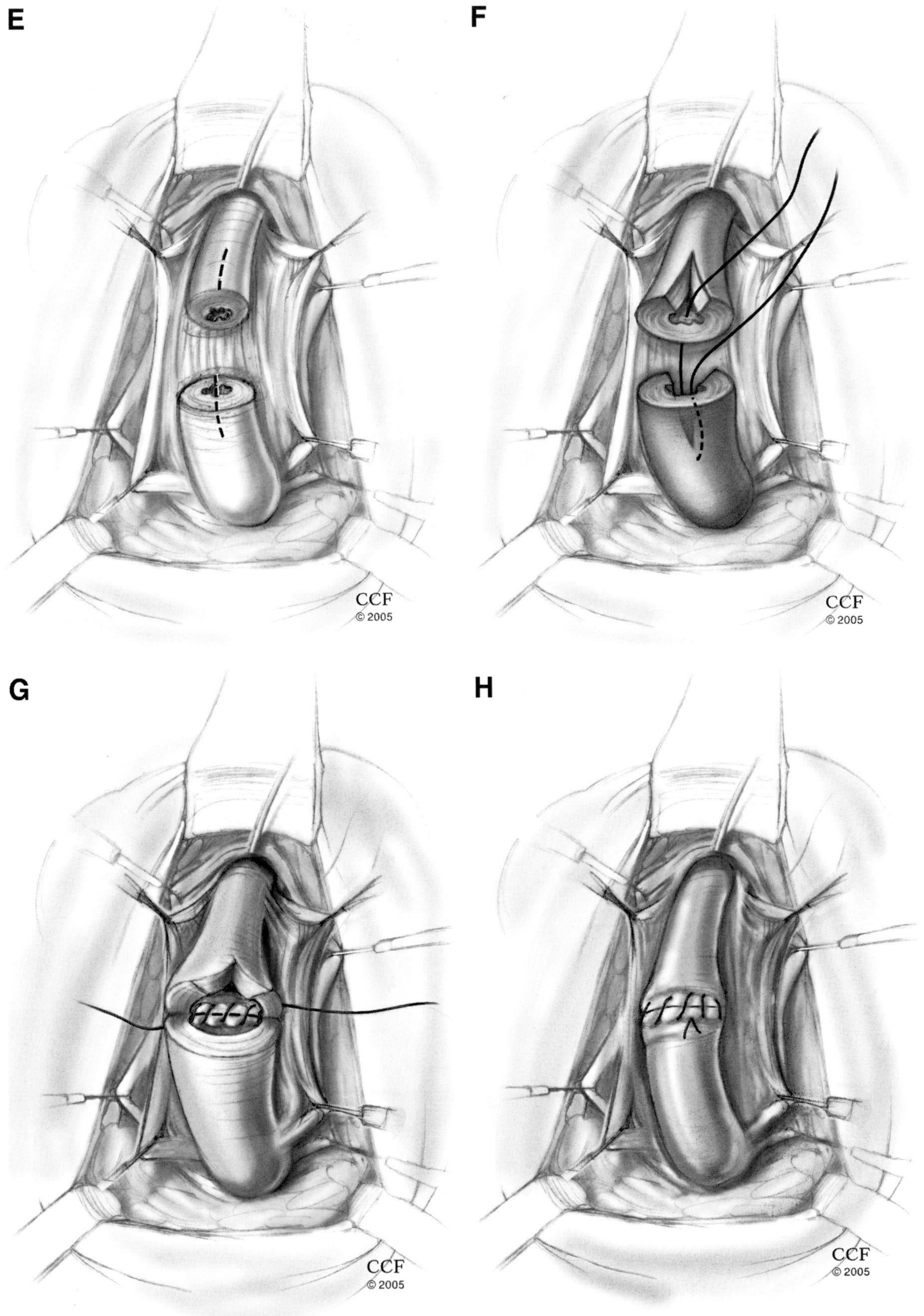


Fig. 40.2 *(Continued)*

I

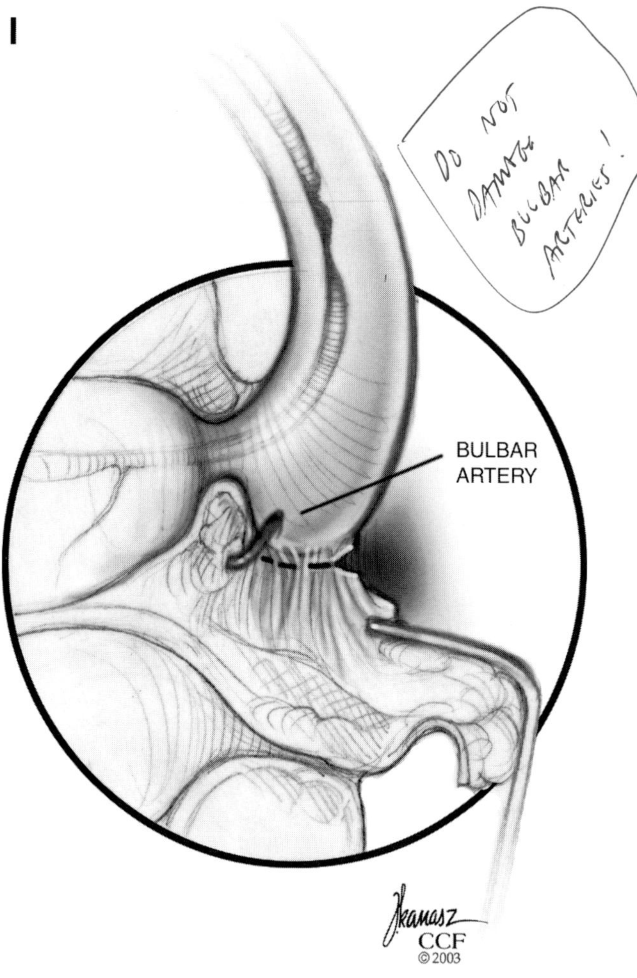


Fig. 40.2 *(Continued)*

urethroplasty and will be the focus of the remainder of this chapter. Buccal mucosa has a thick, nonkeratinized epithelium that makes it easy to handle and suture. The thin, richly vascularized lamina propria leads to excellent graft take, and the donor site morbidity is very acceptable. It is a moist epithelium, and this factor may have implications for long-term success. Although it can be done in other locations, the ideal candidate for a ventral buccal mucosa onlay graft repair is a patient with a bulbous urethral stricture more than 3 cm in length and a fairly healthy corpus spongiosum. Exposure is gained as described above for EPA. The urethra does not have to be mobilized off of the corporal bodies, but I do dissect the corpus spongiosum free laterally on each side to the dorsal most attachments to aid its later closure. A bougie is inserted distally, and a ventral urethrotomy incision is created onto the bougie (Fig. 40.2A). The urethrotomy is continued with tenotomy scissors proximally through the stricture and for at least 1 cm into healthy urethra (Fig. 40.2B). The proximal and distal urethrostomy should accept a 28–30 French bougie. The length of the defect is measured, and attention is turned to the inner cheek.

Exposure is gained with a self-retaining oral retractor with a small additional blade to retract the tongue medially (Fig. 40.4A). A facelift retractor is used on the side of the lip. Stensen's duct is identified opposite the second upper molar and avoided during the dissection. The graft is marked (Fig. 40.4B), and we infiltrate underneath it with 1/2% lidocaine with epinephrine to aid hemostasis. The border of the graft is incised, and it is then elevated off of the underlying muscle with tenotomy scissors. The graft is placed in saline, and meticulous hemostasis is obtained using electrocautery. A dry sponge is left on the donor site until the end of the case. We do not close the donor site and have not seen any significant issues in doing so (Fig. 40.4C). Bilateral grafts may be taken if needed. The graft is then thinned and often reconfigured because it is sometimes necessary to take it in the shape of a rhomboid (wider near the lip and narrowed in the back of the mouth) to get the necessary length. Reconfiguration is done using 5-0 chromic to get a rectangular graft 2.2–2.5 cm in width.

The graft is then sutured to the urethral mucosa distally and proximally using five to seven interrupted sutures of 4-0 or 5-0 PDS with the epithelial surface facing inward toward the lumen (Fig. 40.5). The lateral closure is then done using running 5-0 PDS in a watertight fashion (Fig. 40.5A). The corpus spongiosum is then closed over the top of the graft using running 4-0 PDS (Fig. 40.5B). An 18 French soft silicone catheter is inserted with subsequent closure and drainage as described an EPA. For graft procedures, however, I do place a diverting suprapubic catheter at the end of the case after the patient is placed supine. The urethral catheter is then plugged and taped to the lower abdomen without tension.

Although the first choice for a distal penile urethral stricture is a penile island flap repair, a ventral buccal mucosa onlay graft can be used if there is insufficient penile skin for a flap (Fig. 40.6). With the patient supine, a ventral midline penile incision is made and carried through the glans penis if necessary. The urethrotomy is continued proximally through the stricture and at least 1 cm into healthy urethra (Fig. 40.6A). Glans wings are dissected sufficiently to allow them to be brought around the reconstruction with a urethral meatus of at least 24 French in caliber. An appropriate buccal mucosa graft is harvested and sutured to the urethral mucosa using a few interrupted 5-0 PDS sutures proximally and running 5-0 PDS laterally (Fig. 40.6B). The deep layer of the glans is reapproximated using interrupted 4-0 PDS. The urethral meatus is sutures using interrupted 4-0 or 5-0 chromic, and the more proximal glans is closed in the same fashion.

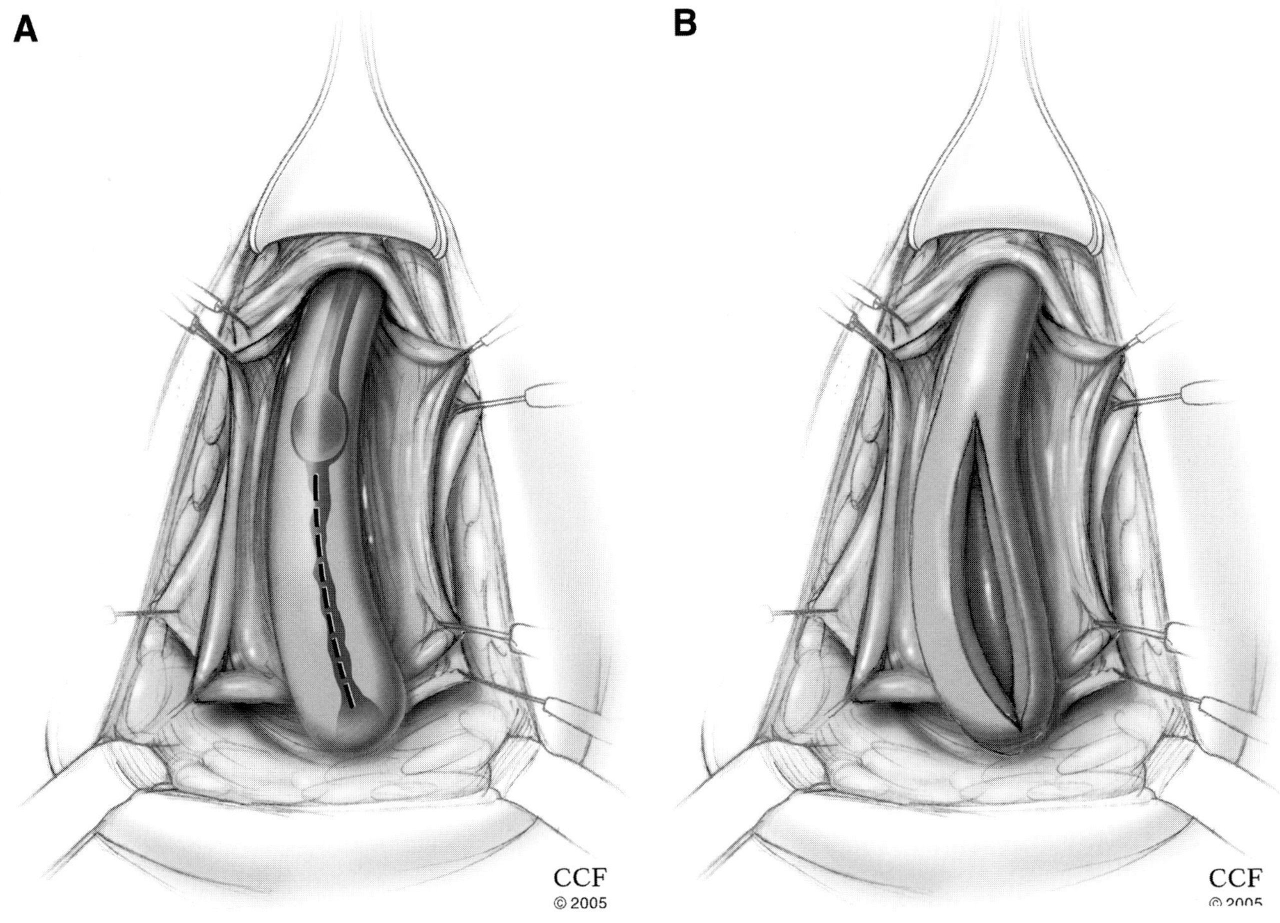


Fig. 40.3

Proximal to the glans, the overlying dartos fascia is quilted to the graft laterally using 4-0 or 5-0 chromic every 1 cm and with the interrupted 4-0 PDS used to close the dartos fascia in the midline. The skin is closed using interrupted 4-0 chromic and a urethral stent is placed through the repair and sutured to the glans penis (Fig. 40.6C). For this purpose I use a soft silicone catheter and cut off both ends so that it is of appropriate length. A diverting suprapubic catheter is placed, and a clear adhesive dressing is placed around the penis.

## Dorsal Buccal Mucosa Onlay Graft

Substitution urethroplasty with the buccal mucosa graft placed dorsally is preferred for bulbous urethral strictures when the corpus spongiosum is not adequate to cover a ventral graft due to scarring (Fig. 40.7). This is also the case when a stricture extends distally into an area where the corpus spongiosum is not thick enough to cover a ventral graft, such as the distal bulbous, penoscrotal, or penile urethra. Some surgeons primarily use dorsal grafts in all areas for the theoretical advantage of improving graft take and decreasing the incidence of sacculation of the graft. These problems, however, have not been significant in our ventral graft series when used in appropriate patients. When doing a dorsal graft, the urethra is exposed in the same fashion as noted above. If the stricture extends distal to the bulbous urethra, the penoscrotal urethra can be accessed by extending the vertical limb of the lambda incision in the exaggerated lithotomy position. A midline penile incision can be used for strictures in the penile and penoscrotal urethra with the patient supine or in a frog-legged position. The corpus spongiosum is mobilized completely off of the underlying corporal bodies and then rotated 180° so that the urethrotomy incision can be made on the dorsal aspect of the urethra (Fig. 40.7A). The urethrotomy is carried through the stricture and 1 cm into healthy urethra distally and proximally. The defect is measured and a buccal mucosa graft harvested as described above. The graft is then spread and fixed onto the corporal bodies with the epithelial surface facing inward toward the lumen (Fig. 40.7B). It is sutured in place using interrupted 5-0 chromic sutures peripherally, with additional sutures placed in the

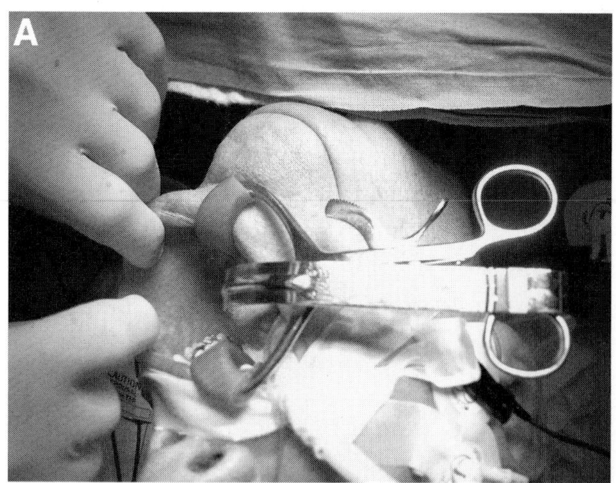

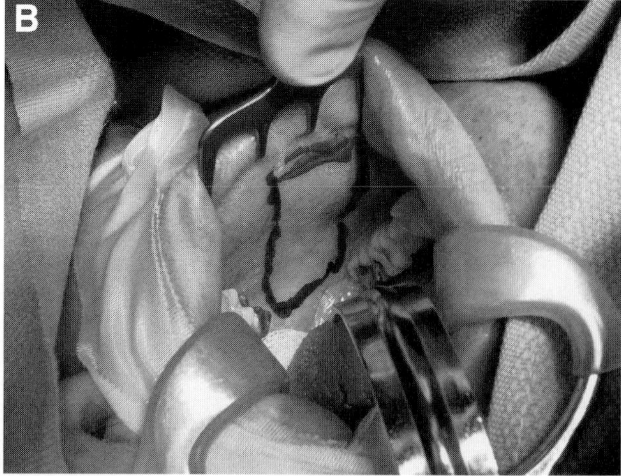

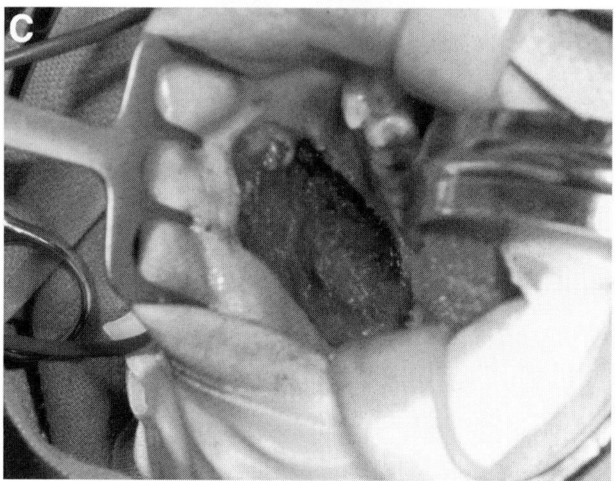

Fig. 40.4

central area of the graft as well. The proximal and distal ends of the graft are sutured to the edge of the corpus spongiosum and urethral mucosa using five interrupted sutures of 5-0 PDS (Fig. 40.7C), with the lateral sutures lines being closed with running 5-0 PDS (Fig. 40.7D). Catheter placement, drainage, and closure are as noted previously.

## Augmented Anastomotic Repair Using Ventral Buccal Mucosa

It is not uncommon for a lengthy stricture to have an area that is more narrow and dense than the remainder of the stricture (Fig. 40.8). This may at times be the result of an initial short stricture that has been instrumented multiple times leading to adjacent wider caliber stricture from the manipulation. In this setting it is advantageous to excise the dense narrow stricture and to anastomose the urethra ventrally or dorsally to improve the urethral plate, shorten the length of graft needed, and optimize graft take. This excision can be done partial thickness or full thickness. After exposing the corpus spongiosum as for a ventral graft, a ventral urethrotomy is made in standard fashion. One can then observe the urethral plate to see if there is an area of particular narrowing or scar that would be amenable to excision (Fig. 40.8A). If it is 1 cm or less in length and not associated with full-thickness spongiofibrosis, the urethral mucosa and the scarred underlying spongiosum can be excised partial thickness leaving some healthy spongiosum in place. The urethral mucosa is sutured together using interrupted sutures of 5-0 PDS with the knots buried. If the narrowed portion is longer or there is full-thickness spongiofibrosis, the urethral is fully mobilized off of the corporal bodies from the suspensory ligament distally to the departure of the urethra from the bulb proximally. The stricture is then excised full thickness (Fig. 40.8B). Buck's fascia is dissected off of the distal urethral segment if needed to aid extensibility and the intracrural space can be developed as well. Dorsal wall anastomosis is done using interrupted 4-0 PDS posteriorly (Fig. 40.8C), initially in one layer and then converting to a two-layer closure as one proceeds laterally with 4-0 PDS on the spongiosum and 5-0 PDS on the ure-

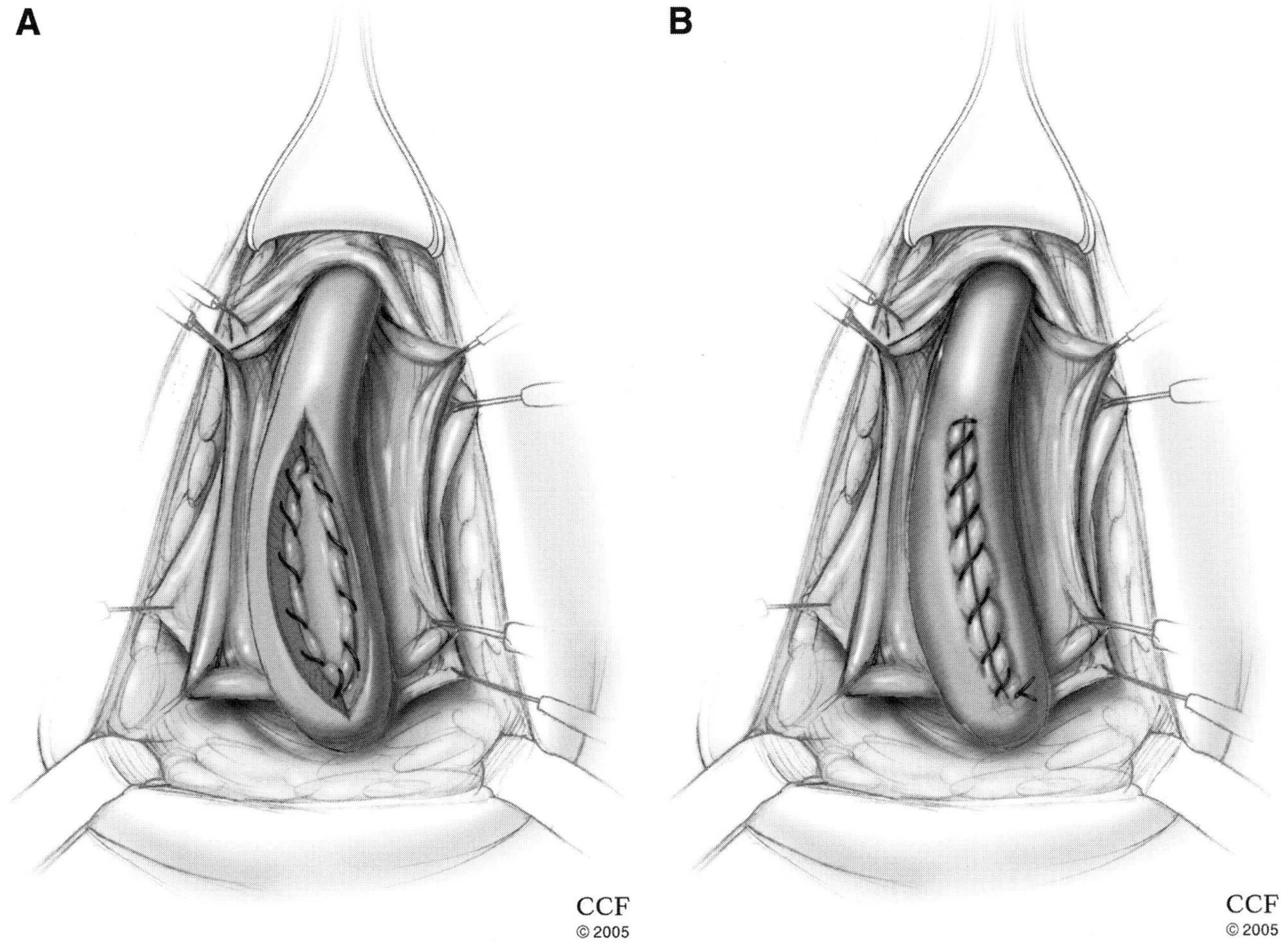


Fig. 40.5

thral mucosa (Fig. 40.8D). The repair proceeds as described for a ventral buccal mucosa onlay graft (Fig. 40.8E,F).

## Augmented Anastomotic Repair Using Dorsal Buccal Mucosa

In similar fashion, the augmented anastomotic repair can be done for a bulbous urethral stricture using a dorsal graft (Fig. 40.9). After full mobilization of the bulbous urethra off of the corporal bodies, the urethra is rotated 180° (Fig. 40.9A,B) and a dorsal urethrotomy incision performed. The problematic area is excised as noted above (Fig. 40.9C). In this setting it is helpful to spread fix the graft onto the corporal bodies before doing the ventral urethral anastomosis as there is better exposure to the area (Fig. 40.9C). Once the graft is in place, the urethra is sutured together ventrally (Fig. 40.9D) and the repair is completed as described above for a dorsal onlay procedure (Fig. 40.9E,F).

## Combination Repairs

Panurethral strictures are those that extensively involve the penile and bulbous urethra (Fig. 40.10). One approach used in these situations is the combination of a proximal buccal mucosa graft and a distal penile or penoscrotal island flap. In this technique, the procedure starts in the exaggerated lithotomy position, and most commonly a standard ventral buccal mucosa onlay graft procedure is done through a perineal incision (Fig. 40.10A). After completion of the urethral work and without closing the incision, the patient is repositioned into low lithotomy for the remainder of the procedure. This is an important step to minimize the chance of a positioning related complication as these procedures can be of long duration. At this point we have most commonly used a longitudinal penile or penoscrotal island flap based on the lateral dartos fascia. The incision is made to the right or left on the midline, depending on which side one wants to base the dartos pedicle, and continued to the upper scrotum. This area is then connected to the perineal work area under the scrotum, and the upper end of the proximal repair is identified. The urethrotomy incision is continued distally as far as is necessary. Glans wings are dissected if needed. The cut edge of the urethral mucosa is sutured to the

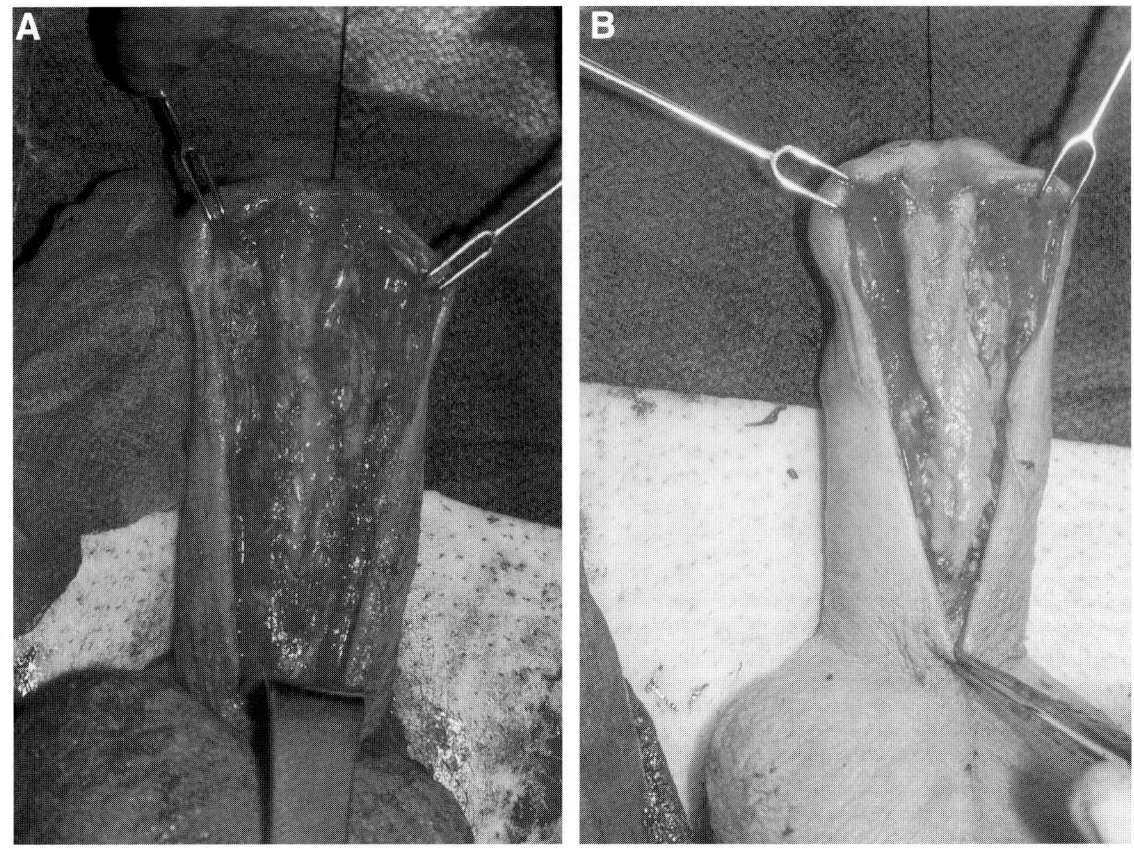


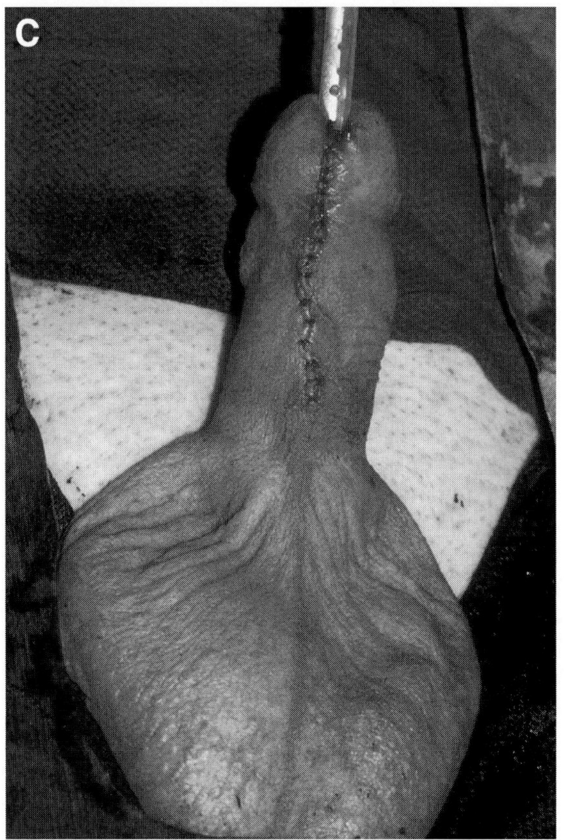


Fig. 40.6

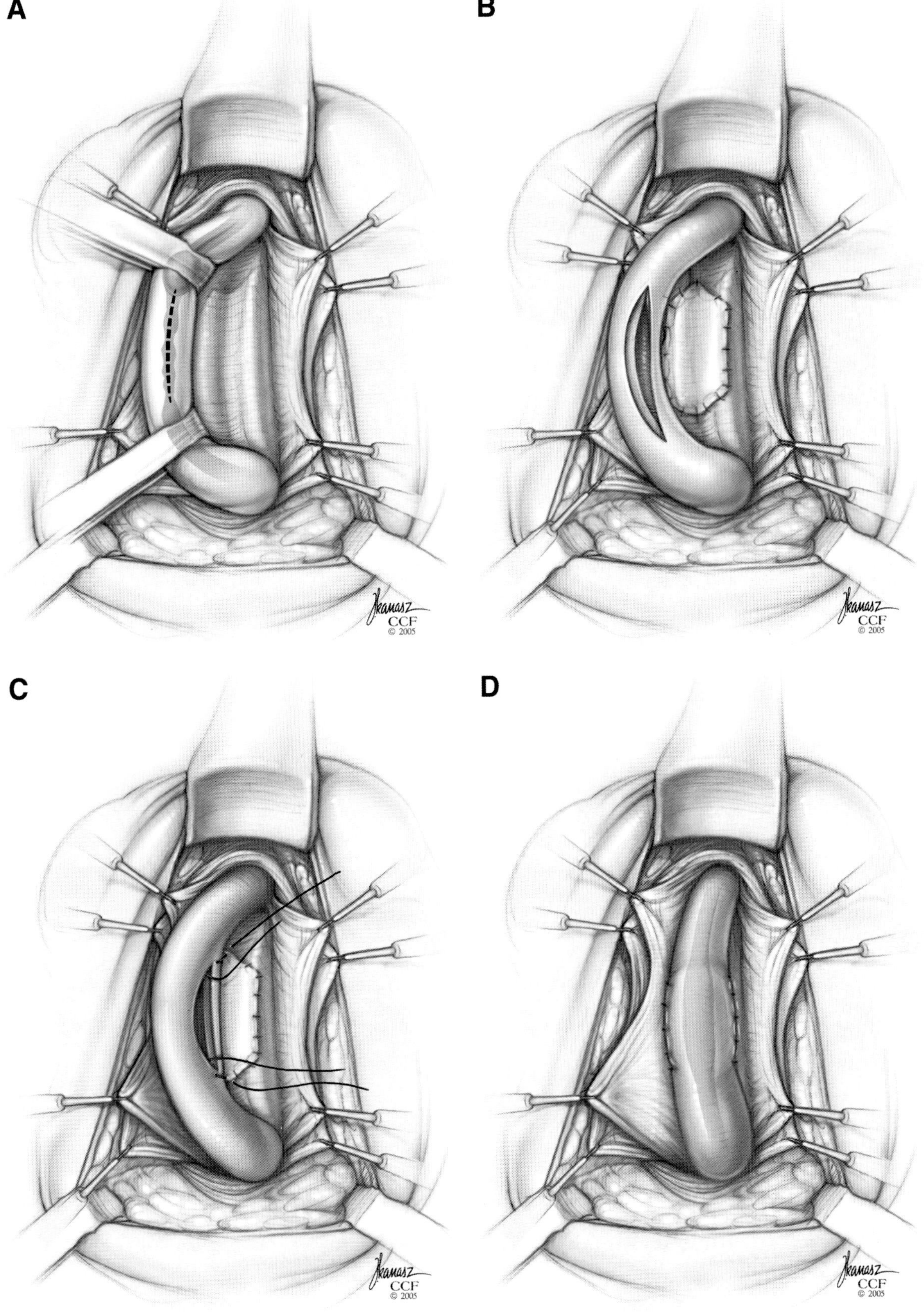
A
B
C
D
Kramasz CCF © 2005
Kramasz CCF © 2005
Kramasz CCF © 2005
Kramasz CCF © 2005

Fig. 40.7

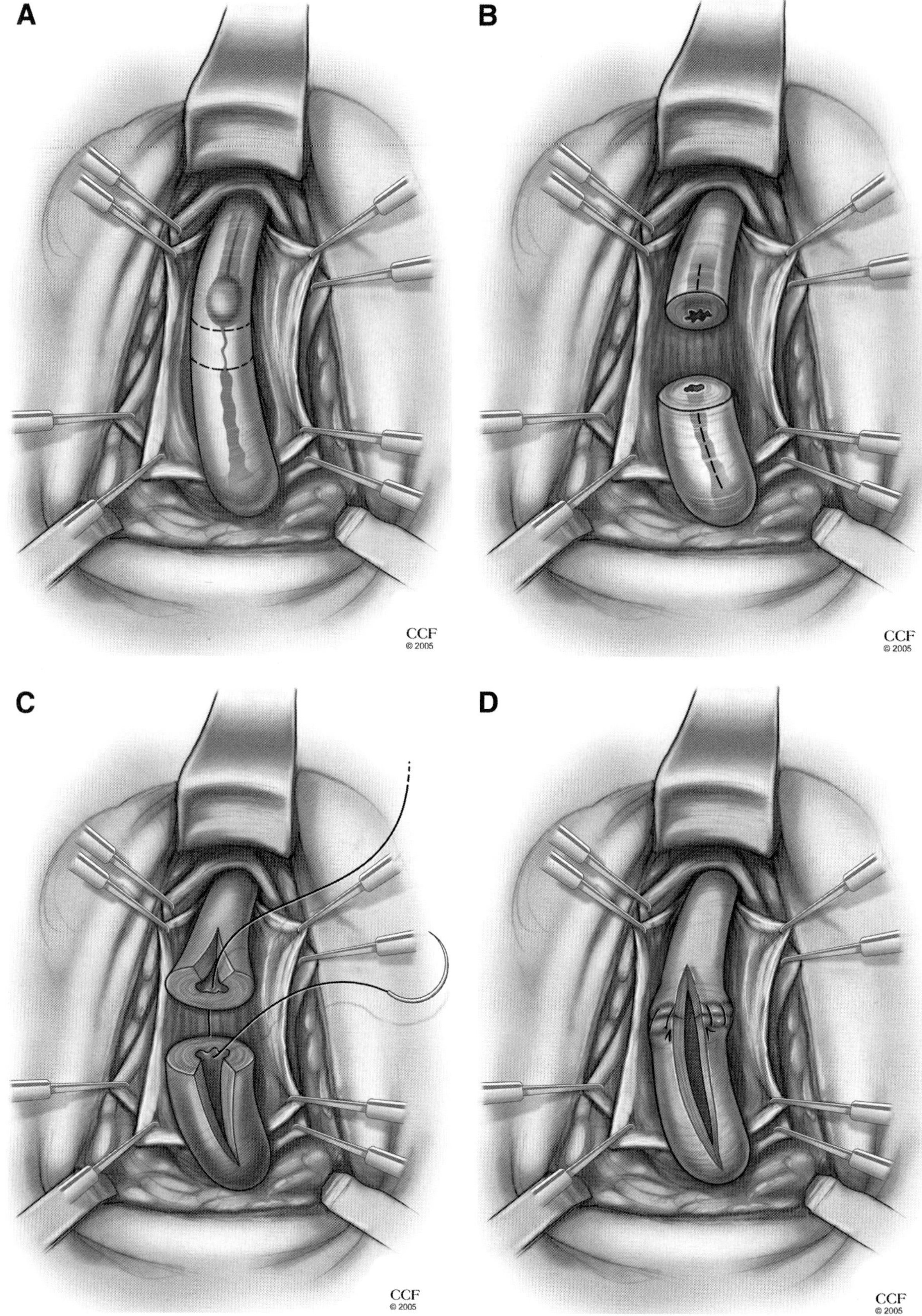


Fig. 40.8

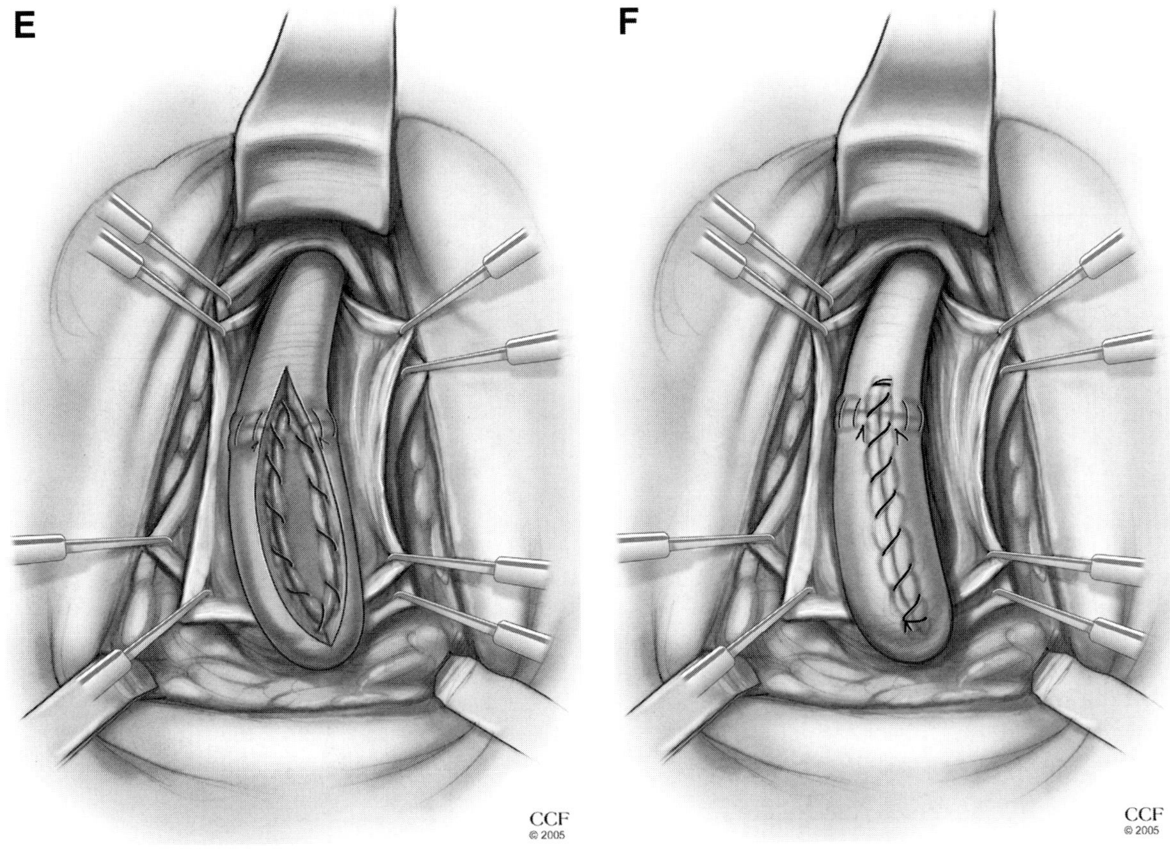


Fig. 40.8 *(Continued)*

adjacent edge of the spongiosum using a running suture of 5-0 chromic. The defect is measured, and the necessary skin island is marked with a pen. The skin island is constructed to achieve a urethral lumen of approx 28 French. The periphery of the skin island is incised just through the dermal layer, preserving the underlying dartos. Tenotomy scissors are used to dissect in the plane between the dartos fascia supplying the skin island and the overlying penile skin. This is done until the skin island will rotate easily into the urethrotomy defect (Fig. 40.10B). Meticulous hemostasis is maintained using bipolar cautery. The skin island is then sutured to the distal end of the buccal graft repair with interrupted 4-0 or 5-0 PDS, being sure to include both the buccal mucosa and the overlying corpus spongiosum in the sutures. The skin island is secured distally, and the glans is managed as described in Fig. 40.6. Lateral closure is done using running 5-0 PDS (Fig. 40.10C). An 18 French soft silicone catheter is placed. A layer of dartos fascia is sutured over the anterior suture line, and a small suction drain is placed adjacent to the repair. The penile skin is closed using interrupted 4-0 chromic (Fig. 40.10D), and a clear adhesive dressing is placed around the penis. The perineal incision is closed in standard fashion, and a suprapubic catheter is placed.

## Staged Buccal Mucosa Graft Urethroplasty

Patients who have undergone multiple previous penile operations for hypospadias may have recurrent stricture disease and insufficient penile tissues for a flap procedure or for one-stage graft reconstruction. In this setting, staged repair provides optimal results. Another situation that may favor staged reconstruction is stricture in the setting of balanitis xerotica obliterans. These strictures are usually very dense and associated with meatal stenosis and variable lengths of stricture proximal to the meatus. There has been some controversy as to whether the urethra needs to be completely excised in association with staged repair, or whether a one-stage approach using buccal mucosa or even a skin island is adequate. In either event, the ability to do a one-stage repair will depend on the availability of normal penile skin for a possible island flap or for good buccal graft coverage, and therefore it may be most suitable to individualize the type of reconstruction based on the appearance of the penile and glanular tissues.

In the first stage of the repair, the urethra is opened ventrally through the skin until healthy urethra is entered (Fig. 40.11A). In the setting of multiple previous hypospadias repairs, this is often at the point where the native ure-

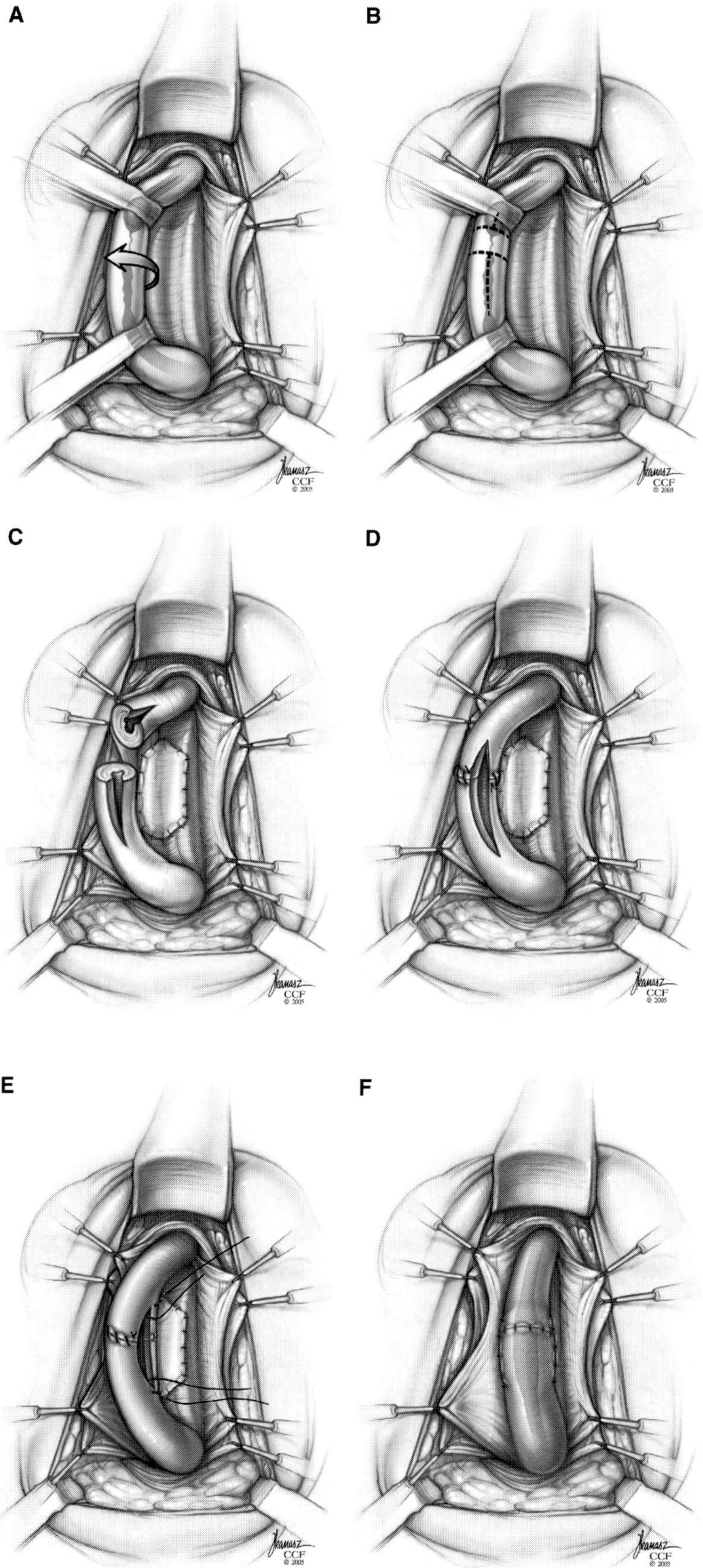


Fig. 40.9

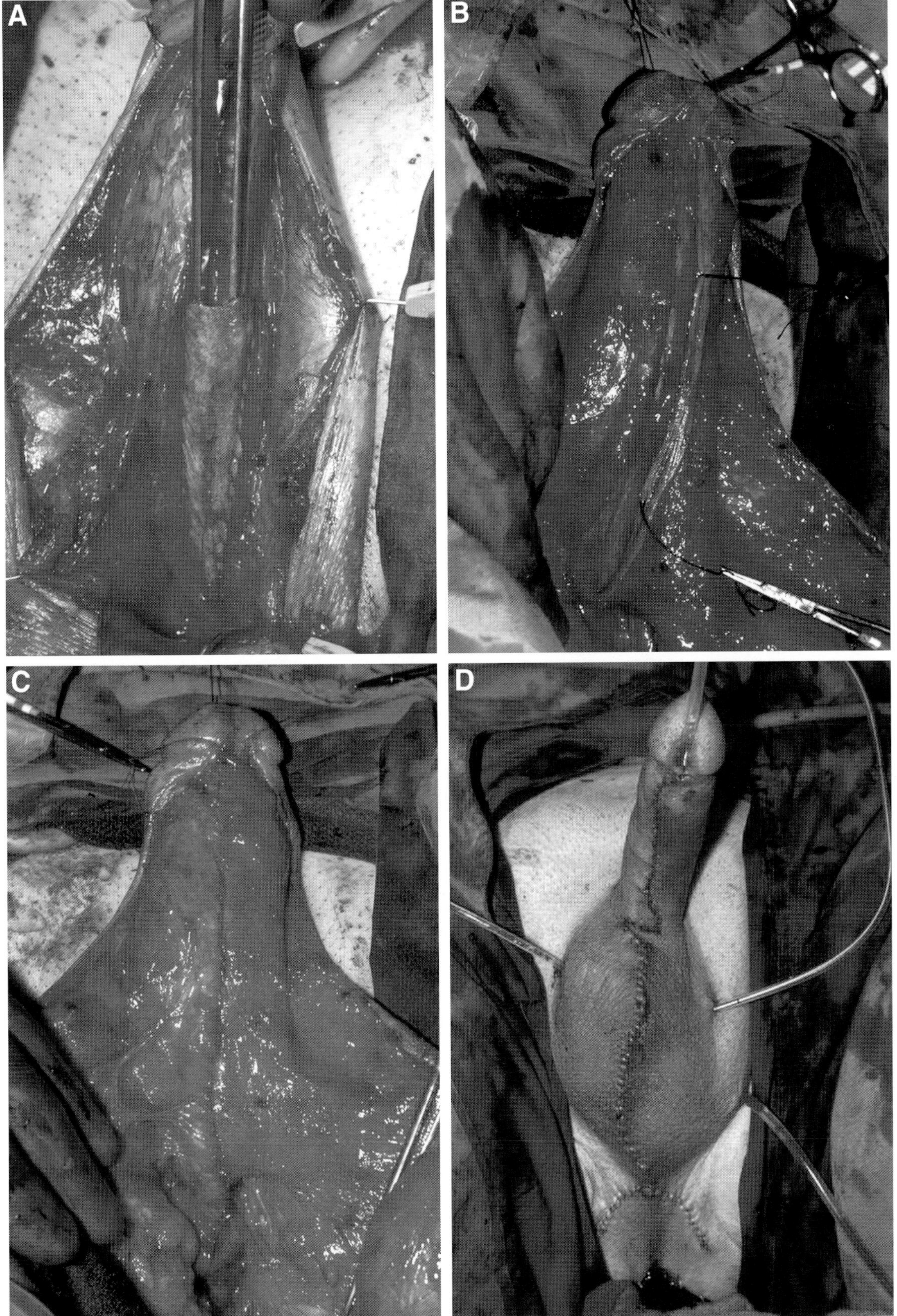


Fig. 40.10

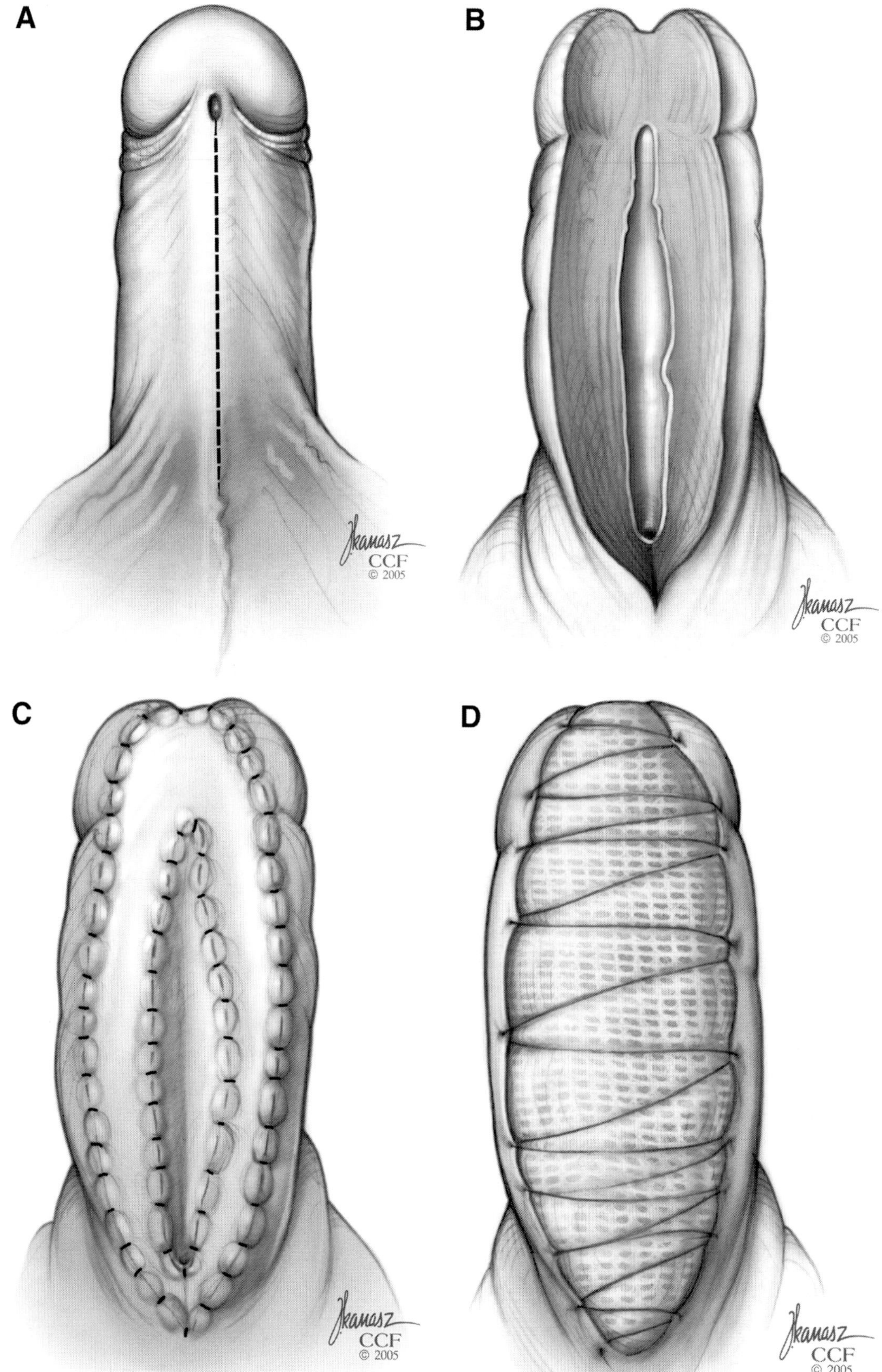


Fig. 40.11

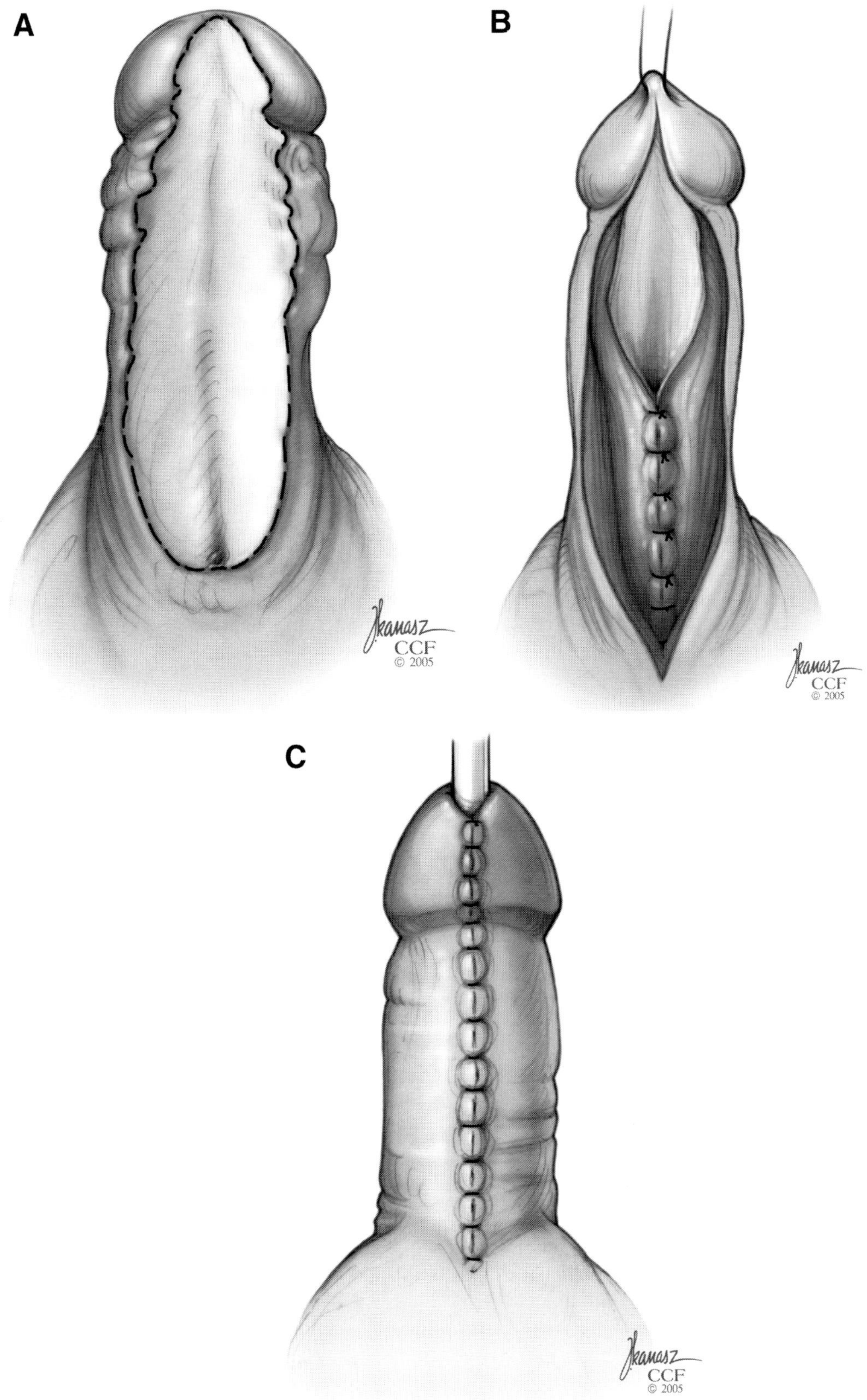


Fig. 40.12

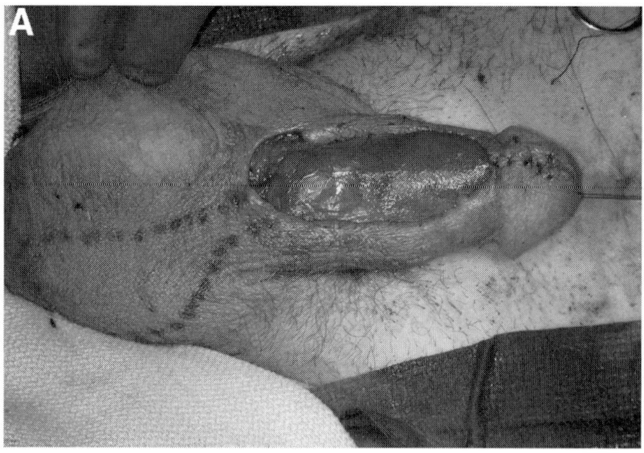


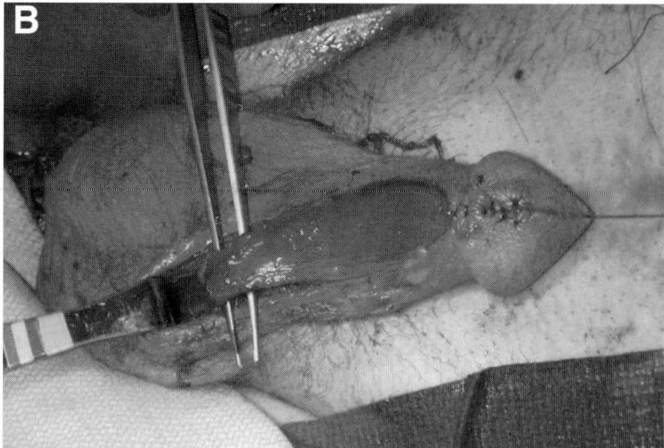


Fig. 40.13

thra begins. If there is a glanular meatus, glans wings are developed. If the existing urethral meatus is subcoronal in location, one can open the glans penis in the ventral midline back to a point where the posterior aspect of the meatus would normally reside (Fig. 40.11B). If necessary, the dartos fascia adjacent to the urethral plate can be quilted into position using small chromic sutures to provide a better graft bed. One or two buccal mucosa grafts are then harvested and thinned. They are brought into the graft bed with the epithelial surface facing upward and sutured in place using interrupted 4-0 chromic (Fig. 40.11C). The glans penis is maintained in a spread fashion to make sure that adequate graft is being brought into the area, as this and the subcoronal region are the most difficult to reconstruct at the second stage and the most prone to fistula. Some scrotal or proximal penile skin is usually sutured to the urethra along the ventral aspect of the penoscrotal urethrostomy, although it is not always included in the final repair. A soft silicone urethral catheter is placed. Xeroform gauze is placed over the graft, followed by a bolster of artificial cotton (batting) that has been soaked in a mixture of mineral oil and saline. The bolster is secured in place using tie over sutures of 3-0 chromic (Fig. 40.11D). A suprapubic catheter is placed. The bolster is removed on postoperative day 5, and the graft is covered with a xeroform gauze dressing for an additional 2 wk. The urethral suprapubic catheters are removed.

After 4–6 mo, second-stage closure may be undertaken (Fig. 40.12). Vertical incisions are made along the lateral edge of the graft and onto the glans penis (Fig. 40.12A). Tenotomy scissors are used to dissect in the plane between the neourethra and the adjacent dartos fascia and glans penis, taking care to preserve its blood supply. Once the edges will reach without tension, the neourethra is closed using a few interrupted 4-0 chromic to align the edges, followed by a running 5-0 PDS (Fig. 40.12B). A second layer of running 5-0 PDS consisting of adjacent dartos fascia is usually possible. The glans penis is closed, as outlined in Fig. 40.6. At this point the penile skin is assessed for thickness and vascularity, and, if felt to be adequate, it is closed in the ventral midline using interrupted 5-0 PDS on the deep or dartos layer and interrupted 4-0 chromic on the skin (Fig. 40.12C).

If the skin appears less healthy and there is concern for fistula formation, a tunica vaginalis flap may be mobilized and rotated over the repair to the level of the proximal subglanular closure (Fig. 40.13A). To do this, the scrotum is entered through the existing incision and the testicle mobilized in its tunic. The tunical vaginalis is then entered and a flap outlined staying away from the epididymis. After the flap is mobilized, hemostasis along the remaining edge of the tunical vaginalis is obtained with running suture or electrocautery, and the testicle is replaced. The tunica vaginalis is mobilized proximally enough to reach the distal repair, but with a broad base and not so much as to compromise its blood supply (Fig. 40.13B). It is sutured into place with small PDS or chromic sutures.

## POSTOPERATIVE CARE

While in the hospital, patients are maintained on intravenous antibiotics. An antibiotic mouthwash is given four times a day, and patients are placed on a full liquid diet for a few days. Prophylactic subcutaneous heparin is administered, and pneumatic compression stockings are used. Following an EPA, the patient returns for a voiding cystourethrogram (VCUG) 10–14 d following surgery, and after a graft procedure the VCUG is done at approx 3 wk. Both catheters are removed if there is no extravasation, and patients are treated with 5 d of a quinolone. A urine culture is done 1 mo later to ensure sterility. Flexible cystoscopy is performed at 6 mo and 1 yr postoperatively. If at 1 yr there is an area that is felt to be at risk for future narrowing, annual cystoscopy is continued until stability is documented. If the repair looks good at 1 yr, the patient follows up with the referring urologist and returns on an as-needed basis.

## SUGGESTED READINGS


1. Albers P, Fichtner J, Bruhl P, Muller SC. Long-term results of internal urethrotomy. J Urol 156:1611–1614, 1996.
2. Andrich DE, Mundy AR. Substitution urethroplasty with buccal mucosal-free grafts. J Urol 165: 1131–1133, 2001.
3. Angermeier KW, Jordan GH, Schlossberg SM. Complex urethral reconstruction. Urol Clin North Am 21: 567–581, 1994.
4. Barbagli G, Selli C, Tosto A, Palminteri E. Dorsal free graft urethroplasty. J Urol 155:123–126, 1996.
5. Berglund R, Angermeier KW. Combined buccal mucosa graft and genital skin flap for reconstruction of extensive urethral strictures [abstr]. J Urol 171: 1168, 2004.
6. Devine CJ, Jr., Devine PC, Felderman TP, et al. Classification and standardization of urethral strictures. Abstract #325, Annual Meeting of the American Urological Association, April 17–21, 1983.
7. Elliott SP, Metro MJ, McAninch JW. Long-term followup of the ventrally placed buccal mucosa onlay graft in bulbar urethral reconstruction. J Urol 169:1754–1757, 2003.
8. Guralnick ML, Webster GD. The augmented anastomotic urethroplasty: indications and outcome in 29 patients. J Urol 165:1496–1501, 2001.
9. Jordan GH. Management of anterior urethral stricture disease. Problems Urol 1:199–225, 1987.
10. Jordan GH. Management of anterior urethral stricture disease. In: Webster GD, Kirby R, King LR and Goldwasser B, eds. Reconstructive Urology. Boston: Blackwell Scientific Publications, 1993:703–723.
11. Morey AF, McAninch JW. When and how to use buccal mucosal grafts in adult bulbar urethroplasty. Urology 48:194–198, 1996.
12. Pansodoro V, Emiliozzi P. Internal urethrotomy in the management of anterior urethral strictures: long-term followup. J Urol 156:73–75, 1996.
13. Venn SN, Mundy AR. Early experience with the use of buccal mucosa for substitution urethroplasty. Br J Urol 81:738–740, 1998.
14. Webster GD, Koefoot RB, Sihelnik SA. Urethroplasty management in 200cases of urethral stricture: a rationale for procedure selection. J Urol 134:892–898, 1985.
15. Wessels H, McAninch JW. Use of free grafts in urethral stricture reconstruction. J Urol 155:1912–1915, 1996.

# 41 Hypospadias Repair

*Jonathan Ross and Robert Kay*

## INTRODUCTION

Hypospadias represents a maldevelopment of the ventrum of the penis (Fig. 41.1). In its fullest form, the urethra, glans, corpora cavernosa, subcutaneous tissues, and skin are all involved. But each case is unique, and some penile elements may be more or less affected in any given case. The urethral anomaly is most obviously expressed in the ectopic urethral meatus located anywhere from the perineum to the proximal glans. But the spongy covering of the urethra may also be abnormal proximal to the meatus. Typically, the spongy tissue covers the proximal urethra, but splits somewhere proximal to the meatus and lies on either side of the urethral plate converging with the glans distally. This leaves a thin uncovered portion of urethra, which may be only a few millimeters long or may extend quite proximal to the hypospadiac meatus. In most cases of hypospadias, the glans is flattened, reflecting the divergent spongiosa distally. The foreskin is incomplete in 95% of cases, being deficient ventrally; the ventral penile skin is often thin and short, tethering the penis and contributing to the frequently seen ventral chordee. Dense fibrous subcutaneous tissue — "chordee tissue" — may also contribute to this ventral curvature. In more severe cases of ventral chordee, the corpora cavernosa themselves may be bent due to a deficiency and subsequent shortening of the ventral sides. Hypospadias repair involves addressing each of these issues sequentially in each case.

## ORTHOPLASTY—PENILE STRAIGHTENING

A circumcision incision is made in the mucosal skirt 8–10 mm from the glanular corona. Ventrally this is brought either proximal to the urethra or across the urethral plate. The former approach is preferred because urethroplasties that utilize the preserved urethral plate have a significantly lower complication rate, and the urethral plate itself rarely contributes to ventral chordee. However, in severe cases of hypospadias with an obviously tethering urethral plate, the incision may be brought across it. If a meatal-based flap is to be performed, then the incision is brought proximal to the flap. The skin is then completely degloved, elevating the skin off of the corporal bodies and detaching all chordee tissue from the shaft of the penis. In most cases of distal hypospadias, this maneuver will be sufficient to straighten the penis, which is confirmed by performing an artificial erection. To perform an artificial erection, a small-gauge butterfly needle is inserted into the corporal body and injectable saline is infused with a 10-cc syringe while digital pressure is applied to the base of the corporal bodies over the pubic bone. Alternatively, a tourniquet may be placed around the base of the penis.

If the penis is still bent after degloving, then an additional straightening procedure is required that addresses the intrinsic corporal disproportion (Fig.41.2). In mild to moderate cases, the chordee may be corrected with a dorsal plication. Buck's fascia is incised in the midline and dissected off the tunix of the corporal bodies. A longitudinal incision is then made in the dorsal midline of the erectile bodies at the level of greatest curvature. This incision must be full thickness through the tunix exposing the erectile tissue. The incision may be made slightly off the midline to avoid dissecting deep into the septum without entering either corporal body. Single-prong skin hooks are placed on either side in the middle of the incision and pulled laterally. The incision is then closed with interrupted suture. A permanent 5-0 suture is placed in the middle with the knot buried, and absorbable 5-0 sutures are placed on either side. A repeat artificial erection is performed to confirm a good result.

In more severe cases of chordee the ventrum of the corporal bodies should be lengthened (as opposed to shortening the dorsum with a plication) (Fig.41.3). In these severe cases, the urethral plate has usually been divided. To accomplish the corporal lengthening, a transverse incision is made in the corporal bodies at the

From: *Operative Urology at the Cleveland Clinic*
Edited by: A. Novick et al. © Humana Press Inc., Totowa, NJ

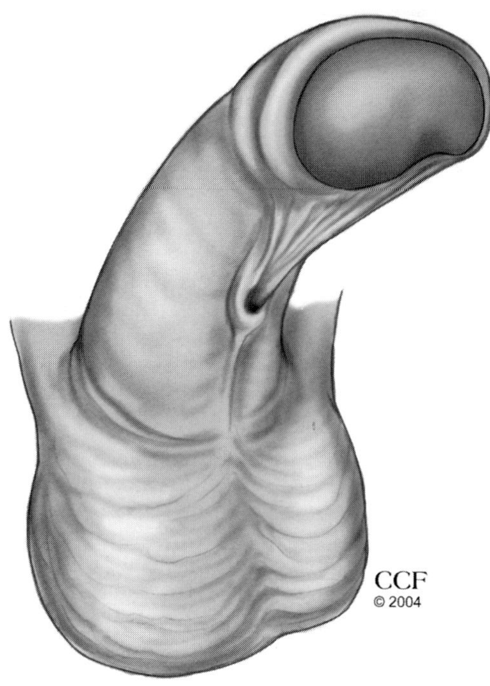


Fig. 41.1

level of greatest curvature, unhinging the penis. It is important that this incision be full thickness through the tunix and extends to the lateral midline of the shaft on either side. In the ventral midline, the septum should be sharply released from the tunix at either edge of the incision to allow complete unhinging of the penis. This incision creates an elliptical defect that is covered with an elliptical graft of dermis or tunica vaginalis. To harvest a tunica vaginalis graft, one of the testes is delivered into the incision with the tunica vaginalis intact. This may require extending the skin incision proximally in the ventral midline onto the scrotum for a short distance. An ellipse of tunica vaginalis is then excised and secured over the elliptical defect. The graft should be placed with the inner tunical epithelium down on the erectile tissue. An absorbable 6-0 suture is placed at the two corners and at the midpoint of the incision superiorly and inferiorly. These four sutures are run along each quadrant, securing the graft in place. An artificial erection is performed, and, if necessary, a small dorsal plication can be performed to augment the effect.

## URETHROPLASTY

After penile straightening, a urethroplasty is performed. The type of repair depends on the degree of hypospadias, the characteristics of the meatus and glans, and whether the urethral plate was divided during chordee correction. In minor glanular hypospadias, the bridge of tissue between the hypospadiac meatus and the glans pit is excised and closed transversely, advancing the dorsal wall of the urethra and preventing a downward deflection of the urinary stream. When the meatus is proximal to the glans, a more involved repair is required.

## MEATAL ADVANCEMENT AND GLANSPLASTY (MAGPI)

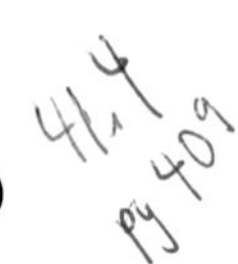

The MAGPI procedure is appropriate for patients with coronal hypospadias, a small meatus, and mobile urethra. When performed in the absence of these criteria, the results are disappointing.

The bridge of tissue between the meatus and the glans "dimple" is incised or wedged out (Fig.41.4). The back wall of the urethral meatus is then advanced up the glans with interrupted 6-0 chromic suture. The ventral lip of the urethral meatus is advanced distally with a traction suture, and nonglans tissue is excised from the margins of the inverted V that is created. The edges of the glans are brought together ventral to the urethral meatus with interrupted 6-0 chromic suture, and the circumcision is closed.

## TUBULARIZED INCISED PLATE (TIP) REPAIR

This modified Thiersch-Duplay repair was popularized by Snodgrass in 1994 and has largely replaced other distal, midshaft, and even proximal repairs in the armamentarium of hypospadiologists. The concept was to expand the application of a simple tubularization to those patients in whom the urethral plate was of inadequate width to accomplish an acceptable urethral diameter. This limitation is overcome by performing a relaxing longitudinal urethral plate incision. Studies have shown that rather than contracting down, the deep tissue thus exposed epithelializes, resulting in a true increase in the ultimate circumference of the urethra. Because the urethral plate is often thin and the repair results in overlying suture lines, it is crucial to interpose a layer of subcutaneous tissue between the urethroplasty and the skin closure.

A urethral catheter is passed to determine if the distal urethra is thin, and a ventral meatotomy is performed down to healthy urethra (Fig. 41.5). A circumcision is performed proximal to the urethral meatus, and an orthoplasty is accomplished. After injecting 1:200,000

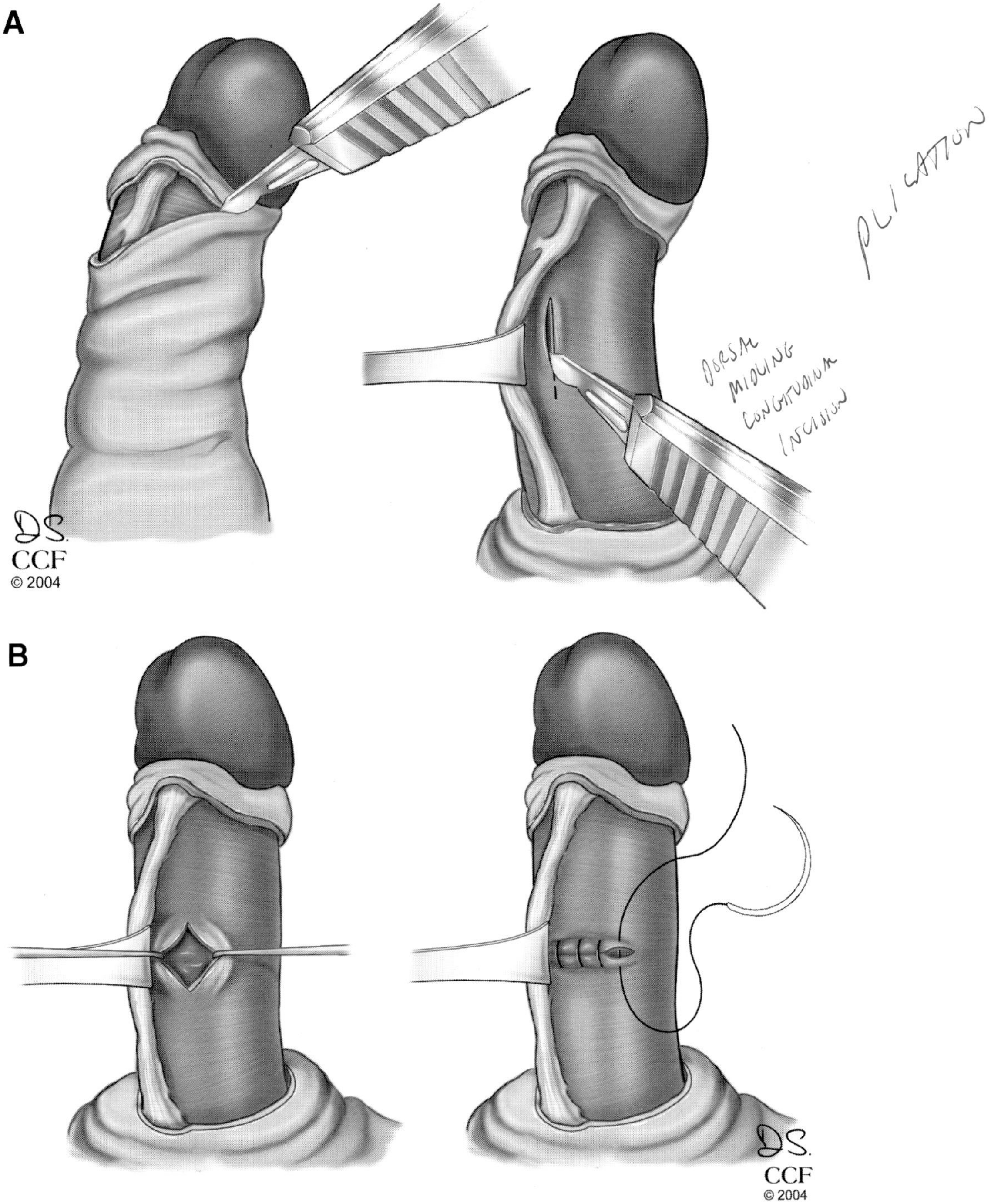

A

B

DS.
CCF
© 2004

Fig. 41.2

epinephrine under the glans ridges, parallel incisions are made on either side of the urethral plate. These incisions are carried deep into the glans, mobilizing the glans wings and urethral plate. A longitudinal incision is made in the urethral plate from the meatus to the end of the glanular urethral plate. This incision should not be carried beyond the urethral plate on to the glans. It is made as deeply as necessary to allow a tension-free closure of the plate over an 8 French catheter. Occasionally, the native urethral plate is wide enough that the TIP maneuver is not necessary. The urethral plate is tubularized over an 8 French catheter with a running absorbable 6-0 suture. A dorsal slit is performed and the apex of that incision secured to the dorsal midline of the mucosal

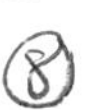

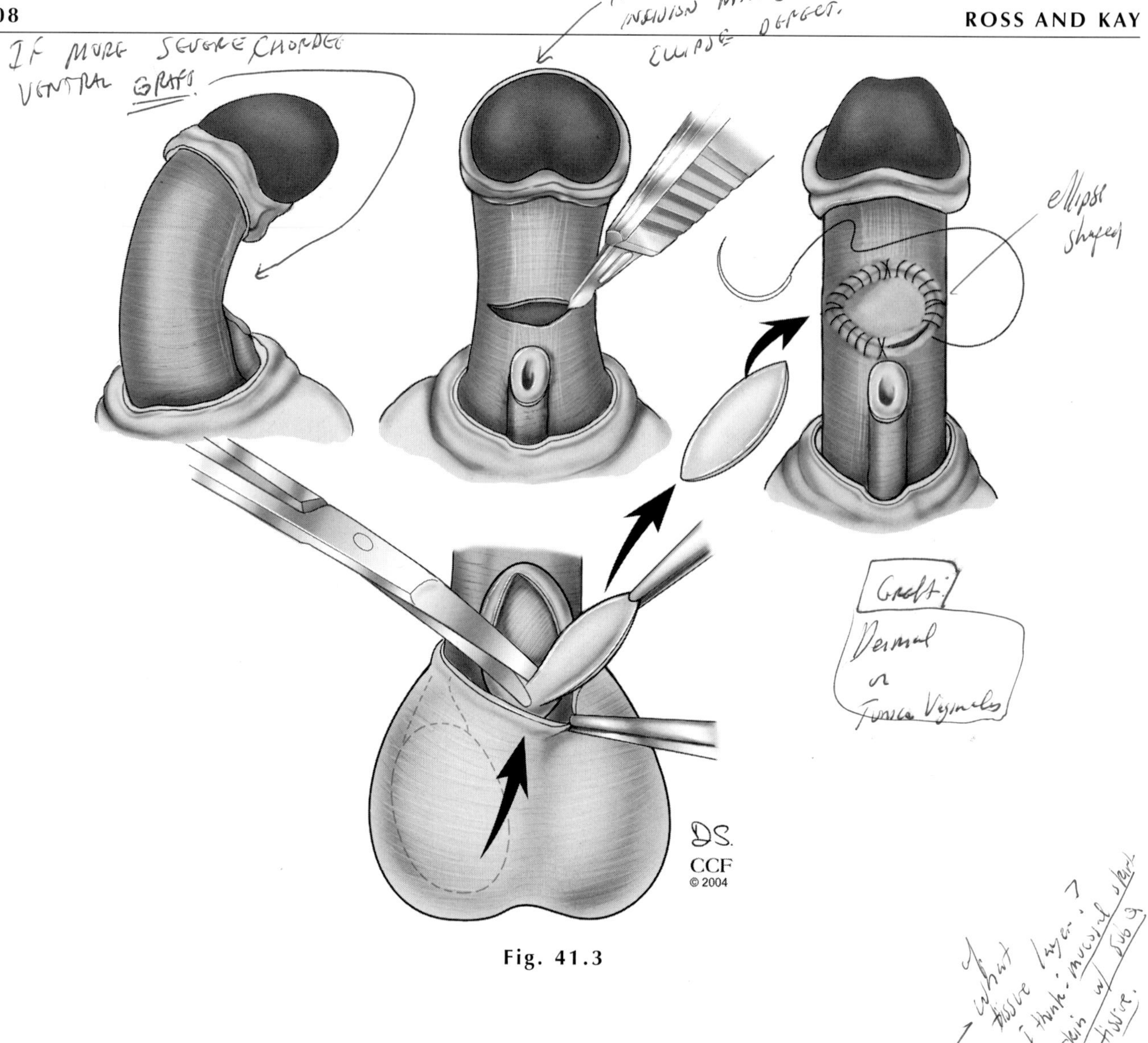


Fig. 41.3

skirt skin with a 6-0 chromic suture. The dorsal skin is then brought around for a ventral midline closure. On one side, the tip of the flap to be excised is de-epithelialized, and on the other side it is simply amputated. The de-epithelialized flap is brought over the urethral plate and secured on either side with 6-0 absorbable sutures. The glans is closed in two layers, and the circumcision and ventral shaft skin are reapproximated with interrupted 6-0 chromic suture.

While some authors have not left a stent postoperatively, we prefer to leave a urethral catheter for 1 wk. With this approach the reoperation rate for distal and midshaft hypospadias is approx 2%.

## MEATAL-BASED FLAP REPAIR (MATHIEU)

This standard distal hypospadias repair has been largely superceded by the TIP repair. However, it is still a useful repair for distal hypospadias with minimal chordee and for reoperations in patients who have meatal retrusion or coronal fistulas.

A ventral meatal-based flap equal in length to the distance of the urethral plate is marked off, and a circumcision and glans wings incisions are performed, preserving the flap (Fig. 41.6). The meatal-based flap is elevated off of the proximal urethra staying in the plane on the spongiosum so that the subcutaneous tissue remains with the flap. A good blood supply to the flap is maintained by minimizing the dissection to the amount necessary to bring the flap up without tension. The flap is secured to the edge of the urethral plate on either side with running absorbable 6-0 suture. The repair should be covered with a deepithelialized flap, if possible. The glans is closed in two layers. The circumcision and ventral shaft skin are closed with interrupted 6-0 chromic suture. A urethral catheter is left for 1 wk.

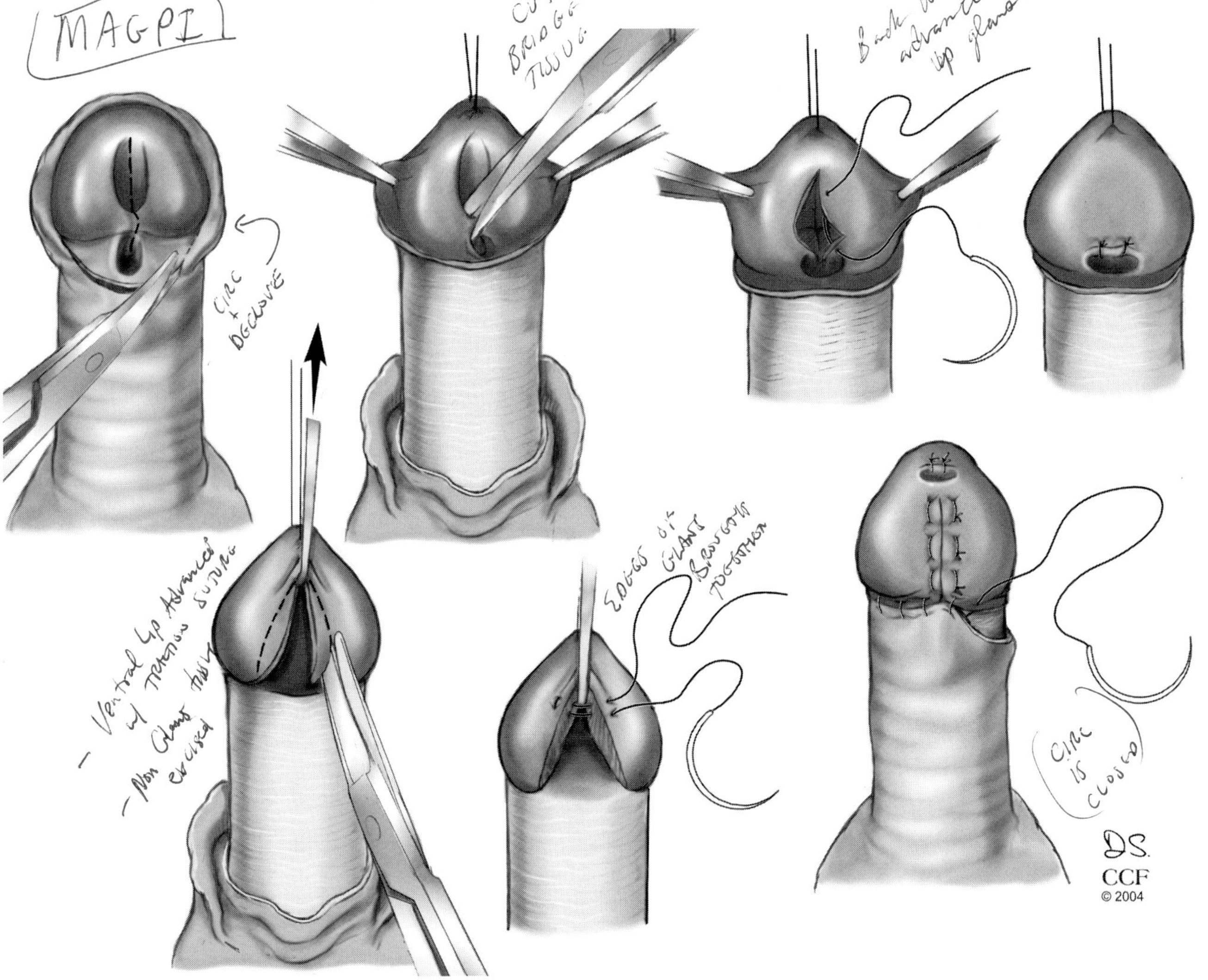

Fig. 41.4

## ISLAND FLAP REPAIR

The island flap repair may be utilized for any degree of hypospadias. It is particularly useful for cases in which the urethral plate is inadequate for tubularization (despite a TIP) and a meatal-based flap is not possible and in cases in which the urethral plate must be divided. It may be used as an onlay or a tube flap.

The initial incisions and glans wing mobilization are the same as for the TIP repair (Fig. 41.7). An orthoplasty is performed. A rectangular flap is marked off on the dorsal inner preputial skin of appropriate dimensions to replace the absent urethra. The plane is then developed between the flap and the dorsal skin, keeping the subcutaneous tissue attached to the flap as its blood supply. The skin will survive on the blood vessels traveling in the dermis.

If the plate has been divided, the flap is tubularized over an 8 French catheter with absorbable suture (Fig. 41.8). It is then secured proximally to the urethral meatus with interrupted sutures and distally to the glans. If the urethral plate is preserved, the flap is brought around and secured as an onlay with running sutures on either side. The glans and skin are closed as described in other repairs. The catheter is left for 7–10 d.

## TWO-STAGE REPAIR

The vast majority of hypospadias repairs may be accomplished in one stage. However, a two-stage approach may be employed for male genitoplasty in patients with ambiguous genitalia. It may also be appropriate in patients with severe hypospadias and marked chordee requiring a ventral patch graft and/or those with marked penoscrotal transposition.

An inverted omega incision is made circumscribing the scrotal tissue dorsally and caudally (Fig. 41.9). Ventrally

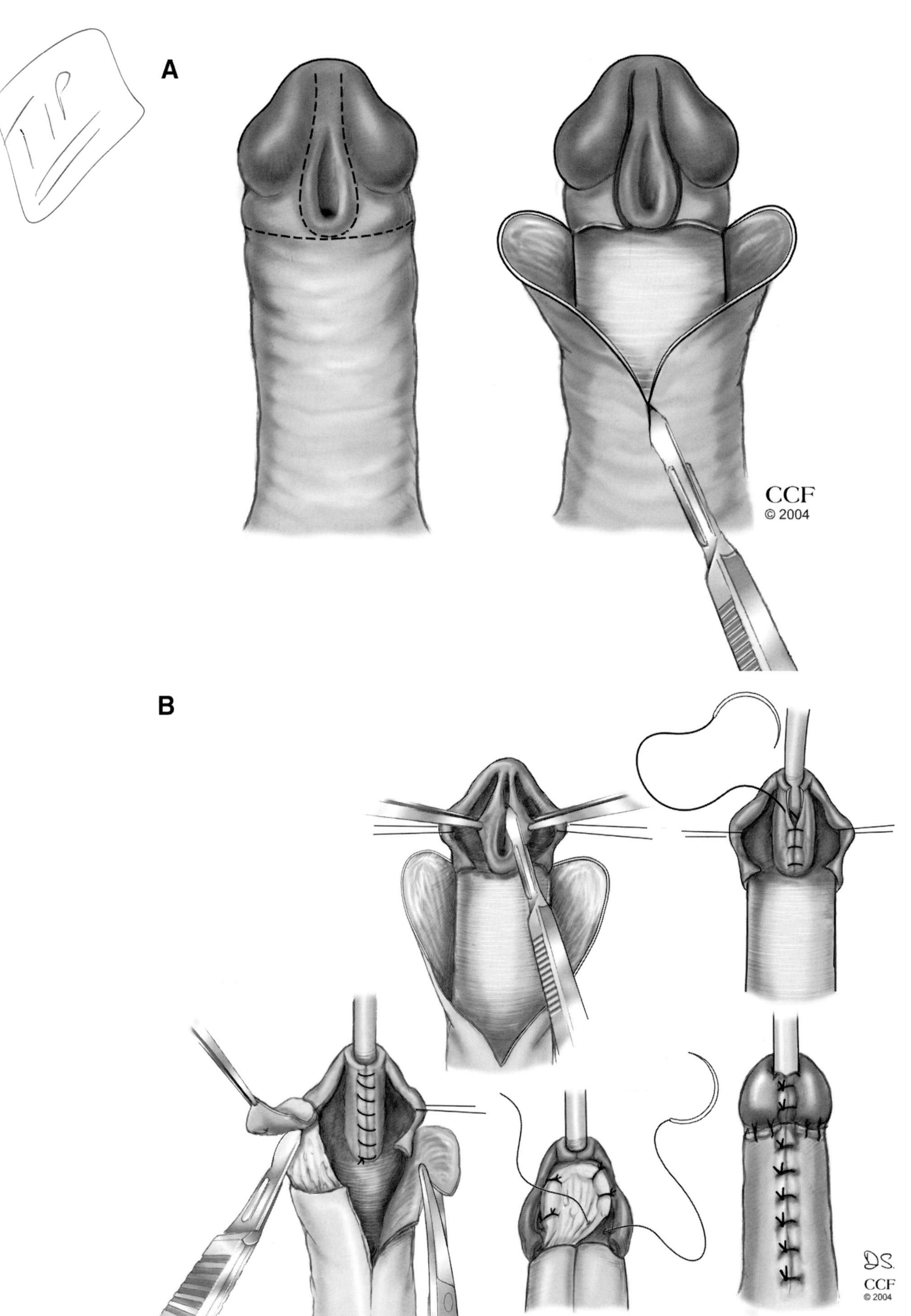


Fig. 41.5

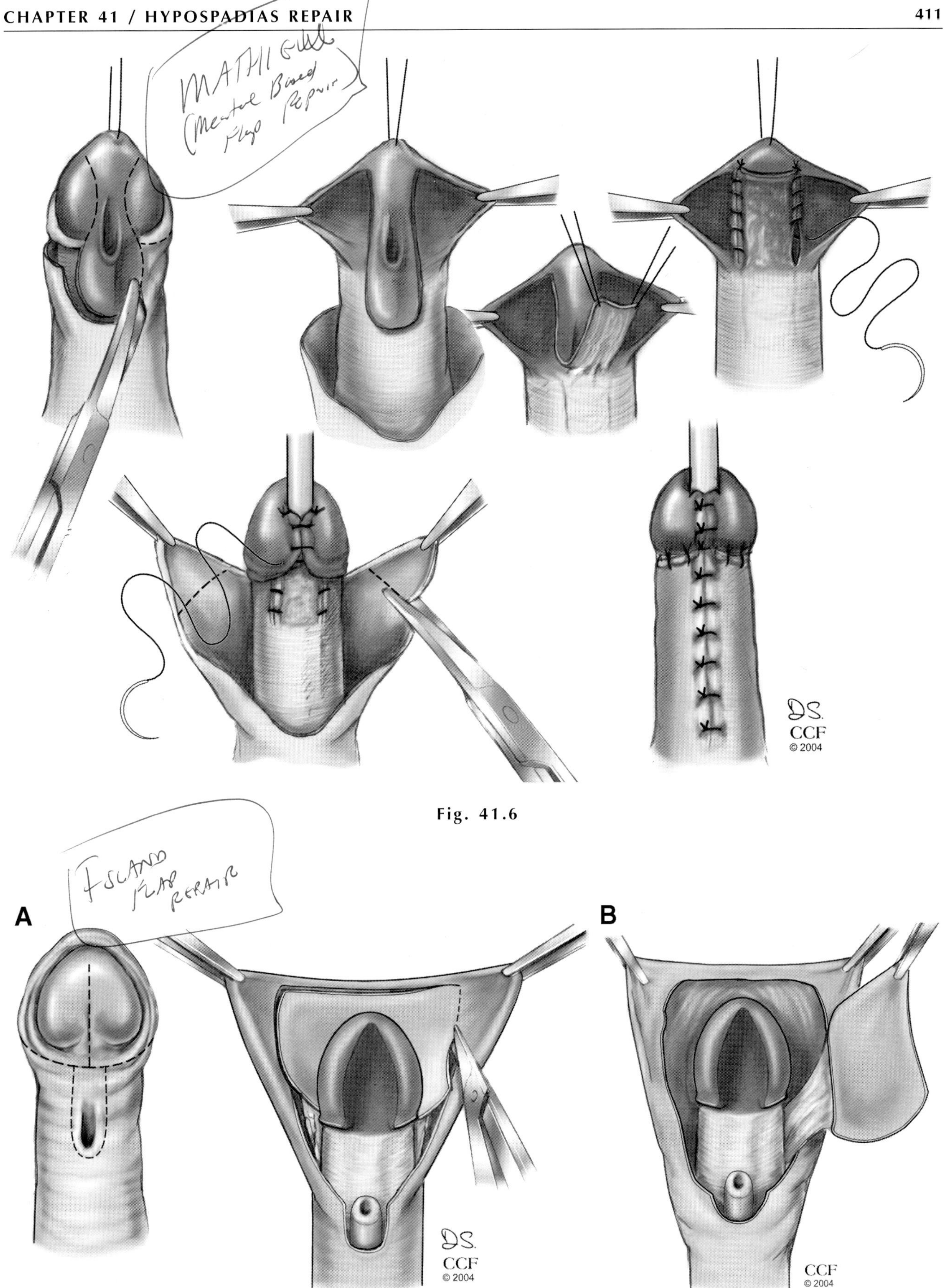


Fig. 41.6

Fig. 41.7

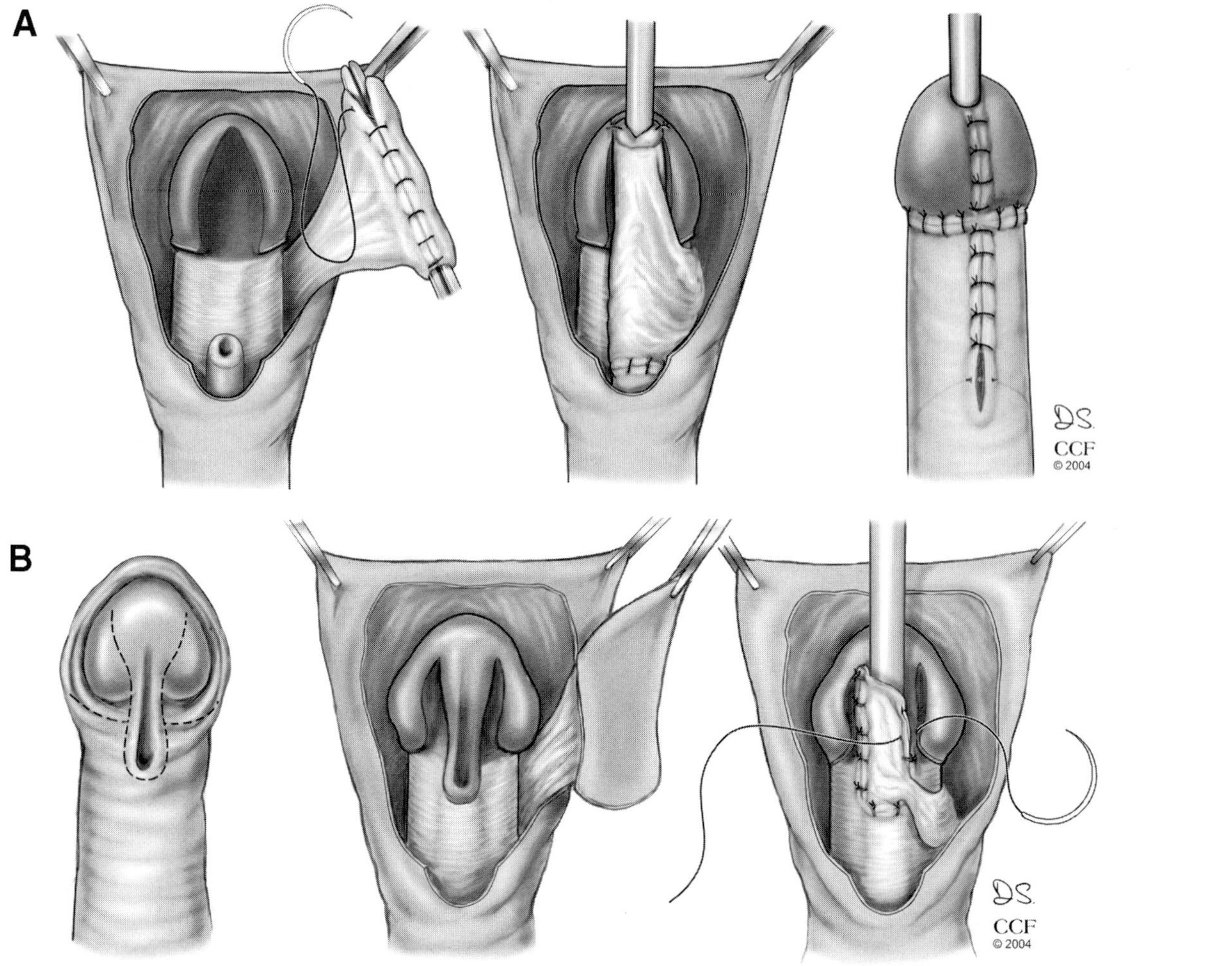

Fig. 41.8

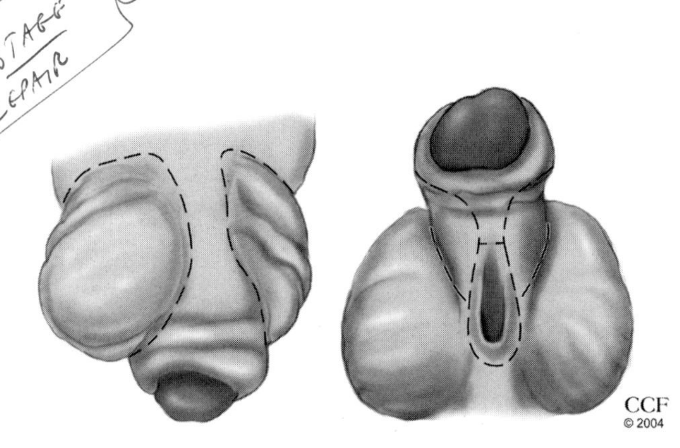


Fig. 41.9

this incision is brought along the urethral plate and proximal to the meatus. A second circumcision incision is brought across the urethral plate. An orthoplasty is performed as previously described.

A dorsal incision is made in the dorsal hood and secured to the dorsal midline of the mucosal skirt skin (Fig. 41.10). The flaps created are brought around for a ventral skin closure. No tissue is excised, and redundant skin is left ventrally to be used for the second-stage urethroplasty. The hemiscrota are mobilized off the proximal urethra and dropped down to a normal location. The various skin flaps are then reapproximated with chromic suture. In the ventral midline, some of the sutures also grasp the tunix of the corporal septum to fix the neourethral plate. The mucosal skirt and glans may be left intact, as shown. If the glans is very small, it may be incised in the midline and the skin flaps placed in the gap to widen the glans for tubularization at the second stage.

At the second stage a simple tubularization urethroplasty is performed (Fig. 41.11). If the glans was left intact at the first stage, then a TIP is performed in the mucosal skirt and glans. The urethroplasty should be covered with a local deepithelialized skin flap and/or a tunica vaginalis flap, prior to skin closure. The catheter is left for 10–14 d.

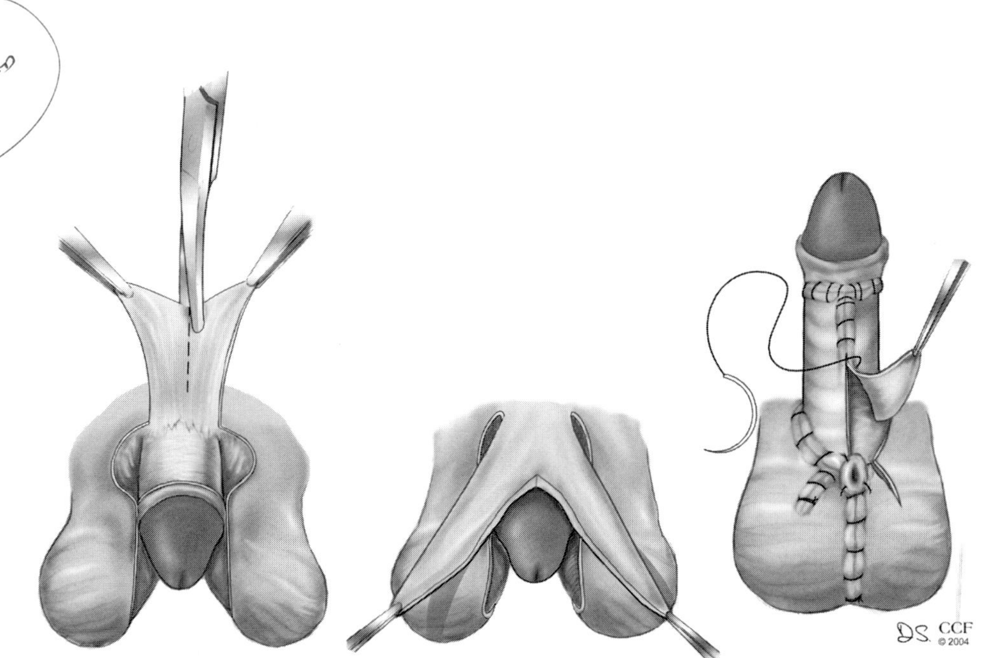


Fig. 41.10

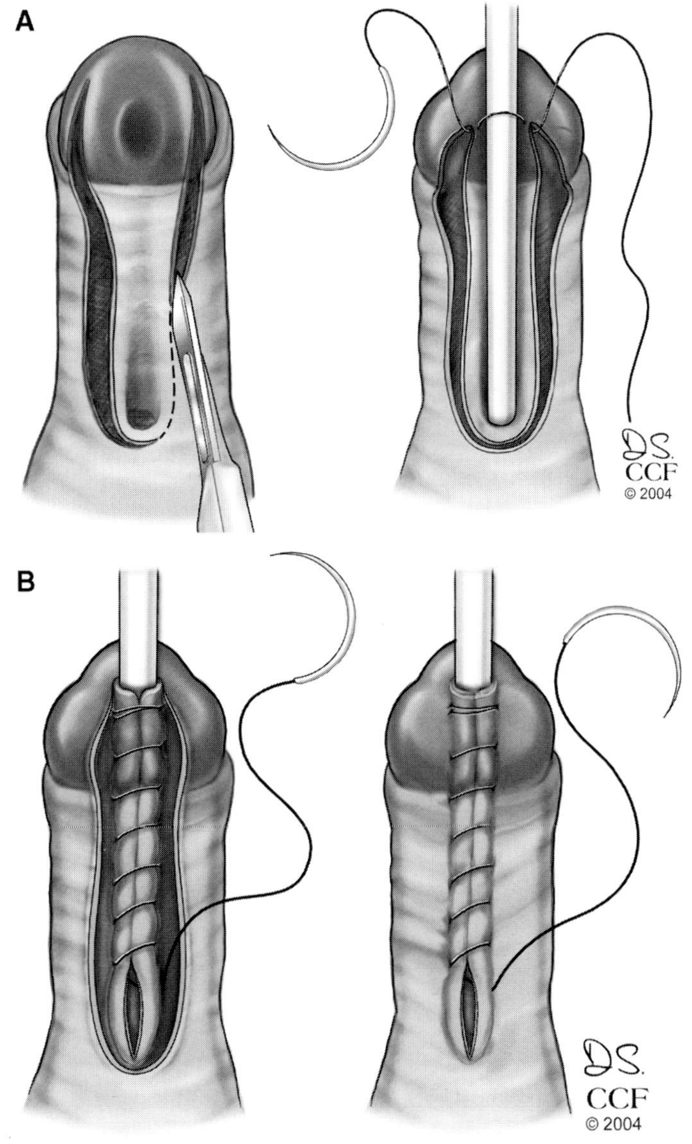


Fig. 41.11

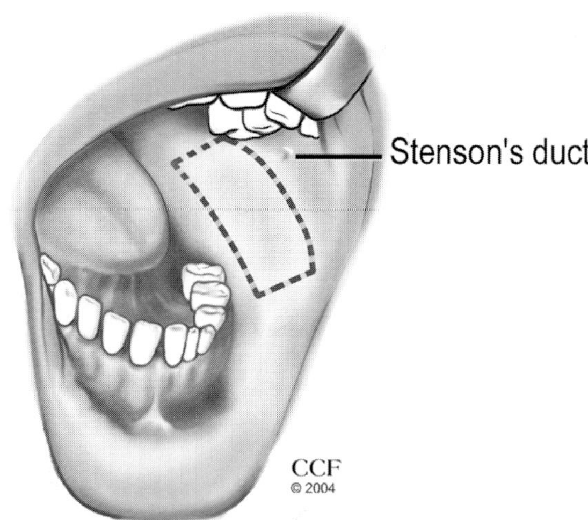


Fig. 41.12

In re-do hypospadias repairs, a free graft may be necessary for urethral reconstruction due to inadequate residual skin following previous repairs (Fig. 41.12). The best material for free grafting is buccal mucosa. A rectangular graft is taken from the inner cheek, avoiding Stensen's duct. It may be extended to the inner lip, if necessary. The donor site need not be closed. The graft is defatted and used as an onlay or tube graft. As with flaps, a tube graft has a higher complication rate than an onlay. In cases where a long length of urethra needs to be replaced and extensive scarring is present, a two-stage repair should be considered. In the first stage the scarred urethra is excised, the glans split, and the buccal graft laid on the penile ventrum and into the glans cleft. It is then tubularized and covered with a tunica vaginalis flap at the second stage.

## POSTOPERATIVE CARE

Patients are generally able to go home on the day of surgery. The catheter is removed 7–14 d later, depending on the extent of the repair. Complications include meatal stenosis, urethrocutaneous fistula, stricture, and urethral diverticulum. The reoperation rate is less than 5% for distal hypospadias repairs and as high as 20–30% for severe degrees of hypospadias.

## SUGGESTED READINGS

1. Baskin LS, Duckett JW, Ueoka K, Seibold J, Snyder HM. Changing concepts of hypospadias curvature lead to more onlay island flap procedures. J Urol 151:91–196, 1994.
2. Belman AB. De-epithelialized skin flap coverage in hypospadias repair. J Urol 140:273–1276, 1988.
3. Churchill BM, Van Savage JG, Khoury AE, McLorie GA. The dartos flap as an adjunct in preventing urethrocutaneous fistulas in repeat hypospadias surgery. J Urol 156:2047–2049, 1996.
4. Duckett JW. MAGPI (meatoplasty and glanuloplasty): a procedure for subcoronal hypospadias. Urol Clin North Am 8:513–520, 1981.
5. Duckett JW. Transverse preputial island flap technique for hypospadias repair. Urol Clin North Am 8:503–511, 1981.
6. Ross J, Kay R. Use of a deepithelialized skin flap in hypospadias repairs accomplished by tubularization of the incised urethral plate. Urology 50:110–112, 1997.
7. Snodgrass W. Tubularized, incised plate urethroplasty for distal hypospadias. J Urol 151:464, 465, 1994.

# 42 Malignancies of the Penis and Urethra

*Mark J. Noble*

## PENECTOMY AND PARTIAL PENECTOMY

### Introduction

Carcinoma of the penis is an uncommon malignancy in the United States. It accounts for less than 1% of all male cancers in America, but it accounts for 10–20% of male malignancies in countries with poor genital hygiene or where neonatal circumcision is rare *(1,2)*. This circumstantial evidence reinforces a belief that neonatal circumcision is protective for the development of squamous cell carcinoma of the penis, and indeed, reports of this disorder in males who were circumcised during the neonatal period are rare. Over the past 20 yr, however, more reports have surfaced indicating that penile cancer is not fully prevented by neonatal circumcision, although its risk is reduced by a factor of between 3.0 and 3.2 *(3,4)*. Other factors that contribute to an increased risk of carcinoma of the penis include smoking (risk increased by factor of 2.8), longstanding phimosis (3.5), chronic balanitis or penile rash or tear (3.9–9.4), a history of human papilloma virus (HPV) infection (5.9), and a history of multiple sexual partners (2.8) *(3,5)*. Clearly, some risk factors overlap with the absence of neonatal circumcision. For example, phimosis and chronic balanitis are virtually never seen in circumcised males, and circumcision provides at least some protection against infection by sexually transmitted diseases, including HPV *(6,7)*.

Aegina, in the seventh century AD, is credited with performing the first penile resection for cancer *(8)*. In 1761, Valsalva completed a partial penectomy utilizing needle and thread to individually ligate vessels, while Cabade achieved successful penectomy with perineal urethrostomy in 1878 *(8)*. A method for combined resection of the penis and inguinal lymph nodes *en bloc* was reported by Hugh Hampton Young in 1931 *(9)*. Over the past 25 yr, carcinoma of the penis has been managed with a variety of procedures depending on a patient's specific clinical circumstance, with variations in the treatment of inguinal lymph nodes as well as the primary tumor. The goal has been to minimize morbidity while at the same time providing an acceptable cure rate. These methods with their indications are summarized here.

### Management of the Primary Penile Lesion

Cancers of the penis may be of any cell type found on the skin, just as is seen elsewhere on the body. By far the most common type of penile cancer is squamous cell carcinoma, which in a series by Banon Perez and coworkers accounted for 82% of those seen *(10)*. Verrucous carcinoma was next most common at 14%, with rare cases of basal cell carcinoma, melanoma, and metastatic lesions also being noted. Because verrucous carcinoma is really a variant of squamous cell carcinoma (it is usually a less aggressive variant), some investigators combine such patients with all experiencing squamous cell carcinoma *(11)*. Sarcoma (epitheliod type) has been quite rarely reported; in most instances it was originally misdiagnosed as Peyronie's disease *(12–15)*. Even more uncommon is penile angiosarcoma, as described by Williams *(16)*. One unusual case of primary adenocarcinoma of the penis has been noted by Van Savage and Carson *(17)*. In their paper, they indicate that a diligent search failed to reveal another primary tumor.

Generally, if adenocarcinoma of the penis is found, urethral origin or a metastatic lesion from the prostate or another organ site should be suspected. In fact, the most common metastatic solid tumor to the penis is prostate cancer, and in such cases the malignancy has a generally poor prognosis and behaves agressively *(18–20)*. Bladder cancer can very rarely metastasize directly to the penis, but most commonly any penile involvement due to bladder cancer results from tumor arising secondarily in the urethra (multifocality) rather than as a manifestation of metastatic spread *(21)*. Systemic cancer, such as lymphoma, can involve various organs including the penis *(22)*. When systemic or metastatic cancer to the penis

From: *Operative Urology at the Cleveland Clinic*
Edited by: A. Novick et al. © Humana Press Inc., Totowa, NJ

occurs, a common symptom can be severe penile pain; in these instances, a penectomy may be needed for palliation despite the usually poor overall outcome *(23,24)*.

Partial or total penectomy is rarely needed in cases of urethral cancer arising as part of the spectrum of bladder cancer; most often urethrectomy suffices, either in conjunction with cystectomy or as a separate procedure. When carcinoma of the anterior urethra presents as a separate entity (from bladder cancer), its location and aggressiveness may preclude local excision, or even penectomy with perineal urethrostomy, and a radical cystectomy may be necessary to completely excise the malignancy.

For squamous cell carcinoma of the prepuce, a circumcision may be the only therapy that is required for both diagnosis and cure. One should be attentive to the proximity of the surgical margin, however, because recurrent tumor has been reported in postcircumcision scar tissue *(25)*. When a cancer arises on the glans or penile shaft, local treatment such as irradiation, laser, 5-fluorouracil cream, or simple excision can be successful for low-grade, superficial lesions, but there is a high recurrence rate (≥40%) for those tumors that are invasive or poorly differentiated *(26–30)*. Thus, if local therapy is contemplated, a biopsy to determine cellular grade and stage is imperative *(31)*. One might think that tumor recurrence following organ-sparing therapy is still salvageable with penile amputation, but in cases where the tumor is of an aggressive cell type, one risks metastatic spread and eventual death by postponing an amputation *(32)*. Also, when radiation has been used, tissue healing can be compromised after amputation. When partial or total penectomy is employed as primary therapy for squamous cell carcinoma, local recurrence rates are low, usually less than 10% *(33–35)*. A 2–3 cm margin of normal tissue is required to minimize the likelihood of local recurrence.

Partial penectomy, when it does not compromise local control of the cancer, enables a better cosmetic result and permits the patient to stand for micturition, as he can usually direct his urinary stream. There is also the possibility for preservation of sexual function, although few reports actually document this *(36)*. To regain length, a pedicle graft with use of a penile prosthesis is generally needed for full reconstruction.

## Management of Regional Lymph Nodes

Regional lymphadenectomy for penile cancer remains a very controversial subject *(36)*. Some groups, such as Heyns and associates, recommend that regional nodes be resected only when grossly involved with cancer, arguing that lymphadenectomy fails to influence long-term survival and the surgical complications and morbidity are high from this additional procedure *(37)*. Other studies such as the report by Fraley et al. suggest that removal of micrometastases to inguinal lymph nodes has therapeutic benefit *(38)*. Few would argue with the premise that metastatic spread of cancer to regional lymph nodes has great prognostic significance (patients with positive lymph nodes have a much-reduced long-term survival, well under 50% at 5 yr, whereas those without positive lymph nodes experience 80–100% 5-yr survival) *(39)*.

Many patients present initially with clinically palpable inguinal nodes, but lymphadenopathy is often the result of the local and regional inflammatory reaction associated with the cancer. For this reason, some recommend removal of the primary lesion (penectomy or partial penectomy, as required) with postoperative treatment for 4–6 wk using a broad-spectrum antibiotic, such as doxycycline *(36)*. If the lymphadenopathy persists, then one can proceed with regional lymph node dissection. Some advocate sentinel lymph node biopsy in patients with nonpalpable inguinal nodes, reserving complete, regional lymphadenectomy for those with positive sentinel biopsies; others maintain that false negatives can be misleading in some of these cases and that a complete node dissection, despite considerable morbidity, is required *(34,35,40,41)*. Morbidity is the rule rather than the exception following ileo-inguinal lymphadenectomy *(42,43)*. Short-term complications include wound infection (15–25%) and sloughing of skin (requiring secondary skin grafting or at least delaying wound closure). Long-term complications include chronic lower extremity lymphedema (30–40%) and increased susceptibility to lymphangitis for the affected extremity (or extremities).

Some studies report that the incidence of chronic lower extremity edema is significantly lowered by sparing the saphenous vein; one must make this decision intraoperatively, but in the absence of bulky lymph node metastases, it is usually feasible from a technical perspective *(42)*. If a patient is not treated initially with node dissection, or if there is a recurrent lesion after node dissection, the local area can be treated with radiation therapy with or without surgery. This can sometimes be used to at least palliate bulky lymph node metastases *(44)*. It is important to provide some method for local control of metastatic lymph nodes because chemotherapy has been found to be only marginally effective for this purpose *(45)*.

## Technique

### Partial Penectomy

To minimize blood loss, a tourniquet is created by wrapping a Penrose drain tightly around the base of the penis, temporarily securing it with a medium curved clamp

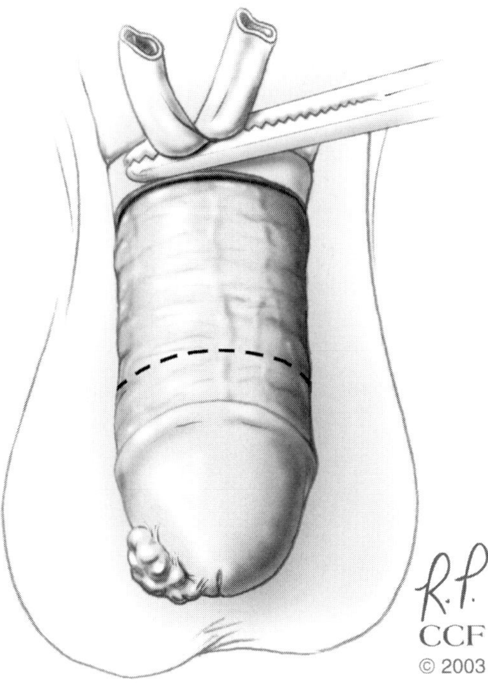


Fig. 42.1

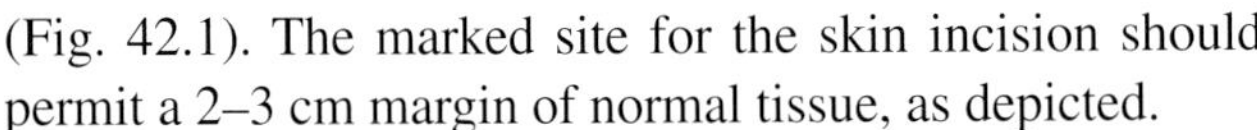

(Fig. 42.1). The marked site for the skin incision should permit a 2–3 cm margin of normal tissue, as depicted.

The lesion may be ulcerated or fungating and may be difficult to sterilize with antiseptic prep solution; in such circumstance it can be covered by securing a sponge around the distal penis with a large silk or an umbilical tape tie (Fig. 42.2). An incision is circumscribed around the penis and is carried down to Buck's fascia. The neurovascular bundle is ligated proximally and distally and divided sharply.

The urethra can be mobilized ventrally to permit a longer stump to facilitate spatulation and creation of a secure urethrostomy (Fig. 42.3). The corpora cavernosa (bilaterally) and then the corpus spongiosum and urethra are divided.

Each corpus cavernosum is closed with running or interrupted suture (Fig. 42.4). One can use either 2-0 or 3-0 monofilament polypropylene nonabsorbable suture with the knots inverted, or one can employ 1-0 or 2-0 polyglycolic acid absorbable suture for this closure. After closure of the corpora, it is important to temporarily release the tourniquet at the base of the penis to be certain these sutures have achieved adequate hemostasis before closure of the skin.

Skin is then closed over the stump with absorbable suture such as 3-0 chromic, and the spatulated urethral neo-meatus is matured to the skin edges with 4-0 chromic suture (Fig. 42.5). A Foley catheter is left in place (not shown) until edema adequately resolves and

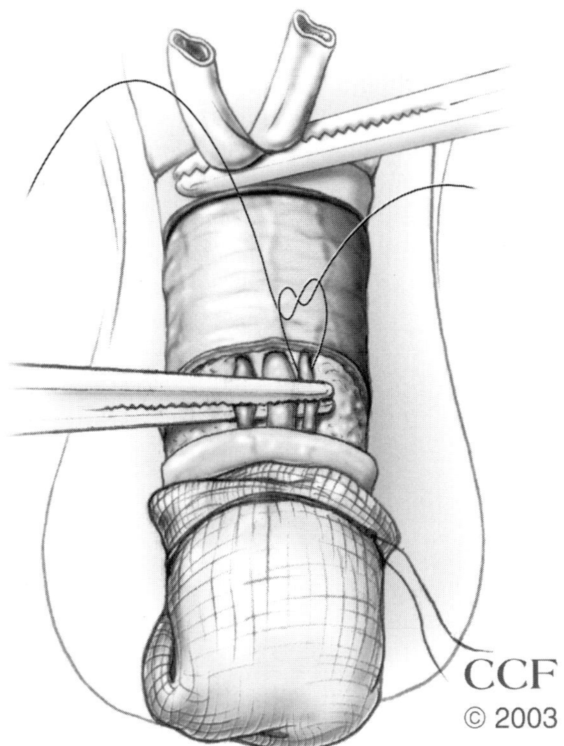


Fig. 42.2

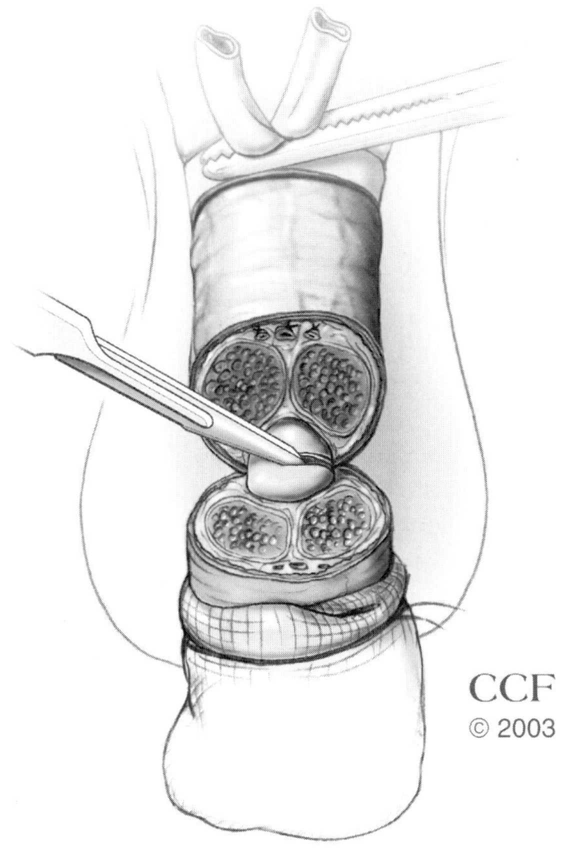


Fig. 42.3

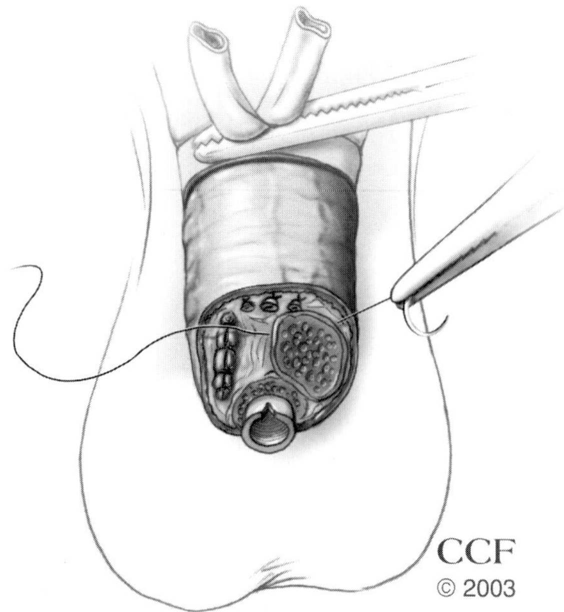


Fig. 42.4

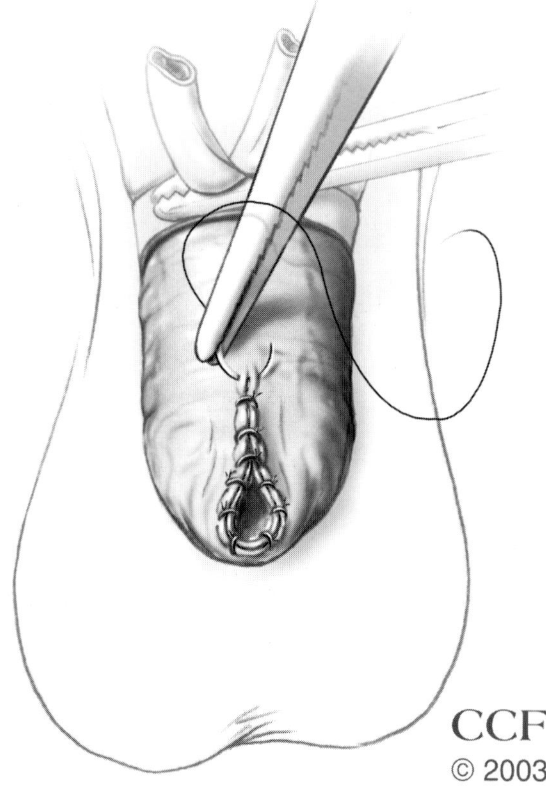


Fig. 42.5

epithelialization is sufficient to enable the patient to begin voiding (usually 3–5 d postoperatively).

## Total Penectomy

An invasive malignancy requiring total penectomy is depicted in Fig. 42.6.

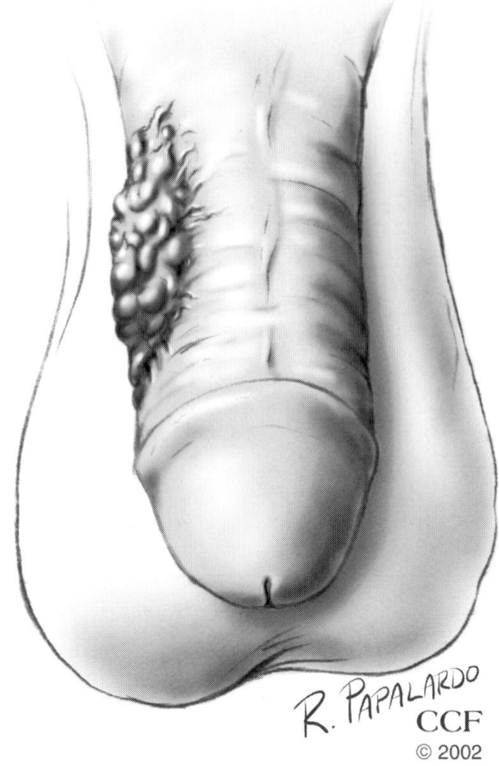


Fig. 42.6

The lesion is covered with a gauze sponge secured with a heavy silk tie or an umbilical tape, as for partial penectomy, to exclude it from the operative field (Fig. 42.7). The skin incision is marked circumferentially around the base of the penis and extending in the midline in both the scrotal and suprapubic direction, as shown.

After incising the skin and subcutaneous tissues, the urethra is dissected from the corpora cavernosa, mobilized by means of traction with a thin Penrose drain, and divided sharply (Fig. 42.8). It is then mobilized proximally toward the urogenital diaphragm.

The dorsal neurovascular bundle is ligated proximally and distally and divided sharply (Fig. 42.9). The penectomy is completed by dividing the corpora cavernosa sharply as proximally as possible (portions of the crura can be freed if necessary) and by dividing any remaining soft tissue at this point.

Each corpus is securely closed with running or interrupted 2-0 polypropylene suture (or polyglycolic acid suture, if preferred) (Fig. 42.10). It is important to obtain good hemostasis at this juncture.

A vertical incision is made in the perineum, and the bulbocavernosus muscles are divided in the midline (Fig. 42.11).

The urethra is mobilized (Fig. 42.12A) and a vertical midline incision created along its length (Fig. 42.12B, inset). This can be facilitated by temporarily placing a

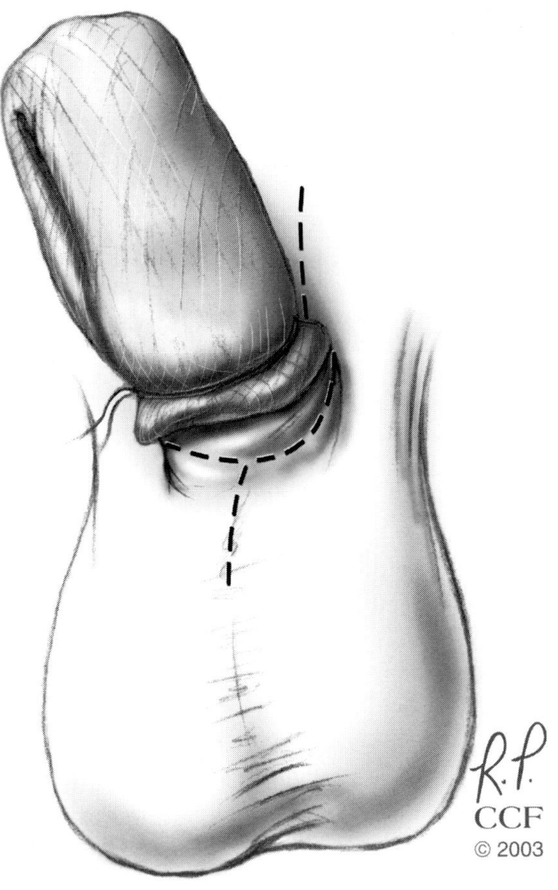


Fig. 42.7

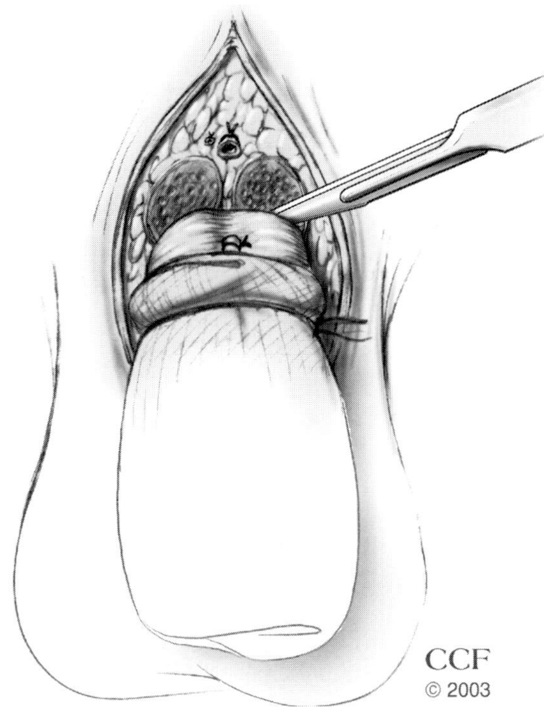


Fig. 42.9

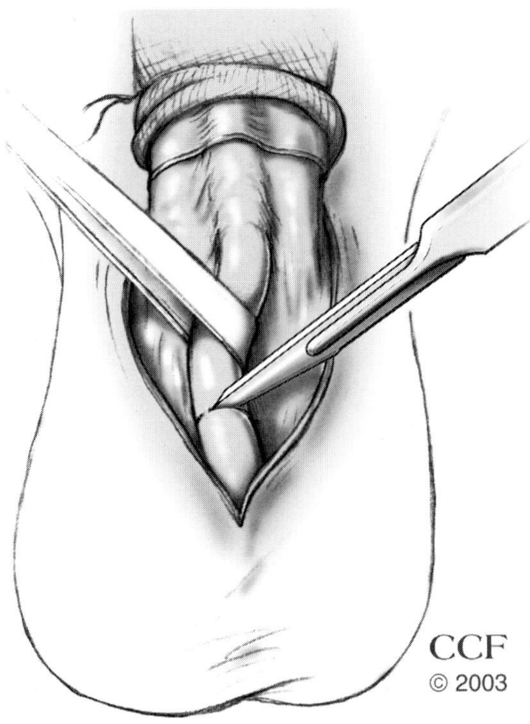


Fig. 42.8

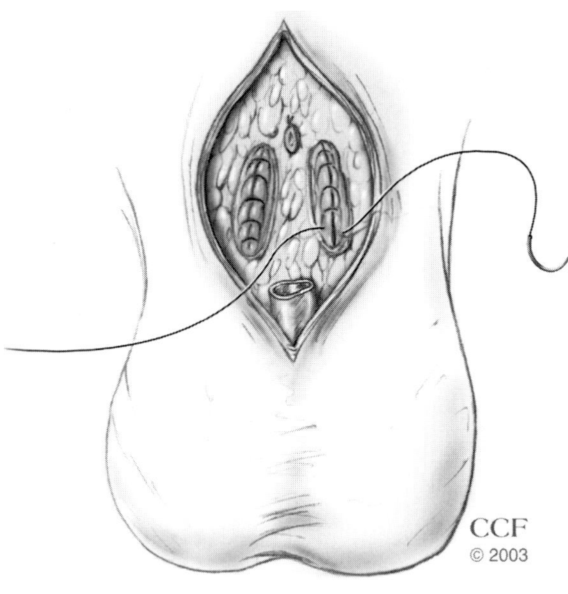


Fig. 42.10

metal sound through the end of the urethral stump. Rather than mobilize the remaining distal urethral stump in order to bring it into the perineal incision for an end cutaneous urethrostomy, blood supply is better preserved if a "loop" cutaneous urethrostomy (analogous to a loop ileostomy) is fashioned. This minimizes any tendency for the urethral meatus to develop stenosis.

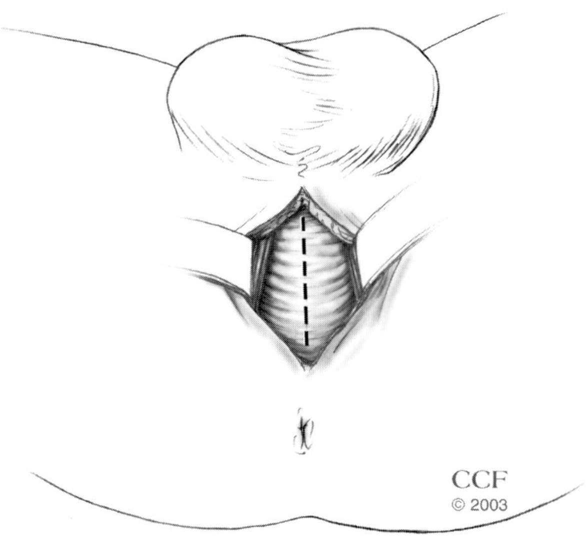


Fig. 42.11

The edges of the urethrostomy are matured to the closed perineal incision with absorbable suture of suitable size (Fig. 42.13). The distal end of the urethra (not shown) is closed with absorbable suture. The scrotum is closed with running or interrupted absorbable suture in one or two layers. A Foley catheter is placed through the urethrostomy until sufficient maturation occurs to permit voiding (usually 3–5 d).

# INGUINAL LYMPHADENECTOMY

## Introduction

Surgical removal of inguinal lymph nodes is usually done in conjunction with pelvic lymphadenectomy (ileo-inguinal lymphadenectomy) in order to remove any regional nodes with metastases in patients with carcinoma of the penis. It is undetermined if lymph node dissection is of therapeutic benefit, but the presence or absence of cancer in inguinal and/or pelvic lymph nodes certainly provides prognostic information and may aid in the decision to consider additional treatment (radiation and/or chemotherapy) *(46)*. Because superficial lymph node metastases nearly always precede deep (pelvic) metastatic spread, some surgeons only perform pelvic lymphadenectomy in patients with positive inguinal lymph nodes, and others are even more selective, removing the "sentinel node" in patients without palpably enlarged inguinal lymph nodes, and only completing a full inguinal lymphadenectomy in those patients with sentinel node positivity *(40)*. The method for complete inguinal lymphadenectomy, illustrated below, is based on several techniques that spare the saphenous vein where possible *(42,47,48)*. Details regarding pelvic node dissection may be found in the chapters on radical prostatectomy and radical cystectomy.

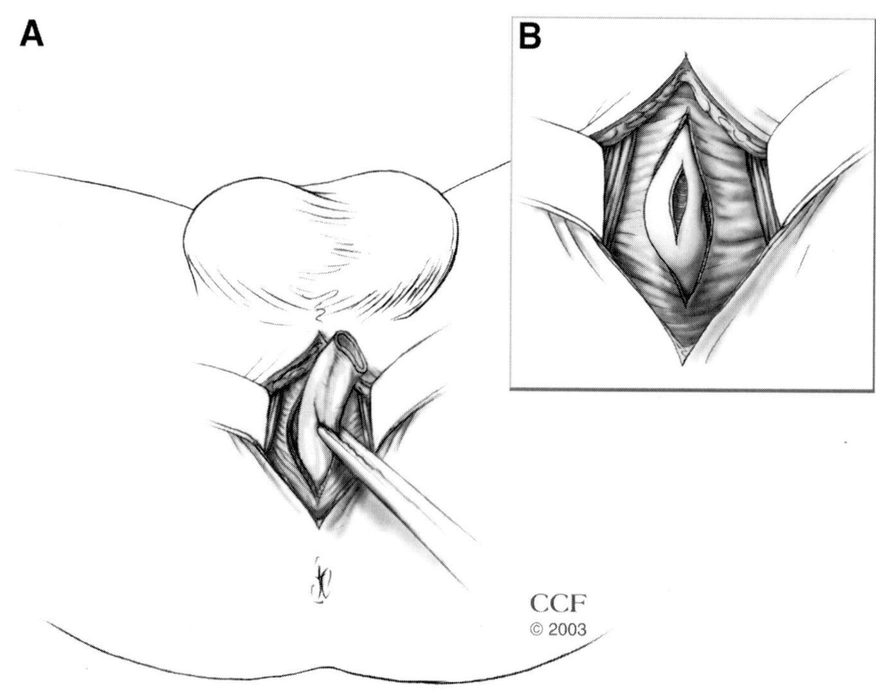


Fig. 42.12

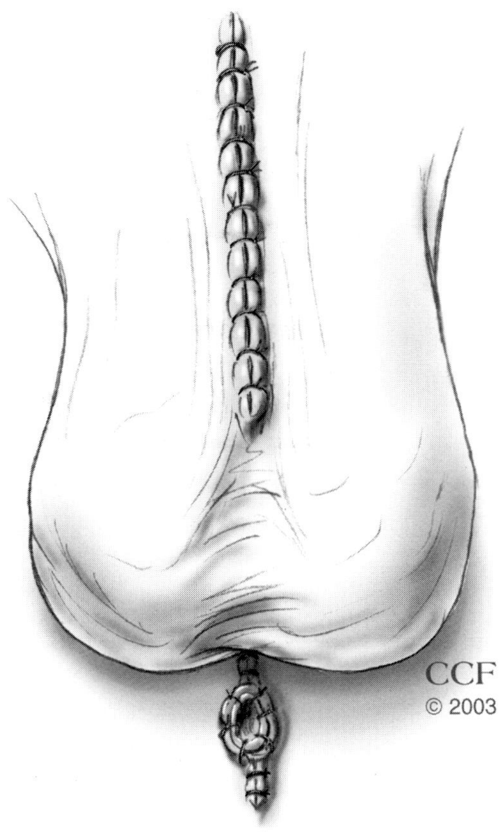


Fig. 42.13

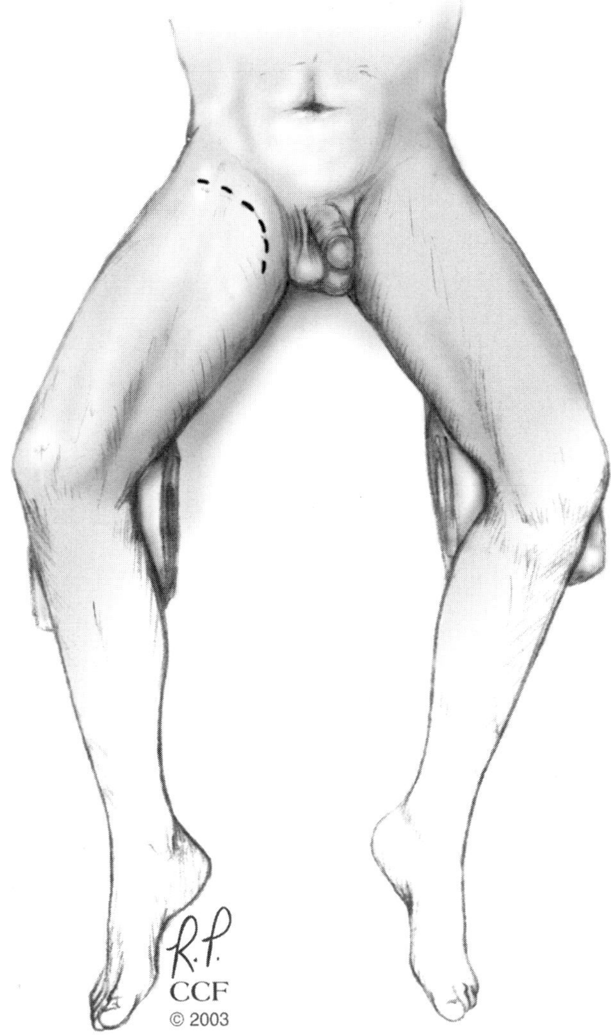


Fig. 42.14

## Surgical Technique

The patient is placed in a modified "frog-leg" position with the legs externally rotated (Fig. 42.14). This aids in exposure and enables better dissection of all adipose and lymphatic tissue from the femoral triangle. A shallow, inverted U-shaped incision can be used. Alternatively, an oblique incision in a skin crease, or even a vertical incision midway along the inguinal ligament, can be used. If the incision is transverse, it should be approx 3 cm below the inguinal ligament.

Skin flaps are created with preservation of a 3- to 4-mm layer of subcutaneum under the skin (Fig. 42.15). This is most easily achieved by dissecting just under Camper's fascia as the skin edge is elevated with skin hooks. This extra fat under the skin flaps will help prevent flap necrosis by preserving better blood supply. Note the demarcation of the adipose and lymph node tissue to be removed; the specimen will have the approximate shape of a quadrilateral with dimensions, as indicated.

One may start either laterally or medially. The adipose and lymphatic tissue is defined by first incising at one edge down to the fascia overlying the thigh muscles (Fig. 42.16). One then dissects and mobilizes beneath the specimen with blunt and sharp technique while avoiding injury to landmarks such as the femoral vessels and nerve. The fascia lata will come out intact under the specimen (except where it is freed around the saphenous vein). The saphenous vein may be followed up to its window of entry into the femoral vein; all lymphatic tissue in the femoral triangle should be removed, thus exposing the femoral vein and artery. Proximal and distal lymphatic communications with the *en bloc* specimen should be ligated or clipped. Classically, the saphenous vein is ligated and a portion removed with the specimen. However, preservation of the saphenous vein (inset) lowers postoperative edema with little likelihood of compromising the lymphadenectomy with respect to prognostic information or even efficacy at removal of micrometastases. One continues to sweep tissue up and to the opposite side. The upper edge of the dissection will be the inguinal ligament, while the lower edge will be approx 15 cm inferior to it. If the saphenous vein cannot be preserved due to technical

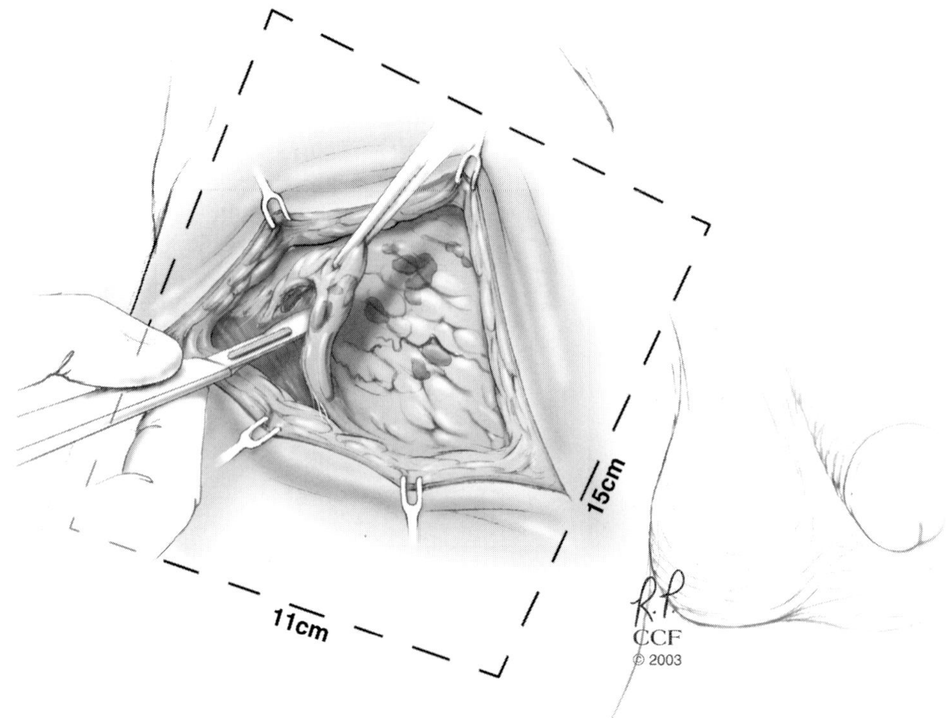


Fig. 42.15

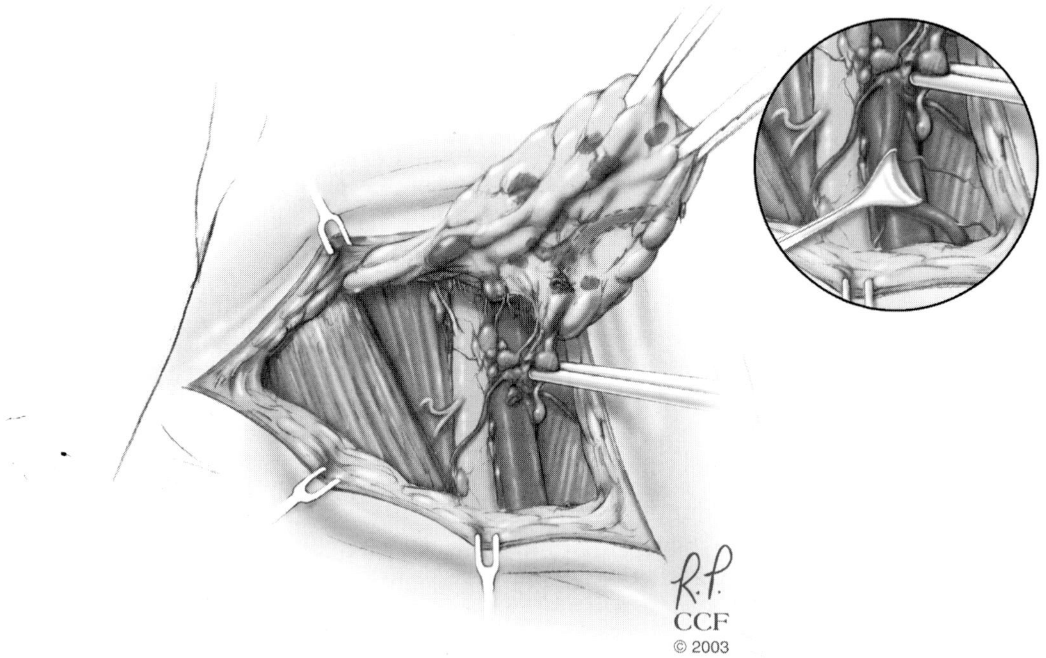


Fig. 42.16

issues, then it must be securely ligated at the proximal and distal limits of the lymphadenectomy quadrilateral; it would not be easy to control were it to retract into its junction with the common femoral vein.

After removal of the specimen, the sartorius muscle is freed from its insertion on the pelvis and crossed over medially to cover and protect the femoral vessels (Fig. 42.17). The incision is carefully closed in layers, using either a 2-0 or a 3-0 polypropylene or polyglycolic acid suture for the subcutaneum and monofilament nylon, subcuticular polyglycolic acid, or skin staples to approximate the skin. An advantage of staples or interrupted

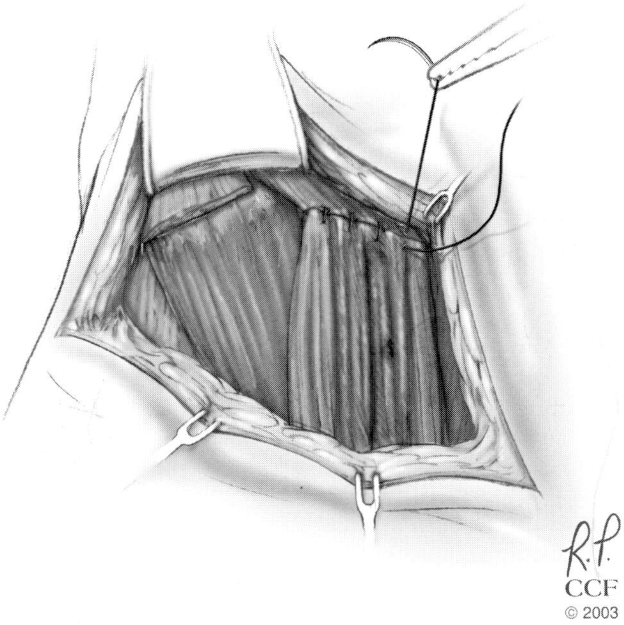


Fig. 42.17

nonabsorbable suture for the skin can be seen if part of the skin edge becomes necrotic; only those sutures or staples in the affected region need be removed, and the remainder of the incision will remain approximated until healed. One or two suction drains in the subcutaneum will help prevent hematoma or seroma, which could lead to infection or other compromise to flap integrity.

## URETHRECTOMY

Total urethrectomy implies removal of the entire urethra in the context of treatment for bladder malignancy in the male patient. Primary urethral carcinoma (in the absence of bladder cancer) is normally treated with partial or total penectomy with or without a cystectomy or, in very limited circumstances, a local resection of the tumor without urethrectomy. Thus, this discussion will be limited to application of urethrectomy to the management of carcinoma of the bladder.

Until 1994, female urethrectomy was always performed as part of cystectomy *(49)*. After a report in 1994 describing the creation of an orthotopic neobladder in a female with good outcome, including urinary continence, salvage of part of the urethra or part of the bladder neck plus urethra has become more common for select cases (where these areas are not involved with foci of bladder cancer or carcinoma *in situ*) *(49–52)*. But in cases of bladder cancer (in females) not meeting appropriate criteria, urethrectomy is performed along with cystectomy and will not be discussed further in this section.

Patients with bladder cancer who do not have a urethrectomy performed at the time of cystectomy have a cumulative risk of developing urethral carcinoma ranging from 3.5 to 22% *(53–61)*. Most series place the risk at roughly 10%, but patients considered at high risk for recurrence in the urethral remnant have already undergone combined cystectomy and urethrectomy in those series, while a study indicating a 22% risk reviewed a group of patients who underwent cystectomy only, no matter what risk factors for urethral recurrence existed. This difference explains, in part, the variation of recurrence risk between various reports. For example, an autopsy study published in 1960 found that 18% of patients dying of carcinoma of the bladder had simultaneous carcinoma *in situ* of the urethra *(62)*.

There is some added operative morbidity associated with performance of urethrectomy at the time of cystectomy *(54)*. Excessive bleeding is rare but certainly can occur. Perineal wound infection occurs in 5–10% of cases. An additional 30–90 min of additional operative time can be required on top of an already lengthy surgical procedure. Finally, total urethrectomy would preclude reconstruction with an orthotopic neobladder for all patients. Because it seems unwarranted for prophylactic (total) urethrectomy to be performed in all males undergoing cystectomy considering that the majority of patients would not be at risk for urethral recurrence, certain indications for urethrectomy at the time of cystectomy have evolved. These include (1) diffuse carcinoma *in situ* of the bladder mucosa, (2) multifocal carcinoma of the bladder, (3) a history of upper tract tumors (this is really another manifestation of multifocality), (4) involvement of the prostatic urethra, and (5) positive transected urethral margin by frozen or permanent section *(63–67)*. If a patient has an extremely poor prognosis or if he is older than 70 yr, many urologists would defer concurrent urethrectomy provided there is no tumor in the prostatic urethra or at the cut urethral margin *(54)*.

One should be clinically suspicious that a patient is experiencing a urethral tumor recurrence if he relates urethral bleeding, penile pain, inguinal lymphadenopathy, or perineal mass *(54,59)*. Unfortunately, some of these patients will not be curable at such presentation (invasive or metastatic disease implies a poor prognosis) *(64)*. Thus, if urethrectomy is deferred, it is important to follow those patients closely to be certain there is no cancer recurrence in the urethral remnant. Perhaps the best method for surveillance of these individuals is a urethral wash cytology every 6 mo; this has been found to be even more sensitive for detection of recurrent cancer than urethroscopy (*in situ* lesions are not always visible) *(68–70)*.

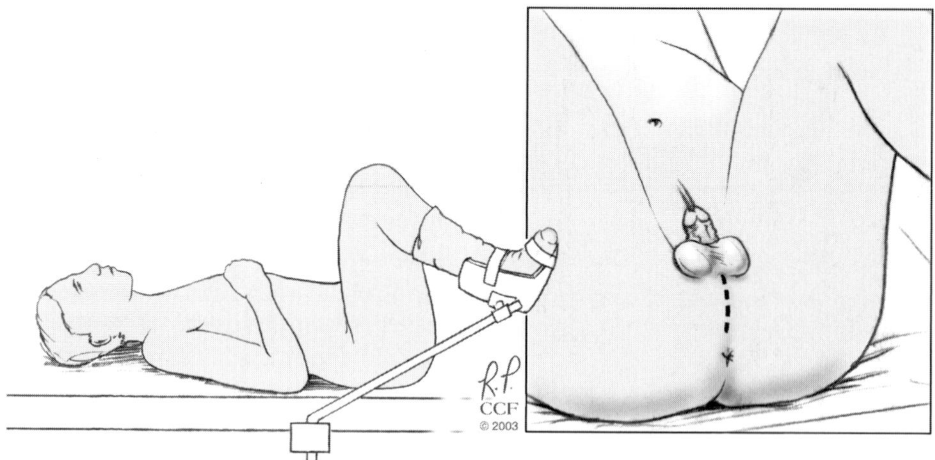


Fig. 42.18

Augmentation of cytology with marker detection such as fluorescent *in situ* hybridization analysis for chromosomal alterations should make the sensitivity even greater, as has been observed with bladder cytology *(71)*.

There are two methods for performing urethrectomy at the time of cystectomy. One can perform an *en bloc* cystectomy and urethrectomy, or one can perform the cystectomy first and then do the urethrectomy secondarily. The latter has the advantage of permitting good hemostasis in the pelvis prior to doing the urethrectomy. Also, one surgeon can perform the urethrectomy while another is constructing the urinary reservoir, thus saving some time. The former provides a theoretically better cancer operation, since there is less likelihood of spillage of tumor cells if there is no transection of the urethra during cystectomy *(53)*. One must say theoretically because no complete study exists describing any differences for either technique in the risk for pelvic or perineal recurrence of tumor *(54)*. The technique of urethrectomy (see below) is fairly standard *(72)*. Please note that it is important that the urethral meatus be excised as part of the specimen, as recurrences at the meatus have been reported *(73)*.

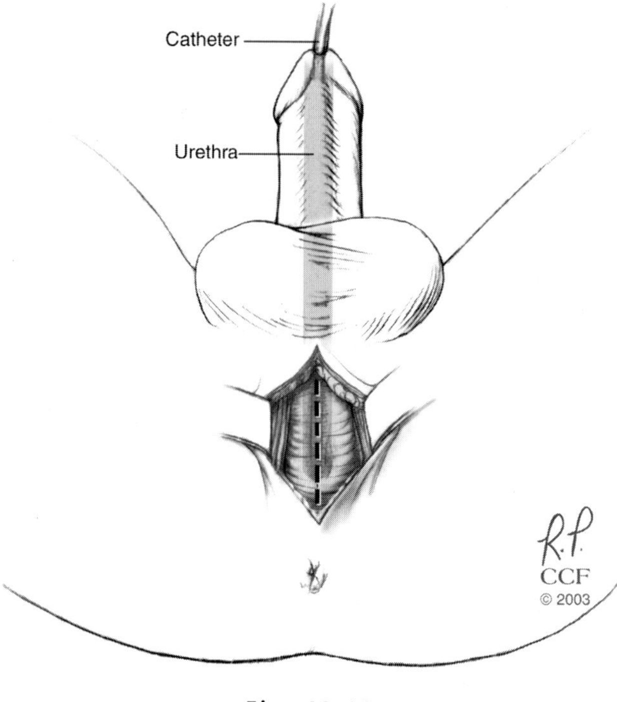


Fig. 42.19

## Surgical Technique

If urethrectomy alone is performed, the patient should be placed in an exaggerated lithotomy position (Fig. 42.18). This maximizes exposure of the perineal structures. If concurrent cystectomy is performed with urethrectomy (not illustrated), a semi-lithotomy position is preferable. In either circumstance, a midline (illustrated) or inverted U-shaped (not illustrated) perineal incision can be made.

A Foley catheter or male urethral sound is placed intraurethrally, and the incision is deepened over this (Fig. 42.19). The bulbocavernosus muscle is identified and incised in the midline and dissected free from the bulbar urethra on either side.

A window is created through Buck's fascia, between the urethra and the corpora cavernosa, using a right-angle clamp (Fig. 42.20).

A Penrose drain is passed dorsal to the urethra and enables the use of traction during dissection (Fig. 42.21). The urethra is mobilized distally by incising Buck's fascia dorsally on each side, as shown. There may be small tributary vessels supplying the urethra that require electrocautery, but major bleeding usually implies entry into

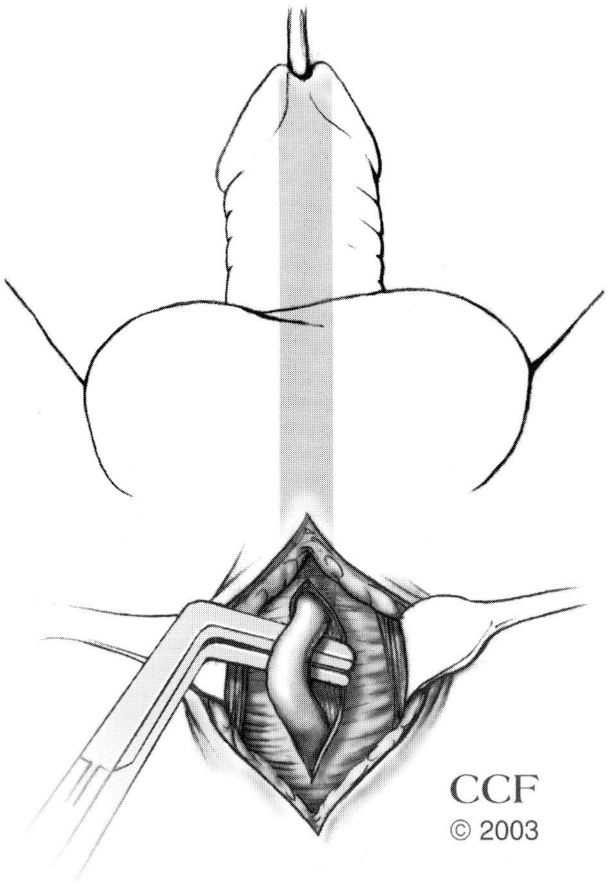

Fig. 42.20

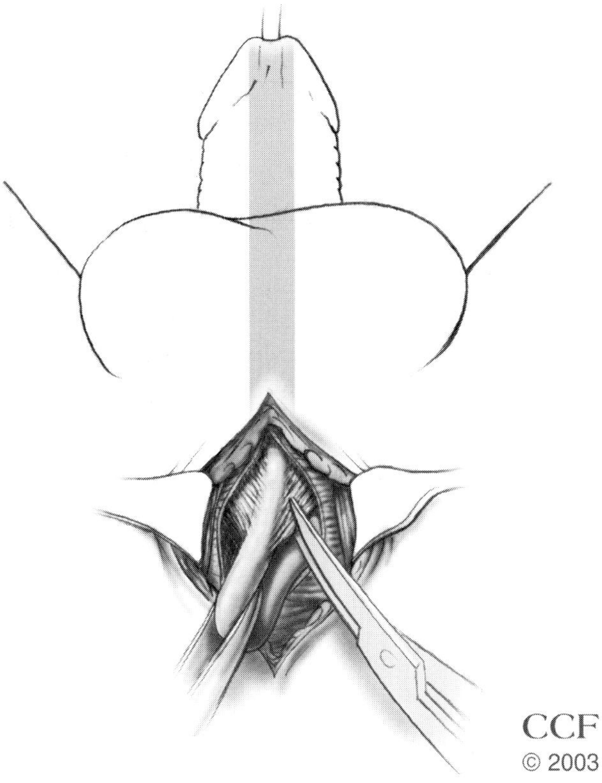

Fig. 42.21

either the corpus cavernosum or corpus spongiosum. Such entry usually requires suturing for control of bleeding.

Further distal dissection is performed, the glans penis is inverted, and the urethra is mobilized to the coronal sulcus (Fig. 42.22).

The penis is returned to its normal orientation. A traction suture may be placed in the glans if desired. A transverse incision is made at the proximal frenulum (Fig. 42.23A), and an umbilical tape or vessel loop is placed around the previously mobilized urethra (Fig. 42.23B). The urethral meatus is then circumscribed sharply, and this incision is connected vertically with the previously made transverse incision at the frenulum (Fig. 42.23B). The urethra is sharply dissected away from glanular tissue, with fine absorbable sutures used as needed to control glanular bleeding.

After the distal urethra is fully freed and brought out through the perineal incision, the glans is reconstructed first with an inner layer of absorbable suture (Fig. 42.24A), and then with a cutaneous layer of fine absorbable suture (Fig. 42.24B). Note the Penrose drain brought out through the proximal portion of the incision.

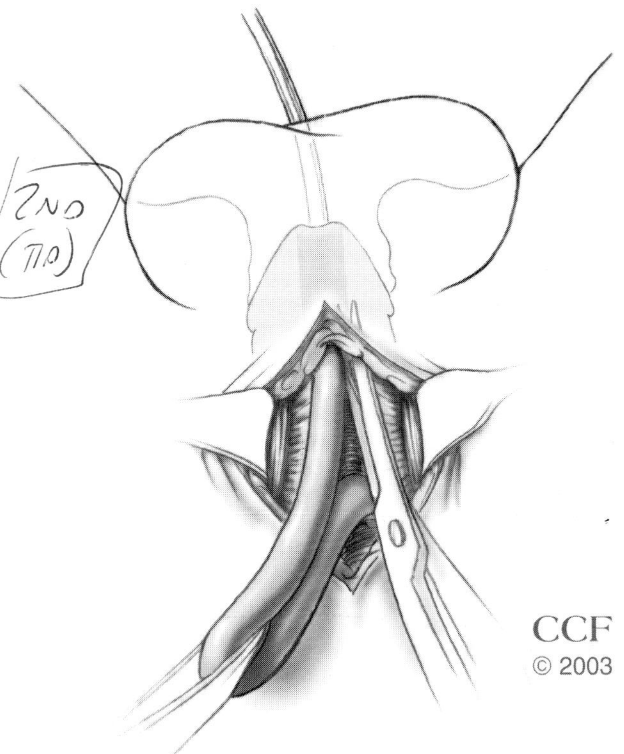


Fig. 42.22

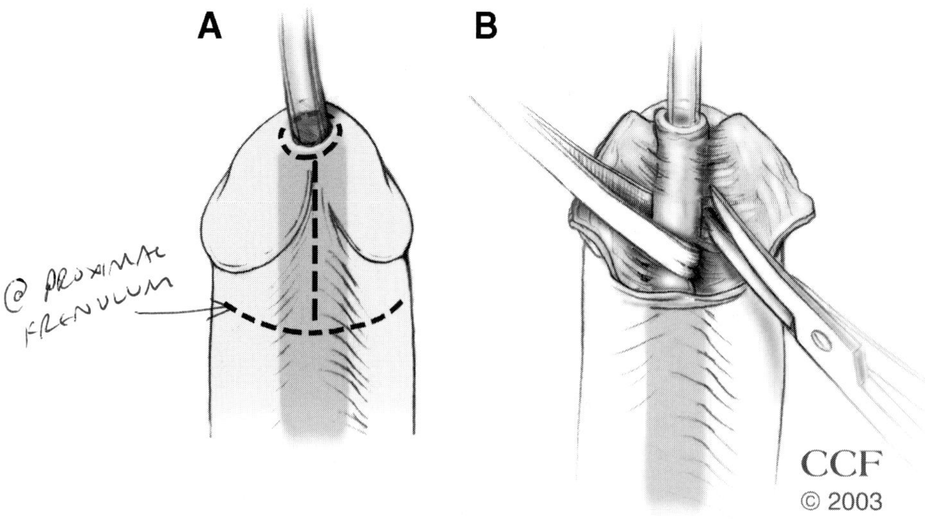


Fig. 42.23

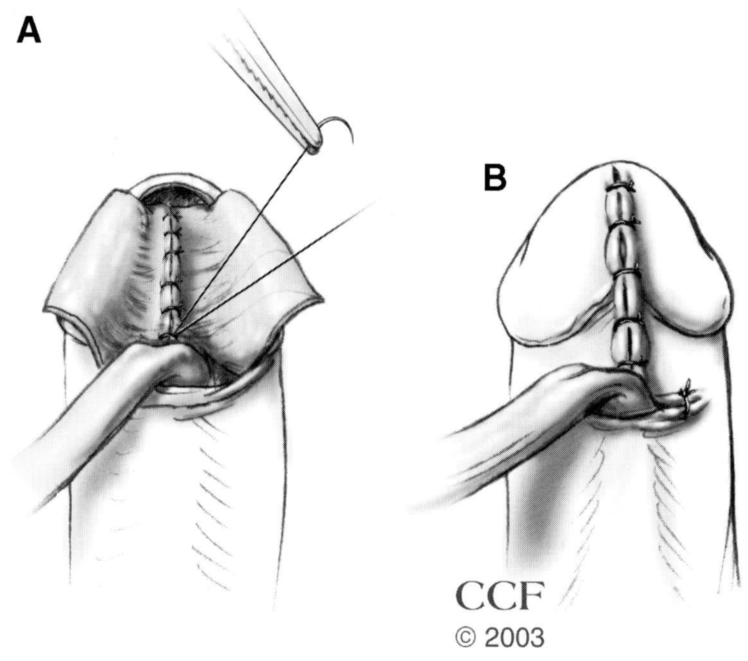


Fig. 42.24

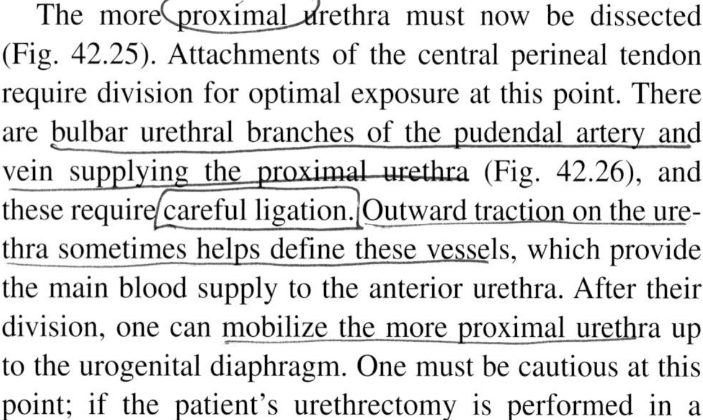

The more proximal urethra must now be dissected (Fig. 42.25). Attachments of the central perineal tendon require division for optimal exposure at this point. There are bulbar urethral branches of the pudendal artery and vein supplying the proximal urethra (Fig. 42.26), and these require careful ligation. Outward traction on the urethra sometimes helps define these vessels, which provide the main blood supply to the anterior urethra. After their division, one can mobilize the more proximal urethra up to the urogenital diaphragm. One must be cautious at this point; if the patient's urethrectomy is performed in a patient who had a prior cystectomy, there may be adhesed loops of bowel in the pelvis that could be injured if the dissection at the membranous urethra is too extensive. If urethrectomy is being performed at the time of cystectomy, then careful dissection of the membranous urethra at the prostatic apex (from above the urogenital diaphragm) with continued dissection of membranous urethra from the perineal incision should enable maintenance of urethral continuity and successful *en bloc* removal of the bladder, prostate, and urethra as an integral specimen.

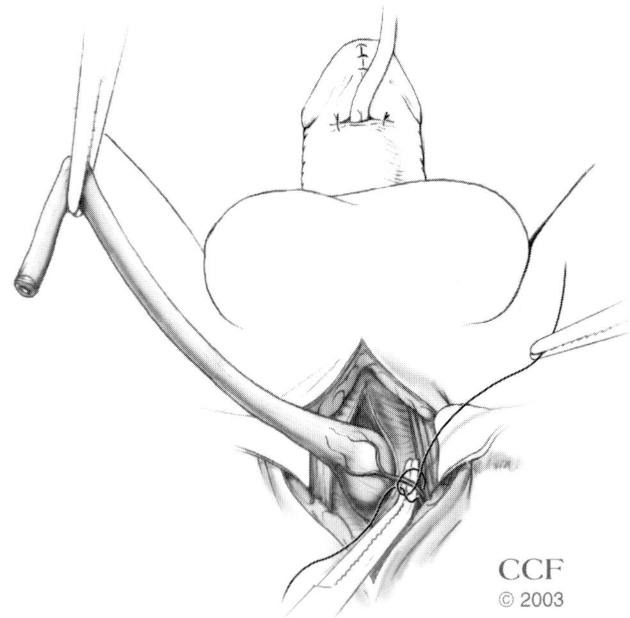


Fig. 42.25

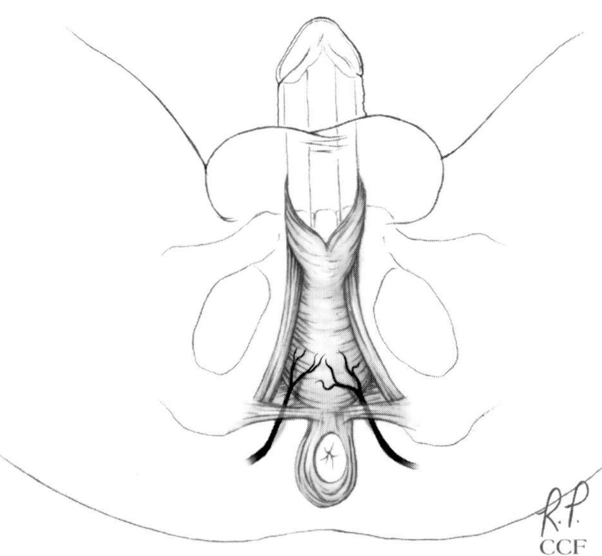


Fig. 42.26

After completion of urethrectomy, hemostasis is carefully achieved and the perineal wound is closed in successive layers (bulbocavernosus muscles, subcutaneous tissue, and skin) (Fig. 42.27). Use of polypropylene monofilament suture for one or more deep layers may reduce the risk of infection and/or dehiscence, although many use absorbable suture with good results as well. The proximal end of the Penrose drain from the penis can be buried, or it can be brought out through the perineal incision

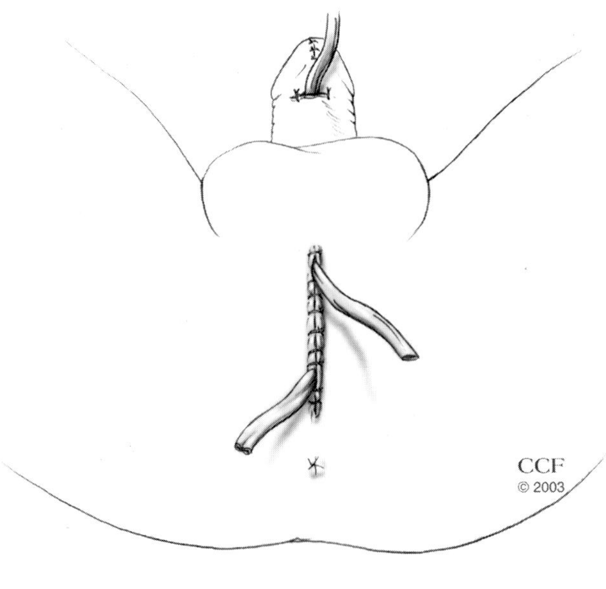


Fig. 42.27

along with another Penrose drain used to drain the bed of the proximal urethra. Alternatively, a suction drain (such as a Jackson Pratt type) may be utilized, although the attached suction bulb can be awkward for the patient. In either case, drains are usually removed at 24–48 h. Penile swelling and/or ecchymosis may occur but is inconsequential and usually resolves in several weeks. Sitz baths followed by use of a blow dryer (on low setting) will often speed healing and minimize fungus or other superficial irritations. As one often observes with hypospadias repair, glanular reconstruction usually results in an excellent cosmetic result, and there is only minor distortion from absence of the urethral meatus.

## REFERENCES

1. Schoeneich G, Perabo FG, Muller SC. Squamous cell carcinoma of the penis. Andrologia 31 (Suppl 1):17, 1999.
2. Kanik AB, Lee J, Wax F, et al. Penile verrucous carcinoma in a 37-year-old circumcised man. J Am Acad Dermatol 37:329, 1997.
3. Maden C, Sherman KJ, Beckmann AM, et al. History of circumcision, medical conditions, and sexual activity and risk of penile cancer. J Natl Cancer Inst 85: 19, 1993.
4. Dillner J, von Krogh G, Horenblas S, et al. Etiology of squamous cell carcinoma of the penis. Scand J Urol Nephrol Suppl:189, 2000.
5. Tsen HF, Morgenstern H, Mack T, et al. Risk factors for penile cancer: results of a population-based

case-control study in Los Angeles County (United States). Cancer Causes Control 12:267, 2001.
6. Lerman SE, Liao JC. Neonatal circumcision. Pediatr Clin North Am 48:1539, 2001.
7. Mallon E, Hawkins D, Dinneen M, et al. Circumcision and genital dermatoses. Arch Dermatol 136:350, 2000.
8. Murphy LJT. The History of Urology. Springfield, IL: Charles C Thomas, 1972:486, 487.
9. Young HH. A radical operation for the cure of cancer of the penis. J Urol 26:285, 1931.
10. Banon Perez VJ, Nicolas Torralba JA, Valdelvira Nadal P, et al. (Malignant neoplasms of the penis). Actas Urol Esp 24:652, 2000.
11. Vesga Molina F, Llarena Ibarguren R, Acha Perez M, et al. (Verrucous carcinoma of the penis: our caseload). Arch Esp Urol 46:23, 1993.
12. Moore SW, Wheeler JE, Hefter LG. Epitheloid sarcoma masquerading as Peyronie's disease. Cancer 35:1706, 1975.
13. Rossi G, Ferrari G, Longo L, et al. Epithelioid sarcoma of the penis: a case report and review of the literature. Pathol Int 50:579, 2000.
14. Huang DJ, Stanisic TH, Hansen KK. Epithelioid sarcoma of the penis. J Urol 147:1370, 1992.
15. Corsi A, Perugia G, De Matteis A. Epithelioid sarcoma of the penis. Clinicopathologic study of a tumor with myogenic features and review of the literature concerning this unusual location. Pathol Res Pract 195:441, 1999.
16. Williams JJ, Mouradian JA, Hagopian M, et al. Hemangioendothelial sarcoma of penis. Cancer 44:1146, 1979.
17. Van Savage JG, Carson CC, 3rd. Primary adenocarcinoma of the penis. J Urol 152:1555, 1994.
18. Lopez de Alda A, Rodriguez Minon Cifuentes JL, Garcia de la Pena E, et al. (Penile metastasis of prostatic carcinoma. Apropos of a case). Actas Urol Esp 14:163, 1990.
19. Kotake Y, Gohji K, Suzuki T, et al. Metastases to the penis from carcinoma of the prostate. Int J Urol 8:83, 2001.
20. Romero Perez P, Amat Cecilia M, Andrada Becerra E. (Metastasis in the glans of prostatic adenocarcinoma. Apropos of a case). Actas Urol Esp 15:284, 1991.
21. Khan MA, Tao W, Mathews P, et al. Penile metastasis arising from transitional cell carcinoma of the urinary bladder. Urol Int 66:162, 2001.
22. Kuwahara Y, Kubota Y, Hibi H, et al. (Malignant lymphoma of the penis: report of two cases). Hinyokika Kiyo 43:371, 1997.
23. Mukamel E, Farrer J, Smith RB, et al. Metastatic carcinoma to penis: when is total penectomy indicated? Urology 29:15, 1987.
24. Buchholz NP, Moch H, Feichter GE, et al. Clinical and pathological features of highly malignant prostatic carcinomas with metastases to the penis. Urol Int 53:135, 1994.
25. Bissada NK. Post-circumcision carcinoma of the penis: II. Surgical management. J Surg Oncol 37:80, 1988.
26. Koch MO, Smith JA, Jr. Local recurrence of squamous cell carcinoma of the penis. Urol Clin North Am 21:739, 1994.
27. McLean M, Akl AM, Warde P, et al. The results of primary radiation therapy in the management of squamous cell carcinoma of the penis. Int J Radiat Oncol Biol Phys 25:623, 1993.
28. Blatstein LM, Finkelstein LH. Laser surgery for the treatment of squamous cell carcinoma of the penis. J Am Osteopath Assoc 90:338, 1990.
29. Chaudhary AJ, Ghosh S, Bhalavat RL, et al. Interstitial brachytherapy in carcinoma of the penis. Strahlenther Onkol 175:17, 1999.
30. Ficarra V, D'Amico A, Cavalleri S, et al. Surgical treatment of penile carcinoma: our experience from 1976 to 1997. Urol Int 62:234, 1999.
31. Agrawal A, Pai D, Ananthakrishnan N, et al. The histological extent of the local spread of carcinoma of the penis and its therapeutic implications. BJU Int 85:299, 2000.
32. Davis JW, Schellhammer PF, Schlossberg SM. Conservative surgical therapy for penile and urethral carcinoma. Urology 53:386, 1999.
33. Sarin R, Norman AR, Steel GG, et al. Treatment results and prognostic factors in 101 men treated for squamous carcinoma of the penis. Int J Radiat Oncol Biol Phys 38:713, 1997.
34. Norman RW, Millard OH, Mack FG, et al. Carcinoma of the penis: an 11-year review. Can J Surg 26:426, 198.
35. Persky L, deKernion J. Carcinoma of the penis. CA Cancer J Clin 36:258, 1986.
36. Montie JE. Penectomy. In: Novick S, Edson Pontes J, eds. Stewart's Operative Urology, Vol. 2, 2nd ed. Baltimore: Williams & Wilkins, 1989: 791–795.
37. Heyns CF, van Vollenhoven P, Steenkamp JW, et al. Carcinoma of the penis—appraisal of a modified tumour-staging system. Br J Urol 80:307, 1997.
38. Fraley EE, Zhang G, Manivel C, et al. The role of ilioinguinal lymphadenectomy and significance

of histological differentiation in treatment of carcinoma of the penis. J Urol 142:1478, 1989.
39. Derakhshani P, Neubauer S, Braun M, et al. Results and 10-year follow-up in patients with squamous cell carcinoma of the penis. Urol Int 62:238, 1999.
40. Dewire D, Lepor H. Anatomic considerations of the penis and its lymphatic drainage. Urol Clin North Am 19:211, 1992.
41. Doehn C, Baumgartel M, Jocham D. (Surgical therapy of penis carcinoma). Urologe A 40:303, 2001.
42. Coblentz TR, Theodorescu D. Morbidity of modified prophylactic inguinal lymphadenectomy for squamous cell carcinoma of the penis. J Urol 168:1386, 2002.
43. Cruz Guerra NA, Allona Almagro A, Clemente Ramos L, et al. (Lymphadenectomy in squamous carcinoma of the penis: review of our series). Actas Urol Esp 24:709, 2000.
44. Magoha GA. Management of carcinoma of the penis: a review. East Afr Med J 72:547, 1995.
45. Germiyanoglu C, Horasanli K, Erol D, et al. Treatment of clinically fixed lymph node metastases from carcinoma of the penis by chemotherapy and surgery. Int Urol Nephrol 25:475, 1993.
46. Fraley EE, Zhang G, Sazama R, et al. Cancer of the penis. Prognosis and treatment plans. Cancer 55:1618, 1985.
47. Catalona WJ. Re: Modified inguinal lymphadenectomy for carcinoma of the penis with preservation of saphenous veins: technique and preliminary results. J Urol 140:836, 1988.
48. Catalona WJ. Modified inguinal lymphadenectomy for carcinoma of the penis with preservation of saphenous veins: technique and preliminary results. J Urol 140:306, 1988.
49. Chiang PH, Huang YS, Wu WJ, et al. Orthotopic bladder substitution in women using the ileal neobladder. J Formos Med Assoc 99:348, 2000.
50. Kakizoe T, Tobisu K. Transitional cell carcinoma of the urethra in men and women associated with bladder cancer. Jpn J Clin Oncol 28:357, 1998.
51. Coloby PJ, Kakizoe T, Tobisu K, et al. Urethral involvement in female bladder cancer patients: mapping of 47 consecutive cysto-urethrectomy specimens. J Urol 152:1438, 1994.
52. De Paepe ME, Andre R, Mahadevia P. Urethral involvement in female patients with bladder cancer. A study of 22 cystectomy specimens. Cancer 65:1237, 1990.
53. Schellhammer PF, Whitmore WF, Jr. Transitional cell carcinoma of the urethra in men having cystectomy for bladder cancer. J Urol 115:56, 1976.
54. Montie JE. Urethrectomy. In: Novick, S, Edson Pontes, J, eds. Stewart's Operative Urology, Vol. 2, 2nd ed. Baltimore: Williams & Wilkins, 1989:726–731.
55. Shinka T, Uekado Y, Aoshi H, et al. Urethral remnant tumors following simultaneous partial urethrectomy and cystectomy for bladder carcinoma. J Urol 142: 983, 1989.
56. Vicini D, Mensi M, Mirando P, et al. (Carcinoma of the urethra in patients having undergone cystectomy for neoplasm of the bladder). Arch Ital Urol Nefrol Androl 61:217, 1989.
57. Yasumoto R, Asakawa M, Yoshihara H, et al. (A clinical study on urethral recurrence observed after cystectomy). Nippon Hinyokika Gakkai Zasshi 81:1525, 1990.
58. Tobisu K, Tanaka Y, Mizutani T, et al. Transitional cell carcinoma of the urethra in men following cystectomy for bladder cancer: multivariate analysis for risk factors. J Urol 146:1551, 1991.
59. Robert M, Burgel JS, Serre I, et al. (Urethral recurrence after cysto-prostatectomy for bladder tumor). Prog Urol 6:558, 1996.
60. Freeman JA, Esrig D, Stein JP, et al. Management of the patient with bladder cancer. Urethral recurrence. Urol Clin North Am 21:645, 1994.
61. Lebret T, Herve JM, Barre P, et al. Urethral recurrence of transitional cell carcinoma of the bladder. Predictive value of preoperative latero-montanal biopsies and urethral frozen sections during prostatocystectomy. Eur Urol 33:170, 1998.
62. Gowing NFC. Urethral carcinoma associated with cancer of the bladder. Br J Urol 32:428, 1960.
63. Raz S, McLorie G, Johnson S, et al. Management of the urethra in patients undergoing radical cystectomy for bladder carcinoma. J Urol 120:298, 197.
64. Richie JP, Skinner DG. Carcinoma in situ of the urethra associated with bladder carcinoma: the role of urethrectomy. J Urol 119:80, 1978.
65. Ahlering TE, Lieskovsky G, Skinner DG. Indications for urethrectomy in men undergoing single stage radical cystectomy for bladder cancer. J Urol 131:657, 1984.
66. Zabbo A, Montie JE. Management of the urethra in men undergoing radical cystectomy for bladder cancer. J Urol 131:267, 1984.
67. Carrion R, Seigne J. Surgical management of bladder carcinoma. Cancer Control 9:284, 2002.
68. Wolinska WH, Melamed MR, Schellhammer PF, et al. Urethral cytology following cystectomy for bladder carcinoma. Am J Surg Pathol 1:225, 1977.
69. Sarosdy MF. Management of the male urethra after cystectomy for bladder cancer. Urol Clin North Am 19:391, 1992.

70. Hickey DP, Soloway MS, Murphy WM. Selective urethrectomy following cystoprostatectomy for bladder cancer. J Urol 136:828, 1986.
71. Dalquen P, Kleibe, B, Grilli B, et al. DNA image cytometry and fluorescence in situ hybridization for noninvasive detection of urothelial tumors in voided urine. Cancer 96:374, 2002.
72. Whitmore WF, Jr., Mount BM. A technique of urethrectomy in the male. Surg Gynecol Obstet 131:303, 1970.
73. Nagata Y, Tanaka M, Nakajima N, et al. (The recurrence of bladder cancer in the glans and fossa navicularis of urethra following cystectomy). Hinyokika Kiyo 34:1043, 1988.

# 43 Surgery for Posterior Urethral Valves

*Jonathan Ross and Robert Kay*

Posterior urethral valves are an uncommon but important cause of prenatally detected hydronephrosis. It often affects both kidneys and may be associated with renal dysplasia and insufficiency. Immediate postnatal evaluation and intervention should be undertaken. A renal ultrasound and voiding cystourethrogram are obtained on the first day of life, and a catheter is placed until intervention is undertaken, usually in the first week of life. Occasionally, boys with posterior urethral valves will present later in life with a urinary tract infection or voiding dysfunction.

## TRANSURETHRAL MANAGEMENT

When possible, transurethral management of valves should be undertaken (Fig. 43.1). If the urethra will accommodate a pediatric resectoscope, then the valves may be incised. The valves typically have a windsail appearance arising from the floor of the prostatic urethra at the utricle and fusing anteriorly, leaving a small posterior opening. They extend distally so that urine egressing from the bladder fills the "sails," causing obstruction. Water flowing through a cystoscope in a retrograde direction may actually flatten the leaflets against the urethral wall, obscuring the diagnosis. With the water off, suprapubic pressure will generate antegrade flow, demonstrating the valves. Once identified, the leaflets may be incised on both sides and, if necessary, at the 12 o'clock position. A sharp hook is the ideal instrument so that the valves may be incised without electric current. However, cutting current may be employed if necessary. If a small resectoscope is not available or is too large, the valves may be fulgurated with a bugbee fulgurator advanced through a pediatric cystoscope. Coagulating current is applied directly to the valve leaflets, which will then regress.

## VESICOSTOMY

If urethroscopic management is not possible, a vesicostomy should be performed. There are contradictory studies regarding the effect of diversion on ultimate bladder function. However, a vesicostomy appears to have less negative impact on ultimate bladder function than do higher diversions.

A 2-cm incision is made halfway between the pubic symphisis and the umbilicus (Fig. 43.2). A U-shaped incision may be employed to reduce the risk of stenosis.

The anterior rectus fascia is opened, and, if necessary, small lateral incisions are made in the rectus muscle on either side (Fig. 43.3).

The bladder is filled and the anterior surface exposed (Fig. 43.4). Dissection is carried superiorly to identify the bladder dome, and the bladder is bluntly mobilized so that it can be brought up to skin level without tension.

A transverse incision is made into the bladder lumen close to the dome (Fig. 43.5). If the incision is made on

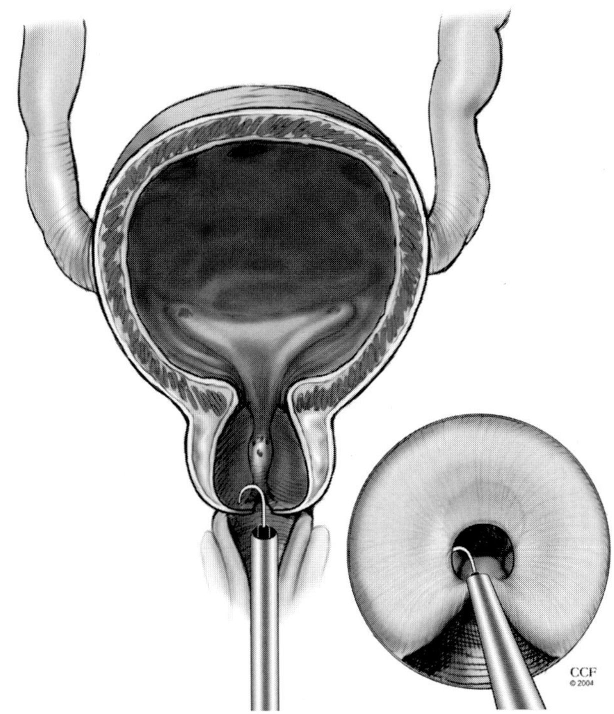


**Fig. 43.1**

From: *Operative Urology at the Cleveland Clinic*
Edited by: A. Novick et al. © Humana Press Inc., Totowa, NJ

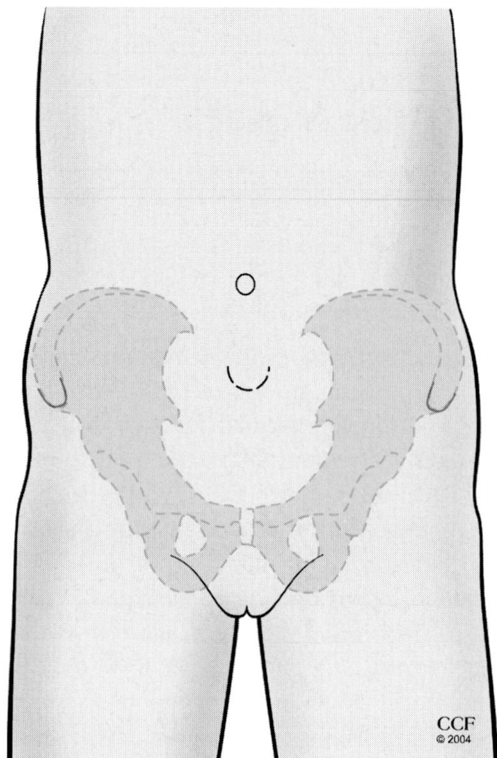


Fig. 43.2

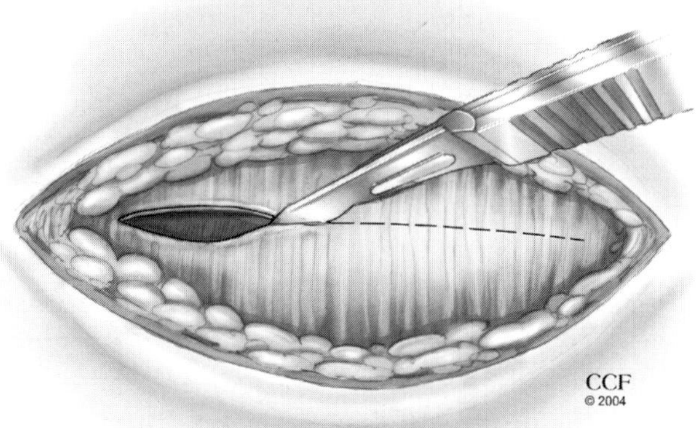


Fig. 43.3

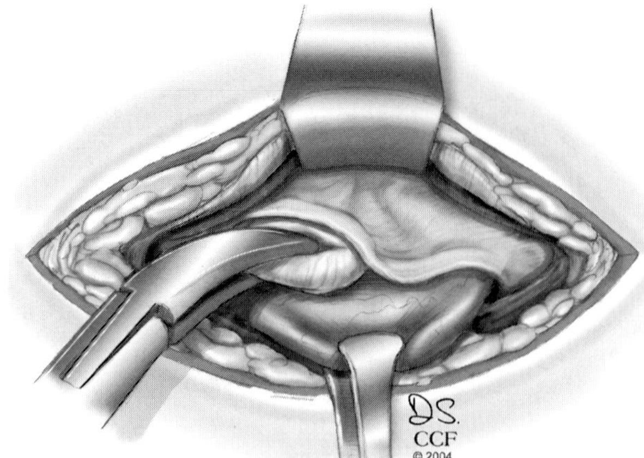


Fig. 43.4

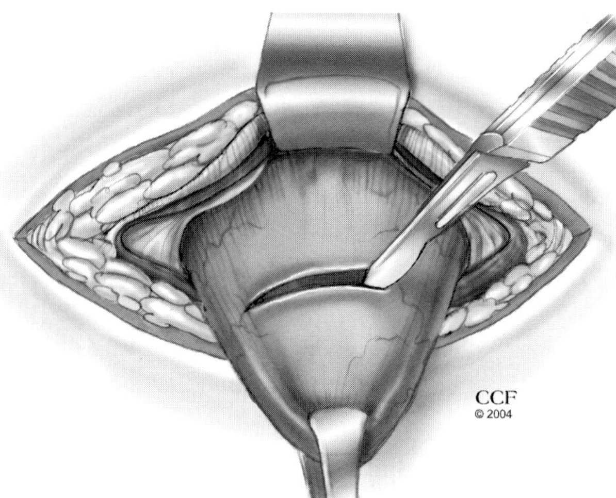


Fig. 43.5

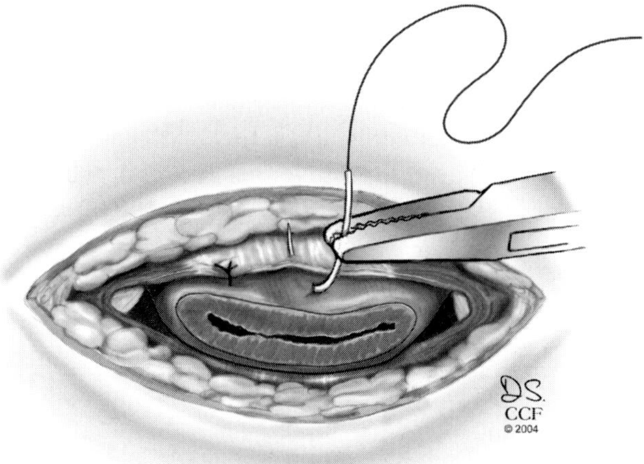


Fig. 43.6

the anterior wall far from the dome, then the risk of postoperative bladder prolapse is increased. The incision may be T'd up superiorly for a short distance to accommodate the U-flap of the skin incision.

Several 4-0 absorbable sutures are placed from the anterior rectus fascial edge to the seromuscular layer of the bladder to keep the bladder at skin level and take tension off the stomal sutures (Fig. 43.6).

The bladder edge is sewn to the skin edge with 4-0 absorbable sutures (Fig. 43.7). If the bladder is very thick, then mucosal bites with only part of the muscle may be employed to avoid bringing the full thickness of the muscular bladder wall into the stoma, which may impair drainage. A 12 French Malecot catheter may be left indwelling for 24–48 h.

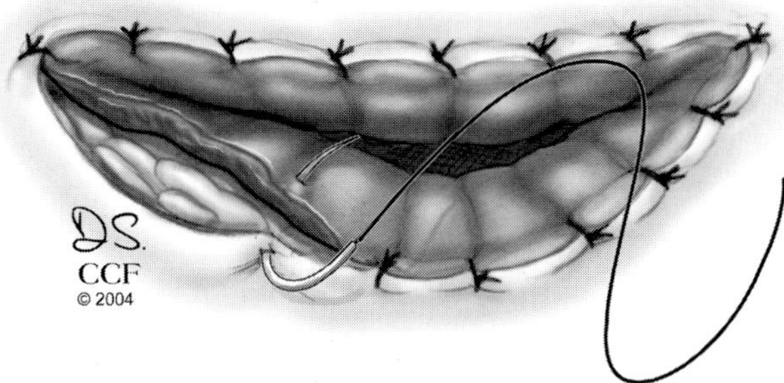


Fig. 43.7

When the child is older and the valves can be definitively treated, the vesicostomy may be taken down. At that time the valves may be treated transurethrally, or they may be incised endoscopically in an antegrade fashion through the vesicostomy just prior to closure (Fig. 43.8).

Patients with a history of posterior urethral valves require life-long urological follow-up. Despite successful relief of the obstruction, many of these boys will develop voiding dysfunction. The typical pattern is of a poorly compliant and/or hyperreflexic bladder in childhood evolving to a hypotonic poorly emptying bladder later in life. To prevent renal damage and/or bladder decompensation, this voiding dysfunction must be diagnosed and, if present, aggressively treated. Some patients may require timed double-voiding and/or anticholinergic medications. If incomplete emptying persists, then intermittent catheterization should be employed. In severe cases, nocturnal catheter drainage or bladder augmentation may eventually be required. However, it is possible that early aggressive treatment of voiding dysfunction may preclude the need for augmentation later in life.

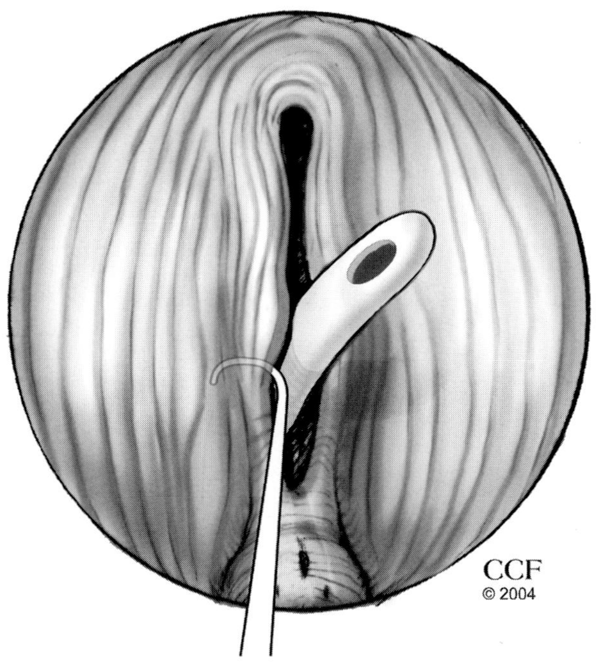


Fig. 43.8

## SUGGESTED READINGS

1. Glassberg KI. The valve bladder syndrome: 20 years later. J Urol 166:1406–1414, 2001.
2. Koff SA, Mutabagani KH, Jatanthi VR. The valve bladder syndrome: pathophysiology and treatment with nocturnal bladder emptying. J Urol 167: 291–297, 2002.
3. Woodhouse CRJ. The fate of the abnormal bladder in adolescence. J Urol 166:2396–2400, 2001.

# 44 Artificial Urinary Sphincter Implantation

*Drogo K. Montague and Kenneth W. Angermeier*

Artificial urinary sphincter (AUS) implantation is most often performed to treat urinary incontinence following radical or subtotal prostatectomy. In these cases, the cuff of the AUS is placed around the bulbous urethra. This device can also be implanted to treat urinary incontinence associated with myelodysplasia in men, women, or children or to treat urinary incontinence caused by intrinsic sphincter deficiency in women. In these cases, the cuff is implanted around the bladder neck. This chapter details the implantation of the AUS with cuff placement around the bulbous urethra.

The AUS has three components: the cuff, a pressure-regulating balloon (PRB), and a pump (Fig. 44.1). As noted, the cuff may be implanted around the bladder neck of men, women, or children. An alternative cuff site is the bulbous urethra of adult males. Above the pump is a deactivation button. This button can be employed to maintain an empty (open) cuff until the device is reactivated. When the device is active, fluid flows from the PRB into the cuff until the cuff and balloon pressures are equal. The PRB is placed into the retropubic space so that pressure increases caused by stress (coughing, lifting, etc.) are transmitted equally to the bladder and the PRB. The pump is implanted in the male scrotum or the female labium majus. When the patient wishes to void, he or she squeezes the pump until it stays flat. This moves cuff fluid back into the PRB. As the patient is voiding, the pressure in the PRB transmits fluid through a delay fill resistor in the top of the pump assembly to the pump until it is full and then through the pump to the cuff until cuff and PRB pressures are equal. PRB pressures, typically in the range of 61–70 cm of water, are safe for normal tissues.

The patient is placed in the lithotomy position (Fig. 44.2). A Foley catheter (18 French) is placed and attached to gravity drainage. A midline incision is made in the perineum.

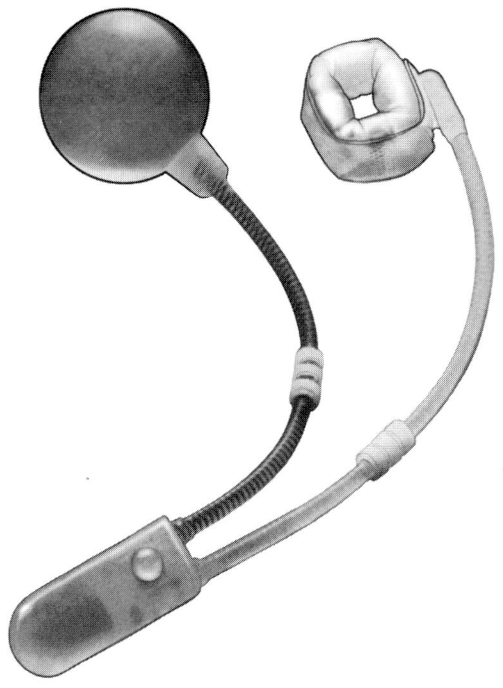

Fig. 44.1

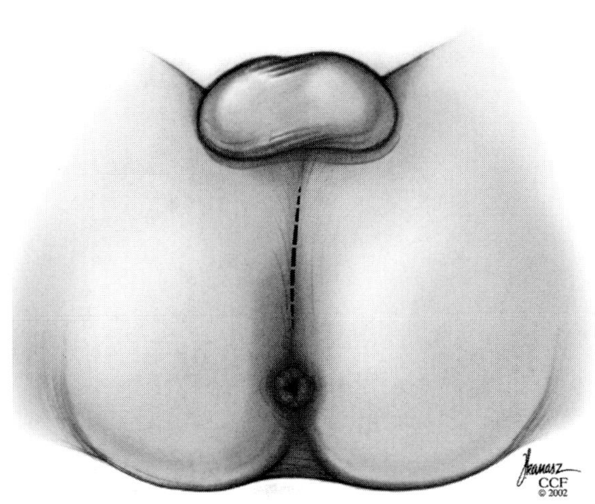

Fig. 44.2

From: *Operative Urology at the Cleveland Clinic*
Edited by: A. Novick et al. © Humana Press Inc., Totowa, NJ

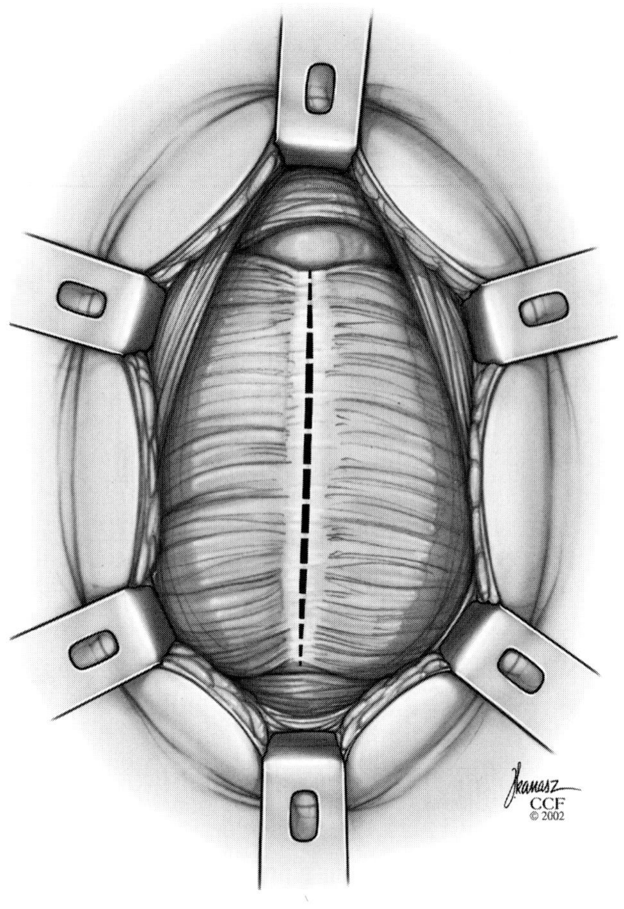


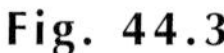
Fig. 44.3

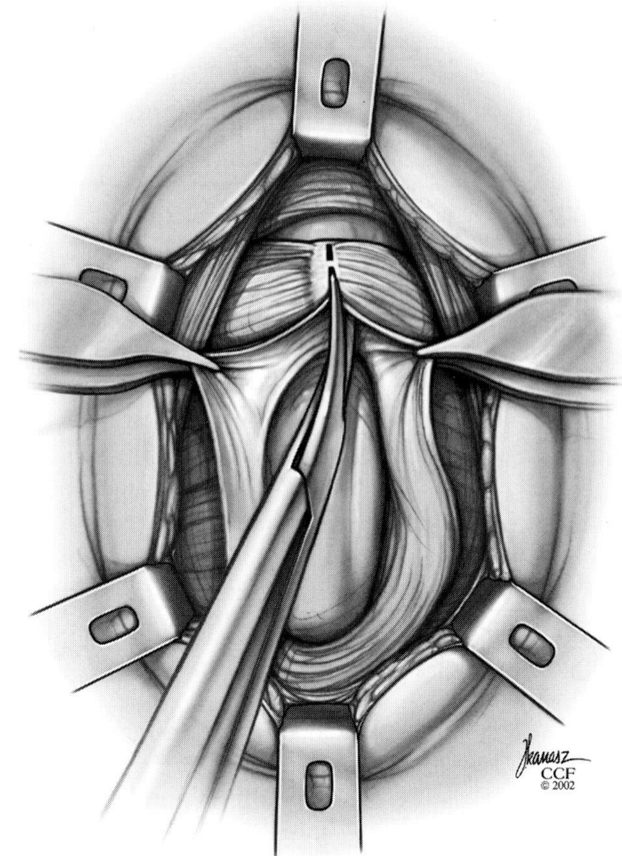


Fig. 44.4

Exposure is maintained with a ring retractor (Fig. 44.3). Dissection in the midline is carried down to the bulbospongiosus muscles.

The bulbospongiosus muscles are divided in the midline (Fig. 44.4).

The bulbocavernosus muscles are dissected off the bulbous urethra (Fig. 44.5).

The bulbous urethra is rotated to one side so that sharp dissection of the posterior attachments of the urethra to the intracrural septum can be performed until direct vision (Fig. 44.6). This is repeated on the opposite side until the bulbous urethra is completely mobilized.

A right-angle clamp is passed behind the mobilized urethra (Fig. 44.7).

This clamp is used to pass a cuff sizer (supplied with the AUS) behind the urethra (Fig. 44.8). The narrow end of the cuff sizer is then passed through a slot in the wide end, and the urethral circumference is determined.

After the cuff size is determined, a solution of isotonic contrast is prepared according to instructions supplied with the device. This is used to fill the pump and to purge air from the cuff and the PRB, both of which are empty when they are implanted. The cuff is then passed behind the urethra, and the cuff tubing is passed through the opening in the opposite end of the cuff (Fig. 44.9 A,B). This opening is then passed over the tubing hub until it slips into a slot beneath the hub. This locks the cuff in place.

A second oblique incision is made over the external inguinal ring on the side of the intended pump placement (Fig. 44.10). This incision is carried down to expose the ring.

The surgeon places his or her index finger in the external ring (Fig. 44.11). If the ring cannot be identified, a point just above the pubic tubercle is chosen. Long blunt scissors are then used to perforate the fascia (the bladder must be empty in order to safely perform this maneuver). The surgeon then advances the index finger through the fascial defect. Correct entry into the retropubic space is confirmed by palpation of the back of the symphysis pubis and the catheter balloon inside the empty bladder. The PRB will later be implanted through this fascial defect.

The cuff tubing is attached to the tubing passer and then passed lateral to the urethra over the pubis to emerge deep to Scarpa's fascia in the inguinal incision (Fig. 44.12).

The bulbospongiosus fascia and muscles are closed over the cuff with a continuous suture of 3-0 Dexon (Fig. 44.13).

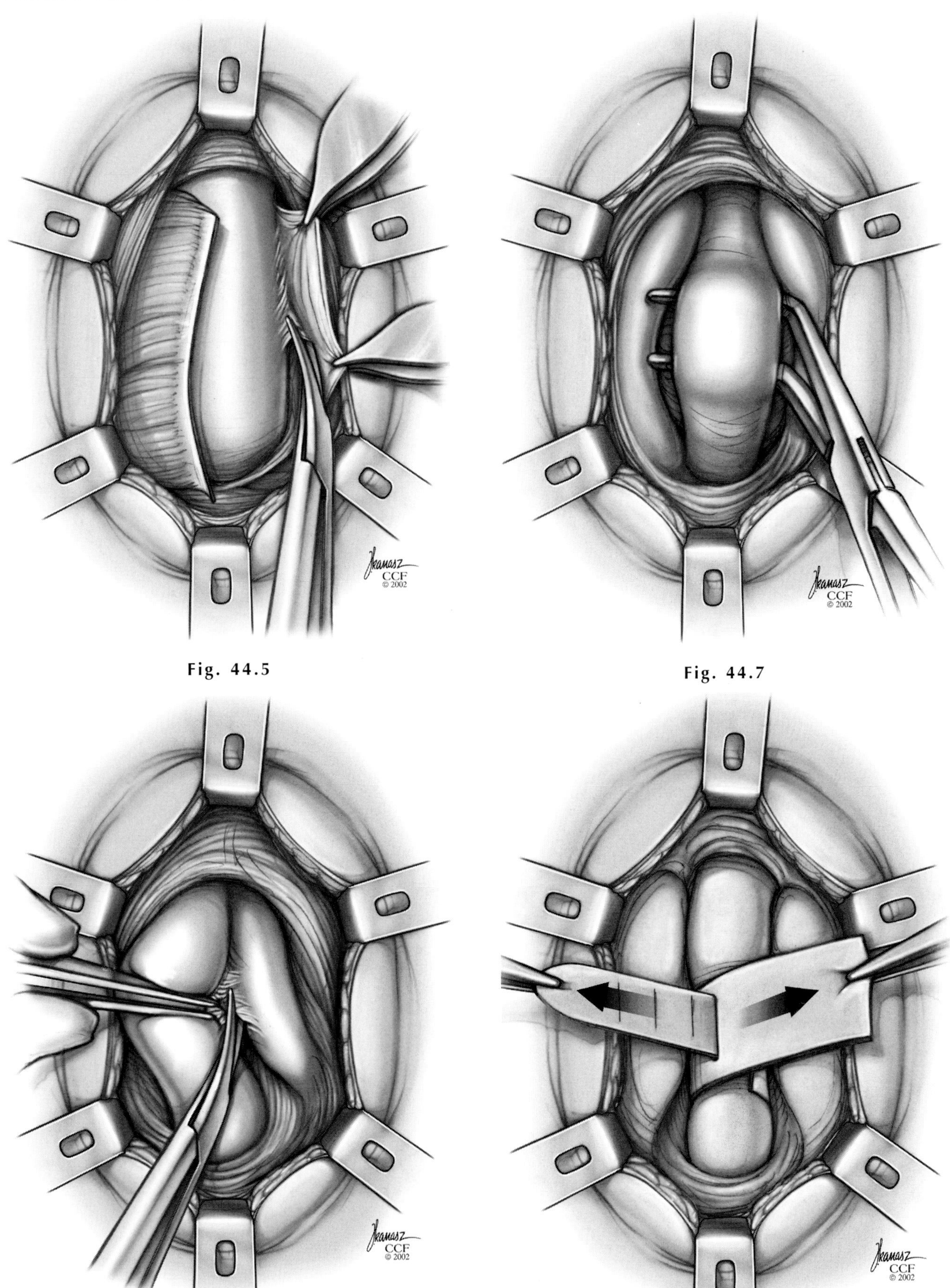


Fig. 44.5

Fig. 44.7

Fig. 44.6

Fig. 44.8

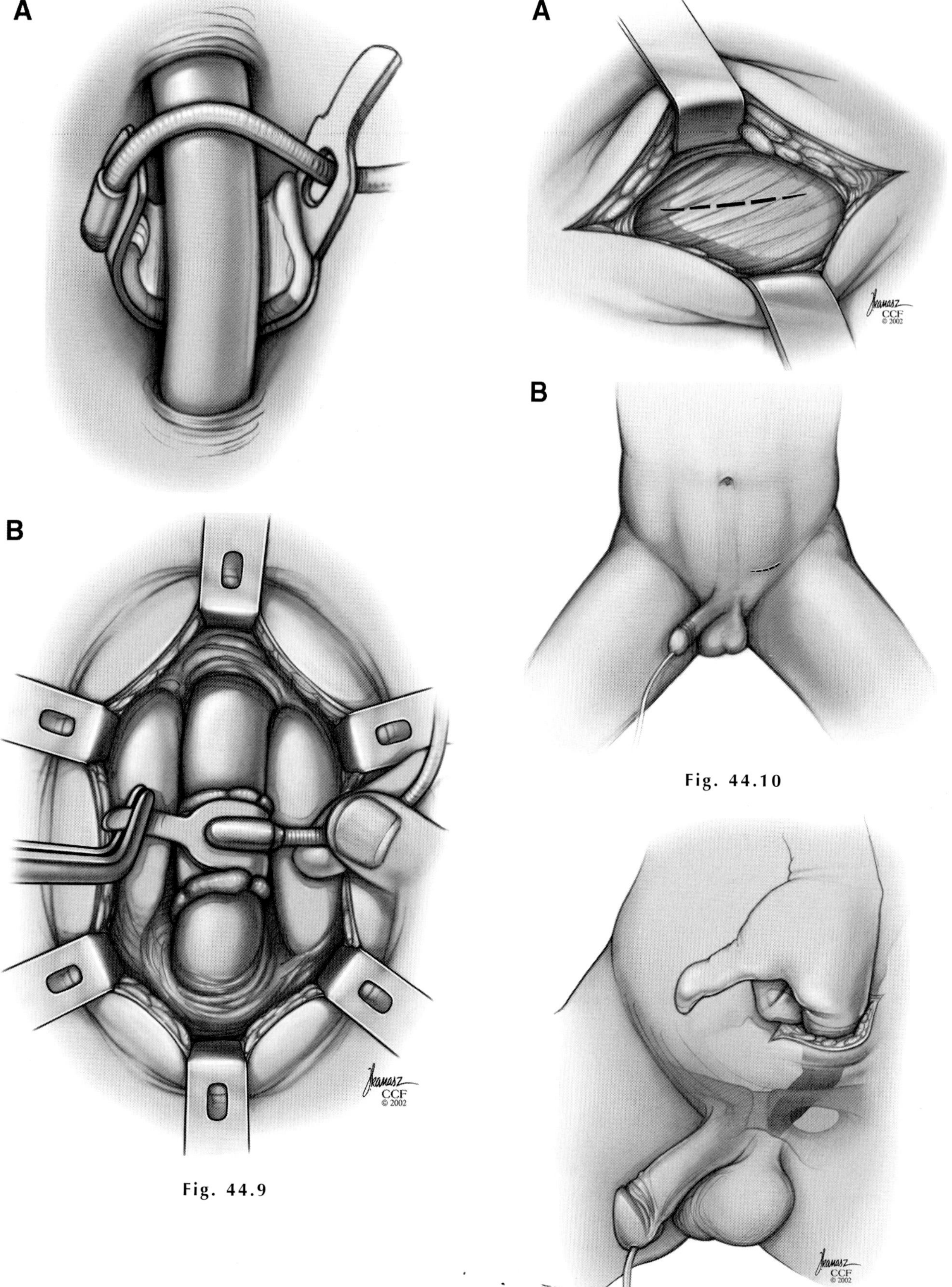


Fig. 44.9

Fig. 44.10

Fig. 44.11

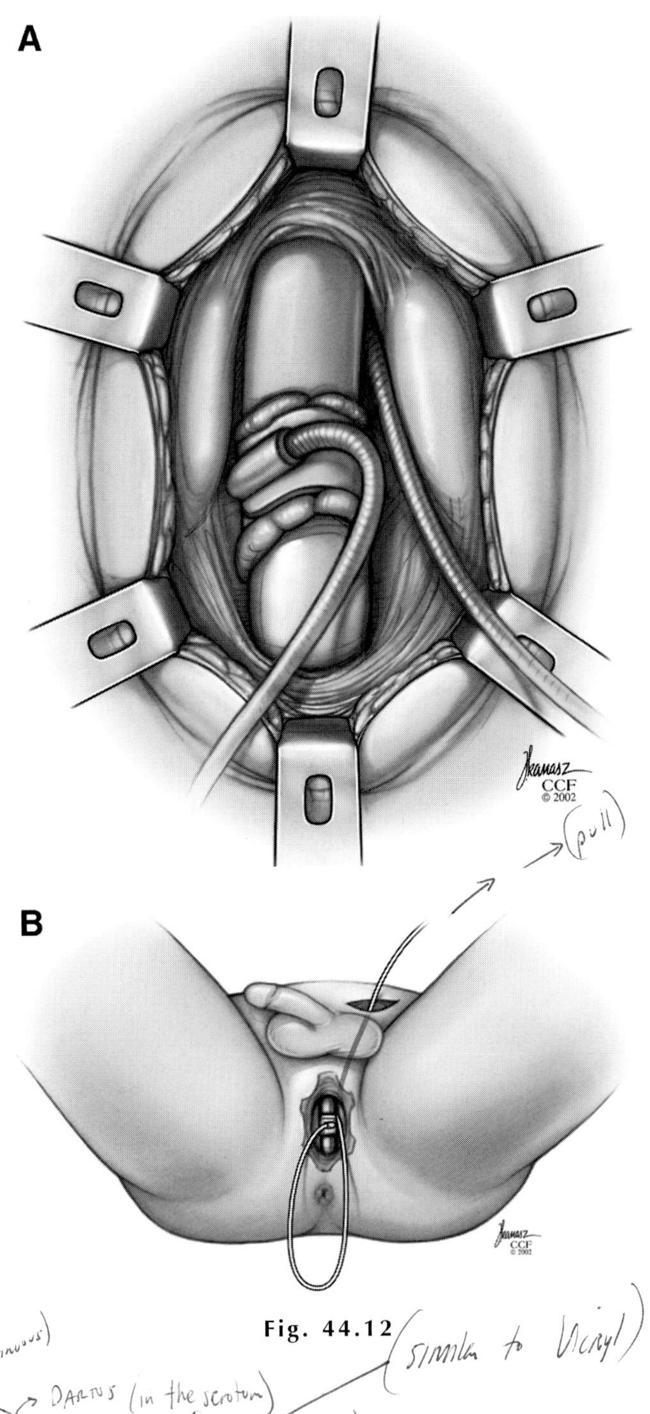


Fig. 44.12

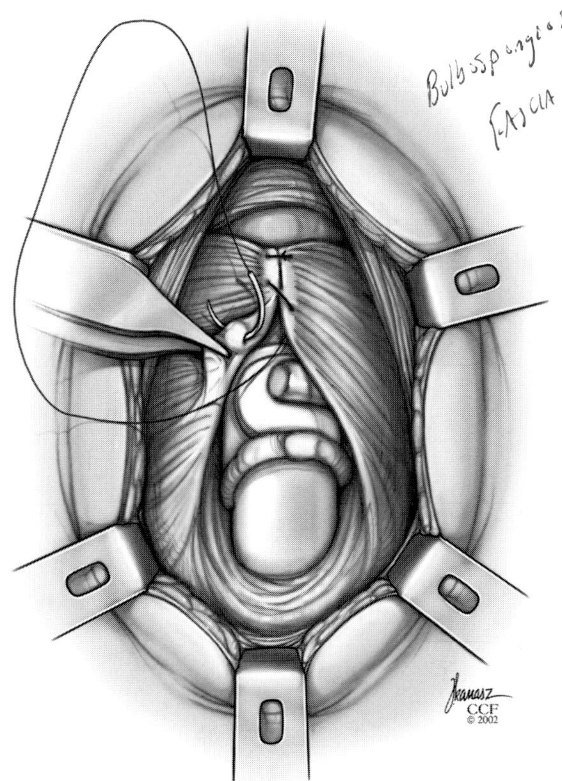

Fig. 44.13

Colles' fascia in the perineum is closed with a continuous suture of 3-0 Dexon (Fig. 44.14).

In the inguinal incision a nasal speculum with long blades is inserted through the previously made fascial defect and used to hold this defect open (Fig. 44.15). The empty PRB is inserted into the retropubic space.

The PRB is filled with 22 mL of isotonic contrast solution (Fig. 44.16).

Ring forceps are introduced beneath Scarpa's fascia to develop a sub-Dartos pouch deep in the scrotum (Fig. 44.17).

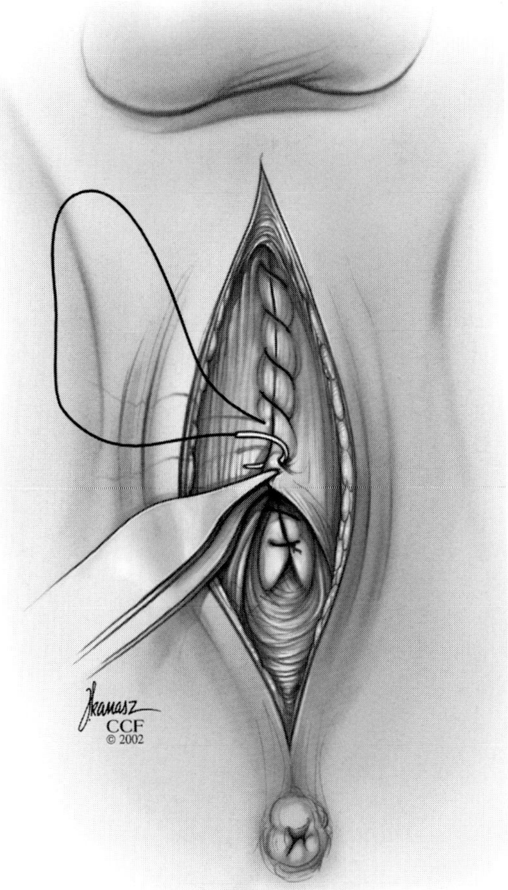

Fig. 44.14

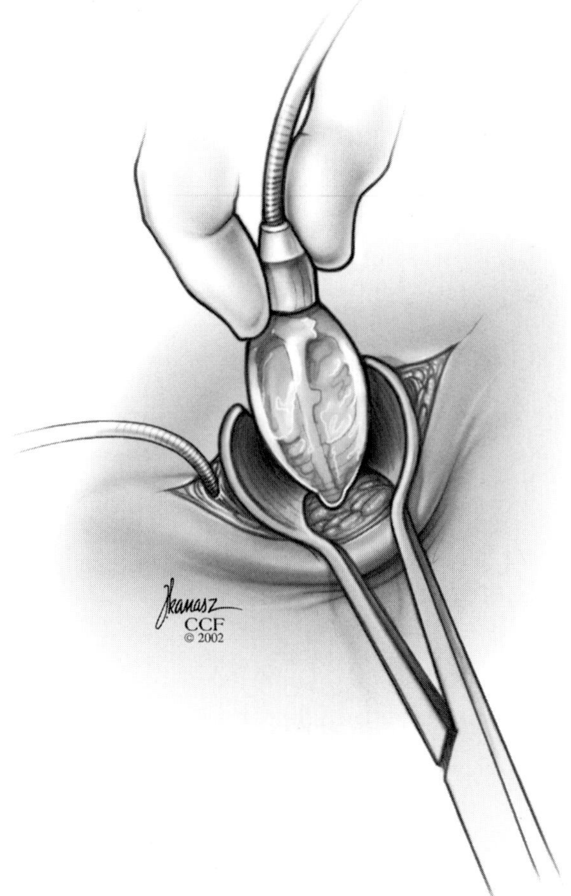


Fig. 44.15

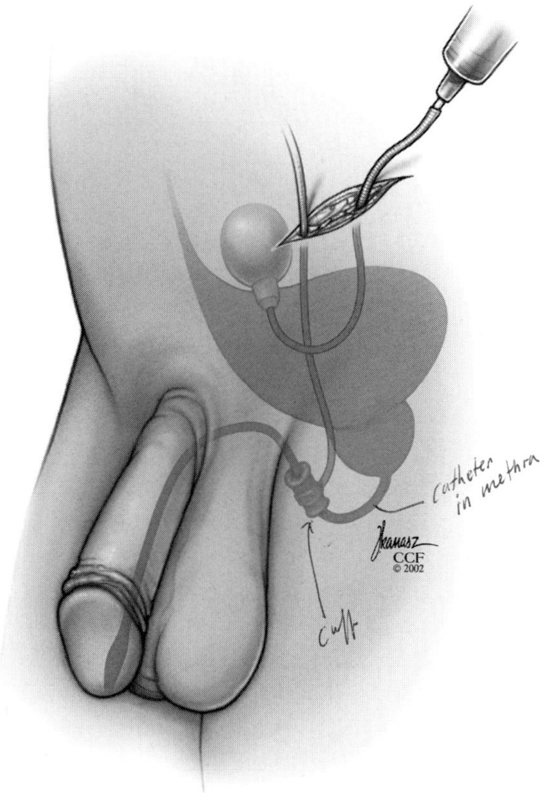


Fig. 44.16

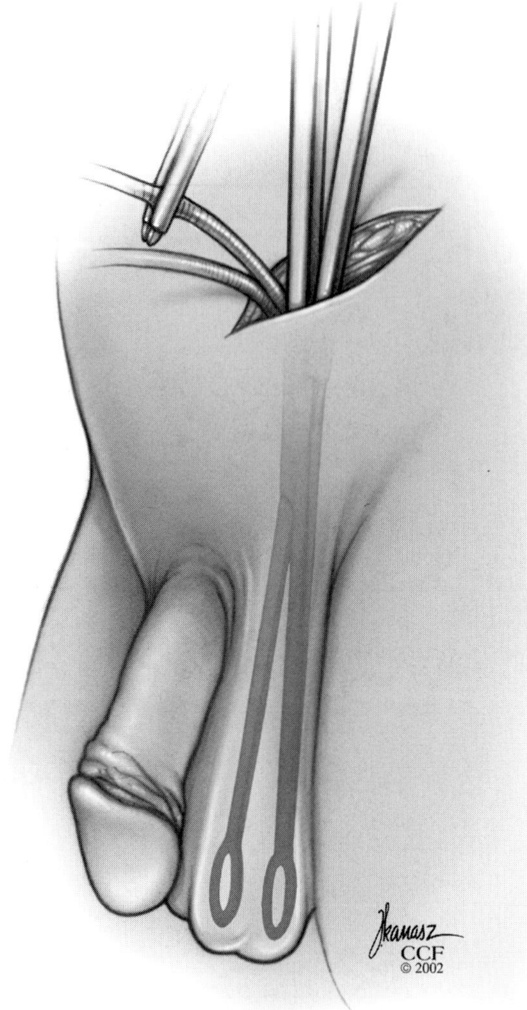


Fig. 44.17

The pump is placed into this sub-Dartos pouch (Fig. 44.18).

Using the Quick Connector™ system, a straight connector connects the PRB tubing to the pump, and a right-angle connector connects the cuff to the pump (Fig. 44.19).

Scarpa's fascia is closed over the tubing and connectors with a continuous suture of 3-0 Dexon (Fig. 44.20).

The pump is cycled until it remains collapsed; this indicates that the cuff is empty (Fig. 44.21). After the pump has almost completely refilled, the deactivation button is pressed; this prevents the cuff from refilling. The skin in each to the incisions is closed with continuous 4-0 Vicryl in a subcuticular fashion.

## POSTOPERATIVE CARE

The Foley catheter is removed on the third postoperative day. Because the device is deactivated, the patient will continue to be incontinent. At a postoperative visit in 6 wk, the AUS is activated by firmly squeezing the pump. The device is now activated and the patient is instructed in its use.

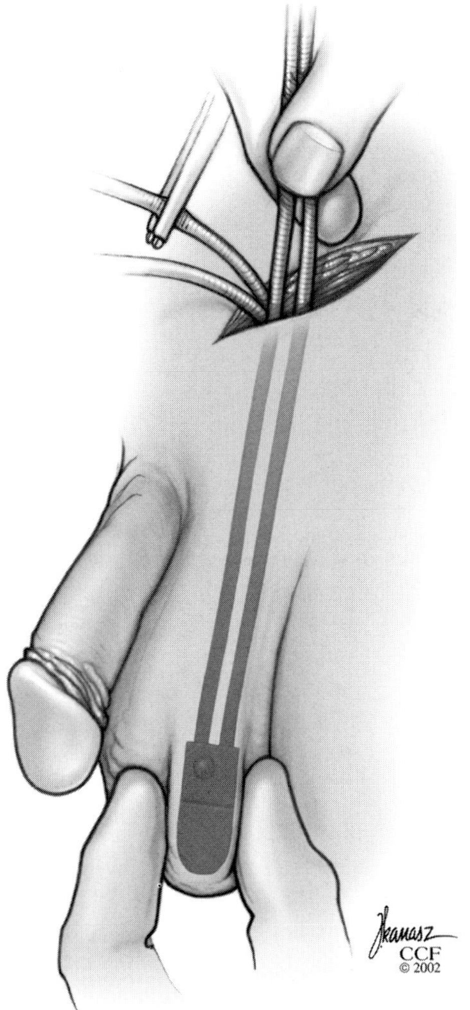


Fig. 44.18

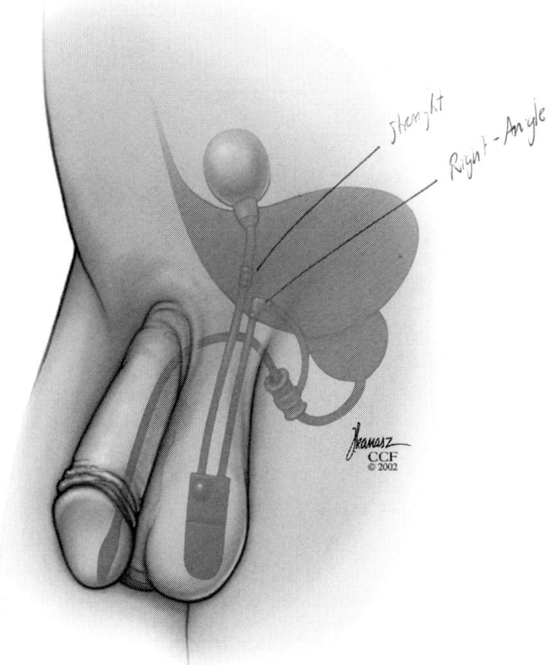


Fig. 44.19

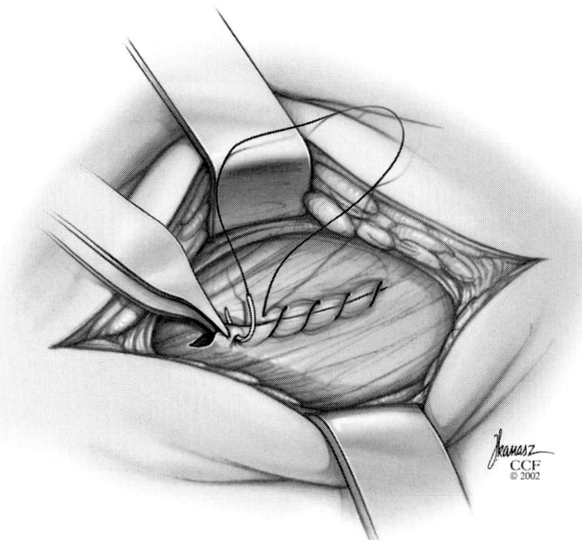


Fig. 44.20

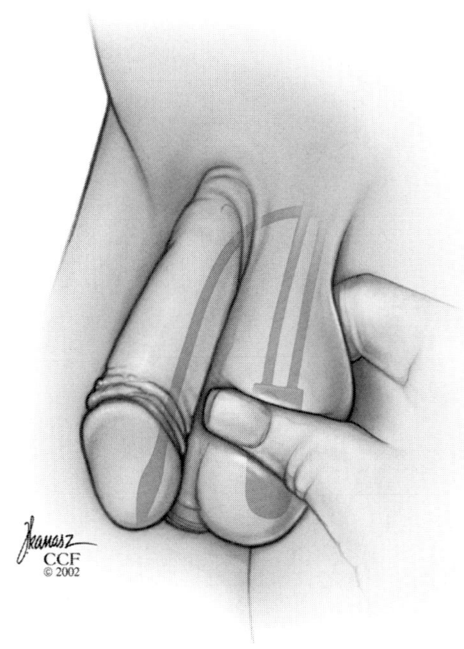


Fig. 44.21

## SUGGESTED READINGS

1. Montague DK. Evolution of implanted devices for urinary incontinence. Cleve Clin Quart 51:405, 1984.
2. Montague DK, Angermeier KW. Artificial urinary sphincter troubleshooting. Urology 58:779, 2001.
3. Montague DK, Angermeier KW, Paolone DR. Long-term continence and patient satisfaction after artificial sphincter implantation for urinary incontinence after prostatectomy. J Urol 166:547, 2001.

# VII THE GENITALIA

# 45 Surgery for Male Infertility

*Antony J. Thomas, Jr.*

## INTRODUCTION

There have been significant refinements in the surgical procedures available for many infertile men. Microsurgery for vasovasostomy and vasoepididymostomy described more than 25 yr ago has been further defined and expanded to include surgery for varicoceles and sperm retrieval from men with obstructive and nonobstructive azoospermia.

This chapter details some of the more frequently performed microsurgical and nonmicrosurgical procedures for the infertile or subfertile male: (1) varicocele ablation, (2) vasovasostomy, (3) vasoepididymostomy, (4) transurethral resection for ejaculatory duct obstruction, and (5) sperm retrieval for obstructive and nonobstructive azoospermia.

## SURGERY FOR VARICOCELE

### Overview

It has been estimated that approximately 15% of men have a varicocele. This dilation of the veins of the pampinaform plexus is caused by gravity in the absence of valves within these testicular veins. Consequently, upon assuming an upright position, the vein(s) stretch creating the palpable cluster of vessels above and often behind the testicle. Very large varicoceles can virtually appear to surround the testis in a cluster, often referred to as a "bag of worms." Approximately 40% of men who seek infertility investigations will have a varicocele on clinical examination. Some but not all of these men will have impairment of their sperm quality. While most affected men will have varicoceles on their left side, more are being identified with bilateral varicoceles, in part as a result of more careful scrutiny and more sophisticated examination with color Doppler ultrasound. There remains controversy among some investigators as to whether correction of the varicocele(s) carries the potential to improve semen parameters. Most of investigators seem to agree that there is sufficient evidence to recommend correcting the varicocele to improve fertility potential, at least in some men who may be affected and have abnormal semen parameters. Men with varicoceles may have marked variations in their semen quality, ranging from being azoospermic to having a completely normal semen analysis. No specific pattern of abnormal parameters is found in the semen of men with varicoceles.

Varicoceles can be identified in some young boys who are going through puberty. When discovered in an adolescent, there is no reason to obtain a semen analysis, but if there is a marked discrepancy in size or growth of the affected testis, this may be an indication for varicocele correction prior to adulthood. There has been reported evidence for "catch-up growth" of the affected testicles in some of these young boys.

### Diagnosis of Varicocele

The presence of a varicocele can generally be ascertained upon routine physical examination (Fig. 45.1). With a man standing in a warm, well-lit room, the distension of the veins within the scrotum should be obvious when a varicocele is moderate or large in size. When placed in a supine position, the dilated veins should

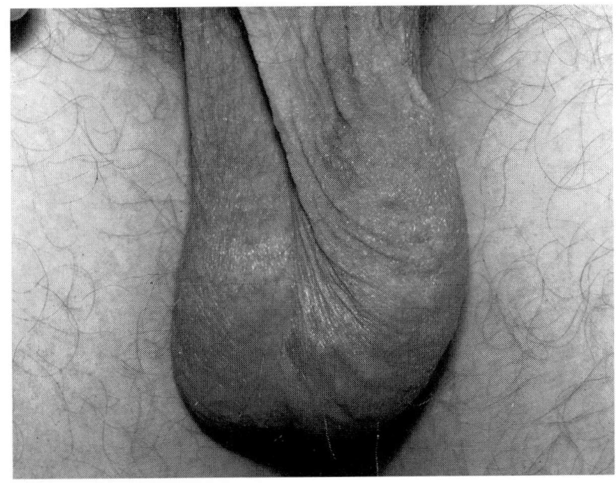

Fig. 45.1

From: *Operative Urology at the Cleveland Clinic*
Edited by: A. Novick et al. © Humana Press Inc., Totowa, NJ

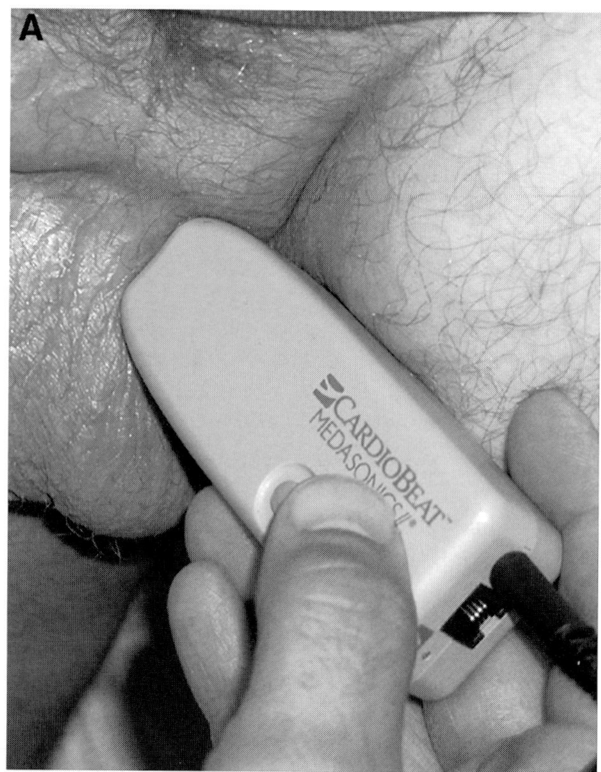


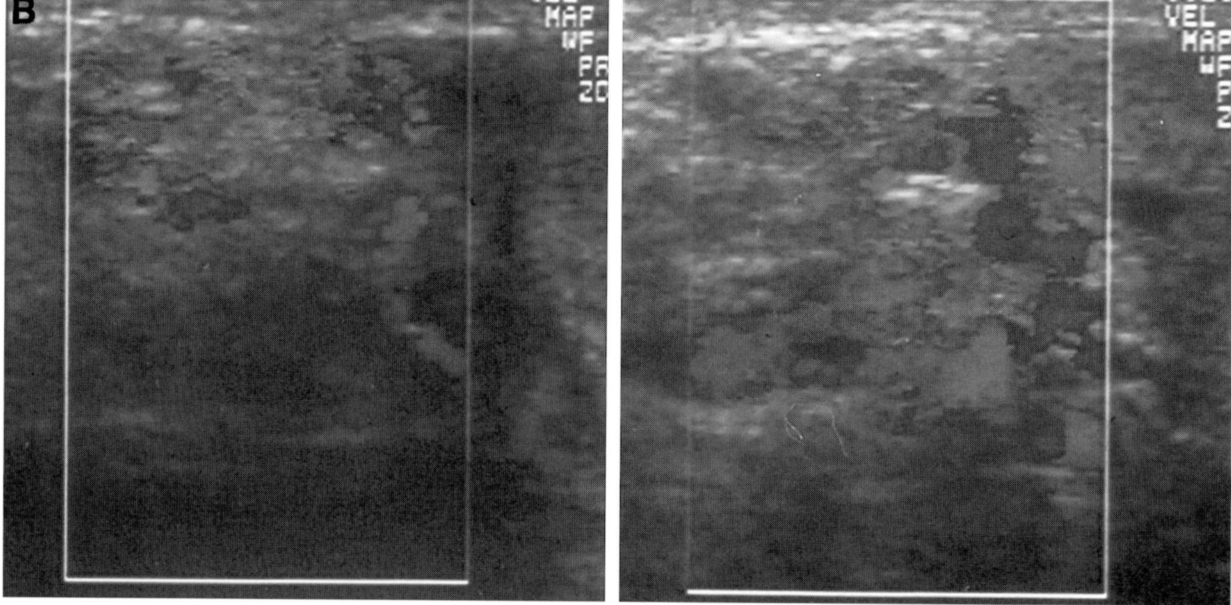


Fig. 45.2

collapse, making the varicocele difficult, if not impossible, to feel. When a small varicocele is suspected, the patient is placed in an upright position and asked to perform a valsalva maneuver while the examiner lightly grasps the cord structures. This will often elicit a palpable "venous impulse."

Additional diagnostic aids for identifying these smaller, clinical varicoceles include the Doppler stethoscope and color Doppler ultrasound (Fig. 45.2). The Doppler stethoscope (Medasonics Cardiobeat, Freemont, CA) can be placed over the spermatic cord and a Valsalva maneuver performed. When a varicocele is present, performing a Valsalva maneuver creates a prominent venous whoosh, heard as the blood flow pattern is altered within these dilated veins. Color Doppler ultrasound will show a change in the size of the veins with Valsalva maneuver, both in a supine and an upright position, when there is a varicocele present.

## Indications for Surgery

Not everyone with a varicocele needs to have it corrected. This determination should be made on a case-by-case basis. In the adolescent, significant discrepancy in testicular size and in the adult abnormal semen parameters, often associated with infertility, are the most common reasons for recommending correction of the varicocele. Other indications that might be considered include an undesirable cosmetic appearance, particularly when the varicocele is extremely large, or chronic and bothersome discomfort associated with a large varicocele.

## Surgical Techniques

Correction of a varicocele can be performed with surgical ligation, transvenous embolization, or laparoscopic clipping of the internal spermatic veins. Many surgeons tend to avoid the laparoscopic technique, because the potential for complications in less-than-experienced hands may be greater with this technique than it is with open surgical ligation or embolization. For surgical ligation, local anesthesia with intravenous sedation or general/regional anesthesia are considered suitable depending on patient and physician preference.

## Subinguinal Approach

Independent investigators have popularized the subinguinal approach to the varicocele with the operating microscope to more accurately identify all the veins in the spermatic cord while assiduously avoiding the testicular artery(ies) and lymphatics. The advantage of this technique is that it requires a small incision with no abdominal muscle or fascia cut. This allows the patient to regain mobility and full range of physical activity more quickly. The disadvantage of this approach is that it requires using the operating microscope to view and carefully dissect the more numerous and smaller veins found distal to the external inguinal ring.

The incision is made just below the level of the external inguinal ring (Fig. 45.3).

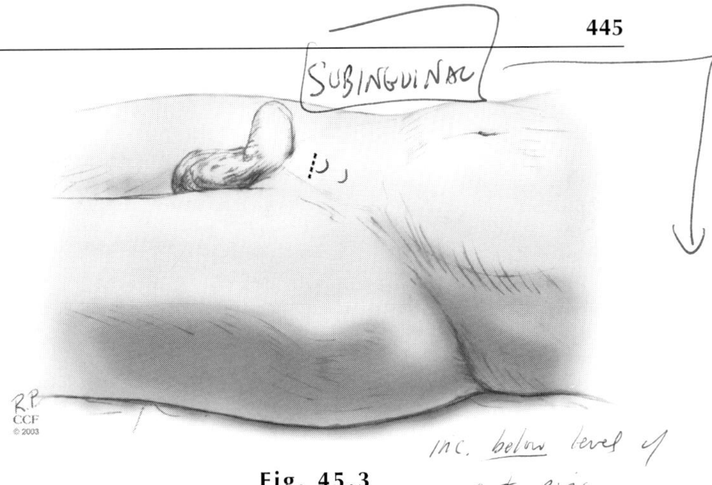


Fig. 45.3

Scarpa's fascia is opened and the loose connective tissue overlying the spermatic cord is visualized and incised (Fig. 45.4). With a small retractor in the inferior portion of the incision, the index finger sweeps superiorly to free the loose connective tissue and expose the cord beneath (Fig. 45.5). The cord is mobilized and lifted out of the incision either with a large Babcock clamp or just manually (Fig. 45.6).

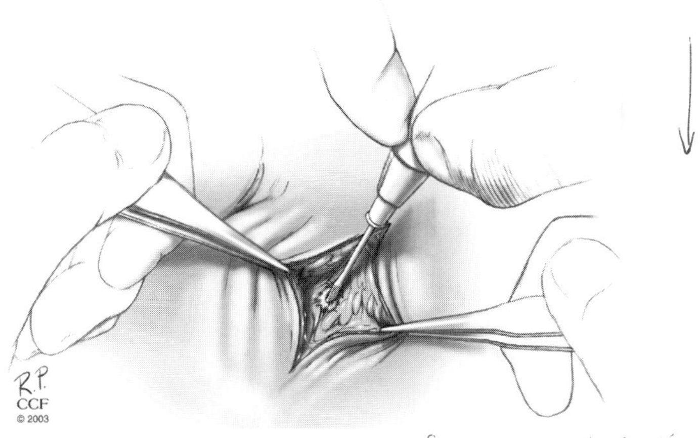


Fig. 45.4

Once the cord is pulled up above the incision two Penrose drains are passed beneath it to hold the cord above skin level by tacking the drains to the drapes with hemostats (Fig. 45.7). The operating microscope is brought to the field, and any large cremasteric veins identified are either ligated or cauterized.

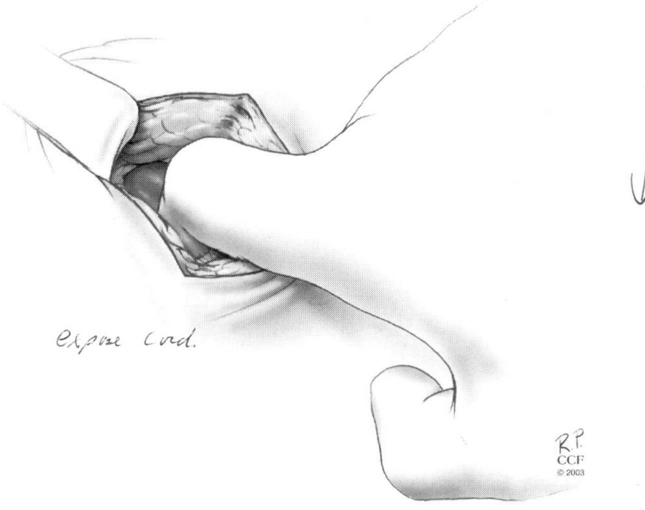


Fig. 45.5

The cremasteric muscle is opened in the direction of its fibers to expose the cord structures below (Fig. 45.8). The position of the testicular artery or arteries is identified

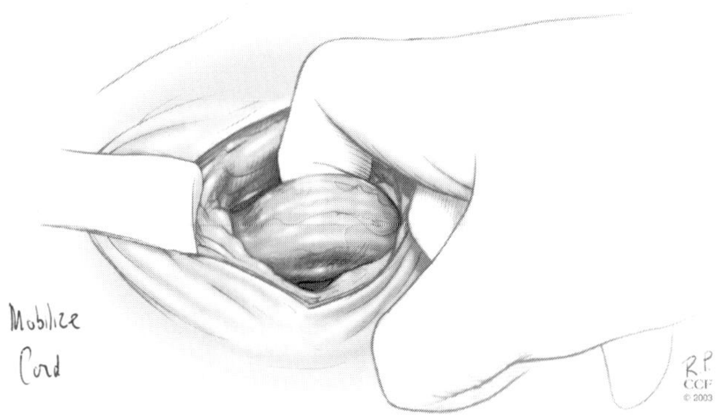

Fig. 45.6

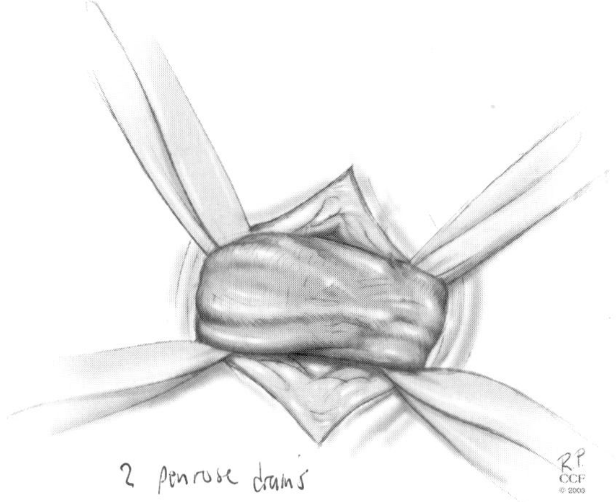

Fig. 45.7

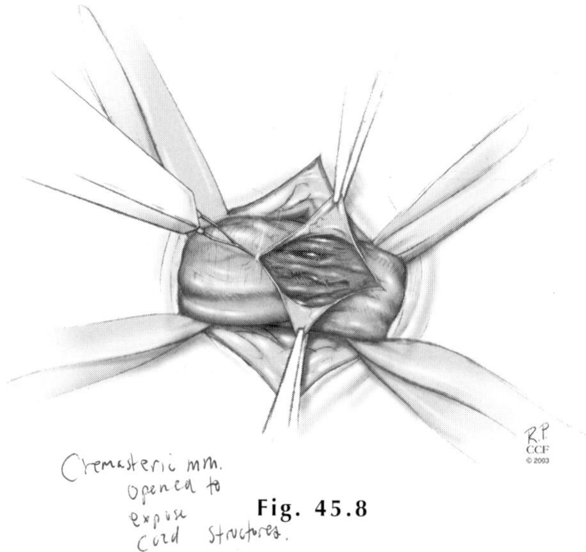

Fig. 45.8

either by direct visualization or with the use of a 2-mm. Doppler probe (Fig. 45.9) (VTI surgical Doppler and a disposable Doppler probe for neurosurgery, manufactured for Mizuho America, Inc. by Vascular Technology, Inc., Lowell, MA).

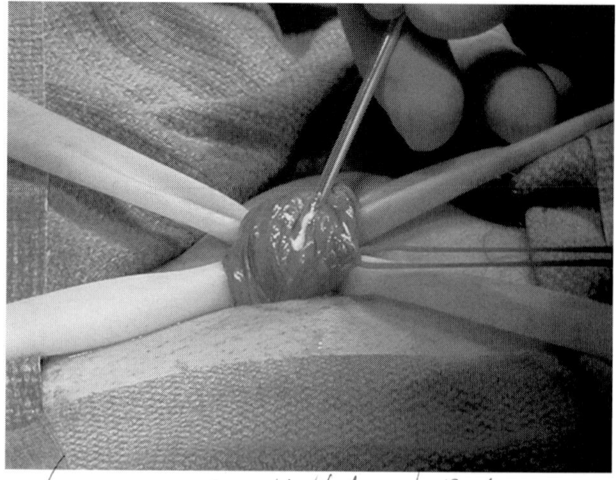

Fig. 45.9

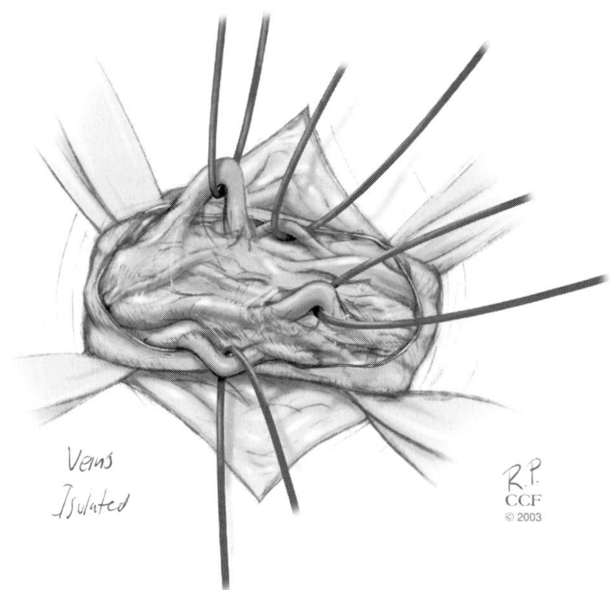

Fig. 45.10

With the exception of the vasal veins, all of the other spermatic veins are methodically isolated from the rest of the cord by moving in a lateral to the medial direction, passing a vessel loop around each vein as they are encountered (Fig. 45.10). No attempt is made to enter into the compartment of the vas deferens or manipulate its associated vessels. There are instances in which veins are found to be adherent to an artery and need to be carefully dissected off in order to completely obliterate the varicocele while preserving the integrity of the artery. If a vein appears too tightly adherent to the artery to allow for safe dissection, it is helpful to explore the cord more proximally toward the external inguinal ring, tugging the cord in a caudal direction with one of the Penrose drains positioned beneath the cord. The veins often coalescence at a more proximal level to form larger veins apart from the

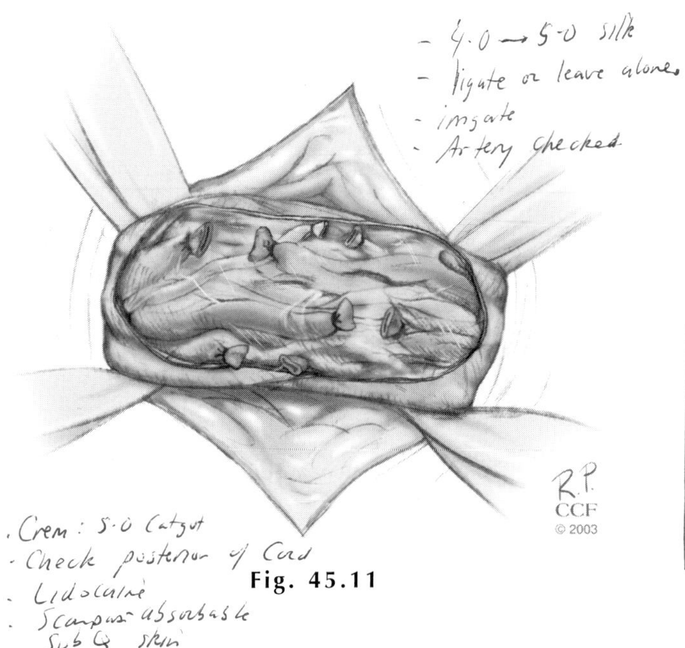


Fig. 45.11

artery. This higher dissection may present less risk to the artery when isolating the vein.

Once all of the veins and arteries are identified, each vein is individually double-ligated with a permanent suture (4-0 or 5-0 silk) and can then be transected or left as is (Fig. 45.11). The cord is then thoroughly irrigated, and the integrity of the artery(ies) is again assessed using the Doppler probe. The cremasteric muscle is reapproximated over the cord with 5-0 plain catgut. The whole cord is then lifted in an anterior direction using the Penrose drains to examine posterior to the cord for large, perforating veins that may be contributing to the varicocele. If identified, they are also ligated. The cord is then placed back into its normal position and the subcutaneous tissue and skin infiltrated with an equal mixture of 1% lidocaine HCl and 0.25% bupivacaine HCl. Scarpa's fascia is reapproximated with absorbable suture, and a subcuticular suture is used for the skin closure.

## The Inguinal Approach

This approach for ligation of the dilated venous plexus can be used in almost any patient. It allows for mobilization of the cord, identification of any large veins within the cremasteric muscle, and identification of veins perforating the posterior inguinal canal that might be contributing to the varicocele.

A skin crease incision is made between the internal and external inguinal ring or alternatively, parallel to the inguinal ligament as one would do for a standard inguinal hernia repair (Fig. 45.12). Once the external oblique fascia is identified and exposed, it is incised in the direction of its fibers (Fig. 45.13). Care is taken to identify and preserve the ileoinguinal nerve. The incision should extend from the level of the internal ring through the external ring so that the spermatic cord can be fully mobilized. Large, ectatic cremasteric veins are either cauterized or ligated, depending on their size. Similar to the subinguinal approach, the cremasteric muscle fibers covering the cord are opened longitudinally and the spermatic vessels are exposed. A Penrose drain is placed beneath the cord, lifting it to the surface of the incision, where the vessels can be more easily isolated.

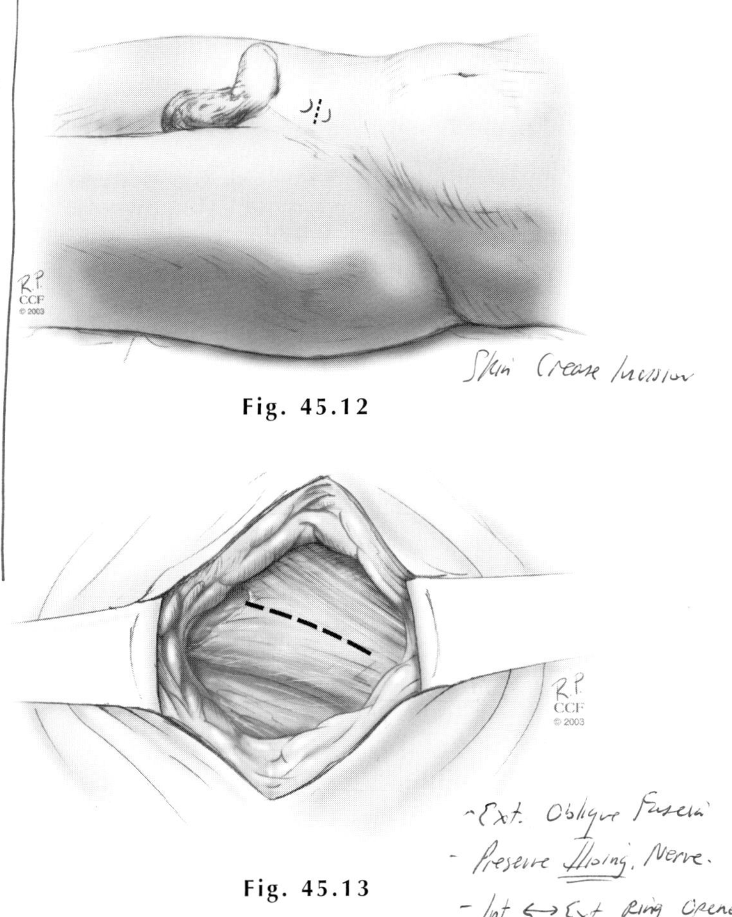


Fig. 45.12

Fig. 45.13

The larger veins comprising the varicocele are identified, and the loose, areolar tissue surrounding them is swept aside as each vein is identified and isolated with a vessel loop (Fig. 45.14). With the use of optical magnification—either loops or the operating microscope—the testicular artery can usually be identified and kept out of harm's way. If not readily identified or in spasm, dripping a dilute solution of papaverine HCl (30 mg/mL [1 mL: 10 mL saline]) over the cord will relax the arterial wall and enhance the pulsations of the artery(ies). A Doppler probe is useful in identifying and preserving the arteries. The clear lymphatics are also preserved. By dissecting the cord structures parallel to the vessels, it is easier to avoid transecting the lymphatics. After all of the veins have been identified and isolated (there are usually only three or four large veins at the level of the internal inguinal ring), they are double-ligated with 4-0 silk sutures and can be divided. After all the

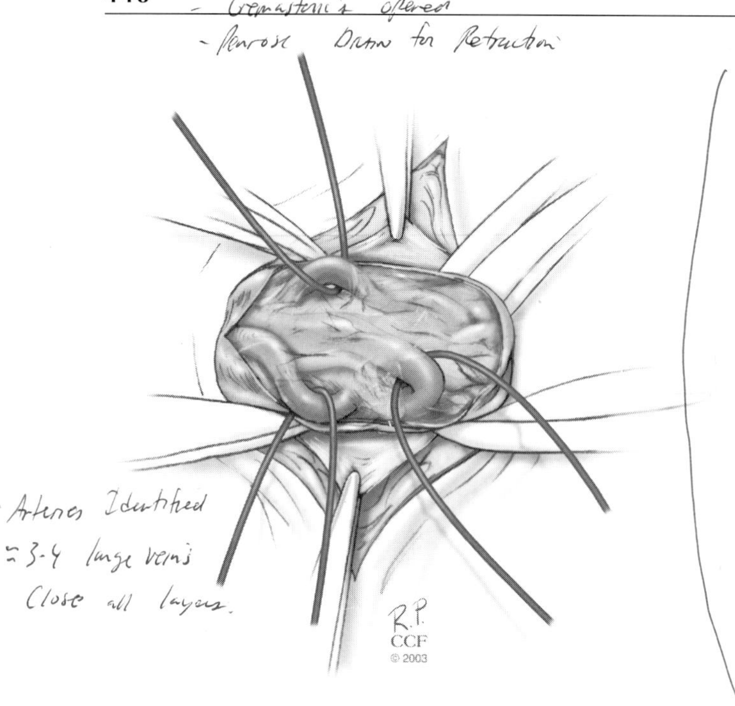


Fig. 45.14

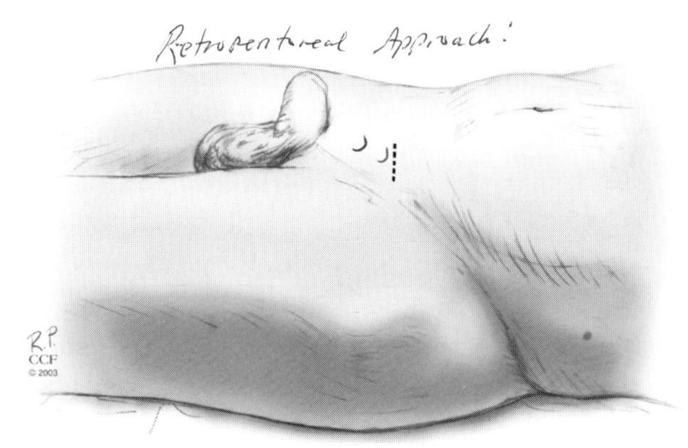


Fig. 45.15

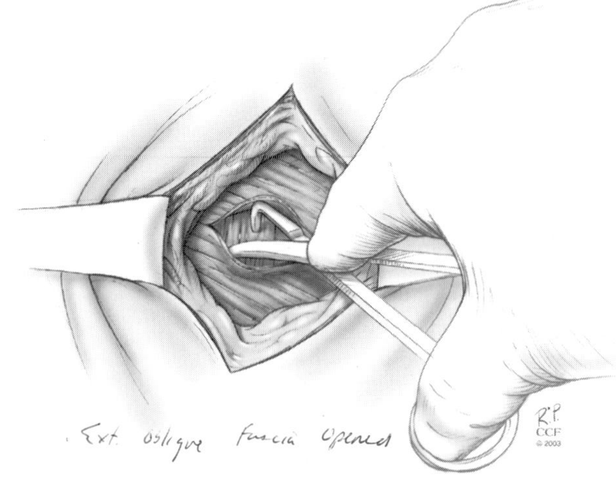


Fig. 45.16

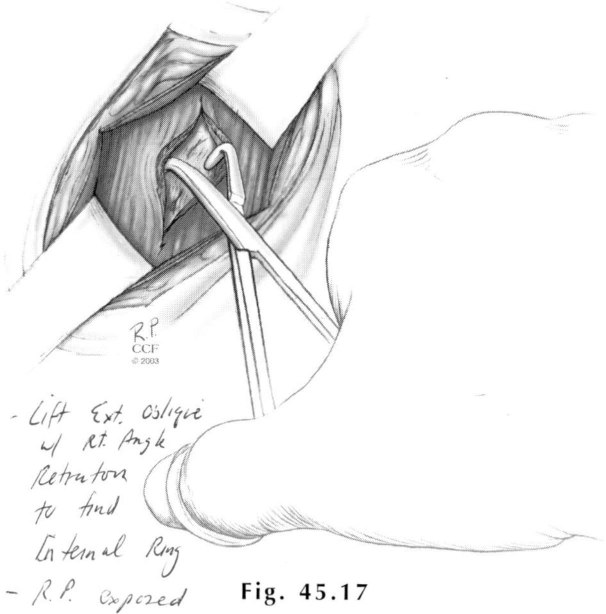


Fig. 45.17

veins have been ligated, the cremasteric muscle is closed over the spermatic cord and the cord is placed in its normal, anatomical position. The external oblique fascia is closed with interrupted 2-0 absorbable sutures, recreating a generous-sized external inguinal ring so as not to compromise blood flow to or from the testis. Subcutaneous tissue and skin are closed in a standard fashion.

## Retroperitoneal Approach

The retroperitoneal approach to the testicular veins is more easily accomplished in the thinner patient, although it can be done for any size individual, necessitating a larger incision for a bigger patient. With the patient in a supine position, a horizontal incision is made medial and inferior to the anterior iliac crest approximately 2 cm superior to the position of the internal inguinal ring (Fig. 45.15).

The incision is carried down through the subcutaneous tissues to the external oblique fascia that is opened in the direction of its fibers (Fig. 45.16). By placing small right-angle retractor at the inferior portion of the incision and lifting up the external oblique fascia, one can identify the internal inguinal ring.

Using a Kelly clamp or similar blunt-tipped instrument, the internal oblique and transversalis muscles are entered and the fibers spread apart, exposing the retroperitoneum at a level just above the internal inguinal ring (Fig. 45.17).

With gentle traction, the muscles are pulled apart along the line of their fibers, exposing the retroperitoneal space (Fig. 45.18). The spermatic vessels generally lie against the peritoneal reflection and can be followed to the internal ring. They are joined at this level by the vas deferens coming from the inferior aspect of the retroperitoneum.

Once the vessels are identified, the veins are individually isolated and double-ligated with permanent suture material

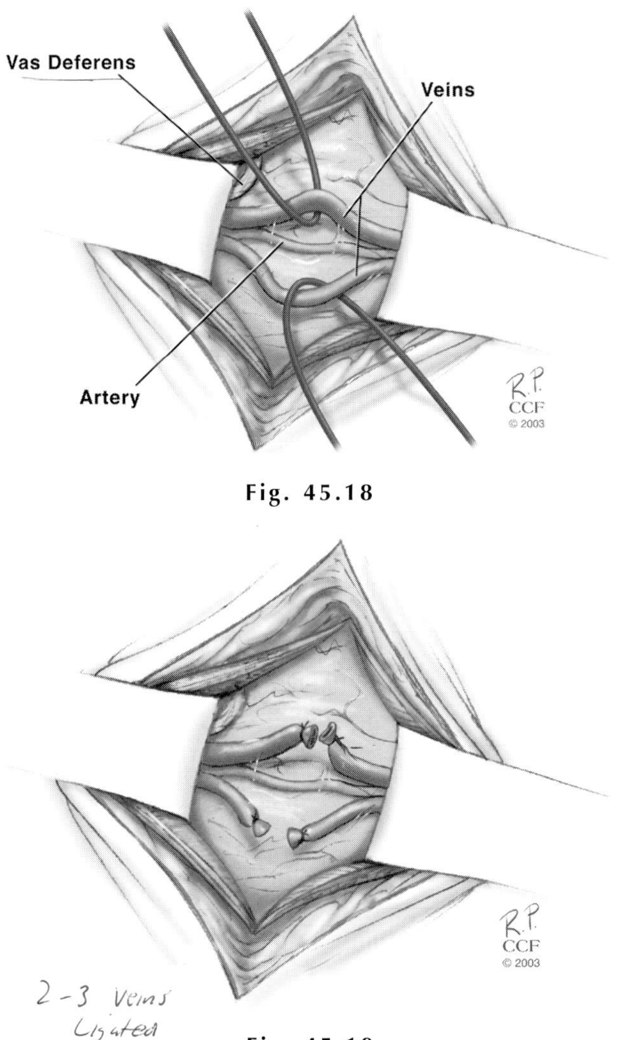


Fig. 45.18

Fig. 45.19

(Fig. 45.19). The testicular artery can often be identified between two large veins, and appropriate care is taken to maintain its integrity. Generally two or three large veins need to be ligated in this area. Once the veins have been ligated and cut, the area is irrigated with saline and the transversalis muscle and internal oblique are brought together with 2-0 chromic catgut or other absorbable suture. The external oblique is closed in a similar fashion using interrupted absorbable suture. Subcutaneous tissue and skin are closed in the usual manner.

## Complications of Varicocele Ligation

The more common complications of varicocele ligation include the persistence of the varicocele and secondary hydroceles that may result from obstruction of the lymphatics. These complications can generally be avoided by careful dissection of all the significant veins within the cord and careful preservation of lymphatic vessels. Injury to the testicular arterial blood supply is a potential risk and can lead to testicular atrophy. If the injury is noted during surgical procedure, attempts can be made to reanastomose the artery end-to-end, but in at least 40% of cases other arterial vessels allow the testis to survive.

## Transvenous Embolization of Varicocele

This technique can be recommended to patients only if there is a skilled interventional radiologist available to perform the procedure. It is then a valid alternative to open surgery. There are inherent advantages and disadvantages to the embolization technique. It allows for rapid return to normal, even strenuous activities. A venogram can act as a roadmap, identifying all the veins that need to be occluded. It can be an effective means of occluding a varicocele after a failed ligation procedure.

This method does require a skilled interventional radiologist experienced in embolization techniques. A rare patient may have an adverse reaction to the contrast material used to identify the varicocele. A coil used for embolization may dislodge from the vein during deployment and be carried through the heart to the lung. If there is bilateral or only a right-sided varicocele, it may be difficult for the radiologist to catheterize the right gonadal vein from the femoral vein approach because of the acute angle of the vein with the vena cava. Some of the lower collateral vessels and perforating veins posterior to the cord may not be accessible to the radiologist. Nevertheless, it is a valid technique for many men.

The procedure involves canulization of the right femoral vein with a 7 French guiding catheter directed into the left gonadal vein, monitoring passage by fluoroscopic imaging (Fig. 45.20). A smaller 4 French guiding catheter is passed through the 7 French catheter to the midportion of the gonadal vein. Nonionic contrast is injected to identify the varicocele and the venous collaterals.

The tip of the catheter is positioned at the level of the sacroiliac, and Gianturco coil(s) (Fig. 45.21, arrowheads) are passed through the catheter into the vein. The catheter is withdrawn upward, and further coils are placed to occlude the vein. A few milliliters of 70% dextrose are injected into the vein after the thrombogenic coils are placed to further promote thrombus formation.

A final injection of contrast confirms adequate occlusion of the veins (Fig. 45.22).

# VASOVASOSTOMY

The most common cause for obstruction of the vas deferens is the purposeful vasectomy performed for elective sterilization. It is not surprising, then, that the most frequently given indication to perform a vasovasostomy

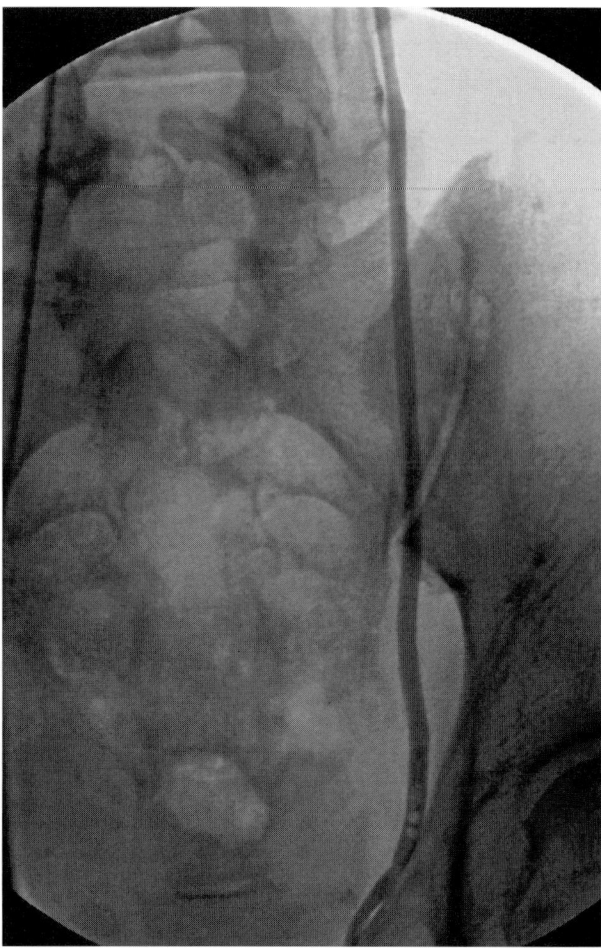

Fig. 45.20

is to reverse a prior vasectomy to restore the man's fertility. The most frequent cause for nonpurposeful vasal obstruction is inadvertent injury during the performance of a hernia repair. This more commonly occurs when the hernia is corrected in infancy.

Elective vasectomy is usually performed through a scrotal incision, and the obstruction occurring during hernia repair generally occurs in the groin. Regardless of where the obstruction is found, the basic principles that should to be considered to optimize the chance for success are the same:

1. There needs to be sufficient mobilization of both ends of the vas deferens so that there will be no tension on the anastomosis.
2. The blood supply within the perivasal adventitia must remain intact. It is tempting to strip away the adventitia immediately surrounding the cut ends of the vas deferens to gain better visualization and less troublesome oozing at the site of the anastomosis. If this is done, however, it can risk a higher rate of secondary scarring and obstruction at the anastomotic site.
3. Precise lumen-to-lumen approximation is imperative. Inaccurate approximation of the luminal edges of the vas deferens leads to sperm leakage outside the suture line and the formation of a sperm granuloma, resulting in a partial or total obstruction at the anastomotic site. While a perfect, leak-proof anastomosis is not necessary, careful apposition of the luminal edges will allow proper healing and minimal chance for sperm leakage.

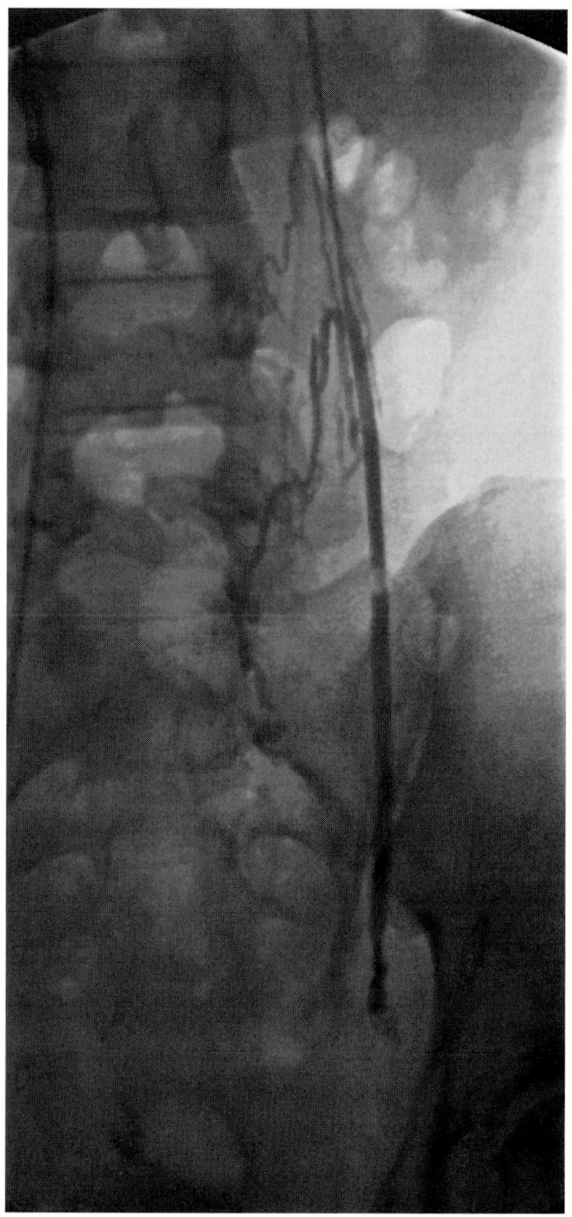

Fig. 45.21

## Anesthetic Considerations

Most men requesting vasectomy reversal are healthy and able to tolerate either a general, regional, or local anesthesia. There are some patients, however, who may have pulmonary or cardiovascular problems for which, for one reason or another, a specific type of anesthesia is preferred. For the vast majority of patients, monitored intravenous sedation and local anesthesia using an equal

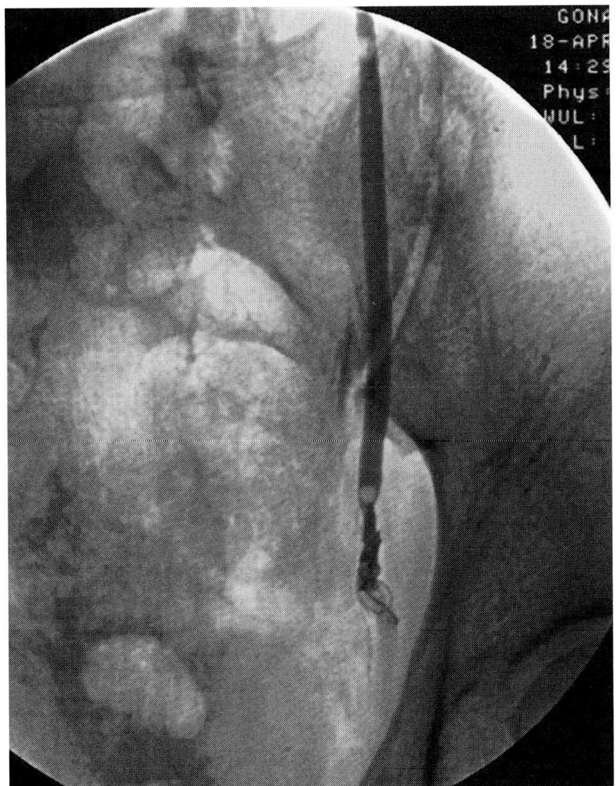

Fig. 45.22

mixture of 1% lidocaine hydrochloride and 0.25% bupivacaine seems to work quite well. If the procedure is prolonged (>3 h), the level of patient anxiety is high, or there is a need for extensive vasal or epididymal mobilization, a general or regional anesthetic may be best.

## Preparation of Vas Deferens for Scrotal Vasovasostomy

With the patient supine, the vas deferens is palpated through the skin to identify the area above the vasectomy site (Fig. 45.23). When using local anesthesia, the skin is infiltrated with the anesthetic solution and the vas deferens is isolated between thumb and forefinger with the vas held medial to the spermatic cord. The vas is grasped with a towel clamp, and a generous amount of local anesthesia is placed in the skin, after which a 1- to 2-cm incision is made.

Only the vas needs to be exposed, the testis remaining in the scrotum. Once the vas is isolated, dissection is carried out to free proximal and distal to the site of the prior vasectomy (Fig. 45.24).

The vas is held up with a towel clamp and the cord effectively blocked by injecting approximately 2–4 mL of the lidocaine/bupivacaine mixture into the perivasal adventitial space using a 30-gauge needle (Fig. 45.25). This effectively blocks the sensory nerves of the cord without risk of injuring the vessels of the spermatic cord.

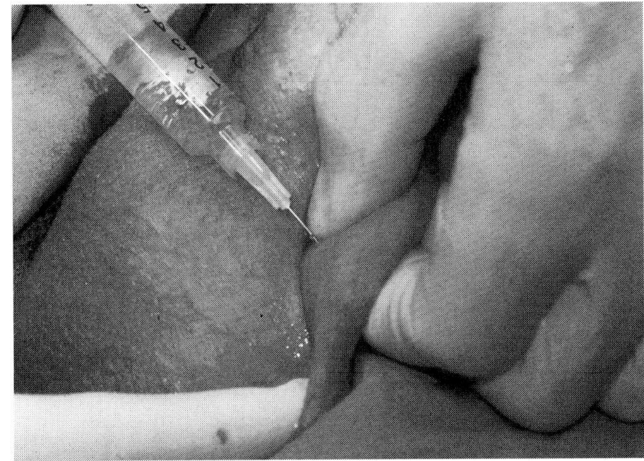

Fig. 45.23

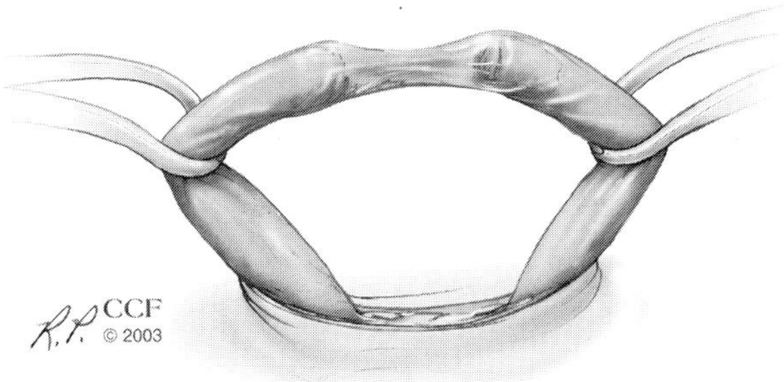


Fig. 45.24

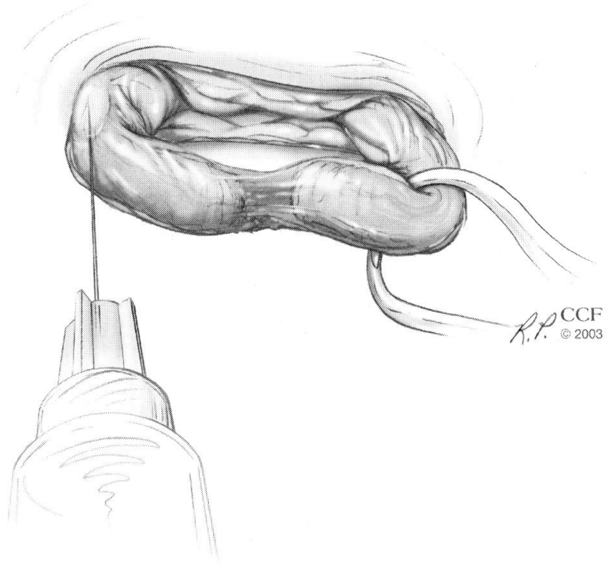


Fig. 45.25

Once sufficient lengths of the proximal and distal segments of the vas deferens are isolated, a 6-0 Prolene suture is passed through the muscularis of each end of the vas at the level where they exit the skin (Fig. 45.26). These sutures will later be tacked to the drapes that will

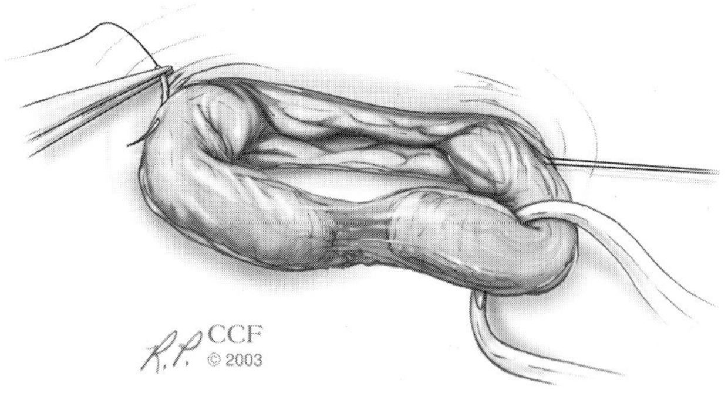


Fig. 45.26

hold the cut ends of the vas deferens above the incision in position where the anastomosis can easily be performed. Once the stay sutures are placed, isolation of the contralateral vas is carried out on the opposite side in a similar fashion.

Some surgeons prefer to use a clamp (Microspike Approximator Clamp, ASSI #3678, Accurate Surgical and Scientific Instruments Corporation, Westbury, NY) rather than the suture method to hold the vas deferens in position for suturing (Fig. 45.27A,B). Whichever method is preferred, sufficient length of both ends of the vas with its associated blood supply must be isolated to perform the surgery without tension.

The operating microscope is used at this point in the procedure. The vas deferens is transected at a right angle above and below the site of obstruction with a sharp scalpel blade over a tongue depressor or flat blade handle (Fig. 45.28). The vas should be cut at a level where the lumen and muscularis appear to be normal. The transected vasal vessels at the cut end of the cut vas are secured with 7-0 Prolene suture. The sutures used by the author for the actual lumen anastomosis of the vas or epididymis are the Sharpoint 10-0, $2^1/_2$ cm nylon double armed, 70 μm needle (3/8 circle 135 M.E.T., Surgical Specialties Corporation, Reading, PA) and the 9-0 Ethilon, VAS-100 needle manufactured by Ethicon (Johnson and Johnson Co.).

Fluid from the proximal (testicular) end of the vas deferens is expressed and placed onto a sterile glass slide to be examined under a light microscope. If there are sperm or sperm parts (sperm heads, sperm with partial tails in opaque fluid and in large numbers) or the fluid is clear and copious with no sperm seen, vasovasostomy is generally indicated. If the fluid is thick, pasty, and devoid of sperm or contains only a few sperm heads, vasoepididymostomy should be considered.

## Multilayer Vasovasostomy

The multilayer anastomosis is begun by placing two 9-0 sutures at the 5- and 7-o'clock positions through the adventitia and muscularis of each side of the vas deferens (Fig. 45.29). It is important that these sutures not be placed too close to the edge of the lumen, as they will prevent proper placement of the first lumenal suture.

A double-armed 10-0 suture is passed at the posterior 6-o'clock position (Fig. 45.30). This suture is tied and cut.

The second and third sutures are placed on either side of the first in an inside-out fashion using double-armed 2.5-cm sutures (Fig. 45.31). Neither suture is tied until both are placed.

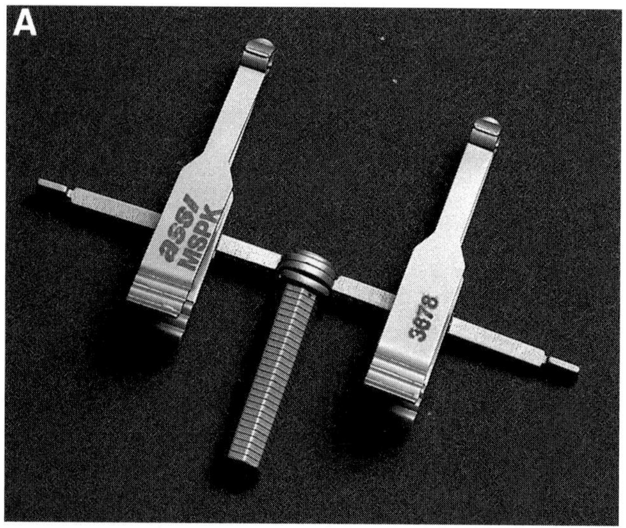


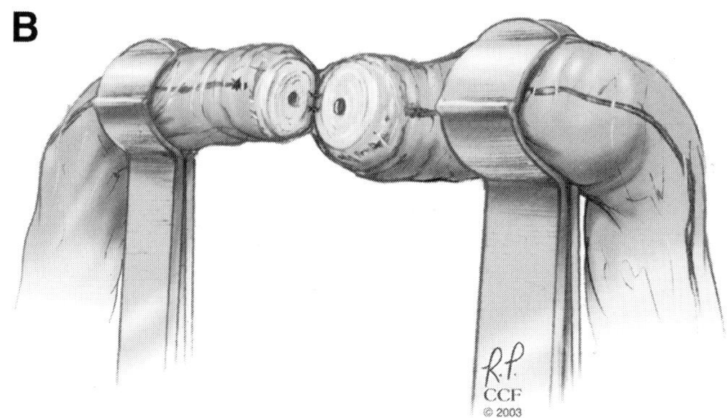


Fig. 45.27

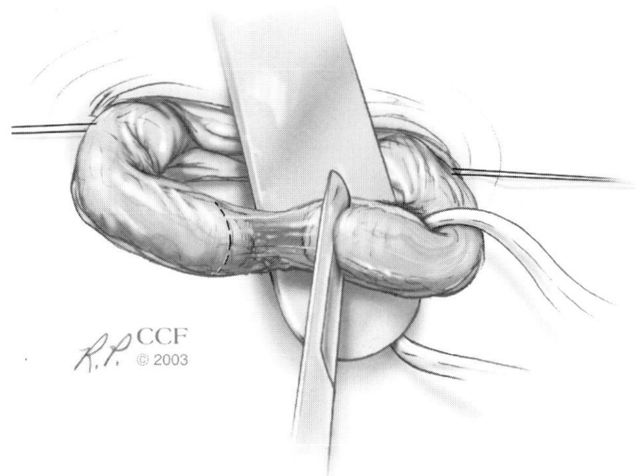


Fig. 45.28

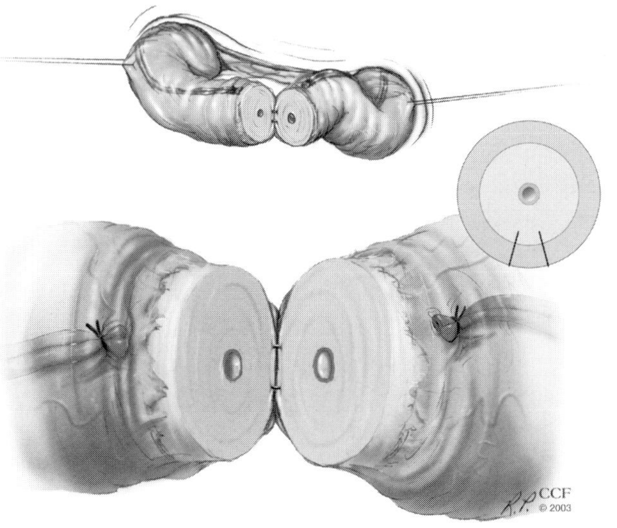


Fig. 45.29

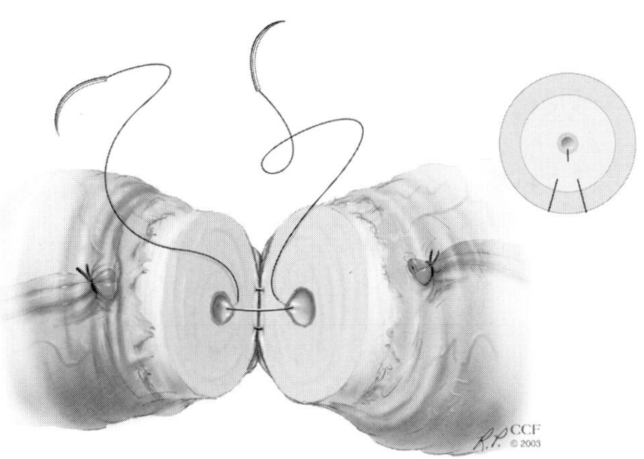


Fig. 45.30

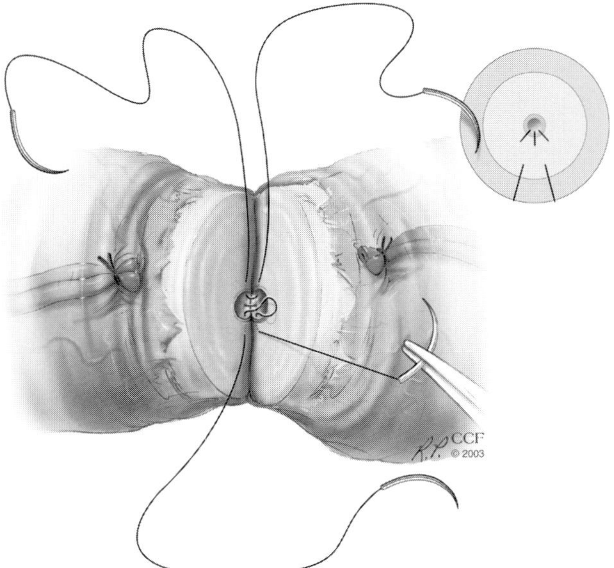


Fig. 45.31

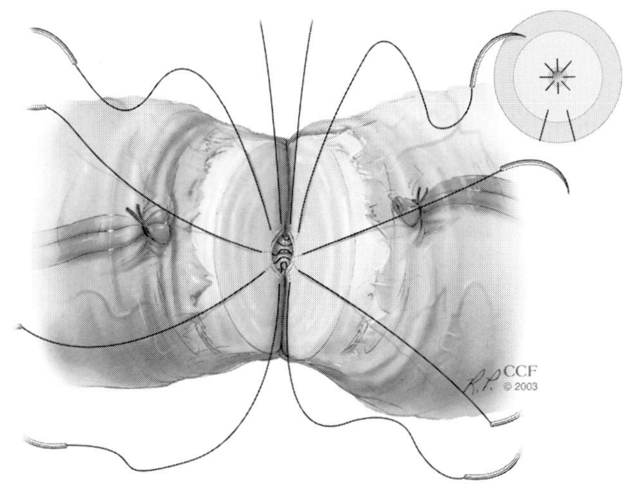


Fig. 45.32

Three to five more equidistant sutures are placed in the remainder of the lumen, leaving all untied (Fig. 45.32). Once all the sutures have been placed, they are tied, beginning with the lateral most sutures and ending with the most superior or 12-o'clock suture.

After the anastomosis of the lumen is complete, a 9-0 suture is passed at the 12-o'clock position (Fig. 45.33). This is placed to prevent unnecessary tension on the lumen while the muscularis is approximated.

Beginning on the side where the very first adventitia-muscularis sutures were placed on the posterior wall, 9-0 sutures are passed just through the muscularis until the 12-o'clock suture is met (Fig. 45.34). The same procedure is carried out on the opposing side of the vas.

A third layer of adventitial sutures is then added again, beginning at the 12-o'clock position, then on either side to

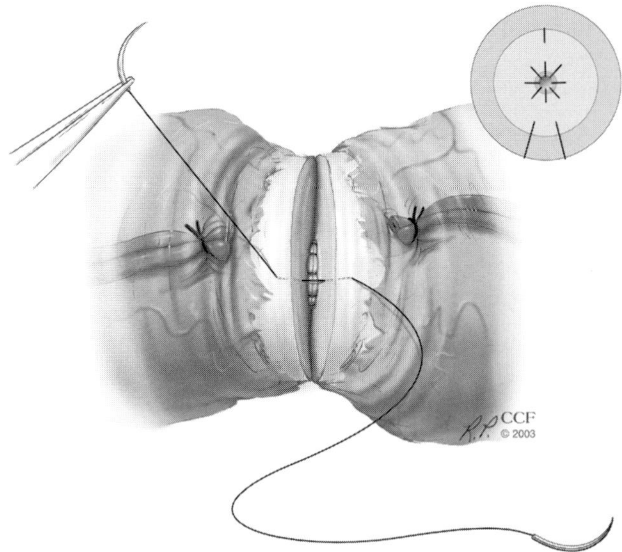


Fig. 45.33

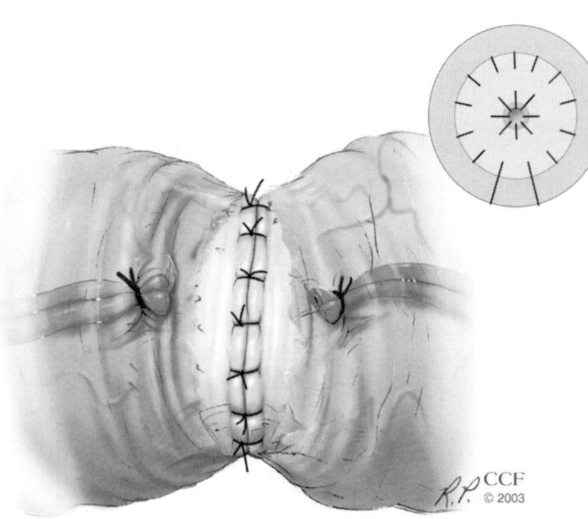


Fig. 45.34

meet the initially placed two sutures, which completes the anastomosis (Fig. 45.35A,B).

## Modified One-Layer Anastomosis

Some investigators have reported that a modified one-layer microsurgical anastomosis is as effective with respect to patency and pregnancy as the multilayer anastomosis. Some surgeons prefer this method because it is simpler, uses fewer sutures, and requires less intensive microsurgical skills. Nonetheless, the technique is precise and in order to be successful must be performed in the same exacting fashion as the multilayer anastomosis.

Using the operating microscope, a double-armed 10-0 suture is passed full thickness through the edge of the proximal and distal lumen, bringing the needles out through the outer wall of the vas (Fig. 45.36). Two more sutures are then passed in this fashion at the 4- and 8-o'clock positions and secured (Fig. 45.37). The last three sutures are passed full thickness at the 10-, 12- and 2-o'clock positions and then tied (Fig. 45.38). The muscularis is bolstered with two sutures of 9-0 placed in between each of the full-thickness sutures (Fig. 45.39). The adventitia can be approximated separately if not previously incorporated within the muscularis sutures (Fig. 45.40).

## Inguinal Vasovasostomy

Obstruction of the vas deferens within the inguinal canal is most often related to a prior hernia repair, frequently one performed in infancy, but can occur after any inguinal procedure where the vas and cord are manipulated. The diagnosis is suspected when examination reveals the testis to be normal size, the epididymis is full and firm, and the vas may be thickened with the convoluted portion more prominent to palpation.

Having proven that there is active spermatogenesis, a vasogram is performed, that reveals the vas lumen to be dilated and obstructed at the level of the inguinal canal (Fig. 45.41).

An inguinal incision is made, and the proximal (testicular) vas is isolated and held with a vascular loop (Fig. 45.42). In some instances there is a strip of scar tissue connecting the two ends of the vas so that tracing the tagged vas cephalad, toward the internal inguinal ring, the other end of the vas can be found.

Once the distal end is isolated, it is freed sufficiently from the surrounding tissue to ensure no tension on the anastomosis (Fig. 45.43). The vasovasostomy is carried out as described above using a modified single or multilayer technique.

## Postoperative Considerations

Almost all men can be discharged from the hospital the same day as their surgery. Those requiring extensive inguinal dissection may need to be kept overnight. It is recommended that patients undergoing scrotal vasovasostomy or vasoepididymostomy wear snug-fitting briefs or scrotal support for 2 wk. They are instructed not to have intercourse or perform any strenuous activities for 3 wk. A semen sample is examined 1 mo following surgery and every 3 mo thereafter for the first year. If no sperm appears in the semen by 6 mo after vasovasostomy, the surgical procedure is considered a failure.

The majority of pregnancies after vasovasostomy occur within 1 yr to 18 mo. The overall pregnancy rate ranges from 50 to 60%, depending on the series reviewed. There is a strong correlation between the occurrence of a pregnancy and the years of obstruction. The Vasovasostomy

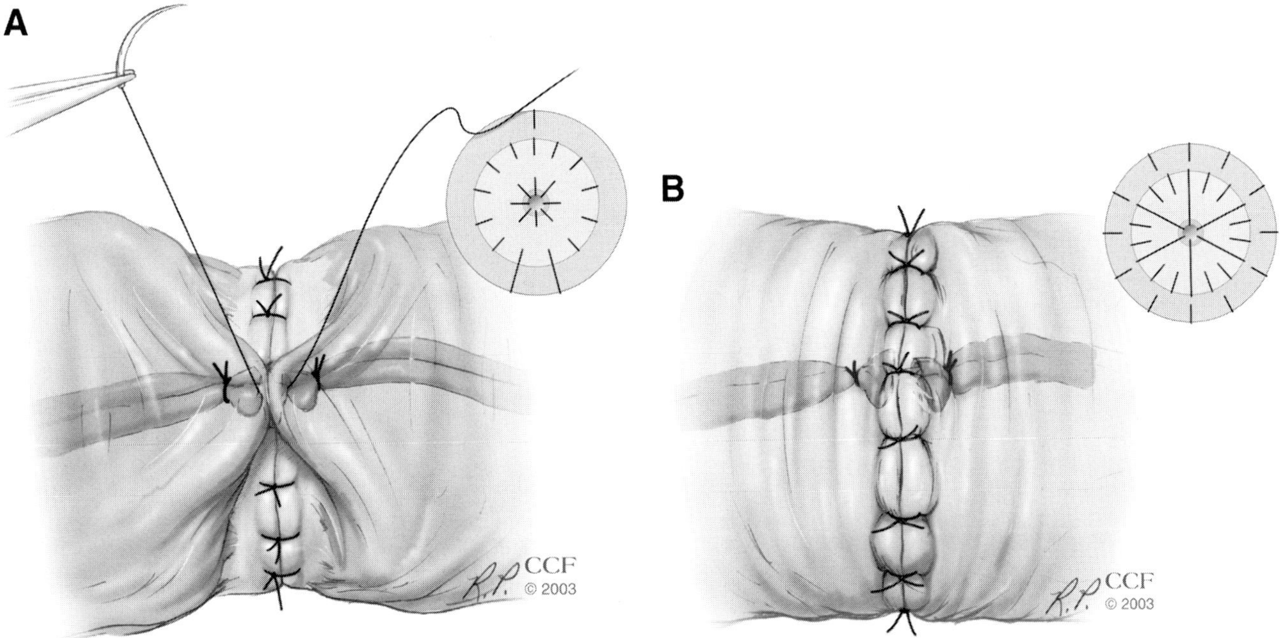


Fig. 45.35

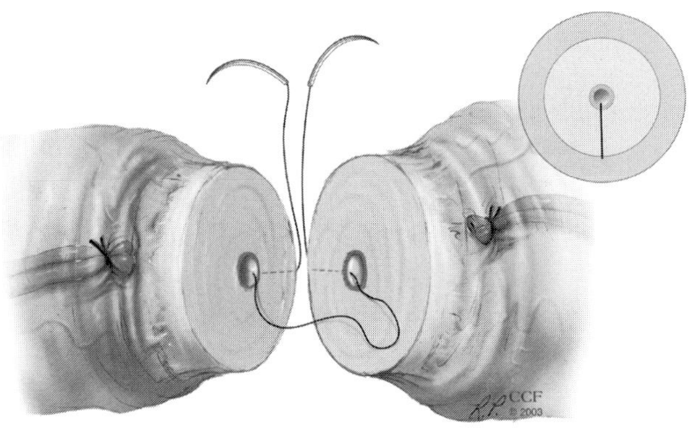


Fig. 45.36

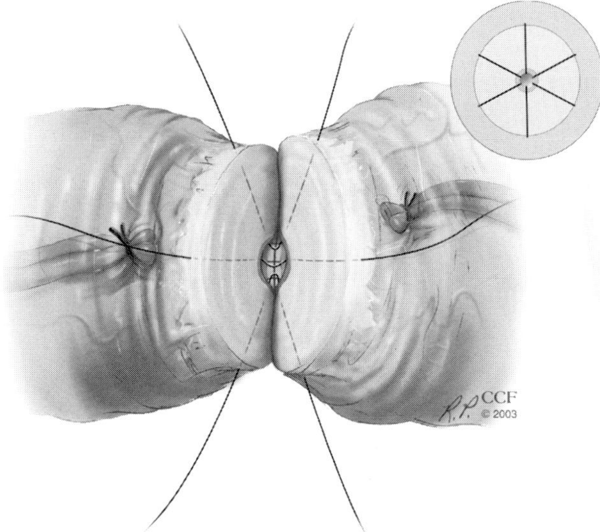


Fig. 45.38

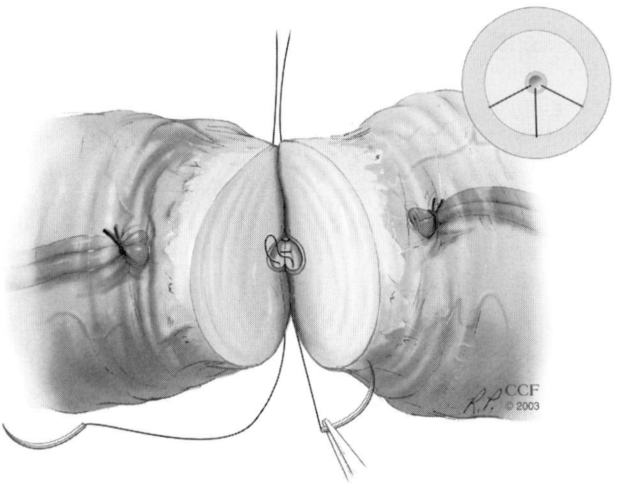


Fig. 45.37

Study Group reported that if a vasectomy was reversed within 3 yr, approximately 74% of patients established a pregnancy with their spouse. When the vasectomy was performed between 3 and 8 yr, 54% of patients established a pregnancy. Between 9 and 14 yr, 44% of patients established a pregnancy. After 14 yr the pregnancy rate was reported to be 30%. This report dealt almost exclusively with vasovasostomy without the performance of vasoepididymostomy. Recent studies have indicated that if a vasoepididymostomy is performed by an experienced micorsurgeon, as indicated by the proximal vassal fluid, in patients with an obstruction interval or more than 14 yr,

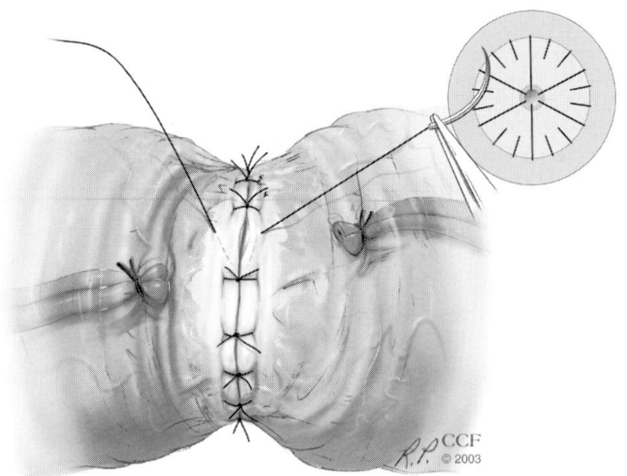


Fig. 45.39

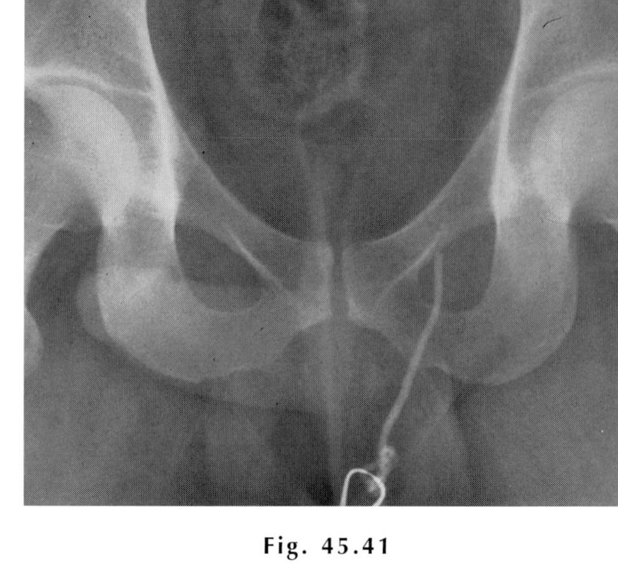

Fig. 45.41

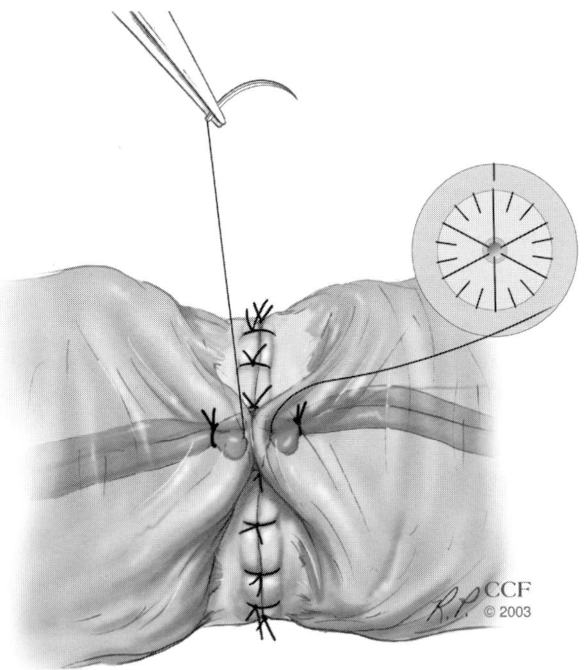


Fig. 45.40

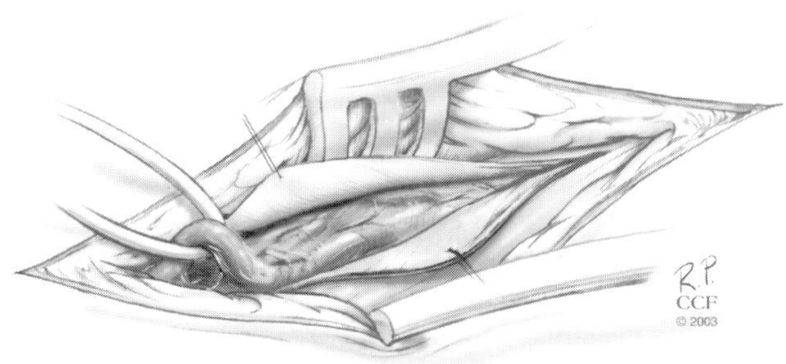


Fig. 45.42

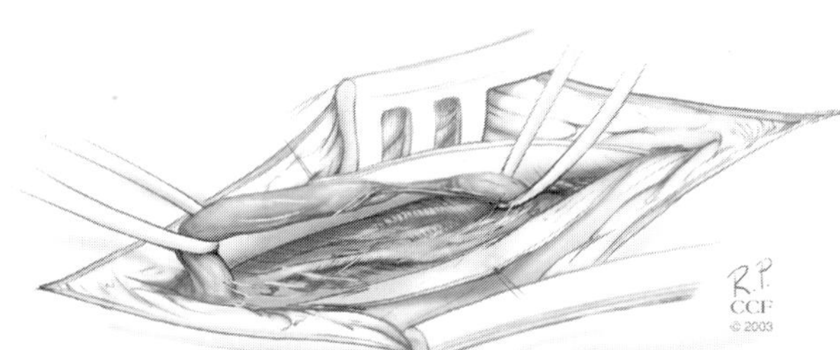


Fig. 45.43

pregnancy rates are better than 40% if the spouse is less than 40 yr of age.

## VASOEPIDIDYMOSTOMY

Obstruction of the epididymis can result from a congenital, inflammatory, traumatic, or postvasectomy cause. Men presenting with epididymal obstruction will be azoospermic and have a normal semen volume and palpable vas deferens. Some men who have had a vasectomy for sterilization and are requesting reversal may have a secondary obstruction within the epididymis due to a high-pressure "blowout." This is more common in men who have had their vasectomy for a long period of time (e.g., 8–10 yr) but it can occur at any time. Recently, Fuchs and Bert reported that 62% of men having vasectomies for more than 15 yr required a vasoepididymostomy on one or both sides when a vasectomy reversal was performed. The characteristics of the

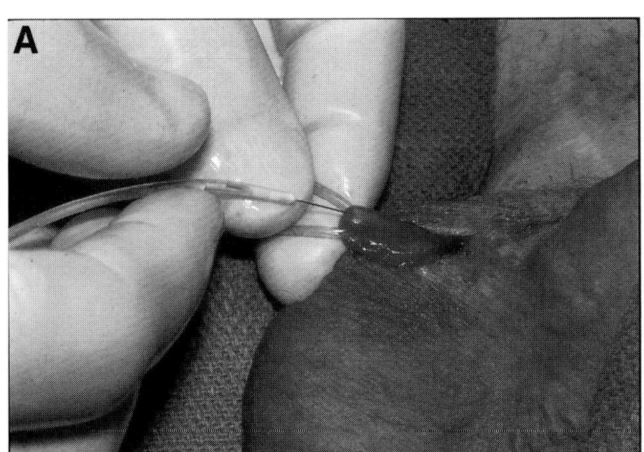


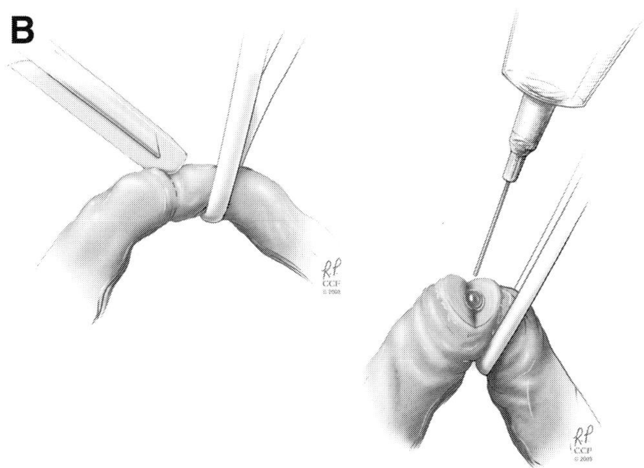


Fig. 45.44

proximal vasal fluid that would necessitate consideration for vasoepididymostomy after vasectomy would be that it is thick, creamy or pasty, devoid of sperm, or containing only a few sperm heads. The absence of sperm in the fluid in and of itself is not always an indication for vasoepididymostomy, as pointed out by a study performed by Sharlip, but rather a combination of the type of fluid and the absence of sperm.

With the exclusion of postvasectomy patients, the diagnosis of bilateral epididymal obstruction should not be difficult. These patients are normal with respect to testicular size, gonadotropin levels, semen volume, and palpable vas deferens. The epididymis may be palpably prominent and at times indurated and nodular.

## Methods of Vasoepididymostomy

A testis biopsy can be performed as a separate procedure preceding the vasoepididymostomy or, as this author prefers, at the time of the planned reparative surgery. A frozen section is sent for pathological examination and confirmation of active spermatogenesis. This author finds it useful to take a small piece of the testicular tissue and tease it apart on a sterile glass slide. A drop of saline is placed over this and a cover slip compressed against the tissue. This tissue can be looked at in the operating room under a light microscope, and if there is normal spermatogenesis, sperm can be easily identified, often with some motility.

Over the past 15 yr, three techniques that have been described for performing a microsurgical vasoepididymal anastomosis. Each method has been reported to have a fairly high degree of success when performed by an experienced microsurgeon. These are the end-to-end anastomosis, originally described by Silber, the end-to-side anastomosis, reported by this author and Fogdestam et al., and, recently, the end-to-side intassusception technique, as described by Berger.

## Vasography

Once active spermatogenesis is ascertained, a vasogram is performed, isolating the straight portion of the vas deferens and passing a 30-gauge lymphangiogram needle directly into the lumen (Fig. 45.44). Alternatively, the vas can be hemi transected and a 24-gauge plastic angiocatheter inserted into the vas lumen and the contrast injected.

A one-to-one mixture of Renografin 60® and saline is injected into the vas deferens and a radiograph taken (Fig. 45.45). This will confirm patency of the vas deferens, seminal vesicles, and ejaculatory ducts. After a vasogram has been performed the vas deferens is further dissected and freed up down to the level of the convoluted vas. The vas is cut at this level, and the associated vasal vessels are ligated with 7-0 permanent sutures (Prolene) at the cut end. The testicular end of the vas deferens and the associated vessels are ligated and secured. The distal vas deferens is freed sufficiently to bring it lateral to the epididymis keeping it within the tunica vaginalis. The anastomosis should be done at the most distal portion of the epididymis where motile or nonmotile normal-appearing sperm are found. The sutures used by this author for vasoepididymostomy are the Sharpoint 10-0, $2^1/_2$-cm suture double-armed, 70-μm needle, 3/8 circle, 135 M.E.T., (Surgical Specialties Corporation, Reading, PA) and the 9-0 Ethilon, VAS-100 needle manufactured by Ethicon (Johnson and Johnson Co.).

## End-to-End Anastomosis

The success of his procedure is based on the fact that the body and tail of the epididymis are a single continuous tubule.

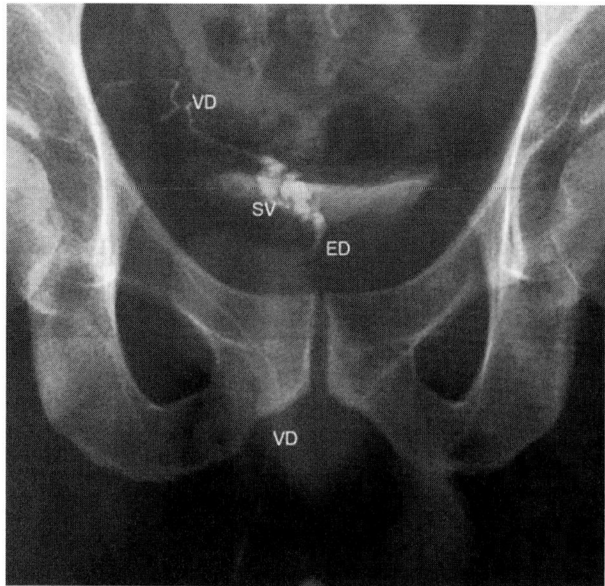


Fig. 45.45

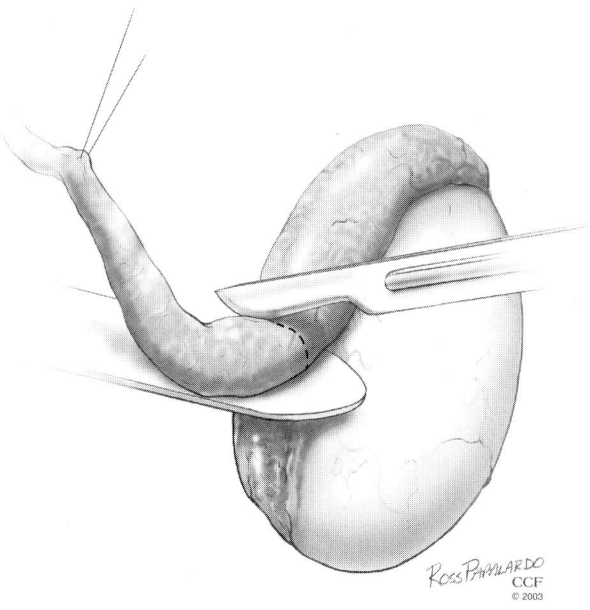

Fig. 45.46

Once the testis and cord structure have been exposed and vasal patency confirmed, the vas deferens with its blood supply is isolated and the vas cut at the level of the mid-convoluted portion. At the cut ends, the blood vessels are secured with 6-0 Prolene sutures.

Careful inspection of the epididymis will sometimes give a clue as to the site of the obstruction. In some instances there is a blue-brown discoloration just below the epididymal tunic, indicating a point of sperm extravasation and obstruction. The epididymis should be explored from the most caudal portion and move cephalad to be certain the anastomosis is performed in the most distal, patent portion of the epididymis.

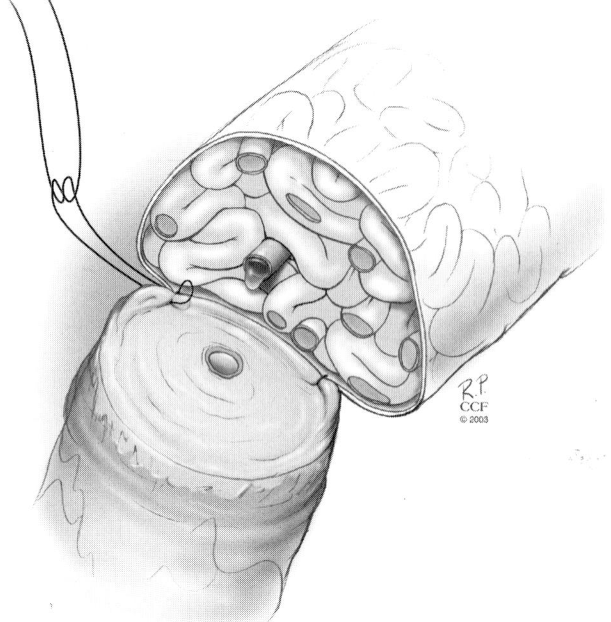

Fig. 45.47

The epididymal tail is dissected away from the inferior aspect of the testis and the epididymis is transected at its distal end (Fig. 45.46). When the epididymis is cut above the level of the obstruction, there will be a continuous flow of sperm-laden fluid exiting from only one opened epididymal tubule. The presence of sperm is confirmed by aspirating fluid from the end of the cut tubule and examining it under a light microscope. If no sperm are found, another transecting cut is made approximately $^1/_2$ cm higher toward the head of the epididymis until normal-appearing motile or nonmotile sperm are identified.

Once the cut tubule exuding sperm is identified, two 9-0 nylon sutures are passed through the edge of the epididymal tunic and into the adventitia and muscularis of the vas deferens to bring the two structures into close approximation (Fig. 45.47). The lumen of the vas deferens is then anastomosed to the cut open tubule exuding sperm.

Four equally spaced double-armed 10-0 sutures are placed into the edge of the epididymal tubule, inside-out, and then through the vas lumen beginning at the 6-o'clock position (Fig. 45.48). The first suture is tied, but the 3-, 9- and 12-o'clock positioned sutures are not tied until all three are placed.

Once the two lumens are approximated, the muscularis and adventitia of the vas deferens are secured to the tunic of the epididymis with interrupted 9-0 sutures (Fig. 45.49).

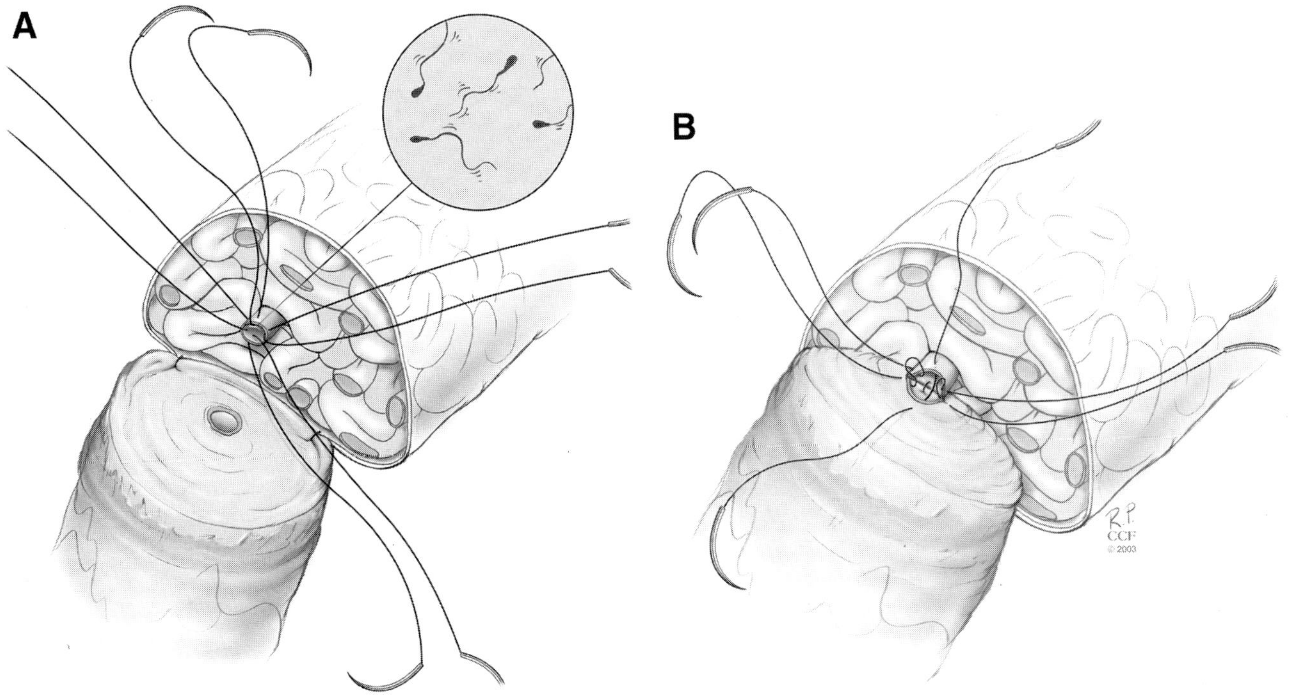


Fig. 45.48

## End-to-Side Technique

After the vas is prepared in the manner described above for the end-to-end anastomosis, the epididymis is examined with the operating microscope and a 1-cm incision is made in the tunic of the epididymis, usually beginning at the caudal level (Fig. 45.50). Using a round-tip microscissor, a small window is created in the tunic, exposing the loops of the intact epididymal tubule below.

By gently compressing the sides of the epididymis with thumb and forefinger, the loops will bulge through the opened tunic, and a single loop can be isolated from the surrounding connective tissue (Fig. 45.51). This anterior surface of this loop is incised with a micro knife, creating an opening of approximately 0.5 mm. The fluid exuding from this loop is aspirated, placed on a glass slide and examined for sperm. If normal-appearing sperm are found, this is the level at which the anastomosis is performed. If motile sperm are to be cryopreserved, they are aspirated as they flow from the opened loop, placed into an appropriate medium, and sent to the cryopreservation laboratory for processing. If no sperm or only sperm parts are found coming from the epididymal tubule, the tunic is incised more cephalad and the same procedure repeated until normal-appearing spermatozoa are identified.

When the proper loop is identified and incised, three 10-0 double-armed sutures are placed (inside-out) in a triangular fashion equidistant from one another (Fig. 45.52).

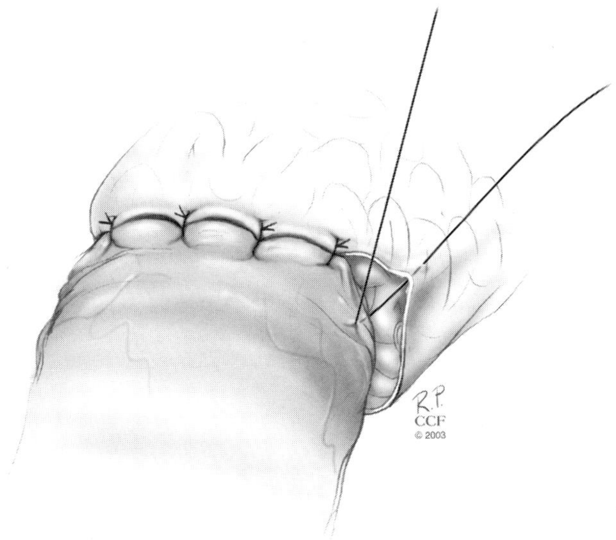


Fig. 45.49

The cut end of the vas deferens is brought to the epididymis just next to the area of the opened tubule (Fig. 45.53). Two 9-0 sutures are passed through the adventitia of the epididymal tunic and into the muscularis and adventitia of the vas deferens at the 5-o'clock and 7-o'clock positions to secure the vas deferens to the epididymal tunic and prevent tension while the lumens are approximated. The 6-o'clock suture that was passed in to the epididymal lumen is now passed in to the lumen of the

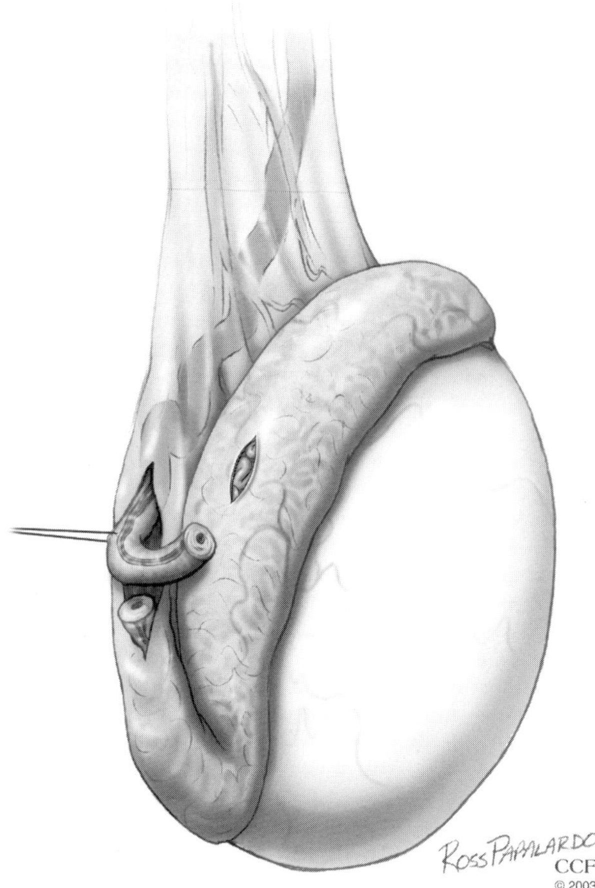


Fig. 45.50

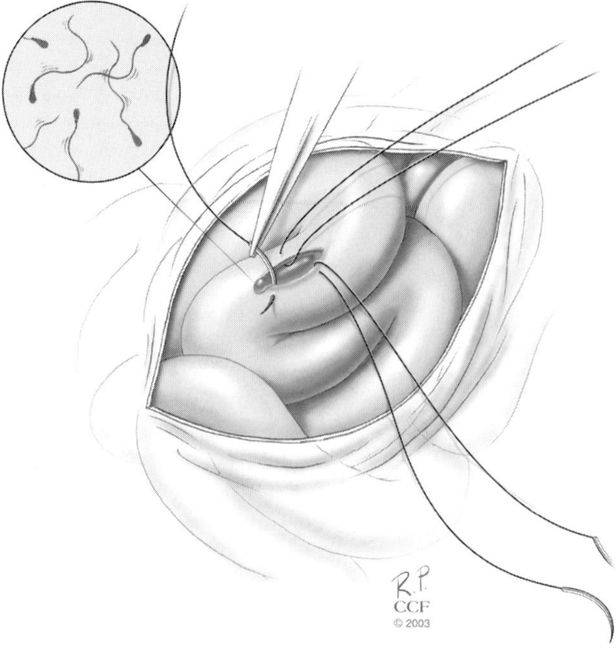


Fig. 45.52

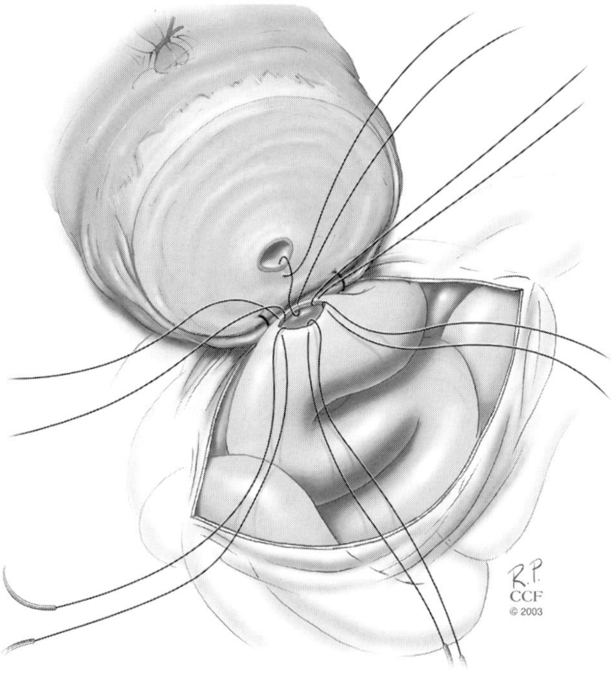


Fig. 45.53

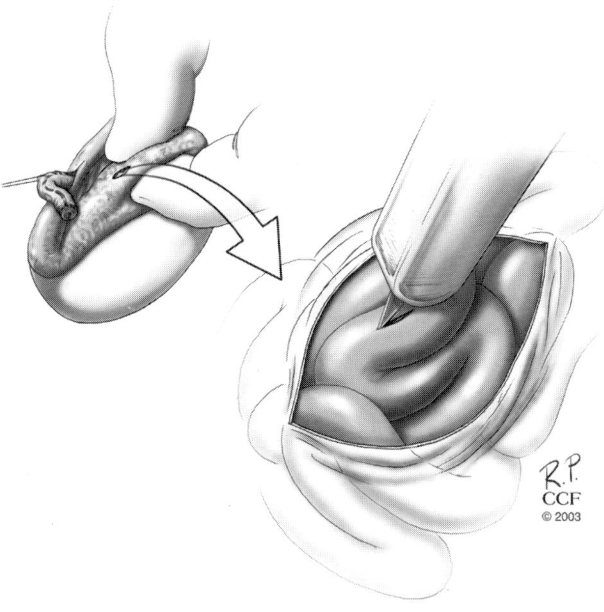


Fig. 45.51

vas deferens and tied. This splays opens up the epididymal lumen and allows for easier passage of two new sutures at the 4- and 8-o'clock positions into the epididymal lumen and the vas (Fig. 45.54). Once properly placed, they are tied.

The two sutures that were initially passed into the epididymal lumen with the 6-o'clock suture are placed into

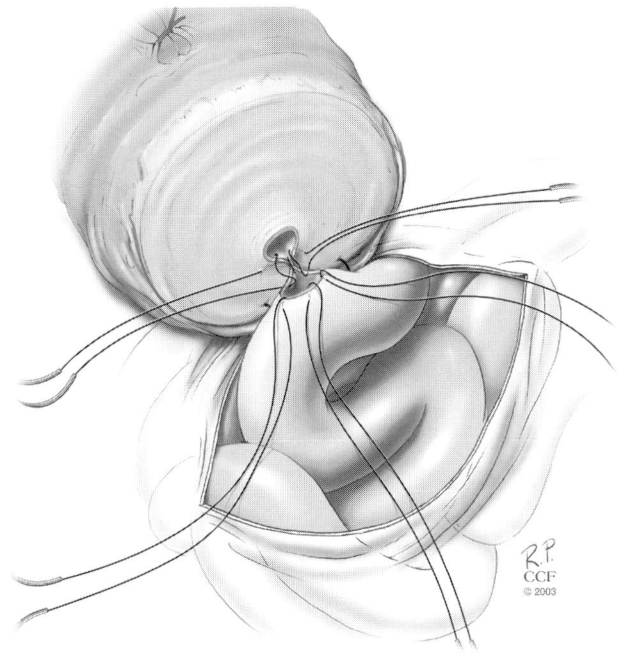


Fig. 45.54

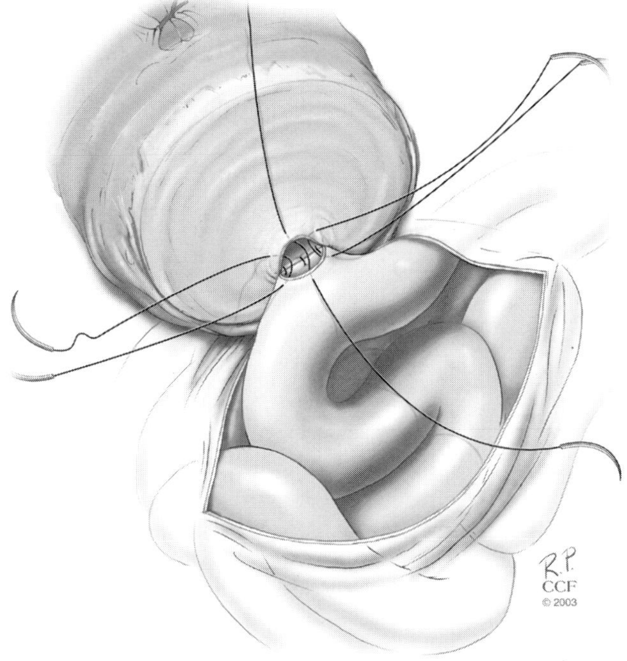


Fig. 45.55

the vasal lumen but not tied (Fig. 45.55). A final 10-0 suture is passed at the 12-o'clock position through the epididymal lumen and into the vasal lumen. Once these last three sutures are properly positioned, they are tied in sequence, tying the 12-o'clock suture last.

The muscularis and adventitia of the vas deferens are approximated to the epididymal tunic, in a circumferential fashion, with 8–10 9-0 sutures (Fig. 45.56).

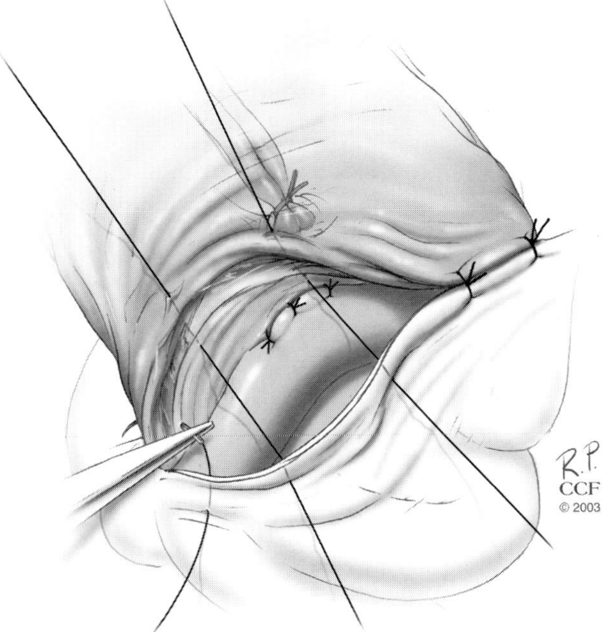


Fig. 45.56

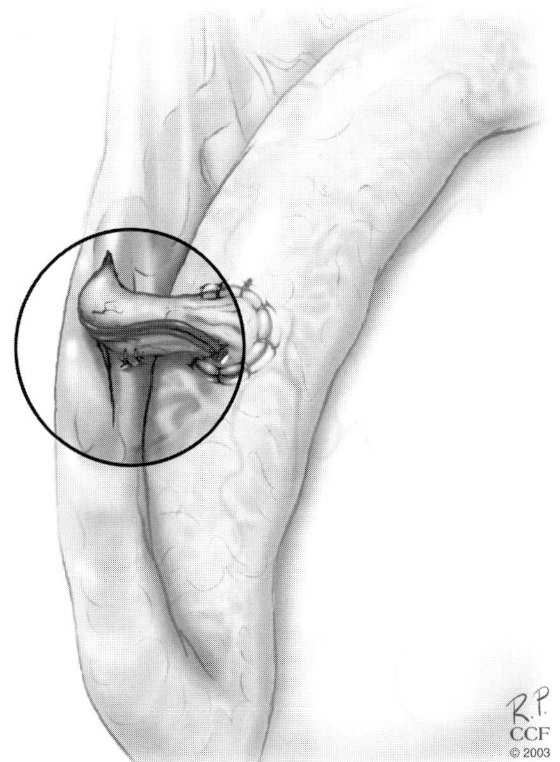


Fig. 45.57

Bolstering sutures are placed along the side of the vas attaching to the visceral tunic (Fig. 45.57). These sutures can prevent any undue stress on the actual anastomosis as the testis is repositioned in the scrotum.

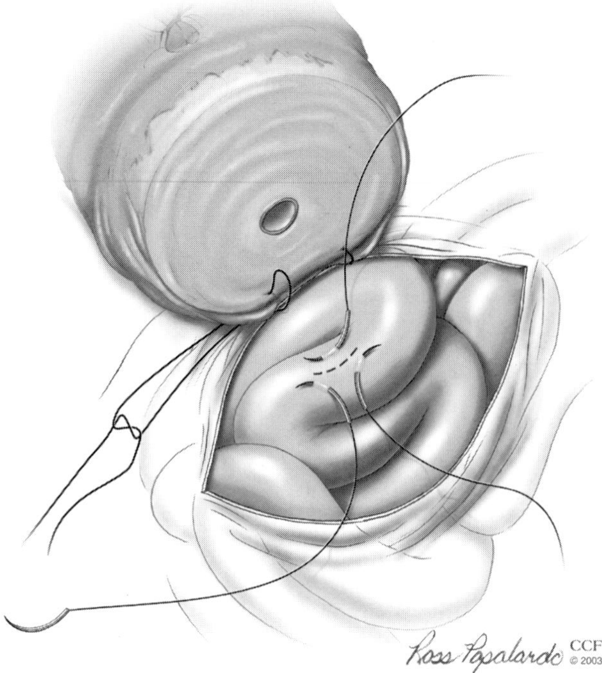


Fig. 45.58

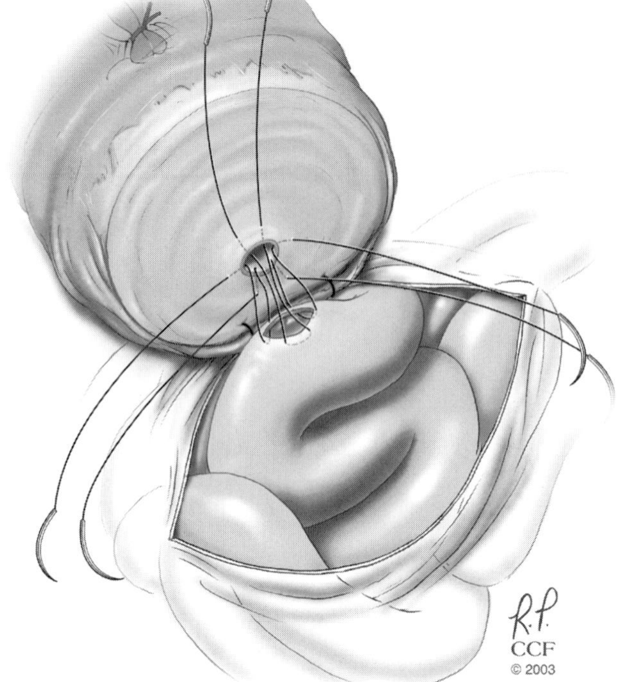


Fig. 45.59

## Intussusception Technique

The difference in this technique over the standard end-to-side technique is that the lumen is not opened until the sutures are placed in the epididymal loop and the opened loop is drawn into the vasal lumen rather than approximated to it. The epididymal loop must be freed from any connective tissue sufficient to allow it to be pulled into the vasal lumen.

Once the vas is cut and an appropriate epididymal loop is isolated, as in the standard end-to-side technique, the vas deferens is approximated to the tunic (Fig. 45.58). Three double-armed 10-0 sutures are passed in a triangular fashion, leaving the center open for incision. With only the needles placed into the lumen of the tubule, an incision is made between the three needles and the fluid that exudes is examined. If normal-appearing sperm are found, the needles are drawn through and left intact. If there are no sperm, the needles can be removed and used again in another epididymal loop.

The two needles attached to the suture closest to the vas are passed into the vas lumen and brought out just through the muscularis (Fig. 45.59). The other two sutures are positioned in a similar fashion. The most posterior suture is tied first followed by the others, in sequence.

As the sutures are tied, the epididymal loop intussuscepts into the vas lumen (Fig. 45.60). The adventitia and muscularis of the vas deferens are then sutured to the tunic of the epididymis, as in the end-to-side technique.

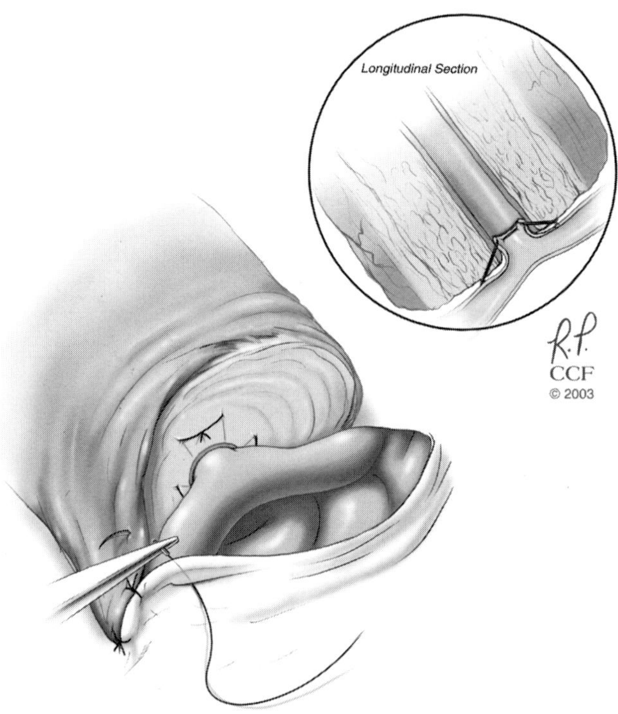


Fig. 45.60

With all procedures, the anastomosis should be within the tunica vaginalis, which can be closed over the testis at the end of the procedure.

**Table 1**
**Results of Microsurgical Vasoepididymostomy**

| *No. of patients* | *Patent (%)* | *Pregnant (%)* | *Source* |
|---|---|---|---|
| 23 | — | 9(39) | McLoughlin, 1982 |
| 46 | 18(39) | 6(13) | Dubin and Amelar, 1984 |
| 41 | 35(85) | 15(37) | Fogdestam et al., 1986 |
| 139 | (78) | (56) | Silber, 1989 |
| 39 | (60) | (36) | Fuchs, 1991 |
| 137 | 108(79) | 47(50)[a] | Thomas, 1992 |
| 107 | 64(70) | 28(35)[b] | Schlegel and Goldstein, 1993 |
| 100 | (65) | (21) | Matthews et al., 1995 |
| 89 | (56) | — | Jarow et al., 1995 |
| 31 | 11 | 3 | Boeckx and Van Helden, 1996 |
| 55 | (85) | 20(44)[c] | Kolettis and Thomas, 1997 |
| 49 | (61) | — | Berardinucci et al., 1998 |
| 24 | 13(54) | 4(17) | Hibi et al., 2000 |

[a]Based on 94 patients with follow-up of >1 yr or those who established a pregnancy before 1 yr (9 patients).
[b]Based on 81 couples without female factor infertility with follow-up of at least 1 yr.
[c]All patients had undergone prior vasectomy.

### Postoperative Care

Postoperative instructions for patients undergoing vasoepididymostomy are similar to those for vasovasostomy. Restriction from heavy lifting, strenuous activity, and intercourse for 3 wk is recommended. Semen analysis is performed at 4 wk, and every 3 mo thereafter for 1 yr. It may take up to 1 yr for sperm to appear in the semen, although most men have sperm in the semen by 6 mo.

In the last 15 yr new microsurgical techniques have been devised that have improved both patency and pregnancy rates. The level at which the vasal epididymal anastomosis is performed plays a crucial role with regard to subsequent maturation and fertilization potential of ejaculated sperm. The results of various authors' reports for microsurgical vasoepididymostomy are included in Table 45.1.

## EJACULATORY DUCT OBSTRUCTION

Complete obstruction of the ejaculatory ducts results in azoospermia. The cause can be either congenital or acquired. Whatever the etiology, the manifestation of obstruction is the same:

1. Azoospermia
2. Small-volume semen (<1.5 mL)
3. Semen is acidic and fructose is absent or low
4. Postejaculatory urine devoid of sperm
5. Gonadotropin levels normal if active spermatogenesis is present
6. Testicles normal in size and consistency, often with palpably thickened epididymides and vasa deferentia

Confirmation of the diagnosis is made based on the above findings, normal spermatogenesis on biopsy, and the dilation of the seminal vesicles and ejaculatory ducts with or without ejaculatory duct cyst (Fig. 45.61, arrowhead) within the substance of the prostate (arrows) when examined using transrectal ultrasound or magnetic resonance imagery of the pelvis.

Effective treatment depends on the ability to reach the ejaculatory ducts or midline cyst with a resectascope loop (Fig. 45.62). If there is no dilation within the prostatic substance, in this author's opinion it is not advisable to try to resect through the prostate and beneath the bladder neck. If, however, there is dilatation of the ejaculatory ducts (Fig. 45.62a) or a midline cyst (Fig. 45.62b), resection to open the ducts/cyst can be accomplished in most instances.

Most of the men who present with ejaculatory duct obstruction are young, and their prostates are small as compared to those of older men with hypertrophy. Because of the relative thinness of the prostate, this author found that a regular 24 French resectascope loop (Fig. 45.63a) was large and cumbersome, as it tended to cut more tissue than needed. Consequently, a modification (Fig. 45.63b) of the loop (Storz # GS27050, Karl Storz, Inc., Tuttlingen, Germany) was made, which allows for smaller strips of tissue to be taken with less risk of resecting more tissue than necessary.

### Method of Resection

With the patient in lithotomy position, a vasogram (if needed) can be performed through a small incision in the scrotum. The vas deferens is isolated, a 30-gauge

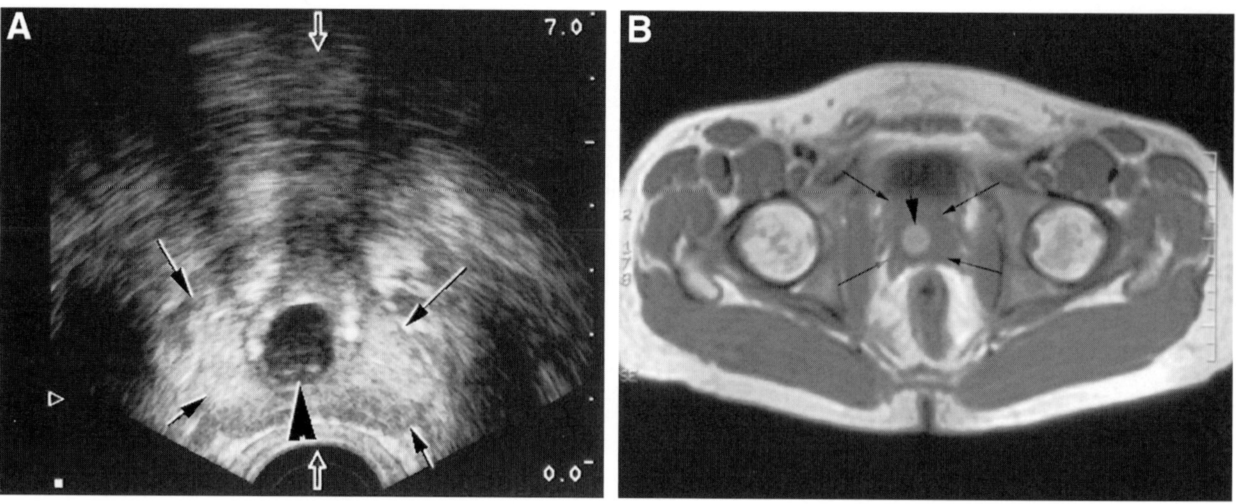


Fig. 45.61

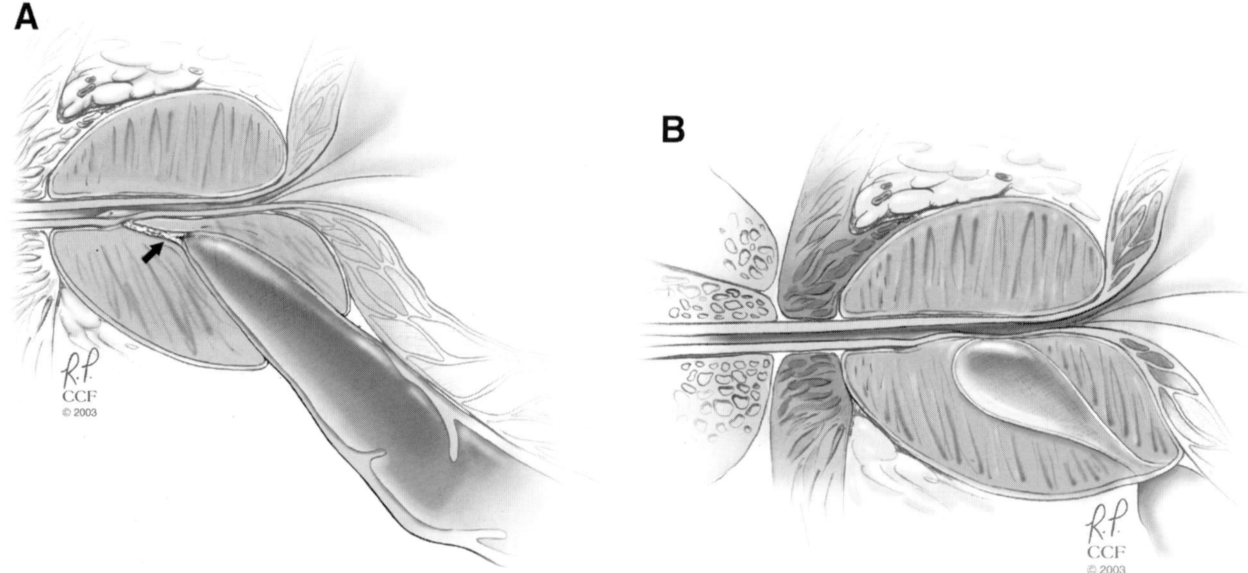


Fig. 45.62

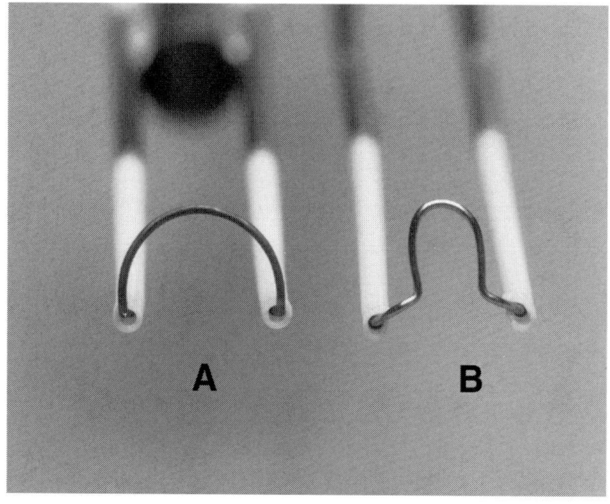


Fig. 45.63

lymphangiogram needle is passed into the dilated lumen, and the fluid in the lumen is aspirated and examined for the presence of sperm. If no sperm are identified, there may be an associated secondary epididymal obstruction similar to that found after long-term vasectomy. Even when no sperm are found in the vasal fluid, the ejaculatory duct obstruction should be corrected followed by the epididymal obstruction once the ejaculatory ducts are opened and the semen volume returned to normal.

After aspirating the vasal fluid, a 1:1 solution of Renographin 60® and saline mixed with a small amount of indigo carmine is injected into the vas and an x-ray is taken to confirm the point of obstruction. The addition of blue indigo carmine will allow the ejaculatory duct to be more easily seen, when opened.

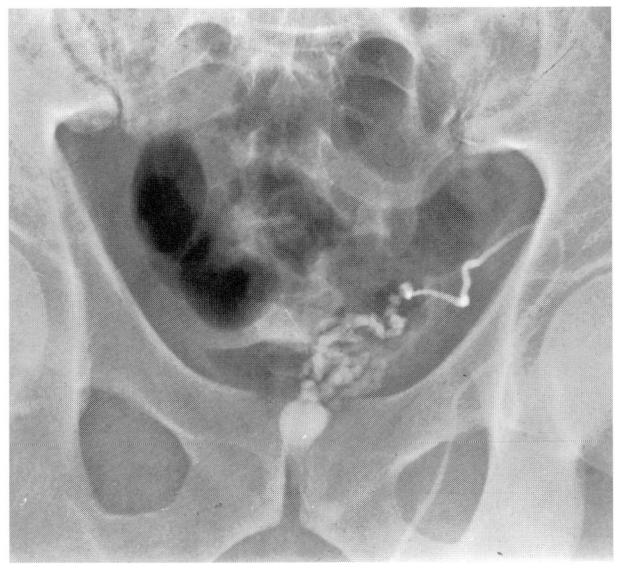

Fig. 45.64

Intraoperative transrectal ultrasound may be helpful at times to identify the point of obstruction and aid in the resection. If there is a midline cyst no attempt is made to unroof the whole cyst as it may create a large prostatic cavity, which can cause urine to mix with the semen at ejaculation. The presence of the acidic urine mixed with the semen may actually impair sperm motility.

Using the small resectoscope loop, one or two swipes are taken of the top of the cyst just proximal to the veru montanum (Fig. 45.65). There is no need to resect the entire veru although the most proximal portion may be involved with the cyst.

A postresection vasogram shows evidence of a collapsed cyst (Fig. 45.66, arrow) and free flow of contrast out of the cyst and into the bladder.

When there is not a cyst and the ejaculatory ducts are obstructed, resection of the prostate tissue on the proximal side of the veru montanum is performed. The point of

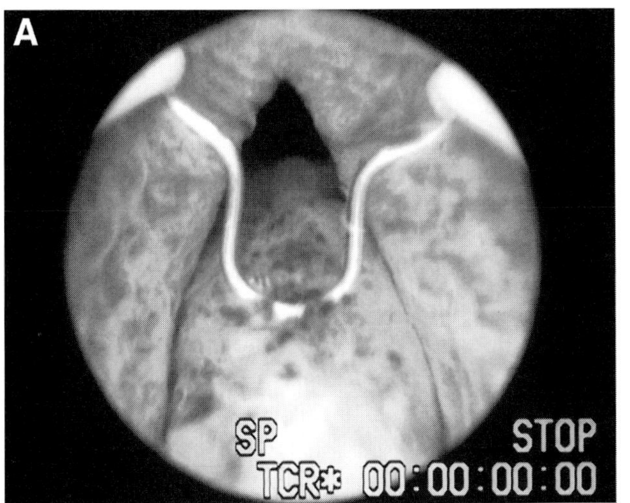


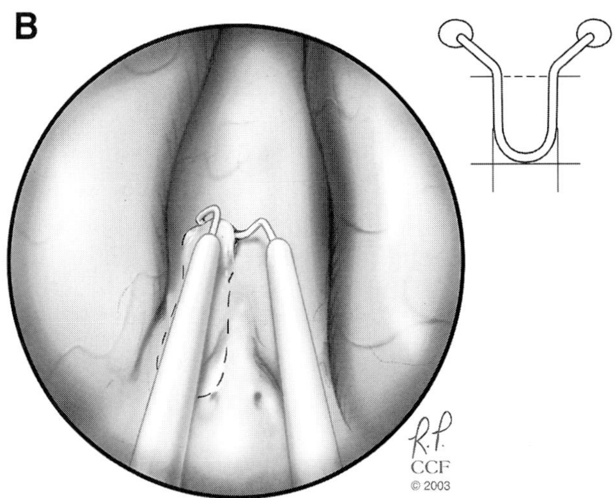


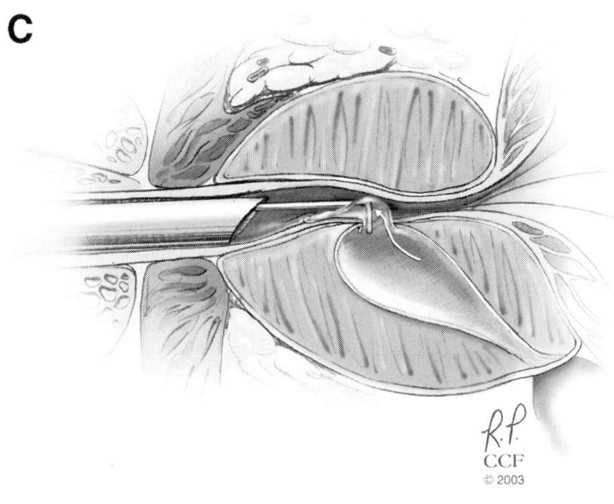


Fig. 45.65

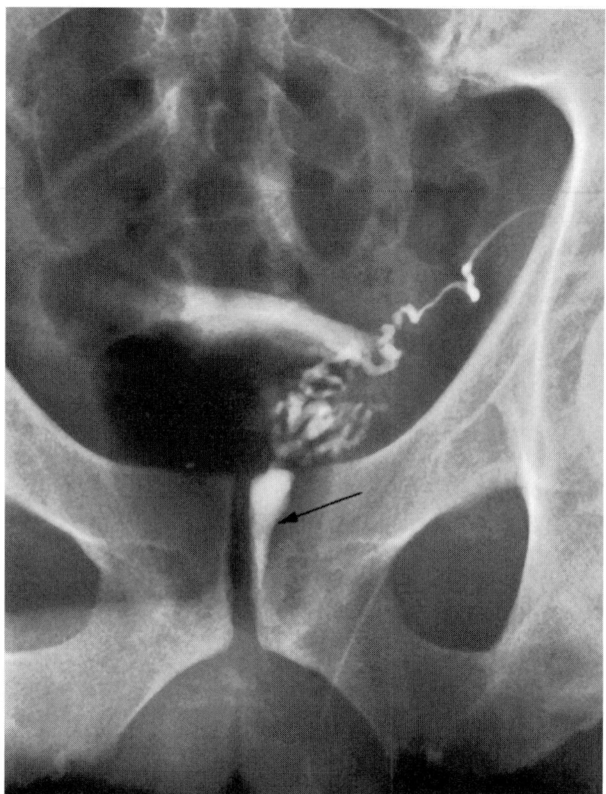

Fig. 45.66

incision may be guided by intraoperative transrectal ultrasound. If indigo carmine has been injected in the vas, the dark blue dye is evident when the patent portion of the duct is opened.

Whether opening a midline cyst or obstructed duct, minimal cauterization is used in order to prevent subsequent scarring and obstruction. After bleeding has been controlled, a 16 or 18 French catheter is placed and kept in the bladder overnight and removed the next morning if the urine is free of blood. If minimal cutting was needed to open the ejaculatory ducts, patients may resume sexual activity after 1 wk. With more extensive resection, it may be appropriate to wait longer.

A semen sample is examined at 1 and 3 mo to determine if there is sperm present. If the semen volume increases to normal but the patient remains azoospermic and there was no sperm in the vas fluid when the procedure was done, there may be a secondary epididymal obstruction that will need to be corrected.

The most common complication of ejaculatory duct resection is bleeding. Judicious use of cautery and an indwelling catheter kept in overnight can minimize the chance that this will occur. Other complications may involve problems from overzealous resection of the ejaculatory ducts, such as perforation of the prostate, undermining the bladder neck, or subsequent urethral stricture from urethral trauma or injury.

## SPERM ACQUISITION

With the advent of in vitro fertilization (IVF) and intracytoplasmic sperm injection (ICSI), reproductive specialists finally had a means of assisting not only subfertile men but even those previously considered sterile, who would have been advised to give up their hopes of having their own biological child, choosing either donor insemination, adoption, or remaining childless. Using a single, viable sperm per egg meant that very few sperm were needed whether obtained from the testis, the excurrent ductal system, or the ejaculate. Fertilization, pregnancy, and a live birth could potentially occur.

There are a variety of methods by which sperm can be recovered from many but not all azoospermic men. Because there is a higher rate of genetic abnormality in azoospermic or severely oligospermic men, there are some specific genetic tests recommended for these men based on the etiology of their azoospermia. The results of these tests may allow a couple to make a more informed decision as to whether they wish to proceed to sperm acquisition and ICSI. These tests are summarized in Table 45.2 and elaborated upon in the recommended readings at the end of this chapter.

There are many different situations in which a patient will request that sperm be obtained for use with (IVF)/ICSI. Sometimes sperm are cryopreserved at the time of corrective surgery for azoospermia as a safeguard in the event of surgical failure. At other times, corrective surgery is not possible, and the option of obtaining sperm from the testis or excurrent ducts is the only one available if a man wants to try and have his own biological offspring. A diagram of the possible choices available for sperm acquisition is shown in Fig. 45.67.

With the use of testicular sperm for ICSI, the testis biopsy is no longer just a diagnostic procedure. Sperm can be isolated from the seminiferous tubules and used fresh or cryopreserved and thawed for use with ICSI.

### Open Testis Biopsy

A standard testis biopsy is still useful to determine the status of spermatogenesis and can be performed using local anesthesia with or without intravenous sedation.

The testis to be biopsied is held postioning the epididymis posterior (Fig. 45.68). The skin is pulled taut over the surface of the testis without pulling the testis up away from the patient, as this will cause discomfort. A few milliliters of 1% lidocaine HCl are injected with a

**Table 2**
**Recommended Genetic Tests Based on Presumed Diagnosis**

| *Presumed diagnosis* | *CFTR* | *Peripheral blood karyotype* | *Y-Chromosome deletion* |
|---|---|---|---|
| Obstructive azoospermia | | | |
| Vasectomy or iatrogenic vasal, epididymal injury | No | No | No |
| Epididymal obstruction | Yes | No | No |
| Ejaculatory duct obstruction | Yes | No | No |
| Congenital absence of vas deferens | Yes | Yes | Optional |
| Nonobstructive azoospermia | | | |
| Hypospermatogenesis | Optional | Yes | Yes |
| Incomplete maturation arrest | Optional | Yes | Yes |
| Spermatogenic failure: Sertoli only, Klinefelter syndrome, etc. | Optional | Yes | Yes |

CFTR: Cystic fibrosis transmembrane conductor regulator gene.

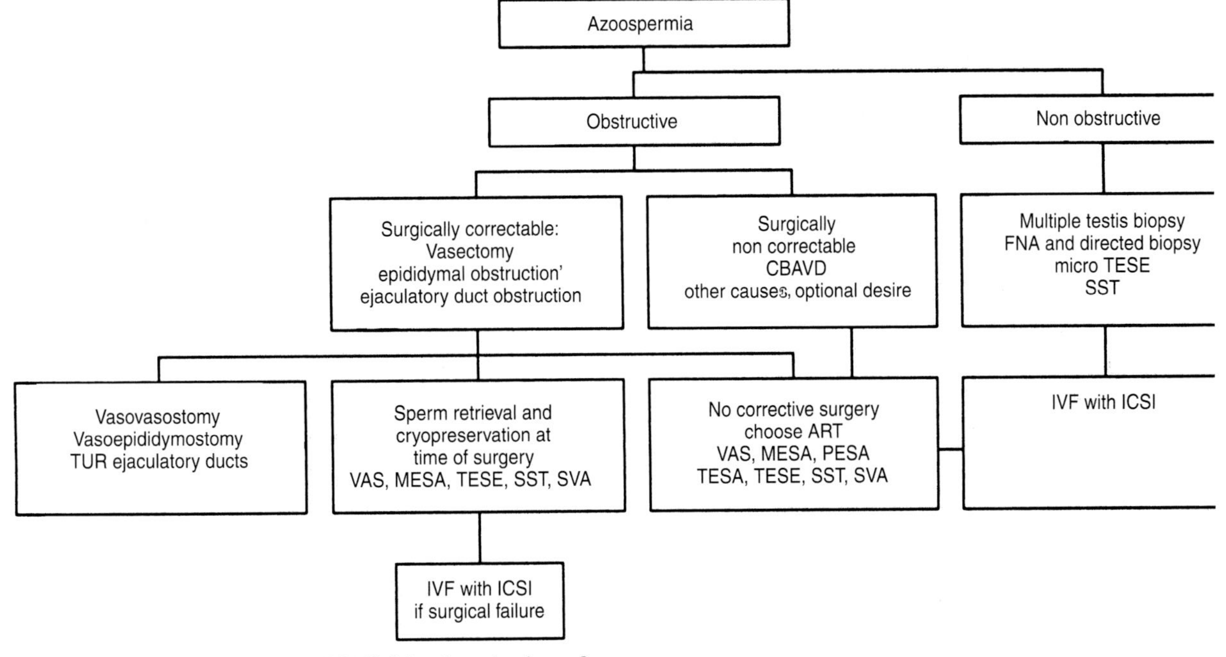


VAS: Vasal aspiration of sperm
MESA: Microsurgical Epididymal Sperm Aspiration
TESE: Testicular Sperm Extraction (Testis biopsy)
SST: Single Seminiferous Tubule Biopsy
SVA: Seminal Vesicle Aspiration of Sperm
PESA: Percutaneous Epididymal Sperm Aspiration
FNA: Fine Needle Aspiration
Micro TESE: Microsurgical Testicular Sperm Extraction

**Fig. 45.67**

Sperm Aquisition for the Azoospermic Male

30-gauge needle raising a wheal 2–3 cm in length across the scrotum.

The 1.5- to 2-cm. incision is made and the tunica vaginalis is opened (Fig. 45.69). An eyelid retractor is used to keep the edges of the tunic apart, exposing the anterior surface of the testis. This area is anesthetized by dripping 1% lidocaine HCl over the surface of the tunica albuginea.

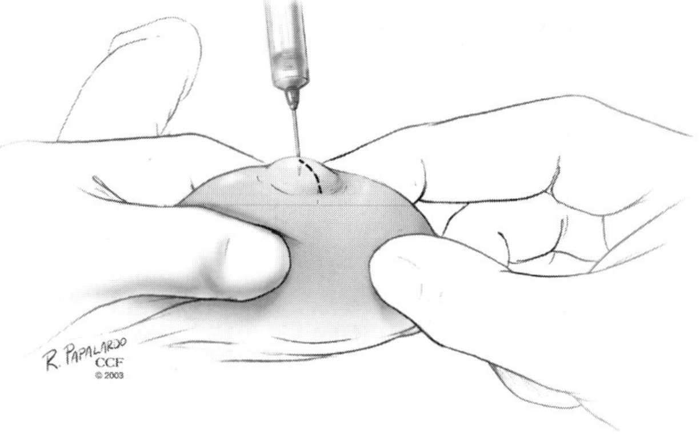


Fig. 45.68

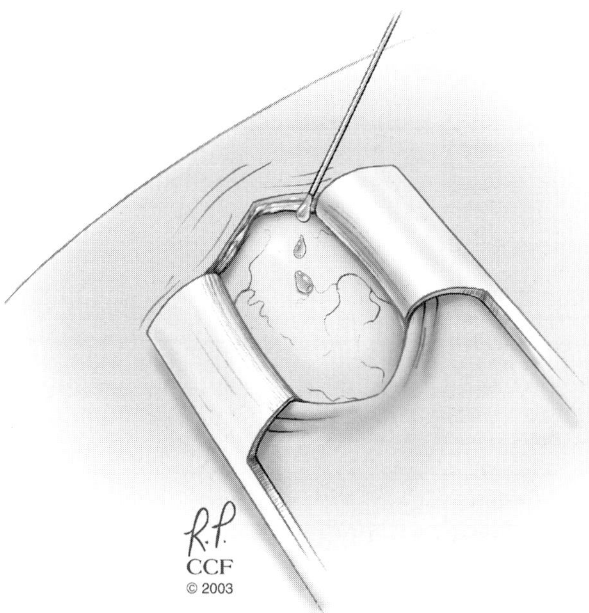


Fig. 45.69

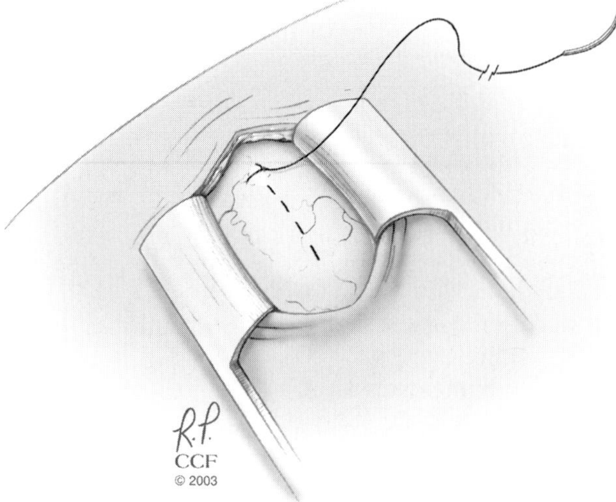


Fig. 45.70

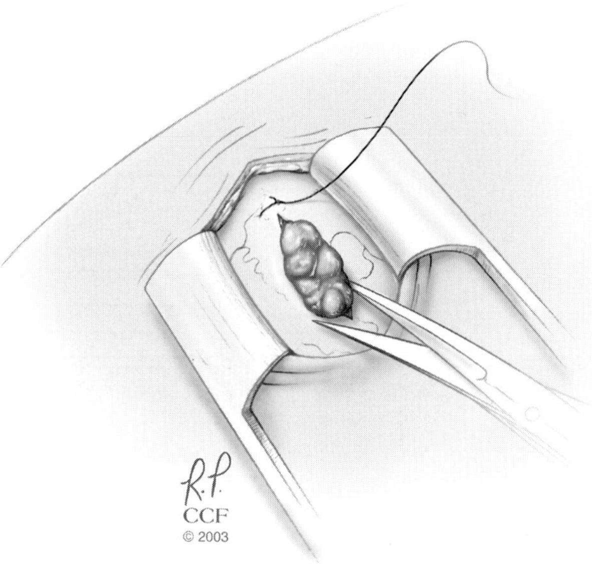


Fig. 45.71

A 5-0 Prolene suture is passed into the tunica albuginea in an area in which there does not appear to be any large blood vessels beneath the tunic (Fig. 45.70). This suture is tied with a 4- to 5-in. tail that is tagged with a hemostat while the needle end kept intact to be used to close the incision after the biopsy is taken. The tag acts as a holding suture if the biopsy site slips from ones grasp and needs to be pulled back into view.

A 1-cm. horizontal incision is made in the tunica, and with gentle pressure exerted on the testis, a cluster of seminiferous tubules are extruded out of the incision and sharply excised with a small scissors (Fig. 45.71). This tissue can be sent for standard histological evaluation, placing it in a preservative such as Bouin's, Zenker's, or Hollande's solution to preserve its cellular architecture. Formalin is not used because it distorts the normal architecture. Tissue with sperm that is meant to be cryopreserved should be placed in an appropriate sperm nutrient medium to maintain sperm viability. Multiple small ($2 \times 4$ mm) pieces can be removed from a single incision if normal or mild hypospermatogenesis present.

The incision in the tunica albuginea is closed with a running interlocking suture (Fig. 45.72). The tunica vaginalis, dartos muscle and skin are closed with absorbable 4-0 sutures.

## Microsurgical Epididymal Sperm Aspiration

This method is ideally suited for the obstructed patient with normal spermatogenesis. It offers the advantage of being able to collect large numbers of motile sperm for IVF/ICSI. The numbers and quality make it more certain

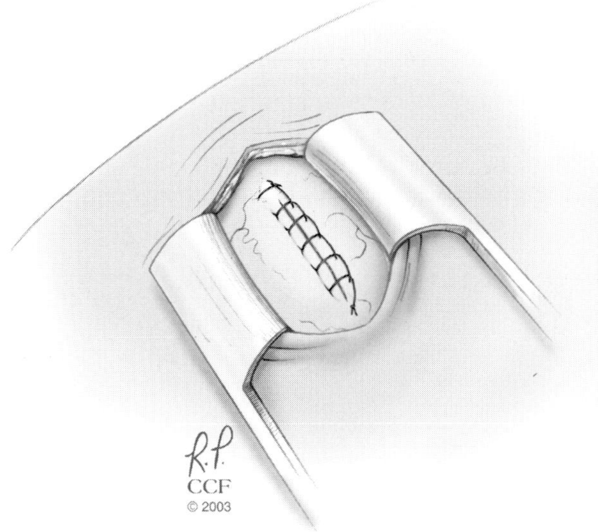


Fig. 45.72

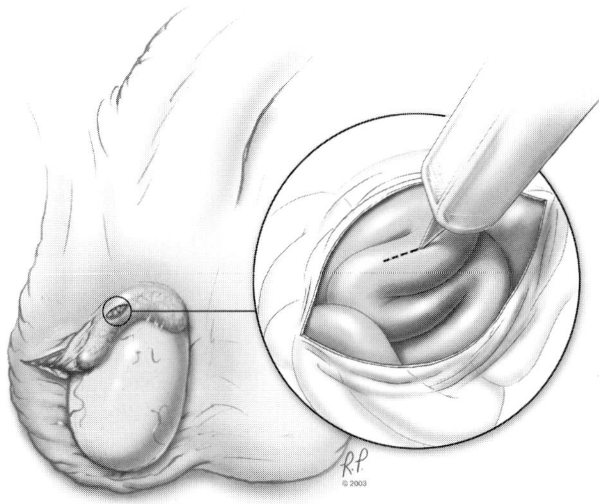

Fig. 45.73

that there will be sufficient sperm in the postthaw sample (if cryopreserved) to be available for ICSI. Disadvantages are that it involves a surgical procedure requiring an operating microscope and consequently increases the cost for the couple also requiring IVF.

The testis is exposed through a scrotal incision, and the epididymis examined under the operating microscope to identify an area in which the epididymal tubule is more dilated (Fig. 45.73). An incision is made in the epididymal tunic, exposing the tubules below similar to preparing to perform a vasoepididymostomy.

Using a micro-knife, one loop of the tubule is incised and the fluid from it is aspirated with a 24-gauge angiocatheter connected to a 1-mL tuberculin syringe (Fig. 45.74). The aspirate is mixed with sperm nutrient medium (i.e.,

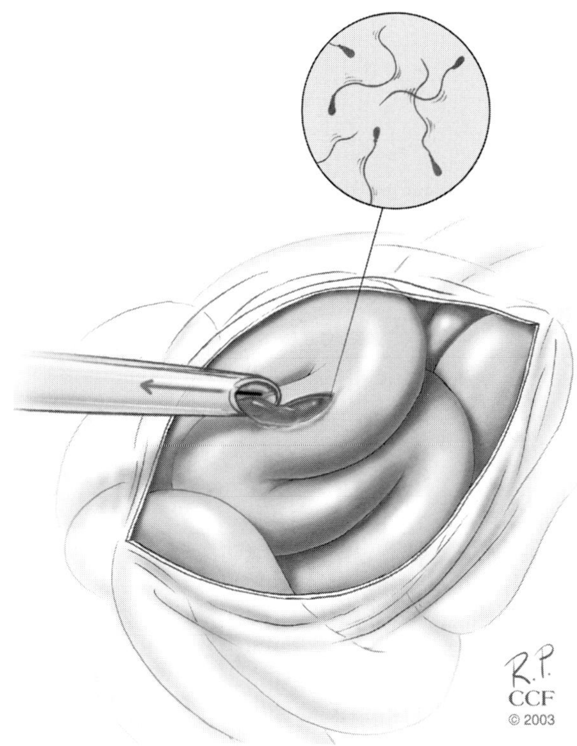


Fig. 45.74

Quinn's® Sperm Washing Medium, SAGE BioPharma, Bedminster, NJ) or other appropriate medium and placed in 1-mL Eppendorfh tubes. The fluid is examined for the presence of motile sperm, and if sperm are found, more fluid is collected and saved to be used then or to be cryopreserved for later use with IVF/ICSI. If no motile sperm are found, another incision is made in the tunic more cephalad and the same procedure carried out until motile sperm are found. The tubules and tunic are closed with 10-0 nylon suture.

## Vasal Aspiration of Sperm

This procedure has been used for men who have ejaculatory dysfunction associated with a spinal cord injury or a functional deficit resulting from the complications of such diseases as diabetes, multiple sclerosis, and neurosarcoidosis, who do not respond to vibratory stimulation or if electroejaculation is not available or not wanted by the patient. The method is simple but does require the surgeon to carefully hemi-transect the vas and, after aspiration of sperm, to close the vasotomy with a fine microsutures.

The vas and its associated vessels are isolated through a small scrotal incision and a plastic loop (tubing cut from a "butterfly" needle works well) passed behind it to act as a holder, preventing it from slipping into the scrotum (Fig. 45.75).

With the loop holding the vas just distal to the point of incision, the anterior surface in cut being mindful to

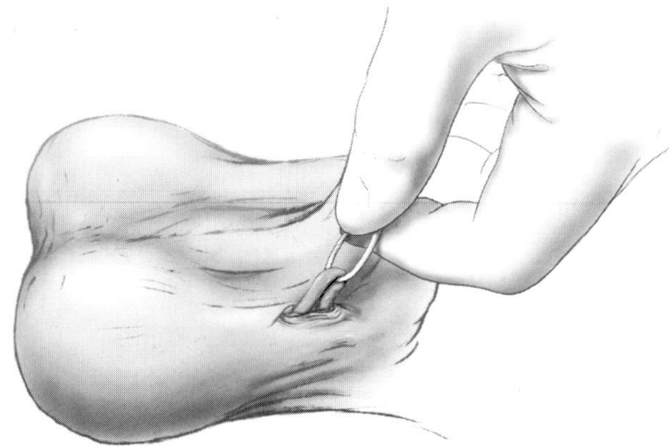

Fig. 45.75

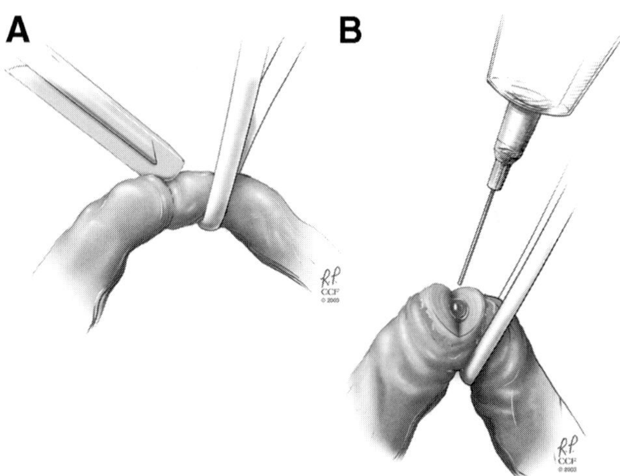


Fig. 45.76

preserve the blood supply, which courses in a longitudinal direction along the side of the vas (Fig. 45.76A). The proximal vas is "milked" toward the opened end and the fluid aspirated with a 24-gauge angiocatheter attached to a 1-mL tuberculin syringe (Fig. 45.76B).

After successful aspiration, the vasotomy is closed with three through-and-through 9-0 nylon sutures using the operating microscope or high-power ocular loops (Fig. 45.77).

## Seminal Vesicle Aspiration of Sperm

Another method of obtaining sperm from men with ejaculatory dysfunction is by direct aspiration of the seminal vesicles guided by transrectal ultrasound.

Similar to performing a prostate biopsy under ultrasound guidance, a long 18-gauge needle is passed through the probe into the seminal vesicle and the fluid aspirated (Fig. 45.78). It is important that the patient be given prophylactic antibiotics before and after the procedure, as one would do for a prostate biopsy, as well as a cleansing enema prior to the procedure to clear the lower colon and

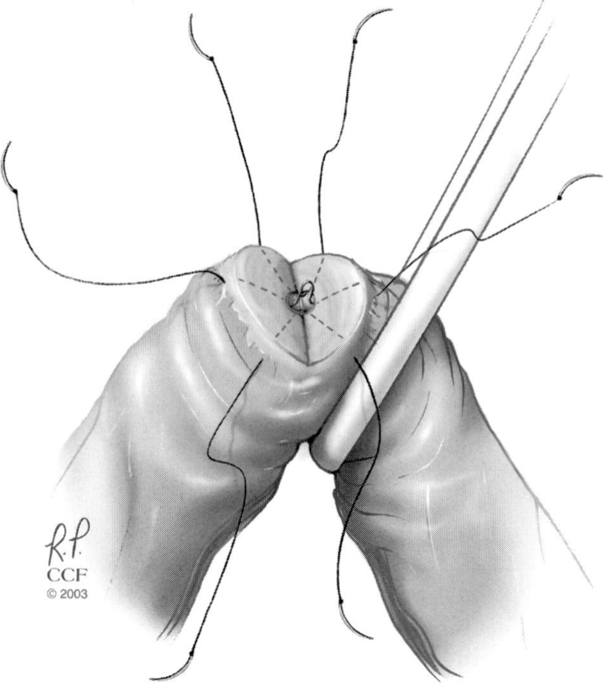


Fig. 45.77

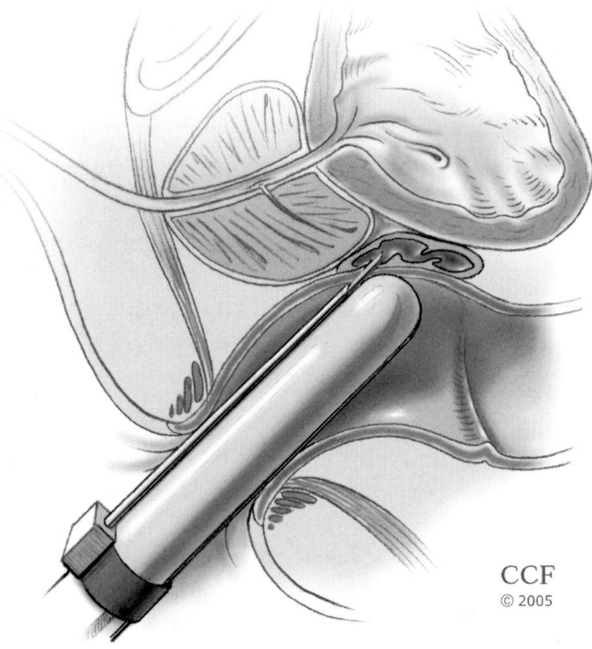


Fig. 45.78

minimize the risk of infection or contamination of the sample. Unfortunately, the quality of the sperm is poor and not always suitable for insemination. Other methods such as vibratory stimulation or electroejaculation may result in somewhat better quality sperm without the risk of infection for some of these patients.

## Testicular Aspiration of Sperm

Smaller numbers of usable sperm can be obtained by less invasive methods than open biopsy or open aspiration from the vas deferens or epididymis. These methods can potentially diminish both morbidity and cost to the patient while still allowing adequate sperm for the IVF/ICSI procedure.

Belker and associates described a quick and efficient method of aspirating sperm from the testis in men with both obstructive and nonobstructive azoospermia. They were more successful in the obstructed men (100% sperm retrieved) as opposed to those with nonobstructive azoospermia (27%). A 1.5-in., 20-gauge needle attached to a 20-mL syringe connected to the appropriate size pistol-grip device (Comeco® syringe holder) is used for the aspiration procedure.

After washing and draping the genitalia in a steile fashion, a cord block is given (Fig. 45.79). Some men may still need oral or intravenous sedation; others can be done with only local anesthesia. The testis is held by the surgeon using the nondominant hand, bringing the anterior surface of the testis tightly against the scrotal skin. A small amount of 1% lidocaine is infiltrated into the skin at the site of the aspirating needle puncture. Holding the aspirating needle device in the dominant hand, the anterior surface of the testis is punctured, and negative pressure is exerted on the syringe by pulling the pistol grip as far back as it will go. With steady negative pressure held, the needle is moved back and forth four to five times in different directions, never removing the needle from the site of puncture. The pressure in the syringe is then gradually reduced by allowing the plunger to return to its original down position over a period of 30–60 s. This slow release prevents the aspirated tissue from being pushed from the needle back into the testis. Once there is no pressure in the syringe, the needle is withdrawn from the testis, and any tubules protruding from the puncture site are cut off and transferred to a 1-mL Eppendorf tube prefilled with sperm nutrient medium. Mild pressure on the puncture site is applied to minimize the risk of a hematoma.

The needle is carefully removed from the syringe and the syringe filled with 5–10 cc of air and the needle reattached. The needle is flushed clear with the air into an Eppendorf tube containing 50 μL of sperm nutrient medium.

## Percutaneous Epididymal Sperm Aspiration

This is a relatively quick, simple, and inexpensive means of obtaining sperm from a man with epididymal or vasal obstruction. It is more easily and successfully performed when there is palpable epididymal fullness as opposed to a soft, thin epididymis that is more difficult to puncture and aspirate.

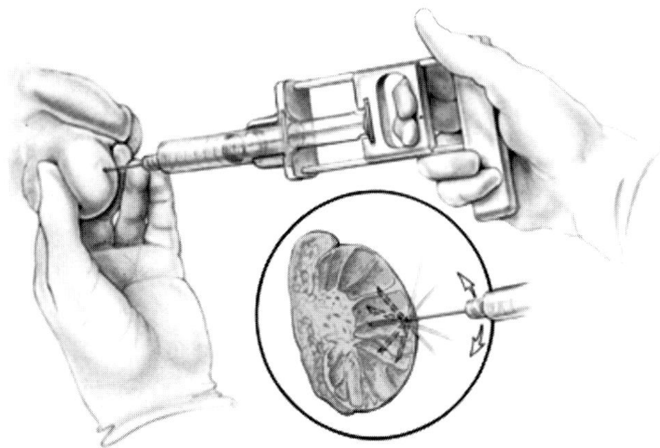

Fig. 45.79

The materials needed are:

23-gauge butterfly needle
10-cc syringe
Small hemostat
Sperm nutrient medium
1% lidocaine HCl
3-cc syringe with 30-gauge needle

Having prepared and draped the genitalia in a sterile fashion, a cord block may or may not be performed. The side to be aspirated is held in the surgeon's nondominant hand holding the head of the epididymis between thumb and forefinger with the scrotal skin snug against the epididymis (Fig. 45.80). One-half milliliter of 1% lidocaine is injected into the skin at the point where the aspirating needle will be inserted. The 23-gauge butterfly needle is attached to the 10-cc syringe previously flushed with sperm nutrient medium, then flushed with air to simply moisten the needle. The needle is inserted 0.5 cm into the caput along its long axis. An assistant pulls back on the syringe to 5 cc of negative pressure and holds it. The needle is then gently moved back and forth a few millimeters within the epididymis while gentle squeezing the caput epididymis with thumb and forefinger to "milk" the sperm into the needle. When a small amount of fluid is aspirated and seen in the clear tubing of the needle just above the needle hub, the tubing is clamped tightly with the hemostat to prevent the fluid from returning to the epididymis and the negative pressure in the syringe is slowly released (30 s) to its original position. The needle is then withdrawn from the epididymis, and gentle pressure is placed on the puncture site to prevent bleeding and hematoma formation.

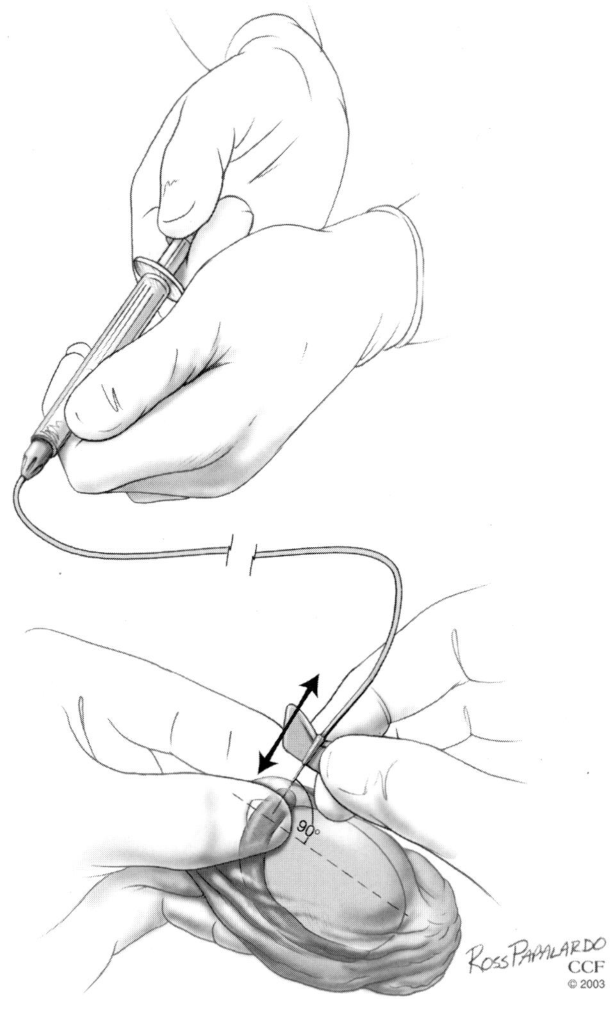


Fig. 45.80

The needle is placed in an Eppendorf tube, and the tubing is flushed with 1 mL of sperm nutrient media entering the Eppendorff tube along with the aspirate. The fluid and aspirate are immediately examined to determine if there are sufficient motile sperm to be cryopreserved or used fresh for ICSI. If insufficient, limited further attempts may be made.

## Single Seminiferous Tubule Sperm Extraction

A relatively minimally invasive method of obtaining sperm from the testis has been described by Shah. His method can be used for men with both obstructive and nonobstructive azoospermia. It can be done using local, regional, or general anesthesia.

With the surface of the testis exposed, either completely or within the opened scrotum, a 26-gauge needle is inserted a couple of millimeters through the tunica albuginea in an area where there is no obvious superficial blood vessel beneath the tunic (Fig. 45.81). One tip of a microforceps is inserted into the needle tract to mildly dilate it (Fig. 45.82).

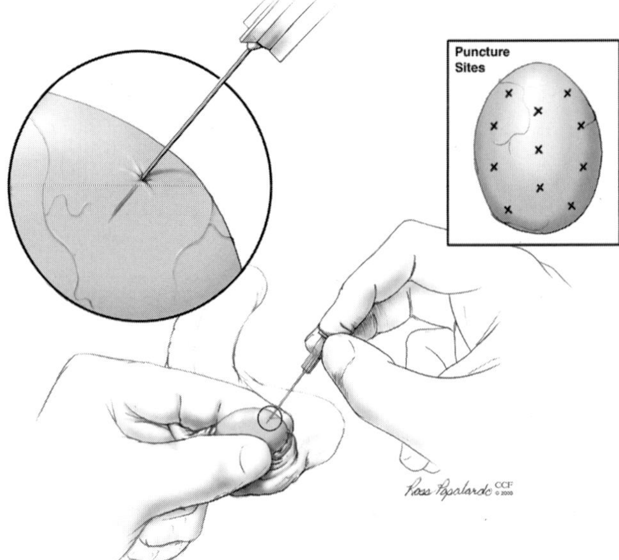


Fig. 45.81

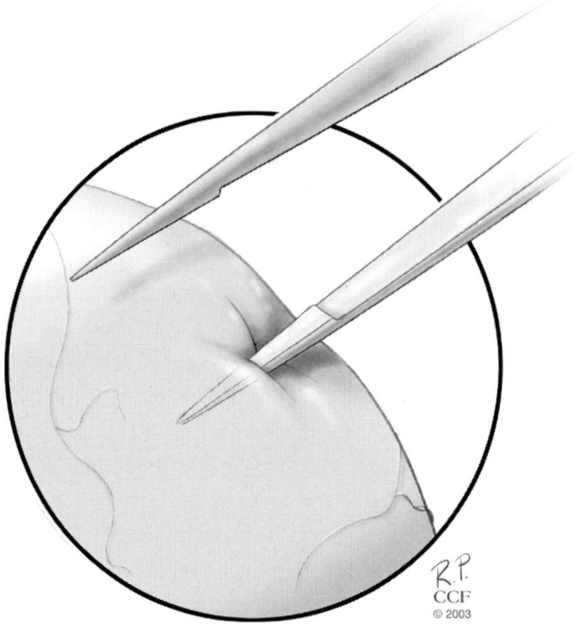


Fig. 45.82

If a seminiferous tubule does not protrude out of the opening, the tips of the microforceps are inserted just beneath the surface and a seminiferous tubule is grasped and pulled out (Fig. 45.83). Gentle pulling at the surface of the testis allows the tubule to extrude and collect in a small pile. When enough length of the tubule(s) has been collected, it is cut at the surface of the testis and placed in a microwell (in vitro fertilization 4-well plate, Becton-Dickinson Labware #35-3654, Franklin Lakes, NJ) with sperm nutrient medium. The tissue is sent to the

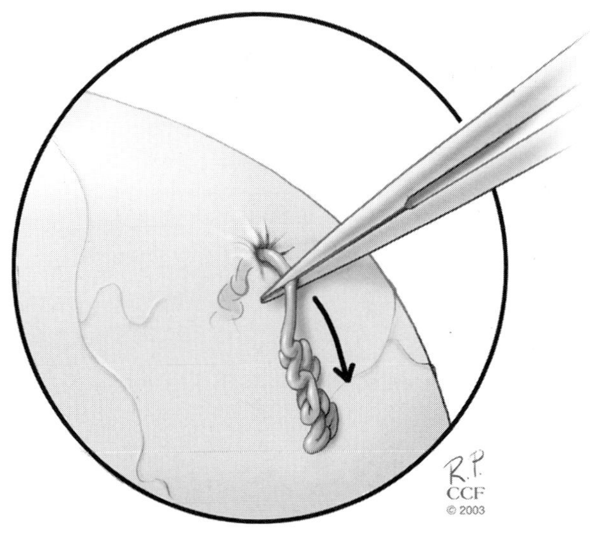


Fig. 45.83

embryologist for examination and isolation of sperm, if present.

Multiple sites can be sampled. If the tubules are fibrotic or sclerotic, they will not pull out of the testis easily, and therefore that site is abandoned.

## Testicular Sperm Extraction

Men with nonobstructive azoospermia (Sertoli cell only syndrome, Klinefelter syndrome, complete maturation arrest, etc.) represent a challenge for the urologist to find sperm usable for ICSI. It is well recognized that some men who are azoospermic may make a few sperm in their testicles but show nothing in the semen. If enough areas of the testis are sampled, sperm may be found in 25–50% of men with nonobstructive azoospermia. The difficulty encountered is in not minimizing the exploration while still preserving the integrity of the testis in order to cause no further compromise in size or hormone function.

Since the major vessels run in a radial fashion beneath the tunica albuginea, one method of testicular sampling to find seminiferous tubules containing sperm is to take multiple samples from different areas of the testis using small horizontal incisions (Fig. 45.84). The first extruded tissue is cut and placed in sperm nutrient medium, after which, with gentle pressure on the testis, tissue from beneath this first sample is forced into the opened incision, sharply excised, and sent to be examined for sperm. Each incision is closed with a running interlocking 5- or 6-0 Prolene, as this type of suture will prevent adhesions to the tunica vaginalis.

The seminiferous tubules of men with Sertoli cell only syndrome, sclerosis associated with Klinefelter syndrome, testicular atrophy, or prior orchitis are generally smaller than tubules containing the full complement of cells associated with normal sperm production. Using the operating microscope to carefully examine the seminiferous tubules, these fuller tubules can be identified and individually picked up.

A generous horizontal incision is made in the mid-testis carried approximately two-thirds the circumference of the testis (Fig. 45.85). Arteries and large veins are carefully preserved. As the two cut halves of the testis are gently opened, the lobules of seminiferous tubules are visualized with the operating microscope, using high magnification

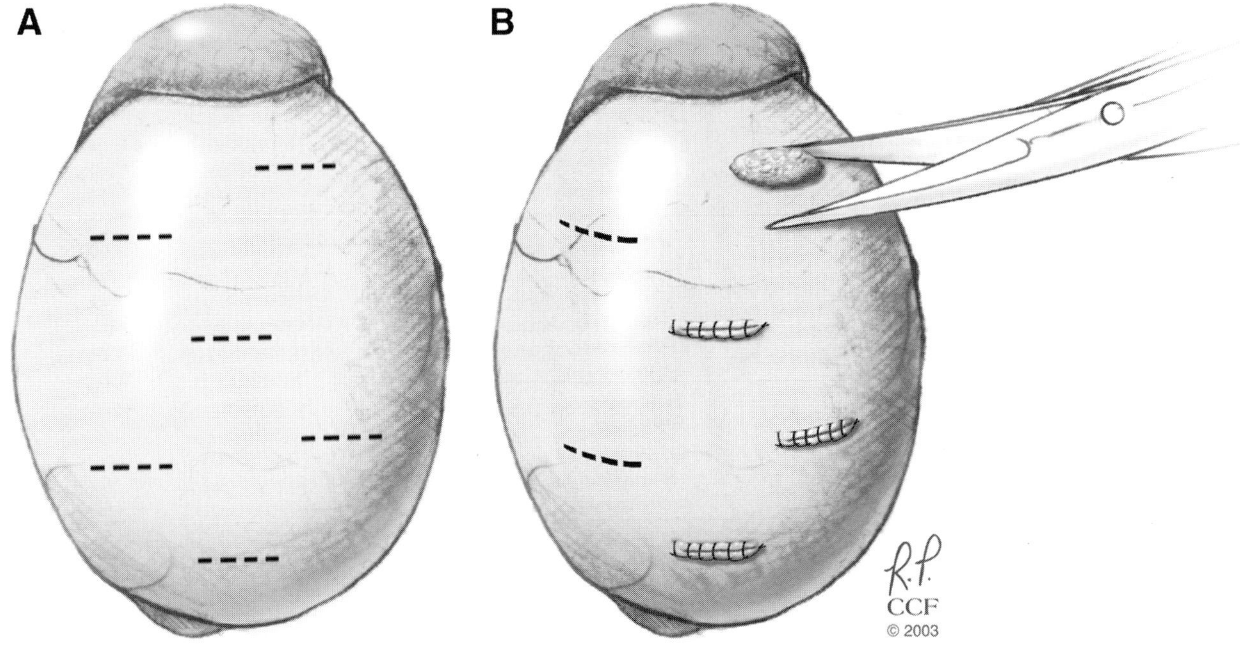


Fig. 45.84

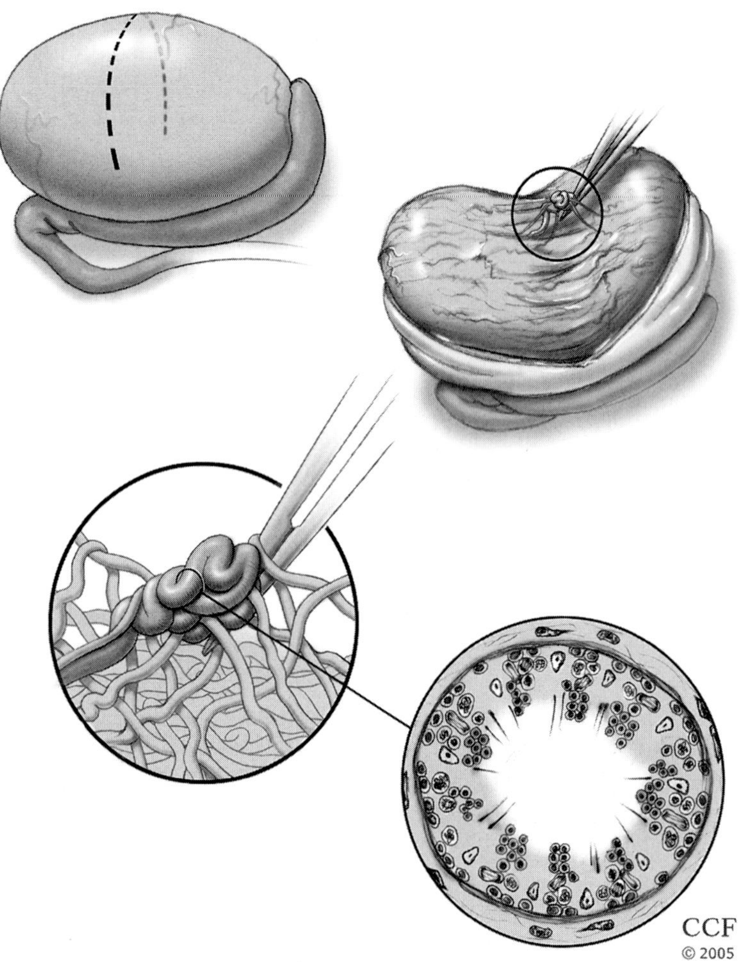


Fig. 45.85

to identify and isolate these tubules, which may have sperm present. The center portion is examined first. Then, by carefully teasing the clusters of lobules apart and examining each segment, single, larger tubules thought to contain sperm are sampled. Each tubule(s) is place in a collecting well and examined by an embryologist or technician trained to tease the tissue apart and examine for sperm. When enough sperm is found or adequate sampling has not resulted in sperm being found, the procedure is terminated and the incision(s) closed with 5- or 6-0 prolene. It has been this author's practice to thoroughly examine the midportion of the testis by open examination, and the periphery of the testis is sampled using the single seminiferous tubule sperm extraction method described above.

## SUGGESTED READINGS

1. Beck EM, Schlegel PN, Goldstein M. Intraoperative varicocele anatomy: a macroscopic and microscopic study. J Urol 148(4):1190–1194, 1992.
2. Belker AM. Principles and techniques of microsurgery. In: Thomas AJ, Nagler HM, eds. Atlas of Surgical Management of Male Infertility New york: Igaku-Shoin Medical Publishers, 1995:43–54.
3. Belker AM, Sherins RJ, Dennison-Lagos L, Thorsell LP, Schulman JD. Percutaneous testicular sperm aspiration: a convenient and effective office procedure to retrieve sperm for in vitro fertilization with intracytoplasmic sperm injection. J Urol 160(6 Pt. 1):2058–2062, 1998.
4. Belker AM, Thomas AJ, Jr., Fuchs EF, et al. Results of 1,469 microsurgical vasectomy reversals by the Vasovasostomy Study Group. J Urol 145(3):505, 1991.
5. Berardinucci D, Zini A, Jarvi K. Outcome of microsurgical reconstruction in men with suspected epididymal obstruction. J Urol 159(3):831–834, 1998.
6. Berger RE. Triangulation end-to-side vasoepididymostomy. J Urol 159(6):1951–1953, 1998.
7. Boeckx W, Van Helden S. Microsurgical vasoepididymostomy in the treatment of occlusive azoospermia. Brit J Urol 77(4):577–579, 1996.

8. Chan PT, Li PS, Goldstein M. Microsurgical vasoepididymostomy: a prospective randomized study of 3 intussusception techniques in rats. J Urol 169(5): 1924–1929, 2003.
9. Craft I, Khalifa Y, Boulos A, Pelekanos M, Foster C, Tsirigotis M. Factors influencing the outcome of in-vitro fertilization with percutaneous aspirated epididymal spermatozoa and intracytoplasmic sperm injection in azoospermic men. Human Reprod 7: 1791–1794, 1995.
10. Dewire DM, Thomas AJ. Microsurgical end-to-side vasoepididymostomy. In: Goldstein M, ed. Surgery of Male Infertility Philadelphia: W.B. Saunders Company,:1995:128–134.
11. Dewire DM, Thomas AJ, Jr., Falk RM, Geisinger MA, Lammert GK. Clinical outcome and cost comparison of percutaneous embolization and surgical ligation of varicocele. J Androl 15 (Suppl):38S–42S, 1994.
12. Dubin L, Amelar RD. Varicocelectomy: 986 cases in a twelve-year study. Urology 10(5):446–449, 1977.
13. Dubin L, Amelar RD. Varicocelectomy: twenty-five years of experience. Int J Fertil 33(4):226–228, 231–235, 1988.
14. Fisch H, Kang YM, Johnson CW, Goluboff ET. Ejaculatory duct obstruction. Curr Opin Urol 12(6):509–515, 2002.
15. Fogdestam I, Fall, Nilsson S. Microsurgical epididymovasostomy in the treatment of occlusive azoospermia. Fertil Steril 46:925–930, 1986.
16. Fuchs EF, Burt RA. Vasectomy reversal performed 15 years or more after vasectomy: correlation of pregnancy outcome with partner age and with pregnancy results of in vitro fertilization with intracytoplasmic sperm injection. Fertil Steril 77(3):516–519, 2002.
17. Goldstein M. Vasovasostomy: surgical approach, decision making, and multiplayer microdot technique. In: Goldstein M,ed. Surgery of Male Infertility Philadelphia: W.B. Saunders Company, 1995:46–60.
18. Goldstein M. Surgical management of male infertility and other scrotal disorders. In: Walsh P, Retik A, Vaughn D, Wein A, eds. Campbell's Urology,8th ed. Philadelphia: Saunders, 2002:1547–1557.
19. Goldstein M, Gilbert BR, Dicker AP, Dwosh J, Gnecco C. Microsurgical inguinal varicocelectomy with delivery of the testis: an artery and lymphatic sparing technique. J Urol 148(6):1808–1811, 1992.
20. Hendry WF. Disorders of ejaculation: congenital, acquired and functional. Br J Urol 82(3):331–341, 1998.
21. Hibi H, Yamada Y, Honda N, et al. Microsurgical vasoepididymostomy with sperm cryopreservation for future assisted reproduction. Int J Urol 7(12):435–439, 2000.
22. Jarow JP. Diagnosis and management of ejaculatory duct obstruction. Techniques Urol 2(2):79–85, 1996.
23. Jarow JP. Varicocele repair: low ligation. Urology 44(4):470–472, 1994.
24. Jarow JP, Ogle A, Kaspar J, Hopkins M. Testicular artery ramification within the inguinal canal. J Urol 147(5):1290–1292, 1992.
25. Jarow JP, Sigman M, Buch JP, Oates RD. Delayed appearance of sperm after end-to-side vasoepididymostomy. J Urol 153(4):1156–1158, 1995.
26. Jones TR, Zagoria RJ, Jarow JP. Transrectal US-guided seminal vesiculography. Radiology 205(1): 276–278, 1997.
27. Kolettis PN, Thomas AJ, Jr. Vasoepididymostomy for vasectomy reversal: a critical assessment in the era of intracytoplasmic sperm injection. J Urol 158(2): 467–470, 1997.
28. Levine LA, Dimitriou RJ, Fakouri B. Testicular and epididymal percutaneous sperm aspiration in men with either obstructive or nonobstructive azoospermia. Urol 62(2):328–332, 2003.
29. McCallum S, Li PS, Sheynkin Y, Su LM, Chan P, Goldstein M. Comparison of intussusception pull-through end-to-side and conventional end-to-side microsurgical vasoepididymostomy: prospective randomized controlled study in male Wistar rats. J Urol 167(5):2284–2288, 2002.
30. McLoughlin MG. Vasoepididymostomy: the role of the microscope. Can J Surg 25(1):41–43, 1982.
31. Marmar JL, DeBenedictis TJ, Praiss D. The management of varicoceles by microdissection of the spermatic cord at the external inguinal ring. Fertil Steril 43(4):583–588, 1985.
32. Marmar JL, Kim Y. Subinguinal microsurgical varicocelectomy: a technical critique and statistical analysis of semen and pregnancy data. J Urol 152(4):1127–1132, 1994.
33. Matthews GJ, Schlegel PN, Goldstein M. Patency following microsurgical vasoepididymostomy and vasovasostomy: temporal considerations. J Urol 154(6): 2070–2073, 1995.
34. Nagler HM, Rotman M, Zoltan E, Fisch H. The natural history of partial ejaculatory duct obstruction. J Urol 167(1):253, 254, 2002.
35. Nguyen HT, Etzell J, Turek PJ. Normal human ejaculatory duct anatomy: a study of cadaveric and surgical specimens. J Urol 155(5):1639–1642, 1996.

36. Ohl DA, Menge AC, Jarow JP. Seminal vesicle aspiration in spinal cord injured men: insight into poor sperm quality. J Urol 162(6):2048–2051, 1999.
37. Ozgok Y, Tan MO, Kilciler M, Tahmaz L, Kibar Y. Diagnosis and treatment of ejaculatory duct obstruction in male infertility. Eur Urol 39(1):24–29, 2001.
38. Sabanegh E, Thomas AJ. Modified resectoscope loop for transurethral resection of the ejaculatory ducts. Urology 44(6):909, 910, 1994.
39. Schlegel PN. Testicular sperm extraction: microdissection improves sperm yield with minimal tissue excision. Human Reprod 14:131–135, 1999.
40. Schlegel PN, Goldstein M. Microsurgical vasoepididymostomy: refinements and results. J Urol 150(4): 1165–1168, 1993.
41. Shah R. Practical aspects of operative sperm retrieval. In: Beyond the Boundaries of Endoscopic Surgery, Infertility-IVF, Practical Sonography-Color Doppler, Vaginal Hysterectomy, Urogynecology. Mumbai, India: Prakash Trivedi, 2003:445–670.
42. Sharlip ID. Microsurgical vasovasostomy: modified one-layer technique. In: Goldstein M, ed. Surgery of Male Infertility Philadelphia: W.B.Saunders Company,1995:47–74.
43. Sharlip ID. The significance of intravasal azoospermia during vasovasostomy: answer to a surgical dilemma. Fertil Steril 38(4):496–498, 1982.
44. Sheynkin YR, Ye Z, Menendez S, Liotta D, Veeck LL, Schlegel P. Controlled comparison of percutaneous and microsurgical sperm retrieval in men with obstructive azoospermia. Human Reprod 13(11):3086–3089, 1998.
45. Silber SJ. Microscopic vasoepididymostomy: specific microanastomosis to the epididymal tubule. Fertil Steril 30(5):565–571, 1978.
46. Silber SJ. Results of microsurgical vasoepididymostomy: role of epididymis in sperm maturation. Human Reprod 4(3):298–303, 1989.
47. Silber SJ. Vasectomy and its microsurgical reversal. Urol Clin North Am 5(3):573–579, 1978.
48. Thomas AJ. Vasoepididymostomy. Urol Clin North Am 14(3):527–538, 1987.
49. Thomas AJ, Jr., Geisinger MA. Current management of varicoceles. Urologic Clin of North Am 17(4):893–907, 1990.
50. Tsirigotis M, Pelekanos M, Beski S, Gregorakis S, Foster C, Craft IL. Cumulative experience of percutaneous epididymal sperm aspiration (PESA) with intracytoplasmic sperm injection. J Assist Reprod Genet 13(4):315–319, 1996.
51. Wood S, Thomas K, Sephton V, Troup S, Kingsland C, Lewis-Jones I. Postoperative pain, complications, and satisfaction rates in patients who undergo surgical sperm retrieval. Fertil Steril 79(1):56–62, 2003.

# 46 Penile Prosthesis Implantation

*Drogo K. Montague and Kenneth W. Angermeier*

A variety of treatment options for erectile dysfunction (ED) exist. For initial treatment in most men with ED, systemic therapy in the form of a phosphodiesterase inhibitor, such as sildenafil citrate, is appropriate. If systemic therapy is either contraindicated or unsuccessful, men and their partners should be offered second-line therapies that include the use of a vacuum erection device, intraurethral prostaglandin, or penile injections. If these second-line treatment options prove unsatisfactory or are rejected, then penile prosthesis implantation should be considered.

Ideally, penile prosthesis implantation should provide its recipient with a flaccid and erect penis that comes as close as possible to the naturally flaccid and erect states. Of the devices available today, the three-piece inflatable penile prostheses come closest to this ideal. These implants consist of paired penile cylinders, a small scrotal pump, and a large abdominal fluid reservoir. The American Medical System (AMS) three-piece inflatable penile prosthesis product line has three models that differ primarily in their cylinder properties (Table 46.1).

Most men will receive maximum benefit if the AMS Ultrex penile prosthesis is implanted because this is the only device that provides both girth and length penis expansion *(1,2)*. The other two models, however, are useful in special circumstances, as shown in Table 46.2 *(3)*.

Three-piece inflatable penile prostheses are implanted by either an infrapubic or a penoscrotal approach. We prefer the penoscrotal approach because it offers the following advantages: avoidance of dorsal penile nerve sensory injury, better corporeal exposure, and the ability to anchor the scrotal pump. The only advantage of the infrapubic approach is the ability to implant the fluid reservoir under direct vision.

## IMPLANTATION OF THE AMS THREE-PIECE INFLATABLE PENILE PROSTHESIS

The AMS three-piece inflatable penile prosthesis (Fig. 46.1) consists of paired cylinders (Table 46.1), a scrotal pump and deflation mechanism, and an abdominal fluid reservoir.

A 3- to 4-cm transverse incision in made at the penoscrotal junction (Fig. 46.2).

In cases where corporeal dilation is difficult, this incision can be extended in an inverted T fashion to the distal penile shaft (Fig. 46.3). This, combined with the proximal exposure obtained later (see Fig. 46.7), allows the surgeon to have access to almost the entire length of each corpus cavernosum.

The incision is carried down through Dartos fascia (Fig. 46.4). Exposure of the urethra and the corpora is maintained with a ring retractor.

A 2-cm corporotomy is marked (Fig. 46.5).

After a full-thickness incision is made through the tunica albuginea, horizontal mattress sutures of 2-0 polydioxanone (PDS) are placed (Fig. 46. 6) *(4)*.

**Table 1**
**Cylinder Properties of AMS Three-Piece Inflatable Penile Prostheses**

| Model | Deflated cylinder diameter (mm) | Inflated cylinder diameter (mm) | Cylinder length expansion |
|---|---|---|---|
| AMS 700CXM | 9.5 | 14.2 | No |
| AMS 700CX | 12 | 18 | No |
| AMS Ultrex | 12 | 18 | Yes |

From: *Operative Urology at the Cleveland Clinic*
Edited by: A. Novick et al. © Humana Press Inc., Totowa, NJ

**Table 2**
**AMS Three-Piece Inflatable Penile Prosthesis Model Selection**

| *Model* | *Cavernous fibrosis* | *Small penis* | *Penile curvature* | *Long penis* | *All others* |
|---|---|---|---|---|---|
| AMS 700CXM | + | + | + | | |
| AMS 700CX | | | + | + | |
| AMS Ultrex | | | | | + |

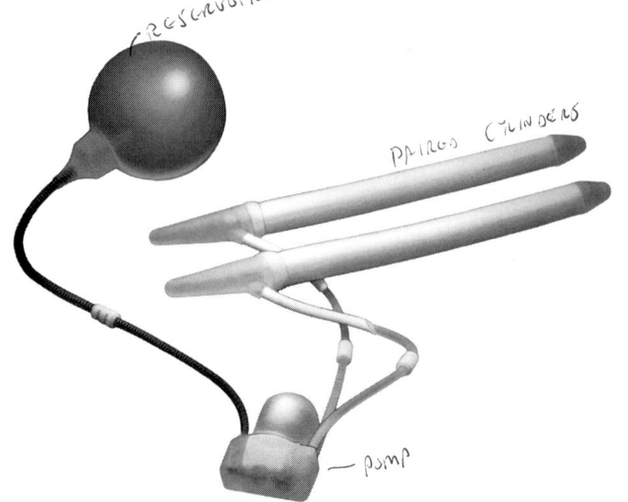

Fig. 46.1

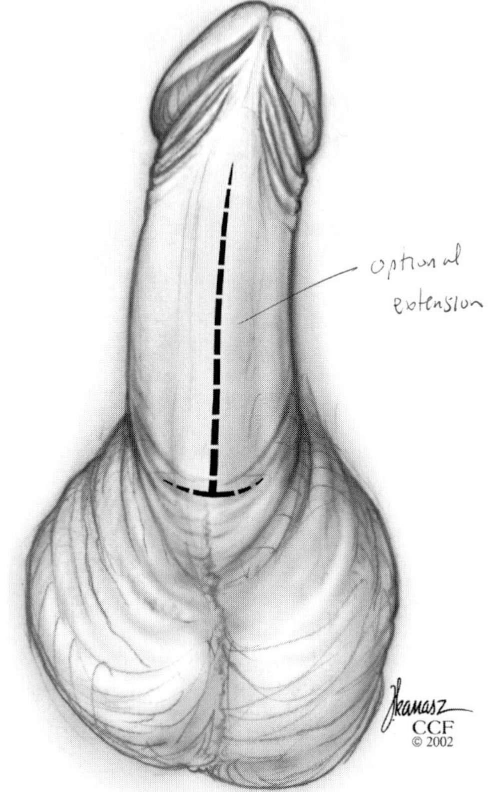


Fig. 46.3

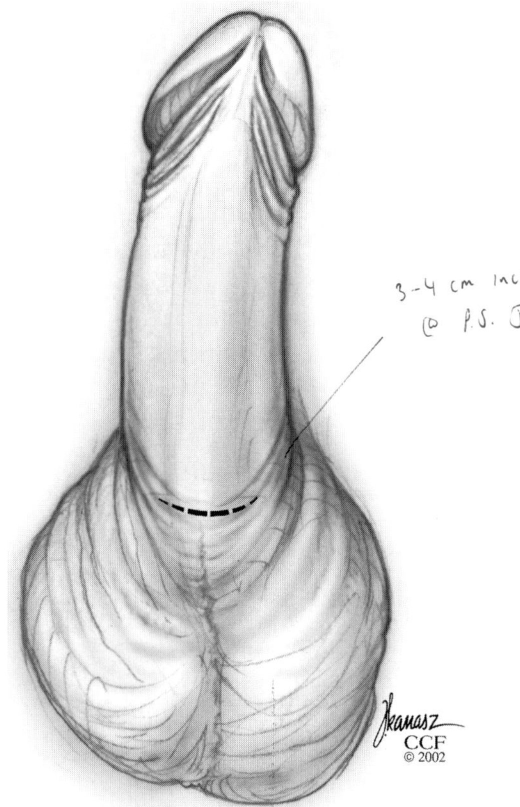


Fig. 46.2

Dilation proximally is carried out with Hegar dilators to 16 mm for the AMS 700CX or AMS Ultrex prosthesis. If this degree of dilation cannot be achieved, implantation of the smaller diameter AMS 700CXM prosthesis should be considered. With this transverse penoscrotal approach, the proximal corpus cavernosum (crus) can be exposed nearly to its attachment to the ischial tuberosity (surgeon's finger in Fig. 46.7).

Distal dilation with Hegar dilators is carried out to 14 mm for Ultrex or CX cylinders; if this degree of dilation is not possible, then implantation of CXM cylinders should be considered (Fig. 46.8).

Palpation through the glans ensures that the dilator has reached the distal limits of the corpus cavernosum (Fig. 46.9).

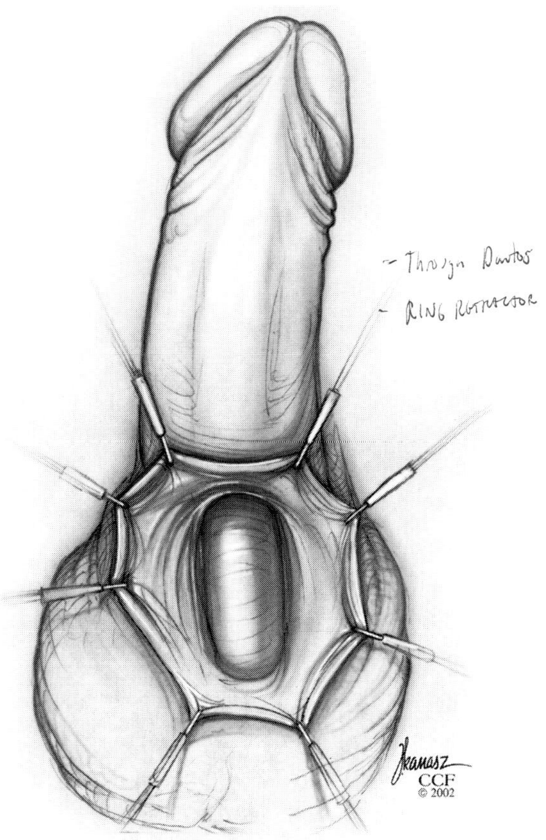


Fig. 46.4

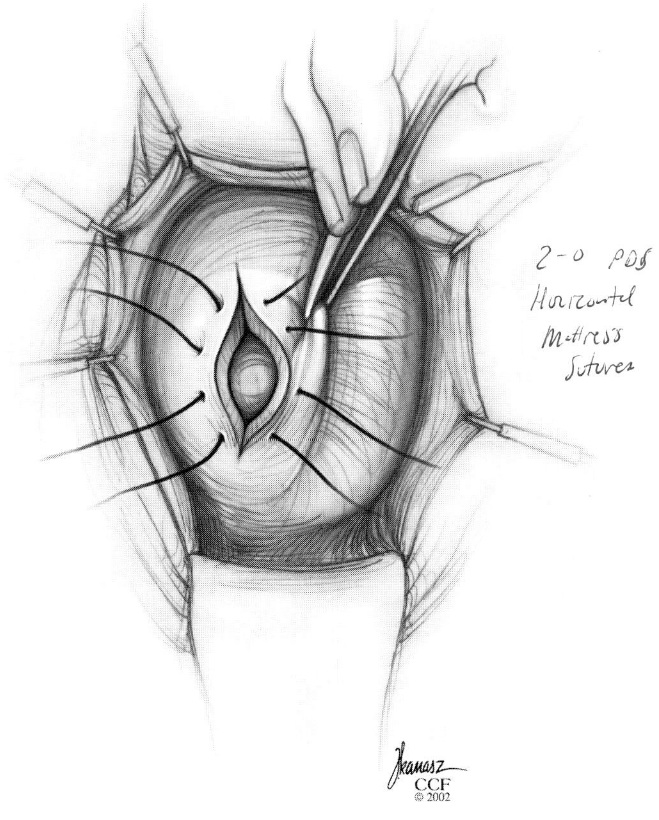


Fig. 46.6

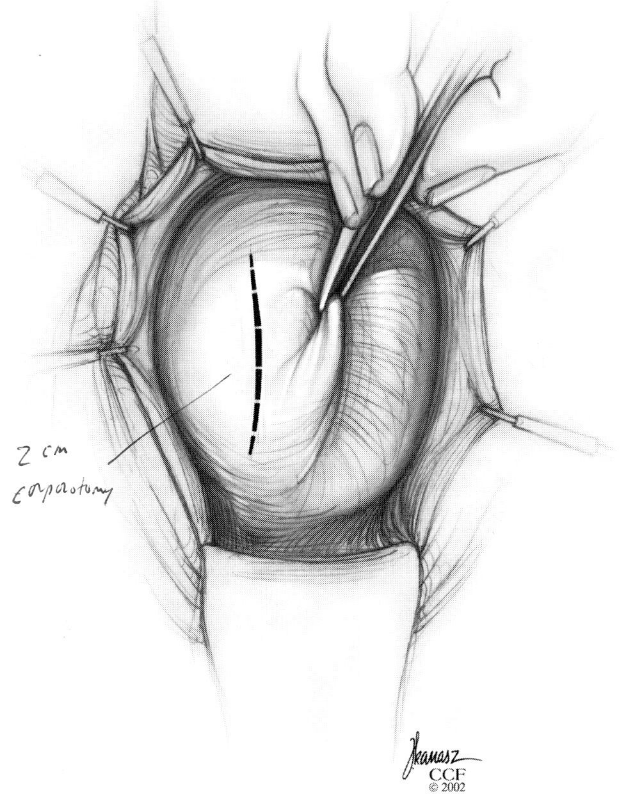


Fig. 46.5

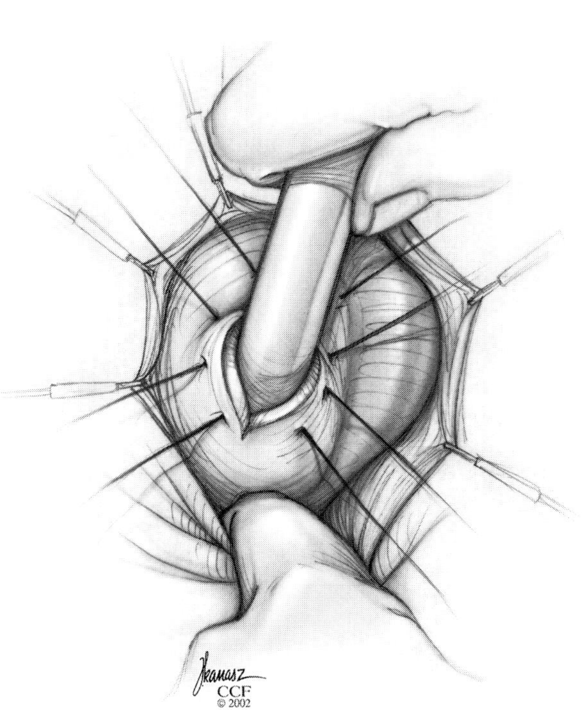


Fig. 46.7

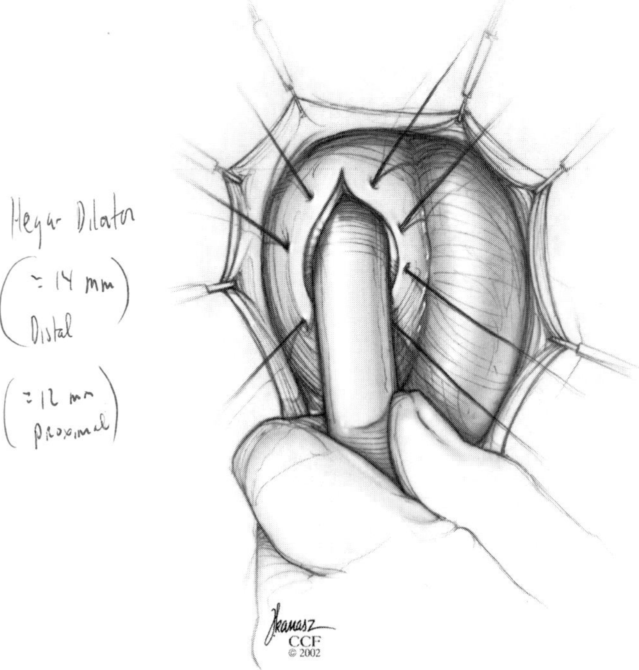


Fig. 46.8

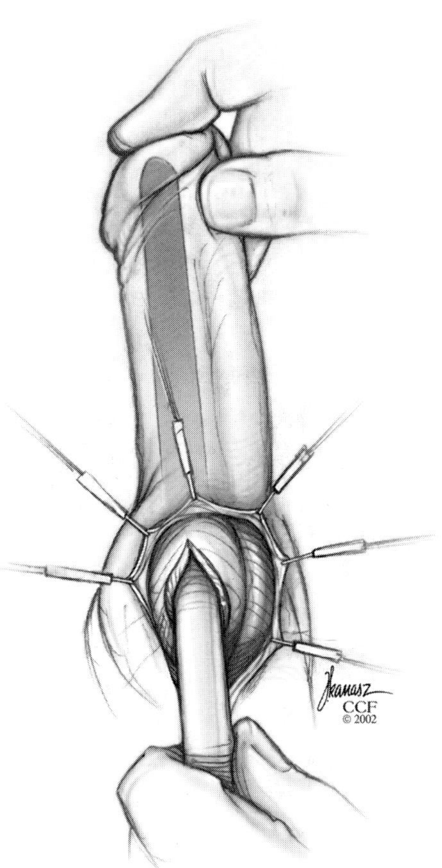


Fig. 46.9

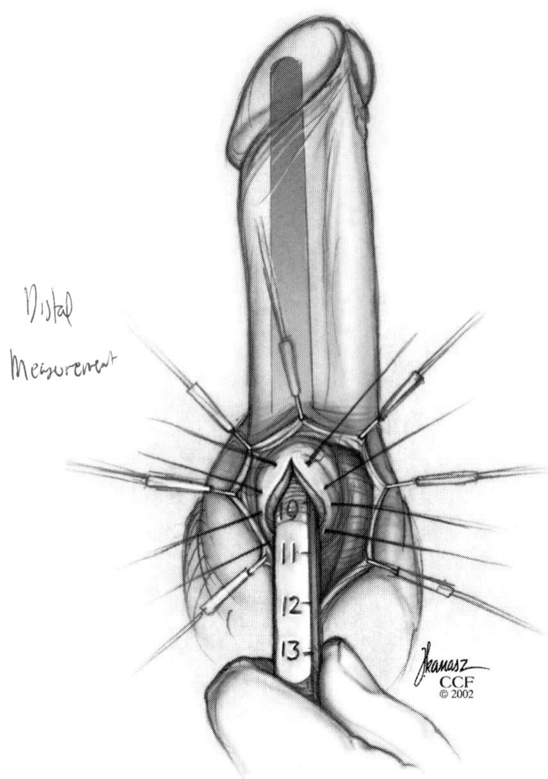


Fig. 46.10

A measurement is made distally, with the reference point being the distal end of the corporotomy. In this case the measurement would be 9 cm (Fig. 46.10).

The proximal measurement reference point is the proximal end of the corporotomy (Fig. 46.11). In this case the measurement would be 8 cm. The distal and proximal measurements are added together to determine the cylinder length (17 cm). The 2-cm corporotomy is not included in the measurement because this measurement technique tends to over estimate corporeal length by approx 2 cm.

The Furlow cylinder insertor is used to drive a straight needle through the distal corporeal tip and the glans (Fig. 46.12). This needle contains a suture that is threaded through the cylinder tip.

This suture is used to pull the cylinder into the distal corpus cavernosum (Fig, 46.13).

If rear tip extenders are needed to adjust cylinder length, they are added now. The proximal portion of the cylinder is then inserted into the proximal corpus cavernosum (crus) (Fig. 46.14).

Once the cylinder is placed, it should lie flatly inside the corpus cavernosum as viewed through the corporotomy (Fig. 46.15). Cylinders that are too long bulge through the corporotomy. This may lead to premature cylinder failure or, in the case of the length expanding Ultrex cylinder, the so-called S-shaped cylinder deformity *(5)*.

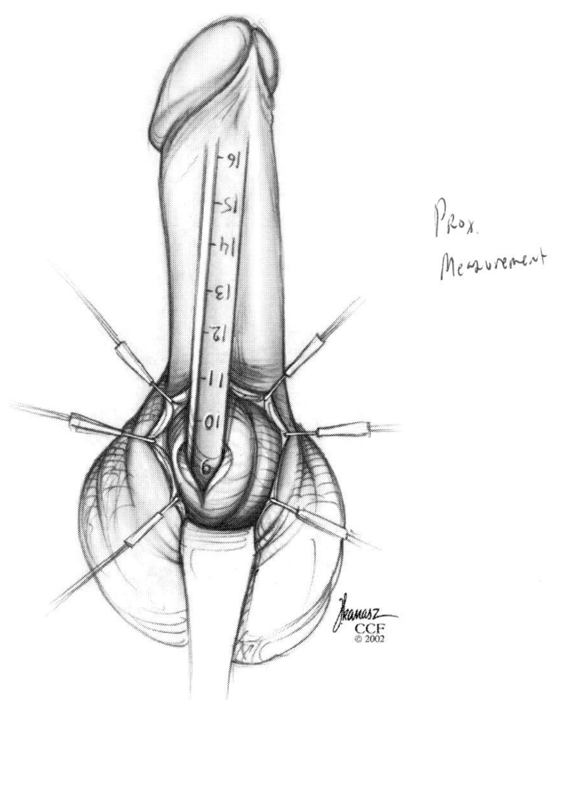


Fig. 46.11

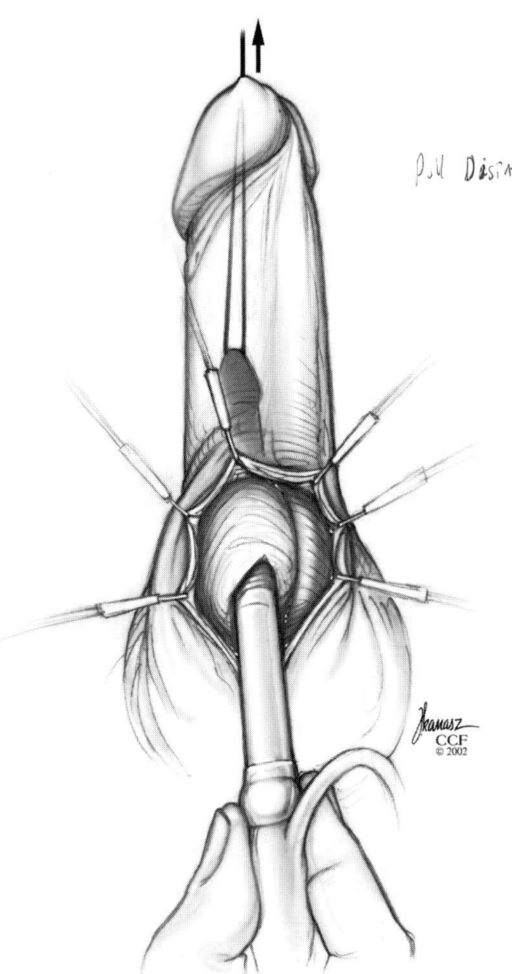


Fig. 46.13

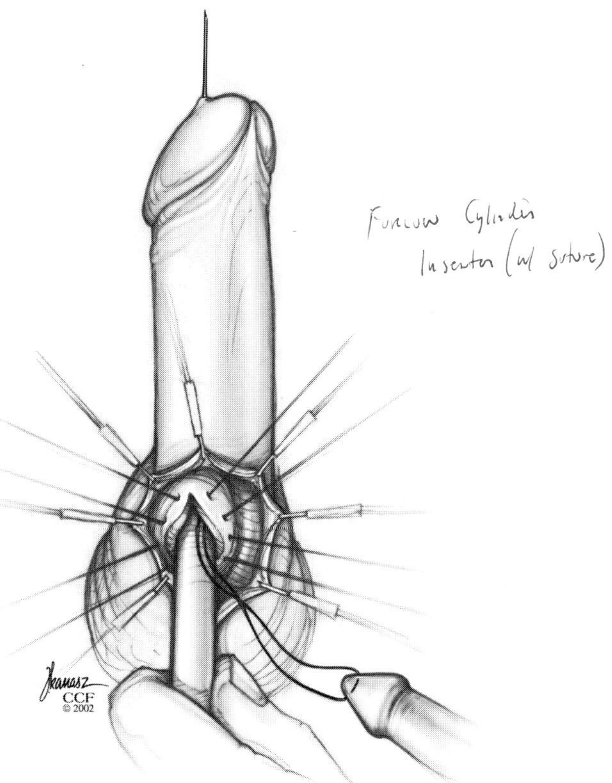


Fig. 46.12

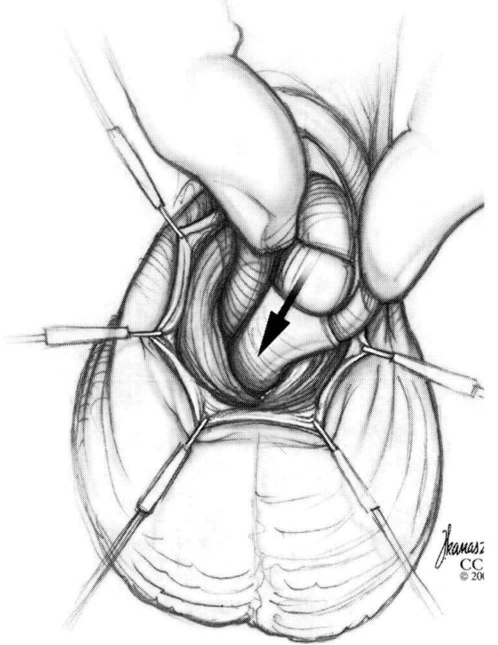


Fig. 46.14

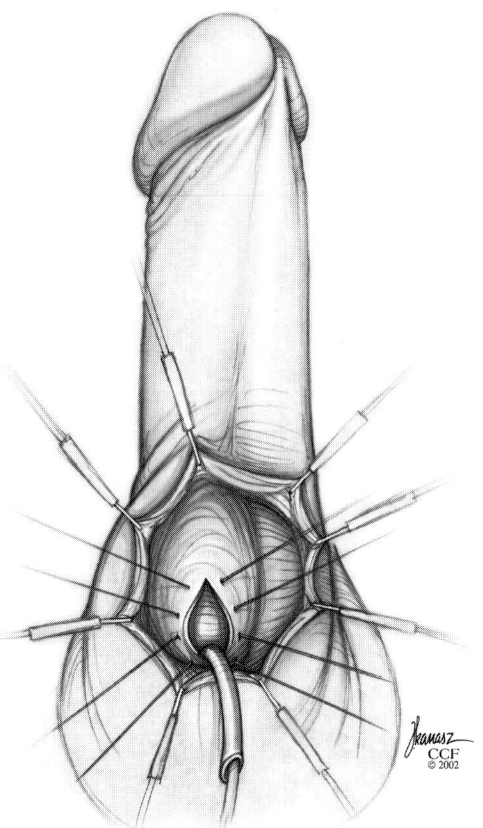


Fig. 46.15

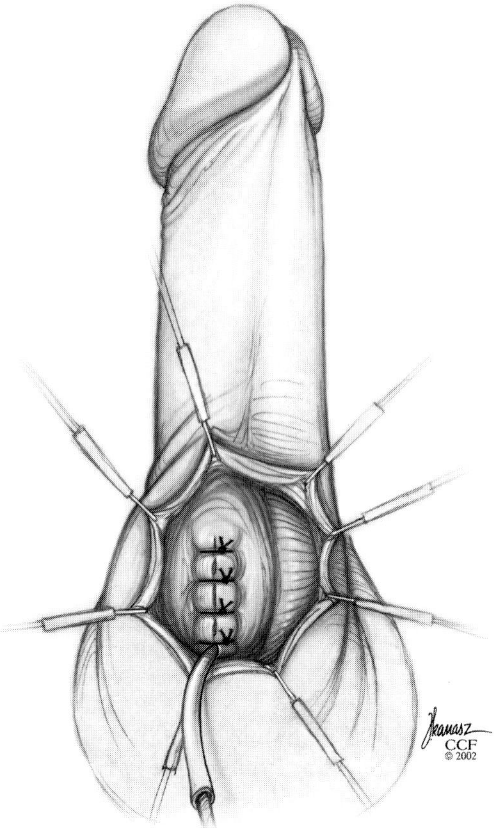


Fig. 46.16

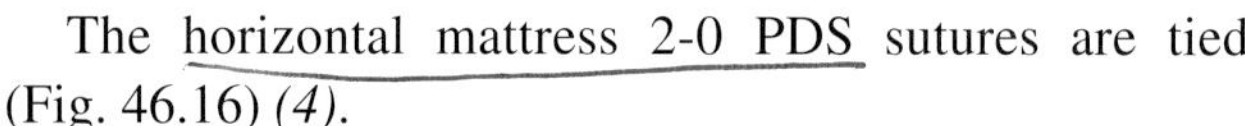

The horizontal mattress 2-0 PDS sutures are tied (Fig. 46.16) *(4)*.

Cylinder implantation on the other side is done in a similar manner (Fig. 46.17).

The distal strands of opposing sutures are tied and pulled down, and then the proximal strands are tied (Fig. 46.18) *(4)*.

This figure shows the completion of the corporotomy closure (Fig. 46.19).

Excess polytetrafluoroethylene covering is removed from the cylinder tubing (Fig. 46.20). This covering prevents the tubing from rubbing against the cylinder inside the corpus cavernosum.

Figure 46.21 shows the completion of the cylinder implantation. Note how the transverse penoscrotal approach allows proximal placement of the corporotomies such that no tubing will be visible or palpable subcutaneously at the base of the penis.

A second midline vertical incision through Dartos fascia is outlined for the pump placement (Fig. 46.22).

Ring forceps are introduced through this incision (Fig. 46.23).

The ring forceps are spread to produce a sub-Dartos septal pouch for the pump (Fig. 46.24).

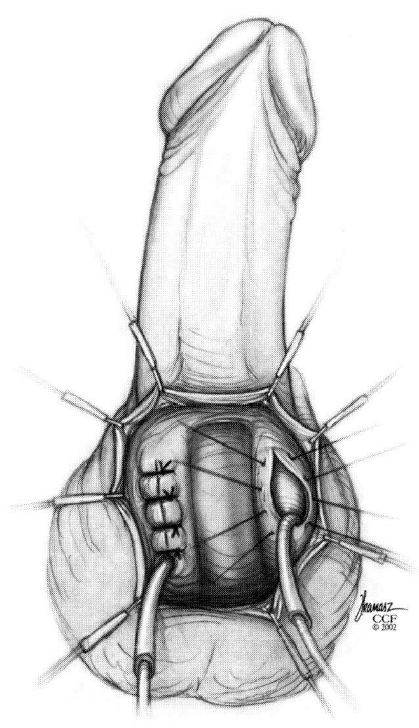


Fig. 46.17

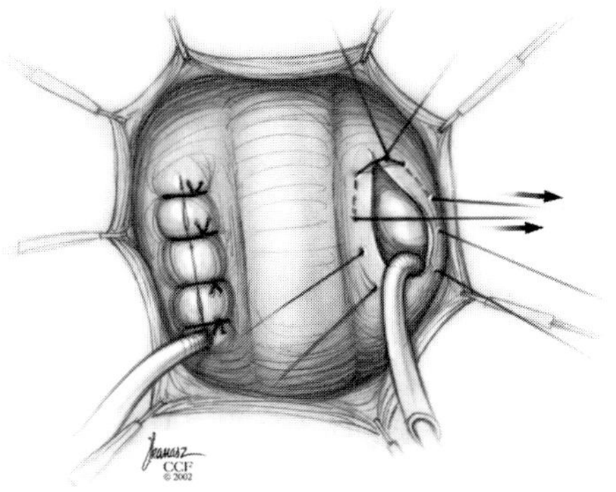


Fig. 46.18

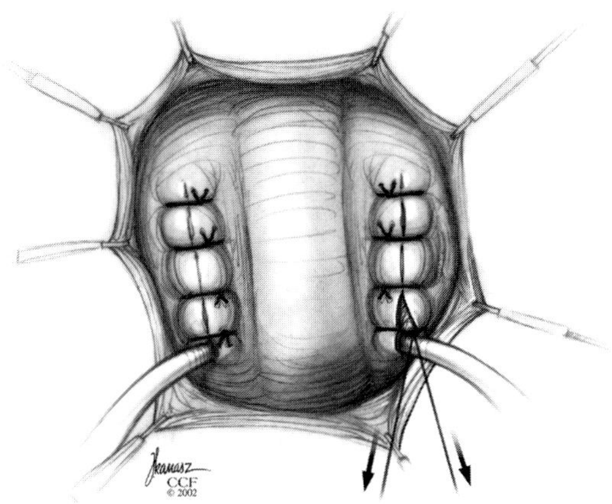


Fig. 46.19

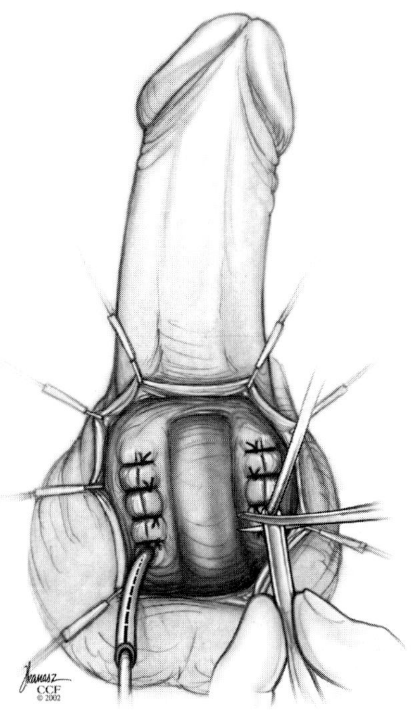


Fig. 46.20

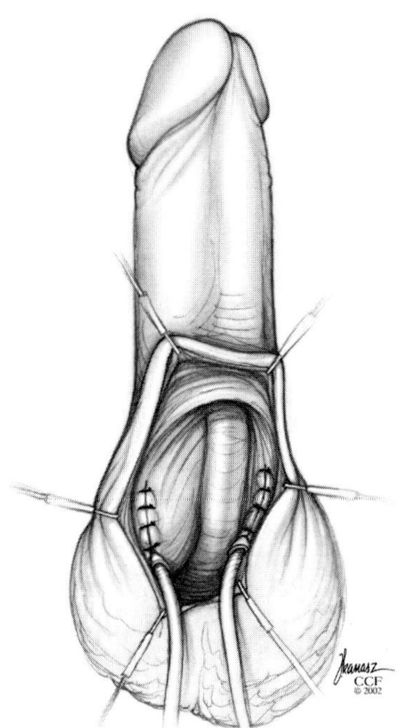


Fig. 46.21

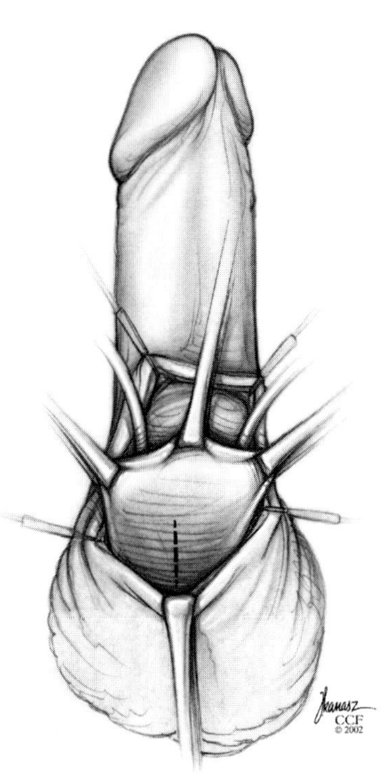


Fig. 46.22

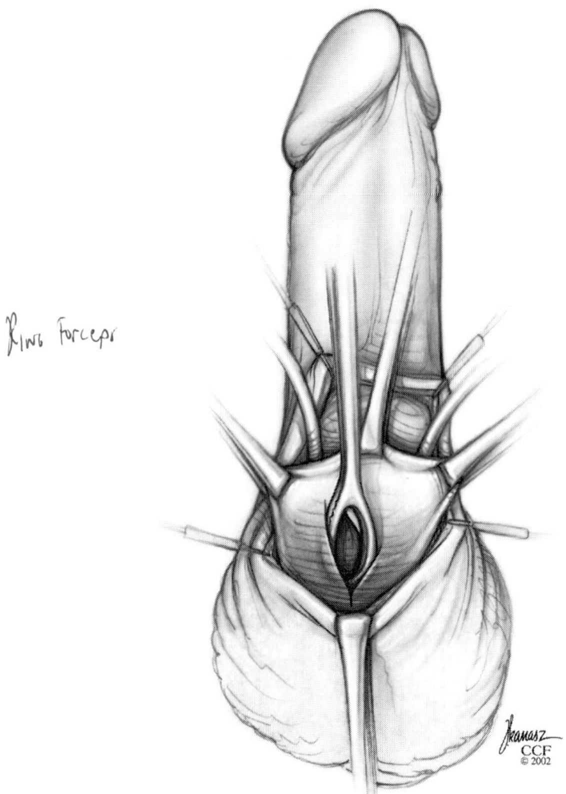


Fig. 46.23

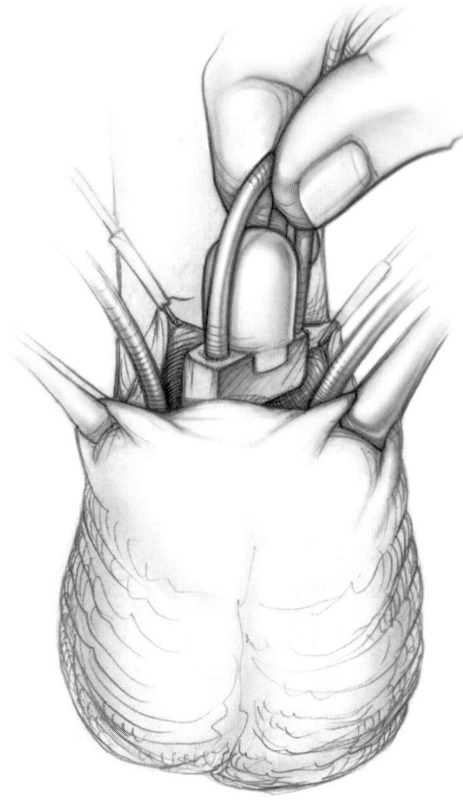

Fig. 46.25

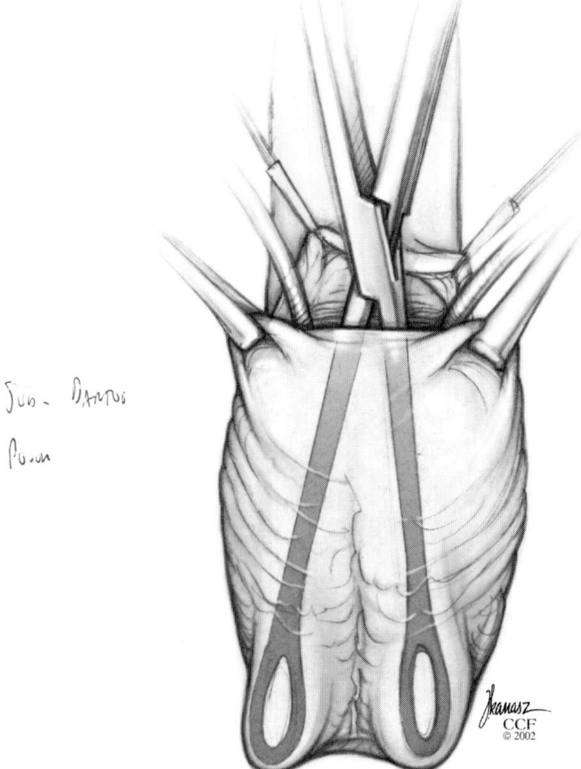


Fig. 46.24

The pump is introduced into this pouch (Fig. 46.25).

The pump is placed so that the deflation button is anterior and at the bottom of the pouch (Fig. 46.26).

All three tubings from the pump are passed via separate stab incisions through the back wall of the pouch (Fig. 46.27). This helps anchor the pump deep within the pouch.

The opening at the top of the pouch is closed with a running 3-0 Dexon suture (Fig. 46.28).

Connections between the pump and the cylinders are made with the Quick Connector system using the straight connectors (Fig. 46.29).

A syringe containing 50 mL of normal saline is attached to the reservoir tubing from the pump (Fig. 46.30). This syringe will serve as a surrogate reservoir to allow testing of the prosthesis by repeated inflation and deflation of the cylinders.

Figure 46.31 depicts the penis in the flaccid (deflated) state.

Figure 46.32 shows the penis in the erect (inflated) state. This cycle of inflation and deflation is repeated three times, checking the location of the cylinder tips under the glans penis and checking the quality and straightness of the erection.

In Fig. 46.33, the penis is left deflated. A Foley catheter attached to gravity drainage is inserted. The

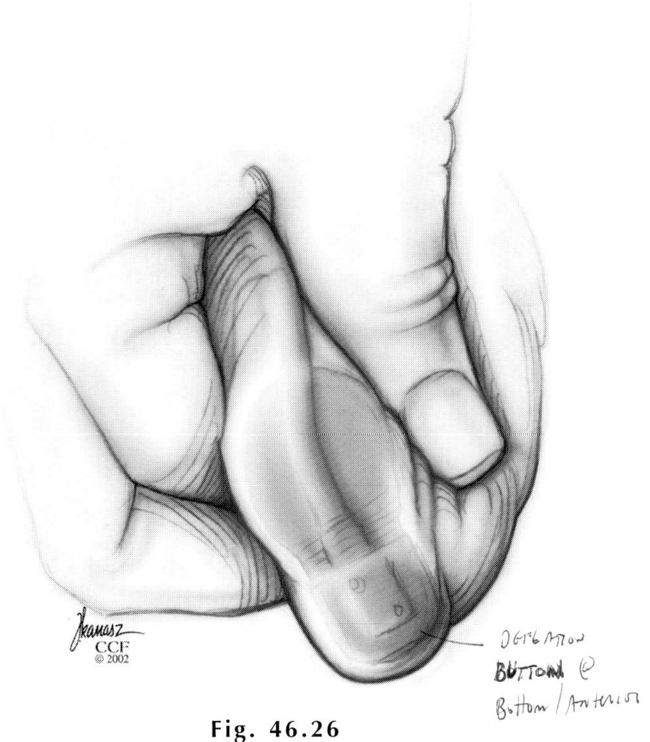


Fig. 46.26

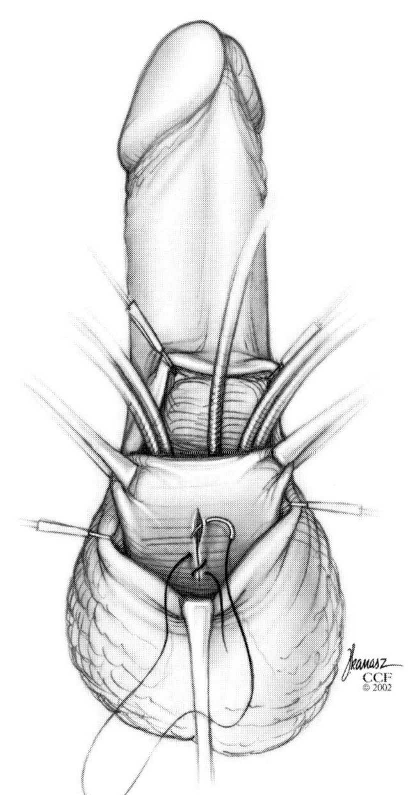


Fig. 46.28

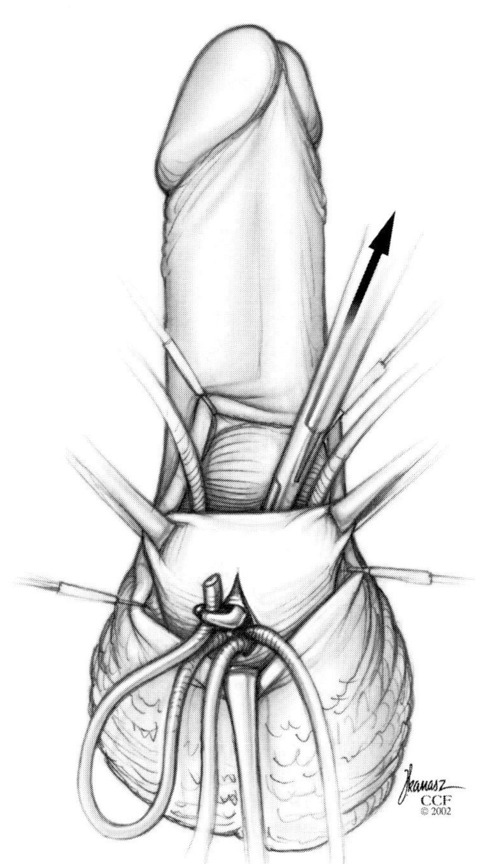


Fig. 46.27

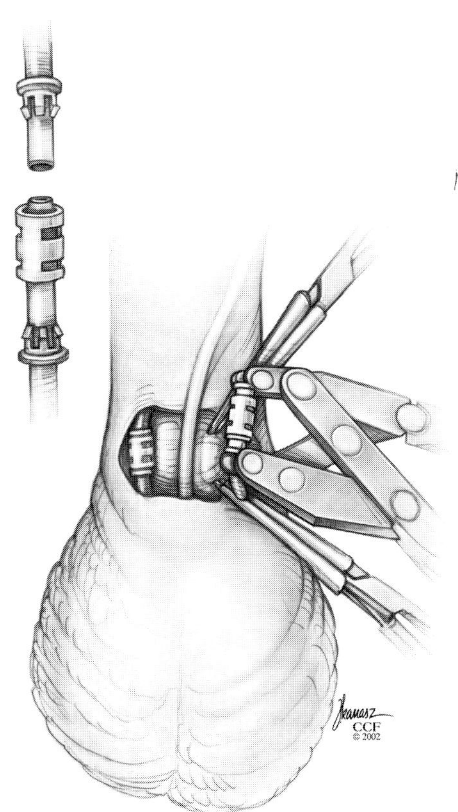


Fig. 46.29

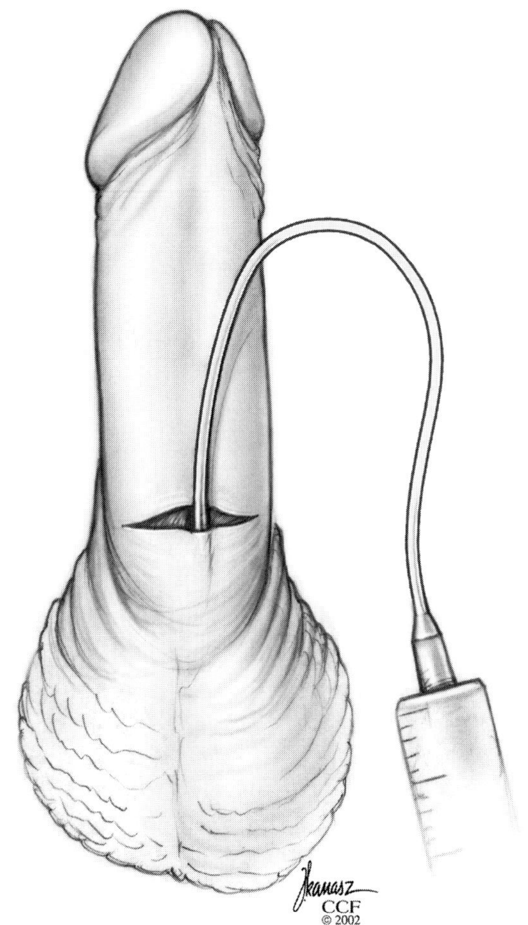

Fig. 46.30

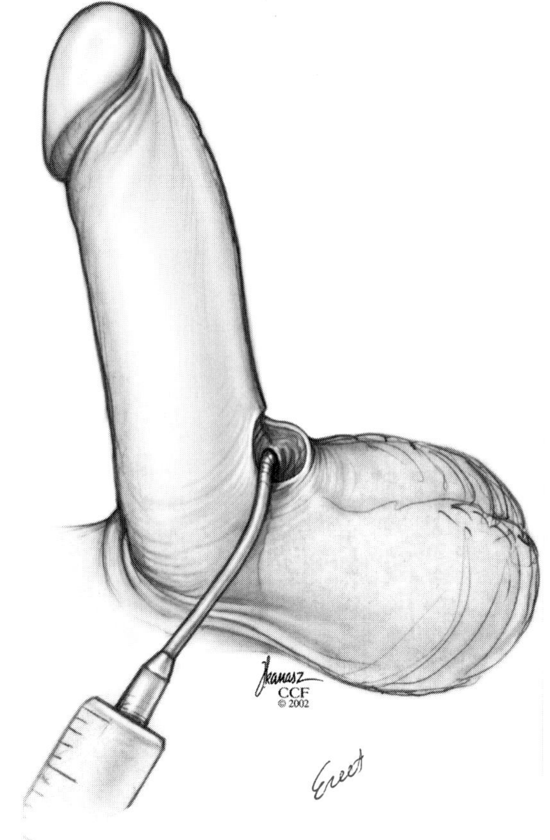

Fig. 46.32

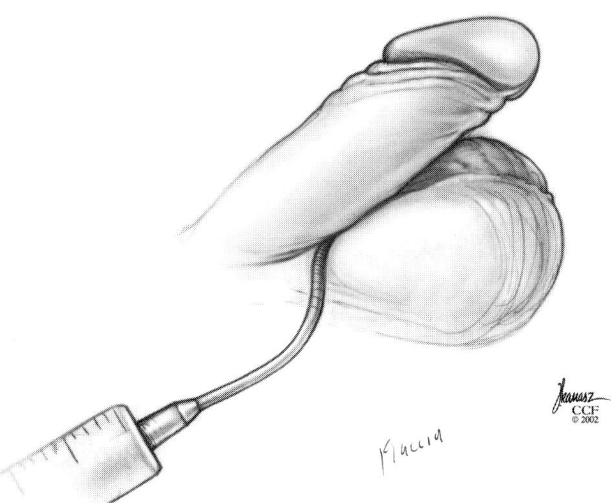

Fig. 46.31

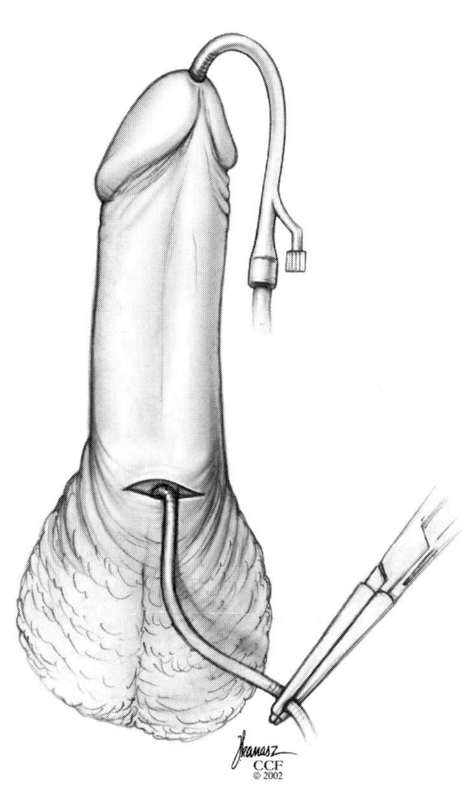

Fig. 46.33

bladder must be completely empty before the reservoir is placed.

The surgeon introduces his or her finger through the incision and moves it up until he or she can palpate the external inguinal ring (Fig. 46.34). In the process of doing

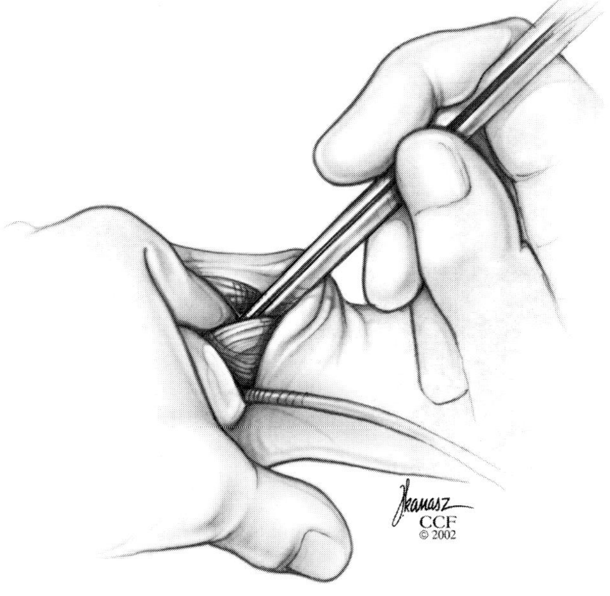


Fig. 46.34

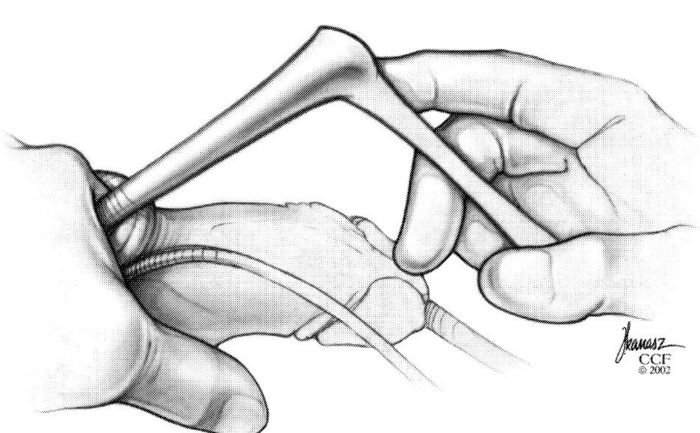


Fig. 46.35

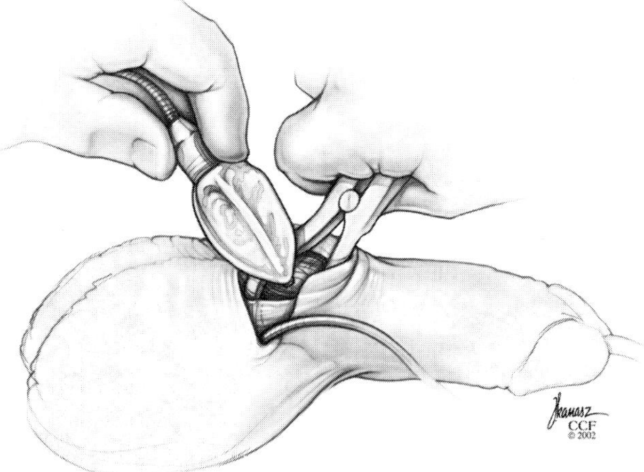


Fig. 46.36

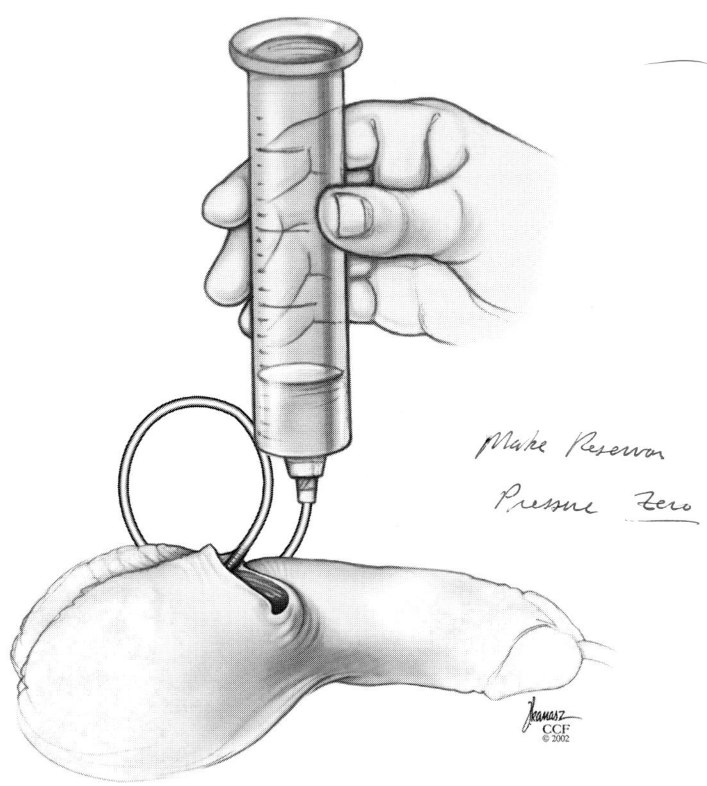


Fig. 46.37

this, the surgeon sweeps away the superficial fascia. If the external ring cannot be palpated, then a point just above the pubic tubercle is chosen. Long blunt Metzenbaum scissors are used to perforate the transversalis fascia enough so that the surgeon's index finger can be slipped into the retropubic space. Entry into the retropubic space is confirmed by palpating the back of the symphysis pubis and the Foley balloon inside the empty bladder.

A nasal speculum with long blades is introduced through the transversalis defect and spread (Fig. 46.35).

The empty reservoir is introduced into the retropubic space (Fig. 46.36).

The reservoir is filled to its capacity with normal saline. There are three reservoir sizes: 50, 65, and 100 mL. After the reservoir is filled, the surgeon palpates to confirm that the reservoir is beneath the transversalis fascia and that the tubing exits directly through the fascial defect. A 50-mL syringe without its plunger is used to permit fluid flow from the reservoir into the syringe until the reservoir pressure is zero (Fig. 46.37). This helps prevent autoinflation of the prosthesis.

The final connection between the pump and reservoir is made (Fig. 46.38).

A 7-mm Blake drain is placed through a stab incision and brought down to line on top of the cylinder connections beneath the transverse scrotal incision (Fig. 46.39). The incision is then closed with running 3-0 Dexon suture

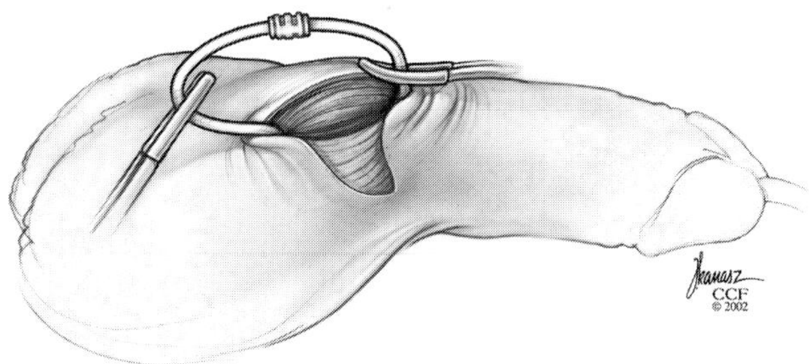


Fig. 46.38

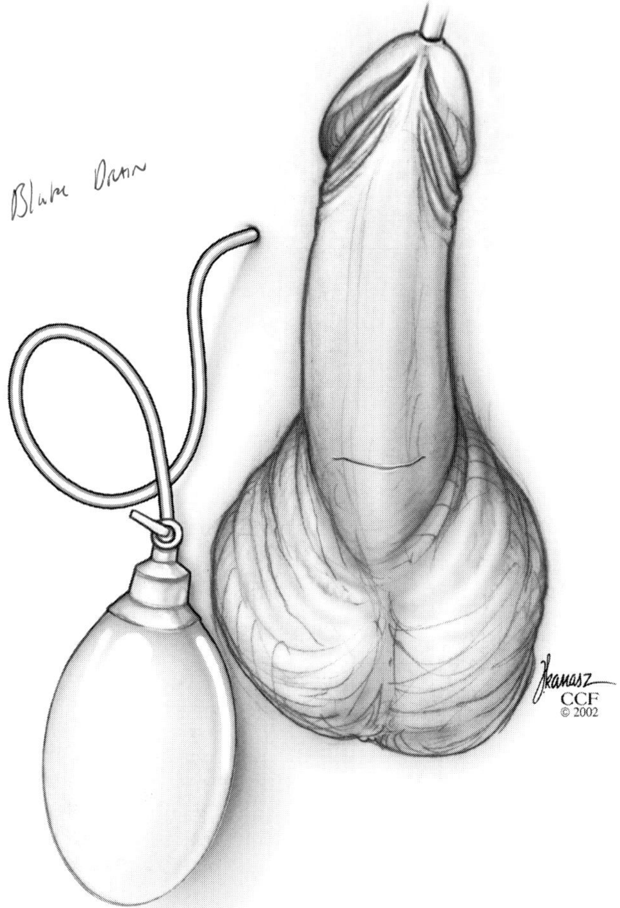


Fig. 46.39

to Dartos fascia and running 4-0 Vicryl subcuticular suture to the skin.

## POSTOPERATIVE CARE

The Foley catheter and drain are removed on the first postoperative morning and the patient is discharged in less than 24 h. The patient is advised to try to keep the penis up on the lower abdomen pointing to the umbilicus while healing is taking place. This avoids ventral curvature of the penis, which may occur if the penis is worn down during the early postoperative period.

Patient instruction in the use of the prosthesis and permission for coitus is usually possible 4–6 wk after surgery. Using water-soluble lubricant initially avoids vaginal dryness, which might result from anxiety associated with the first use of the prosthesis. The couple is also cautioned that if foreplay is not adequate to produce arousal, failure to achieve orgasm is likely.

## REFERENCES

1. Montague DK, Lakin MM. Early experience with the controlled girth and length expanding cylinder of the American Medical Systems Ultrex penile prosthesis. J Urol 148:1444, 1992.
2. Milbank AJ, Montague DK, Angermeier KW, et al. Mechanical failure with the AMS Ultrex inflatable penile prosthesis: pre- and post-1993 structural modification. J Urol 167:2502, 2002.
3. Montague DK, Angermeier KW, Lakin MM, et al. AMS 3-piece inflatable penile prosthesis implantation in men with Peyronie's disease: comparison of CX and Ultrex cylinders [see comments]. J Urol 156:1633, 1996.
4. Montague DK. Penile prosthesis corporotomy closure: a new technique. J Urol 150:924, 1993.
5. Wilson SK, Cleves MA, Delk JR, 2nd. Ultrex cylinders: problems with uncontrolled lengthening (the S-shaped deformity). J Urol 155:135, 1996.

# 47 Priapism

*J. Stephen Jones and Drogo K. Montague*

They (patients with priapism) are not at all relieved (of the erect member) by . . . repeated acts of sexual intercourse. . . . For the most part the patients die on the seventh day *(1)*.

—Arataeus the Cappadocian, first century AD

Priapism is a prolonged, painful erection in the absence of ongoing sexual excitement. The corpora cavernosae are engorged while sparing the corpus spongiosum. Permanent damage to the erectile tissues may occur if priapism is not reversed. The condition may be classified as arterial low flow (ischemic) or high flow (nonischemic). The former is considered a urological emergency, whereas the latter is not and will often resolve without treatment. Arteriography and embolization or surgical ligation are performed only if nonischemic priapism fails to respond to conservative management.

Little or no cavernous flow and abnormal cavernous blood gases characterize ischemic priapism. Initial management includes injection of sympathomimetic agents and therapeutic aspiration. The agent of choice is phenylephrine diluted in saline to a concentration of 100–500 mg/mL injected intracorporeally every 3–5 min for approx 1 h. Children and high-risk adults should be managed with appropriately adjusted doses and concentrations.

If nonsurgical measures fail, a corporoglanular shunt may be performed under local or general anesthesia. Failure to respond to a distal shunt may require performance of a proximal shunt.

## DISTAL SHUNTS

The Winter shunt is a minimally invasive corporoglanular shunt based on creating a fistula between the corpora cavernosae and the glans penis (Fig. 47.1). Usually performed under local anesthesia, multiple small openings are created in the tip of the corporal bodies using either a no. 11 scalpel blade or a Tru-Cut® biopsy needle. This is successful in a minority of cases.

An Al-Ghorab shunt is a more involved version of the corporoglanular shunt. An incision is made in the glans penis just distal to the corona under anesthesia (Fig. 47.2).

A wedge of the joined corpora cavernosae is removed (Fig. 47.3), allowing blood from the corpora cavernosae to shunt into the glans penis (inset). The skin of the glanular incision is then closed to allow shunting from the corporae into the glans.

## PROXIMAL SHUNTS

If the simpler distal shunts are not successful, many patients will ultimately require a proximal shunt in order to reverse the priapism. The saphenous vein shunt (Grayhack)

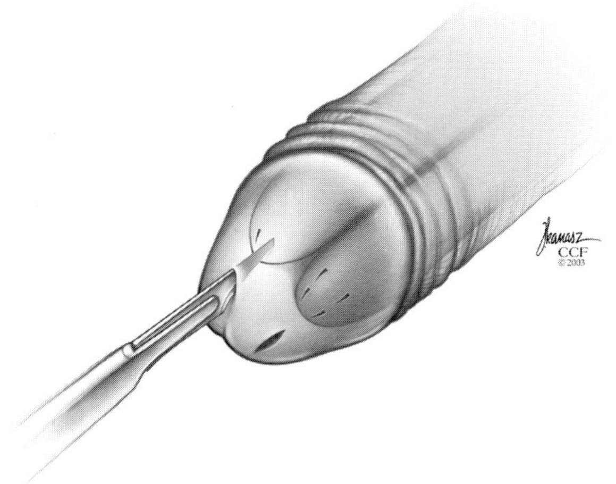


Fig. 47.1

From: *Operative Urology at the Cleveland Clinic*
Edited by: A. Novick et al. © Humana Press Inc., Totowa, NJ

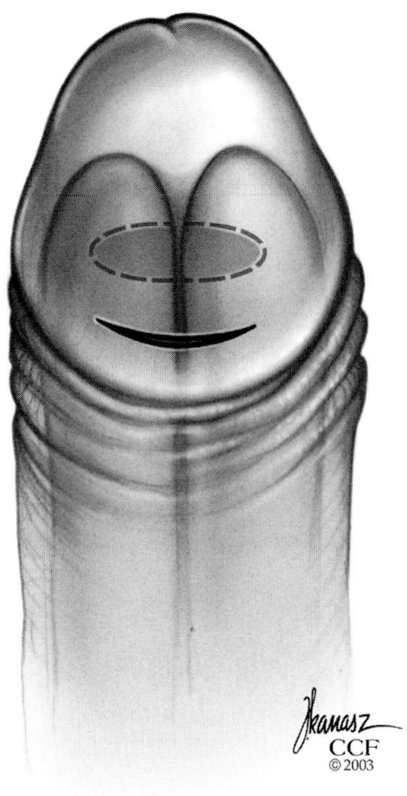


Fig. 47.2

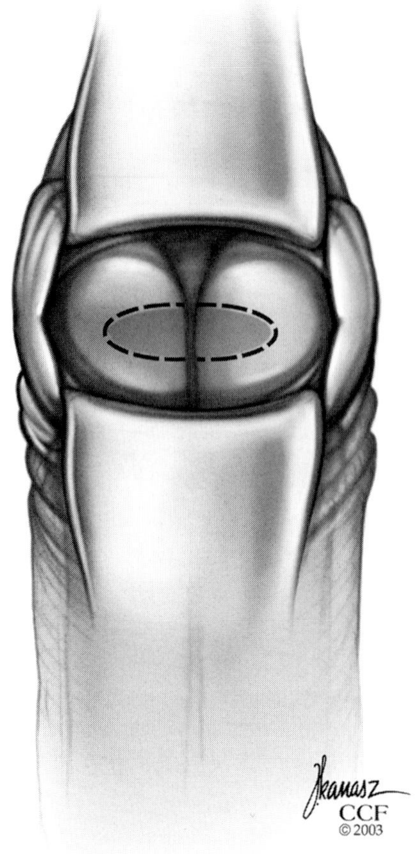


Fig. 47.3

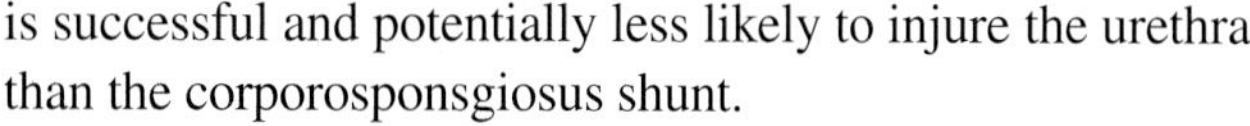

is successful and potentially less likely to injure the urethra than the corporosponsgiosus shunt.

A corporospongiosus shunt (Quackles) is created through a perineal incision. The base of the corporal crura is exposed. Matching 1-cm elliptical excisions are created in the medial crura and the lateral spongiosum adjacent to that site. The openings are sutured together in order to establish communication between the two bodies (Fig. 47.4, inset).

The saphenous vein shunt (Grayhack) allows release of corporal blood through the saphenous vein. Two incisions are used (Fig. 47.5). A longitudinal incision is created at the lateral base of the penis to expose the midportion of the corpus cavernosum. The saphenous vein is exposed through a separate incision, and a tunnel is created between these two incisions to allow the transected saphenous vein to be brought through to the penile incision.

An elliptical opening in the corpus cavernosum at this level is created laterally (Fig. 47.6). The spatulated saphenous vein is anastomosed to the tunica albuginea, establishing free flow out of the corporal body.

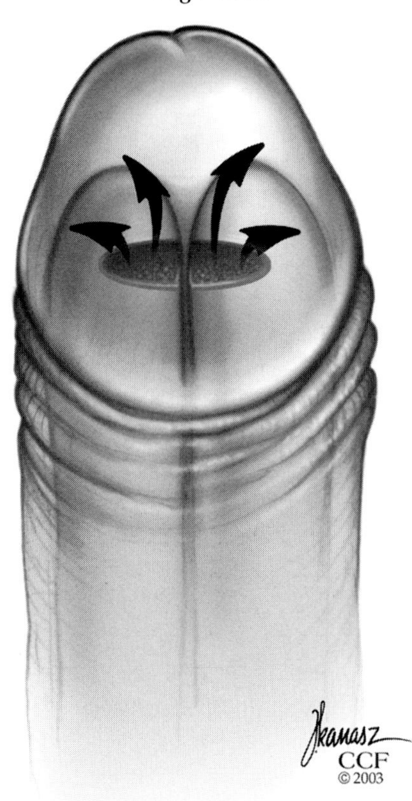


Fig. 47.3 (Inset)

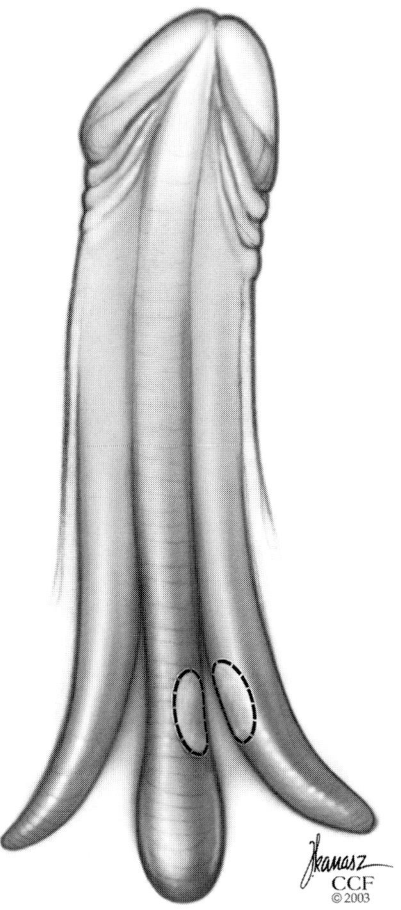


Fig. 47.4

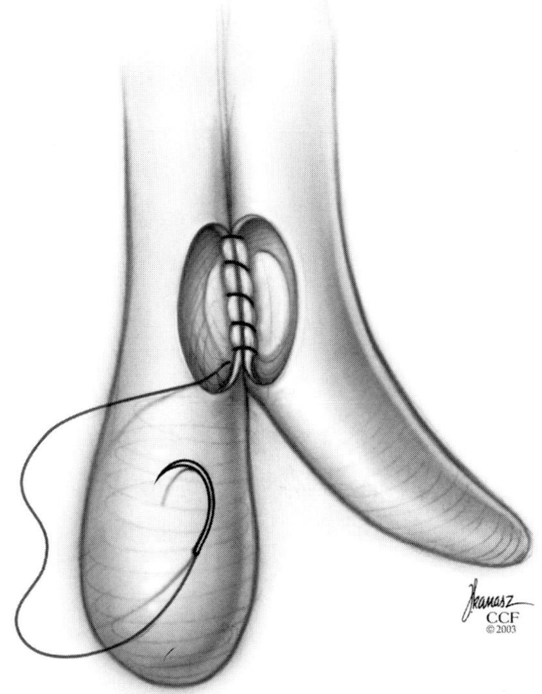


Fig. 47.4 (Inset)

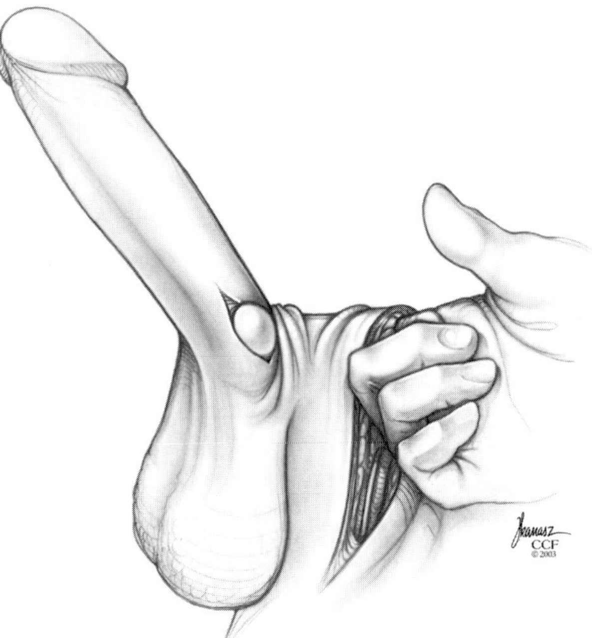


Fig. 47.5

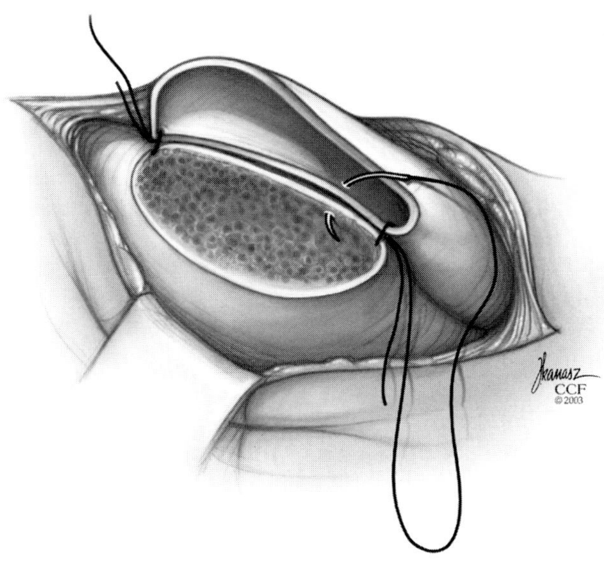


Fig. 47.6

## REFERENCE

1. Adams F, ed. The Extant Works of Arataeus the Cappadocian, Book II, Ch. XII. Birmingham, AL: Classics of Medicine Library, 1990:288, 289.

# 48 Peyronie's Disease and Congenital Penile Curvature

*Kenneth W. Angermeier*

## CONGENITAL PENILE CURVATURE

Congenital curvature is usually seen in young men who report the onset following puberty. The urethral meatus is in a normal location, and the fascial layers and corpus spongiosum of the penis are normally developed. Erect and stretched penile lengths are often greater than normal. It has been suggested that the curvature is related to overall hypercompliance of the tunica albuginea associated with relative shortness of one aspect of the tunica. The curvature is most commonly in a ventral or lateral direction. Erectile rigidity and maintenance are usually normal. A photograph helps to document the degree and direction of curvature prior to surgery. Patients with curvature that significantly interferes with sexual intercourse are surgical candidates and are usually best suited for tunical plication based on their anatomy.

## PEYRONIE'S DISEASE

Peyronie's disease is characterized by the development of a fibrotic lesion within the tunica albuginea of the corpora cavernosa. This scar or plaque restricts the elasticity of the involved tunical segment and may lead to erectile curvature or other deformity.

The most accepted etiology at this time is that repetitive penile trauma is responsible for the tunical injury, leading to fibrosis. During erection the penis remains relatively straight as the symmetrically elastic corpora cavernosa fill with blood. The septal strands become taut between the dorsal and ventral tunica albuginea, providing much of the axial rigidity of the penis. When the erect penis is subjected to loading and some degree of bending occurs, stress is focused at the junction of the septal strands and tunica albuginea. Bending of the penis during intercourse may be exaggerated by age-related changes in erectile function and rigidity. In addition, it has been shown that the concentration of elastic fibers within the tunica albuginea decreases with time. This decrease in the modulus of elasticity with aging may interfere with the ability of the tunica to withstand tissue distortion. It has been theorized that the above factors may lead to delamination of the inner circular and outer longitudinal layers of the tunica albuginea at the site of attachment of the septal strands, resulting in hemorrhage and local inflammation. Fibrin may remain trapped within the relatively hypovascular tunica, leading to persistent inflammation and subsequent fibrosis. The process can extend laterally, leading to a more extensive or even circumferential plaque. Obviously, there are many more patients with penile trauma than those with clinical Peyronie's disease, indicating that some inherent predisposition to excessive scar formation may exist. This is supported by the association of Peyronie's disease with Dupuytren's contracture in 10% of patients and noncontractile Dupuytren's contracture in up to 40%.

Although some patients may recall a distinct episode of buckling trauma to the penis during intercourse, most do not. The disease process begins with an inflammatory phase, which may be associated with pain and tunical induration. Over a period of 12–24 mo, the tunical lesion remodels and matures, with resolution of discomfort in the majority of cases. Variable degrees of erectile curvature may occur as a result of this process and may change over time. Once the scar has matured, there will be no further change in the configuration of the penis. Calcification of the plaque occurs in 20% of patients and indicates a mature lesion. Erectile curvature is due to tethering by the inelastic, fibrotic tunica and is in the direction of the most predominant lesion. Opposing plaques may balance each other such that the erect penis is relatively straight, although often foreshortened. Relative flaccidity distal to the level of the plaque may be present in some patients as well. The exact cause of this disparity in erection is

From: *Operative Urology at the Cleveland Clinic*
Edited by: A. Novick et al. © Humana Press Inc., Totowa, NJ

unclear, as Doppler studies have shown that intracavernosal arterial flow is maintained in these patients. Restriction of full expansion of the tunica albuginea and the intracavernosal fibrous network may mechanically limit erectile rigidity or possibly contribute to localized corporeal veno-occlusive dysfunction.

As in most instances, evaluation of the patient with Peyronie's disease begins with a detailed history. It is important to accurately document the onset of the initial symptoms and the evolution of those symptoms over time. Some patients first notice penile pain during erection or palpate a nodule or firmness along the penile shaft. Others describe the presence of curvature as their initial evidence of disease. Patients should be asked whether an episode of penile buckling or trauma preceded the condition. Symptoms may evolve slowly or occur rapidly, with patients describing the onset of curvature "overnight" in some instances. When present, pain will eventually resolve in most cases as inflammation diminishes. Configuration and stability of the erect penis is documented by history and with the aid of photographs.

A detailed sexual history is also elicited, because erectile function is an important factor in deciding upon the most appropriate form of treatment. Patients are asked about their sexual function prior to and following the onset of disease. We record the frequency of intercourse, erectile rigidity, and maintenance and the integrity of orgasm, ejaculation, and libido. The presence and nature of any curvature prior to the development of Peyronie's disease is documented.

Physical examination involves grasping the glans and stretching the penis to allow for accurate palpation between the index finger and thumb. One should be able to define the extent and location of the plaque, including dorsal, lateral, and ventral components, when present. A simple plain film of the penis may be considered if one wishes to document the presence of calcification within the scar. More advanced imaging studies do not seem to contribute significant additional information in our experience.

After complete maturation of the tunical scar, patients with mild to moderate penile curvature who remain functional should be followed conservatively. If erectile rigidity or maintenance is a problem, they can be treated with standard treatments for impotence such as an oral agent, vacuum erection device, injection therapy, or a penile prosthesis. In patients with erectile curvature precluding or significantly interfering with sexual intercourse, surgical treatment may be considered. In general, curvature tends to become problematic when it exceeds 45° dorsally, or 30° laterally or ventrally. To confirm stability of the patient's situation prior to surgery, we wait until the disease has been present for at least 1 yr and erectile configuration stable for 6 mo before proceeding. Some patients undergo a duplex ultrasound of the penis following pharmacological injection prior to surgery. The ultrasound allows one to obtain information with regard to cavernosal arterial inflow and veno-occlusion and provides an opportunity to visualize the erectile configuration if photographs are not available. In addition, the presence of collateral vessels from the dorsal artery of the penis to the cavernosal arterial system is documented because these vessels may be compromised during surgical mobilization of the neurovascular bundles (NVBs), although this is uncommon in our experience.

There are two ways to surgically straighten a curved erection: shorten the long side (tunical plication) or lengthen the short side (tunical incision/excision with grafting). In patients with Peyronie's disease, we take several factors into consideration when counseling patients about selection of the surgical technique:

## Erectile Function

Postoperative erectile dysfunction has been observed in approx 10–30% of patients following plaque incision or excision with grafting. In a group of patients assessed by dynamic infusion cavernosometry prior to surgery, it was shown that there is a correlation between preoperative erectile function and postoperative success following plaque excision and dermal graft inlay. Preoperative evaluation of erectile function with nocturnal penile tumescence monitoring or duplex ultrasonography has also been reported in patients undergoing plaque incision using dermis or alternative grafts. These studies suggest that postoperative results are optimal in patients with normal subjective and objective erectile function preoperatively. Based on this information, patients with below normal but adequate erectile function with or without a phosphodiesterase inhibitor may wish to consider plication as long as other factors are favorable. With this procedure, there is less disruption of the erectile tissue and subtunical venous network. The risk of erectile deterioration following plication at our institution has been very low, and this is consistent with other reports using similar techniques.

## Penile Length

Plication procedures result in further shortening of erectile length, as the longer side of the penis is shortened to match the opposite side. Although this provides excellent penile straightening, some additional decrease in erectile length occurs. This must be clearly explained to the patient prior to surgery. Patients with greater baseline penile length are less likely to be functionally affected by this. One can estimate the length of the erection after plication by manually stretching the penis in the flaccid state, as the stretched length is limited by the short side. Plaque incision or excision with graft inlay tends to preserve remaining length by expanding the "short" aspect of the penis for straightening. Patients should be cautioned, however, that erectile length will not be restored in most cases to their premorbid status, even following plaque incision or excision.

### Degree of Curvature

If curvature is severe, tunical plication will need to be more extensive and may result in excessive penile shortening. Therefore, plaque incision or excision may be preferred in this situation.

### Location of Curvature

In the setting of dorsal curvature, plaque incision requires mobilization of the NVBs to expose the tunical scar. In experienced hands this can be readily and safely accomplished. This maneuver may result in a temporary change in sensation of the glans penis. Ventral curvature necessitates mobilization of the corpus spongiosum, which carries a low risk of urethral injury. Depending on the technique, tunical plication may require total, partial, or no mobilization of the neurovascular bundles to correct ventral curvature. Correction of dorsal or lateral curvature requires no special maneuvers relative to the NVBs or urethra. This decreases operative time and lessens the chance of alterations in glans sensation postoperatively.

### Local Erectile Deformity

Patients with Peyronie's disease may develop significant constriction or indentation of the penis at the site of the tunical scar. Tunical plication will generally not change the appearance of this lesion despite penile straightening. If the plication results in mild indentation of the tunica albuginea opposite the scar deformity, there could be some instability or hinging of the erection in this area. In this setting, therefore, a graft procedure may be preferred in order to correct the local deformity.

In the setting of Peyronie's disease, both tunical plication and plaque incision or excision with graft inlay are discussed with the patient in relation to the above factors, and a mutual decision is made as to how to proceed.

## SURGICAL PROCEDURES

### Plication

Plication procedures may be categorized according to the manner in which the tunica albuginea is manipulated to achieve shortening of the long side of the corpora cavernosa.

#### Tunical Excision

The technique described by Nesbit begins most commonly by degloving the penis through a circumcising incision (Fig. 48.1A). Prior to any penile procedure, it is important to discuss circumcision status with the patient to make sure that it is clear what will be done in this regard at the time of surgery. If an uncircumcised patient wishes to avoid circumcision, the ventrum of the penis can be approached through a ventral midline incision or a lateral curvature may be corrected using a lateral longitudinal incision. For dorsal exposure, a sigmoid incision is preferred to minimize scar contracture. After the penis is exposed, an artificial erection is performed to assess the curvature and plan the site for tunical excision. Buck's fascia is incised longitudinally just above the level of the corpus spongiosum and elevated at the appropriate location opposite the site of maximal curvature (Fig. 48.1B). Larger circumflex veins should be ligated and divided between 4-0 Vicryl ties with control of smaller vessels using bipolar cautery. In the setting of lateral or dorsal curvature, this part of the procedure is relatively straightforward as the dorsal NVBs do not come into play. For ventral curvature, however, these structures are elevated by dissecting in the plane between the tunica albuginea and Buck's fascia beginning ventrolaterally and working toward the midline (Fig. 48.1C). This is done very meticulously, using loupe magnification and bipolar cautery for hemostasis. Nesbit did not carry this dissection across the midline, but only far enough to expose the dorsolateral aspects of the corpora cavernosa. Once the tunica albuginea in the area of interest is exposed, we prefer to simulate the plication using a number of Allis clamps on the tunica at the site of each proposed site of plication as described by Kelami. An artificial erection is performed, and the clamps can be adjusted to get the desired effect. The marks of the clamps on the tunica are then used as a guide to excise transversely oriented ellipses of tunica, taking great care to preserve the underlying erectile tissue (Fig. 48.1D). In the setting of lateral curvature, one column of ellipses is usually sufficient. For dorsal or ventral curvature, paired ellipses on either side of the midline are used. The elliptical defects are then closed transversely, effectively shortening the long side of the penis (Fig. 48.1E). A variety of sutures have been used in the past to close these defects. The options include a 2-0 or 3-0 nonabsorbable monofilament, 3-0 PDS, or a combination of these. We favor an interrupted 3-0 Prolene with the knot buried at the midpoint of the ellipse, followed by final

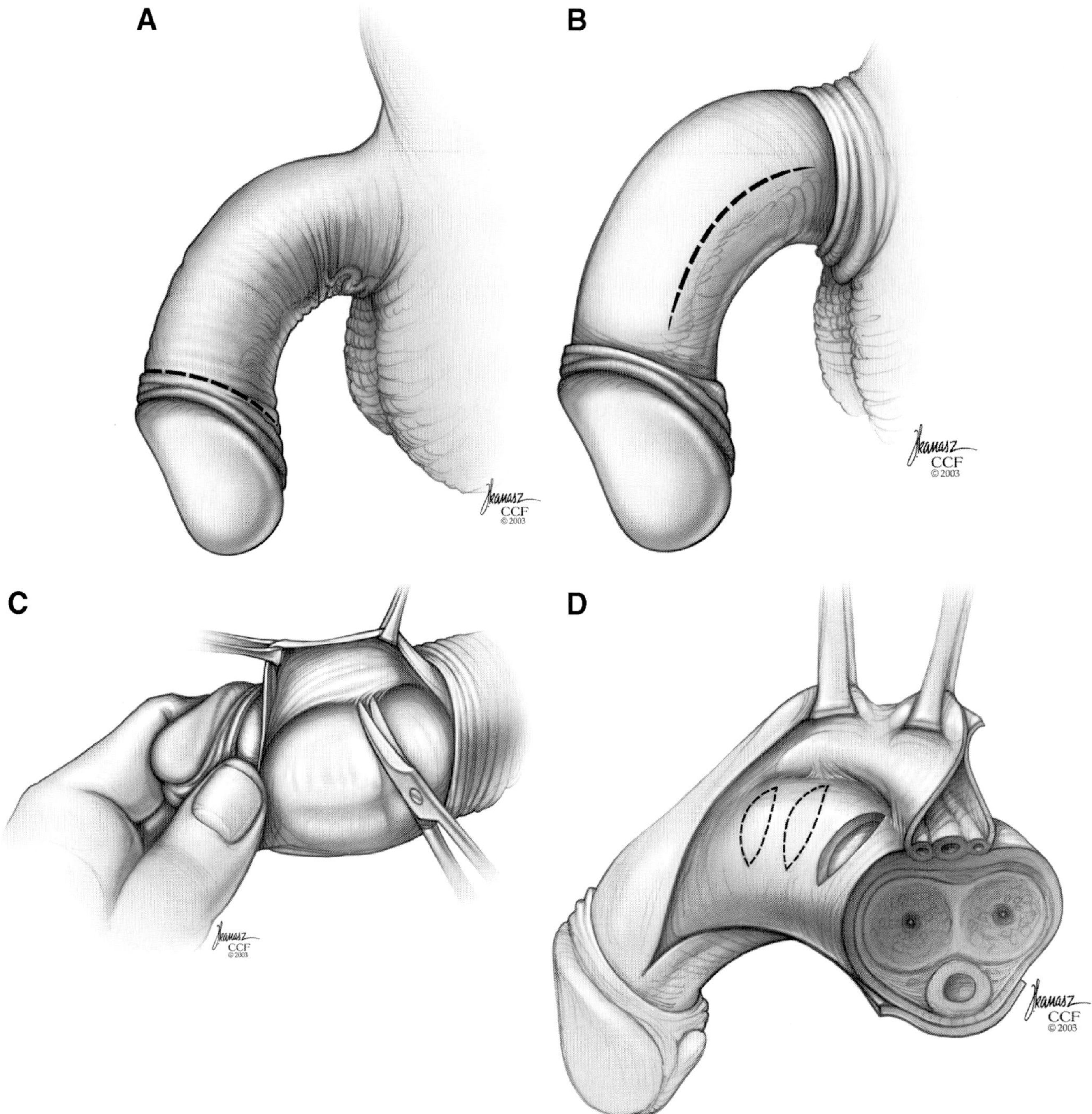


Fig. 48.1

closure with running 3-0 PDS. One should be careful to not make the ellipses wider than approx 1–1.5 cm each to avoid secondary distortion of the erection. The artificial erection is repeated, and additional ellipses can be added as needed until adequate straightening is obtained. Two to three pairs of ellipses are usually sufficient in our experience. Buck's fascia is approximated over the plication sites using interrupted absorbable 5-0 sutures (Fig. 48.1F). A small suction drain may be placed in the sub-dartos space as needed. The dartos layer and skin are closed in standard fashion (Fig. 48.1G). In our experience this technique is applicable to all patients with Peyronie's disease and those with congenital lateral or dorsal curvature.

Pryor and Fitzpatrick reported their modification of Nesbit's procedure in 1979. They advocated the excision of a single tunical ellipse opposite the point of maximum curvature. The tunica albuginea is exposed with complete mobilization of NVBs when necessary depending on the

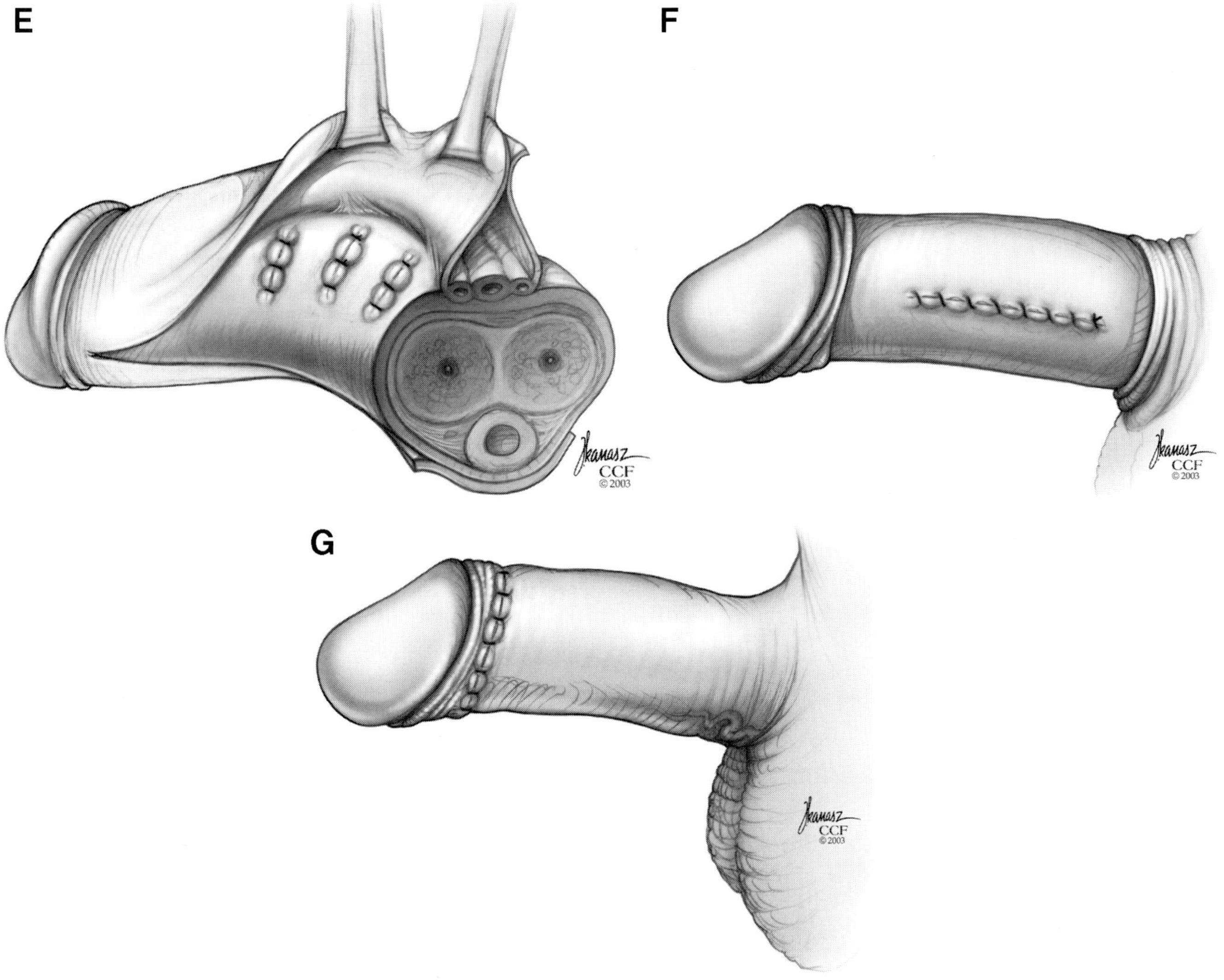


Fig. 48.1 (*Continued*)

direction of curvature (Fig. 48.2A,B). This can be done through a lateral approach or with a dorsal approach through the bed of the dorsal vein of the penis. Planning of the ellipses may be aided by using interrupted sutures to imbricate the tunica and assess straightening or with the use of Allis clamps. The edges of the ellipse are then marked and used as a guide for excision after the sutures or clamps are removed (Fig. 48.2C). The ellipse is generally 0.5–1 cm wide and half the circumference of the penis, and the resulting defect is closed transversely (Fig. 48.2D). Further ellipses may be added if necessary following repeat artificial erection. We close the tunica with three evenly spaced interrupted sutures of 3-0 Prolene with the knots buried, with final closure using a running 3-0 PDS locking every other suture. This method of plication is our preferred technique for men with congenital ventral curvature, as it seems to be more durable than other less invasive techniques. The mechanical forces imparted upon the dorsal aspect of the corpora in this setting may be greater than those seen in lateral curvature or in men with Peyronie's disease and account for this finding.

### Tunical Incision

We have also used a technique described by Yachia, who combined the use of Allis clamps with transverse closure of longitudinal tunical incisions. In this technique (Fig. 48.3), the penis is degloved and artificial erection performed, as described previously (Fig. 48.3A). After marking the site of maximal curvature, the tunical albuginea at the corporotomy site is exposed by elevating Buck's fascia. This can be done focally at each planned incision site, but we favor longitudinal incision and dissection of Buck's fascia for dorsal (Fig. 48.3B) and lateral curvature and partial mobilization of the NVBs through a lateral or dorsal approach to expose

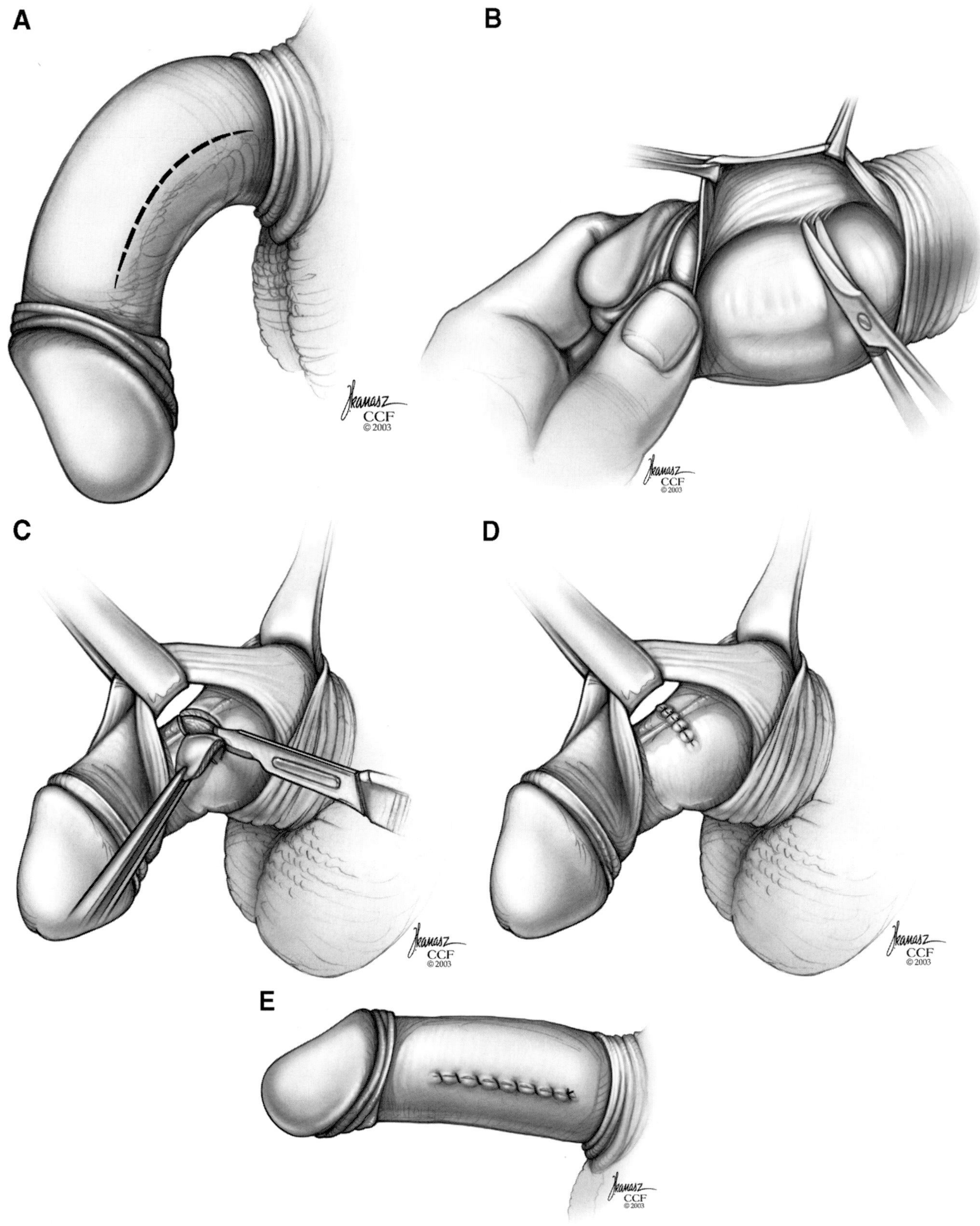


Fig. 48.2

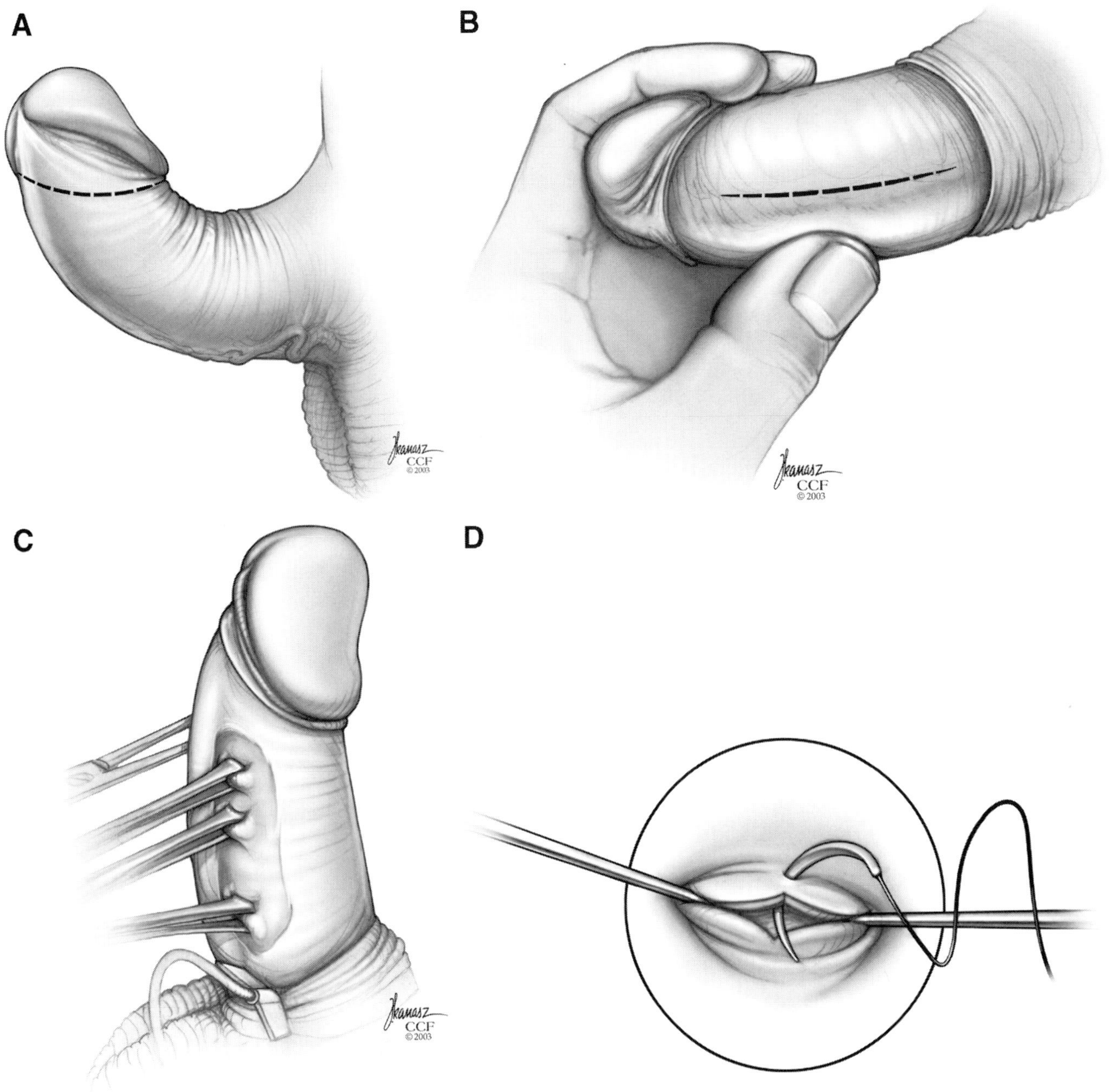


Fig. 48.3

the dorsolateral aspect of the corpora for ventral curvature. Allis clamps are then applied to the tunica albuginea to simulate the plication in either a single column for lateral curvature or paired columns on each side of the midline for ventral or dorsal curvature (Fig. 48.3C). After the clamps have been adjusted to obtain adequate straightening, as documented by artificial erection, the first clamp is removed and the tunica albuginea is incised longitudinally between the marks of the clamp using a #11 blade. Care is taken not to incise into the underlying erectile tissue. Single skin hooks are used to draw the incision transversely. Yachia described closure using running 3-0 PDS, although running 3-0 Prolene has also been reported (Fig. 48.3D). We favor an interrupted suture of 3-0 Prolene with the knot buried at the midpoint of the incision, followed by final closure using running 3-0 PDS. This is repeated at each corporotomy site, and the final result is assessed with repeat artificial erection (Fig. 48.3E,F).

### No Tunical Incision

After reviewing Nesbit's procedure and the results of Pryor and Fitzpatrick, Essed and Schroeder developed a

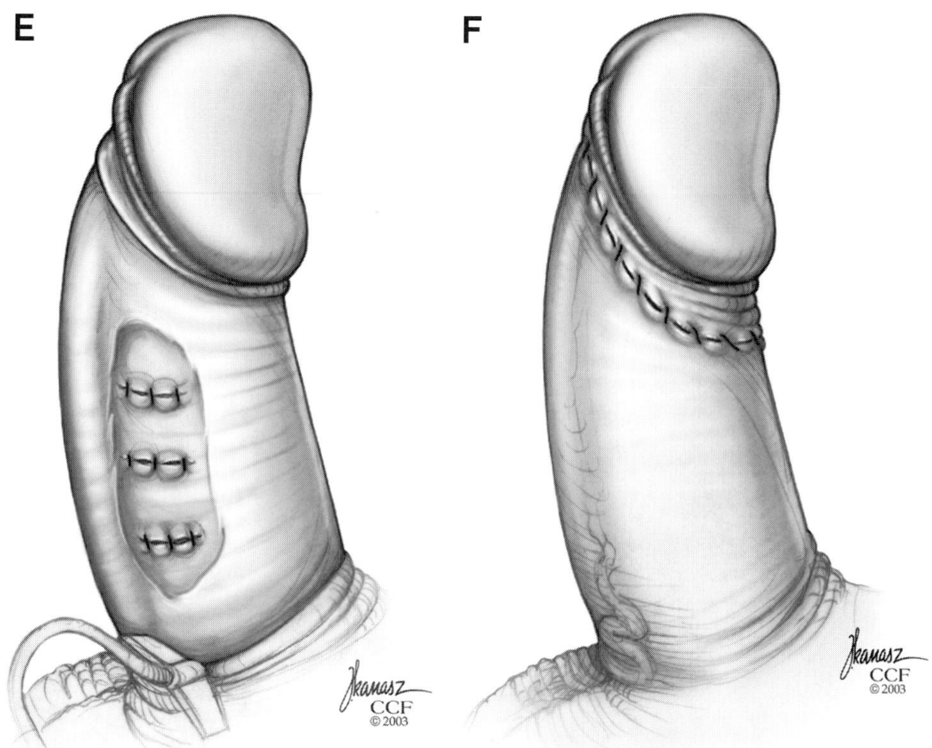


Fig. 48.3 (*Continued*)

technique of tunical plication without tissue excision or incision (Fig. 48.4). They felt that this eliminated unnecessary corporeal trauma and avoided damage to underlying erectile tissue. The procedure starts by degloving the penis and then performing an artificial erection to identify the site of maximal curvature. In the setting of dorsal curvature, the urethra is circumferentially mobilized off of the corpora cavernosa to expose their ventral aspect (Fig. 48.4A). Alternatively, the NVBs within Buck's fascia are dissected off of the dorsal tunica albuginea to treat ventral curvature. Two or four single skin hooks are inserted into the tunica and pulled crosswise to simulate the plication. When straightening is achieved using the hooks, the points of insertion are marked and then connected. This usually results in an ellipse opposite the tunical scar. Nonabsorbable 3-0 multifilament sutures are placed to approximate the marked tunica albuginea and close the ellipse transversely (Fig. 48.4B,C). This maneuver results in shortening of the convex side of the penis and overall straightening. Eight sutures are usually required. The urethra is then sutured back in place along the corporal bodies, and closure commences in standard fashion. Knispel et al. modified this procedure slightly by using interrupted sutures of 2-0 Prolene with the knots inverted, resulting in a low incidence of palpable knots.

In 1992 Donatucci and Lue described a less invasive procedure for suture plication that obviates the need for mobilization of the NVBs or the corpus spongiosum (Fig. 48.5). After the induction of anesthesia, an intracavernosal injection of papaverine or alprostadil is given. Depending on the direction of curvature, the corpora may be exposed through a lateral, ventral, or circumcising incision. After the site opposite the area of maximal curvature is exposed, the proposed suture entry sites are marked with a pen. Two or three pairs of 2-0 Ticron or Tevdex plicating sutures are used in order to minimize suture tension and postoperative discomfort. In order to correct dorsal curvature, the sutures are perispongiosal in location (Fig. 48.5A). In the setting of ventral curvature, the sutures are placed into the tunica albuginea between the dorsal vein and the dorsal arteries (Fig. 48.5B). The sutures are tied one row at a time, and the degree of correction can be continuously monitored as a result of the pharmacological erection. After penile straightening, the erection is reversed using intracavernosal phenylephrine, if necessary.

## Plaque Incision or Excision With Graft Inlay

For dorsal or dorsolateral curvature, a circumcising incision is made and the penis is degloved (Fig. 48.6 A,B). An artificial erection establishes the location and severity

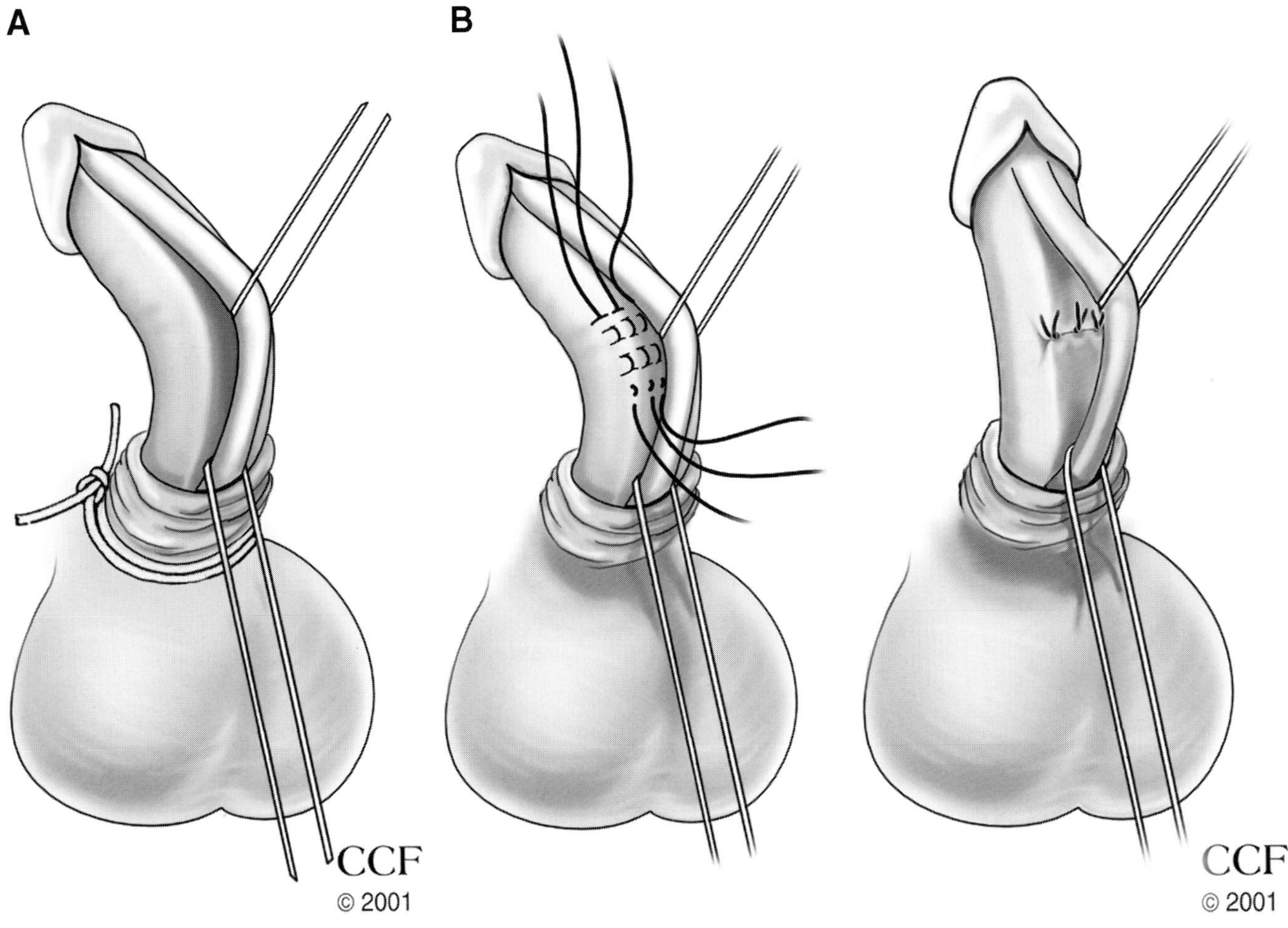


Fig. 48.4

of curvature. Buck's fascia along with the dorsal NVBs is then mobilized off of the underlying tunical albuginea. This can be done in two ways. The first is the lateral approach. In this technique, longitudinal incisions through Buck's fascia are made bilaterally just above the level of the corpus spongiosum (Fig. 48.6C). Circumflex veins are ligated and divided near the corpus spongiosum. The dissection takes place from lateral to medial on both sides in the plane right on the tunical albuginea, elevating Buck's fascia and its contents (Fig. 48.6D). Once across the midline, small retractors or a vessel loop are used to gain exposure to take the dissection distally and proximally as needed (Fig. 48.6E). Stay sutures in the tunica help to keep the NVBs out of the way during the remainder of the procedure. It may be necessary to dissect under the proximal glans penis distally to gain adequate exposure. Small emissary veins encountered during the dissection are controlled with bipolar cautery. Once the dissection is complete, stay sutures are placed in the tunica beyond the tunical scar distally, proximally, and laterally to maintain exposure.

A second method to elevate NVBs is the dorsal midline approach, which is started by performing an abbreviated penile vein ligation (Fig. 48.7). Buck's fascia is incised over the deep dorsal vein of the penis, and the vein is then dissected free and excised from the retrocoronal plexus to the base of the penis (Fig. 48.7A). The deep layers of Buck's fascia in the bed of the excised dorsal vein are incised in the midline, and tenotomy scissors are used to dissect in the plane between the tunica albuginea and Buck's fascia, which encompasses the neurovascular structures. The dissection is carried from medial to lateral and is continued well around the circumference of the penis until normal tunica is identified (Fig. 48.7B).

When performing plaque incision, the point of maximal erectile curvature is marked during an artificial erection, and the tunical incision is then made at that site (Fig. 48.8). We prefer to carry the incision around to the lateral corporal body and to release tension with inward pointing V on either end (Fig. 48.8A), which results in a rectangular tunical defect (Fig. 48.8B). The edges of the

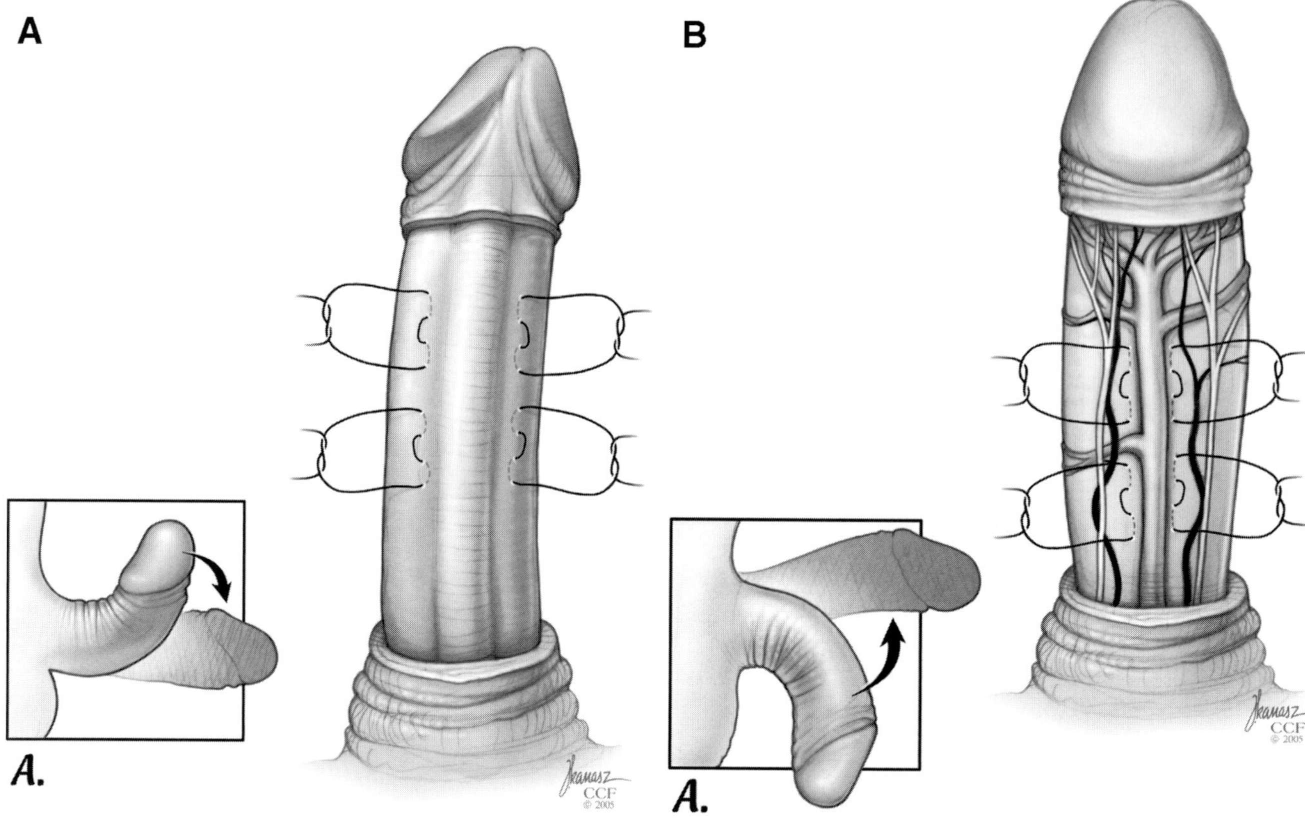


Fig. 48.5

tunica are carefully undermined a bit circumferentially, and the septal strands are divided off of the tunica in the midline for a short distance both distally and proximally. The defect is measured to calculate the size of the graft needed.

When excising a dense or calcified plaque, the tunical scar is defined by palpation and marked, and a scalpel is used to incise the tunica albuginea around the periphery of the plaque (Fig. 48.9A). The plaque is then sharply dissected from the underlying erectile tissue. Septal strands in the midline must be divided. The edges of the tunica are undermined slightly, and four to six lateral darting incisions are then made to expand the edges of the defect, which generally ends up much larger than the size of the excised plaque (Fig. 48.9B). The length and width of the defect are then recorded.

If using dermis, a graft 25–30% larger than the corporotomy defect is measured on the lateral lower abdomen just above the iliac crest in a nonhirsute area (Fig. 48.10A). We prefer to remove the epidermis freehand using a no.10 scalpel blade (Fig. 48.10B). The dermal graft is then harvested, and the undersurface is carefully defatted (Fig. 48.10C). The donor site is closed primarily. The dermal graft is placed into the tunical defect with the fat side down and initially secured into place using interrupted sutures of 4-0 PDS at the apices and along the darting incisions. The graft is carefully tailored, and the septum is attached to the midline of the graft using interrupted 4-0 PDS sutures. The periphery of the graft is closed in watertight fashion using a running locking suture of 4-0 or 5-0 PDS (Fig. 48.10D). After irrigating and achieving hemostasis, Buck's fascia is reapproximated in the dorsal midline using interrupted 5-0 PDS if dorsal mobilization of the NVBs was performed or along both ventrolateral incisions following a lateral approach. Care must be taken to avoid injury to the dorsal arteries and nerves of the penis. An artificial erection is repeated to confirm penile straightening. One or two small suction drains are placed superficial to Buck's fascia and deep to the dartos fascia along the shaft of the penis. The skin incision is then closed.

Cadaveric pericardium has also been reported for use as a graft inlay during these procedures and acts as a scaffold for tissue ingrowth. After tunical incision or excision, the graft is rehydrated in normal saline for 10–15 min (Fig. 48.11A). It is generally sized about 10% larger than the tunical defect and sutured in place using interrupted and running 4-0 PDS on a taper needle (Fig. 48.11B,C).

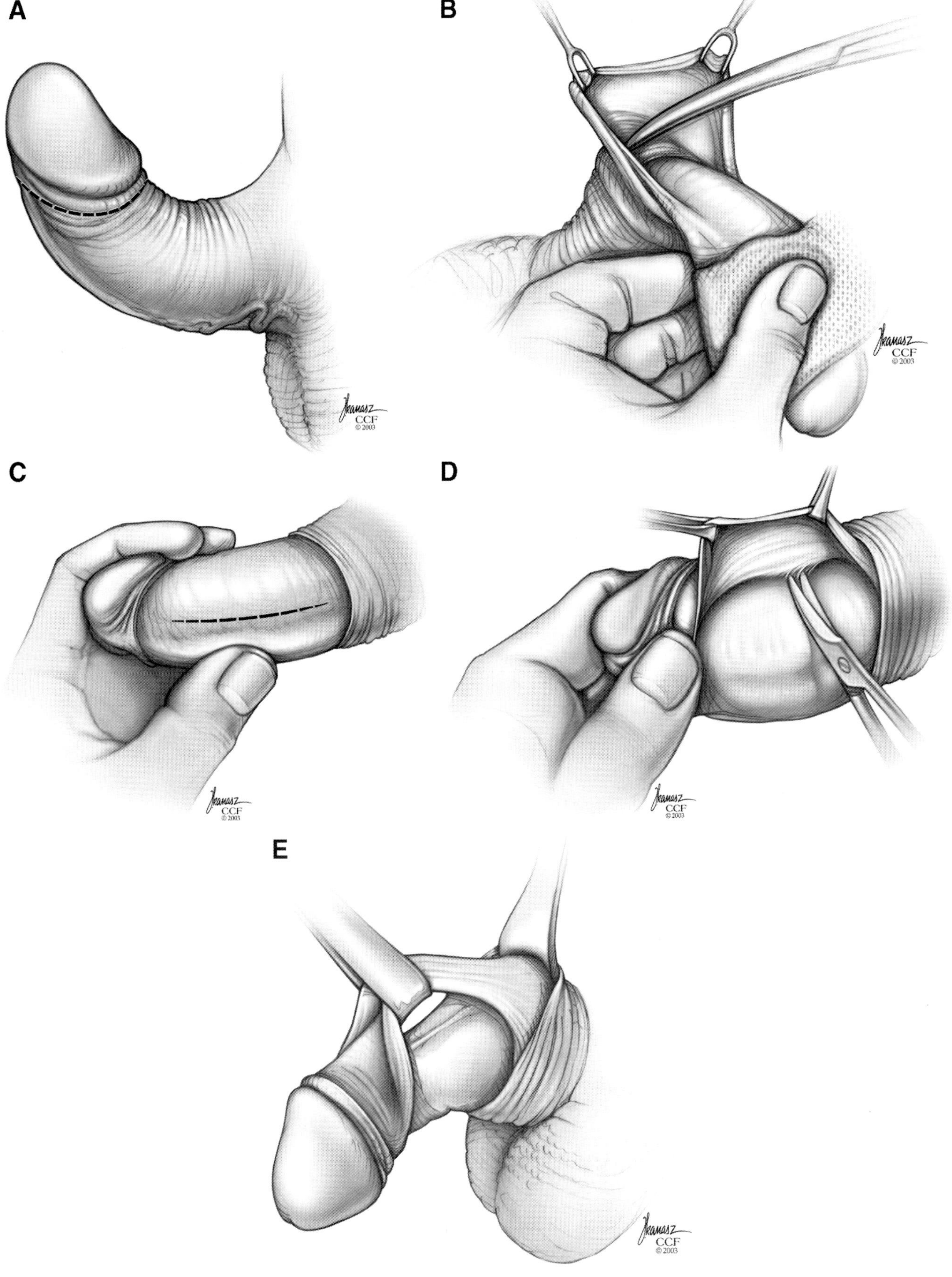


Fig. 48.6

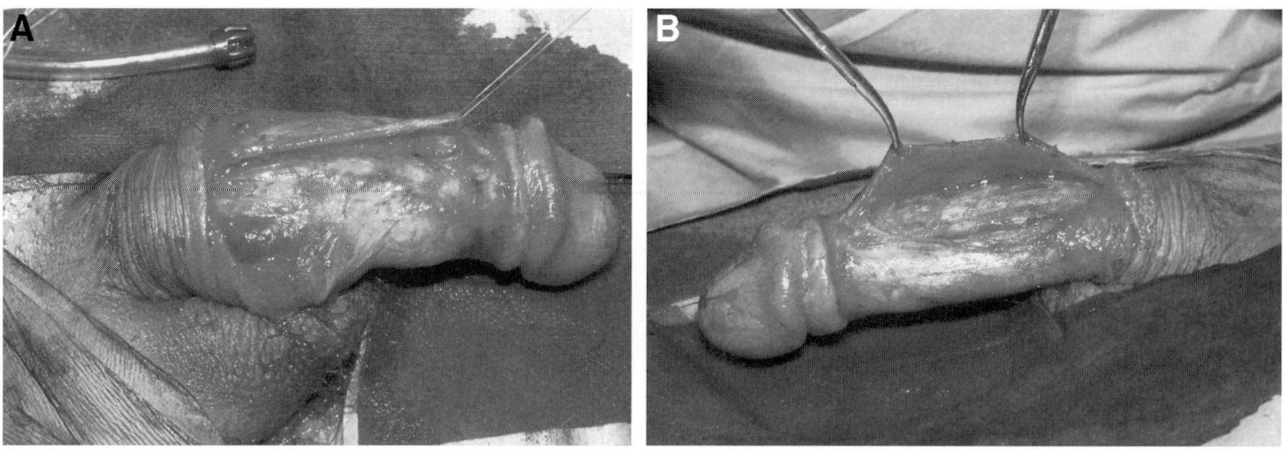


Fig. 48.7

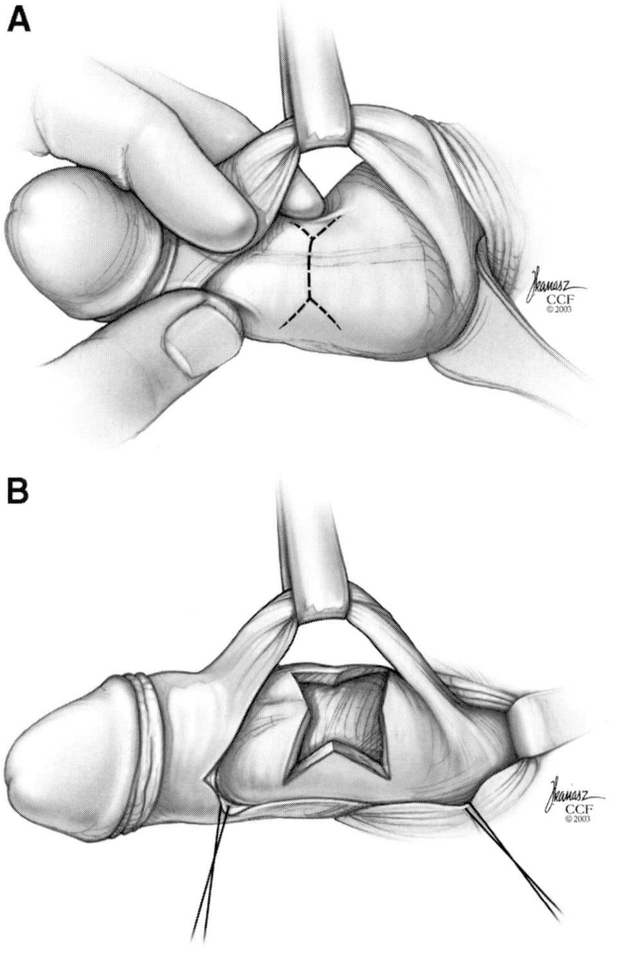

Fig. 48.8

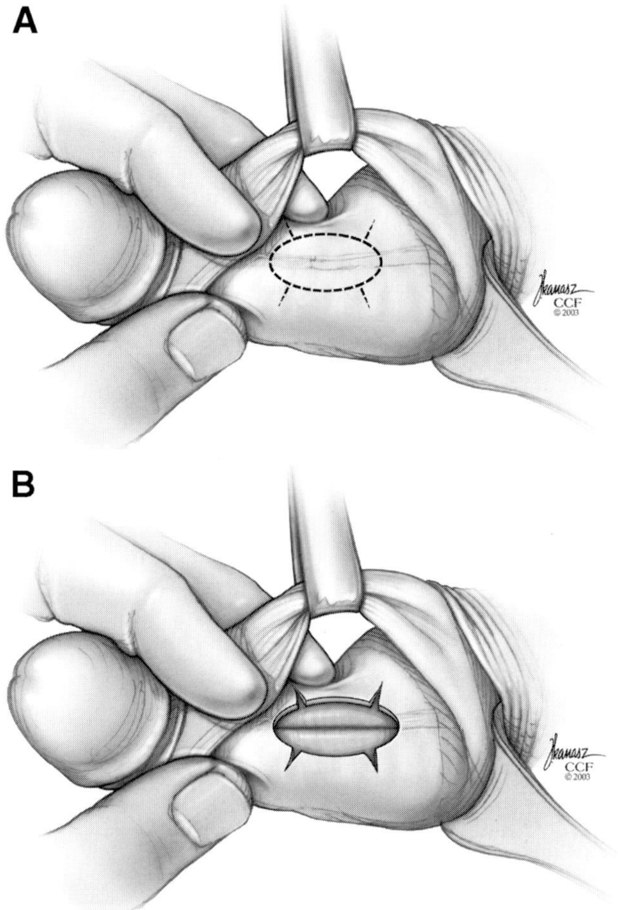

Fig. 48.9

We have not had personal experience with other reported graft materials such as vein, tunica vaginalis, or small intestinal submucosa.

The surgical procedure varies slightly for a ventral tunical plaque. The skin incision may be made in the ventral midline of the penis or through a circumcision (Fig. 48.12). Buck's fascia is incised longitudinally on either side of the urethra, and any circumflex or periurethral veins are ligated and divided. The corpus spongiosum is dissected and elevated from the underlying tunica albuginea and scar

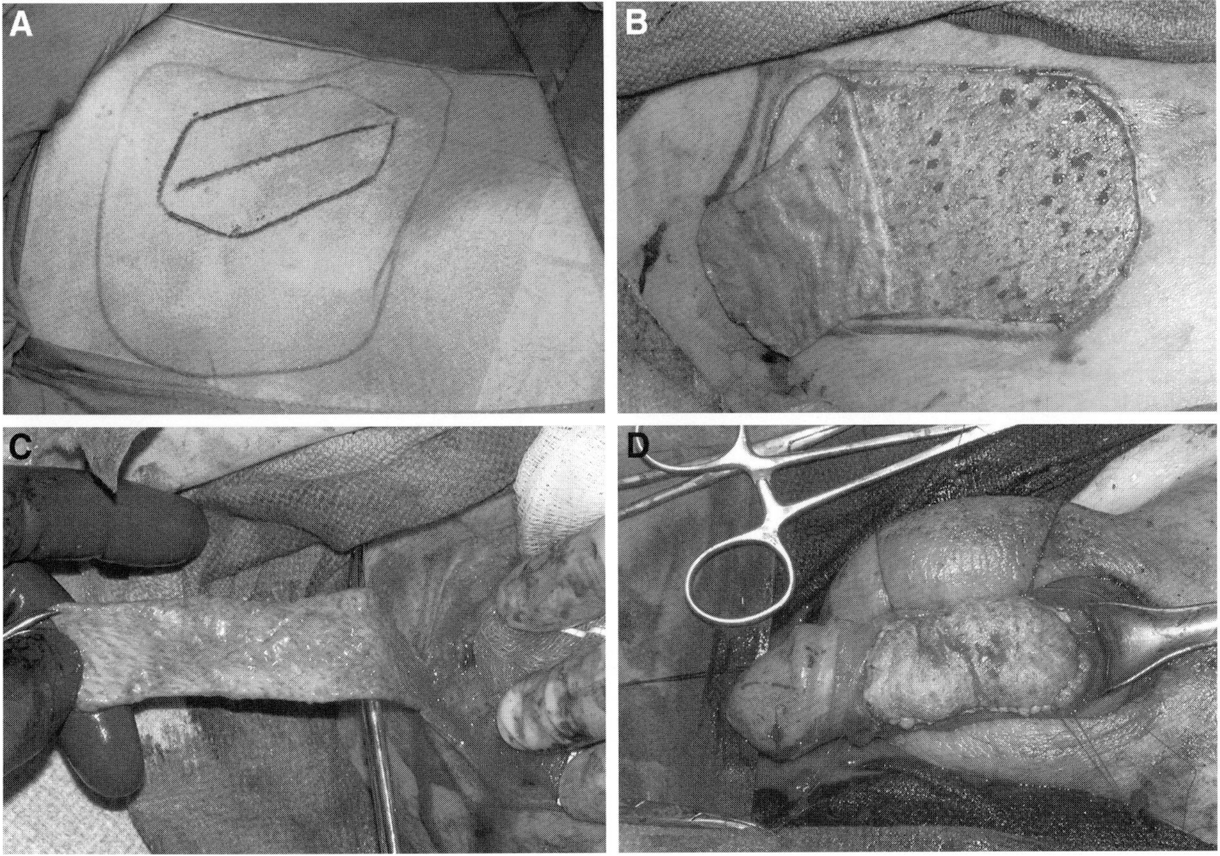


Fig. 48.10

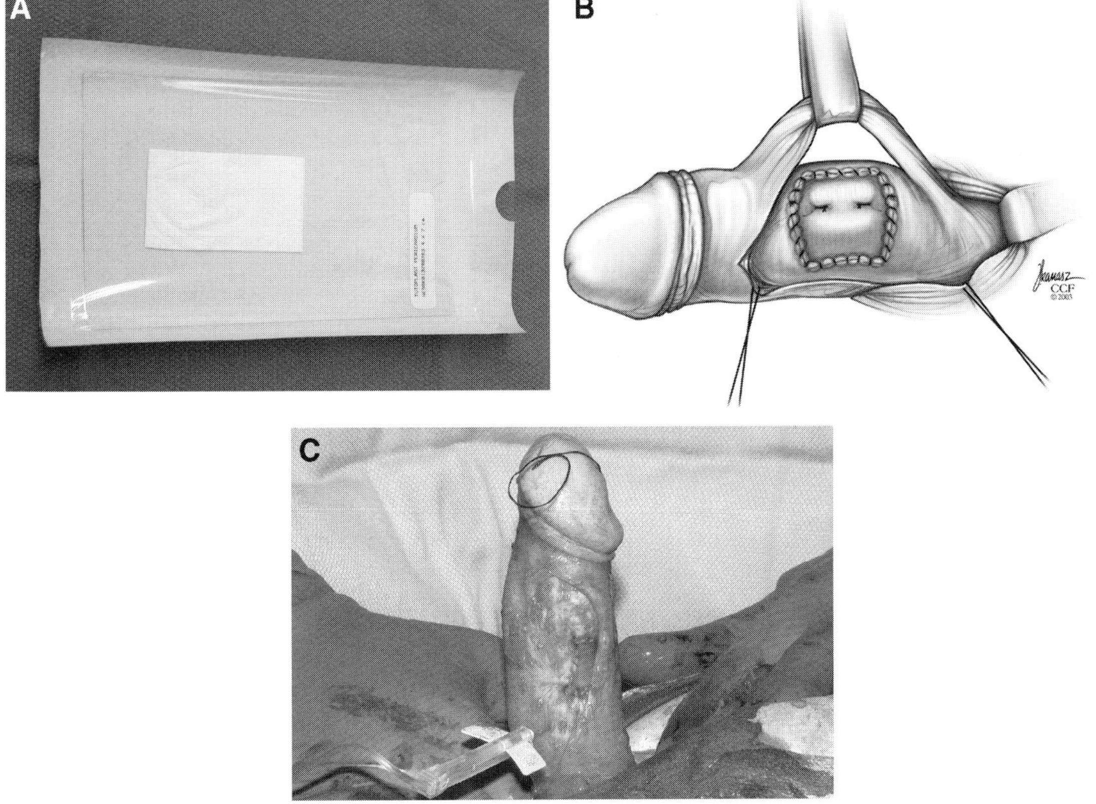


Fig. 48.11

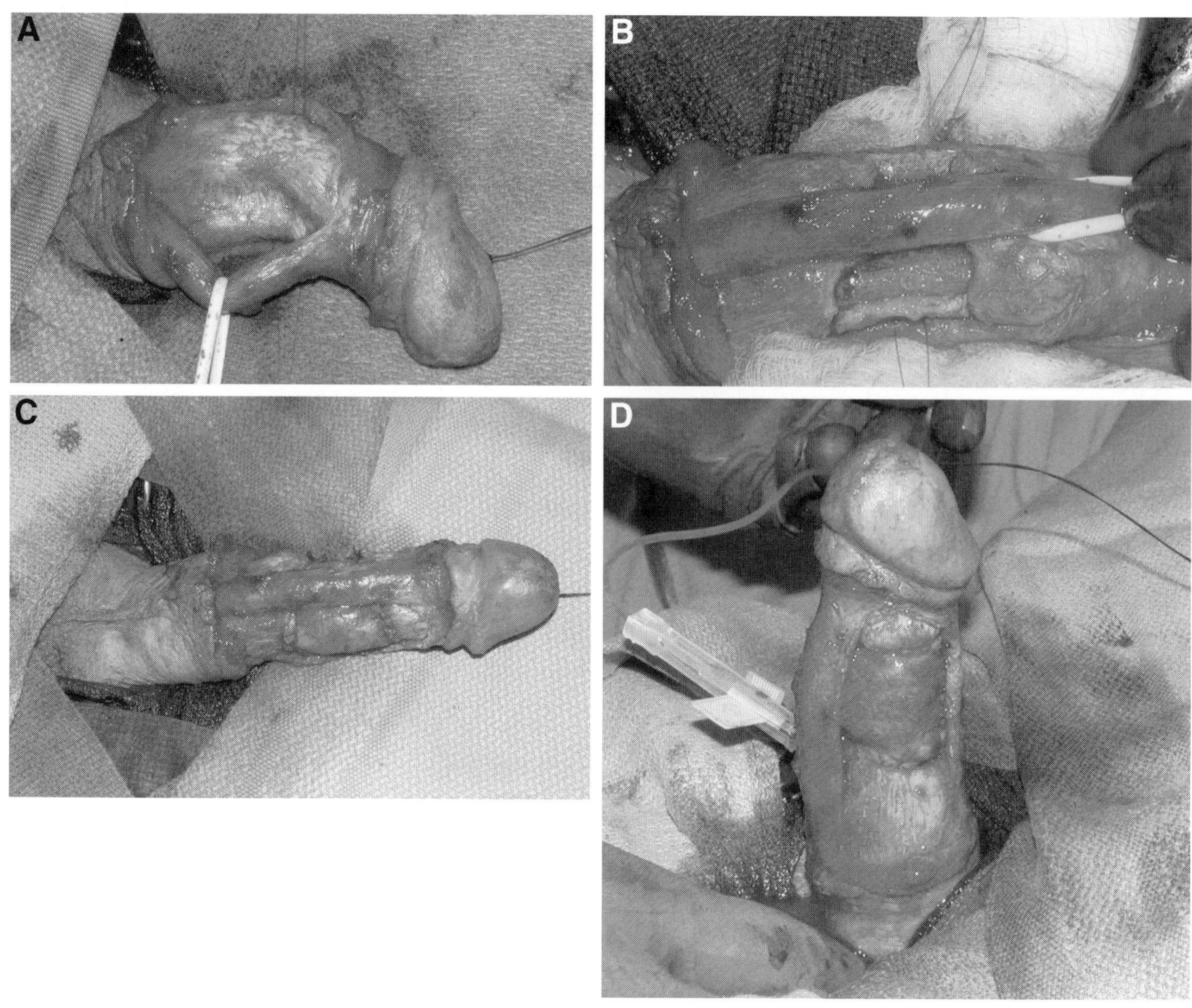


Fig. 48.12

(Fig. 48.12A). Incision or excision of the plaque and grafting proceed as described above (Fig. 48.12B–D). During closure, dartos flaps may be dissected from the overlying skin and passed between the graft and the corpus spongiosum. The flaps are sutured together to maintain their position. The skin is closed in standard fashion.

After closure, a 16 French Foley catheter is inserted, and a clear adhesive dressing is placed on the penis.

## POSTOPERATIVE CARE

Postoperative care following the above procedures varies slightly. All are done on an outpatient basis, although patients undergoing a graft procedure are kept overnight for 23-h observation. In these patients the urethral catheter and the drain are removed the next morning prior to discharge. All patients are instructed to remove the dressing in the shower 4–5 d following surgery. Painful erections can be minimized with the use of diazepam at bedtime and amyl nitrite capsules as needed for the first 7–10 d. Approximately 2 wk after surgery, patients undergoing a graft procedure are encouraged to promote erections with gentle noncoital stimulation to aid the graft-healing process. In all patients, sexual intercourse is allowed at approx 6 wk postoperatively, as this is when sufficient healing has generally occurred with resolution of pain and edema.

## SUGGESTED READINGS

1. Akkus E, Carrier S, Baba K, Hsu GL, Padma-Nathan H, Nunes L, Lue TF. Structural alterations in the tunica

albuginea of the penis: impact of Peyronie's disease, ageing and impotence. Brit J Urol 79:47–53, 1997.
2. Chun JL, McGregor A, Krishnan R, Carson CC. A comparison of dermal and cadaveric pericardial grafts in the modified Horton-Devine procedure for Peyronie's disease. J Urol 166:185–188, 2001.
3. Daitch JA, Angermeier KW, Montague DK. Modified corporoplasty for penile curvature: long-term results and patient satisfaction. J Urol 162:2006–2009, 1999.
4. Devine CJ, Jr., Blackley SK, Horton CE, Gilbert DA. The surgical treatment of chordee without hypospadias in men. J Urol 146:325–329, 1991.
5. Devine CJ, Jr., Somers KD, Jordan GH, Schlossberg SM. Proposal: trauma as the cause of the Peyronie's lesion. J Urol 157:285–290, 1997.
6. Donatucci CF, Lue TF. Correction of penile deformity assisted by intracavernous injection of papaverine. J Urol 147:1108–1110, 1992.
7. Essed E, Schroeder FH. New surgical treatment for Peyronie disease. Urology 25:582–587, 1985.
8. Gelbard MK, James K, Dorey, F. The natural history of Peyronie's disease. J Urol 144:1376–1379, 1990.
9. Hellstrom WJ, Reddy S. Application of pericardial graft in the surgical management of Peyronie's disease. J Urol 163:1445–1447, 2000.
10. Jordan GH. Peyronie's disease and its management. In: Krane RJ, Siroky MB, Fitzpatrick JM, eds. Clinical Urology. Philadelphia: JB Lippincott Co., 1994: 1282–1297.
11. Jordan GH, Angermeier KW. Preoperative evaluation of erectile function with dynamic infusion cavernosometry/cavernosography in patients undergoing surgery for Peyronie's disease: correlation with postoperative results. J Urol 150:1138–1142, 1993.
12. Jordan GH, Schlossberg SM. Surgery of the penis and urethra. In: Walsh PC, Vaughan ED, Retik AB, Wein AJ, eds. Campbell's Urology, 8th ed. Philadelphia: WB Saunders, 2002:3886–3954.
13. Kelami A. Congenital penile deviation and its treatment with the Nesbit-Kelami technique. Br J Urol 60:261–263, 1987.
14. Knispel HH, Gonnermann D, Huland H. Modified surgical technique to correct congenital and acquired penile curvature. Eur Urol 20:107–112, 1991.
15. Levine LA, Lenting EL. A surgical algorithm for the treatment of Peyronie's disease. J Urol 158:2149–2152, 1997.
16. Licht MR, Lewis RW. Modified Nesbit procedure for the treatment of Peyronie's disease: a comparative outcome analysis. J Urol 158:460–463, 1997.
17. Nesbit RM. Congenital curvature of the phallus: report of three cases with description of corrective operation. J Urol 93:230–232, 1965.
18. Pryor JP, Fitzpatrick JM. A new approach to the correction of the penile deformity in Peyronie's disease. J Urol 122:622, 623, 1979.
19. Yachia D. Modified corporoplasty for the treatment of penile curvature. J Urol 143:80–82, 1990.

# 49 Inguinal Surgery in Children

*Jonathan Ross and Inderbir Gill*

## INTRODUCTION

The inguinal incision is employed for common pediatric problems such as undescended testicle, hydrocele, and hernia. It is also used for less common problems such as testicular tumor. An understanding of inguinal anatomy in the normal and abnormal setting is crucial for treating these disorders with a minimum of complications.

## INGUINAL INCISION

An incision is made along Langer's lines extending from just above the pubic tubercle laterally for approx 2 cm (Fig. 49.1).

Scarpa's fascia is exposed and incised with a scissors down to the external oblique aponeurosis (Fig. 49.2). Scarpa's is then opened parallel to the incision sharply or with cautery. The superficial epigastric vein may be encountered in the lateral corner of the incision and should be controlled with cautery before dividing. By a combination of sharp and blunt dissection, the fine attachments to the surface of the external oblique aponeurosis are divided until the inguinal ligament is identified. Dissection is then carried in a scrotal direction along the inguinal ligament until the external ring is identified.

An incision is made in the external oblique aponeurosis in the lateral portion of the incision (Fig. 49.3A). The external oblique aponeurosis is then opened along the length of its fibers, exposing the inguinal canal (Fig. 49.3B,C). Care must be taken to avoid injuring the ilioinguinal nerve running just below the aponeurosis.

After completing the inguinal operation, the incision is closed in layers. The external oblique aponeurosis is closed with a running 3-0 polidioxanone suture starting laterally. The closure should be stopped before the neo-external ring is too tight. Scarpa's fascia is reapproximated with fine chromic suture, and the skin is closed with a running subcuticular suture such as 5-0 plain gut.

## UNDESCENDED TESTICLE

Undescended testis is one of the most common congenital genitourinary anomalies. The incidence of undescended testis is 3% in term infants and 30% in premature infants. Many undescended testes will descend spontaneously in the first months of life, and the incidence at 1 yr of age is 0.8%.

Men with a history of an undescended testis are at risk for infertility and testicular tumors. The incidence of infertility is only slightly increased in cases of unilateral cryptorchidism, but is 40–70% in men with a history of bilateral undescended testis. There is circumstantial evidence to suggest that early orchidopexy (at 6–12 mo of age) may improve ultimate fertility.

The risk of testicular cancer in men with a history of cryptorchidism is 5–10 times that in the general population. This increased risk is greater for intraabdominal than for inguinal testes. Carcinoma *in situ* occurs in 2–3% of men with a history of cryptorchidism, and 20% of testis tumors in these men occur in the normally descended contralateral testis. There is no direct evidence that orchidopexy reduces the tumor risk, but it puts the testicle in a location where tumors are more easily palpated and therefore detected earlier. All men with a history of an undescended testis should perform routine testicular self-exam after puberty.

An undescended testis is defined as a testis that has become arrested in its descent through the normal pathway. This is distinguished from the rarer ectopic testis, which is a testis that has deviated from the normal pathway of descent. The most common location for undescended testes is the inguinal canal. Other sites include the high scrotum, pubic tubercle, superficial inguinal pouch, and the abdomen. Ectopic testicles may be found in the femoral canal, perineum, prepubic space, or the contralateral scrotum.

Because most undescended testes are located in the inguinal canal, they can be evaluated on clinical exam.

From: *Operative Urology at the Cleveland Clinic*
Edited by: A. Novick et al. © Humana Press Inc., Totowa, NJ

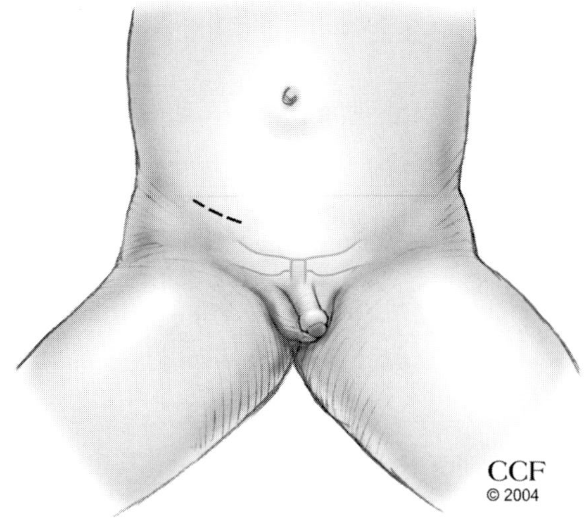


Fig. 49.1

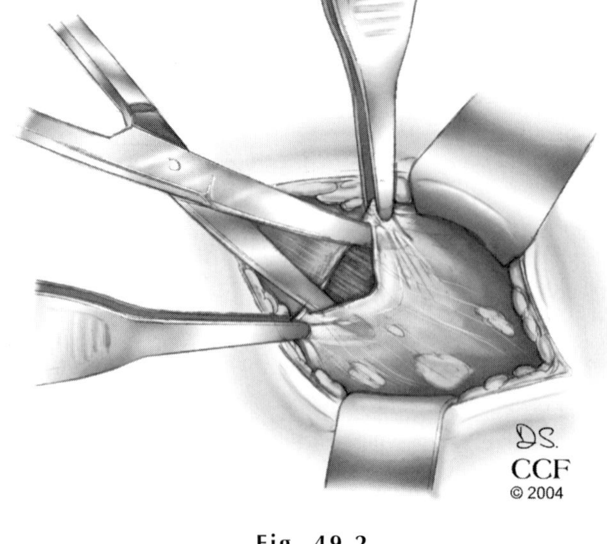


Fig. 49.2

Impalpable testes present a more challenging problem and require a more extensive evaluation. In a boy with bilateral impalpable testes, the question arises whether the testes are intraabdominal or are absent. Bilateral anorchia can be diagnosed biochemically with a human chorionic gonadotropin (HCG) stimulation test. This is accomplished by administering three doses of 1500 units of HCG on alternate days. If there is no rise in serum testosterone and baseline gonadotropin levels are elevated, then the child has anorchia and no further evaluation is necessary. If there is a rise in testosterone after the administration of HCG, then the child has at least one functioning testis—presumably intraabdominal. Occasional boys with low testosterone levels but normal gonadotropin levels will have testicles present—hence the dual requirement of a negative HCG stimulation test and elevated baseline gonadotropins.

In the boy with a unilateral impalpable testis, an HCG stimulation test is obviously of no value. In these boys, and in boys with bilateral impalpable testes and a positive HCG stimulation test, further evaluation is indicated. Several radiological tests are available to identify an intraabdominal testis. Ultrasound, computerized tomography, and magnetic resonance imaging have all been used. The overall accuracy of these tests in localizing an undescended testis is 80–90%. However, the majority of testes in reported series are inguinal. The accuracy of these imaging studies for localizing an intraabdominal testis is less than 25%. Gonadal venography is more accurate and able to locate or confirm the absence of an intraabdominal testis in 75% of cases. However, this modality requires heavy sedation or anesthesia in children, is invasive, and is technically difficult in patients younger than 6 yr.

Because the readily available tests are insensitive for detecting an intraabdominal testis, they are of little benefit. In the minority of cases when a radiological study identifies an intraabdominal testis, then an operation to bring the testicle down will be required. However, the failure of any of these tests to identify a testis does not mean the testis is absent—each test has a significant false-negative rate. Therefore, a negative study also mandates an operation to locate an intraabdominal testis or prove definitively that it is absent. Because the results of radiological tests will not alter the management, there is little value in performing them. A possible exception is the child whose body habitus makes physical examination of the inguinal region difficult. If ultrasound can identify an inguinal testis in such a child, then the child will be spared laparoscopy.

Approximately 50% of boys with a unilateral impalpable testis will in fact have an absent testis on that side. Because of the inability of radiological studies to reliably identify an intraabdominal testis, an operation is required to determine the presence or absence of an impalpable testis. Historically, this has been approached through an inguinal incision, which could be extended into the abdomen if necessary. While open exploration is still an accepted approach, the addition of laparoscopy to the operative armamentarium has reduced the morbidity of these explorations. Prior to a formal operative incision, laparoscopy is performed through a supra- or infraumbilical incision. If an intraabdominal testis is identified, then an orchidopexy is performed. This can usually be accomplished laparoscopically with the addition of two working ports. For high intraabdominal testes, a first-stage Fowler-Stephens may be performed laparoscopically.

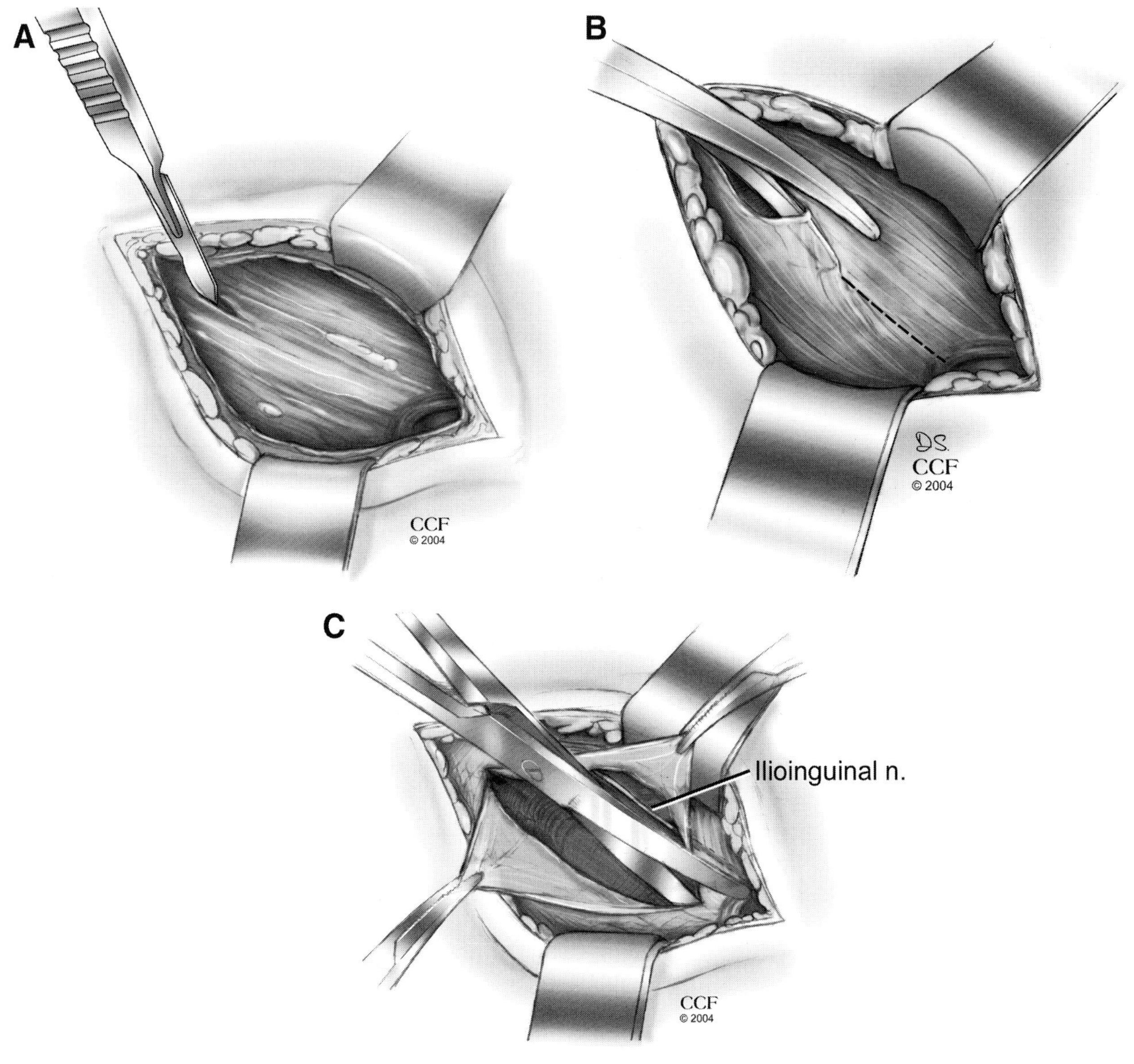


Fig. 49.3

If blind-ending vessels are identified in the abdomen, the procedure is terminated. If vessels are seen entering the inguinal canal through a closed ring, a scrotal exploration is undertaken. A hemosiderin-laden nubbin is usually identified and excised. If vessels are seen entering the canal through an open ring, an inguinal exploration is undertaken. This allows repair of the hernia and excision of a nubbin, if present. In some cases the inguinal exploration will reveal a viable testis that was missed on physical exam.

## ORCHIDOPEXY

In most cases, once an inguinal incision is made, the hernia sac is immediately apparent in the inguinal canal. The testis and cord structures are so intimately attached to the hernia that dissection outside the hernia sac will prevent injury to the vas or vessels. The hernia sac (with the testis inside) is completely mobilized within the inguinal canal up to the internal ring. Many attachments can be taken down bluntly, although cremasteric fibers should be cauterized to minimize staining of the operative field with blood. The distal gubernacular attachments usually need to be divided sharply or with cautery. Even distal to the testis, care must be used to remain outside the hernia sac because the vas may loop distal to the testis within the sac.

The hernia sac is opened over the testis and the opening extended just distal to the internal ring (Fig. 49.4).

The back wall of the hernia sac is directly on top of the vessels and vas, which are actually retroperitoneal structures. This back wall of the hernia is dissected bluntly

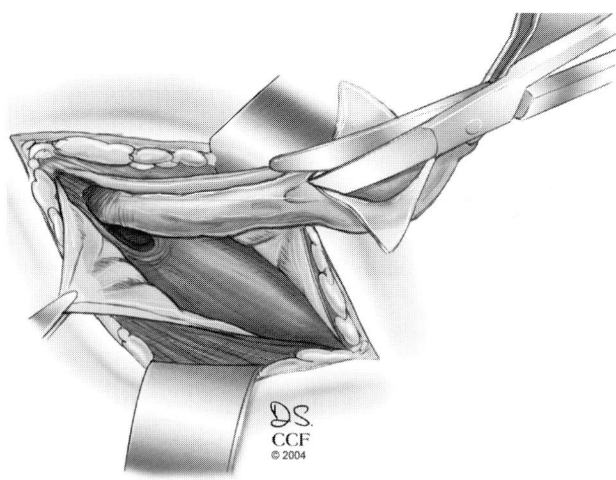


Fig. 49.4

with a blunt-tipped scissors (Fig. 49.5). The scissors is introduced into the plane from one edge with the blades parallel to the floor. It is then turned 90º and gently spread, separating the back wall from the cord. The back wall is then divided with a scissors just above the internal ring.

Once divided, the back wall is mobilized off the cord toward the internal ring with blunt dissection (Fig. 49.6). Occasional tight bands may need to be divided sharply. The hernia sac is closed with a fine running absorbable suture.

Using blunt and sharp dissection, the attachments between the cord and the peritoneum are separated, as are lateral attachments to the cord in the retroperitoneum (Fig. 49.7). A retractor may be placed between the sac (peritoneum) and the cord elevating the hernia off the cord above the internal ring to facilitate this dissection. If necessary, the internal oblique may be opened from the internal ring cranially to provide higher exposure for this dissection. If inadequate length is obtained, the cord may be moved medial to the inferior epigastric vessels giving a straighter course to the scrotum. This can be accomplished by dividing the inferior epigastric vessels or by bluntly dissecting medial to them through the floor of the canal. Care must be taken to avoid entering the peritoneum. The cord is then passed medial to the vessels.

A tract is developed bluntly over the pubic tubercle into the hemiscrotum, and an incision through the skin is made over a finger in the scrotum (Fig. 49.8). A scissors is used to bluntly develop a dartos pouch deep to the scrotal skin. A tonsil clamp is passed through the scrotal incision up into the inguinal incision and the peritesticular tissue is

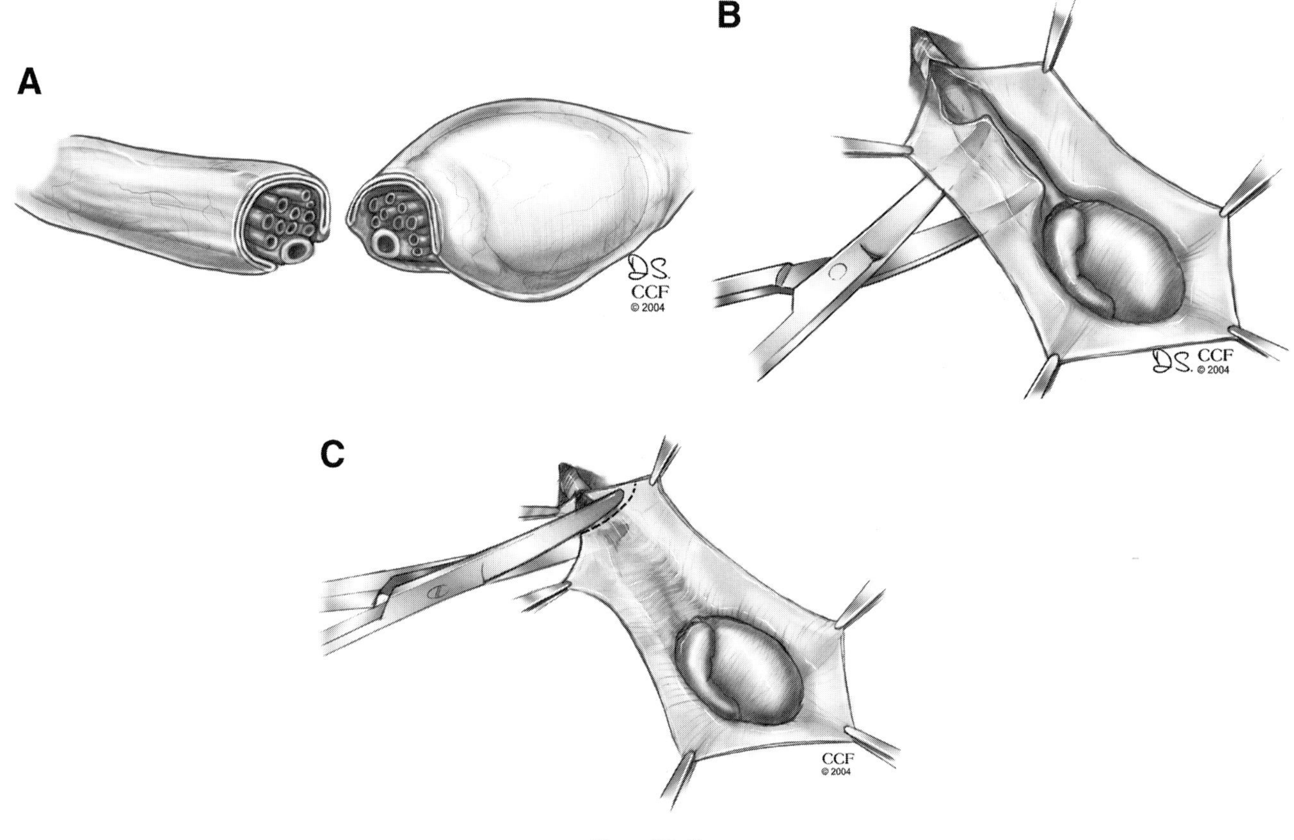


Fig. 49.5

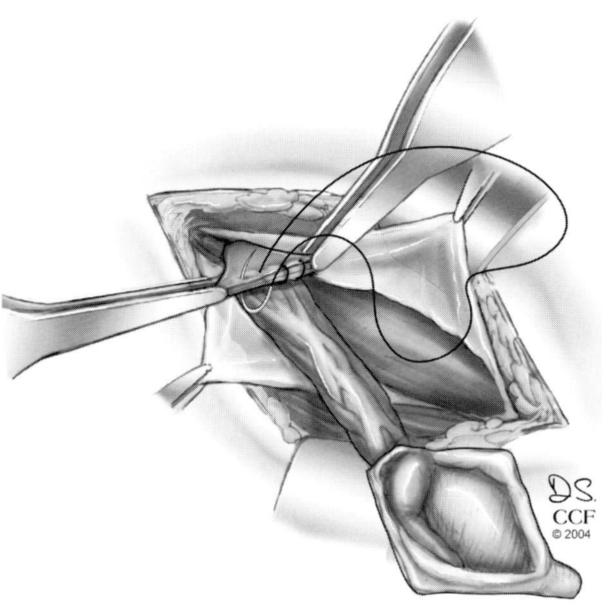


Fig. 49.6

grasped and drawn down, bringing the testis through the scrotal incision.

A 4-0 chromic suture is placed on either side of the scrotal incision through the dartos and the tunix of the testis, securing the testis in place (Fig. 49.9). The testis is then put in the dartos pouch, and the scrotal incision is closed with interrupted 4-0 chromic suture.

## LAPAROSCOPIC ORCHIDOPEXY

Laparoscopy has become a standard technique in the approach to an impalpable testis. If blind-ending vessels are identified, anorchia is confirmed. If vas and vessels are seen entering the internal ring, an inguinal or scrotal exploration is undertaken to rule out an inguinal testis or remove a remnant. If an intraabdominal testicle is identified, then it may be managed with a laparoscopic orchidopexy.

After draping the operative field, the bladder is drained with a urethral catheter, and a 3-mm stab incision is made in the superior umbilical crease (Fig. 49.10). A 2-mm needlescopic port is then introduced using a closed technique. Two pops can be felt as the instrument passes through the fascia and peritoneum. Needloscopy is performed in the Trendelenburg position. This allows the intestines to fall out of the pelvis. The vas and vessels on the normal side will be seen entering a normal closed internal ring. If the intraabdominal testis is within 2 cm of the internal ring, it should be possible to bring it into the scrotum in one stage. Two additional 2-mm ports are placed on either side of the rectus muscles at the level of

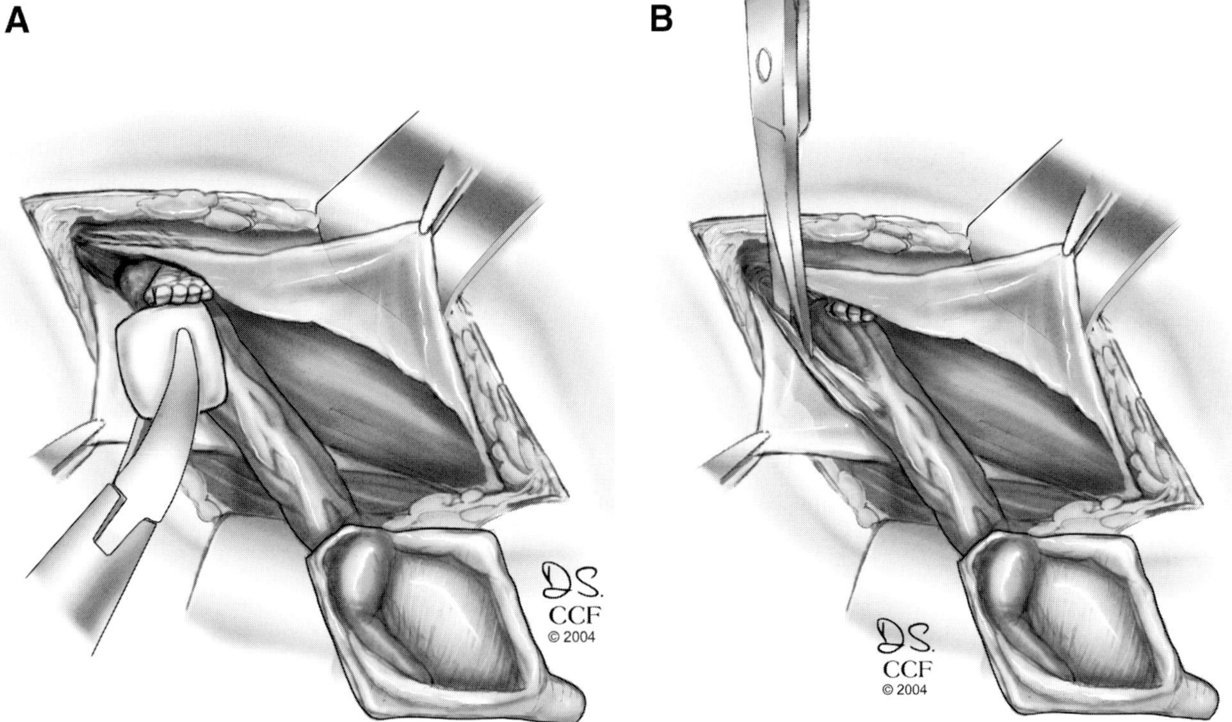


Fig. 49.7

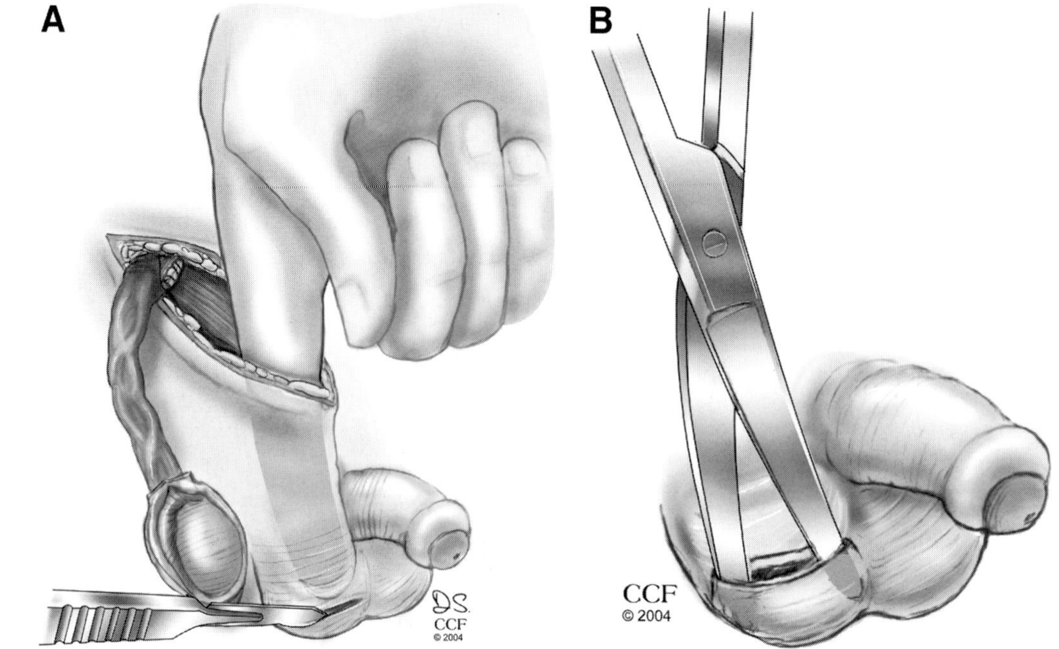

A
B
DS.
CCF
© 2004
CCF
© 2004

Fig. 49.8

A
B
C
DS.
CCF
© 2004
CCF
© 2004
CCF
© 2004
DS.

Fig. 49.9

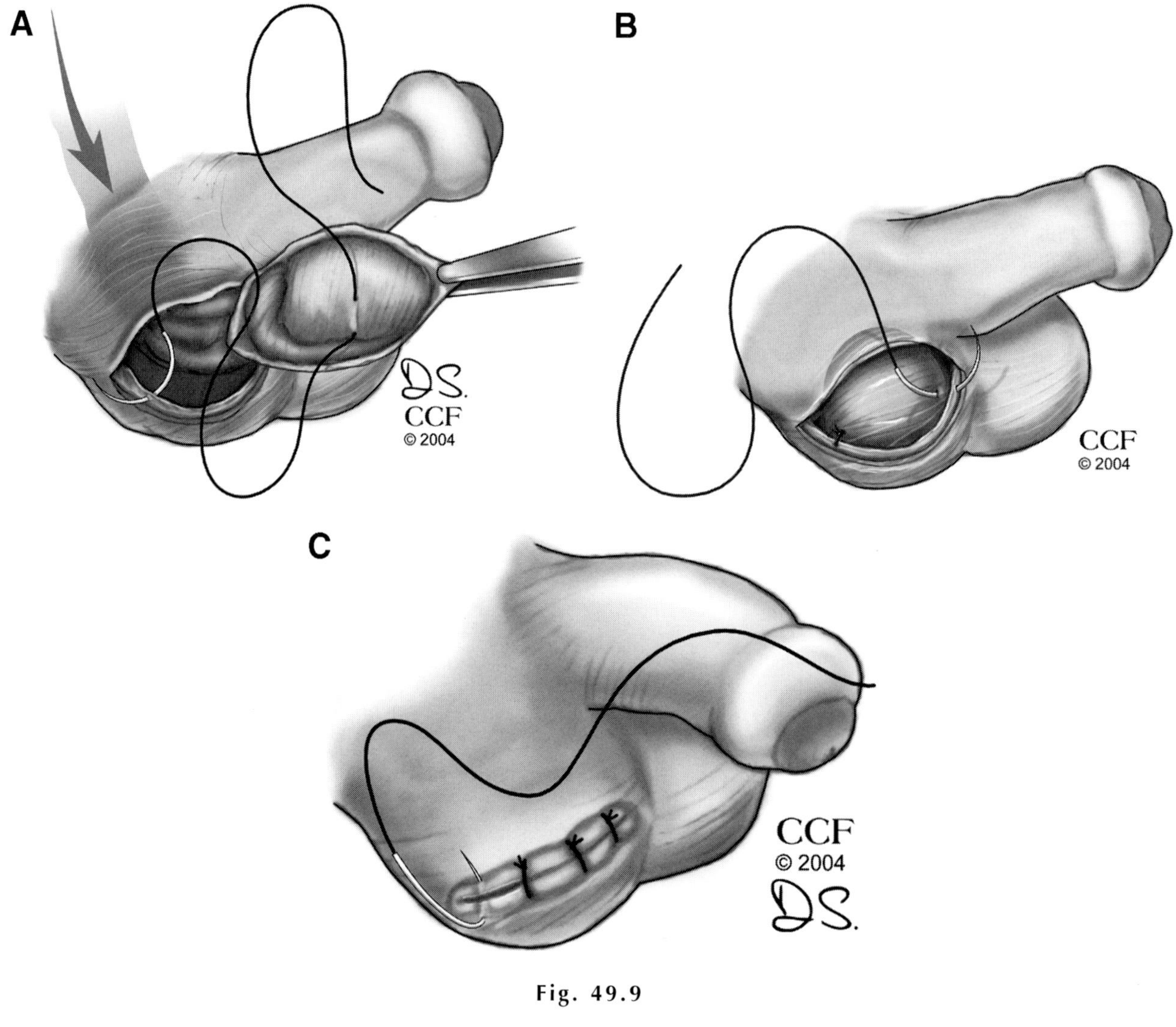

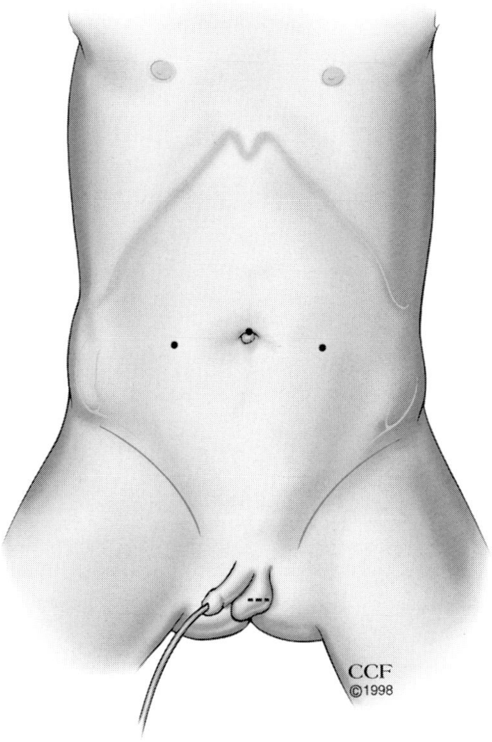


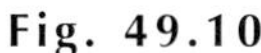
Fig. 49.10

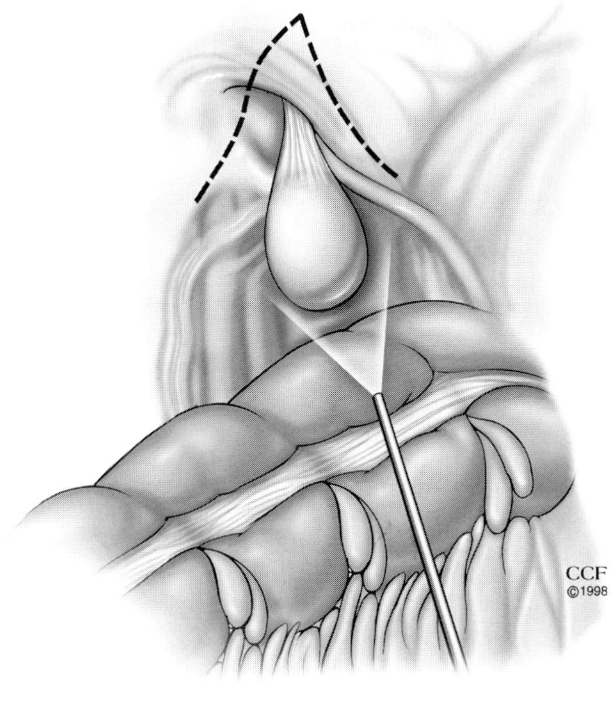


Fig. 49.11

the umbilicus. No incisions are needed. These ports are placed under direct vision with the needlescope. The 2-mm umbilical port may be replaced with a 5-mm trochar for better visualization.

The operation is performed with a needlescopic grasper and electrocautery scissors passed through the lateral ports (Fig. 49.11). The operating table is rotated 30º to elevate the ipsilateral side. This allows the intestines to drop out of the operative field. An inverted V peritoneotomy is made over the internal ring, encompassing the vas deferens and spermatic vessels and preserving the peritoneum between them.

The body of the testicle is then grasped near its upper pole (Fig. 49.12). The vas is easily identified, as are the testicular vessels. The testis is retracted into the abdominal cavity, placing its distal gubernacular attachments on stretch. The taut gubernaculum is meticulously divided with electrocautery. Extreme care is taken to preserve the vas, which may loop distal to the testicle.

The liberated testicle is retracted anteromedially, and the posterior and lateral attachments of the testicular vessels are divided (Fig. 49.13). Dissection is carried out along the pelvic sidewalls, preserving perivascular and perivasal tissue. With the needlescopic approach this can be accomplished beyond the iliac vessels with minimal traction on the cord.

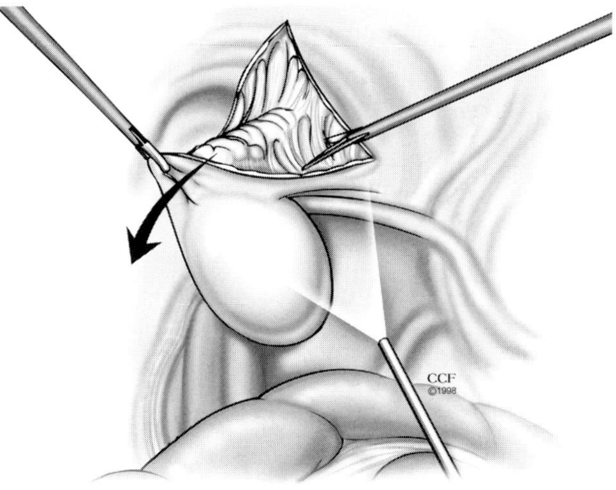


Fig. 49.12

Dissection is continued until the testicle is adequately mobilized (Fig. 49.14). This is usually the case if the testicle can be brought to the contralateral ring.

A scrotal incision is made, and a dartos pouch is created (Fig. 49.15). A tonsil or Kelly clamp is passed through this incision and over the pubic tubercle. Under needlescopic guidance the clamp is passed through an edge of the medial umbilical ligament. This can be done

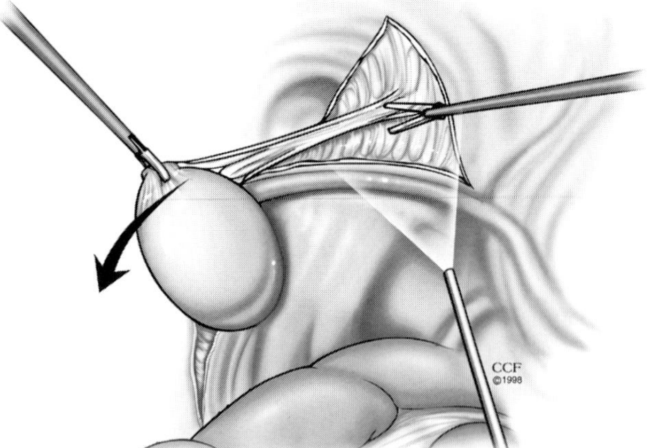


Fig. 49.13

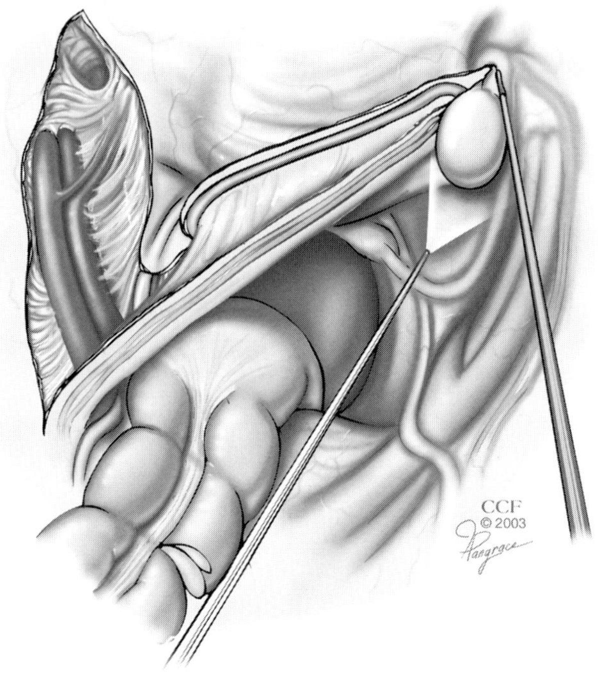


Fig. 49.14

just medial to the ligament, taking care to stay lateral to the bladder, or the clamp may be passed just lateral to the ligament. Gentle spreading creates an adequate tunnel. Some of the pneumoperitoneum is now lost, but it can be easily restored by placing a surgical sponge over the scrotal incision. The testis is passed to the clamp with the needlescopic forceps, and it is drawn down into the scrotum. If the testis is felt to be under tension, additional needlescopic dissection can be undertaken at this time. Gentle manual traction on the testis at the scrotal level helps to identify attachments that still need to be divided. If necessary, the parietal peritoneum may be dissected off

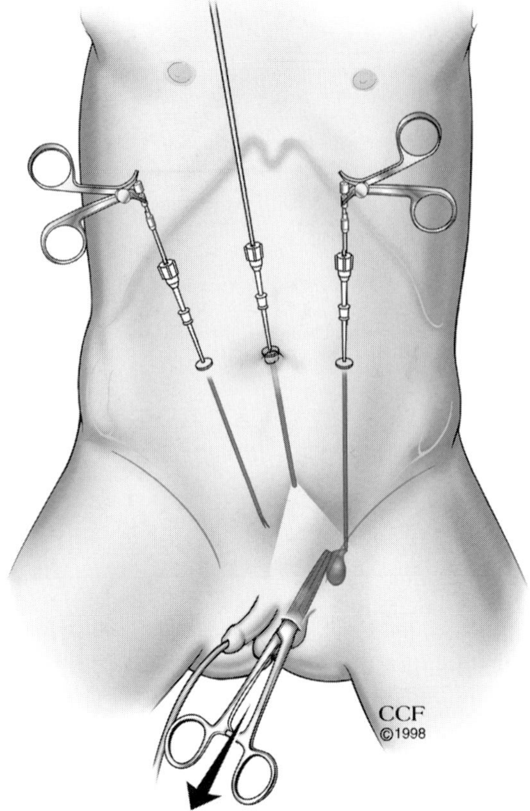


Fig. 49.15

the cord structures and divided to gain additional length. When the dissection is completed, the testis is secured in the scrotum in a standard fashion and the scrotum is closed with interrupted chromic suture. The needlescopic incisions do not require any formal closure. If a 5-mm port is employed, the fascia is approximated with 4-0 absorbable suture, and the skin closed with a subcuticular 5-0 plain gut suture.

## FOWLER-STEPHENS ORCHIDOPEXY

High intraabdominal testes offer a particular challenge. There is often inadequate vascular length to bring these testicles into the scrotum. To facilitate mobilization, the vessels may be divided high in the abdomen and the testis brought down on the pedicle of vasal vessels and collaterals in the peritoneum between the vas and distal spermatic vessels (Fig. 49.16). When performed in a single stage, the success rate is approx 67%. Alternatively, the vessels may be divided *in situ* without testicular mobilization. Collateral vessels are then allowed to develop in the peritoneum between the vessels and the vas. Six months later the testicle is mobilized on the vasal pedicle and brought to the scrotum. When performed in two stages, the

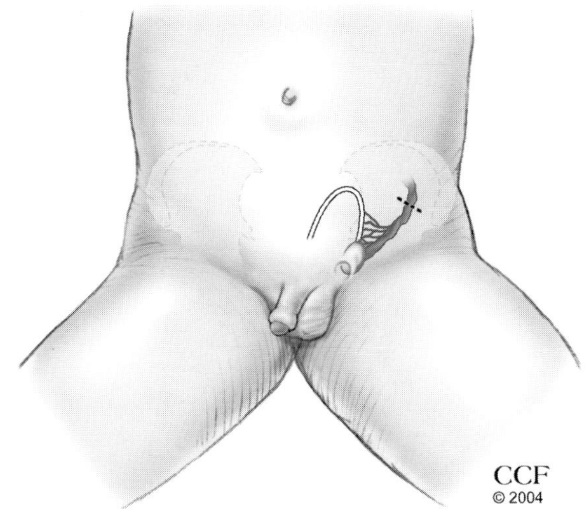


Fig. 49.16

success rate has been approx 77%. The collaterals between the vasal artery and the distal spermatic vessels are felt to facilitate survival of the mobilized testicle. This peritoneum should be left intact (as opposed to a one-stage orchidopexy, in which it would be dissected off of the cord). The first-stage ligation may be performed laparoscopically. The second stage is performed in the same way as a one-stage laparoscopic orchidopexy; except the vessels are divided at the previous ligature site and the peritoneum over the distal cord is preserved.

For high intraabdominal testicles, an autotransplantation may be considered as an adjunct to the Fowler-Stephens orchidopexy. Following division of the vessels and mobilization of the testicle, a microvascular anastomosis is performed between the testicular vessels and the inferior epigastric vessels (Fig. 49.17). Whether this time-consuming maneuver adds significantly to testicular survival is controversial.

## HYDROCELE/HERNIA

Hydroceles and hernias present as inguino-scrotal swellings. Hydroceles are nontender and transilluminate. A normal testis should be palpable. In equivocal cases an ultrasound is diagnostic. Most infant hydroceles resolve by 1 yr of age. Persistent hydroceles should be repaired to prevent the development of a hernia. Hernias do not transilluminate and can usually be palpated up to the inguinal ring. Bowel sounds may be auscultated. Again, ultrasound is helpful in equivocal cases. Hernias should be corrected when diagnosed.

Pediatric hernias and hydroceles differ from their adult counterparts. In children, these entities are due to persistence of the tongue of peritoneum that descends with the testis—the patent processus vaginalis. This allows fluid (hydrocele) and/or intraabdominal contents (hernia) to move back and forth into the scrotum. Repair of both focuses on high ligation of this patent processus (Fig. 49.18). A muscular repair of the anatomical hernia is rarely required except in older children.

A standard inguinal incision is made (Fig. 49.19). The cremasteric fibers are opened along the length of the

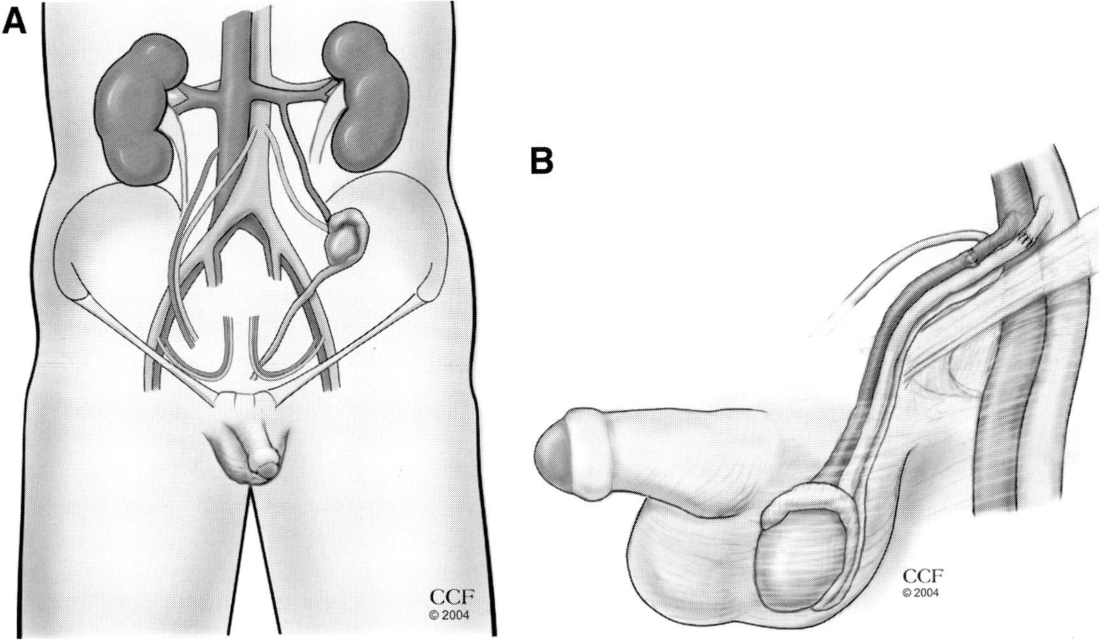


Fig. 49.17

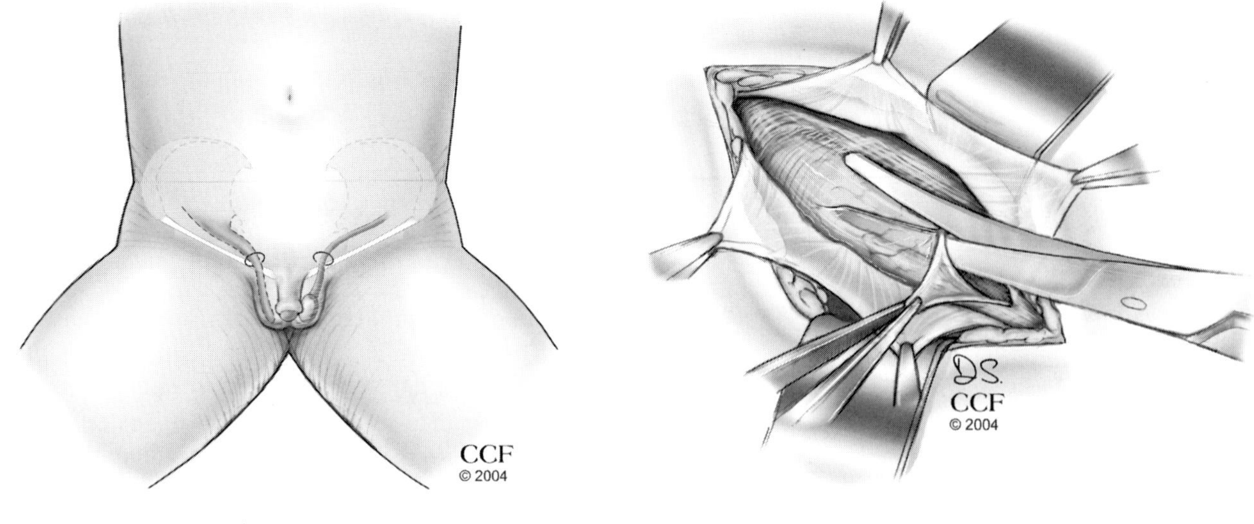


Fig. 49.18

Fig. 49.19

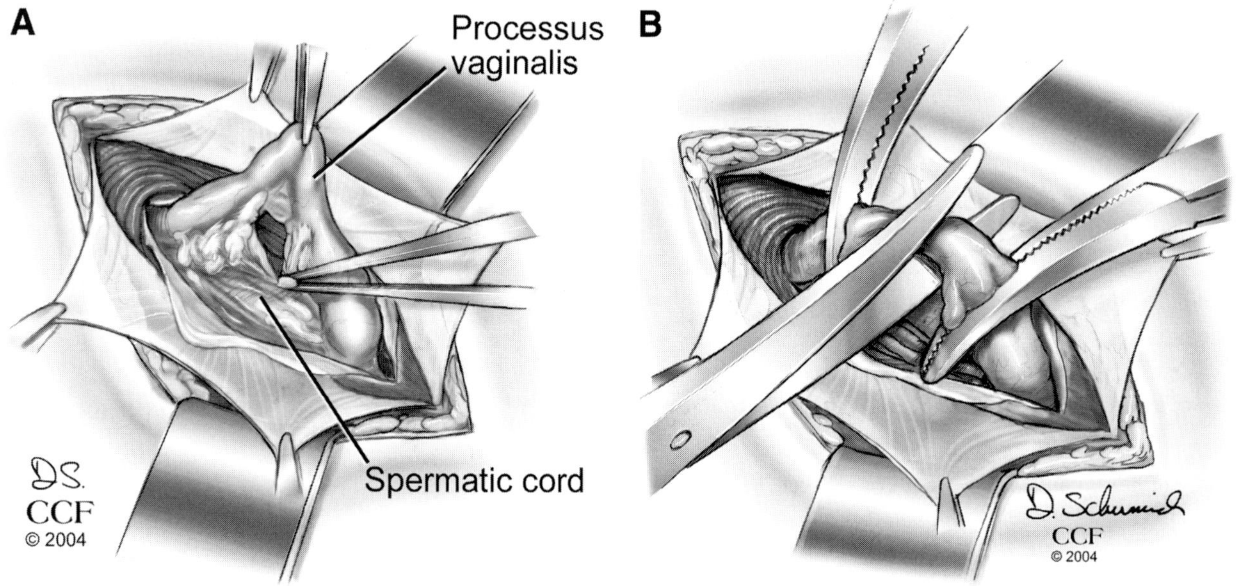


Fig. 49.20

inguinal canal. This exposes the hernia/patent processus vaginalis on the anteromedial aspect of the cord.

If the patent processus is relatively small, it may be grasped with forceps and dissected off of the cord structures by bluntly pushing the cord structures down off of the processus (Fig. 49.20). Once a window is created, the processus is doubly clamped and divided.

The processus is mobilized by blunt dissection to the internal ring, where it is suture-ligated with a 4-0 polydioxanone suture and divided (Fig. 49.21). If the hernia is large, it may be opened so that bowel or omentum in the hernia can be reduced before closing the hernia at the internal ring. Closure may be accomplished with a running suture, if necessary. If the hernia is large, it may be opened down to just distal to the internal ring and the back wall dissected off the cord structures just as described for an orchidopexy. It should then be closed just above the internal ring. Usually no muscular closure is necessary in children as the hernia is a result of the patent processus and not an intrinsic weakness at the internal ring. However, a large hernia may dilate the internal ring, and in that instance the internal ring should be reinforced. This is accomplished by sewing the superior edge of the internal oblique just distal to the internal ring to the

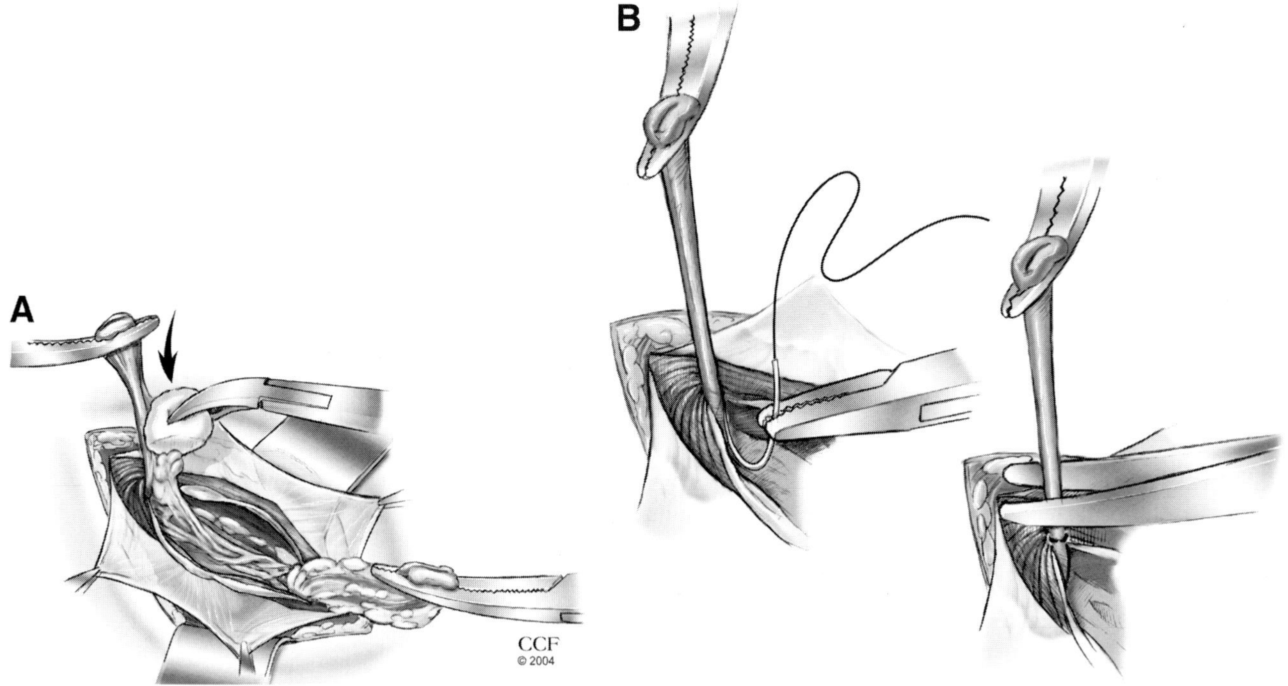


Fig. 49.21

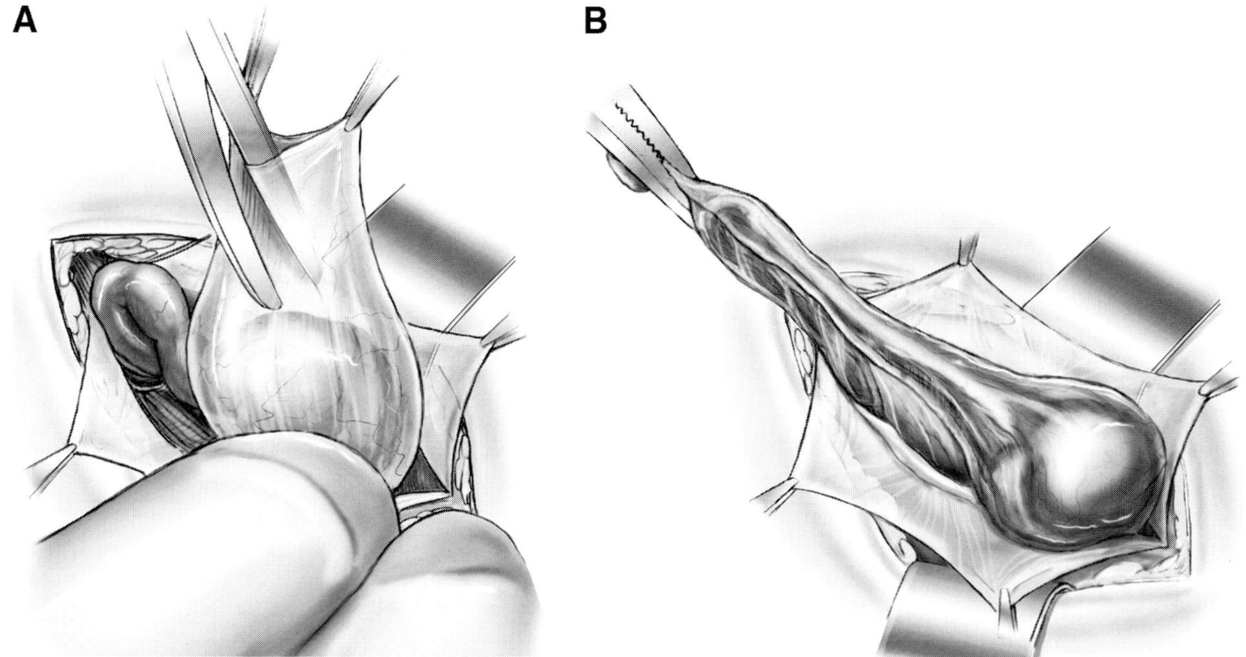


Fig. 49.22

underside of the inguinal ligament. Usually one or two interrupted sutures are sufficient.

Following high ligation of the processus, the distal end of the patent processus is opened widely on the anterior surface, taking care to avoid injuring the vas or testicular vessels (Fig. 49.22). If the processus is large, the testis is eventually delivered into the inguinal surgical field. The appendix testis is removed, and redundant processus may be excised. No attempt is made to remove the back wall of the processus that is adherent to the cord structures.

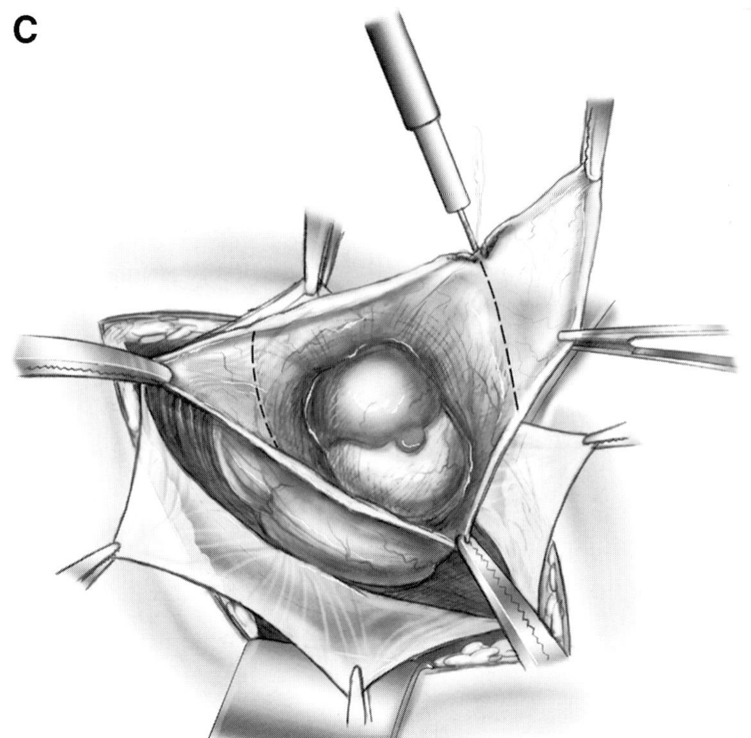


Fig. 49.22 (*Continued*)

## PREPUBERTAL TESTIS TUMORS

A large proportion of prepubertal testis tumors is benign, including teratoma, epidermoid cyst, and most stromal tumors. The primary malignant tumor—yolk sac— is associated with an elevated α–fetoprotein (AFP) level in more than 90% of cases. It is important to keep in mind that AFP levels are quite high in normal infants and cannot be interpreted in patients younger than 8 mo. Unless there is great suspicion that a tumor is malignant, the operation starts with an excisional biopsy, as described below. Benign tumors can safely be treated with enucleation. Yolk sac tumors should be treated with inguinal orchiectomy. Retroperitoneal lymph node dissection plays no role in the routine management of prepubertal testis tumors. If a yolk sac tumor is present, it is treated with observation or platinum-based multiagent chemotherapy. Even in the presence of metastatic disease, the cure rate is very high.

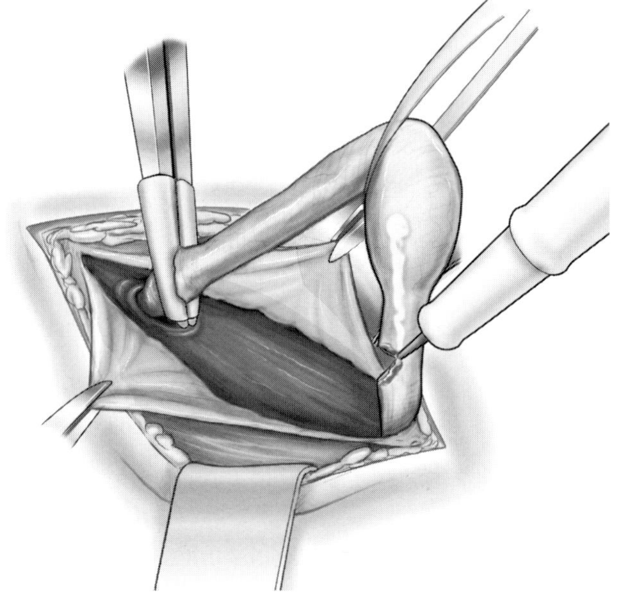

Fig. 49.23

## INGUINAL EXPLORATION FOR TESTICULAR TUMORS

An inguinal incision is performed, and the testis is completely mobilized into the inguinal incision within the tunica vaginalis (Fig. 49.23). If the tumor is likely malignant (i.e., elevated AFP in a child older than 1 yr of age) or completely replaces the testis on ultrasound, then the spermatic cord is ligated and divided at the internal ring with a silk suture.

If a benign tumor might be present, the cord is clamped with a rubber-shod clamp and the operative field draped off (Fig. 49.24). The tunica vaginalis is opened, and the tumor is enucleated or excised with a margin of normal testicular tissue. Frozen section is obtained, and if a benign tumor is

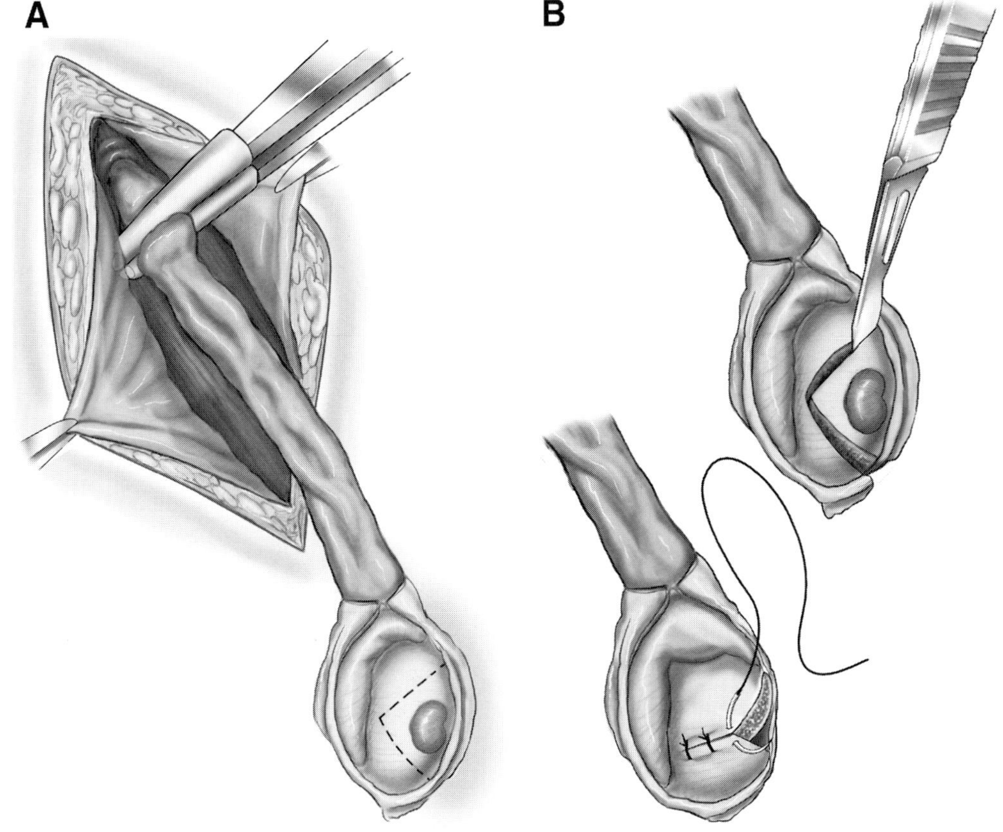


Fig. 49.24

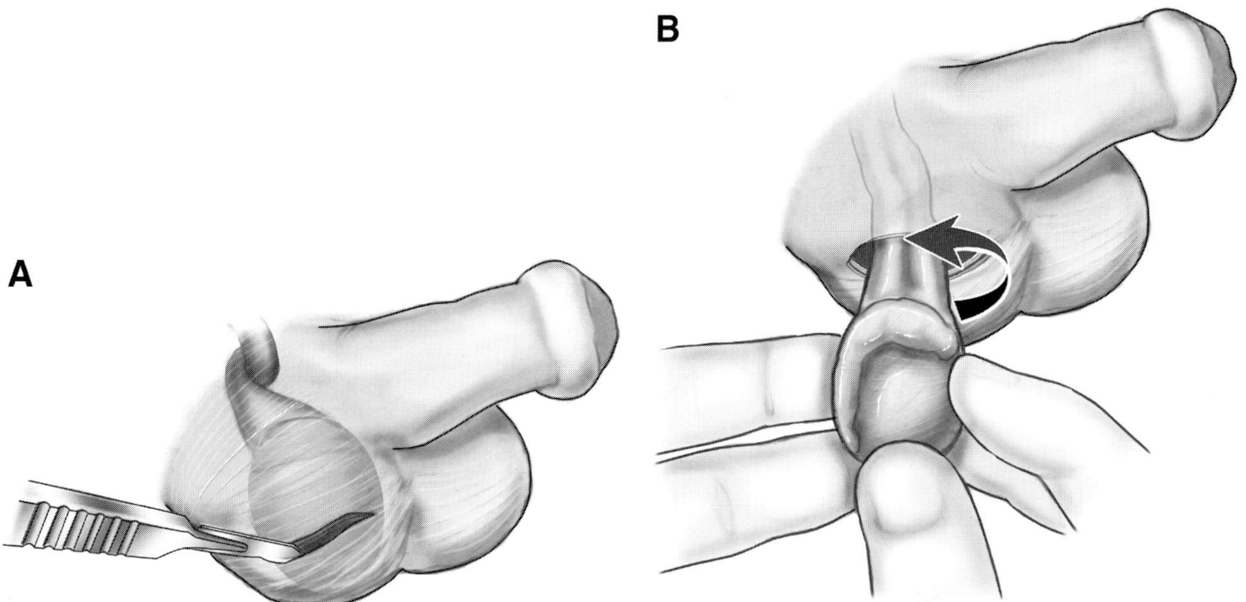


Fig. 49.25

confirmed, the testis is closed with a running 5-0 chromic suture. The testis is returned to the scrotum, and the inguinal incision is closed. If the frozen section is positive for malignancy or equivocal, the testis is removed as described.

## TESTICULAR TORSION

The most common entities presenting as an acute scrotum are testicular torsion, torsion of the appendix

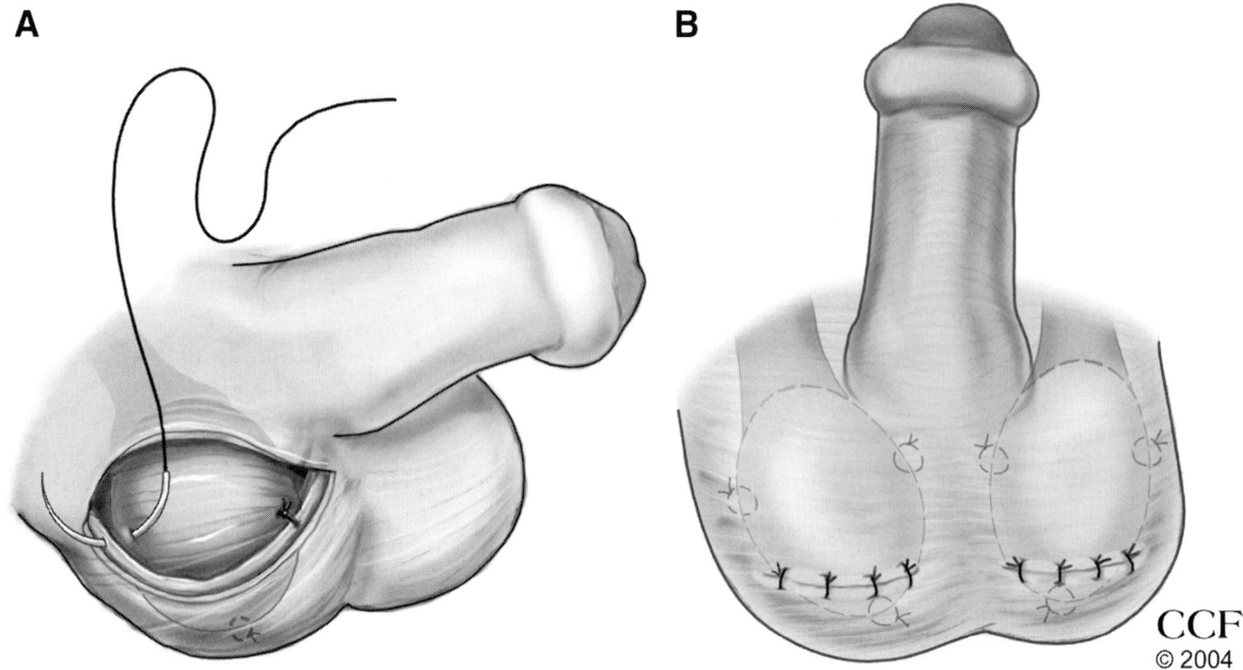


Fig. 49.26

testis, and epididymitis. Testicular torsion typically presents with severe sudden pain and swelling. Children with torsion of the appendix testis usually have milder pain of longer duration at presentation. Often the torsed appendix can be felt as a tender hard nodule at the upper pole of the testis. The urinalysis is typically positive in children with epididymitis. In equivocal cases a Doppler ultrasound can be obtained. However, if a testicular torsion is likely, immediate surgical exploration should not be delayed.

The testis is delivered through a transverse scrotal incision (Fig. 49.25). It is detorsed and observed.

If the testis is clearly necrotic, it is excised. If viable, it is fixed to the deep scrotal tissues at three points with permanent suture (Fig. 49.26). Whether the involved testis is removed or preserved, a contralateral orchidopexy is performed.

## SUGGESTED READINGS

1. Cendron M, Huff D, Keating MA, et al. Anatomical, morphological and volumetric analysis: a review of 759 cases of testicular maldescent. J Urol 149: 570–573, 1993.
2. Cisek LJ, Peters CA, Atala A, et al. Current findings in diagnostic laparoscopic evaluation of the nonpalpable testis. J Urol 160:1145–1149, 1998.
3. Hrebinko RL, Bellinger MF. The Limited Role of Imaging Techniques in managing children with undescended testes. J Urol 150:458–460, 1993.
4. Kass EJ, Stone KT, Cacciarelli AA, Mitchell B. Do All Children With an Acute Scrotum Require Exploration? J Urol 150:667–669, 1993.
5. Ross JH, Gill IS, Kay R. Needlescopic approach to the nonpalpable testis. Pediatr Endosurgery and Innovative Tech, 4:195–200, 2000.
6. Ross JH, Rybicki L, Kay R. Clinical behavior and contemporary management algorithm for prepubertal testis tumors: Summary of the Prepubertal Testis Tumor Registry. J Urol 168:1675–1679, 2002.
7. Rushton HG, Belman AB, Sesterhenn I, et al. Testicular sparing surgery for prepubertal teratoma of the testis: a clinical and pathological study. J Urol 144:726, 1990.

# 50 Adult Scrotal Surgery

*Gerard A. Deoreo and J. Stephen Jones*

## INTRODUCTION

Scrotal operations are among the most common operations performed by urologists. Postoperative scrotal complications may have significant morbidity for the patient, with time to full resolution often measured in weeks to months. Therefore, it is important to adhere to surgical principles that minimize potential morbidity. These surgical principles include excellent hemostasis, sufficient debridement of inflammatory lesions, and drainage where indicated.

## HYDROCELECTOMY

Perhaps the most common scrotal lesion presenting to the urologist for surgical evaluation is the hydrocele. Size, local discomfort, and cosmetic disfigurement play major roles in deciding when operative intervention is warranted. A scrotal ultrasound is often helpful to rule out associated scrotal pathology, especially to rule out an unexpected testicular neoplasm. In the uncomplicated hydrocele, however, which transilluminates well and in which the testicle is easily palpable, the ultrasound may be unnecessary. Associated hernias must be ruled out. Communicating hydroceles in children are discussed elsewhere in this book.

The hydrocele arises in the potential space created by the visceral and parietal layers of the tunica vaginalis. More fluid is secreted than is absorbed, thus the formation of this fluid-filled space. When the hydrocele approaches the size of an orange or when it starts to envelop the penis, surgical consideration for intervention becomes warranted. A patient may choose elective repair for any size lesion if he finds it cosmetically disturbing.

The general principles governing hydrocelectomy include adequate excision of the redundant tunica vaginalis, excellent hemostasis, and suturing of the excised edges to prevent hydrocele recurrence. Whether or not to place a Penrose drain is decided at the end of the procedure. If generalized oozing is present and the possibility of postop hematoma is significant, a Penrose drain may be placed for 24–48 h. Excisional and plication procedures are illustrated below. Figure 50.1 shows a typical gross anatomical appearance of a 15- to 20-cm hydrocele.

A transverse incision is made, and the intact hydrocele is delivered out of the scrotal vault. The sac is gently mobilized and freed of adherent tissues with moist gauze and sharp dissection. Cautery may be used liberally for hemostasis.

The sac is opened and the fluid aspirated (Fig. 50.2). Care is taken to inspect the testicle, epididymis, and vas. It may or may not be necessary to separately isolate the internal spermatic vessels and vas to prevent their injury during dissection.

The opened and mobilized tunica vaginalis is then excised by cautery or sharp dissection, leaving 2 cm of residual sac for simple over-sewing using 3-0 or 4-0 chromic suture (Fig. 50.3).

Alternately, the excised margins may be folded backwards on themselves (bottleneck procedure) (Fig. 50.4) behind the epididymis and cord structures and then loosely sutured together such that the secretory surfaces are now "outside," facing the dartos fascia, making recurrence improbable. The suture line should be left loose so as not to cause vascular compromise of the cord structures. If a Penrose drain is felt necessary, it is brought out the most dependent portion of the scrotum and tacked loosely to the skin with a 2-0 silk suture. The drain is removed in 24–48 h.

### Simple Plication Technique

For small, thin-walled sacs, the placation (Lord) technique may be more appropriate (Fig. 50.5). A transverse incision is made over the hydrocele, the sac is pushed up with digital pressure, and the sac opened and drained. In this procedure, no or very minimal tissue is excised.

From: *Operative Urology at the Cleveland Clinic*
Edited by: A. Novick et al. © Humana Press Inc., Totowa, NJ

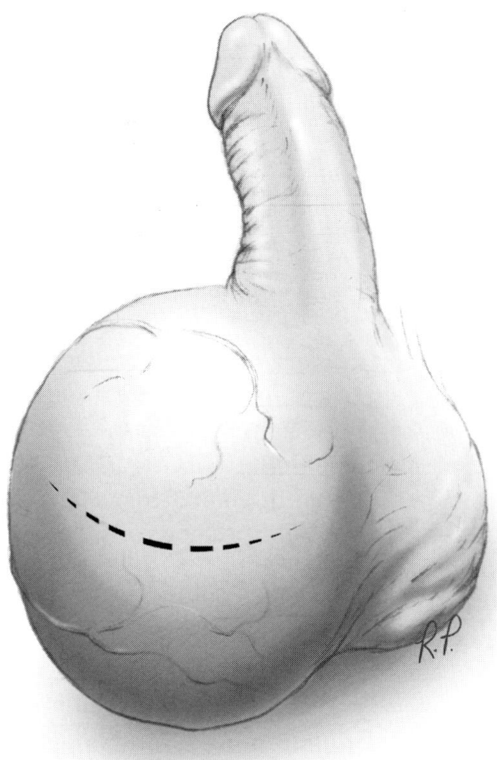


**Fig. 50.1**

A typical gross anatomical appearance of a 15- to 20-cm hydrocele. A transverse incision is made and the intact hydrocele is delivered out of the scrotal vault. The sac is gently mobilized and freed of adherent tissues with moist gauze and sharp dissection. Cautery may be used liberally for hemostasis.

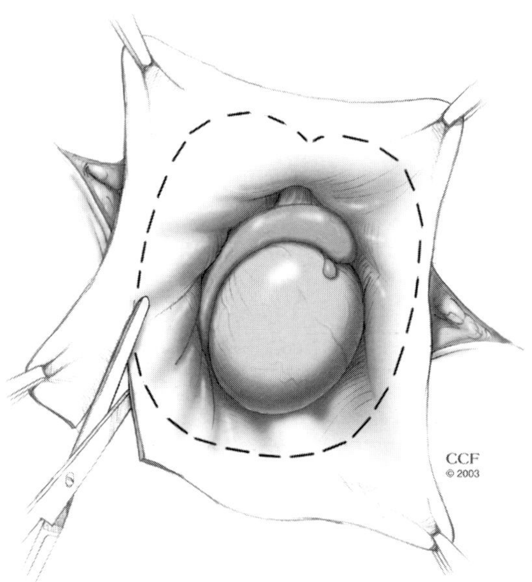


**Fig. 50.2**

The sac is opened and the fluid aspirated. Care is taken to inspect the testicle, epididymis, and vas. It may or may not be necessary to separately isolate the internal spermatic vessels and vas to prevent their injury during dissection.

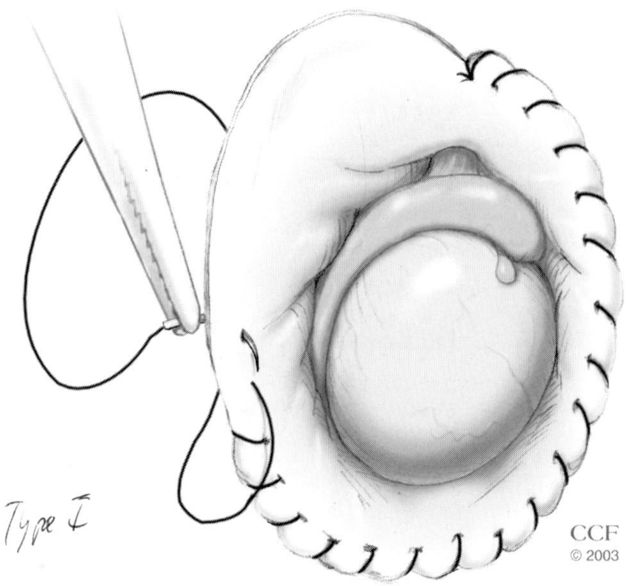


**Fig. 50.3**

The opened and mobilized tunica vaginalis is then excised by cautery or sharp dissection, leaving 2 cm of residual sac for simple oversewing using 3-0 or 4-0 chromic suture.

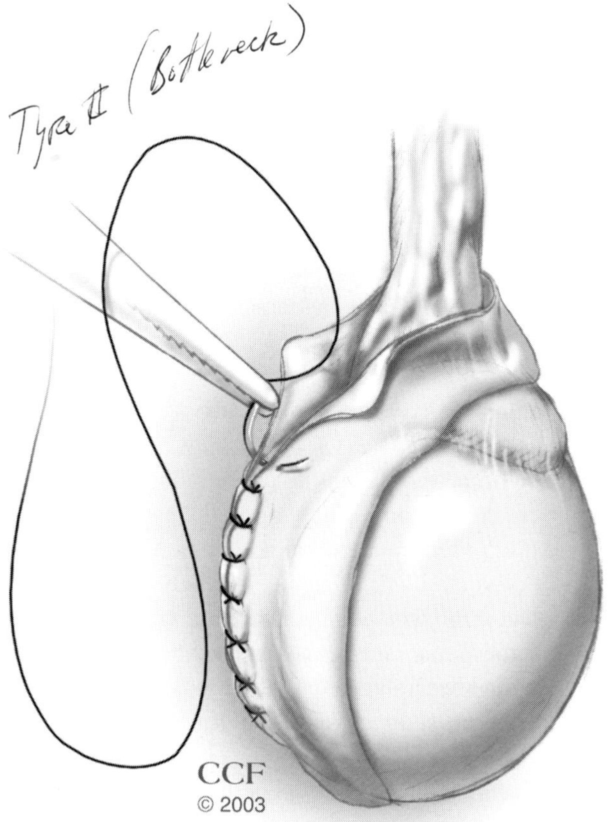


**Fig. 50.4**

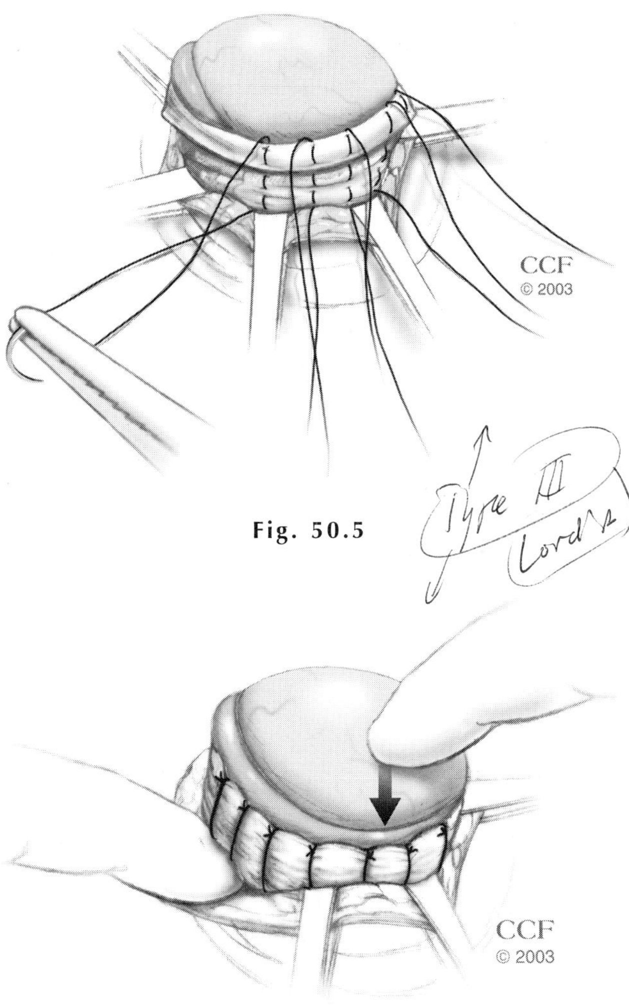


Fig. 50.5

Fig. 50.6

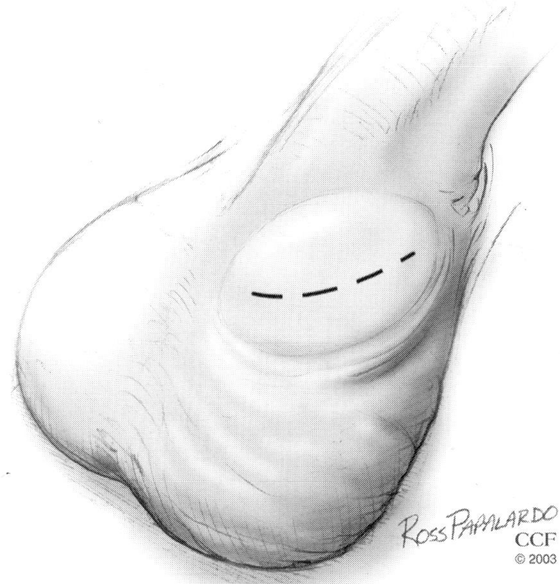


Fig. 50.7

The free ends of the sac are pushed down and plicated at the level of the inferior testicle and the redundant sac oversewn to bunch up the tunic and obliterate the potential space (Fig. 50.6).

## Postoperative Care

Collodion may be applied to the incison, and then a small piece of telfa gauze over the collodian. Fluff gauze is then bunched in a pair of elastic briefs ("mesh panties"). Ice packs and rest are recommended until swelling and any drainage have subsided. Routine use of antibiotics is not necessary. Resumption of normal activities is based on patient comfort and degree of postoperative swelling.

## SPERMATOCELECTOMY

Spermatoceles are very common benign cysts of the epididymis. They usually are small and typically arise from the head of the epididymis. They will transilluminate easily and can be palpated as a discrete lesion, demonstrably separate from the testicle. Most commonly they are asymptomatic and 2–3 cm in size when clinically noticeable.

If they are larger and present painful symptoms or are cosmetically disfiguring, excision may be warranted. When excising the spermatocele, care must be taken to not injure the epididymis at the point of the tubular attachment. This could cause tubular obstruction, preventing sperm migration toward the more distal tubules. When excising the lesion, it is best not to place sutures in the epididymis at the site of origin of the spermatocele because these, too, can create tubular obstruction. Based on the size of the lesion, it can be excised either by delivering the testicle from the scrotal vault or merely mobilizing the lesion while leaving the testicle *in situ*.

The spermatocele is approached through a transverse scrotal incision just over the lesion (Fig. 50.7).

The spermatocele is mobilized intact by careful, sharp dissection until it is completely isolated and the small tubular stalk on which it arises is identified (Fig. 50.8). This stalk is then ligated with 4-0 absorbable suture and the cyst is delivered intact.

Closure of a small layer of fascia over the epididymal defect will aid in hemostasis and also prevent possible sperm extravasation and spermatic granuloma (Fig. 50.9).

The wound is closed in layers and a small fluff dressing and scrotal support applied (Fig. 50.10). Other postoperative considerations will be similar to those noted for hydrocele above.

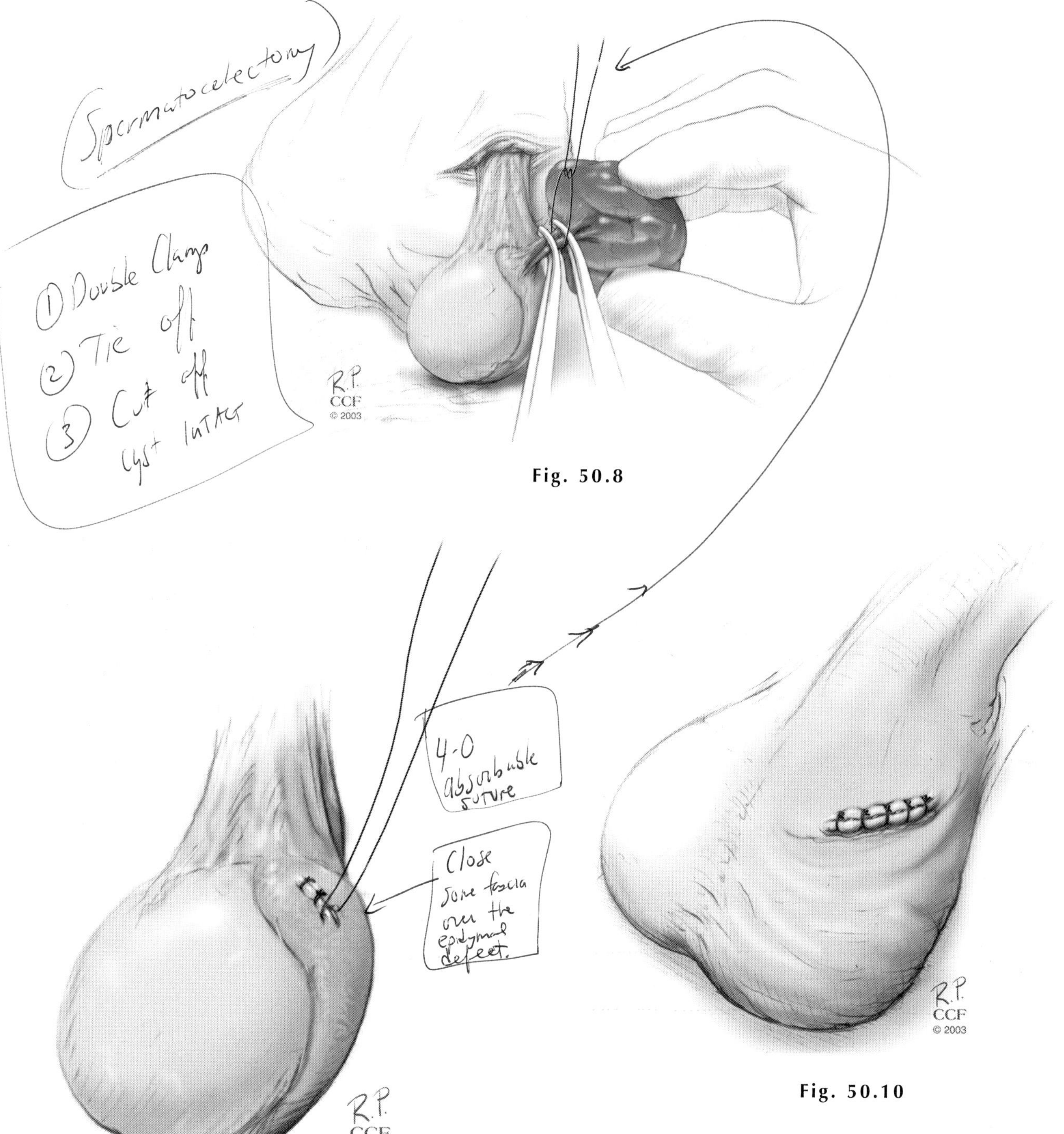


Fig. 50.8

Fig. 50.9

Fig. 50.10

## INCISIONAL VASECTOMY

Vasectomy is a very common and well-tolerated procedure done almost exclusively for voluntary sterilization. Unless the patient specifically requests general anesthesia, the procedure is typically done in the office under local anesthesia. The patient and his partner should be counseled that vasectomy should be considered an irreversible procedure, although some discussion of vaso-vasostomy may be appropriate. A correctly done procedure should produce sterility at confidence levels approaching 100%. There are no documented systemic long-term side effects from vasectomy except the possibility of a spermatic granuloma (<1%). Short-term side effects would include orchalgia, some swelling, and the possibility of postoperative hematoma. Hemostasis with a cautery unit during the procedure can minimize this risk. If a hematoma does occur, scrotal compression dressing, scrotal elevation, and the application

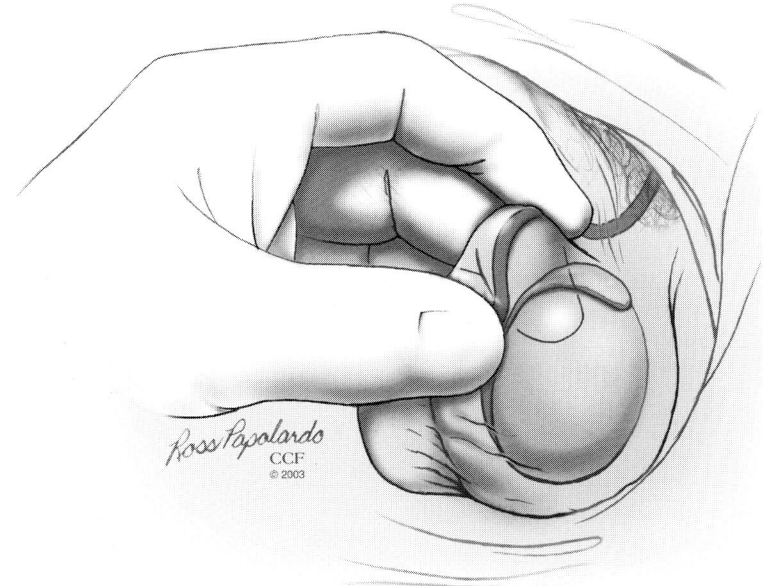


Fig. 50.11

of ice pack can usually manage it. Rarely is surgical evacuation of the hematoma required. The patient must continue contraception until a postvas semen analysis shows zero sperm in the ejaculate.

## TRADITIONAL VASECTOMY

The procedure may be performed in the supine or lithotomy position (Fig. 50.11). If done with the patient supine, it is convenient to stand on the ipsilateral side and move to the other side of the table to perform the contralateral vasectomy. The skin is prepped with betadine, and the mid-portion of the vas is isolated under the skin between thumb and middle finger of the nondominant hand. An effort is made to mobilize the vas away from the other cord structures for later ease in delivery of the vas. A skin wheel is infiltrated with 1% plain lidocaine, and more lidocaine is injected along the proximal vas, approximately 2 cc on each side of the vas.

A 1- to 2-cm incision is made longitudinally just over the vas and deepened until the vas comes into view (Fig. 50.12). It may be helpful to spread the adjacent tissues with a small curved hemostat.

The vas is grasped with a single-tooth tenaculum and elevated out of the scrotal vault (Fig. 50.13). This maneuver may cause groin or testicular pain, and therefore more lidocaine along the vas may be helpful.

An incision is made directly over the vas with a no. 15 blade until the vas is free of all cremasteric attachments (Fig. 50.14).

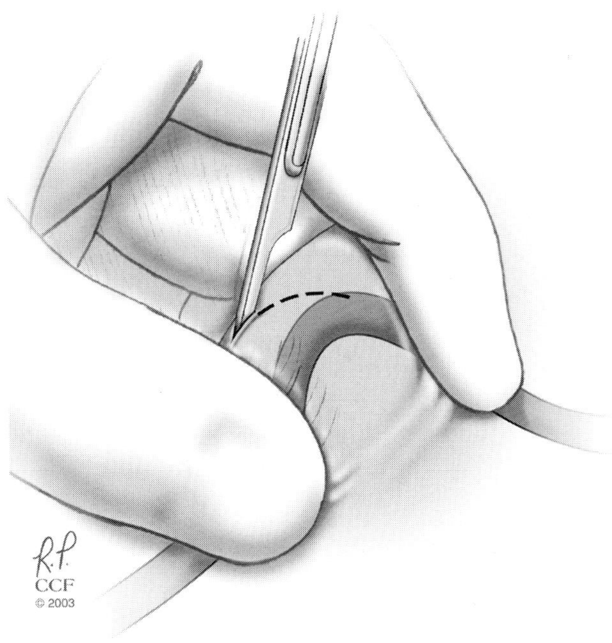


Fig. 50.12

A curved hemostat is used to develop this plane and then spread under the vas for about 2 cm (Fig. 50.15). This will free up the vas as an isolated structure. It is helpful to then place this hemostat on the fascial bridge just created under the loop of vas. This will secure the structures were the patient to move and prevent the vas from falling back into the scrotum. An assistant should securely hold the two ends of the vasal loop with thumb forceps.

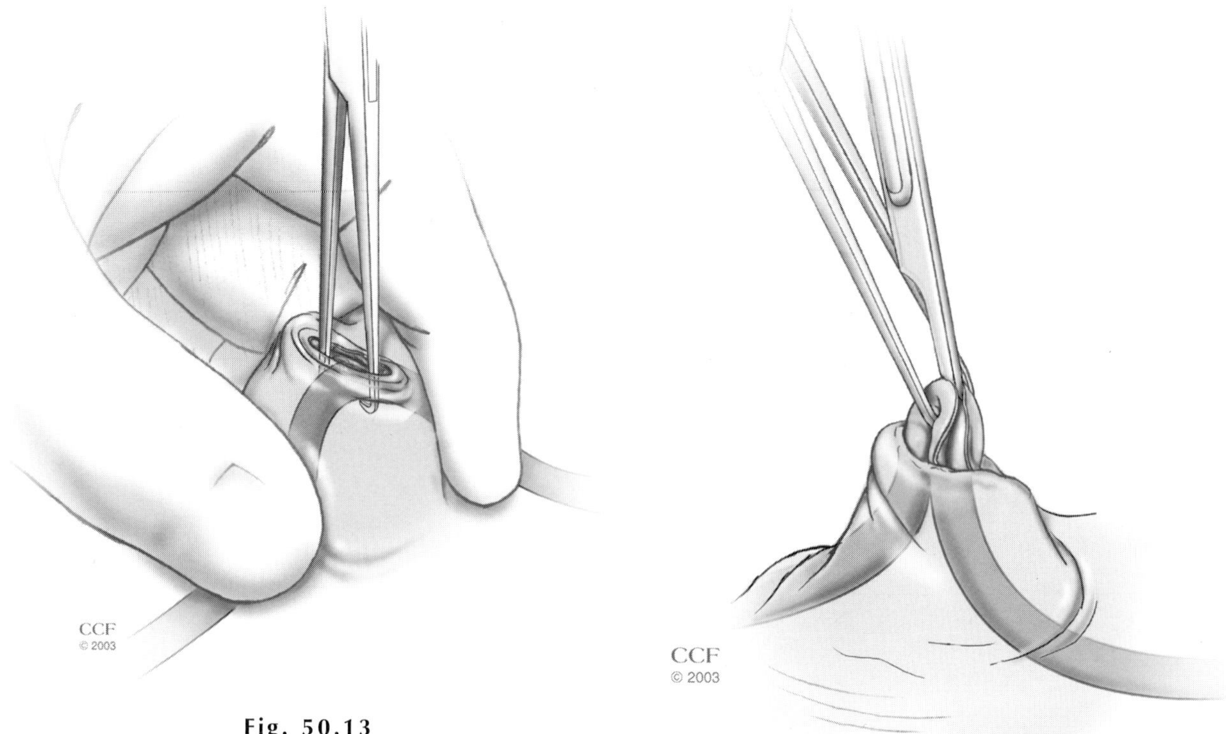


Fig. 50.13

Fig. 50.14

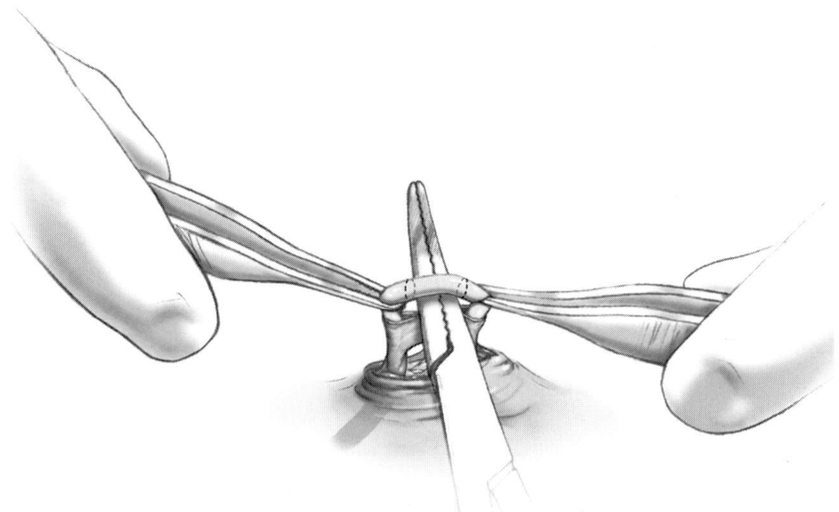

Fig. 50.15

Ten millimeters of vas is excised and then the two ends are cauterized with a needle electrode, passing the electrode at least 5 mm into the vasal lumen (Fig. 50.16). The raw end and any visible vascular bleeders are cauterized.

The testicular end of the vas is allowed to fall back under the cremasteric fascia, and this fascia is oversewn this with 4-0 chromic (Fig. 50.17). This will create a tissue layer between the two cut ends to keep them in separate tissue planes and further guarantee against recanalization.

The skin is closed with an everting vertical mattress suture of 4-0 chromic (Fig. 50.18). Usually a couple of 4 × 4s packed into a pair of jockey shorts is all that is

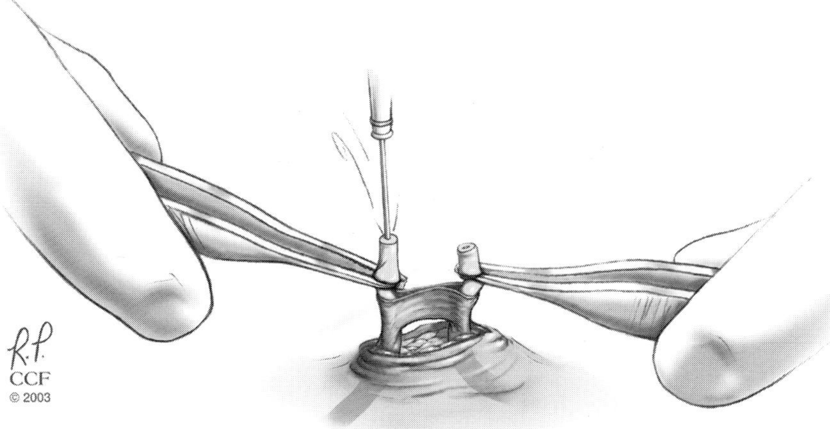


Fig. 50.16

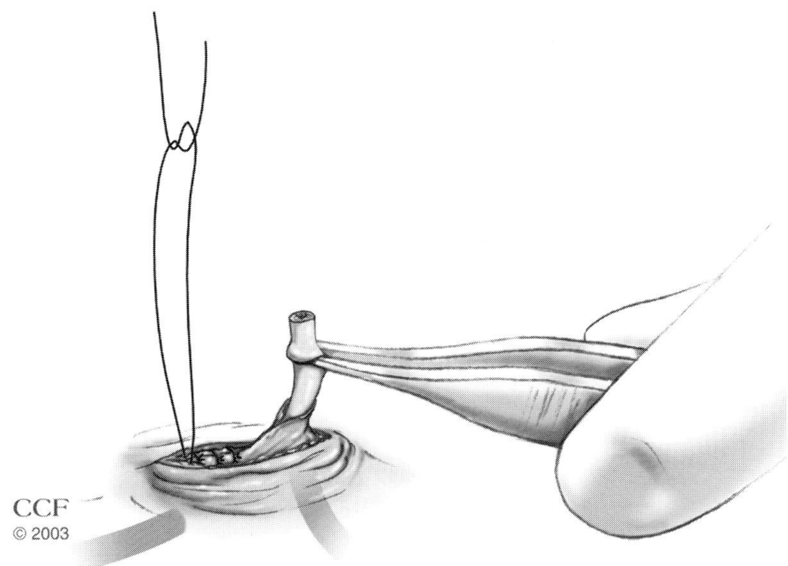


Fig. 50.17

needed for postoperative wound op care. Alternatively, a small collodian topical application may be used.

## PERCUTANEOUS VASECTOMY

Using the no-scalpel vasectomy instruments in percutaneous fashion, vasectomy may be performed in the office setting without fixation of the vas to skin using the ring tenaculum. Warming the previously shaved, prepped, and draped scrotum with a warm towel relaxes the dartos and cremasteric muscles so the vas is readily palpable. This should be as warm as will be tolerated by the patient. The skin puncture may need no sutures. Postoperative care and semen analyses are similar as for the incisional vasectomy. The percutaneous approach is fast, effective, and perhaps somewhat less painful than the standard incisional techniques.

The nondominant thumb is placed at the raphe and used to trap the vas between the first and second fingers in a tripod grasp (Fig. 50.19). The vas is isolated by gently "kneading" all cord structures away so the vas is isolated between thumb and fingers. With vas held to skin using the tripod grasp, 1% plain lidocaine is injected through a 25- or 27-gage, 1/2-in. needle while advancing through skin into the vasal sheath. This dissects the vas sheath and other cord structures away from the vas. Multiple needle passes are avoided.

The tripod grasp is maintained to secure the vas, and then the ulnar (right side for right-handed surgeon) prong

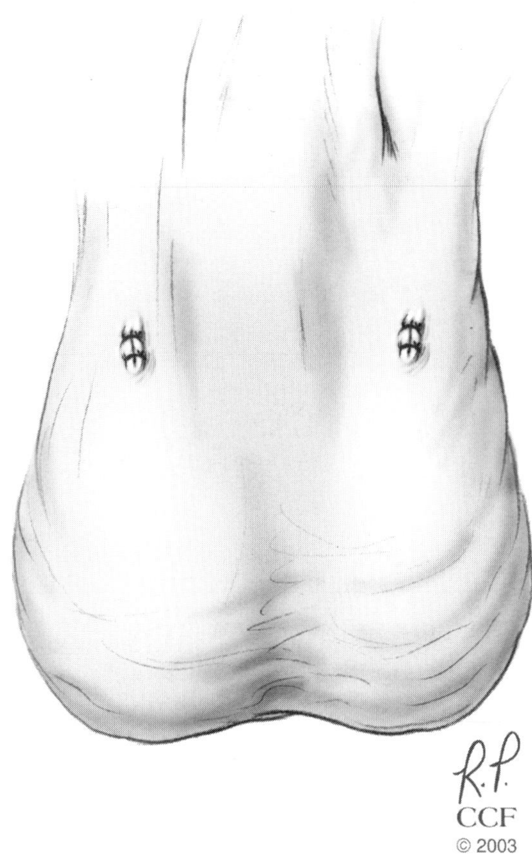


Fig. 50.18

of the sharp no-scalpel hemostat is placed through the skin all the way to vas while continuing to hold the vas securely in the tripod grasp (Fig. 50.20). This clamp is then closed, placed through the incision, and spread to expose the vas.

The exposed aspect of the vasal sheath is grasped with the ringed tenaculum and elevated out of the scrotum (Fig. 50.21). It is incised with a scalpel longitudinally. Cutting slightly into the vas wall assures that the sheath is opened completely so that the vas extrudes through the sheath. The vas is regrasped with another ringed tenaculum, and the sheath falls away to expose a 1- to 3-cm mobile section of vas. Following vasal excision and occlusion by the surgeon's method of choice, the procedure is repeated on the contralateral vas from the opposite side of the table through a second hemostatic puncture.

## ORCHIECTOMY

### Radical Inguinal Approach

If there is preoperative concern that a neoplasm of the testicle, epididymis, or cord structures could be present, the inguinal approach to the testicle is mandated. All cord structures can be delivered into the inguinal incision for inspection, biopsy, or reconstruction. A rubber-shod clamp should be placed across the cord, allowing time for inspection or biopsy, if appropriate. If a diagnosis of testicular neoplasm is established by either biopsy or gross inspection, then a strong curved Kelley clamp is placed across the cord at the internal inguinal ring level. The cord structures are dissected below this clamp into two smaller segments and doubly clamped, suture-ligated with 0-silk, and divided. The testicle and cord are then dissected free and

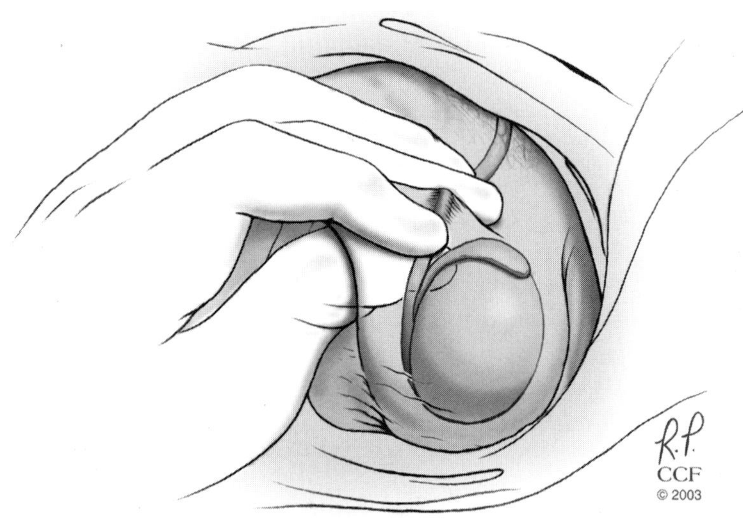


Fig. 50.19

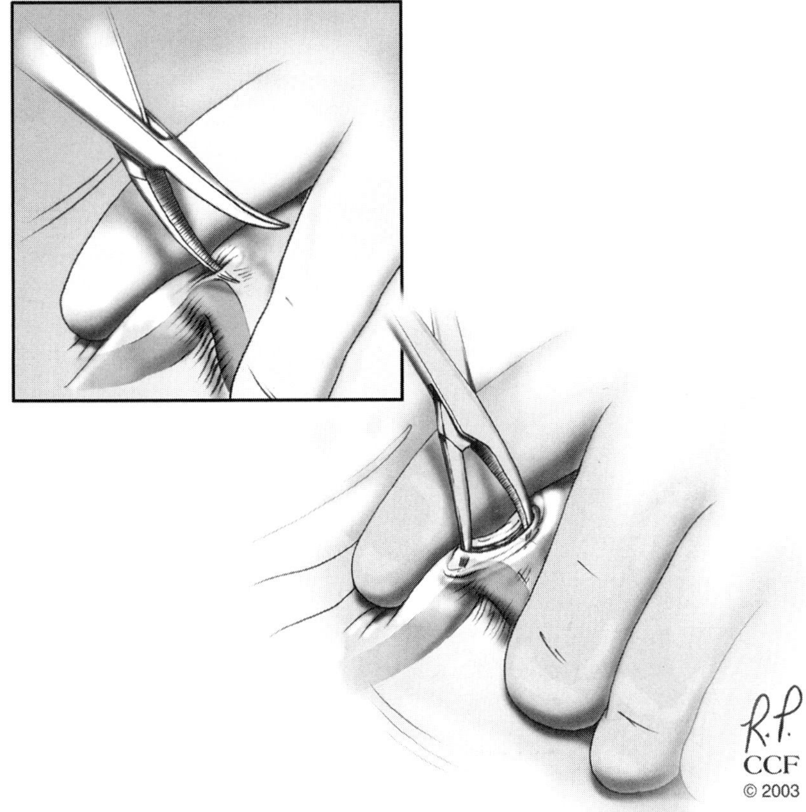


Fig. 50.20

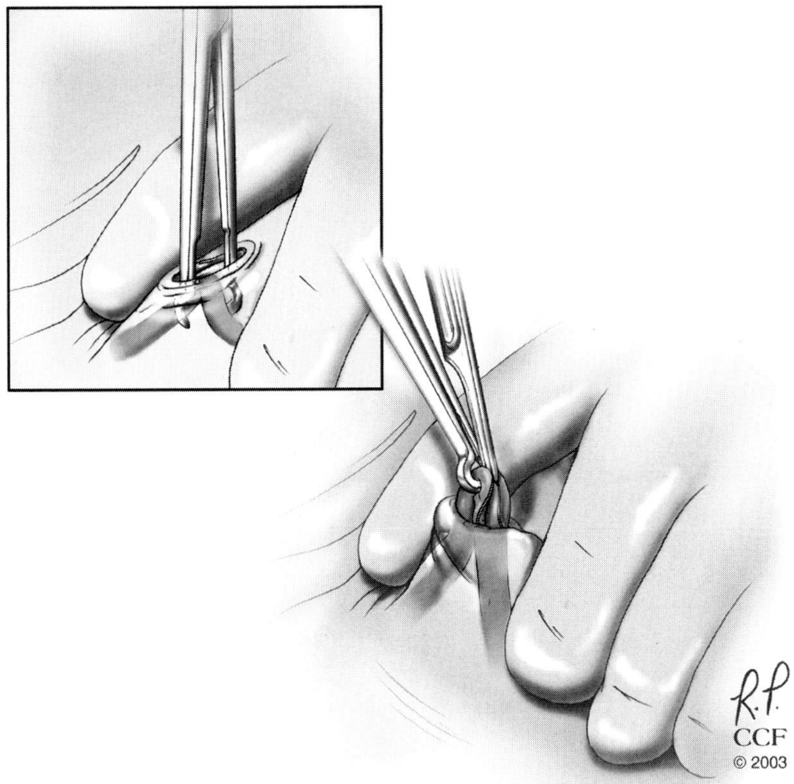


Fig. 50.21

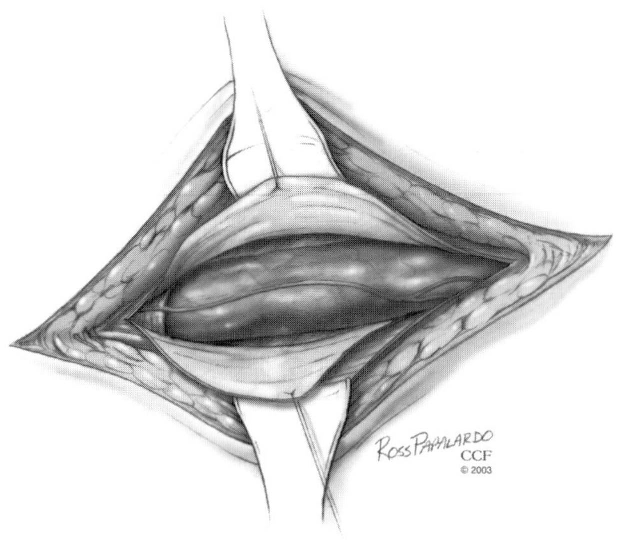


Fig. 50.22

removed. The testicle should not be biopsied or otherwise incised near the operative field for fear of tumor seeding.

If the procedure is being done for an epididymal lesion or paratesticular lesion or lesion of the spermatic cord, one would use this inguinal approach and then decide on the procedure of choice based on biopsy with frozen section of the paratesticular neoplasm.

Examples of these would include adenomatoid tumors and cystadenomas of the epididymis, paratesticular meso-thelioma, rhabdomyosarcoma, and leiomyosaracoma of the spermatic cord. Other mesenchymal tumors of cord include liposarcoma, benign lipomas, and fibrosarcomas.

A standard oblique inguinal incision is made paralleling the inguinal ligament (Fig. 50.22). The length of the incision will be dictated by the size of the testicular mass; it should be long enough for easy delivery of the testicle and cord structures. The fascia of the external oblique is opened in the direction of its fibers. The ileo-inguinal nerve is mobilized out of the field, and the cord structures are bluntly dissected just enough to allow placement of the rubber-shod clamp.

With the rubber-shod clamp securely in place, the testicle is mobilized out of the scrotum and dissected off the gubernacular attachment, and these structures are brought into the operative field (Fig. 50.23). If there is any chance

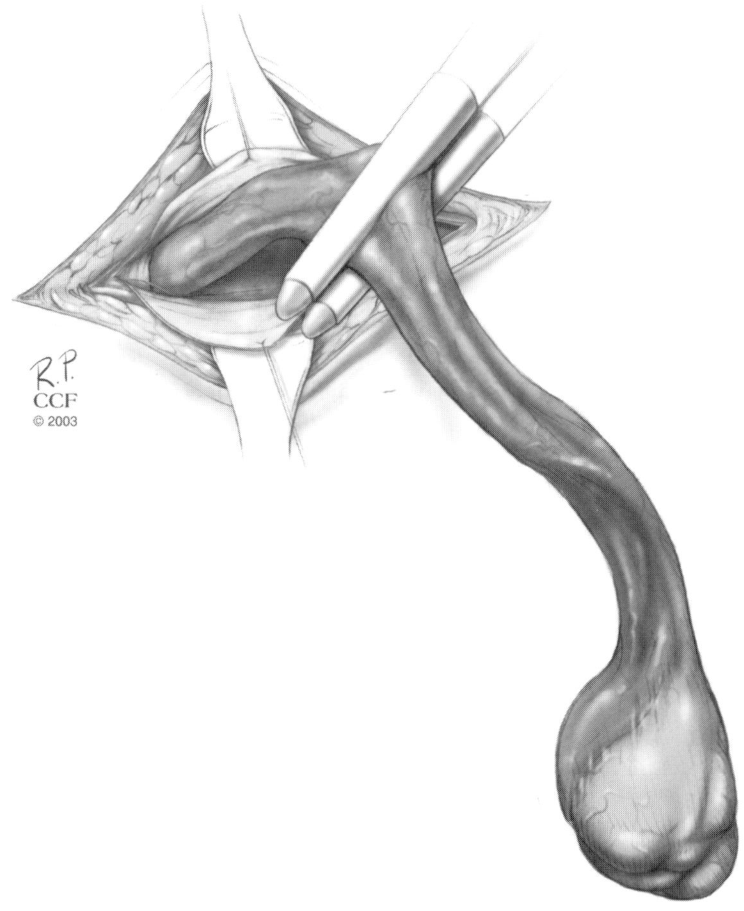


Fig. 50.23

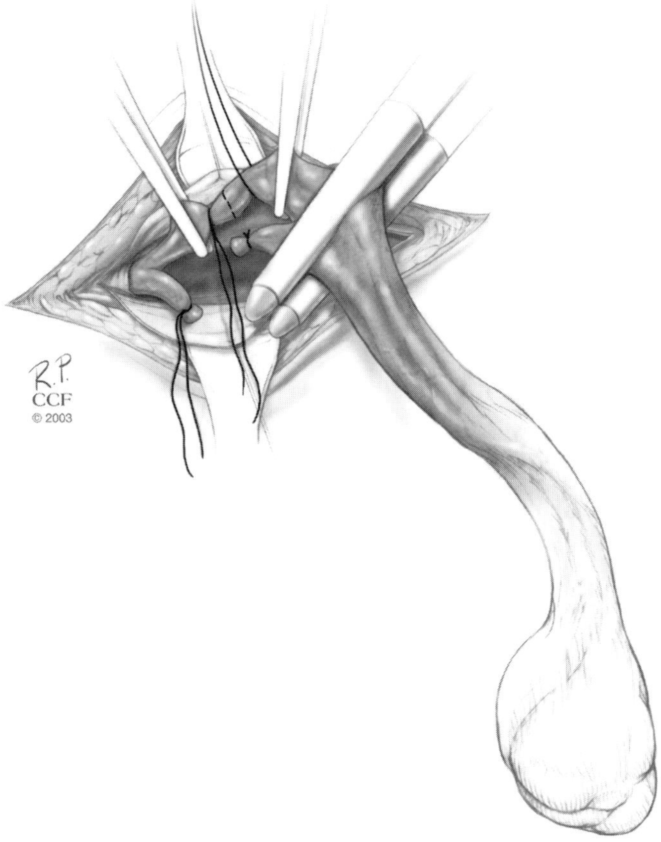


Fig. 50.24

of malignancy, the operative field should be redraped to protect it from the scrotal contents.

When orchiectomy is to be performed, the cord structures are sharply divided into two segments: one with the vas and cremasteric fibers and the other with the internal spermatic vessels (Fig. 50.24). These segments are individually clamped, suture-ligated with 0-silk, and divided. (Leaving several inches of suture as a tag on the proximal cord segment will facilitate retrieving and removing the proximal cord if later retroperitoneal lymphadenectomy is required.) The specimen is sent to pathology. Preliminary information from a frozen section may be helpful to counsel the concerned family immediately following surgery. The wound is closed in layers—the skin with a subcuticular suture, if appropriate.

## SIMPLE SCROTAL ORCHIECTOMY

The most common reason to perform this procedure is for the hormonal management of prostatic carcinoma. Because of the widespread use of luteinizing hormone-releasing hormone agonists, this procedure is now less commonly done, but it still represents a cost-effective technique for the hormonal management of prostatic carcinoma. Certain patients may find the procedure convenient in that it obviates the need for regular office visits, injections, and the supplemental costs often incurred. Other indications would be for refractory inflammatory conditions or perhaps a painful atrophic testicle from a high-riding incompletely descended testicle or missed testicular torsion. In doing a bilateral orchiectomy, two separate high scrotal incisions are preferred. In this way there is less tissue mobilization required and therefore less chance for postoperative hematoma. Alternately, a low transverse or midline raphe incision may also be used. Drainage is seldom required.

An oblique incision is made over the upper portion of the cord (Fig. 50.25). This incision is made only as long as needed to safely deliver the testicle and cord structures. Because there is no concern about replacing the testicle, one can extrude it through a small incision by digital pressure. The tunica vaginalis is opened and the testicle and cord structures mobilized free. At a convenient level on the cord, the structures are separated into two segments and doubly clamped. These are then doubly ligated with 0 chromic suture ligatures and divided. Hemostasis

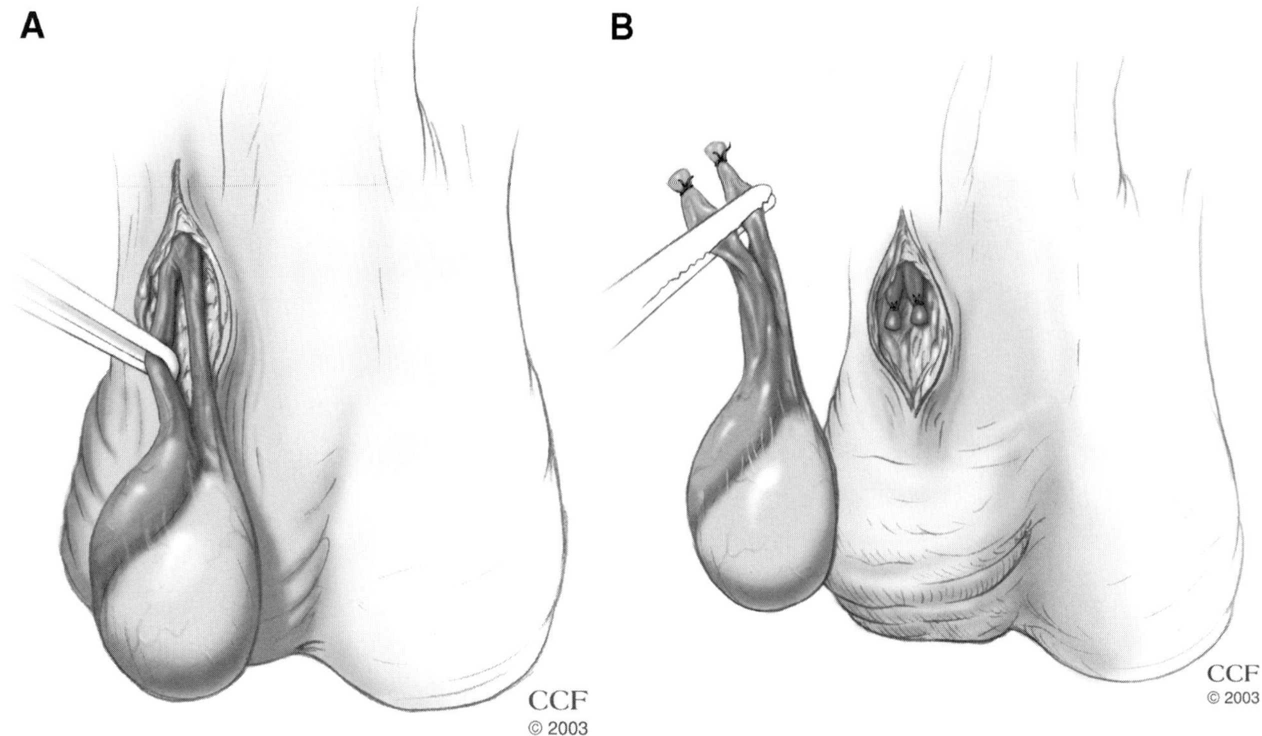


Fig. 50.25

is accomplished with the bovie and the wound closed in two layers with 2-0 chromic.

## EPIDIDYMECTOMY

In the modern era of effective antibiotics and antituberculous medications, this procedure is rarely indicated. Indications would include a chronic, painful, and refractory epididymitis or the concern that an epididymal mass could be a neoplasm rather than inflammation. Scrotal ultrasound is often of little help in this differential diagnosis. Granulomatous, suppurative tuberculous epididymitis with sinus tract formation is a clear indication, but this is rarely seen. The most common tumor involving the epididymis is an adenomatoid tumor. This is a benign tumor. Epididymal surgery is not indicated for chronic orchalgia.

The testicle is exposed as described for simple scrotal orchiectomy (Fig. 50.26). The tunica vaginalis is opened and the vas identified and cut across as high as convenient. The inguinal portion of the vas is cauterized with a needle electrode. Care must be taken to only ligate/cauterize the artery of the epididymis and avoid the internal spermatic vessels supplying the testicle.

Using the vas for countertraction, the epididymis is elevated and sharply dissected off the surface of the tunica albugenia (Fig. 50.27). Hemostasis with the needle electrode is important.

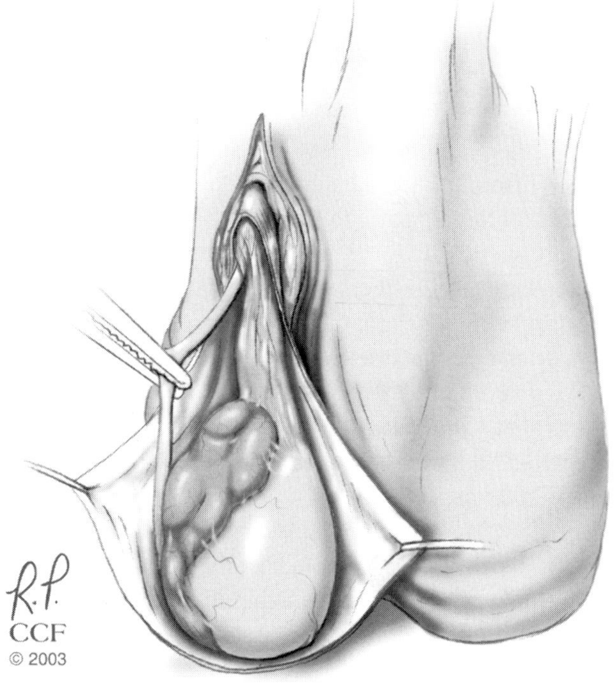


Fig. 50.26

The bed of the epididymis is oversewn with 4-0 chromic, taking small bites of the remaining tunica albugenia (Fig. 50.28). The testicle is repositioned in its anatomical position

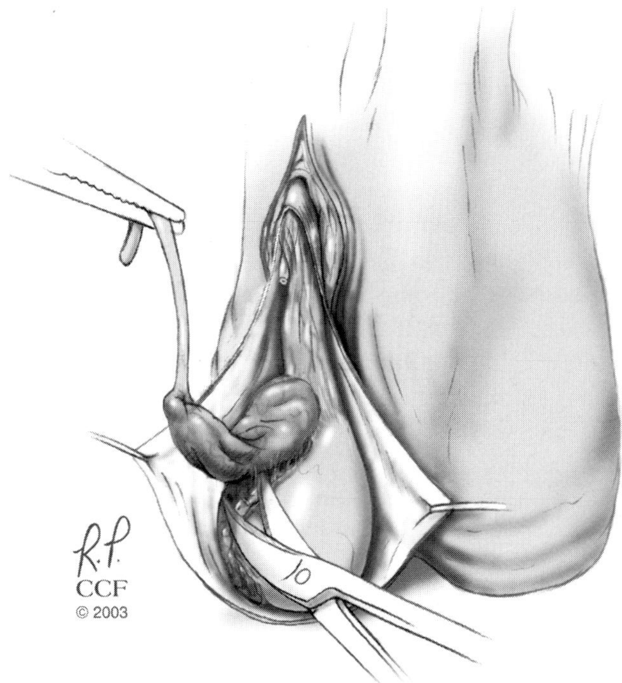


Fig. 50.27

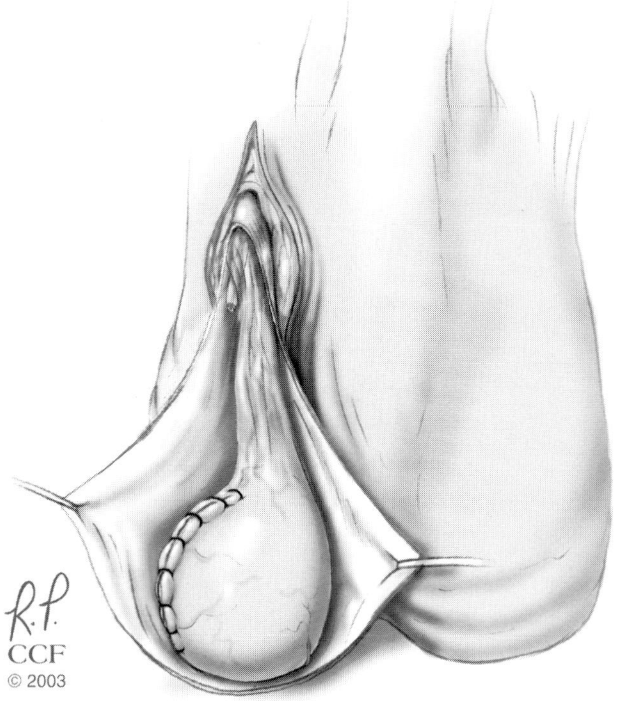


Fig. 50.28

and the scrotum closed in layers with chromic suture. As the tissue planes are often a bit vascular, a small Penrose drain and a fluff pressure dressing with mesh panties will provide good postoperative comfort and hemostasis.

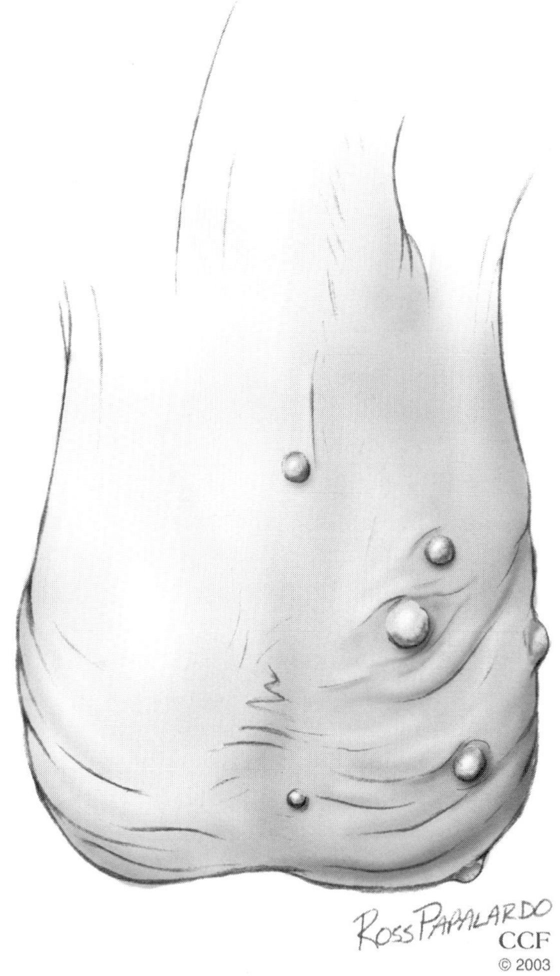


Fig. 50.29

## SCROTAL WALL CYSTS AND INFECTIONS

Often called sebaceous cysts, these common cystic lesions of the scrotal wall are sometimes cosmetically disfiguring. Pathologically they are epithelial inclusion cysts comprised of a dense capsule and filled with a cheesy epithelial secretion. They can also present as an infected, draining, superficial scrotal abscess. If the lesion is infected and draining, it cannot be removed intact because it has already opened to form the draining sinus tract. In this case the lesion is opened, the suppurative and sebaceous material debrided, and as much as possible of the residual capsule removed. A small drain may or may not be required. This incision is left open to granulate closed with time. A short course of appropriate antibiotics may be advisable, especially in diabetics.

Epithelial cysts may present as a separated cluster of similar lesions ranging from 5 to 15 mm in diameter (Fig. 50.29). To effectively remove them and prevent recurrence, each must be excised individually.

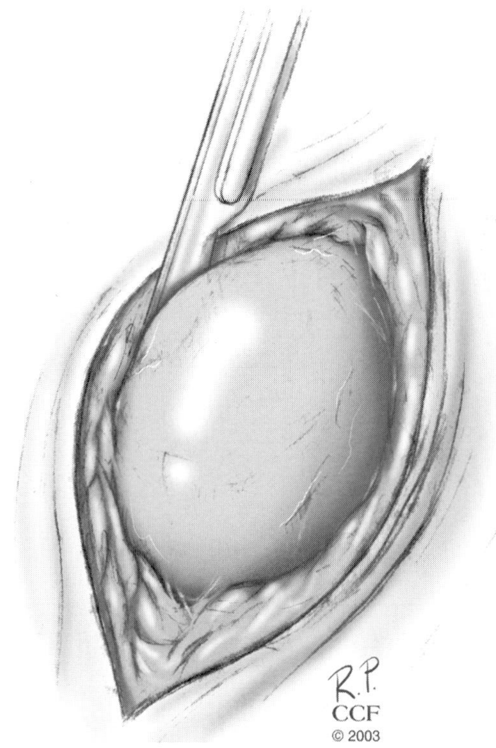


Fig. 50.30

The surgical goal is to remove the cyst intact in order to ensure complete excision of the lesion and obviate recurrence at that site (Fig. 50.30). After suitable prep and local anesthesia, an incision is made just over the lesion until the capsule of the cyst is identified. Using a pointed hemostat and/or a blade, the cyst is freed from the dartos fascia.

With gentle upward countertraction, the lesion can be delivered intact and removed (Fig. 50.31). The procedure is repeated for the other lesions, and the small scrotal incisions are closed with 4-0 or 5-0 chromic vertical mattress sutures. Usually no dressing other than a drop of collodion is required.

If the multiple lesions cluster in close proximity to each other, it is more efficient to do a limited scrotal wall resection and take the scrotal skin off intact with the lesions untouched (Fig. 50.32). This can be done with sharp dissection of the skin and subcutaneous tissues.

Typically there is adequate scrotal skin redundancy so that a limited subcutaneous dissection will mobilize the edges to be easily closed with a 4-0 chromic vertical mattress suture (Fig. 50.33).

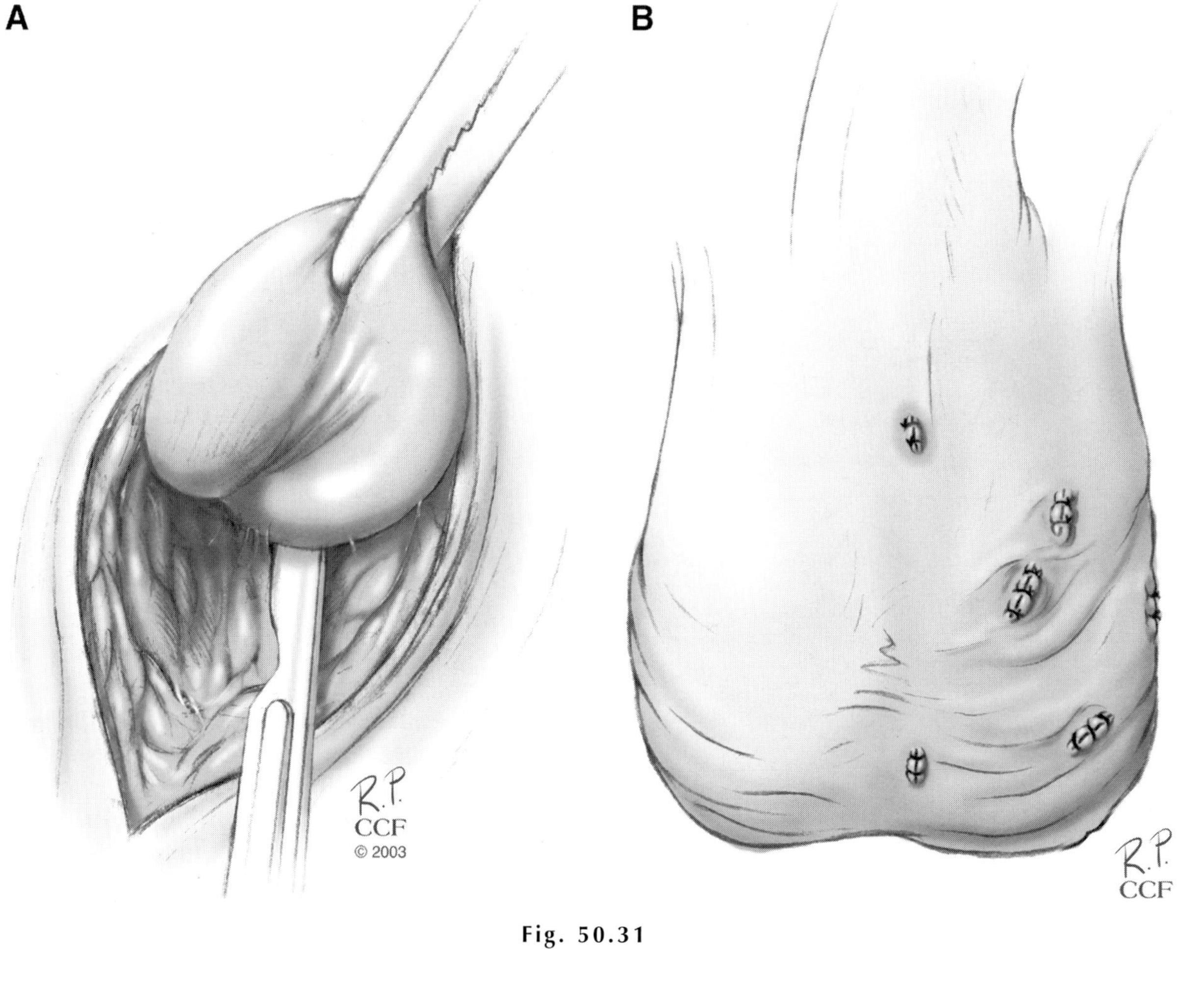

Fig. 50.31

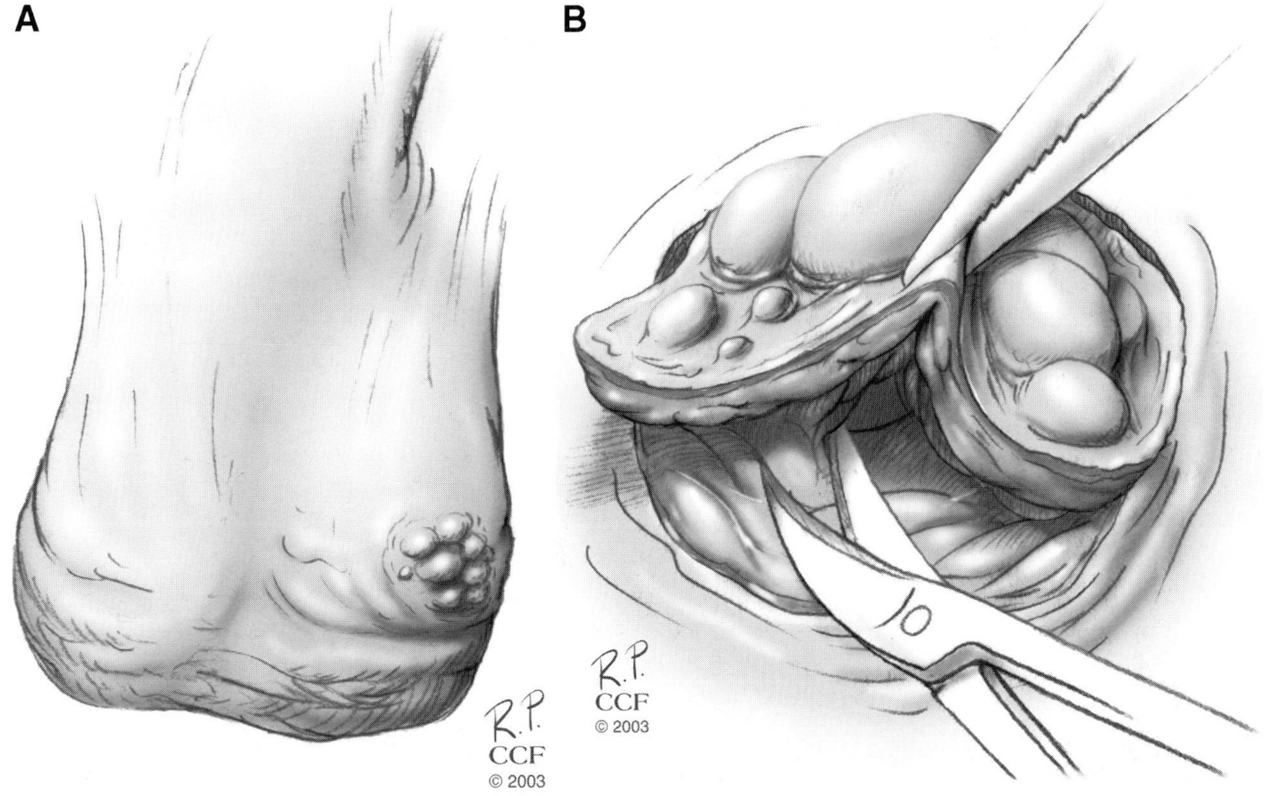


Fig. 50.32

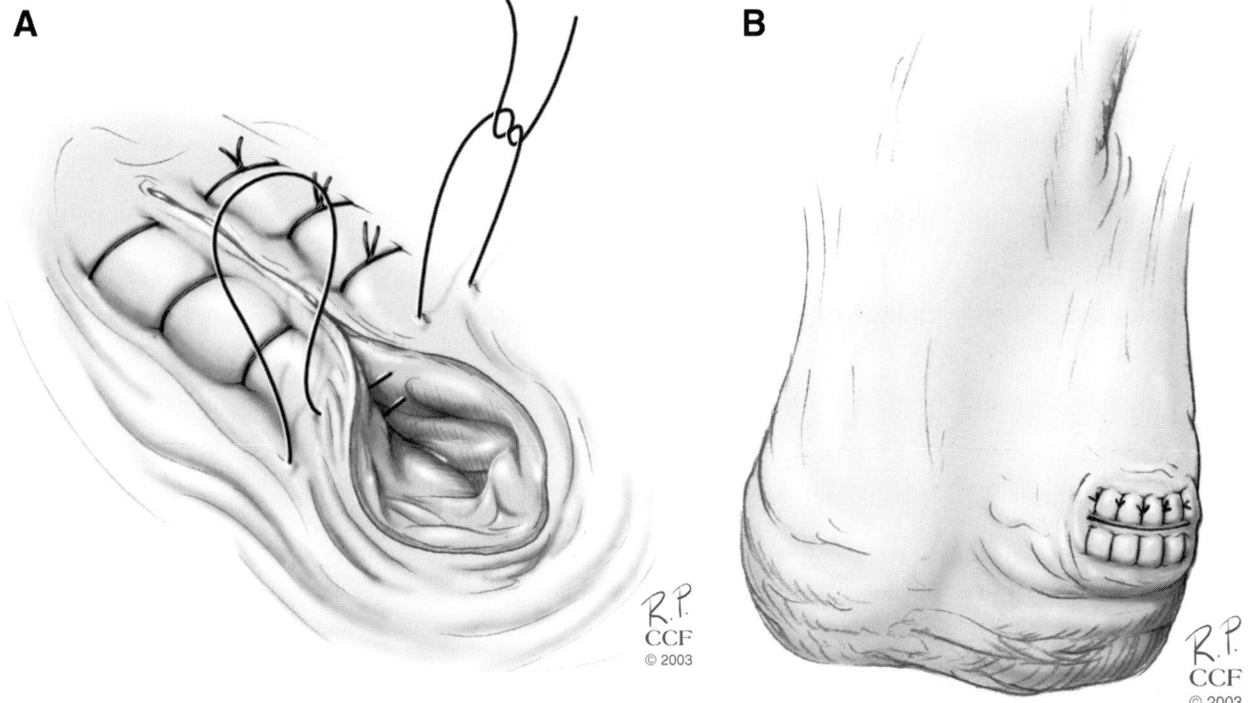


Fig. 50.33

## MANAGEMENT OF SCROTAL INFECTIONS

The scrotum can be the source of localized infections such as carbuncles or furuncles. These can be incised and drained with either a Penrose drain or an iodoform gauze wound pack. Deeper infections, which extend below the dartos fascia or even into the scrotal vault, require more aggressive incision and drainage in addition to careful postoperative wound care, dressing changes, and appropriate antibiotics. One should be alert to the possibility that the etiology is an infected urethral diverticulum or a periurethral abscess or perirectal abscess. Cystoscopy or retrograde uretrhogram may be helpful to rule out this etiology. Sigmoidoscopy in the operating room also may be beneficial, especially if there is any concern of Fournier's gangrene being imminent.

The most severe condition in this category is Fournier's gangrene, also referred to as synergistic gangrene, because numerous organisms, both aerobic and anaerobic, are involved, each with an additive effect to create the progressive necrotizing fasciitis encountered. This disease may be fatal, depending on the degree of involvement, the time from onset to surgical intervention, and the comorbidities present. Scrotal gangrene is often seen in elderly, poorly cared for individuals who are obese, and most especially in diabetics. The inflammatory process may involve a periurethral or perirectal abscess and may extend under the scrotal fascia and up to the inguinal ligament. The gas gangrene can also extend up along the lateral abdominal wall and track up to the axilla. Extensive loss of scrotal and penile skin can occur.

Fournier's gangrene requires immediate and urgent operative intervention, often with a general surgical or plastic surgical colleague. An infectious disease consult is also advisable. This disease should not be observed on antibiotics alone. This is a fulminant gangrenous infection, which spreads rapidly, literally in hours, to destroy full-thickness skin and fascial planes in spite of appropriate antibiotics.

Incision and drainage are not adequate for this disease. All questionable tissue must be debrided and full-thickness tissue planes excised. If there is any doubt as to tissue viability, this tissue should be resected. If the scrotal vault is extensively involved, there is no compelling reason to salvage the testicle and cord. They should be removed, ligating the cord as high as possible. This makes for a more manageable wound defect for postoperative packing and wound care. Often the testicle and cord will overlie necrotic tissue, which cannot be adequately debrided if they are left *in situ*. Typically these patients will require several trips back to the operating room for secondary debridement and partial wound closure. Intensive postoperative wound management with whirlpool baths, hydrogen peroxide wound packing, and frequent dressing changes will be required. When the process has been arrested and good granulation tissue is starting to form, further procedures will be required to now close the defects created by the inflammatory process and the subsequent surgical interventions. These may include delayed closure of the remaining wound defects, with or without split thickness tissue grafting of larger defects not suitable for complete healing by secondary granulation.

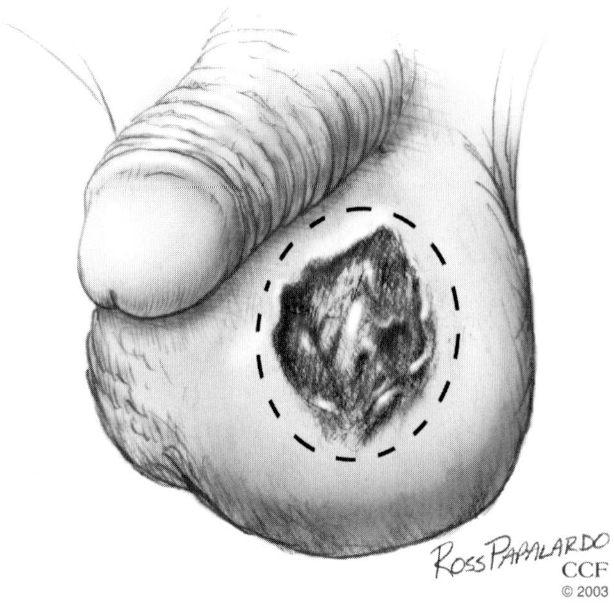


**Fig. 50.34**

This early necrotic lesion is still localized to the scrotal vault and not yet tracking proximal to the external ring (Fig. 50.34). The skin is a shiny gray color with associated peripheral cellulitis.

Wide excision of the inflammatory process is undertaken using the cautery current to dissect all questionable nonviable tissue (Fig. 50.35).

The flap of necrotic tissue is grasped with allis clamps as necessary and then liberally debrided with electrocautery (Fig. 50.36). This debridement should be deep enough to expose pink, viable, and well-vascularized tissue.

When the scrotal vault is clean and the dissection is down to pink, well-vascularized tissue, the wound cavity is packed open with iodoform gauze, which is irrigated with hydrogen peroxide and changed three times a day

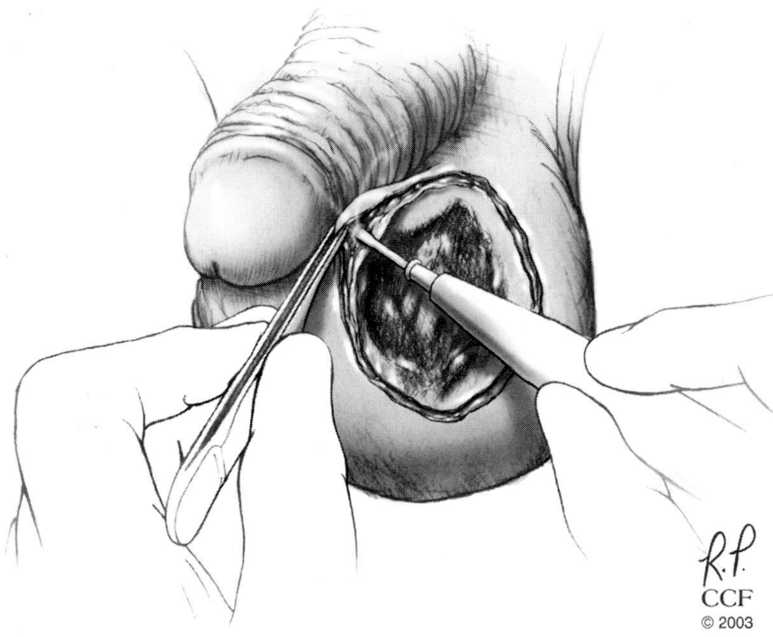


Fig. 50.35

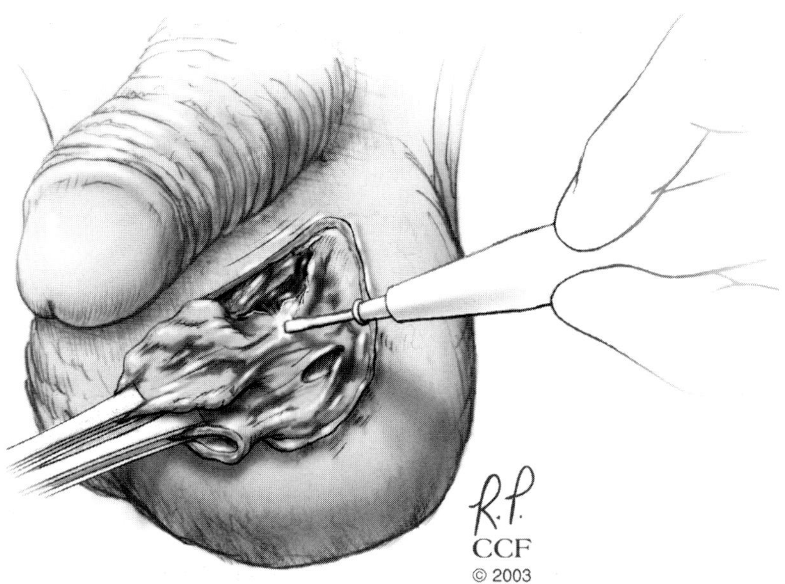


Fig. 50.36

(Fig. 50.37). Whirlpool treatments can follow the removal of the wound packing with the packing replaced after the hydrotherapy.

The necrotizing gangrene may be quite advanced at presentation (Fig. 50.38). The gas gangrene is clearly extensive, involving the entire left scrotum, left medial thigh, and extending well above the external ring. This lesion, left untreated for any length of time, will result in fatal sepsis.

Wide scrotal dissection and debridement are carried out (Fig. 50.39). The testicle is mobilized to be removed with as much cord as possible. Alternately, if the testicle and cord are felt salvageable, they may be buried in a subcutaneous flap in the medial thigh to be repositioned later as healing progresses. The incision and debridement then progress up the scrotum, over the inguinal ligament and external ring with the proximal extent of the dissection to be decided by the apparent viability of the tissues.

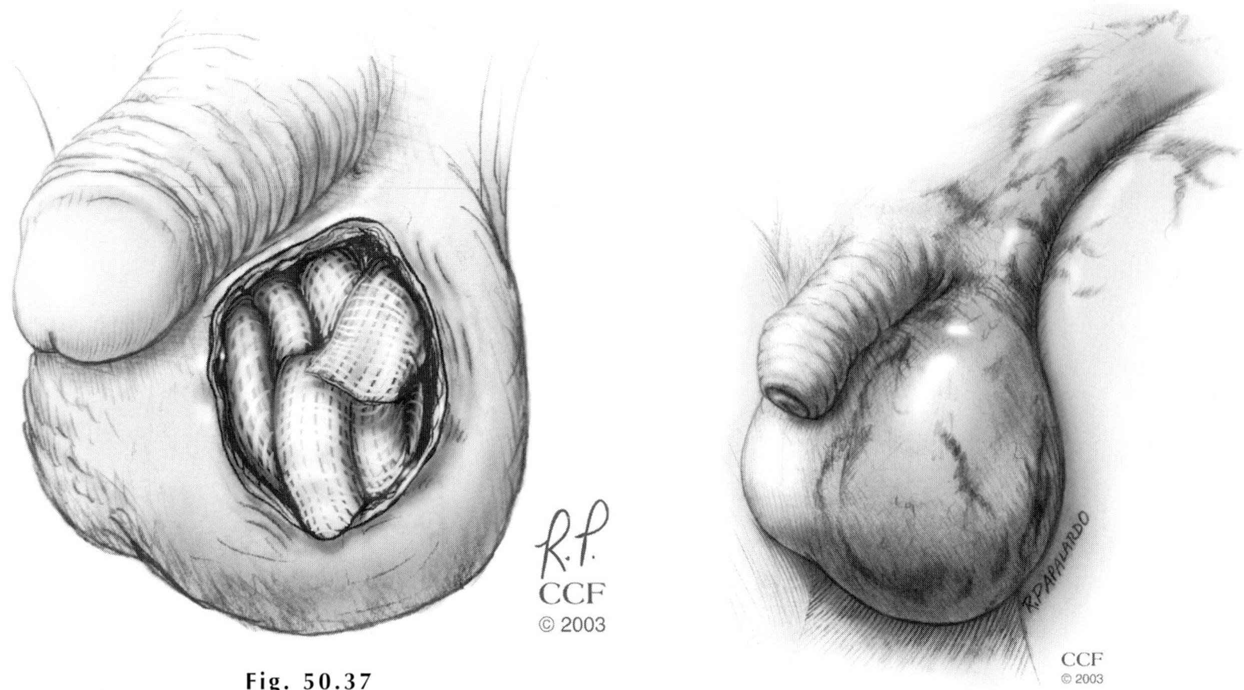


Fig. 50.37

Fig. 50.38

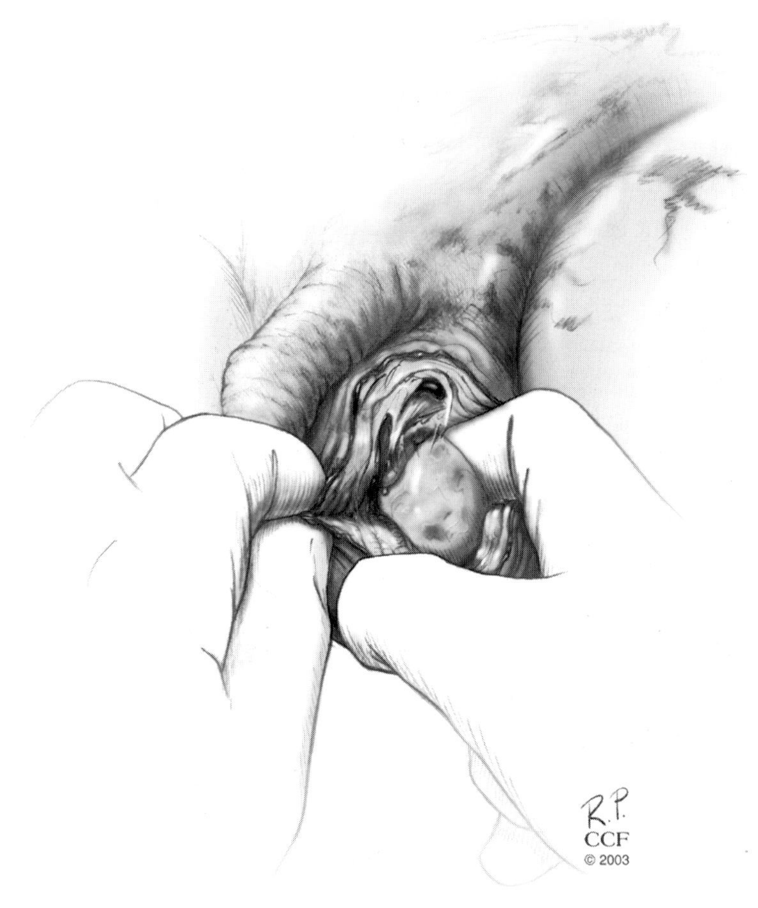


Fig. 50.39

Tunneling under the tissues of the thigh may be necessary to place appropriate drains. In this case, a return trip to the operative room may be necessary to ensure that the initial debridement and drainage has been sufficient.

## SUGGESTED READINGS


1. Eke N. Fournier's gangrene: a review of 1726 cases. Br J Surg 87:718–728, 2000.
2. Fillo J, Cervenakov I, Labas P, et al. Fournier's gangrene: can aggressive treatment save life? Int Urol Nephrol 33:533–536, 2001.
3. Goldstein M. Surgical management of male infertility and other scrotal disorders. In: Walsh PC, ed. Campbell's Urology, 8th ed., Vol. 2. Philadelphia: Saunders, 2002:1532–1587.
4. Hinman F, Jr. Testis: Excision. In: Atlas of Urologic Surgery. Philadelphia: Saunders, 1998:373–410.
5. Jordan GH. Scrotal trauma and reconstruction. In: Graham SD, Jr., ed. Glenn's Urologic Surgery, 5th ed. Philadelphia: Lippincott-Raven, 1998:539–550.
6. McAninch JW. Disorders of the testis, scrotum & spermatic cord. In: Tanagho EA, ed. Smith's General Urology, 15th ed. New York: Lange Medical Books/McGraw-Hill, 2000:684–693.
7. Morpurgo E, Galandiuk S. Fournier's gangrene. Surg Clin North Am 82:1213–1224, 2002.
8. Nisbet AA, Thompson IM. Impact of diabetes mellitus on the presentation and outcomes of Fournier's gangrene. Urology 60:775–779, 2002.
9. Norton KS, Johnson LW, Perry T, Perry KH, Sehon JK, Zibari GB. Management of Fournier's gangrene: an eleven year retrospective analysis of early recognition, diagnosis, and treatment. Am Surg 68:709–713, 2002.
10. Olsofka, JN, Carrillo EH, Spain DA, Polk HC, Jr. The continuing challenge of Fournier's gangrene in the 1990's. Am Surg 65:1156–1159, 1999.
11. Siegel SW. Surgery of the scrotum. In: Novick AC, ed. Stewart's Operative Urology, 2nd ed., Vol. 2. Baltimore: Williams & Wilkins, 1989:746–754.
12. Spirnak JP. Scrotum and its contents. In: Current Therapy in Genitourinary Surgery, 2nd ed. St. Louis: B.C. Decker, 1992:391–397.
13. Vick R, Carson CC, 3rd. Fournier's disease. Urol Clin North Am 26:841–849, 1999.

# Index

TO LEARN:

- Retractor Types + Advantages/Uses.